Cardiac CT Imaging

Matthew J. Budoff • Jerold S. Shinbane
Editors

Cardiac CT Imaging

Diagnosis of Cardiovascular Disease

Third Edition

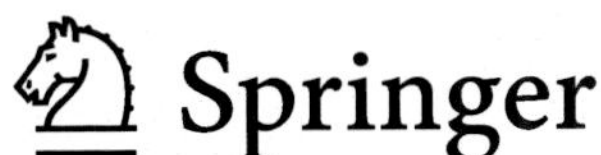

Editors
Matthew J. Budoff
Division of Cardiology
Harbor-UCLA Medical Center
Torrance, CA
USA

Jerold S. Shinbane
Keck School of Medicine
University of Southern California
Los Angeles, CA
USA

Additional material to this book can be downloaded from http://extras.springer.com.

ISBN 978-3-319-28217-6 ISBN 978-3-319-28219-0 (eBook)
DOI 10.1007/978-3-319-28219-0

Library of Congress Control Number: 2016934867

Springer Cham Heidelberg New York Dordrecht London

Printed on acid-free paper

Springer International Publishing AG Switzerland is part of Springer Science+Business Media (www.springer.com)

Foreword to the Second Edition

Cardiac CT has finally come of age. After nearly 30 years of development and growth, tomographic X-ray is being embraced by cardiologists as a useful imaging technology. Thirty years ago, Doug Boyd envisioned a unique CT scanner that would have sufficient temporal resolution to permit motion-artifact-free images of the heart. In the late 1970s, I had the good fortune to work closely with Dr. Boyd, Marty Lipton, and Bob Herkens who had the vision to recognize the potential of CT imaging for the diagnosis of heart disease. In the early 1980s, when electron beam CT became available, others, including Mel Marcus (deceased), John Rumberger, Arthur Agatston, and Dave King (deceased), were instrumental in making clinical cardiologists aware of the potential of cardiac CT.

In 1985, several investigators recognized the potential of cardiac CT for identifying and quantifying coronary artery calcium. Now, 20 years later, there is wide recognition of the value of coronary calcium quantification for the prediction of future coronary events in asymptomatic people. It has been a long and arduous road, but finally, wide-spread screening may significantly reduce the 150,000 sudden deaths and 300,000 myocardial infarctions that occur each year in the United States as the first symptom of heart disease

In the late 1970s, it was thought that a 2.4-s scan time was very fast CT scanning. With the development of electron beam technology, scan times of 50 ms became possible, giving rise to terms such as fast CT, ultrafast CT, and RACAT (rapid acquisition computed axial tomography). Now, with the development of multidetector scanners capable of 64, 128, 256, and beyond simultaneous slices, spatial resolution is approaching that of conventional cineangiography, and the holy grail, noninvasive coronary arteriography, appears attainable.

In this book, Drs. Matthew Budoff and Jerold Shinbane, preeminent leaders in the field of cardiac CT, have described the many and varied uses of the technology in the diagnosis of cardiovascular disease. The book clearly documents that cardiac CT has not only arrived but has become a very valuable and potent diagnostic tool.

Bruce H. Brundage, MD, MACC
Heart Institute of the Cascades, Bend, OR, USA
UCLA School of Medicine, Los Angeles, CA, USA

Preface

It is a testament to the intellect and diligence of the physician-scientists and engineers involved in the field of cardiovascular computed tomography that a third edition of this text is necessary in so short a time since this field was created. Our first cardiac CT angiogram was performed in January 1995, over 20 years ago. The trials and tribulations that we faced over the introduction of this modality are reminiscent of a quote by the philosopher Arthur Schopenhauer:

> All truth passes through three stages.
> First, it is ridiculed.
> Second, it is violently opposed.
> Third, it is accepted as being self-evident.

Cardiovascular CT has now matured into a firmly established subspecialty of radiology and cardiovascular medicine with a multidisciplinary society with 4000 members, a board examination, dedicated journals, numerous scientific statements from leading national societies, focused national and international meetings, and clear education and training pathways. The foundation has been provided by a sound medical literature, which continues to grow at an astounding pace. We hope that research maintains the same forward momentum fueled by the intellectual curiosity and passion to increase the understanding of the cardiovascular system and improve patient care. As we look ahead, we also continue to look back and acknowledge our debt to the pioneers of this technology who dedicated their careers to forwarding this discipline, who persevered the ridicule and violent opposition, and may or may not be enjoying the current acceptance and utilization in this "self-evident" era of cardiac CT.

Cardiovascular CT has become a powerful risk stratifying tool for the early detection of atherosclerosis, used as a calcium score to identify asymptomatic persons at risk of CVD. It has also developed into the de facto noninvasive angiogram, a measure of coronary stenosis, a substitute for coronary angiography or noninvasive exercise testing in certain clinical situations, and a powerful tool to image the heart for congenital heart disease, trans-aortic valve procedures, perfusion imaging, and coronary anomalies. There has been a paradigm shift in its role related to cardiovascular therapies, with progress from pre- and postprocedure assessment to use in the actual guidance of a variety of invasive procedures.

Advances in CT scanners, imaging techniques, postprocessing workstations, and interpretation for diagnostic and therapeutic applications have now made the field relevant to the entire spectrum of physicians who diagnose and treat cardiovascular disease. As such, a thorough knowledge of cardiovascular CT is required for the thoughtful and individualized application in patient care. We hope that this text will provide the substrate for a detailed understanding of the art and science of this technology.

Torrance, CA, USA

Matthew J. Budoff, MD
Jerold S. Shinbane, MD, FACC, FHRS, FSCCT

Contents

Contributors

Stephan Achenbach, MD University of Erlangen, Erlangen, Germany

Anas Alani, MD Department of Medicine, University of Florida – Gainesville, Gainsville, FL, USA

Los Angeles Biomedical Research Institute at Harbor-UCLA, Torrance, CA, USA

Chesnal Dey Arepalli, MBBS, DNB Department of Radiology, St. Paul's Hospital, Vancouver, BC, Canada

Reza Arsanjani, MD Departments of Imaging and Medicine, Cedars-Sinai Medical Center and the Cedars-Sinai Heart Institute, Los Angeles, CA, USA

Craig J. Baker, MD, FACS Department of Surgery, Keck Hospital of the University of Southern California, Los Angeles, CA, USA

Daniel S. Berman, MD Departments of Imaging and Medicine, Cedars-Sinai Medical Center and the Cedars-Sinai Heart Institute, Los Angeles, CA, USA

Philipp Blanke, MD Department of Medicine, St. Paul's Hospital, Vancouver, BC, Canada

Matthew J. Budoff, MD David Geffen School of Medicine at UCLA, Los Angeles Biomedical Research Institute, Torrance, CA, USA

Phillip M. Chang, MD Department of Medicine, Keck Medical Center of USC/Keck School of Medicine at USC, Los Angeles, CA, USA

Leonardo C. Clavijo, MD, PhD, FACC, FSCAI, FSVM Department of Medicine, Division of Cardiovascular Medicine, Department of Clinical Medicine, University of Southern California, Los Angeles, CA, USA

Patrick M. Colletti, MD Department of Radiology, University of Southern California, Los Angeles, CA, USA

Stephen C. Cook, MD, FACC Adult Congenital Heart Disease Center, Heart Institute, Children's Hospital of Pittsburgh of UPMC, Pittsburgh, PA, USA

Mark J. Cunningham, MD Department of Surgery, Keck Hospital of the University of Southern California, Los Angeles, CA, USA

Damini Dey, PhD Departments of Imaging and Medicine, Cedars-Sinai Medical Center and the Cedars-Sinai Heart Institute, Los Angeles, CA, USA

Rahul N. Doshi, MD, FACC, FHRS Department of Medicine, Keck Medical Center of USC, Los Angeles, CA, USA

Joachim Eckert, MD Department of Cardiology, Cardioangiologisches Centrum Bethanien, Frankfurt, Hessen, Germany

John D. Friedman, MD Departments of Imaging and Medicine, Cedars-Sinai Medical Center and the Cedars-Sinai Heart Institute, Los Angeles, CA, USA

Leticia Fernández Friera, MD Department of Medicine, Division of Cardiology, Mount Sinai Medical Center, New York, NY, USA

Centro Nacional de Investigaciones Cardiovasculares, Madrid, Spain

Mario Jorge Garcia, MD, FACC, FACP Division of Cardiology, Montefiore Medical Center, Bronx, NY, USA

Guido Germano, PhD Departments of Imaging and Medicine, Cedars-Sinai Medical Center and the Cedars-Sinai Heart Institute, Los Angeles, CA, USA

Ilan Gottlieb, MD, MSc, PhD Casa de Saude Sao Jose, Rio de Janeiro, RJ, Brazil

Swaminatha V. Gurudevan, MD, FACC Department of Medicine, Healthcare Partners Medical Group, Pasadena, CA, USA

Rory Hachamovitch, MD Department of Nuclear Medicine, Cleveland Clinic, Heart and Vascular Institute, Cleveland, OH, USA

Sean W. Hayes, MD Departments of Imaging and Medicine, Cedars-Sinai Medical Center and the Cedars-Sinai Heart Institute, Los Angeles, CA, USA

Harvey S. Hecht, MD, FACC, FSSCT Department of Medicine, Icahn School of Medicine at Mount Sinai, New York, NY, USA

Mount Sinai Medical Center, New York, NY, USA

Antreas Hindoyan, MD Division of Cardiovascular Medicine, Department of Internal Medicine, Keck School of Medicine of the University of Southern California, Los Angeles, CA, USA

Muhammad Aamir Latif, MD Department of Medicine, Center for Healthcare Advancement and Outcomes, Baptist Health South Florida, Miami, FL, USA

Kai H. Lee, PhD Associate Professor of Clinical Radiology, Department of Radiology, Keck School of Medicine, University of Southern California, Los Angeles, CA, USA

Jonathon A. Leipsic, MD, FRCPC, FSCCT Department of Radiology, St. Paul's Hospital, Vancouver, BC, Canada

João A.C. Lima, MD Division of Cardiology, Johns Hopkins Hospital, Baltimore, MD, USA

Songshou Mao, MD Department of Medicine, Los Angeles Biomedical Research Institute, Los Angeles, CA, USA

Suresh Maximin, MD Department of Radiology, University of Washington, Seattle, WA, USA

Bradley S. Messenger, MD Division of Cardiology, Department of Medicine, Harbor-UCLA Medical Center, Torrance, CA, USA

James K. Min, MD, FACC Department of Radiology, Dalio Institute of Cardiovascular Imaging, Weill Cornell Medical College and the NewYork Presbyterian Hospital, New York, NY, USA

Rine Nakanishi, MD, PhD Department of Medicine, Cardiac CT, Los Angeles Biomedical Research Institute at Harbor-UCLA, Torrance, CA, USA

Christopher Naoum, MBBS, FRACP Department of Radiology, St. Paul's Hospital, Vancouver, BC, Canada

Khurram Nasir, MD, MPH Department of Medicine, Center for Healthcare Advancement and Outcomes, Baptist Health South Florida, Miami Beach, FL, USA

Ronald J. Oudiz, MD Department of Medicine, Los Angeles Biomedical Research Institute, The David Geffen School of Medicine at UCLA, Harbor-UCLA Medical Center, Torrance, CA, USA

Priya Pillutla, MD Adult Congenital Heart Disease Program, Harbor-UCLA Medical Center, Torrance, CA, USA

Paolo Raggi, MD Department of Medicine, Mazankowski Alberta Heart Institute, University of Alberta, Edmonton, AB, Canada

Asim Rizvi, MD Department of Radiology, Dalio Institute of Cardiovascular Imaging, Weill Cornell Medical College and the NewYork Presbyterian Hospital, New York, NY, USA

Alan Rozanski, MD Division of Cardiology, Mt. Sinai Saint Luke's and Roosevelt Hospitals, New York, NY, USA

John A. Rumberger, PhD, MD Cardiac Imaging, The Princeton Longevity Center, Princeton, NJ, USA

Javier Sanz, MD Department of Medicine, Division of Cardiology, Mount Sinai Medical Center, New York, NY, USA

Leslie A. Saxon, MD Department of Medicine, USC Center for Body Computing, Keck Medical Center of USC, Los Angeles, CA, USA

Axel Schmermund, MD Department of Cardiology, Cardioangiologisches Centrum Bethanien, Frankfurt, Hessen, Germany

Marco J.M. Schmidt, MD Department of Cardiology, Cardioangiologisches Centrum Bethanien, Frankfurt, Hessen, Germany

Jeffrey M. Schussler, MD, FACC, FSCAI, FSCCT, FACP Division of Cardiology, Department of Internal Medicine, Baylor University Medical Center, Dallas, TX/Jack and Jane Hamilton Heart and Vascular Hospital, Dallas, TX, USA

Division of Cardiology, Department of Medicine, Texas A&M College of Medicine, Dallas, TX, USA

Nada Shaban, MD Department of Medicine, Division of Cardiology, North Shore University Hospital, Manhasset, NY, USA

Ravi K. Sharma, MD Division of Cardiology, Johns Hopkins Hospital, Baltimore, MD, USA

Leslee Shaw, PhD Department of Medicine, Emory Clinical Cardiovascular Research Institute, Emory University School of Medicine, Atlanta, GA, USA

Jerold S. Shinbane, MD, FACC, FHRS, FSCCT Division of Cardiovascular Medicine, Department of Internal Medicine, Keck School of Medicine of the University of Southern California, Los Angeles, CA, USA

Jabi E. Shriki, MD Department of Radiology, Puget VA Health System, University of Washington, Seattle, WA, USA

Piotr Slomka, PhD Departments of Imaging and Medicine, Cedars-Sinai Medical Center and the Cedars-Sinai Heart Institute, Los Angeles, CA, USA

Vaughn A. Starnes, MD H. Russell Smith Foundation, Cardiovascular Thoracic Institute, Keck Hospital of the University of Southern California, Los Angeles, CA, USA

Gale L. Tang, MD Department of Surgery, University of Washington, Seattle, WA, USA

Louise E.J. Thomson, MBChB Departments of Imaging and Medicine, Cedars-Sinai Medical Center and the Cedars-Sinai Heart Institute, Los Angeles, CA, USA

Thomas Voigtländer, MD Department of Cardiology, Cardioangiologisches Centrum Bethanien, Frankfurt, Hessen, Germany

Wm. Guy Weigold, MD, FACC, FSCCT Department of Medicine, Department of Medicine (Cardiology), Cardiac CT, MedStar Washington Hospital Center, Washington, DC, USA

Cardiac CT Core Lab, MedStar Health Research Institute, Washington, DC, USA

MedStar Cardiovascular Research Network, Washington, DC, USA

Part I

Overview

1 Computed Tomography

Matthew J. Budoff

Abstract

Cardiac CT scanners are rapidly improving, each major vendor has introduced a state of the art scanner every 2–3 years. The basic applications, terminology and acquisition has not changed dramatically, however, improvements in hardware and software continue to reduce radiation exposure, scan times, artifacts and improve image quality. This chapter outlines the basic CT terminology, functions and background behind the current state of CT scanners for cardiac applications. It reviews spatial, temporal and contrast resolution limits of the CT scanners. An overview of common terms, radiation exposure and protocols are included. This acts as an introductory chapter to be expanded by subsequent chapters that will each go into more details on specific topics. Comparison to magnetic resonance for image quality and functionality, and dose comparisons to mammography, nuclear and fluoroscopy are included.

Keywords

Cardiac CT • Angiography • MDCT • MRI • Coronary calcium • Protocols • Radiation • Spatial resolution • Temporal resolution

Overview of X-ray Computed Tomography

The development of computed tomography (CT), resulting in widespread clinical use of CT scanning by the early 1980s, was a major breakthrough in clinical diagnosis across multiple fields. The primary advantage of CT was the ability to obtain thin cross-sectional axial images, with improved spatial resolution over ultrasound, nuclear medicine, and magnetic resonance imaging. This imaging avoided superposition of three-dimensional (3-D) structures onto a planar 2-D representation, as is the problem with conventional projection X-ray (fluoroscopy). CT images, which are inherently digital and thus quite robust, are amenable to 3-D computer reconstruction, allowing for ultimately nearly an infinite number of projections. From a cardiac perspective, the increased spatial resolution is the reason for its increase in sensitivity for atherosclerosis, plaque detection and coronary artery disease (CAD). With CT, smaller objects can be seen with better image quality. Localization of structures (in any plane) is more accurate and easier with tomography than with projection imaging like fluoroscopy. The exceptional contrast resolution of CT (ability to differentiate fat, air, tissue and water), allows visualization of more than the lumen or stent, but rather the plaque, artery wall and other cardiac and non-cardiac structures simultaneously.

The basic principle of CT is that a fan-shaped, thin X-ray beam passes through the body at many angles to allow for cross-sectional imaging. The corresponding X-ray transmission measurements are collected by a detector array. Information entering the detector array and X-ray beam itself is collimated to produce thin sections while avoiding unnecessary photon scatter (to keep radiation exposure and

M.J. Budoff, MD
David Geffen School of Medicine at UCLA, Los Angeles Biomedical Research Institute, Torrance, CA, USA
e-mail: mbudoff@labiomed.org

M.J. Budoff, J.S. Shinbane (eds.), *Cardiac CT Imaging: Diagnosis of Cardiovascular Disease*,
DOI 10.1007/978-3-319-28219-0_1

Table 1.1 Typical Hounsfield unit values

Air ~ −1000 HU
Fat −100 to −40
Water – zero
Non-enhanced myocardium and blood – 40–60
Contrast enhanced myocardium 80–140
Calcium >130 (to about 1000)
Enhanced blood pools (lumen, aorta, LV) 300–500
Metal >1000

image noise to a minimum). The x-ray tub and detector array rotate around the patient separated by 180°, allowing continuous acquisition of data. The data recorded by the detectors are digitized into picture elements (pixels) with known dimensions. The gray-scale information contained in each individual pixel is reconstructed according to the attenuation of the X-ray beam along its path using a standardized technique termed "filtered back projection." Gray-scale values for pixels within the reconstructed tomogram are defined with reference to the value for water and are called "Hounsfield units" (HU; for the 1979 Nobel Prize winner, Sir Godfrey N. Hounsfield), or simply "CT numbers." These CT numbers are the attenuation or brightness of the individual pixel (smallest definable unit on CT) of data. A three dimensional pixel is called a voxel. Typical pixel values for studies commonly seen on cardiac CT are listed in Table 1.1.

Dr Hounsfield is credited with the invention of the CT scanner in late 1960s. Since CT uses X-ray absorption to create images, the differences in the image brightness at any point will depend on physical density and the presence of atoms with a high difference in anatomic number like calcium, and soft tissue and water. The absorption of the X-ray beam by different atoms will cause differences in CT brightness on the resulting image (contrast resolution). Blood and soft tissue (in the absence of vascular contrast enhancement) have similar density and consist of similar proportions of the same atoms (hydrogen, oxygen, carbon). Bone has an abundance of calcium and is thus brighter on CT. Fat has an abundance of hydrogen. Lung contains air which is of extremely low physical density and appears black on CT (HU −1000). The higher the density, the brighter the structure on CT. Calcium is bright white, air is black, and muscle or blood is gray. There are over 5000 shades of this gray scale represented on CT, centered around zero (water-gray). Computed tomography, therefore, can distinguish blood from air, fat and bone but not readily from muscle or other soft tissue. The densities of blood, myocardium, thrombus, and fibrous tissues are so similar in their CT number, that non-enhanced CT cannot distinguish these structures. Thus, the ventricles and other cardiac chambers can be seen on non-enhanced CT, but delineating the wall from the blood pool is not possible (Fig. 1.1). Investigators have validated the measurement of "LV size" with cardiac CT, which is the sum of both left ventricle (LV) mass and volume [1]. Due to the thin wall which does not contribute significantly to the total measured volume, the left and right atrial volumes can be accurately measured on non-contrast CT [2].

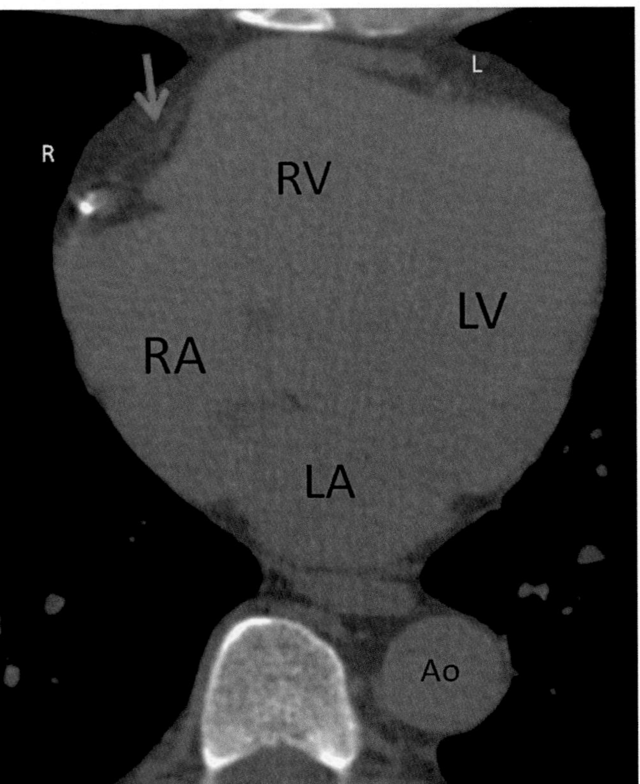

Fig. 1.1 A non-contrast CT scan of the heart. Quite a bit of information can be garnered without contrast. The pericardium is visible as a thin line just below the R and L. The coronary arteries can be seen, and diameters and calcifications are present. The right coronary artery is seen near the R, the left anterior at the L, and the circumflex at the C. The four chambers of the heart are also seen, and relative sizes can be measured from this non-contrast study. The interatrial septum is clearly seen (*red arrow*). The ascending aorta is also present on this image and can be evaluated. *Ao* aorta, *L* left anterior descending artery, *LA* left atrium, *LV* left ventricle, *RA* right atrium, *RV* right ventricle

Because contrast resolution uses attenuation or density to visualize structures in gray scale, limitations of contrast resolution exist even on contrast enhanced studies. These include differentiating the cardiac vessels from cardiac cavities with same density (such as when the arteries run become intra-myocardial), and differentiating non-calcified plaque from surrounding low density structures, including thrombus. Even with good contrast enhancement, differentiating different types of plaque (lipid-laden and fibrous) can sometimes be challenging, although it is always easy to differentiate the bright white plaques (calcified) from non-calcific plaques.

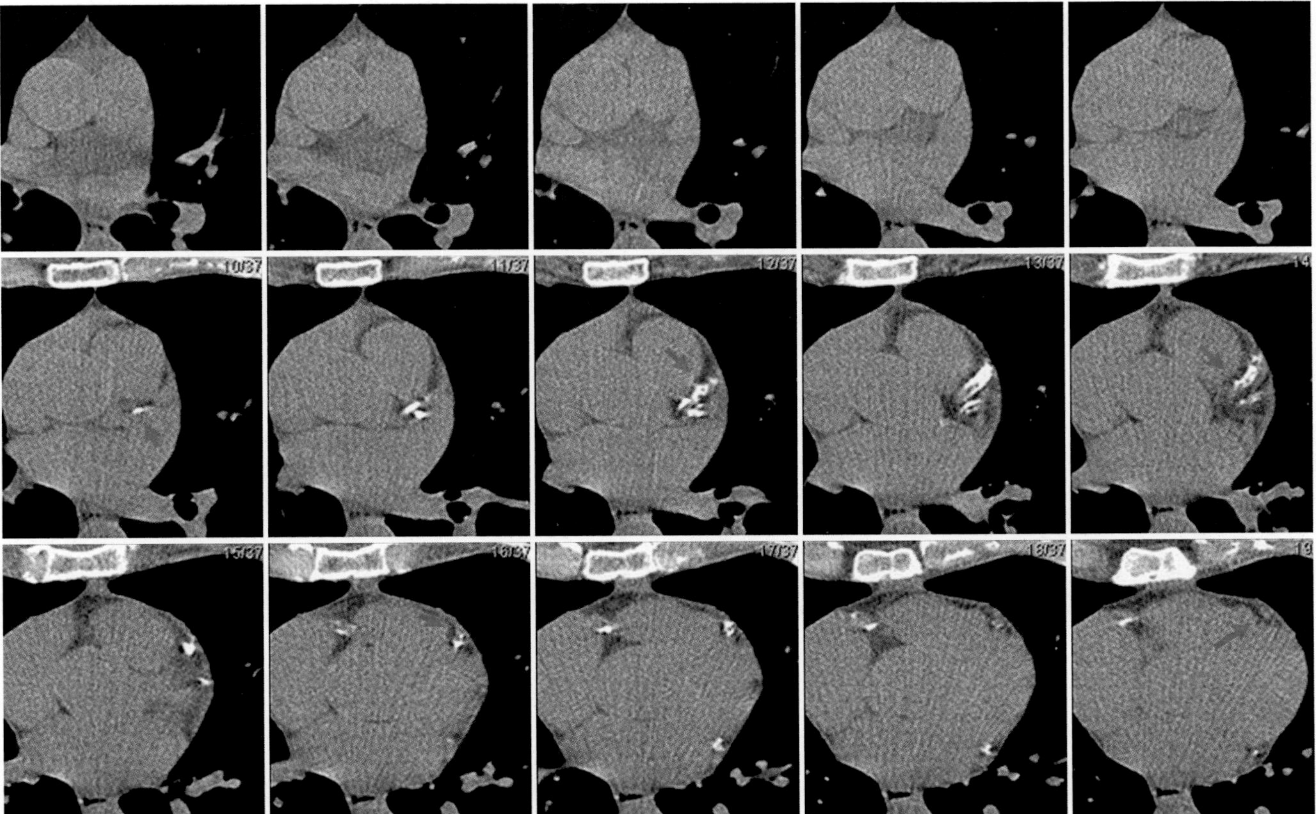

Fig. 1.2 Sequential 3 mm slices from a non-contrast CT scan study (calcium scan). This study depicts the course and calcifications of the left anterior descending (LAD) artery. The white calcifications are easily seen (*red arrows*) and quantitated by the computer to derive a calcium score, volume or mass with high inter-reader reproducibility

The higher spatial resolution of CT allows visualization of coronary arteries both with and without contrast enhancement. The ability to see the coronary arteries on a non-contrast study depends upon the fat surrounding the artery (of lower density, thus more black on images), providing a natural contrast between the myocardium and the epicardial artery (Fig. 1.1). Usually, the entire course of each coronary artery is visible on non-enhanced scans (Fig. 1.2). The major exception is bridging, when the coronary artery delves into the myocardium and cannot be distinguished without contrast. The distinction of blood and soft tissue (such as the left ventricle, where there is no air or fat to act as a natural contrast agent) requires injection of contrast with CT. Similarly, distinguishing the lumen and wall of the coronary artery also requires contrast enhancement. The accentuated absorption of X-rays by elements of high atomic number like calcium and iodine allows excellent visualization of small amounts of coronary calcium as well as the contrast-enhanced lumen of medium-size coronary arteries (Fig. 1.3). Air attenuates the X-ray less than water, and bone attenuates it more than water, so that in a given patient, Hounsfield units may range from −1000 HU (air) through 0 HU (water) to above +1000 HU (bone cortex), Table 1.1. Coronary artery calcium in coronary atherosclerosis (consisting of the same calcium phosphate as in bone) has CT number >130 HU, typically going as high as +1000 HU. It does not go as high as the bony cortex of the spine due to the smaller quantity and mostly inhomogeneous distribution in the coronary artery plaque. Metal, such as that found in valves, wires, stents and surgical clips, typically have densities of +1000 HU or higher.

Cardiac CT

Cardiac computed tomography (CT) provides image slices or tomograms of the heart. CT technology has significantly improved since its introduction into clinical practice in 1972. Current conventional scanners used for cardiac and cardiovascular imaging now employ either a rotating X-ray source with a circular, stationary detector array (spiral or helical CT) or a rotating electron beam (EBCT). The attenuation map recorded by the detectors is then transformed through a filtered back-projection into the CT image used for diagnosis. The biggest issue with cardiac imaging is the need for

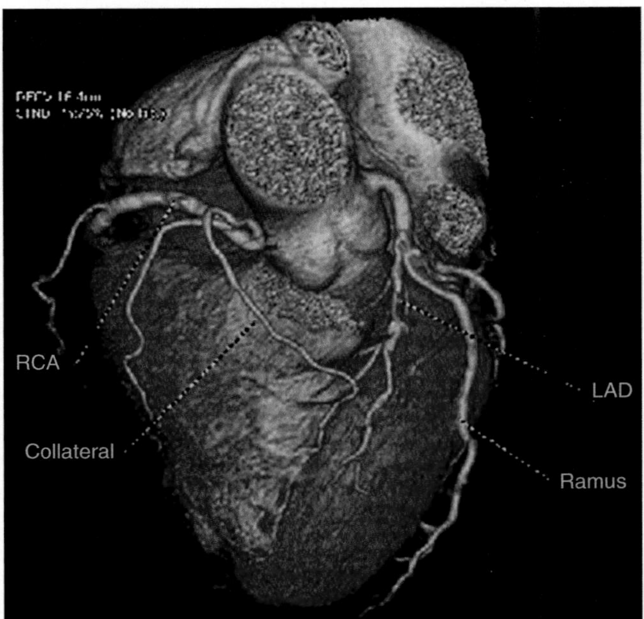

Fig. 1.3 A contrast-enhanced CT of the coronary arteries, with excellent visualization of a high-grade stenosis in the mid-portion of the LAD. A large collateral vessel is seen from the RCA, but this is quite rare, as usually the collaterals are too small to be well seen on cardiac CT. A large ramus intermedius is well visualized, and the dominant RCA is present. This is but one view of many that can be visualized with cardiac CT, allowing for near-complete visualizations of the coronary tree

both spatial and temporal resolution. Cardiac magnetic resonance (MR) has been an emerging technique for almost two decades, making little progress toward widespread utilization over this time. Temporal resolution (how long it takes to obtain an image) is inversely related to spatial resolution with cardiac MR. Improving the MR spatial resolution requires prolonging the imaging time. This greatly limits the ability to focus with precision on moving objects, as the viewer needs to settle for either a high resolution image plagued by cardiac motion, or a low resolution image with no motion artifacts. Cardiac CT does not suffer from this inverse relationship, and allows for both high spatial and temporal resolution simultaneously. Multidetector CT (MDCT), with improved spatial resolution, allows for rotation speeds now on the order of 130–220 ms. The most distinct advantage of cardiac CT over cardiac MR is the improved spatial resolution and thinner slice thickness achievable with current systems. CT has the ability to image every 0.5 mm (submillimeter slices), providing high z-axis (through plane resolution). In-plane resolution is dependent upon the number of pixels that can be seen by a given detector array. Resolution of current CT systems uses a matrix of 512×512, allowing x- and y-axis (in plane) resolution down to 0.35 mm. MR systems use a matrix of 256×256, and flat plate technology currently used in advanced fluouroscopy labs and cardiac catheterization labs use 1024×1024 matrix resolution. The best resolution reported by a cardiac MR study (using the 3 Tesla magnet) demonstrated resolution in the *x*-, *y*- and *z*-axes of 0.6 × 0.6 × 3 mm [3]. The best resolution offered by cardiac CT is 0.35 × 0.35 × 0.5 mm, which is almost a factor of 10 better spatial resolution and approaching the ultimate for 3-D tomography of nearly cubic (isotropic) "voxels" – or volume elements (a three dimensional pixel). As we consider non-invasive angiography with either CT or MR, we need to remember that both spatial and temporal resolution is much higher with traditional invasive angiography (discussed in more detail below).

Reconstruction algorithms and multi-"head" detectors common to both current electron beam and spiral/helical CT have been implemented enabling volumetric imaging, and multiple high-quality reconstructions of various volumes of interest can be done either prospectively or retrospectively, depending on the method. The details of each type of scanner and principles of use will be described in detail.

MDCT Methods

Sub-second MDCT scanners use a rapidly rotating X-ray tube and several rows of detectors, also rotating. The tube and detectors are fitted with slip rings that allow them to continuously move through multiple 360° rotations. The "helical" or "spiral" mode is possible secondary to the development of this slip-ring interconnect. This allows the X-ray tube and detectors to rotate continuously during image acquisition since no wires directly connect the rotating and stationary components of the system (i.e., no need to unwind the wires). This slip-ring technology was considered the most fundamental breakthrough for CT, allowing advancement from conventional CT performing single slice scanning in the 1980s to rapid multislice scanning in the 1990s. With the gantry continuously rotating, the table moves the patient through the imaging plane at a predetermined speed (table speed). The relative speed of the gantry relative to the rotation of the detectors is the scan pitch. Pitch is calculated as table speed divided by collimator width. The collimator width is simply the number of detectors multiplied by the detector width. A typical 64 detector system with 0.625 mm detectors will thus have a collimation width of 64 × 0.625 mm = 40 mm. Thus, each rotation of the detector array will 'cover' 40 mm of the body. If the pitch is 1, than the table is moving at 40 mm and the coverage is 40 mm, allowing for no overlapping data and acquisition of 0.625 mm data per slice. Moving the table faster will lead to wider slices, as a pitch of 1.5 will infer that the table is moving at 60 mm/rotation, while the detector array only covers 40 mm, so each of the 64 detectors will be responsible for almost 1 mm of the 60 mm that was covered during the rotation. A low pitch (low table speed, typically used in cardiac imaging) allows for over-lapping data from adjacent detectors. A typical pitch for cardiac CT is 0.25, meaning that the table is moved at 10 mm per rotation, while the detectors cover 40 mm, allowing thin slice acquisition and overlapping datasets. The heart is literally moved only ¼ of the way through the detector array each rotation, so it takes 4 rotations to completely cover any portion of the heart. The pitch is varied based upon the heart rate of the patient, to allow optimal timing of image acquisition. Most commonly, physicians use a low table speed and thin imaging, leading to a lot of images, each very thin axial slices which are of great value for visualizing the heart with the highest resolution. The downside is that the slower the table movement (while still rotating the X-ray tube), the higher the radiation exposure (See Chap. 3).

The smooth rapid table motion or pitch in helical scanning allows complete coverage of the cardiac anatomy in 5–25 s, depending on the actual number of multi-row detectors. The current generation of MDCT systems complete a 360° rotation in about 3 tenths of a second (300 ms) and are capable of acquiring 64–640 sections of the heart simultaneously with electrocardiographic (ECG) gating in either a prospective or retrospective mode. MDCT differs from single detector-row helical or spiral CT systems principally by the design of the detector arrays and data acquisition systems, which allow the detector arrays to be configured electronically to acquire multiple adjacent sections simultaneously. For example, in 64-row MDCT systems, 64 sections can be acquired at either 0.5–0.75 or 1–1.5 mm section widths or 16 sections 2.5 mm thick (commonly used for calcium scoring).

In MDCT systems, like the preceding generation of single-detector-row helical scanners, the X-ray photons are generated within a specialized X-ray tube mounted on a rotating gantry. The patient is centered within the bore of the gantry such that the array of detectors is positioned to record incident photons after traversing the patient. Within the X-ray tube, a tungsten filament allows the tube current to be increased (mA), which proportionately increases the number of X-ray photons for producing an image. Thus, heavier patients can have increased mA, allowing for better tissue penetration and decreased image noise. One of the advantages of MDCT is the variability of the mA settings, thus increasing the versatility for general diagnostic CT in nearly all patients and nearly all body segments. The other variable on the acquisition is the voltage, commonly expressed as killivoltage (kv or kVp). The voltage was not varied on cardiac CT for the first 20 years of use, but more recently it has been noted that by reducing the kV, exponential reduction in radiation exposure can be achieved. As the kV goes down, image noise goes up, so it is important that the kV only be reduced on thinner patients. While 120 kV was most typical, now increasingly 100 kV and even 80 kV studies are being reported, especially in children, where radiation issues are much more acute.

For example, the calcium scanning protocol employed in the National Institutes of Health (NIH) Multi-Ethnic Study of Atherosclerosis is complex [4]. Scans were performed using prospective ECG gating at 50 % of the cardiac cycle, 120 kV, 106 mAs, 2.5 mm slice collimation, 0.5 s gantry rotation, and a partial scan reconstruction resulting in a temporal resolution of 300 ms. Images were reconstructed using the standard algorithm into a 35 cm display field of view. For participants weighing 100 kg (220 lb) or greater, the milliampere (mA) setting was increased by 25 %.

However, the kV is typically not currently reduced for calcium scoring for two reasons. First, the radiation dose of calcium scoring is generally low (approximately 0.7 milliSieverts), similar to mammography (0.75 milliSieverts) and lower than annual background radiation (3–6 milliSieverts per year). Secondly, as the kV is lowered, calcium and contrast appear brighter, and this would change the calcium scores, which up until this point, have only been obtained using 120 kV acquisitions. As more data is available on the algorithms for scoring with lower kV scans, calcium scoring may undergo a radiation reduction of up to 40 % by lowering the kV from 120 to 100 for the acquisition. This will require new thresholds for definitions of calcium (for example- 147 HU instead of 130 HU as the definition of calcium, and 228 instead of 200 HU for the next threshold, etc.). The exact thresholds will have to be developed for each CT system prior to use. Thus, while calcium score dose can be reduced by iterative reconstruction, use of 100 kVp will need to wait for further validation. This is not an issue with CT angiography, as lower kVp will brighten the contrast, raising the signal to noise quality of the study.

MDCT systems can operate in either the sequential (prospective triggered) or helical mode (retrospective gating). These modes of scanning are dependent upon whether the patient on the CT couch is stationary (axial, or sequential mode) or moved at a fixed speed relative to the gantry rotation (helical mode). The sequential mode utilizes prospective ECG triggering at predetermined offset from the ECG-detected R wave analogous to EBCT and is the current mode for measuring coronary calcium at most centers using MDCT, and increasingly being used for CT angiography when heart rates are stable and slow. This mode utilizes a "step and shoot modality," which reduces radiation exposure by "prospectively" acquiring images, as compared to the helical mode, where continuous radiation is applied (and thousands of images created) and images are "retrospectively" aligned to the ECG tracing. In the sequential mode, a 64-slice scanner can acquire 64 simultaneous data channels of image information gated prospectively to the ECG. Thus a 64-channel system (with 0.625 mm detectors) can acquire, within the same cardiac cycle, 40 mm in coverage per heartbeat (collimation). The promise of improved cardiac imaging from the 64–640 slice scanners is mostly larger volumes of coverage simultaneously (up to 160 mm of coverage per rotation with a 320 slice scanner with 0.5 mm detectors), allowing for less *z*-axis alignment issues (cranial–caudal), and improved 3-D modeling with only 2–5 s of imaging, although each vendor has a different array of detectors, with different slice widths and capabilities (Table 1.2). As coverage speeds increase, breath-hold and contrast requirements will also diminish.

Modern MDCT systems have currently an X-ray gantry rotation time of less than 500 ms. The fastest available rotation time is 260 ms, by using half scan reconstruction (discussed below), lowers this to 130 ms acquisitions. This remains suboptimal in faster heart rates (>70 bpm), as imaging during systole (or atrial contraction during late diastole) will be plagued by motion artifacts. Reconstruction algorithms have been developed that permit the use of data acquired during a limited part of the X-ray tube rotation (e.g., little more than one half of one rotation or smaller sections of several subsequent rotations) to reconstruct one cross-sectional image (described below). Simultaneous recording of the patient ECG permits the assignment of reconstructed images to certain time instants in the cardiac cycle. Image acquisition windows of approximately 200 ms can be achieved without the necessity to average data acquired over more than one heartbeat (Fig. 1.4). This may be sufficient to obtain images free of motion artifacts in many patients if the data reconstruction window is positioned in suitable phases of the cardiac cycle, and the patient has a sufficiently low heart rate. Motion-free segments on four-slice MDCT decrease from approximately 80 to 54 % with increasing heart rates [5], and similar observations have been made with both 16- and 64-detector systems. Dual source CT, utilizing two x-ray tubes and two detector arrays moving simultaneously around the body, can utilize partial images from each detector array to effectively 'half' the temporal resolution, allowing motion free images up to heart rates of 70 bpm or more. However, the system is limited by 32 detectors, so collimation or coverage is only 19.2 mm per rotation (32 × 0.6 mm).

Table 1.2 Sample protocols for MDCT angiography: contrast-enhanced retrospectively ECG-gated scan

4-Slice scanner: 4 × 1.0 mm collimation, table feed 1.5 mm/rotation, effective tube current 400 mAs at 120 kV. Pitch =1.5/4.0 collimation =0.375. Average scan time =35 s
16-Slice scanner (1.5 mm slices): 16 × 1.5 mm collimation, table feed 3.8 mm/rotation, effective tube current 133 mAs at 120 kV. Pitch =3.8/24 mm collimation =0.16. Average scan time =15–20 s
16-Slice scanner (0.75 mm slices): 16 × 0.75 mm collimation, table feed 3.4 mm/rotation, effective tube current 550–650 mAs at 120 kV. Pitch =3.4/12 mm collimation =0.28. Average scan time = 15–20 s
64-Slice scanner (0.625 mm slices): 64 × 0.6.25 mm collimation, table feed 10 mm/rotation, effective tube current 685 mAs at 120 kV. Pitch =10/40 mm collimation =0.25. Average scan time=5 s
Dual Source scanner (0.6 mm slices): 32 × 0.6 mm collimation, table feed 6 mm/rotation, effective tube current 685 mAs at 120 kV. Pitch =6/19.2 mm collimation =0.3. Average scan time=10–12 s
320-Slice scanner (0. 5 mm slices): 320 × 0.5 mm collimation, table feed 12 mm/rotation, effective tube current 685 mAs at 120 kV. Pitch =12/40 mm collimation =0.3. Average scan time=2–3 s

MDCT Terminology

Isotropic Data Acquisition

The biggest advance that the newest systems provide is thinner slices, important for improving image quality as well as diminishing partial volume effects. The current systems

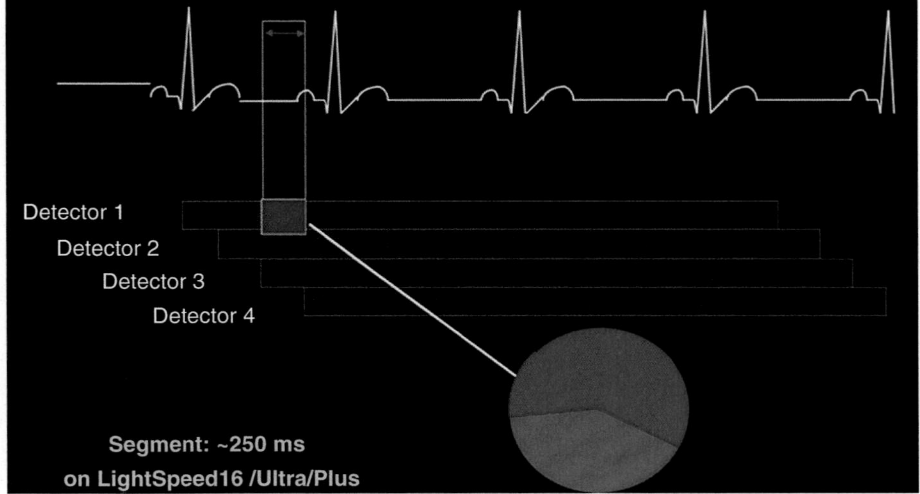

Fig. 1.4 A typical acquisition using the "halfscan" method on multidetector CT (Light-Speed16, GE Medical Systems, Milwaukee Wisconsin). This demonstrates an acquisition starting at approximately 50 % of the R-R interval. A scanner with a rotation speed of 200 ms takes approximately 250 ms to complete an image, as depicted

allow for slice thick-nesses between 0.5 and 0.625 mm (depending on manufacturer and scan model). Thus, the imaging voxel is virtually equal in size in all dimensions (isotropic). The spatial resolution of current CT systems is 0.35 × 0.35 mm, and has always been limited by the z-axis (slice thickness). Current systems theoretically allow for isotropic resolution (as reconstructed images can be seen at 0.4 mm), allowing for no loss of data by reconstructing the data in a different plane. This is very important for imaging the coronary, peripheral, and carotid arteries, as they run perpendicular to the imaging plane (each slice only encompasses a small amount of data) and to follow these arteries, one must add multiple slices together in the z-axis. The old limitations of CT (better interpretation for structures that run within the plane it was imaged, i.e., parallel to the imaging plane) are no longer present. There is now no loss of data with reformatting the data with multiplanar reformation (MPR) or volume rendering (VR). This differs significantly from MR, which due to thick slice acquisition (still > 1 mm), does not allow free rotation of the resultant in-plane images. Thus, acquisition for CT is quite simple, obtaining axial slices through the area of interest, with the ability to reconstruct a three-dimensional image that can be free rotated. MR requires acquisition of data within the plane of interest, so if a short axis image of the left ventricle is required, it must be obtained in that plane, not reconstructed from the axial data. Furthermore, the thinner slice imaging allows for less partial volume artifacts (different densities overlying one another, causing a mixed picture of brightness on the resultant scan) and less streaking and shadowing, prevalent from dense calcifications and metal objects (such as bypass clips, pace-maker wires, and stents).

Pitch

In the helical or spiral mode of operation, a 64-MDCT system can acquire 64 simultaneous data channels while there is continuous motion of the CT table. The relative motion of the rotating X-ray tube to the table speed is called the scan pitch and is particularly important for cardiac gating in the helical mode. Increased collimator coverage allows for decreasing the pitch, without losing spatial resolution. The definition of pitch for the multidetector systems is the distance the table travels per 360° rotation of the gantry, divided by the dimension of the exposed detector array (the collimation, which is the slice thickness times the number of imaging channels). For example, a 64-slice system, with 64 equal detectors each of 0.625 mm, gives a collimation of 40 mm. Thus, if the table is moving at 40 mm/rotation, the pitch is 1.0. The pitch remains 1.0 if the table moves at 60 mm/rotation and the slices are thicker (0.975 mm each), or if the number of channels (detectors utilized) increases. Moving the table faster will lead to thicker slices, which will decrease resolution and lead to partial volume effects. If there is no overlap, the pitch is 1. If 50 % overlap is desired, the pitch is 0.5, as the table is moved slower to allow for overlapping images. This is necessary with multisector reconstruction. Typical pitch values for cardiac work are 0.25–0.4, allowing for up to a 4-fold overlap of images. If the collimation with 64-row scanners increases to 40 mm, the table can move four times faster than the 16-slice scanner, without affecting slice thickness. Thus, the coverage with increased numbers of detectors can go up dramatically over a short period of scanning time, by imaging more detectors and increasing the speed of table movement in concert.

Field of View

Another method to improve image quality of the CT angiograph (CTA) is to keep the field of view small. The matrix for CT is 512 × 512, meaning that is the number of voxels in a given field of view. This is significantly better than current MR scanners, accounting for the improved spatial resolution. If the field of view is 15 cm, than each pixel is 0.3 mm. Increasing the field of view to 45 cm (typical for encompassing the entire chest) increases each pixel dimension to 0.9 mm, effectively reducing the spatial resolution of each data-point 3-fold.

Contrast

Finally, the high scan speed allows substantial reduction in the amount of contrast material. The high speed of the scan allows one to decrease the amount of contrast administered; by using a 64-channel unit with a detector collimation of 0.625 mm and a tube rotation of 0.35 s (typical values for a 64-detector coronary CTA), the acquisition interval is around 5–6 s, which allows one to reduce the contrast load to approximately 50 mL. For a faster acquisition protocol, the contrast delivery strategy needs to be optimized according to the scan duration time. Use of a 320 detector scanner (which currently has 0.5 mm slices), covers the entire heart with one rotation, further reducing the contrast needs (although some minimal amount of contrast will be required to fill the heart and arteries in question). The general rule is the duration of scanning (scan acquisition time) equals the contrast infusion time. So, if an average rate of 4 mL/s is used, a 15-s scan acquisition would require 60 mL of contrast. With volume scanners (64- and greater detector systems), the scan times are reduced to 5–8 s, and contrast doses are subsequently reduced as well.

Prospective Triggering

The prospectively triggered image uses a "step and shoot" system, used for calcium scoring for years, now widely available for all MDCT scanners. This obtains images at a certain time of the cardiac cycle (see Chap. 2), which can be chosen in advance, and then only one image per detector per cardiac cycle is obtained. This reduces (radiation) requirements, and does allow for CT angiographic images only when heart rates are slow, as motion artifacts may plague these images. When performing prospective gating, the temporal resolution of a helical or MDCT system is proportional to the gantry speed, which determines the time to complete one 360° rotation. To reconstruct each slice, data from a minimum of 180° plus the angle of the fan beam are required, typically 210° of the total 360° rotation. For a 64-row system with 0.35-s rotation, the temporal resolution is approximately 0.20 s or 200 ms. By reducing the display field of view to the 20 cm to encompass the heart, the number of views can be reduced to further improve temporal resolution to approximately 200 ms per slice. The majority of MDCT systems now have gantry rotation speeds of 250–330 ms and temporal resolution of 83–167 ms per image when used for measuring coronary calcium or creating individual images for CT angiography. Although physically faster rotational times may be possible in the future, this is still rotation of an X-ray source (with or without attached detectors) within a fixed radius of curvature. This is subject to the forces and limitations of momentum. While interpretation can be limited by the phase chosen (i.e.- 75 % of the R-R interval), there is an ability to add padding. Padding allows for additional phases to be imaged, but is dependent upon the heart rate. With slower heart rates, padding can be increased, to typically include an additional 10–15 % of the cardiac cycle on each side of the phase chosen (allowing for phases from 60 to 85 % to be acquired), so acquisition may be widened to allow extra phases to allow for some correction of motion artifacts. However, the more padding applied, the higher the radiation exposure.

Retrospective Gating

The ECG is used to add R peak markers to the raw data set. A simultaneous ECG is recorded during the acquisition of cardiac images. The ECG is retrospectively used to assign source images to the respective phases of the cardiac cycle (ECG gating). The best imaging time to minimize coronary motion is from 40 to 80 % of the cardiac cycle (early to mid-diastole).

The interval between markers determines the time of each scanned cardiac cycle. Retrospective, phase-specific, short time segments of several R-R intervals are combined to reconstruct a "frozen axial slice." During helical scanning, the patient is moved through the CT scanner to cover a body volume (i.e., the heart). An advantage of the helical acquisition mode is that there is a continuous model of the volume of interest from base to apex, as opposed to the sequential/cine mode in which there are discrete slabs of slices which have been obtained in a "step and shoot" prospective fashion. The obvious detriment to the helical acquisition is the increase in radiation dose delivered to the patient, as continuous images are created, and then "retrospectively" aligned to the ECG tracing to create images at any point of the R-R interval (cardiac cycle). This allows for all phases (1–100 %) to be recreated as needed, allowing for many phases to overcome motion artifacts, correct for stair-step (misalignment) artifacts, and calculate ejection fraction and wall motion. However, radiation doses are higher than prospective imaging, even when using dose modulation.

Halfscan Reconstruction

A multislice helical CT halfscan (HS) reconstruction algorithm is most commonly employed for cardiac applications. Halfscan reconstruction using scan data from a 180° gantry rotation (180–250 ms) for generating one single axial image (Fig. 1.4). The imaging performances (in terms of the temporal resolution, *z*-axis resolution, image noise, and image artifacts) of the heartscan algorithm have demonstrated improvement over utilizing the entire rotation (full scan). It has been shown that the halfscan reconstruction results in improved image temporal resolution and is more immune to the inconsistent data problem induced by cardiac motions. The temporal resolution of multislice helical CT with the halfscan algorithm is approximately 60 % of the rotation speed of the scanner. The reason it is not 50 % of the rotation speed is that slightly more than 180° is required to create an image, as the fan beam width (usually 30°) must be excluded from the window (Fig. 1.4). Thus approximately 210° of a rotation is needed to reconstruct an entire image. Central time resolution (the point in the center of the image) is derived by the 180° rotation. MDCT using the standard halfscan reconstruction method permits reliable assessment of the main coronary branches (those in the center of the image field) in patients with heart rates below 65 beats/min [6,7]. The necessity of a low heart rate is a limitation of MDCT coronary angiography using this methodology.

With halfscan reconstruction, the proportion of the acquisition time per heartbeat is linearly rising from 20 % at 60 beats/min to 33 % at 100 beats/min. When evaluating the diastolic time, the proportion is much greater. Slower heart rates have longer diastolic imaging. The diastolic time useful for imaging for a heart rate of 60 beats/min is on the order of 400 ms (excluding systole and atrial contraction). Thus, a 250 ms scan will take up 70 % of the diastolic imaging time. Increase the heart rate to 100 beats/min (systole remains relatively fixed) and the biggest change is shortening of diastole. Optimal diastolic imaging times are reduced to approximately 100 ms, clearly far too short for a motion-free MDCT scan acquisition of 250 ms (Fig. 1.5, left panel). Thus, heart rate reduction remains a central limitation for motion-free imaging of the heart using MDCT. This can be partially overcome by multisegment reconstruction, described below.

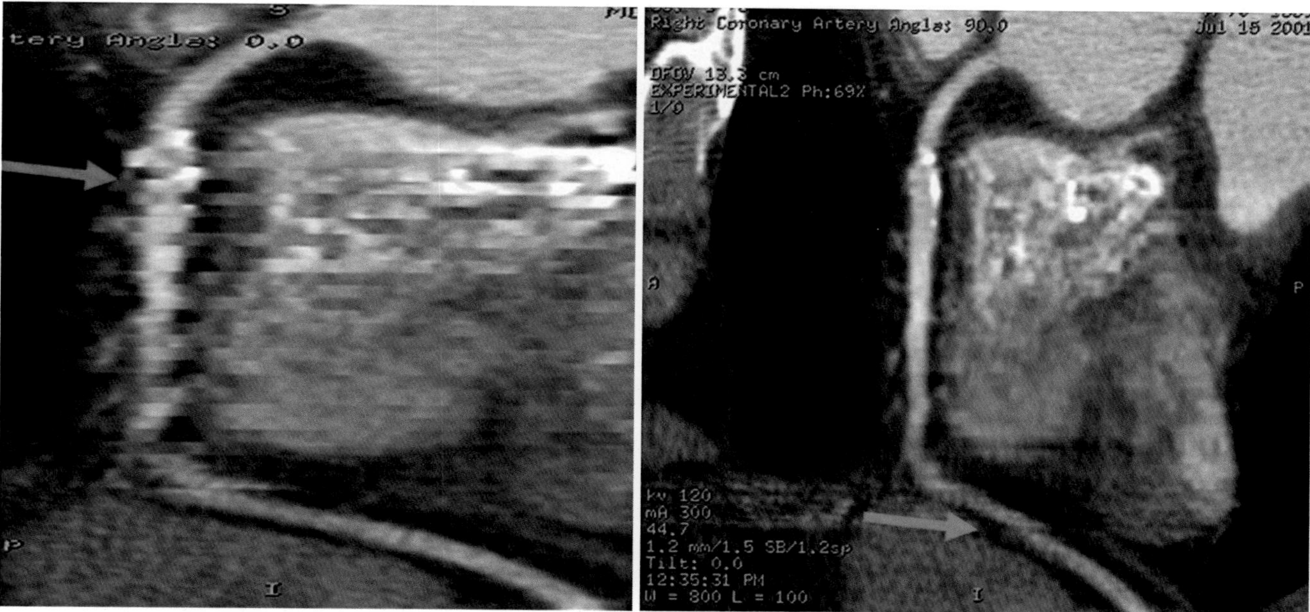

Fig. 1.5 LightSpeed16 CT angiography images. On the left is the halfscan reconstruction. On the right, is a reconstructed image using the same dataset, using multisegment reconstruction. There are still some motion artifacts in the distal right (*green arrow*), but much improved over the halfscan image, which is not interpretable (*red arrow*)

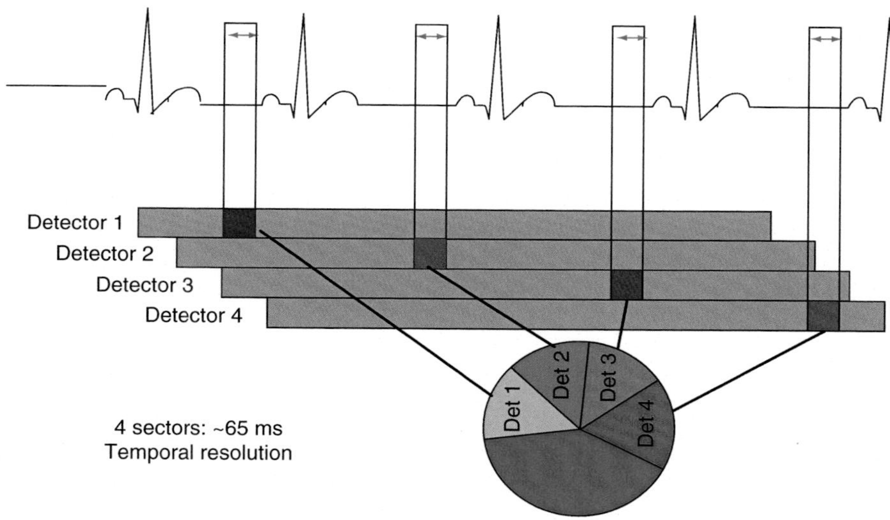

Fig. 1.6 A demonstration of a theoretical image using multisegment reconstruction. The resulting image is constructed of four equal segments from four different detectors. Each is reconstructed from the same point in the cardiac cycle (approximately 50 % in this depiction). Four different detectors, each visualizing the same portion of the heart in the same portion of the cardiac cycle, can be used to add together to create one image. In practice, the segments are not always of equal length, and four images are not always available for reconstruction

Multisegment Reconstruction

The scan window refers to the time when the volume of interest is present in the scan field and is therefore "seen" by the detector. It is the limiting factor for temporal resolution. In multisegment reconstruction, it defines the number of cardiac cycles available and hence the maximum number of segments that can be used to reconstruct one slice. Multisegment reconstruction utilizes a helical scanning technique coupled with ECG synchronization (images are retrospectively aligned to the ECG data acquired to keep track of systolic and diastolic images). Multisegment reconstruction can typically use up 2–4 different segments correlated to the raw data. By using four heartbeats to create an image, the acquisition time can be reduced to a minimum of 65 ms (Fig. 1.6).

During retrospective segmented reconstruction, views from different rotations are combined to simulate one halfscan rotation (approximately 210° of data is needed to create an image). To calculate the number of segments that can be extracted from a scan window, the number of positions available for reconstruction is determined automatically by a workstation. Each position is extended into a wedge so that the combination of all wedges simulates a halfscan tube

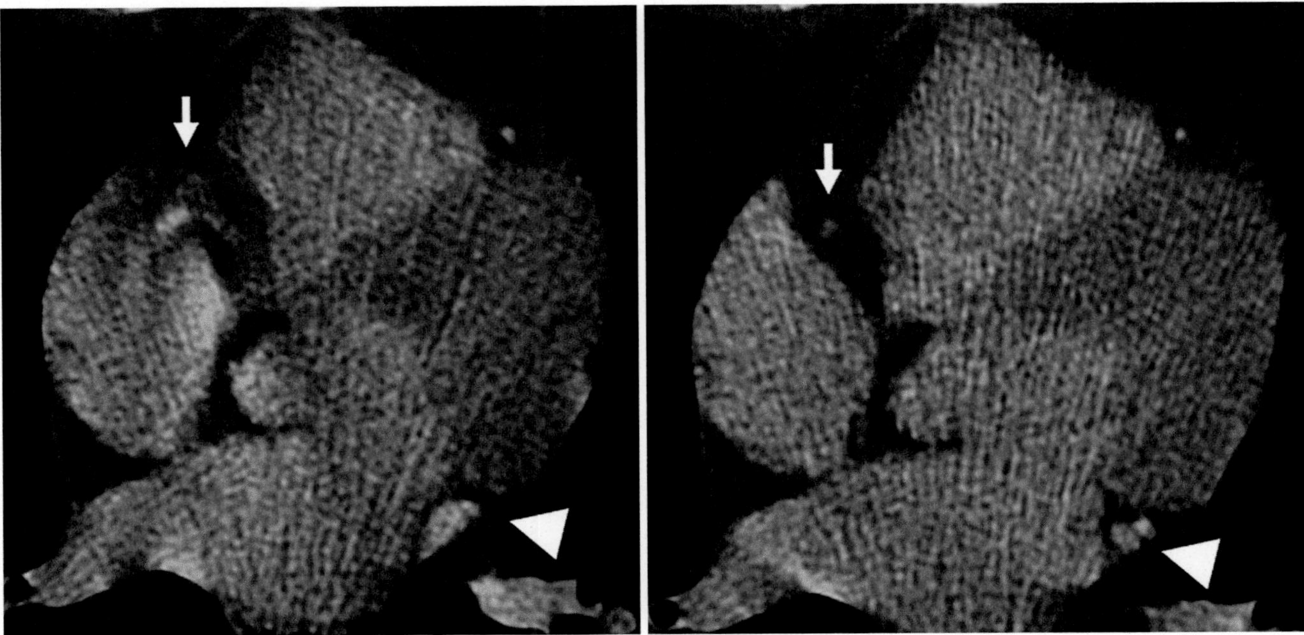

Fig. 1.7 The figure on the left demonstrates a standard halfscan reconstruction with a rotation speed of 400 ms (approximate 260 ms image temporal resolution), with image data acquired on a four-channel MDCT system, 1.25 mm slice collimation, 0.6 gantry speed and a heart rate of 72 beats/min. The image to the right demonstrates the same helical scan data but processed with a two-sector reconstruction algorithm resulting in an effective temporal resolution of 180 ms. Note how the proximal right coronary artery (*white arrows*), as well as the left circumflex and great coronary vein, are now distinguishable (*white arrowhead*) and motion-free on the multisector reconstructed image

rotation. The raw data acquired in this virtual halfscan rotation is sufficient for the reconstruction of one slice. The size of the largest wedge (largest segment) defines the temporal resolution within the image (Fig. 1.6). In other words, the subsegment with the longest temporal data acquisition determines the temporal resolution of the overall image. If the four segments used to create an image were of the following size (65 ms, 65 ms, 50 ms, and 100 ms), then the temporal resolution of the reconstructed image is 100 ms.

The use of multisegment reconstruction has allowed for markedly improved effective temporal resolution and image quality. Just to be clear about how this works, let's use an analogy of a pie. Imagine needing just over half of a pie for a picture. To create an image, you can either add together one small slice from several pies (Fig. 1.6) or you can take one large piece from one pie (Fig. 1.4). The advantage of taking small pieces from each heartbeat is that the temporal resolution goes down proportionally. The difficulty in using this technique is that the pieces of the pie must align properly. Patients with even very slight arrhythmias (especially atrial fibrillation, sinus arrhythmia, or multifocal atrial rhythms), changing heart rates (increased vagal tone during breath-holding, catecholamine response after getting a contrast flush, etc.), or premature beats will cause misregistration (misalignment) to occur. If the heartbeats used are not perfectly regular, the computer will inadvertently add different portions of the cardiac cycle together, making a non-diagnostic image. Thus, there is still need for regular rhythms with CT angiography, although with higher detector systems (i.e., 64–640 detectors), the number of heartbeats needed to cover the entire heart goes down to 1–4, reducing the chance of significant changes in heart rates due to premature beats, breath-holding, vagal or sympathetic tone.

By combining information from each of the detector rows, the effective temporal resolution of the images can *theoretically* be reduced to as low as 65 ms. However, to do this requires four perfectly regular beats consecutively and a fast baseline heart rate, and usual reconstructions allow for two to three images to be utilized, yielding an effective temporal resolution of 130–180 ms per slice (Fig. 1.7), but with a direct proportional increase in radiation exposure to the patient. This method of segmenting the information of one image into several heartbeats is quite similar to the established prospective triggering techniques used for MRI of the coronary arteries [8,9]. With multisegment reconstruction the length of the acquisition time varies between 10 and 20 % of the R-R interval. Since the reconstruction algorithm is only capable of handling a limited number of segments, the pitch (table speed) is often increased for patients with higher heart rates. Thus, fewer images are available with higher heart rates, decreasing the potential success rate with this methodology (see section "Speed/temporal resolution" below).

Multisegment reconstruction has been shown to improve depiction of the coronary arteries as compared to halfscan reconstruction [10,11] (Fig. 1.5). This methodology will improve temporal resolution, but high heart rates will still increase the motion of the coronaries, increasing the likelihood of image blurring and non-diagnostic images (Fig. 1.5, right panel still demonstrating some blurring of the mid-distal right coronary artery with heart rates of 70–75 beats/min). It is fairly common for patients with low heart rates at rest to increase the heart rate significantly at the time of CT angiography. This can occur due to three factors: anxiety about the examination, the breath-hold, or the warmth of the contrast infusion to the patient. Thus, there is still a need for somewhat reduced heart rates during MDCT angiography with all current reconstruction systems.

Studies examining the image quality of multisegment and halfscan reconstruction in CT with four [12] and eight [11] detector rows showed similar image quality in both phantoms and patients. However, Dewey et al. [13] demonstrated that the accuracy, sensitivity, specificity, and rate of non-assessable coronary branches were significantly better using multisegment reconstruction in a 16-slice MDCT scanner. The authors attributed the difference to the higher image quality and resulting longer vessel length free of motion artifacts with multisegment reconstruction. The obvious advantage of multisegment reconstruction is achieved by reducing the acquisition window per heartbeat to approximately 160 ms on average, particularly useful for diagnostic images of the right coronary artery and circumflex artery (the two arteries that suffer the most from motion artifacts) [14]. Therefore, MDCT in combination with multisegment reconstruction does not always require administration of beta blockers to reduce heart rate. This improvement simplifies the procedure and expands the group of patients who can be examined with non-invasive coronary angiography using MDCT. The potential is for even greater application with aligning these multiple segments together with 64+ detector scanners, further improving the diagnostic rate with MDCT angiography, and coverage for more widespread applications such as gating the entire aorta or triple-rule out imaging (imaging the entire chest to evaluate pulmonary embolism, aorta and coronaries simultaneously).

Limitations of Multisegment Reconstruction

Heart rates above 65 beats/min demonstrate the biggest benefit of multisegment reconstructions. The benefit of multisegment reconstruction in low heart rates has not been demonstrated, and some experts recommend avoiding this in lower heart rates to minimize radiation exposure. A drawback of multisegment reconstruction is the effective radiation dose, which is estimated to be 30 % higher than necessary for halfscan reconstruction, resulting from the lower pitch (slower table speed, increasing the time the X-ray beam is on) needed with multisegment reconstruction. The results of studies indicate that multi-segment reconstruction has superior diagnostic accuracy and image quality compared with halfscan reconstruction in patients with normal heart rates (Fig. 1.7). Thus, multisegment reconstruction holds promise to make the routine use of beta blockers to reduce the heart rate before CT coronary angiography less necessary as a routine. One further limitation is that certain heart rates cannot undergo multisegment reconstruction if the R-R interval (in milliseconds) is an even multiple of the scanner rotational speed. If the heart rate and the rotation of the scanner are synchronous, the same heart phase always corresponds to the same angle segment, and a partial-scan interval cannot be divided into smaller segments. Finally, if the heart rate is unexpectedly irregular (i.e., Premature Ventricular Contractions (PVCs) or stress reaction to the dye causing increased heart rate during imaging), multi-segment reconstruction will not be successful and the diagnostic image quality will have to rely on the halfscan reconstruction. Some scanners (Philips Medical Systems is the first to introduce such proprietary software) have intrinsic programs which improve the success rate with multisegment reconstruction at increased heart rates. How well these systems work and how often are clinical questions still being answered.

EBCT Methods

While now discussion is included mostly for historical reasons, it is important to remember that the origins of cardiac imaging with CT lies firmly with the Electron beam computed tomography (GE Healthcare, Waukegan, WI). This is a tomographic-imaging device developed over 25 years ago specifically for cardiac imaging. At Harbor-UCLA, we started performing CT angiography of the coronary arteries in January 1995, literally 10 years earlier than MDCT systems were able to image the coronary tree with similar accuracy. To date, and specifically over the past decade, there has been a huge increase in diagnostic and prognostic data regarding coronary artery imaging. To this day, most of the prognostic and diagnostic work done with coronary artery calcium scanning was done with EBCT. In order to achieve rapid acquisition times useful for cardiac imaging, these fourth-generation CT scanners have been developed with a non-mechanical X-ray source. This allows for image acquisition on the order of 50–100 ms, and with prospective ECG triggering, the ability to “freeze” the heart. Electron beam scanners use a fixed X-ray source, which consists of a 210° arc ring of tungsten, activated by bombardment from a magnetically focused beam of electrons fired from an

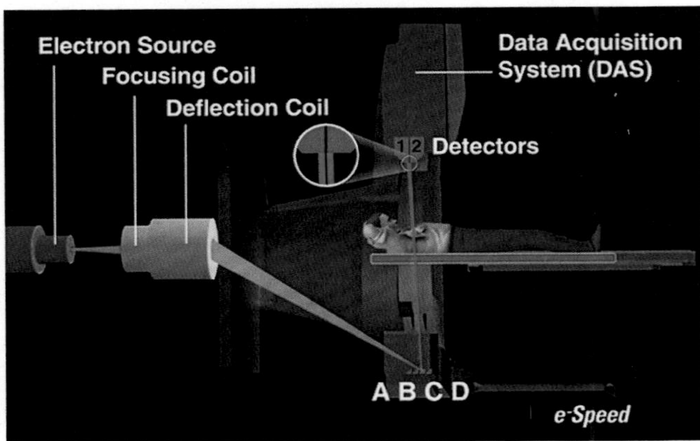

Fig. 1.8 Depiction of the e-Speed electron beam computed tomography scanner. The electron source emits a beam, which is steered magnetically through the detection coil, then reflected to tungsten targets (*A B C D*), where a fan-shaped X-ray beam is created and, after passing through the area of interest, seen by the detectors

electron source "gun" behind the scanner ring. The patient is positioned inside the X-ray tube, obviating the need to move any part of the scanner during image acquisition (Fig. 1.8). EBCT is distinguished by its use of a scanning electron beam rather than the traditional X-ray tube and mechanical rotation device used in current "spiral" single and multiple detector scanners (requiring a physically moving X-ray source around the patient). EBCT requires only that the electron beam is swept across the tungsten targets to create a fan beam of X-ray, possible in as short as 50 ms per image (20 frames/s). The electron beam is emitted from the cathode, which is several feet superior to the patient's head, and then passes through a magnetic coil, which bends the beam so that it will strike one of four tungsten anode targets. The magnetic coil also steers the beam through an arc of 210°. The X-rays are generated when the electron beam strikes the tungsten anode target, then passes through the patient in a fan-shaped X-ray and strikes the detector array positioned opposite the anodes. This stationary multisource/split-detector combination is coupled to a rotating electron beam and produces serial, contiguous, thin section tomographic scans in synchrony with the heart cycle.

There have been four iterations for EBCT since it was introduced clinically in the early 1980s. Since its initial introduction in 1982, it has been known as "rapid CT," "cine CT," "Ultrafast CT©," Electron Beam CT, and "Electron Beam Tomography©." The overall imaging methods have remained unchanged, but there have been improvements in data storage, data manipulation and management, data display, and spatial resolution. The original C-100 scanner was replaced in 1993 by the C-150, which was replaced by the C-300 in 2000. The current EBCT scanner, the e-Speed (GE/Imatron) was introduced in 2003. The e-Speed is a multislice scanner and currently can perform a heart or vascular study in one-half the total examination time required by the C-150 and C-300 scanners. The e-Speed, in addition to the standard 50 and 100 ms scan modes common to all EBCT scanners, is capable of imaging speeds as fast as 33 ms. A major limitation of this modality currently is the slice width, which is limited to 1.5 mm. Current MDCT scanners can obtain images in 0.5–0.75 mm per slice.

Three imaging protocols are used with the EBCT scanner. They provide the format to evaluate anatomy, cardiovascular function, and blood flow. The imaging protocol used to study cardiovascular anatomy is called the *volume scanning mode* and is similar to scanning protocols employed by conventional CT scanners. Single or dual scans are obtained and then the scanner couch is incremented a predetermined distance. For non-contrast studies, the table increment is usually the width of the scan slice, so that there is no overlap imaging of anatomy. For contrast studies, especially those to be reconstructed three-dimensionally, table incrementation is usually less than the slice width, giving overlap of information to improve spatial resolution (see Chaps. 3 and 4). For example, moving the table forward 1 mm, while taking a 1.5 mm slice, gives 33 % overlap per image. Using the older scanners, with slice thickness of 3 mm, moving the table only 1.5 mm gives overlap to improve spatial resolution. This scanning mode is utilized with and without contrast enhancement and provides high spatial resolution of cardiovascular anatomy. This technique provides high resolution axial images, and is ideal for evaluation of the aorta, coronary arteries, and congenital heart disease. A 3-D arteriogram reconstructed from tomographic images has the potential for more complete visualization of the coronary arteries (Figs. 1.3 and 1.9). The end-systolic images can be compared to the end-diastolic images, allowing for accurate measurement of regional wall thickening and motion, myocardial mass (utilizing the known specific gravity of cardiac tissue), global and regional ejection fraction [15]. Importantly, since blood is being injected into the venous system, simultaneous enhancement of the right and left ventricle allows for excellent visualization of all cardiac chambers simultaneously, and measure of both right and left ventricular function and structure [16].

The *flow mode imaging protocol* acquires a single image gated to the electrocardiogram at a predetermined point in the cardiac cycle (e.g., end-diastole (peak of the R-wave)). Images can be obtained for every cardiac cycle or multiples thereof. Scanning is initiated before the arrival of a contrast bolus at an area of interest (e.g., left ventricular (LV) myocardium) and is continued until the contrast has washed in and out of the area. Time density curves from the region of interest can be created for quantitative analysis of flow (Fig. 1.10). The filling of different chambers can be visualized sequentially, allowing for visualization of flow into and out of any area of interest. This was the original methodology

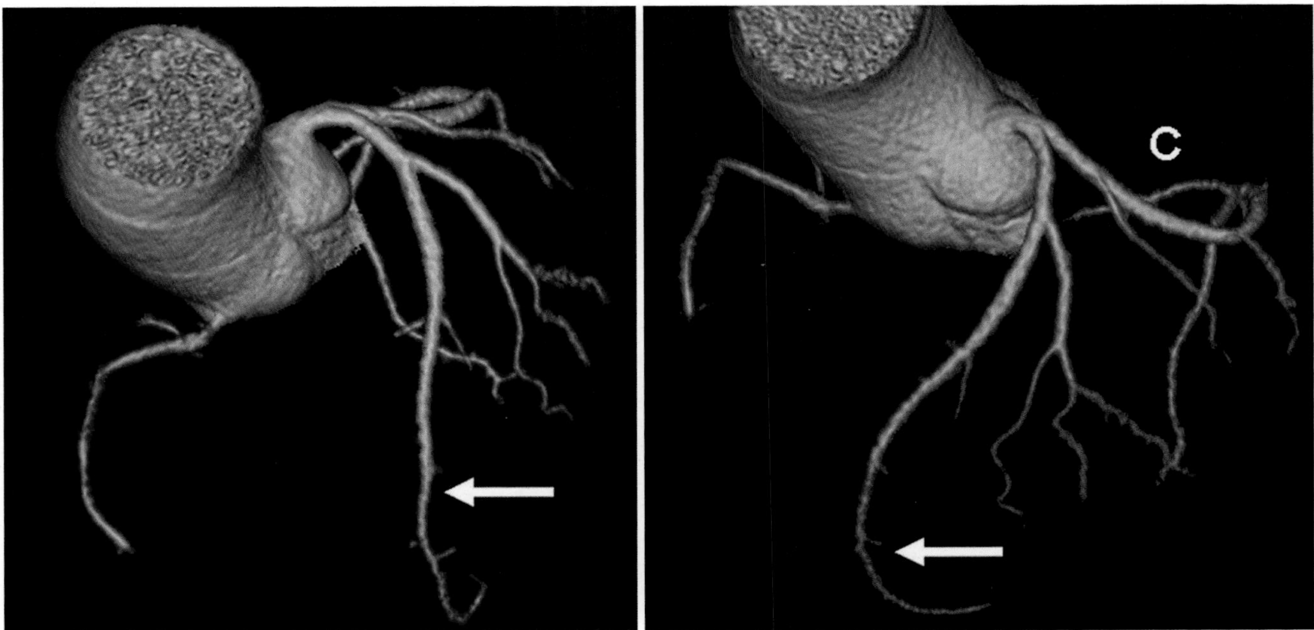

Fig. 1.9 A contrast-enhanced electron beam angiogram demonstrating long segments of the left anterior descending (*arrow*). Images such as seen here can be created which are much more similar to a conventional coronary angiogram, if desired. *C* circumflex artery

employed to assess for graft patency, prior to the ability to create 3-D images. It should be noted that early studies dating back to 1983 have demonstrated saphenous vein graft patency with this technique, achieving an accuracy of approximately 90 % as compared to invasive angiography [17]. This technique is still commonly employed to detect shunts (Chap. 23), as well as to deter-mine the length of time it takes for contrast to travel from the arm vein at the site of injection to the central aortic root (allowing for accurate image acquisition of the high resolution contrast-enhanced images, Chap. 7).

MDCT Scanners Spatial Resolution

Spatial resolution compares the ability of the scanners to reproduce fine detail within an image, usually referred to as the high contrast spatial resolution. Spatial resolution is important in all three dimensions when measuring coronary plaque. Even if limited to the proximal coronary arteries, the left system courses obliquely within the x–y imaging plane, while the right coronary artery courses through the x–y imaging plane. Simply put, one axial image may demonstrate 5 or more centimeters of the left anterior descending, while most images will demonstrate only a cross-section of the right coronary artery. For more on cardiac anatomy with examples, see Chap. 4. The in-plane resolution of MDCT systems are among the best of any imaging modality, higher than echocardiography, nuclear imaging and magnetic resonance imaging. The resolution in z dimension is determined by the detector width in MDCT (this may be thought of as the measurement of the slice width for individual images). This is a "voxel" or volume element and it has the potential to be nearly cubic using MDCT. Current coronary artery calcification (CAC) scanning protocols vary between manufacturers from 2.5 to 3.0 mm for MDCT. For CT angiography, MDCT obtains images with 0.5–0.625 mm per axial slice. Thus, MDCT has a significant advantage in terms of spatial resolution, and results in less partial volume averaging than all other modalities. Also the principles of resolution of say a 1 mm vessel require that the slice width be 1 mm or less. Partial volume averaging occurs when a small plaque has dramatically different CT numbers related to whether it is centered within one slice or divided between two adjacent slices. Thus, thinner slices will have less partial volume averaging. The visualization of smaller lesions is only possible with smaller slice widths (Fig. 1.11). Modern MDCT systems permit simultaneous data acquisition in 64–640 parallel cross-sections with 0.50–0.625 mm collimation each. The in-plane spatial resolution is now as high as 17 line pairs/cm with new high definition detector arrays. However, conventional CT angiography still has higher temporal and spatial resolution, allowing for better visualization of the smaller arteries and collateral vessels. Modern angiographic equipment has a resolution of 40 line pairs per centimeter with a six-inch field of view, the usual image magnification for coronary angiography [18]. Thus, invasive coronary angiography still has a 3–4-fold better resolution than current MDCT systems. It is likely to remain this way until the perfection of flat panel detectors for CT – which would be akin

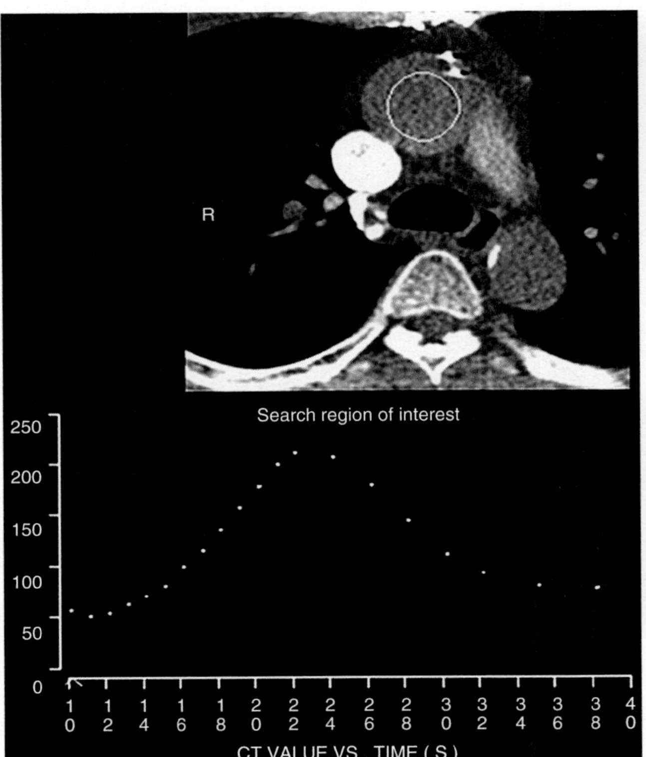

Fig. 1.10 A flow or timing study. This study images the same level over time. A region of interest (in this study, the *circle* is placed in the ascending aorta) defines the anatomy to be measured. The graph below measures the Hounsfield units (HU) of that region of interest on each subsequent image. Initially, there is no contrast enhancement, and the measures are of non-enhanced tissue, around 50–60 HU. Contrast starts to arrive on this study around 16 s, and peaks at 22 s. The *bright white structure* next to the ascending aorta is the superior vena cava, filled with unmixed contrast

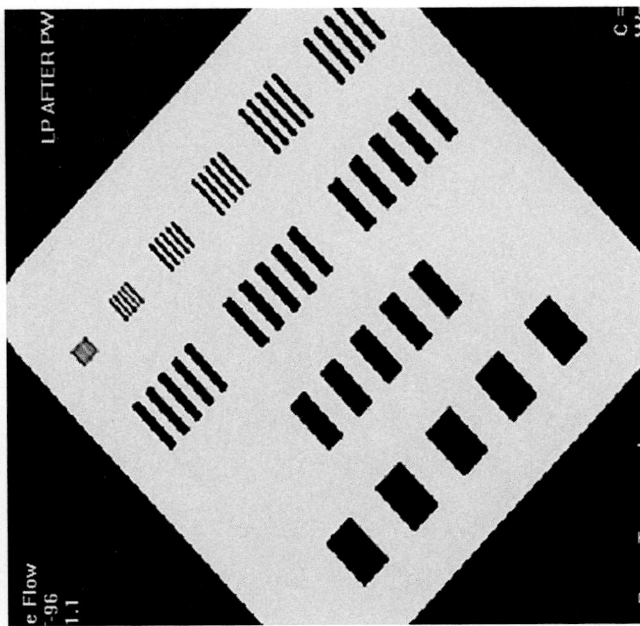

Fig. 1.11 Spatial resolution as measured on computed tomography. A phantom is imaged, and the *smaller line pairs* per centimeter are evaluated. Somewhat similar to an eye chart, the *thinnest lines* clearly seen define the spatial resolution of the scanner

to the current state of the art in conventional angiography devices. However, three dimensional reconstructions and better contrast resolution (ability to see different densities) of CT over fluoroscopy, helps improve diagnostic accuracy of MDCT.

Generally, the higher X-ray flux (mAs = tube current × scan time) and greater number and efficiency of X-ray detectors available with MDCT devices leads to images with better signal-to-noise ratio and higher spatial resolution when compared to earlier scanners. Early detection of calcified plaque is dependent upon distinguishing the plaque from image noise. Newer MDCT systems (64 detector +) have reduced image noise compared to older systems (8–18 noise/HU versus 24 noise/HU). Image noise CT has been shown to have an association with body mass index which may result in falsely identifying noise as calcified plaque or overestimation of true plaque burden. Typical values for mAs for MDCT angiography is on the order of 300–400. While CT scanners have difficulties with the morbidly obese patient, MDCT can increase the mAs (and kV) to help with tissue penetration. Other approaches to overcome image noise in obese patients, beyond increasing mA and kV include reconstructing thicker slices (slice thickness is inversely proportional to image noise) and use of iterative reconstruction (discussed below).

Speed/Temporal Resolution

Cardiac CT is dependent upon having a high temporal resolution to minimize coronary motion-related imaging artifacts. By coupling rapid image acquisition with ECG gating, images can be acquired in specific phases of the cardiac cycle. Studies have indicated that temporal resolutions of 19 ms are needed to suppress all pulmonary and cardiac motion [19]. Interestingly, temporal resolution needs to be faster to suppress motion of the pulmonary arteries than for cardiac imaging. The study by Ritchie et al. demonstrated the need for 19 ms imaging to suppress pulmonary motion (despite breath-holding), while needing 35 ms imaging to fully suppress motion for cardiac structures. This is most likely due to the accordion motion of the pulmonary arteries, whereby the motion of the heart causes the surrounding pulmonary arteries to be pulled in and out with each beat. This has led to some physicians to use cardiac gating during pulmonary embolism studies to improve resolution down to fourth and fifth generation branches of the pulmonary system.

Cardiac MR motion studies of the coronary arteries demonstrate that the rest period of the coronary artery (optimal diastolic imaging time) varies significantly between individ-

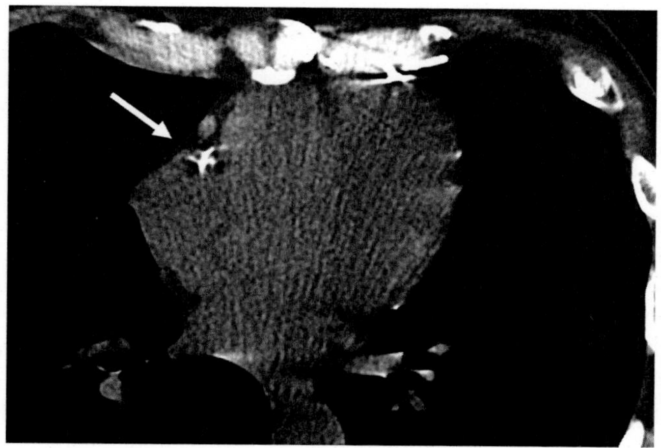

Fig. 1.12 A typical motion artifact seen with calcium scans on MDCT images. The limited reproducibility of this technique is due to the star artifacts seen on this image (RCA, *white arrow*). Prospective gating is done, with halfscan reconstruction techniques. In cases of faster heart rates, motion artifacts seen here are commonplace. To limit radiation to a reasonable level for this screening text, no overlap or retrospective images are obtained, so multisegment reconstruction is not possible

uals with a range of 66–333 ms for the left coronary artery and 66–200 ms for the right coronary artery [20] and that for mapping coronary flow, temporal resolution of 23 ms may be required for segments of the right coronary artery [21,22]. Current generation cardiac CT systems which create images for measuring calcified plaque at 135–220 ms (prospectively gated MDCT) cannot totally eliminate coronary artery motion in all individuals. Motion artifacts are especially prominent in the mid-right coronary artery, where the ballistic movement of the vessel may be as much as two to three times its diameter during the twisting and torsion of the heart during the cardiac cycle (Fig. 1.12). It should be noted that the motion of the coronary artery during the cardiac cycle is a 3-D event with translation, rotation, and accordion type movements. Thus portions of the coronary artery pass within and through adjacent tomographic planes during each R-R cycle. Blurring of plaques secondary to coronary motion increases in systems with slower acquisition speeds. The resulting artifacts tend to increase plaque area and decrease plaque density and thus alter the calcium measurements. The artifacts may make those segments of the CT angiogram non-diagnostic, a problem that plagued up to 70 % of the early four-slice MDCT system studies [5,12].

The image quality achieved with cardiac CT is determined not only by the 3-D spatial resolution but also by the temporal resolution. The spatial resolution is directly related to the scan slice thickness and the reconstruction matrix. The temporal resolution, which determines the degree of motion suppression, is dependent on the pitch factor (which is determined by the table speed), the gantry rotation time, and the patient's heart rate during the examination. As stated above, utilizing more detectors (i.e., 4- versus 8- versus 16- versus 64-detector/channel systems) reduces scan time (i.e., breath-hold time) and section misregistration (misalignment), but has no effect on temporal resolution.

Radiation Dose

Computed tomography utilizes X-rays, a form of ionizing radiation, to produce the information required for generating CT images. Although ionizing radiation from natural sources is part of our daily existence (background radiation including air travel, ground sources, and television), a role of healthcare professionals involved in medical imaging is to understand potential risks of a test and balance those against the potential benefits. This is particularly true for diagnostic tests that will be applied to healthy individuals as part of a disease screening or risk stratification program. In order for healthcare professionals to effectively advise individuals they must have an understanding of the exposure involved. The use of radiological investigations is an accepted part of medical practice, justified in terms of clear clinical benefits to the patient which should far outweigh the small radiation risks. Diagnostic medical exposures, being the major source of man-made radiation exposure of the population, add up to 50 % of the radiation exposure to the population. However, even small radiation doses are not entirely without risk. A small fraction of the genetic mutations and malignant diseases occurring in the population can be attributed to natural background radiation. The concept of "effective dose" was introduced in 1975 to provide a mechanism for assessing the radiation detriment from partial body irradiations in terms of data derived from whole-body irradiations. The effective dose for a radiological investigation is the weighted sum of the doses to a number of body tissues, where the weighting factor for each tissue depends upon its relative sensitivity to radiation-induced cancer or severe hereditary effects. It thus provides a single dose estimate related to the total radiation risk, no matter how the radiation dose is distributed around the body. Adoption of the *effective dose* as a standard measure of dose allows comparability across the spectrum of medical and non-medical exposures. "The effective dose is, by definition, an estimate of the uniform, whole-body equivalent dose that would produce the same level of risk for adverse effects that results from the non-uniform partial body irradiation. The unit for the effective dose is the sievert (Sv)" (www.fda.gov/cdrh/ct/rqu.html). Although it has many limitations, the effective dose is often used to compare the dose from a CT examination, a fluoroscopic examination, and the background radiation one experiences in a year. Units are either millirem (mrem) or millisievert (mSv); 100 mrem equals 1 mSv. The estimated dose from chest X-ray is 0.04 mSv, and the average annual

Table 1.3 Common tests with estimated radiation exposures

Test	Radiation dose (mSv)	
1 Stress MIBI	6	
1 LC spine	1.3	
1 Barium enema	7	
1 Upper GI	3	
1 Abdominal X-ray	1	
1 Dental X-ray	0.7	
1 Cardiac catheterization	2.5–10	
	Radiation dose for MDCT (mSv)	**Radiation dose for EBCT (mSv)**
Calcium scan	1–1.5	0.6
CT angiography	8–13	1–1.5
CTA dose modulation	5–8	–
Lung CT	8	1.5
Abdomen/pelvis	10	2
Body scan	12	2.6
Virtual colon	8–14	2–3

back-ground radiation in the United States is about 300 mrem or 3 mSv [23]. Table 1.3 shows the estimated radiation doses of some commonly used tests.

The Food and Drug Administration (FDA) in describing the radiation risks from CT screening in general used the following language (www.fda.gov/cdrh/ct/risks.html):

In the field of radiation protection, it is commonly assumed that the risk for adverse health effects from cancer is proportional to the amount of radiation dose absorbed and the amount of dose depends on the type of X-ray examination. A CT examination with an effective dose of 10 millisieverts (abbreviated mSv; 1 mSv =1 mGy in the case of x rays) may be associated with an increase in the possibility of fatal cancer of approximately 1 chance in 2000. This increase in the possibility of a fatal cancer from radiation can be compared to the natural incidence of fatal cancer in the US population, about 1 chance in 5. In other words, for any one person the risk of radiation-induced cancer is much smaller than the natural risk of cancer. Nevertheless, this small increase in radiation-associated cancer risk for an individual can become a public health concern if large numbers of the population undergo increased numbers of CT procedures for screening purposes.

Since CT is the most important source of ionizing radiation for the general population, dose reduction and avoidance is of the utmost importance, especially for the asymptomatic person undergoing risk stratification, rather than diagnostic workup. Already, 50 % of a person's lifetime radiation exposure is due to medical testing, and this is expected to go up with increased exposure to nuclear tests and CT scanning. Used as a tool in preventive cardiology, cardiac CT is increasingly being performed in the population of asymptomatic persons, a priori healthier individuals, where use of excessive radiation is of special concern.

The other variable involved in dose is the protocol used. The lowest radiation and most commonly applied is acquired by prospective triggering; that is, the X-rays are only on during the acquisition of data that will be used for the image. MDCT, however, can use prospective triggering or retrospective gating, 120 or 140 kilovolts (kV) (with protocols possible with lower kV depending upon future research and tube current improvements), and a wide range of mA. Retrospective gating means that the X-rays are on throughout the heart cycle. One drawback of MDCT is the potential for higher radiation exposure to the patient, depending on the tube current selected for the examination. The X-ray photon flux expressed by the product of X-ray tube current and exposure time (mAs). For example, 200 mA with 0.5 s exposure time yields 100 mAs in MDCT. In millisieverts, calcium scanning leads to an approximate dose of 0.9 mSv for MDCT (similar to the dose of another screening test, mammography – 0.7 mSv). This is in comparison to a conventional coronary angiogram, with mean doses of 8 mSv [23].

There are primary three factors that go into radiation dosimetry. The X-ray energy (kV), tube current (mA), and exposure time. The distance of the X-ray source from the patient is a fourth source, but, unlike fluoroscopy, this distance is fixed in all current CT scanners. Since MDCT angiography at the time utilized retrospective imaging, and since radiation is continuously applied while only a fraction of the acquired data is utilized, high radiation doses from retrospective CT studies (doses of 6–10 mSv/study) still play a role in decisions to utilize this modality in heart failure and atrial fibrillation, where retrospective studies are largely required [24–26]. The American Heart Association wrote a scientific statement for radiation doses [23] from cardiac studies and cited the following doses: retrospective CTA with dose modulation – 9 mSv; prospective triggered CTA – 3 mSv; stress-rest Sestamibi – 9 mSv; FDG PET scan 14 mSv and invasive coronary angiogram – 7 mSv [23]. Doses have come down dramatically with MDCT due to multiple approaches, including lower kVp (i.e. 100), dose modulation, and prospective triggering, now averaging 2.1 mSev for MDCT angiography in clinical practice [24]. Since the publication by Choi et al. [24], new detectors, iterative reconstruction and more aggressive use of 'fast-pitch' imaging has further reduced doses. It is conceivable that mean doses will dip below 1 mSv once use of these new techniques becomes widespread.

Theoretically, since narrow collimation (beam widths) causes "overbeaming," the dose efficiency is lower with four-slice scanners than with more detectors. Estimated efficiency goes from 67 % with 4 slices (1.25 mm, 5 mm coverage) to 97 % with 16 slices (at 1.25 mm, covering 20 mm). However, obtaining thinner slices will offset this gain, as obtaining more images will lead to higher radiation doses. Typical studies with four-slice MDCT scanners obtained 600 images, while 16-slice scanners typically produce about 1200 scans, and 64-detector scanners are reporting over 2000 images produced per study. Newer MDCT studies report continue to show dramatic radiation reductions from the early 4-slice MDCT scanners and even from the more recent 64-MDCT studies [27].

The energy used can be altered in MDCT studies, and while typical imaging is done in the range of 120–140 kV, this can be varied with MDCT. The attenuation (densities) of calcium and iodine contrast agents increases with reduced X-ray energy (reduced kV settings). This can reduce the X-ray exposure, as the X-ray power emitted by the tube decreases considerably with reduced kV settings. To compensate for the lower power (and resultant increased noise of the image), the tube current (mA) can be increased. Scans with less than 120 kV tube voltage (i.e., 80 kV) can potentially maintain contrast-to-noise ratios that have been established for coronary calcium and CT angiography images, and significant lower radiation expo-sure. Preliminary experiments have demonstrated a reduction in radiation exposures of up to 50 % with use of 80 kV. Jakobs et al. demonstrated that the radiation dose for CAC scoring with use of 80 kV may be as low as 0.6 mSv [28]. As the noise will go up with 80 kV imaging, this may be too low for CT angiography in larger patients, but for children and slim adults, this affords a sub-millisievert dose for the first time with CTA. CT angiography protocols are much more common with 100 kV protocols, providing a reduction in radiation of 40 %, as the dose reduction from kV reduction is exponential, so a 20 % kV reduction affords a 40 % dose reduction. A very low kV (i.e.- 80) is most often used for pediatric patients. Similarly, for obese patients, where penetration is important, a kV of 135 or 140 can be utilized, but the dose will go up exponentially, so this is not widely employed. The power (mAs) used is directly proportional to the radiation dose. Higher mAs results in lower image noise, following the relationship: noise is inversely proportional to the square root of the mAs. Thus, limiting mAs can result in lower radiation, but higher noise. It is important to remember that reducing mAs too much to save radiation will increase noise to the point where the scan is non-diagnostic. Most centers use either an "automatic" mAs system, which adjusts the mAs based upon the image quality, or leave the mAs relatively fixed.

Prospective triggering or "sequential" mode is typically used and strongly recommended for coronary calcium assessment with MDCT, due to the lower radiation doses to which the patient is exposed. However, the drawback of using MDCT prospective triggering is the inability to perform overlapping images, and longer image acquisition times. Thus, all CT vendors currently recommend retrospective image acquisition in the "helical" mode for performance of MDCT angiography, despite the higher radiation doses. This is due to the requirement during retrospective imaging for slower table movement to allow for oversampling, for gap-less and motion-reduced imaging, as well as the possibility of multisegment reconstruction. Retrospective imaging allows the clinician to have multiple phases of the cardiac cycle available for reconstruction, to find the portion of the study with the least coronary motion. Many clinicians utilize multiple phases for reconstruction, with different phases used for different coronary arteries. However, constant irradiation is redundant, as most images are reconstructed during the diastolic phases of the heart cycle. Thus, a new method for reducing radiation dose with MDCT is to implement tube current modulation. Tube current is reduced during systole, when images are not utilized for reconstruction of images for MDCT angiography, by 80 %, and then full dose is utilized during diastole. Depending upon the heart rate, this may reduce radiation exposure by as much as 47 % [28], but with slower heart rates, this reduction will be less, as systole encompasses a shorter and shorter fraction of the cardiac cycle. Dose modulation protocols reduce radiation doses with MDCT by attempting to decrease beam current during systole, when images are not used for interpretation, and should be employed whenever possible [29]. Most of these protocols turn down the beam current (mA) during systole, so that diagnostic images are still available from roughly 40–80 % of the R-R interval (cardiac cycle).

Dose modulation widely, but not universally employed, as it is harder to use with very fast heart rates, as the time to ramp up and ramp down the radiation dose becomes significant, and the ever shortening diastole becomes a smaller target. Also, irregular heart rates (frequent premature beats or atrial fibrillation) makes anticipation of the next R-R interval challenging, so most often dose modulation is turned off in this setting. The routine use of beta blockers makes even more sense in this setting, given the increased ability to use dose modulation more effectively and frequently with lower heart rates. A misconception is the potential loss of wall motion and other functional data with dose modulation. If dose modulation is used, there are systolic images, and while they are somewhat noisier (harder to read plaque), the image quality is still excellent for wall motion and ejection fraction assessment. An image from end-systole (early diastole) and end-diastole can be compared to calculated wall thickening, ejection fraction, and cardiac motion.

Another method to decrease radiation exposure is to increase the pitch. The pitch is usually very low, on the order of 0.20–0.25 for CT angiography cases, and usually 1 for coronary calcium scanning. This low pitch raises radiation exposure, but is partially compensated by the more efficient dose of using the larger collimation available with increased detectors. For individuals with different heart rates, different pitches can be used to obtain similar datasets. Thus, for those with slower heart rates, a faster pitch may allow for some reduction in cardiac exposure during these studies, and thus proportionally less radiation with dose modulation than for those with higher heart rates. The newest scanners available in 2014 now allow for the first time, acquisition of retrospective imaging with 'fast-pitch' acquisitions, moving the gantry very fast during the cardiac cycle and acquiring multiple datasets with a much lower radiation profile and improved resolution. This likely represents the next great breakthrough in cardiac CT imaging, allowing for full datasets to calculate ejection fraction, wall motion and plaque with radiation doses of <1 milliSievert.

One must be careful and cognizant of the dose being given. In one study using 16-slice MDCT, the pitch was reduced based upon the patient being able to hold their breath for 20 s, so very high overlap was obtained (very small pitch). The mean irradiation dose received by the patients during this MDCT angiography study was 24.2 mSv [30]. Understanding the physics and implications of higher mAs and kV and thinner slices will help the clinician choose the necessary parameters, without over-irradiating the patient. This concept, called "information/ milliSv," causes one to think about the benefit garnered from each mSv given.

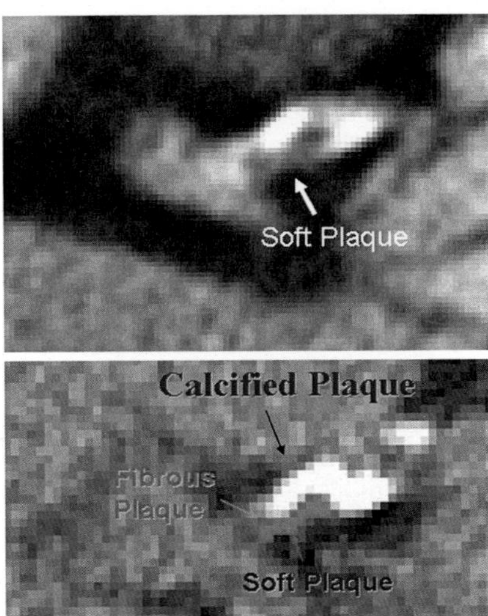

Fig. 1.13 A contrast-enhanced (*top image*) and non-contrast study (*bottom image*) of the left main and proximal LAD. The soft plaque is visible (*dark region*, representing fat density) with calcified plaque (*white regions*). A computer program can be applied (AcuImage, San Francisco, CA) to the individual pixels to measure lower density (*pink squares*, fat density), intermediate density (*red squares*, fibrous density), and high density (*white squares*, calcified plaque). This can theoretically quantitate the volume of soft plaque, fibrous plaque, and calcified plaque in any given CT image

Clinical Applications of Cardiovascular CT

Cardiac CT has several unique diagnostic capabilities applicable to the many facets of CAD, worth the radiation exposures and time needed to learn these applications. Each will be discussed at length in chapters throughout this book. The presence of coronary calcium is invariably an indicator of atherosclerosis [31,32]. Non-contrast studies can accurately identify and quantify coronary calcification (a marker of total plaque burden) [33], while contrast-enhanced studies can define ventricular volumes, ejection fraction, and wall motion and wall thickening with high accuracy [34]. Studies can be performed at rest, and during exercise can identify reversible ischemia [35].

Coronary angiography during cardiac catheterization is the clinical gold standard for definitive diagnosis and determination of coronary lesions. Pathologic studies have demonstrated that the severity of coronary stenosis is underestimated by visual analysis during clinical coronary angiography [36–39]. This may result from the limitations of resolution based upon fluoroscopy and the 2-D imaging inherent in coronary angiography, as well as the inability to see beyond the lumen with conventional angiography. The true promise of cardiovascular CT is to visualize the coronary artery, including the lumen and wall. Three-dimensional digital coronary images may provide more accurate representation of coronary artery anatomy and be more amenable to quantitation, thereby improving the diagnosis and treatment of CAD [40]. There is rapidly accumulating data with MDCT to visualize the coronary arteries accurately and reliably (CT angiography) [41–44]. Looking beyond the lumen by visualizing the wall and its constituents (including fat, calcium, and fibrous tissue) is now possible with cardiac CT (Fig. 1.13). Coronary plaque composition evaluation is being actively investigated [45,46]. This so-called "soft plaque" or 'high-risk plaque' evaluation has demonstrated to have prognostic significance over coronary calcium or risk factors alone, as well as helping to target revascularization better than luminography alone [46].

Future of CT and MR

The strengths of magnetic resonance cardiovascular imaging include greater definition of tissue characteristics, perfusion, valvular function, lack of X-ray radiation, and lack of need for potentially nephrotoxic contrast media, compared to CT technologies. Several studies have been reported comparing this modality to coronary angiography [47–49]. Limited temporal and spatial resolution [50], partial volume artifacts (due

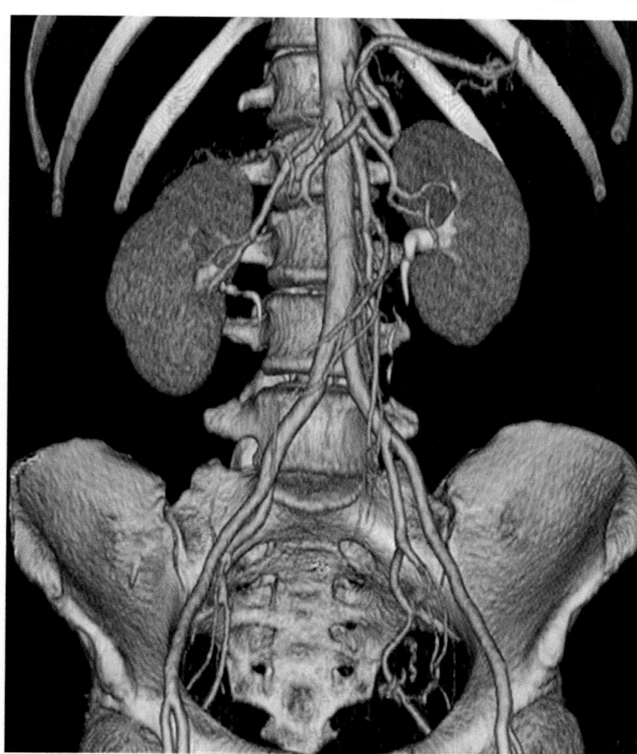

Fig. 1.14 A contrast-enhanced study demonstrating the abdominal aorta, renal arteries and kidneys, and iliac circulation. This study can be done with 40 cm^3 of iodinated contrast, taking between 5 and 10 s depending on the scanner used. Highly diagnostic vascular imaging is quite routine with CT scanners

to slice thickness limitations) [51], reliance on multiple breath-holds, and poor visualization of the left main coronary artery [52] all reduce the clinical applicability of MR angiography. Reported sensitivities for MR angiography range from 0 to 90 % [9,47]. MR angiography remains a technically challenging technique with certain limitations hindering its clinical use. CT angiography offers advantages over MR angiography, including single breath-hold to reduce respiratory motion, higher spatial resolution, reduced slice thickness and overall study time of 35–50 s with CT techniques as compared to 45–90 min for MR angiography [9]. The rapidity and ease with which CT coronary angiography can be performed suggest possible cost advantages compared with MR angiography and selective coronary angiography [53]. Thus, for most applications (in the absence of renal insufficiency or contrast allergy), CT will be the preferred method to evaluate anatomy, be it coronary, renal, carotid or peripheral vascular beds (Fig. 1.14). MR, in the foreseeable future, will remain a better test for intercranial imaging, as the bony structures cause some scatter with CT imaging.

For cardiovascular CT in general, better workstations (ease of use and diagnostic capabilities), as well as improvements in both spatial and temporal resolution will continue to push this diagnostic tool to the forefront of cardiology. For MDCT, increased numbers of detectors will allow for better collimation and spatial reconstructions. Having more of the heart visualized simultaneously will also allow for reductions in the contrast requirements and breath-holding, further improving the methodology. Multisector reconstruction (combining images from consecutive heart beats) and dose modulation (to reduce radiation exposure during systole, when images are not used for reconstruction) are increasingly being applied, which will continue to improve the image quality and diagnostic rate of these machines. Functional data, now being made available with the advent of fractional flow reserve estimates from CT (FFRct) and transluminal attenuation gradients (TAG) will continue to push the frontier of CT angiographic imaging forward quickly [54].

References

1. Mao S, Budoff MJ, Oudiz RJ, Bakhsheshi H, Wang S, Brundage BH. A simple single slice method for measurement of left and right ventricular enlargement by electron beam tomography. Int J Card Imaging. 2000;16:383–90.
2. Budoff MJ, Mao SS, Wang S, Bakhsheshi H, Brundage BH. A Simple single slice method for measurement of left and right atrial volume by electron beam computed tomography. Acad Radiol. 1999;6:481–6.
3. Stuber M, Botnar RM, Fischer SE, et al. Preliminary report of in-vivo coronary MRA at 3 Tesla in humans. Magn Reson Med. 2002;48:425–8.
4. Carr JJ, Nelson JC, Wong ND, et al. Calcified coronary artery plaque measurement with cardiac CT in population-based studies: standardized protocol of Multi-Ethnic Study of Atherosclerosis (MESA) and Coronary Artery Risk Development in Young Adults (CARDIA) study. Radiology. 2005;234:35–43.
5. Nieman K, Rensing BJ, van Geuns RJ, et al. Non-invasive coronary angiography with multislice spiral computed tomography: impact of heart rate. Heart. 2002;88(5):470–4.
6. Ropers D, Baum U, Pohle K, et al. Detection of coronary artery steno-sis with thin-slice multi-detector row spiral computed tomography and multiplanar reconstruction. Circulation. 2003;107:664–6.
7. Nieman K, Cademartiri F, Lemos PA, Raaijmakers R, Pattynama PM, de Feyter PJ. Reliable noninvasive coronary angiography with fast submillimeter multislice spiral computed tomography. Circulation. 2002;106:2051–4.
8. Regenfus M, Ropers D, Achenbach S, et al. Noninvasive detection of coronary artery stenosis using contrast-enhanced three-dimensional breath-hold magnetic resonance coronary angiography. J Am Coll Cardiol. 2000;36:44–50.
9. Kim WY, Danias PG, Stuber M, et al. Coronary magnetic resonance angiography for the detection of coronary stenoses. N Engl J Med. 2001;345:1863–9.
10. Blobel J, Baartman H, Rogalla P, Mews J, Lembcke A. Spatial and temporal resolution with 16-slice computed tomography for cardiac imaging. Fortschr Roentgenstr. 2003;175:1264–71.
11. Lembcke A, Rogalla P, Mews J, et al. Imaging of the coronary arteries by means of multislice helical CT: optimization of image quality with multisegmental reconstruction and variable gantry rotation time. Fortschr Roentgenstr. 2003;175:780–5.

12. Wicky S, Rosol M, Hoffmann U, Graziano M, Yucel KE, Brady TJ. Comparative study with a moving heart phantom of the impact of temporal resolution on image quality with two multidetector electrocardiography-gated computed tomography units. J Comput Assist Tomogr. 2003;27:392–8.
13. Dewey M, Laule M, Krug L, et al. Multisegment and halfscan reconstruction of 16-slice computed tomography for detection of coronary artery stenosis. Invest Radiol. 2004;39:223–9.
14. Mao S, Lu B, Oudiz RJ, Bakhsheshi H, Liu SCK, Budoff MJ. Coronary artery motion in electron beam tomography. J Comput Assist Tomogr. 2000;24:253–8.
15. Baik HK, Budoff MJ, Lane KL, Bakhsheshi H, Brundage BH. Accurate measures of ejection fraction using electron beam tomography, radionuclide angiography, and catheterization angiography. Int J Card Imaging. 2000;16:391–8.
16. Mao SS, Budoff MJ, Oudiz RJ, et al. Effect of exercise on left and right ventricular ejection fraction and wall motion in patients with coronary artery disease: an electron beam computed tomography study. Int J Cardiol. 1999;71:23–31.
17. McKay CR, Brundage BH, Ullyot DJ, et al. Evaluation of early post-operative coronary artery bypass grafts patency by contrast-enhanced computed tomography. J Am Coll Cardiol. 1983;2:312–7.
18. Nissen SE, Gurley GL. Assessment of coronary angioplasty results by intravascular ultrasound. In: Serruys PW, Straus BH, King III SB, editors. Restenosis after intervention with new mechanical devices. Dordrecht: Kluwer; 1992. p. 73–96.
19. Ritchie CJ, Godwin JD. Minimum scan speeds for suppression of motion artifacts in CT. Radiology. 1992;185:37–42.
20. Wang Y, Vidan E. Cardiac motion of coronary arteries: variability in the rest period and implications for coronary MR angiography. Radiology. 1999;213(3):751–8.
21. Hofman MB, Wickline SA. Quantification of in-plane motion of the coronary arteries during the cardiac cycle: implications for acquisition window duration for MR flow quantification. J Magn Reson Imaging. 1998;8(3):568–76.
22. Marcus JT, Smeenk HG. Flow profiles in the left anterior descending and the right coronary artery assessed by MR velocity quantification: effects of through-plane and in-plane motion of the heart. J Comput Assist Tomogr. 1999;23(4):567–76.
23. Gerber TC, Carr JJ, Arai AE, et al. Ionizing radiation in cardiac imaging: a science advisory from the American Heart Association Committee on Cardiac Imaging of the Council on Clinical Cardiology and Committee on Cardiovascular Imaging and Intervention of the Council on Cardiovascular Radiology and Intervention. Circulation. 2009;119:1056–65.
24. Choi TY, Malpeso J, Li D, Sourayanezhad S, Budoff MJ. Radiation dose reduction with increasing utilization of prospective gating in 64-multidetector cardiac computed tomography angiography. J Cardiovasc Comput Tomogr. 2011;5:264–70.
25. Gopal A, Mao SS, Karlsberg D, Young E, Waggoner J, Ahmadi N, Pal RS, Leal J, Karlsberg RP, Budoff MJ. Radiation reduction with prospective ECG-triggering acquisition using 64-multidetector computed tomographic angiography. Int J Cardiovasc Imaging. 2009;25(4):405–16.
26. Mark DB, Berman DS, Budoff MJ, Carr JJ, Gerber TC, Hecht HS, Hlatky MA, Hodgson JM, Lauer MS, Miller JM, Morin RL, Mukherjee D, Poon M, Rubin GD, Schwartz RS. ACCF/ACR/AHA/NASCI/SAIP/SCAI/SCCT 2010 expert consensus document on coronary computed tomographic angiography: a report of the American College of Cardiology Foundation Task Force on Expert Consensus Documents. J Am Coll Cardiol. 2010;55(23):2663–99.
27. Khosa F, Khan A, Nasir K, Shuaib W, Budoff M, Blankstein R, Clouse ME. Influence of image acquisition on radiation dose and image quality: full versus narrow phase window acquisition using 320 MDCT. ScientificWorldJournal. 2013:731590. doi:10.1155/2013/731590.
28. Jakobs TF, Becker CR, Ohnesorge B, et al. Multislice helical CT of the heart with retrospective ECG gating: reduction of radiation exposure by ECG-controlled tube current modulation. Eur Radiol. 2002;12:1081–6.
29. Trabold T, Buchgeister M, Kuttner A, et al. Estimation of radiation exposure in 16-detector row computed tomography of the heart with retrospective ECG-gating. Rofo. 2003;175:1051–5.
30. Leta R, Carreras F, Alomar X, et al. Non-invasive coronary angiography with 16 multidetector-row spiral computed tomography: a comparative study with invasive coronary angiography. Rev Esp Cardiol. 2004;57:217–24.
31. Janowitz WR, Viamonte M, Agatston AS. Comparison of serial quantitative evaluation of calcified coronary artery plaque by ultrafast computed tomography in persons with and without obstructive coronary artery disease. Am J Cardiol. 1991;68:1–6.
32. Blankenhorn DH. Coronary artery calcification: a review. Am J Med Sci. 1961;242:1–9.
33. Breen JF, Sheedy PF, Schwartz RS, et al. Coronary artery calcification detected with ultrafast CT as an indication of coronary artery disease. Radiology. 1992;185:435–9.
34. Lipton MJ, Higgins CB, Boyd DP. Computed tomography of the heart: evaluation of anatomy and function. J Am Coll Cardiol. 1985;5:555–95.
35. Roig E, Chomka EV, Castaner A, et al. Exercise ultrafast computed tomography for the detection of coronary artery disease. J Am Coll Cardiol. 1989;13:1073–81.
36. Marcus ML, Armstrong MD, Heistad DD, Eastham CL, Mark AL. Comparison of three methods of evaluating coronary obstructive lesions: postmortem arteriography, pathologic examination and measurement of regional myocardial perfusion during maximal vasodilation. Am J Cardiol. 1982;49:1688–706.
37. Grondin CM, Dyrda I, Pasternac A, Campeau L, Bourassa MG, Les-perance J. Discrepancies between cineangiographic and postmortem findings in patients with coronary artery disease and recent myocardial revascularization. Circulation. 1974;49:703–8.
38. Thomas AC, Daview MJ, Dilly S, Dilly N, Franc F. Potential errors in estimation of coronary arterial stenoses from clinical coronary arteriography with reference to the shape of the coronary arterial lumen. Br Heart J. 1986;55:129–39.
39. Mintz GS, Painter JA, Pichard AD, et al. Atherosclerosis in angiographically normal coronary artery reference segments: an intravascular ultrasound study with clinical correlations. J Am Coll Cardiol. 1995;25:1479–85.
40. Budoff MJ, Nakazato R, Mancini GBJ, et al. CT angiography for the prediction of hemodynamic significance in intermediate and severe lesions: head-to-head comparison with quantitative coronary angiography using fractional flow reserve as the reference standard. J Am Coll Cardiol Img. 2016. doi:10.1016/j.jcmg.2015.08.021.
41. Budoff MJ, Dowe D, Jollis JG, Gitter M, Sutherland J, Halamert E, Scherer M, Bellinger R, Martin A, Benton R, Delago A, Min JK. Diagnostic performance of 64-detector row coronary computed tomographic angiography of individuals undergoing invasive coronary prospective multicenter ACCURACY (assessment by coronary computed individuals without known coronary artery disease: results from the tomographic angiography for evaluation of coronary artery stenosis in angiography) trial. J Am Coll Cardiol. 2008;52(21):1724–32.
42. Pagali SR, Madaj P, Gupta M, Nair S, Hamirani YS, Min JK, Lin F, Budoff MJ. Interobserver variations of plaque severity score and segment stenosis score in coronary arteries using 64 slice multidetector computed tomography: a substudy of the ACCURACY trial. J Cardiovasc Comput Tomogr. 2010;4(5):312–8.
43. Hamirani YS, Isma'eel H, Larijani V, Drury P, Lim W, Bevinal M, Saeed A, Ahmadi N, Karlsberg RP, Budoff MJ. The diagnostic

accuracy of 64-detector cardiac computed tomography compared with stress nuclear imaging in patients undergoing invasive cardiac catheterization. J Comput Assist Tomogr. 2010;34(5):645–51. PMID: 20861764.
44. Abdulla J, Pedersen KS, Budoff M, Kofoed KF. Influence of coronary calcification on the diagnostic accuracy of 64-slice computed tomography coronary angiography: a systematic review and meta-analysis. Int J Cardiovasc Imaging. 2012;28(4):943–53. doi:10.1007/s10554-011-9902-6.
45. Alani A, Nakanishi R, Budoff MJ. Recent improvement in coronary computed tomography angiography diagnostic accuracy. Clin Cardiol. 2014;37(7):428–33. doi:10.1002/clc.22286. PMID: 24756932.
46. Min JK, Edwardes M, Lin FY, Labounty T, Weinsaft JW, Choi JH, Delago A, Shaw LJ, Berman DS, Budoff MJ. Relationship of coronary artery plaque composition to coronary artery stenosis severity: results from the prospective multicenter ACCURACY trial. Atherosclerosis. 2011;219:573–8. PMID: 21696739.
47. Manning WJ, Li W, Edelman RR. A preliminary report comparing magnetic resonance imaging with conventional angiography. N Engl J Med. 1993;328:828–32.
48. Pennell DJ, Keegan J, Firmin DN, Gatehouse PD, Underwood SR, Longmore DB. Magnetic resonance imaging of coronary arteries: technique and preliminary results. Br Heart J. 1993;70: 315–26.
49. Paschal CB, Haache EM, Adler LP. Coronary arteries: three-dimensional MR imaging of the coronary arteries: preliminary clinical experience. J Magn Reson Imaging. 1993;3:491–501.
50. Duerinckx AJ, Urman MK. Two dimensional coronary MR angiography: analysis of initial clinical results. Radiology. 1994;193: 731–8.
51. Duerinckx AJ, Urman MK, Atkinson DJ, Simonetti OP, Sinha U, Lewis B. Limitations of MR coronary angiography. J Magn Reson Imaging. 1994;4:81.
52. Duerinckx AJ, Atkinson DP, Mintorovitch J, Simonetti OP, Urman MK. Two-dimensional coronary MRA: limitations and artifacts. Eur Radiol. 1996;6:312–25.
53. Chernoff DM, Ritchie CJ, Higgins CB. Evaluation of electron beam CT coronary angiography in healthy subjects. AJR Am J Roentgenol. 1997;169:93–9.
54. Leipsic J, Yang TH, Thompson A, Koo BK, Mancini GB, Taylor C, Budoff MJ, Park HB, Berman DS, Min JK. CT angiography (CTA) and diagnostic performance of noninvasive fractional flow reserve: results from the determination of fractional flow reserve by anatomic CTA (DeFACTO) study. AJR Am J Roentgenol. 2014;202(5):989–94. doi:10.2214/AJR.13.11441.

Cardiovascular Computed Tomography: Current and Future Scanning System Design

2

Rine Nakanishi, Wm. Guy Weigold, and Matthew J. Budoff

Abstract

Since the heart is continually in motion, cardiac computed tomography (CT) has capabilities required to scan the heart with high spatial resolution, high temporal resolution, larger detector coverage and fast scan speed. Recent technology enabled current versions of cardiac CT to display the heart with much fewer artifacts and less radiation dose. In this chapter, we will address the current and future scanning system design of cardiac CT.

Keywords

Cardiac CT • Spatial resolution • Temporal resolution • Detector coverage • Scan speed

Introduction

The heart can be visualized in gross form on any standard chest CT, but for a detailed evaluation of cardiac anatomy exact specifications of scanner hardware and software must be in place because the heart is continually in motion, the structures of interest (i.e., coronary arteries) are small, and their curvilinear course requires multi-planar reformatting for analysis.

For these specifications to be met, the scanner hardware must be robust, the scanner must be fitted with ECG-monitoring equipment, and cardiac-specific software and image reconstruction servers must be installed.

R. Nakanishi, MD, PhD
Department of Medicine, Cardiac CT, Los Angeles BioMedical Research Institute at Habor-UCLA Medical Center, Torrance, CA, USA
e-mail: nakanishi.rine@gmail.com

W.G. Weigold, MD, FACC, FSCCT
Department of Medicine, MedStar Washington Hospital Center, Washington, DC, USA

Cardiac CT Core Lab, MedStar Health Research Institute, Washington, DC, USA

MedStar Cardiovascular Research Network, Washington, DC, USA
e-mail: guy.weigold@medstar.net

M.J. Budoff, MD (✉)
David Geffen School of Medicine at UCLA, Los Angeles Biomedical Research Institute, Torrance, CA, USA
e-mail: mbudoff@labiomed.org

Elements of Scanner Design

The general design of a CT scanner equipped for cardiac imaging is the same as that of any modern scanner: an x-ray tube mounted on a rotating gantry opposite a detector array generates x-rays which are emitted across the bore, are attenuated as they pass through the patient's chest, and are scintillated by the detectors as the gantry rotates around the patient obtaining attenuation data from multiple view angles. These data are transmitted to an image reconstruction server which then computes the axial images. To perform cardiac CT, however, a number of additional capabilities are required, namely, high spatial resolution, high temporal resolution, and fast scan speed, while delivering an acceptable radiation exposure.

M.J. Budoff, J.S. Shinbane (eds.), *Cardiac CT Imaging: Diagnosis of Cardiovascular Disease*,
DOI 10.1007/978-3-319-28219-0_2

Special Design Considerations for Cardiac CT

Spatial Resolution

Spatial resolution is the product of multiple variables including detector characteristics and collimation, sampling rate, and reconstruction methods. State of the art scanners use thin 0.5–0.625 mm collimation. This reduces volume averaging thus increasing image detail of small objects, and allows reconstruction of isotropic datasets, thereby preserving z-axis resolution and permitting multiplanar reformatting necessary for analysis of cardiac anatomy.

GE Healthcare has focused their system development on spatial resolution, developing a new detector scintillation material with a fast decay time (30 ns), minimal afterglow (one-quarter that of conventional Gd_2O_2S crystals), and increased efficiency. This new detector is one element of a multi-pronged approach to increasing image resolution, which also includes new electronics that permit increased sampling, and a new iterative reconstruction algorithm [1] (Fig. 2.1). These innovations increase spatial resolution by 3–4.5 line pairs per cm (lp/cm), which is substantial given that current resolution of systems is approximately 12–15 lp/cm. The enhanced resolution is particularly useful for imaging stented and/or calcified coronary arteries, while lowering radiation requirements.

Temporal Resolution

In order to reconstruct an axial image, attenuation data from multiple view angles that encompass half a rotation around the patient are required. The amount of time needed to obtain this data is the nominal, heart-rate independent temporal resolution of the scanner. Hence, a gantry that requires 330 ms to make one complete rotation has a baseline temporal resolution of 165 ms. This is analogous to shutter speed: just as shutter speed must be sufficiently fast to capture motion-free images of a moving subject, temporal resolution must be sufficiently fast to capture the data needed for image reconstruction within the relatively brief period of cardiac diastasis. If temporal resolution is insufficient, motion artifact occurs (Fig. 2.2). A temporal resolution of 165 ms is relatively slow for cardiac imaging, so systems overcome this by various means: faster gantry rotation, multi-cycle reconstruction, and a second x-ray tube.

Multi-cycle reconstruction combines data from multiple contiguous heart beats to complete the half-scan of views (Fig. 2.3). This technique is heart-rate dependent: it can only be used within certain ranges of heart rates, since the cardiac cycle and gantry rotation must be asynchronous.

An approach adopted by Siemens in 2006 uses two x-ray tubes mounted on the gantry at 90° angles; therefore, only a quarter turn of the gantry is required to collect the 180° of attenuation data. Hence, a most recent dual-source system with a gantry rotation time of 250 ms has a baseline central temporal resolution of approximately 66 ms. This obviates

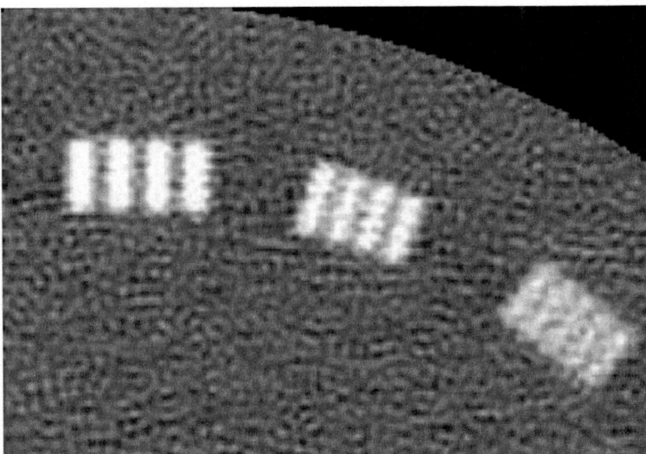

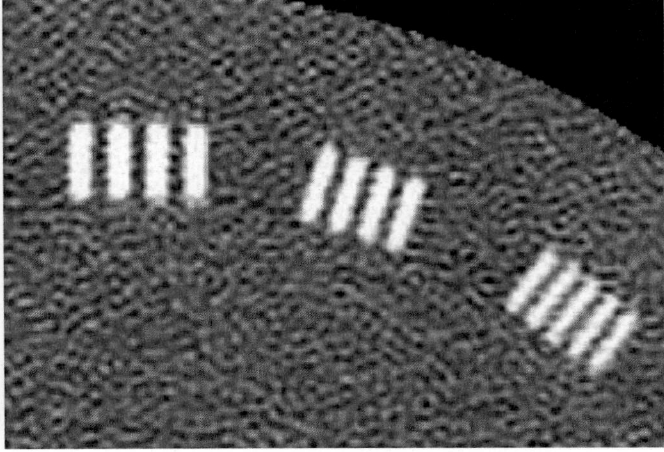

Fig. 2.1 Increased sampling improves image quality. Axial images of line-pair phantom demonstrate improved spatial resolution using increased sampling density (on the *right*) compared to standard sampling frequency (on the *left*). Note the improved edge detail and resolution of the line pairs of the image derived from the high density sampling dataset (Reproduced with permission from Chandra [2])

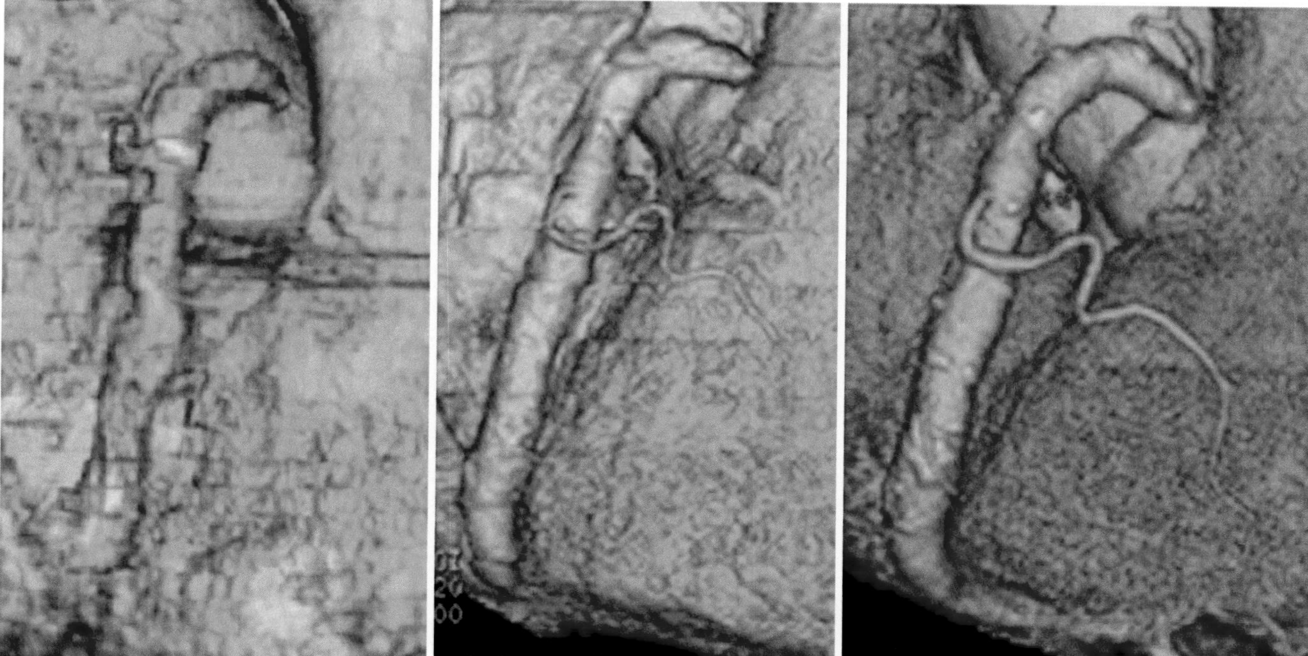

Fig. 2.2 Better temporal resolution improves image quality of moving structures. 3D volume reconstructions of the right coronary artery in 3 CT scans representing 3 generations of CT scanner (4-, 16-, and 64-slice, from *left to right*, respectively), possessing temporal resolution of 400, 250, and 180 ms from *left to right*, respectively. Note that the vessel appears distorted and disjointed, due to motion artifact, when temporal resolution is insufficient (*far left*), while motion artifact is minimally present, and small anatomic details are clearly imaged when temporal resolution is improved (*far right*) (Reproduced with the kind permission of Springer Science + Business Media from Hurlock et al. [3])

the need for multi-cycle reconstruction, making the system less susceptible to variation in heart rate, and providing high heart rate independent temporal resolution. Several reports demonstrated very good image quality [4, 5] and, in a comparison of 64 MDCT and DSCT scans, the dual-source system produced better image quality at higher heart rates [6]. Image quality is still improved, however, by reducing heart rate before scanning. The improvement of temporal resolution is not the only way to solve the issue for motion artifact. As a post image processor, GE currently provides the motion-correction algorithm (Snapshot Freeze; GE Healthcare) which improves image quality using coronary motion artifact and supplements interpretability for diagnostic problems of CAD [7].

Detector Coverage and Scan Speed

The several novel multi-slice CTs have achieved wider z-axis coverage. The scan length is 16 cm, which is mostly enough to scan the whole heart in a single heart beat, avoiding breathing or misalignment artifact. In addition, by increasing coverage or faster temporal resolution, scan times have been recently reduced to just < 1 s, resulting in the minimization of the radiation exposure. The Toshiba's Aquilion One scanner (Aquilion One Dynamic Volume CT; Toshiba Medical System, Tochigi-ken, Japan) has 320 rows of detectors, with 0.5 mm collimation, 16 cm of coverage, and can perform an axial 1-beat acquisition of the entire heart when the rate is well controlled. The GE revolution also demonstrated a wider coverage of 16 cm and 0.23 mm collimation, with gantry rotation 280 mm. The Philips iQon (Philips Healthcare, Cleveland, OH), is a 256-row scanner, which allows axial acquisition of the entire heart in 2 beats.

Radiation Exposure

Traditional cardiac CT uses a helical scan mode and very low pitch to perform retrospective ECG-gated reconstructions. This delivers an undesirably high radiation exposure, so various methods have been designed to reduce radiation exposure.

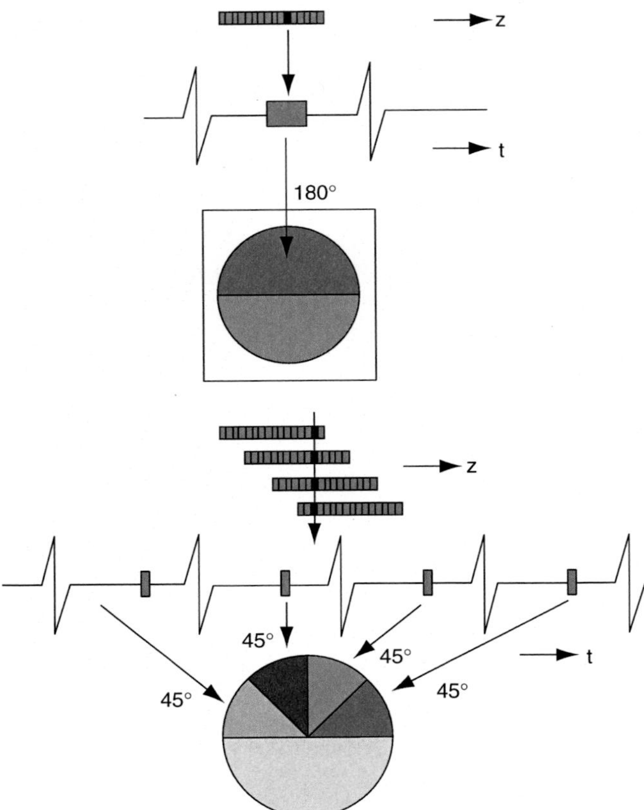

Fig. 2.3 Multi-cycle reconstruction. Single cycle recon (**a**): The duration of the acquisition window (*gray bar*) is approximately equivalent to one-half the gantry rotation time, since this is the time required to obtain 180° of attenuation data. Multi-cycle recon (**b**): When multiple detector rows are present, the axial slice position in the z-position can be imaged at multiple different times, using multiple, shorter, acquisition windows distributed across multiple contiguous beats. This data can then be combined to provide 180° of attenuation data and used to reconstruct the axial image. Temporal resolution of the image is improved because the duration of the each acquisition window is shorter (Reproduced with permission of Wolters Kluwer from Vembar et al. [8])

One of the first was ECG-based tube current modulation, which fluctuates tube current in sync with the heart rate, maintaining high tube current during diastasis and providing the best image quality in that phase, then lowering tube current during other phases when high-resolution detail is not required (Fig. 2.4). This results in a dose savings of approximately 40 %.

A great advance in dose reduction was made with the advent of prospective, ECG-triggered, axial cardiac CT (Fig. 2.5). By keeping the x-ray tube off during most of the scan, and only turning it on during diastasis, as triggered by the ECG, radiation exposure is dramatically reduced. GE first published results using this method [9] with good clinical results and radiation doses of 1–2 mSv [10], and this approach is now offered by all manufacturers. Using a 64-slice system, the entire heart can be covered in 3–4 acquisitions; however this leaves the system vulnerable to fluctuations in heart rate and rhythm during the scan. Larger coverage mitigates this vulnerability by reducing the number of beats required for data acquisition. However, larger coverage lends to higher radiation doses, as the detectors are less efficient when having to expose a wider detector array. Hence, Philips' 128-row iCT system can cover the entire heart in 2 beats, with a reported radiation exposure of 3–5 mSv. Toshiba's 320-row Aquilion One scanner can cover the entire heart in one beat, with a reported radiation exposure of approximately 6 mSv. However, lower radiation doses and dependable coronary scanning using 1-beat acquisition requires heart rate reduction. At higher heart rates (>65 bpm), optimal image quality requires a 2- or 3-beat acquisition (and use of multi-cycle recon) which increases radiation exposure to approximately 13 (2-beat) to 19 (3-beat) mSv [11, 12]. Acquiring with a wide exposure window ("padding") can ensure the capture of motion-free data, but increases radiation exposure (Fig. 2.6). A narrower exposure window can be used with preservation of image quality if heart rate is controlled and reduces radiation exposure.

High Pitch Helical Scanning

Radiation exposure is inversely proportional to pitch in ECG-gated helical CT. Thus, increasing the pitch could dramatically lower radiation requirements in cardiac CT. In 2009, Siemens introduced an innovative scanning method using a high pitch helical mode which takes advantage of the dual-source design [13, 14] (Fig. 2.7). The high pitch (3.2–3.4) would normally produce gaps in the attenuation data using a single-source system, but, in a dual-source system, these gaps are compensated for by gathering data from the second detector. Scan time is less than one second, with radiation exposures now reported less than 1 mSv. Initial studies performed on the first-generation dual-source system proved the feasibility of the method, though the authors noted that these first-generation systems are not suitable for this high pitch technique. High pitch scanning with their new scanner, with faster gantry rotation (250 ms) and larger coverage (96 rows), has been reported to produce very good coronary image quality with radiation exposure of <1 mSv [4, 15, 16], or even lower, with <0.1 mSv [17]. Of note, in this initial investigational phase, low heart rates (<60 bpm) are absolutely required, as the entire data collection takes place within a 250–270 ms acquisition window of one heart beat; hence

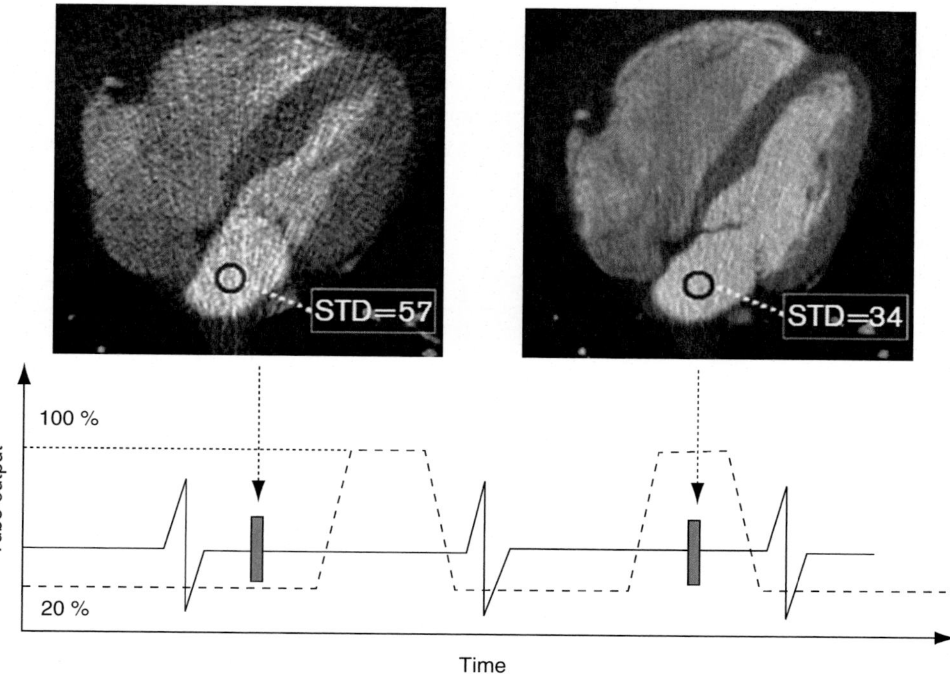

Fig. 2.4 ECG-based tube current modulation reduces radiation exposure. Once the desired acquisition phase is determined, based on heart rate, in this case 75 % phase, scanning proceeds with maintenance of 100 % tube output during that phase, while tube current is reduced outside of that phase. This can reduce effective radiation dose by 40 % or more; however, note that images reconstructed from the low tube output phases (*left image*) will be excessively noisy, and are usually considered unusable for coronary interpretation (Reproduced with permission of Wolters Kluwer from Vembar et al. [8])

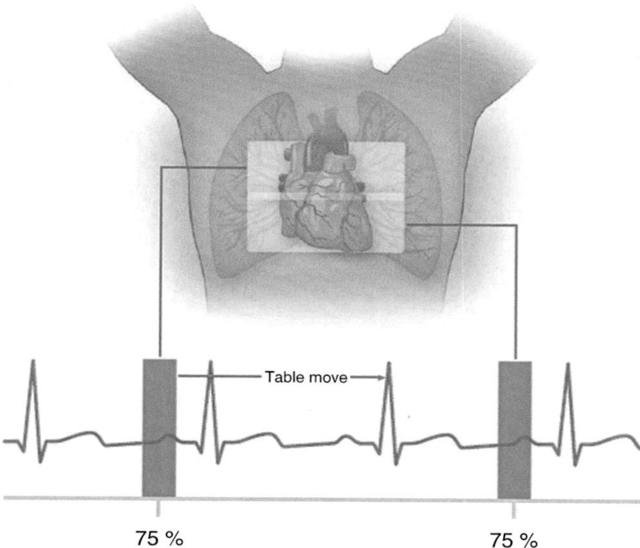

Fig. 2.5 Prospective ECG-triggered acquisition method. Cardiac rhythm is monitored while table remains stationary. When cardiac cycle reaches pre-determined acquisition phase (in this case 75 %, diastolic, phase), x-ray source is briefly turned on (<1 s, *blue bars*) and acquires attenuation data of a length equivalent to the craniocaudal coverage of the detector array, and is then turned off. The table is advanced almost the length of craniocaudal coverage (minus a small amount of overlap), and the process repeats again. Depending on the craniocaudal coverage of the scanner, the entire heart can be scanned in 1–4 acquisitions (Reproduced with the kind permission of Springer Science + Business Media from Weigold et al. [18])

diastasis must be at least this long to provide motion free data acquisition.

The GE Revolution can now utilize the new detector and reconstruction system, along with a fast pitch algorithm, to lower radiation exposure by preserving image quality while scanning with less radiation (<1 mSv), because images are of higher resolution and lower noise than would otherwise be achievable with a low-exposure scan.

Future Directions

Future scanner designs are closely guarded industry secrets, but some concepts have been openly discussed. Flat-panel volume CT systems replace detector rows with a large area detector, and provide coverage of the entire heart in one axial acquisition and extremely high spatial resolution of up to 26 lp/cm, comparable to invasive angiography [19]. However, the contrast resolution is inferior to that of multi-detector CT, a high radiation exposure is needed to achieve a sufficient contrast-to-noise ratio, scintillation times are slow and temporal resolution is insufficient for cardiac imaging.

Dual energy scanning is being developed by all vendors by various means, including rapid fluctuation of tube energy, stacked detectors, or the dual-tube design in which each tube emits photons of different energy levels. Dual energy CT could take the field to a new level of diagnostic power if it can be used for refined tissue characterization, such as differentiating plaque characteristics. This is difficult to do in the coronary arteries, and initial studies have not yielded any breakthroughs, but at the least it has the potential to enhance coronary lumen visualization in heavily calcified vessels by differentiating calcium and iodine [20, 21] (Fig. 2.8). Dual-energy CT may also yield new applications for non-coronary imaging, such as imaging of myocardial perfusion [22].

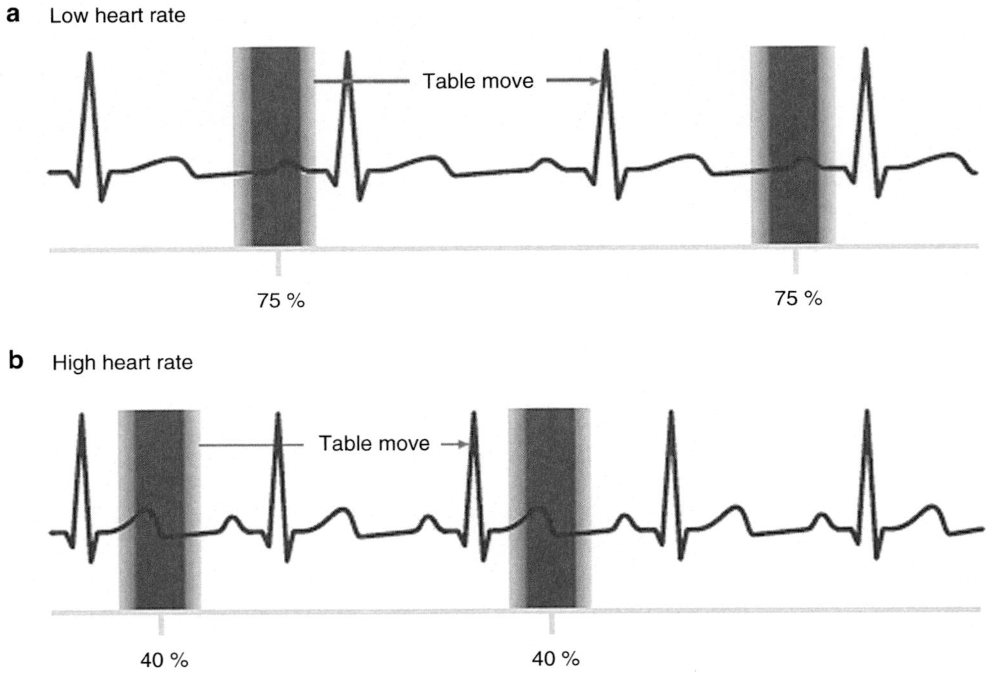

Fig. 2.6 Prospective CCTA phase selection and padding. Acquisition phase and padding depend on heart rate: For low heart rates (**a**), target late diastole (75 % phase) for prospective acquisition, but if heart rate is high (**b**) (>75 bpm), target end-systole (40 % phase) which is more likely to produce motion-free images. By restricting acquisition to the minimum exposure window (*dark gray*), radiation dose is minimized, but ability to reconstruct adjacent cardiac phases is obliterated. Widening the acquisition window ("padding," light gray shading) allows reconstruction of a small number of additional phases, which can help interpretation of motion artifact, but increases the radiation dose (Reproduced with the kind permission of Springer Science+Business Media from Weigold et al. [18])

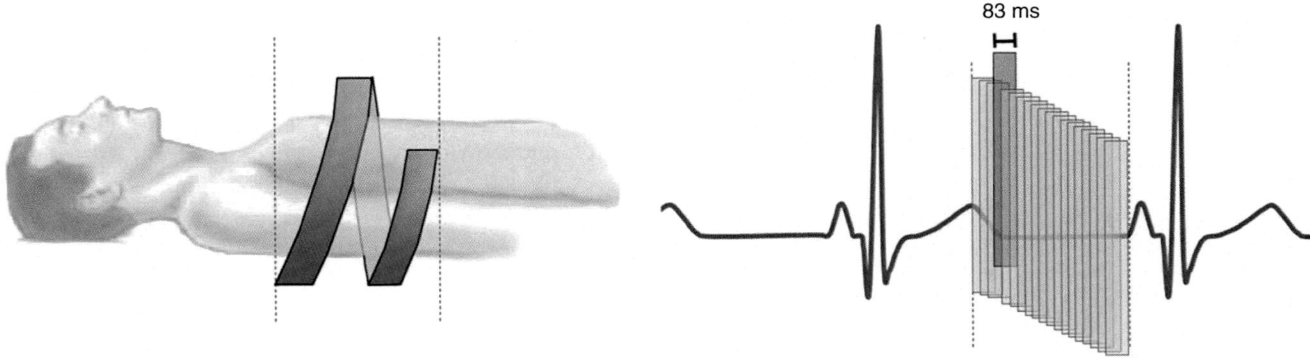

Fig. 2.7 Method of high-pitch coronary CCTA. Single source helical CT requires a pitch ≤ 1.5; a faster pitch results in gaps in the data (*left panel*). A dual-source system can scan at a higher pitch (up to 3.2), using the second x-ray source-detector system to fill in what would otherwise be gaps in the data. Since the table speed is so high, the entire heart can be imaged in a fraction of a second, from data derived from a single heartbeat (*right panel*). If the image acquisition is triggered appropriately to synchronize acquisition with diastasis, and the heart rate is sufficiently low, motion-free images can be obtained with a very low radiation dose (Reproduced with permission of Elsevier from Achenbach et al. [14])

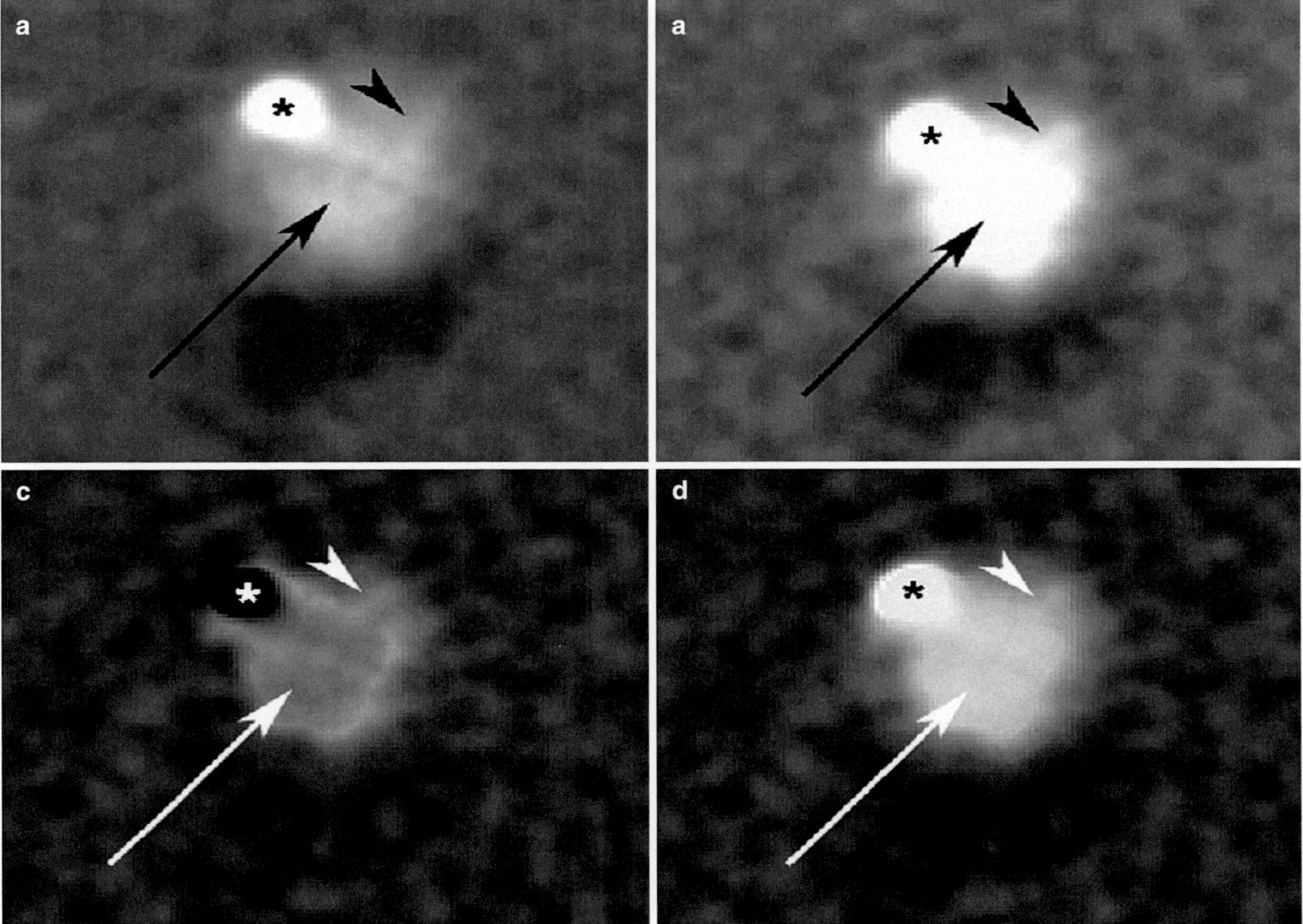

Fig. 2.8 Dual energy CT. Dual energy CT can be used to characterize tissue: Vessel cross sectional images derived from high- (140 keV) and low-energy (90 keV) attenuation profiles (**a** and **b**, respectively) demonstrate the influence of photon energy on photoattenuation. The contrast-filled lumen (*arrow*) exerts greater photoattenuation on low-energy photons, and hence appears brighter in (**b**), while calcification (*asterisk*) appears high-density in both images. In the subtracted image (**c**), dense calcification has been "removed." By adding in the low-energy (90 keV) attenuation data to this subtracted image, depiction of the lumen edge is enhanced (because of reduced contrast blooming), and visualization of a small side branch (*arrowhead*) is improved (**d**) (Reproduced with permission of Wolters Kluwer from Boll et al. [23])

Conclusions

Since the turn of the twenty-first century, there has been an explosion in technological development of cardiac CT systems, with concomitant gain in reliability and accuracy, especially of coronary imaging. The theme has been one of progressively improved spatial and temporal resolution, reduced scan time, and, most recently, a focus on driving down radiation exposure. In appropriately selected patients, using careful technique, it is easily achievable to perform a cardiac CT using less radiation exposure than that of a standard chest CT or an invasive coronary angiogram. The goal of future systems will be to make this more widely achievable in a larger group of patients without requiring patient selection or stringent patient prep. Given the history of rapid technological advancement, we can expect to see this goal achieved in the near future.

References

1. Thibault JB, Sauer KD, Bouman CA, Hsieh J. A three-dimensional statistical approach to improved image quality for multislice helical CT. Med Phys. 2007;34:4526–44.
2. Reproduced with permission from Chandra N. CT sampling technology [white paper]. Waukesha: GE Healthcare; 2008.
3. Hurlock GS, Higashino H, Mochizuki T. History of cardiac computed tomography: single to 320-detector row multislice computed tomography [Review]. Int J Cardiovasc Imaging. 2009;25:31–42.
4. Hell MM, Bittner D, Schuhbaeck A, et al. Prospectively ECG-triggered high-pitch coronary angiography with third-generation dual-source CT at 70 kVp tube voltage: feasibility, image quality, radiation dose, and effect of iterative reconstruction. J Cardiovasc Comput Tomogr. 2014;8:418–25.
5. Achenbach S, Ropers D, Kuettner A, et al. Contrast-enhanced coronary artery visualization by dual-source computed tomography – initial experience. Eur J Radiol. 2006;57:331–5.

6. Achenbach S, Ropers U, Kuettner A, et al. Randomized comparison of 64-slice single- and dual-source computed tomography coronary angiography for the detection of coronary artery disease. JACC Cardiovasc Imaging. 2008;1:177–86.
7. Leipsic J, Labounty TM, Hague CJ, et al. Effect of a novel vendor-specific motion-correction algorithm on image quality and diagnostic accuracy in persons undergoing coronary CT angiography without rate-control medications. J Cardiovasc Comput Tomogr. 2012;6:164–71.
8. Vembar M, Walker MJ, Johnson PC. Cardiac imaging using multislice computed tomography scanners: technical considerations. Coron Artery Dis. 2006;17:115–23.
9. Hsieh J, Londt J, Vass M, Li J, Tang X, Okerlund D. Step-and-shoot data acquisition and reconstruction for cardiac x-ray computed tomography. Med Phys. 2006;33:4236–48.
10. Earls JP, Berman EL, Urban BA, et al. Prospectively gated transverse coronary CT angiography versus retrospectively gated helical technique: improved image quality and reduced radiation dose. Radiology. 2008;246:742–53.
11. Hoe J, Toh KH. First experience with 320-row multidetector CT coronary angiography scanning with prospective electrocardiogram gating to reduce radiation dose. J Cardiovasc Comput Tomogr. 2009;3:257–61.
12. Steigner ML, Otero HJ, Cai T, et al. Narrowing the phase window width in prospectively ECG-gated single heart beat 320-detector row coronary CT angiography. Int J Cardiovasc Imaging. 2009;25:85–90.
13. Hausleiter J, Bischoff B, Hein F, et al. Feasibility of dual-source cardiac CT angiography with high-pitch scan protocols. J Cardiovasc Comput Tomogr. 2009;3:236–42.
14. Achenbach S, Marwan M, Schepis T, et al. High-pitch spiral acquisition: a new scan mode for coronary CT angiography. J Cardiovasc Comput Tomogr. 2009;3:117–21.
15. Gordic S, Desbiolles L, Sedlmair M, et al. Optimizing radiation dose by using advanced modelled iterative reconstruction in high-pitch coronary CT angiography. Eur Radiol. 2016;26(2):459–68.
16. Layritz C, Schmid J, Achenbach S, et al. Accuracy of prospectively ECG-triggered very low-dose coronary dual-source CT angiography using iterative reconstruction for the detection of coronary artery stenosis: comparison with invasive catheterization. Eur Heart J Cardiovasc Imaging. 2014;15:1238–45.
17. Schuhbaeck A, Achenbach S, Layritz C, et al. Image quality of ultra-low radiation exposure coronary CT angiography with an effective dose <0.1 mSv using high-pitch spiral acquisition and raw data-based iterative reconstruction. Eur Radiol. 2013;23:597–606.
18. Weigold W, Olszewski M, Walker MJ. Low-dose prospectively gated 256-slice coronary computed tomographic angiography. Int J Cardiovasc Imaging. 2009;25 Suppl 2:217–30.
19. Gupta R, Cheung AC, Bartling SH, et al. Flat-panel volume CT: fundamental principles, technology, and applications. Radiographics. 2008;28:2009–22.
20. Andreini D, Pontone G, Mushtaq S, et al. Diagnostic accuracy of rapid kilovolt peak-switching dual-energy CT coronary angiography in patients with a high calcium score. JACC Cardiovasc Imaging. 2015;8:746–8.
21. Barreto M, Schoenhagen P, Nair A, et al. Potential of dual-energy computed tomography to characterize atherosclerotic plaque: ex vivo assessment of human coronary arteries in comparison to histology. J Cardiovasc Comput Tomogr. 2008;2:234–42.
22. Ruzsics B, Schwarz F, Schoepf UJ, et al. Comparison of dual-energy computed tomography of the heart with single photon emission computed tomography for assessment of coronary artery stenosis and of the myocardial blood supply. Am J Cardiol. 2009;104:318–26.
23. Boll DT, Hoffmann MH, Huber N, Bossert AS, Aschoff AJ, Fleiter TR. Spectral coronary multidetector computed tomography angiography: dual benefit by facilitating plaque characterization and enhancing lumen depiction. J Comput Assist Tomogr. 2006;30(5):804–11.

Radiation Dosimetry and CT Dose Reduction Techniques

3

Kai H. Lee

Abstract
Increasing radiation exposure to the population from widespread use of multi-row detector CT necessitates efforts to limit the x-rays applied in CT procedures. Options are available on CT scanners to modulate the patient dose. This chapter describes the metrics of radiation dose, and the influence of various technical parameters in the scan and dose modulation options on patient dose and image quality. With that information, practitioners of CT will be better prepared to optimize the scan protocols to reduce the patient dose without sacrificing the image quality necessary for interpretation.

Keywords
CT radiation metrics • Dose modulation • Scanning parameters

Introduction

The ability of modern multi-detector CT scanners with sub-millimeter resolution, sub-second rotation time, and large volume imaging has resulted in widespread use of CT. However, the widespread use of CT has also raised concerns about the risks of radiation to patients. The National Council on Radiation Protection, NCRP Report No. 160, in 2006 [1] reported that radiation exposure to the United States population due to medical sources increased more than seven times in the 20 years between 1986 and 2006. According to the NCRP report, CT constituted about 10 % of the diagnostic examinations that utilize x-rays in 2006, it contributed to nearly 50 % of the population dose. The use of CT continued to rise since publication of NCRP Report 160. Reports in scientific and lay journals found fewer than three million CT examinations done in 1980, which rose to 62 million in 2007, and to 80 million at the end of 2014 [2–4]. Based on our current knowledge of radiation biology, the deleterious effects of radiation are cumulative and medical radiation is increasingly a significant contributor to the amount of radiation accumulated in a person's lifetime [5, 6]. The risk of cancer from radiation exposure is especially worrisome to children and young women who received multiple CT examinations early in their life. For example, studies found that one CT examination of the female chest gives as much radiation as 10 mammograms to each breast [7]. In addition to radiation from CT, cardiac patients may be exposed to radiation from nuclear medicine perfusion studies and coronary angiography. Therefore, the practitioners of CT must be constantly aware of the risks of radiation, and strive toward applying the lowest dose to the patient consistent with the clinical study.

One of the difficulties confronting the clinicians when evaluating the radiation safety of a CT procedure is the plethora of terms used to quantify the amount of radiation given to the patient. Thus, this chapter sets out on two aims. The first aim is to explain the fundamental concepts of radiation dosimetry associated with CT scans. The second aim is to describe the scanning techniques and available technologies to reduce radiation dose to patients.

K.H. Lee, PhD
Associate Professor of Clinical Radiology,
Department of Radiology, Keck School of Medicine,
University of Southern California,
1200 North State Street, Los Angeles, CA 90033, USA
e-mail: kailee@usc.edu

M.J. Budoff, J.S. Shinbane (eds.), *Cardiac CT Imaging: Diagnosis of Cardiovascular Disease*,
DOI 10.1007/978-3-319-28219-0_3

Fundamentals of Radiation Dosimetry

Absorbed Dose

The damaging health effects of radiation are commonly called radiation effects. Our current knowledge of radiation effects was derived from animal studies, atom bomb survivors, and victims of radiation accidents [6]. There were many contributing factors to the observed radiation effects, but the outcomes ultimately depended on the amount of radiation received. The **radiation dose**, or dose in short, is the amount of energy deposited by the ionizing radiation per unit mass of tissue. Radiation **dosimetry** is the field of study which measures and quantifies the radiation dose. Of the bewildering number of terms to quantify radiation dose, there are three related terms fundamental to radiation protection. The three terms are the absorbed dose, the equivalent dose, and the effective dose.

The International System (SI units) of radiation dose measurements is the **Gray** [8]. One Gray (Gy) of radiation is defined as 1 J of energy deposited in 1 kg of tissue, i.e.,

$$\text{Dose}(\text{Gy}) = \frac{1\,\text{joule}}{1\,\text{kg tissue.}}$$

The Gray is a large dose of radiation. When evaluating radiation dose from CT examinations, a sub-unit of the Gray is used. The Gray sub-unit commonly used to quantify radiation dose from CT examinations is the milli-Gray (mGy). One mGy is one thousandth of a Gray. That is,

$$1\,\text{mGy} = 10^{-3}\,\text{Gy}.$$

Equivalent Dose

The severity of biological damage depends not only on the dose of radiation absorbed in tissue, but also on the type of radiation absorbed. For example, 1 mGy of neutron radiation produces far greater tissue damages than 1 mGy of x-rays. We therefore need a unit of measurement that accounts for both the quantity of radiation absorbed in the tissues and the effectiveness of the absorbed radiation in producing biological damages. The **equivalent dose** was devised to incorporate both the physical factors and the effectiveness of the absorbed radiation in producing biological damage. The equivalent dose is a biological scale for measuring the deleterious health effects of radiation. The same biological damage is expected for the same equivalent dose regardless of the type of radiation absorbed in tissue.

The equivalent dose (H) is measured in **Sievert** (Sv). A sub-unit of Sievert is the milli-Sievert (mSv). One milli-Sievert equals to one thousandth of a Sievert. The equivalent dose in mSv is calculated by multiplying the radiation absorbed dose D in mGy by a quality factor Q, also called the biological damage weighting factor W_r [9], for the type of radiation absorbed in tissue, i.e.,

Table 3.1 Biological damage weighting factors

Type of radiation	Weighting factor
X- and gamma rays, electrons, positrons	1
Protons	2
Neutrons	10
Alpha particles	20

$$H(\text{mSv}) = D(\text{mGy}) \times W_r.$$

The biological damage weighting factors for four types of radiation are given in Table 3.1.

The values of W_r are proportional to the density of ionization created by the incident radiation along its path of travel in tissue. For x-rays, gamma rays, beta particles, and electrons from radioactive materials, the density of ionization created in tissue is relatively low. The weighting factor W_r equals 1. Thus, when working with x-rays from CT, the equivalent dose and absorbed dose are numerically equal, i.e., 1 mSv = 1 mGy. For neutrons, the weighting factor $W_r = 10$. The equivalent dose for 1 mGy of neutron absorbed dose equals

$$\begin{aligned} H(\text{mSv}) &= 1(\text{mGy}) \times 10 \\ &= 10\,\text{mSv}. \end{aligned}$$

The above example shows that neutrons are ten times more damaging to the human body than x-rays for the same absorbed dose.

In summary, the absorbed dose in mGy is the quantity of radiation energy deposited per unit mass of tissue. The equivalent dose in mSv is a measure of biological damage equal to the absorbed dose modified by a weighting factor according the relative effectiveness of the absorbed radiation to produce biological damage.

Given this metric to quantify radiation, Table 3.2 lists the average equivalent dose received annually to the total body by workers in various occupations [10–13]. The table also gives the natural background radiation and the regulatory limits on radiation exposure for reference. It is interesting to note that the transcontinental flight crews who are not classified as occupational radiation workers receive an annual equivalent dose from the cosmic rays higher than the nuclear medicine technologists who routinely handle radioactive materials on the job.

Table 3.2 Typical annual whole-body radiation dose

	mSv
Nuclear medicine technologists	1.7
Airline flight crews between Los Angeles and New York City	2.2
Nuclear power plant workers	2.3
Intervention radiologists	18
Cardiologists (catheterization)	16
Natural background radiation at sea level	2.5
Regulatory limit on the occupational workers	50
Regulatory limit on the general public	1

Radiation Effects to the Patient

The goal of protecting patients undergoing radiological procedures is to prevent the occurrence of **deterministic effects**, and to minimize the risk **of stochastic effects**. Deterministic effects are radiation induced somatic injuries. Examples of radiation induced somatic injuries are skin erythema, epilation, and cataracts. The FDA has documented severe deterministic effects such as hair loss and skin necrosis on patients from CT and prolonged fluoroscopy guided procedures. Deterministic effects are preventable. There is ample clinical evidence of threshold doses below which such effects are not seen. Once the threshold dose is reached, severity of the injury increases with the radiation dose.

Stochastic risks are probabilistic occurrences of carcinogenesis and genetic mutations. The current concept of stochastic risks assumes no threshold dose for its occurrence. Exposure to any amount of ionizing radiation is harmful. The probability of the occurrence of stochastic effects, rather than its severity, increases in direct proportion to the radiation absorbed dose. This is in contrast to deterministic effects in which the severity increases as the dose increases above the threshold. This concept of stochastic risks is called linear no threshold model, and is the basis of radiation protection regulations.

Effective Dose

Our knowledge of stochastic risks is based on data collected from total body exposure to radiation. If we wish to estimate the stochastic risks to a person after a partial body exposure such as a chest CT, we must translate the chest CT dose to an equivalent whole-body dose in order to utilize the database for risk estimates. The **effective dose** was devised for this purpose. The effective dose is the dose of radiation that when given uniformly to the whole-body will produce the same stochastic risk as the dose of radiation delivered to only a part of the body, such as the chest dose from a cardiac CT study.

Table 3.3 Tissue/organ sensitivity

Tissue/organ	Weighting factor, Wr
Gonads	0.20
Bone marrow, colon, lung, stomach	0.12
Bladder, breast, liver, esophagus, thyroid	0.05
Skin, bone surface	0.01

The effective dose translates a partial body exposure to an equivalent uniform dose of radiation delivered to the total body. The purpose for calculating the effective dose is to provide a common denominator for the assessment of stochastic risks using our database of whole-body exposures. Unlike the absorbed dose and the equivalent dose, the effective dose is not a physically measurable quantity. The effective dose is an imaginary total body dose. It is calculated from the absorbed dose given to any region or regions of the body.

If we wish to estimate the stochastic risks from CT of the chest, we must translate the partial body irradiation to an equivalent whole-body dose in order to utilize the database for risk estimates. To do so, a mathematical model is used to compute the doses to other organs resulting from radiation scattered from CT of the chest. These computed organ doses are then multiplied by a risk factor according to the susceptibility of each organ to radiation. Summation of the product of these computed organ doses and their associated risk weighting factor is called the effective dose. That is, the effective dose E is computed using the equation

$$\mathbf{E} = \sum \mathbf{H}_i \, \mathbf{w}_i$$

Where **E** is the effective dose
$\mathbf{H}_i$ is the dose equivalent to a given organ
$\mathbf{w}_i$ is the risk weighting factor for that organ.

The effective dose is thus a weighted sum of the computed equivalent doses to all organs in the body. Table 3.3 is a partial list of weighting factors for different body organs published in the International Commission on Radiation Protection Report 103 [14].

One may interpret the effective dose as a calculated equivalent dose of radiation given to the entire body that would be required to produce the same risk of cancer and genetic damage as a dose of radiation delivered to a localized region of the body, such as in a CT examination. In other words, the risk from a part of the body exposed to a given dose of radiation is the same as the total body uniformly receiving the effective dose. The effective dose is an extrapolated whole-body dose from a partial body dose. As such, the effective dose is a computed value rather than a physically measurable quantity. The effective dose is calculated to serve as a common denominator for comparing stochastic risks between different medical or non-medical exposures to radiation. Now that we understand the concept of the absorbed dose, equivalent dose, and effective dose, the next step is to learn how to calculate the effective dose from CT.

CT Dosimetry

CT Dose Metrics

Special dosimetric techniques had to be developed for measuring CT doses because the geometry of the x-ray field in CT scans is very different from conventional radiographic or fluoroscopic exposures. The fundamental metric developed for CT dosimetry is the **Computed Tomography Dose Index** (CTDI). From the CTDI, the **dose-length product** (DLP) is calculated, and is in turn used to derive the effective dose (E) for risk comparison [15–18].

CTDI

The CTDI, or specifically the $CTDI_{100}$, is measured using a dosimeter of 100 mm length in a cylindrical acrylic phantom of 16-cm diameter to simulate a head, or 32-cm diameter to simulate the body (Fig. 3.1).

Four measurements are made in the periphery and one in the center of the phantom. The four peripheral measurements and the central measurement are used to compute the weighted average of the $CTDI_{100}$ in the phantom as follows:

$$CTDI_W = 0.87 * \begin{bmatrix} 2/3CTDI_{100}(\text{periphery}) \\ +1/3CTDI_{100}(\text{center}) \end{bmatrix},$$

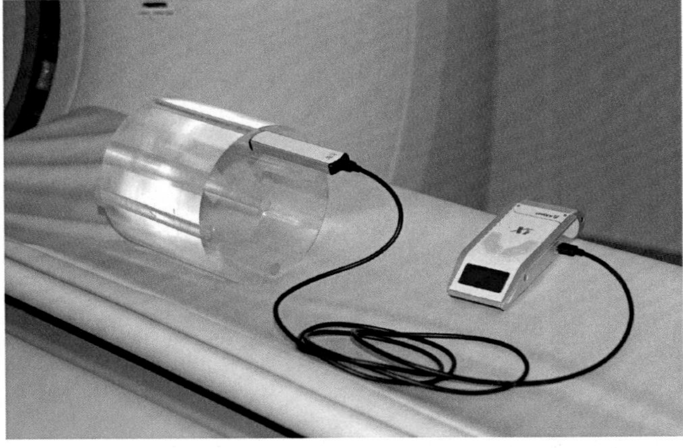

Fig. 3.1 A typical setup of the dosimeter, ionization chamber, and 16-cm diameter acrylic phantom for measuring the CTDI of the head. There are 4 holes 1 cm from the surface, and one hole in the center of the phantom for insertion of the ionization chamber for dose measurements

where $CTDI_w$ is the weighted average of $CTDI_{100}$ in the phantom. The constant 0.87 is a conversion factor to relate dose measured in air to dose in soft tissues. The $CTDI_w$ is interpreted as the average absorbed dose in the cross section of the phantom being measured. The $CTDI_w$ is not the dose to the patient [19]. It is an index of the amount of x-rays used in a CT examination expressed in terms of a dose to a phantom.

$CTDI_w$ was developed during the infancy of CT scanners in the 1970s, when patients were scanned sequentially section by section. This mode of operation is called axial scan. In an axial scan, the x-ray tube rotates 360° around the patient to measure x-rays transmitted through the patient one cross section at a time. The x-ray tube in the early models of CT scanners had to rewind upon completing each rotation to untangle the electrical cables. While the x-ray tube was returning to the starting position, the table advanced the patient to the next section to scan. There was no data acquisition while the patient table was in motion. Axial scans followed a "scan-stop-scan" pattern. The advent of slip ring technology in the early 1990s enabled the development of helical CT scanners. Slip rings are electro-mechanical devices for providing electrical power to the generator, x-ray tube, x-ray detectors, and computers on the gantry from the power source in the building. The rotating x-ray tube, generator, x-ray detectors, and computers draw power from the slip rings much like electric street cars draw power from the stationary overhead cables. The slip rings enable the gantry assembly to rotate continuously for data acquisition without having to rewind and pause after each rotation to untwist the cables, thus eliminating the inter-scan delay and shortening the total examination time.

In a helical scan, the table translates the patient continuously through the gantry during rotation of the x-ray tube and detectors. The scanning motion is called a helical because the x-ray beam paints a spiral or helical pattern around the patient as shown in Fig. 3.2.

The relative motion of the x-ray beam and the patient table is described by the term pitch. Pitch is a dimensionless unit equal to the distance the table moved in one rotation of the x-ray tube divided by the width of the x-ray beam at the axis of rotation. That is,

$$\text{Pitch} = \frac{\text{Distance moved by patient table in one tube rotation}}{\text{X} - \text{ray beam width at axis of rotation.}}$$

The higher the pitch, the faster the patient translates through the gantry, and the greater is the distance of separation between two loops of the x-ray beam. We need a good grasp of the concept of pitch because pitch has a strong influence on the image resolution, noise, and patient dose. In an axial scan, there is no table motion so the pitch equals zero. For helical scans with pitch equals to 1, the patient moved a distance in one rotation of the x-ray tube equal to the width of the x-ray

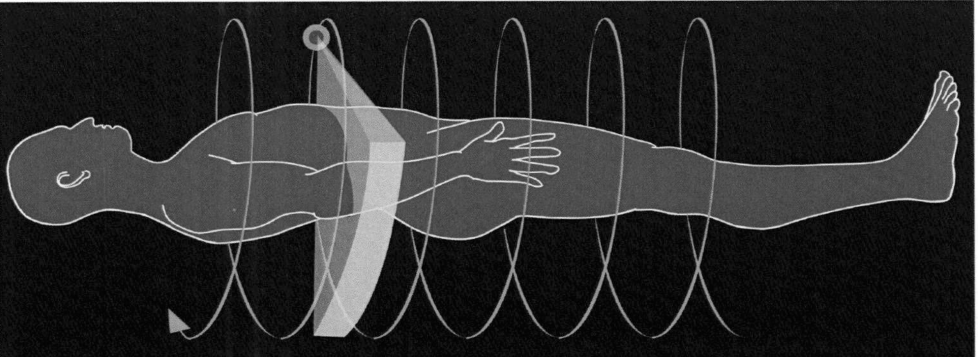

Fig. 3.2 The x-ray beam traces a helical pattern on the patient with the x-ray tube rotating while the patient table translates through the gantry at the same time

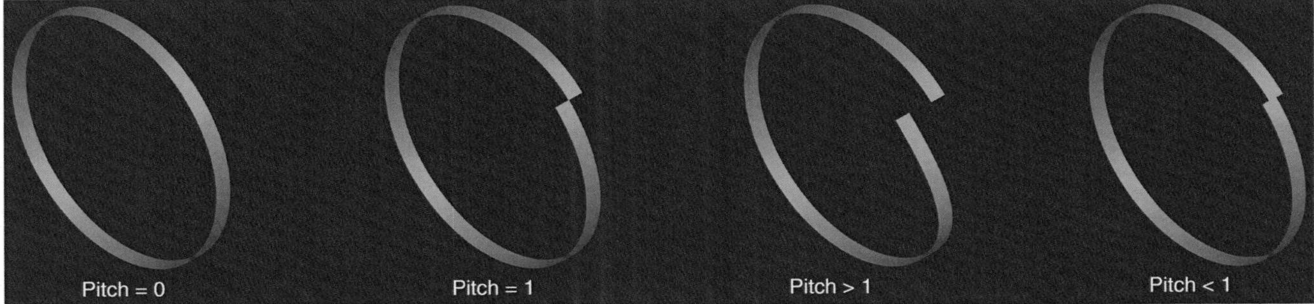

Fig. 3.3 In an axial scan, there is no table motion during tube rotation and the pitch = 0. With a pitch = 1, the loops of x-ray beam are contiguous and abutting each other with each rotation. With a pitch > 1, the beam leaves a gap between rotations. With a pitch < 1, the x-ray beam overlaps between rotations

beam. The borders of the x-ray beams abut each other in successive rotations. If the table moves a distance greater than the width of the x-ray beam in one rotation, the pitch is greater than 1. There is a gap between two loops of the x-ray beam when scanning with a pitch greater than 1. In scans with a pitch less than 1, the patient table moves a distance less than the width of the x-ray beam, and the x-ray beam overlaps in successive loops. The x-ray beam pattern on the patient for different values of pitch is illustrated in Fig. 3.3.

With the development of helical CT, the $CTDI_w$ was modified to account for variable overlaps in the spiral path of the x-ray beam in helical scans. The currently used index of radiation dose to the patient is the $CTDI_{vol}$. The $CTDI_{vol}$ is calculated by dividing the $CTDI_w$ by the pitch, i.e.,

$$CTDI_{vol} = CTDI_w / \text{pitch}.$$

As shown in the above equation, $CTDI_{vol}$ is inversely proportional to the pitch. A higher pitch leads to a lower the $CTDI_{vol}$, as there is less overlapping of the x-ray beam in the scan volume.

Dose-Length Product

One final measurable dosimetric parameter for CT is the dose-length product (DLP). The DLP is proportional to the total amount of x-ray energy deposit in the scan volume. DLP is defined as:

$$DLP = CTDI_{vol} \times \text{scan length}.$$

DLP is an important risk indicator because radiation risks depend not only on the quantity and type of radiation given, but on the volume of tissue irradiated as well. For example, a radiation oncologist could deliver 70 Gy (70,000 mGy) of x-rays to a small region surrounding the prostate gland to cure a patient with prostate cancer. If 70 Gy was delivered over the entire body, the person will most certainly die. For the same dose of radiation the deleterious effects increase with the volume of tissue irradiated. The $CTDI_{vol}$ is an index of the average amount of x-ray energy deposited per unit mass of tissue. It does not provide information regarding the total amount of radiation energy deposited or the volume of tissue irradiated. The value of $CTDI_{vol}$ is unchanged whether the scan length is 1 cm or 100 cm, but the volume of tissue irradiated and the biological effects from the exposure would be quite different. Because it is difficult to measure the mass of tissue irradiated in a CT scan, the $CTDI_{vol}$ is multiplied by the scan length to obtain the DLP as an indirect measure of the irradiated volume and the total amount of x-ray energy deposited in the patient. The two descriptors of CT dosimetry, $CTDI_{vol}$ and DLP, are widely used as indices of the amount of x-rays utilized for a CT scan, the volume of tissue exposed to radiation, and the total amount of energy deposited in the scan volume. Because $CTDI_{vol}$ and DLP are such important indicators of the risks, the values of $CTDI_{vol}$ and DLP are displayed on the control console in all CT systems manufactured since year 2000.

The Effective Dose from CT

The effective dose is not a measured dose, but can be calculated from the DLP using a simple formula developed by the ICRP [20, 21]. The effective dose is conveniently calculated by multiplying the DLP by the corresponding conversion factor shown in Table 3.4, i.e.,

$$E(\mathrm{mSv}) = \mathrm{DLP} \times \mathrm{CF}$$

where CF is the conversion factor for the corresponding CT procedure.

By using the $CTDI_{vol}$, DLP, and conversion factors in Table 3.4, some typical values of the effective dose from different CT procedures are shown in Table 3.5. The effective doses from other radiologic examinations are also shown in the table for comparison [22, 23].

Uses and Misuses of $CTDI_{VOL}$

The CTDI was originally developed to quantify the x-rays used for an axial CT scan in terms of radiation dose to a cylindrical methylmethacrylate (trade names: Acrylic, Lucite, Plexiglas) phantom. The dose metric was later refined to account for helical scans. The $CTDI_{vol}$ as utilized today offers a standardized method to conveniently characterize the x-ray output of a CT scanner for a given CT examination. Because the $CTDI_{vol}$ is highly reproducible and can be easily measured with high degrees of consistency, it is widely used as an index to compare the amount of x-rays used for different scan protocols, and even for comparing scanners made by different manufacturers. However, many users misinterpreted the $CTDI_{vol}$ as the radiation dose the patient received [19]. The misinterpretation can be traced to the $CTDI_{vol}$ and DLP being shown on the computer console as soon as a scan protocol is selected for the patient to be scanned, and some state laws require the two indices be recorded in the patient's examination report. An astute user may notice that the values of $CTDI_{vol}$ and DLP are unchanged so long as the technical parameters for the scan protocol remain the same regardless of the size of patient placed on the table and the section of the body to be scanned. The $CTDI_{vol}$ is only an index of the x-ray output for a given scan protocol, not the actual dose to the patient.

The conversion factors applied to the DLP to calculate the effective dose were based on a mathematical model of a standard man of 70 kg. If the conversion factors were applied to a patient having a body mass index very different from that of a standard man, the calculated effective dose can be very different. For pediatrics there are separate tables of conversion factors for different age groups to account for differences in their body sizes [24]. If the body sizes and other related parameters are carefully adjusted, the calculated effective dose serves as a useful metric to compare the relative risks of different scan protocols and different imaging modalities utilizing ionizing radiation. For example, this metric allows comparison of the relative risks of radionuclide perfusion studies with cardiac CT angiography. The effective doses that the patient received from other imaging modalities can also be added together for assessment of stochastic risks.

Table 3.4 CT effective dose conversion factors

Region of body	Conversion factor
Head	0.0021
Neck	0.0059
Chest	0.0140
Abdomen	0.0150
Pelvis	0.0150

Table 3.5 Typical effective doses of radiological examinations

Radiologic examination	Typical effective dose (mSv)
Head/neck CT	2–5
Chest CT	5–7
Abdomen/pelvis CT	3–7
Coronary CT angiogram	5–15
Coronary bi-plane angiogram	3–10
MIBI cardiac stress/rest per 1.3 GBq	10.6
PA chest x-ray	0.02
Skull x-ray	0.07
Lumbar spine	1.3
I.V. urogram	2.5
Upper GI	3.0

Updating the $CTDI_{VOL}$

The CTDI was developed when CT scans were performed using a narrow beam of x-rays to scan the patient axially one slice at a time. CT technologies and its applications have since advanced far beyond the scan pattern on which the CTDI was developed 30 years ago. For example, a 320-row CT scanner has an axial scan length of 160 mm. The 100 mm length ionization chamber used to measure the $CTDI_{vol}$ is too short even to intercept the x-ray field from edge to edge, much less the tail ends of the beam in adjacent sections. The assumption that all the primary and scattered x-rays were collected by the ionization chamber is clearly not valid for the large cone beam and multi-row CT systems. The latest proposed paradigm adopts the dosimetric techniques utilized in radiation oncology to measure the equilibrium dose as an index of the x-ray output from a CT scan [25, 26]. The equilibrium dose methodology can be used to quantify x-ray output for axial, helical, narrow or broad beam scanning in air or in phantom with or without table translation. Perhaps due to its drastic departure from the $CTDI_{vol}$ concept and lack of a standardized procedure to measure the equilibrium dose, the new metric has not gained wide acceptance to replace the conventional $CTDI_{vol}$ as an index of the x-ray output from CT scans.

Methods to Reduce CT Dose

Dose Reduction Techniques

A number of studies reported that radiation dose from CT examinations can be reduced by more than 50 % simply by modifying the basic technical parameters in the scanning protocols [27–31]. The parameters selectable by the users for dose reduction include the scan length, x-ray tube voltage, x-ray tube current, acquisition thickness, pitch, ECG gating, and image reconstruction algorithms.

Limiting the Scan Length

Users have the tendency to liberally scan beyond the region of interest just to be sure nothing is missed. However, the effective dose to a patient is proportional to the dose-length-product DLP which in turn is proportional to the craniocaudal length being scanned. Hence, it is essential to establish scanning protocols to limit the scan length to include only the region of interest. A study [32] reported use of the scan for calcium score as a guide to determine the minimum scan length for the individual patient in CT angiography studies. Prior to CT angiography, the patient was given a pre-scan using the calcium score protocol. The beginning of the scan was determined from the calcium score images at 1 cm above the visualized most cranial aspect of the coronary arteries and the end of the scan at 1 cm below the posterior descending artery. The dose savings from limiting the scan length more than offsetting the dose from the calcium score scan. The effective dose was reported to be reduced by as much as 30 %.

Reducing the Tube Voltage

The intensity of x-rays emitted from an x-ray tube is approximately proportional to the square of the kilovoltage (kV) applied to it. Using a lower tube voltage would result in applying less x-rays to the patient for the study, however there are negative aspects of using lower kV x-rays. Use of a lower tube voltage must take in consideration of the patient's body mass to counter the potential negative effects on image quality. One of the negative effects is the increase in image noise and reduction of the soft tissue image contrast due to less x-rays passing through the patient. In fact, applying lower kV x-rays to a large patient could actually increase the patient dose. The reason is because low energy x-rays are more easily absorbed in the patient and unable to reach the image receptor. The user then applies a higher beam current or a longer scan time to compensate for the reduced transmission of x-rays to the detectors in order to keep the image noise to an acceptable level. This results in negating the dose reduction benefits of using lower kV. With that caution in mind, several studies reported that for coronary CT angiography of patients weighing 185 lb or less, reducing the voltage from 120 to 100 kV reduces the effective dose by 30–40 % to the range 5–12 mSv from 9 to 17 mSv without degrading the diagnostic accuracy [27–32]. Other studies have shown that for thin patients, the tube voltage can be further reduced to 80 KV with a dose savings as high as 80 % [33, 34]. The above studies demonstrated that considerable dose savings can be achieved with overall preservation of image quality when tube voltage reduction is matched with the size of the patient.

Reducing the tube voltage for CT angiography has a bonus advantage in addition to lowering the patient dose. Contrast agents have higher probability of interaction with low energy x-rays by photoelectric effect. Arterial vessels containing contrast agent attenuate the x-rays more strongly and show up with higher contrast against the soft tissue background in spite of more noise in the overall image.

Modulating the Tube Current and Time Product

Radiation dose to the patient is directly proportional to the product of the tube current measured in mA and the tube rotation time in seconds (mAs). While options for varying the tube rotation time are limited for cardiac CT, there is great latitude in the choice of tube current. Similar to reducing the tube voltage, there is a delicate balance between the desire to lower the mA for dose reduction, and the need to apply sufficient mA to keep the subsequent increase in image noise from interfering with clinical interpretation. When the mA is reduced, the intensity of the x-ray beam passing through the patient is lessened, resulting in decreased patient dose. Reducing the mA has the undesirable effect of increasing the image noise and reducing the overall quality of the images because less x-rays, and therefore less data, are received by the detectors to reconstruct the images. The question becomes one of deciding the optimum mA to minimize dose to the patient without compromising the image quality for accurate diagnosis. Answer to this question depends on the comfort level of the interpreting physician to image noise, and this subjectivity obviously varies from physician to physician.

CT manufacturers responded to this question by incorporating dose modulation options into their system to assist the users in making the trade-off between the patient dose and image quality. The dose modulation options in various trade names are actually different implementations of the automatic exposure control (AEC) technique that has been in use for decades in fluoroscopy and radiography. In a nutshell, AEC controls dose to the patient by modulating the x-ray beam intensity according to the patient's anatomy to produce the desired image quality. The intensity of the x-ray beam emitted from the x-ray tube and subsequently sent through the patient is directly proportional to the mA across the tube. By modulating the electron current mA according to the thickness of tissues that the x-ray beam must pass through, the desired image quality can be maintained without imparting unnecessary radiation to the patient. For example, the CT scanner could automatically raise the mA to produce a more intense x-ray beam to pass through the abdomen, and reduce qthe mA to produce a less intense x-ray beam to pass through the lungs.

There are three conditions under which the AEC can be called upon to modulate the tube current (mA) to produce the desire image quality, and in the process reduce unnecessary radiation to the patient. First, the AEC could be programmed to adjust the mA along the long axis of the patient so that the mA is reduced when the x-ray beam passes through large volume of air in the thorax, and is raised when the beam goes through the more attenuating soft tissues in the abdomen and pelvis. Second, the mA is adjusted in the transverse plane of the patient according to the tube angle during its rotation around the patient. That is, the mA is reduced when the x-ray beam is passing through the patient in the thinner AP and PA directions, and increased in the thicker lateral directions. Third, the overall tube current is adjusted according to the patient's size such that a lower mA would be used on pediatric than adult patients, and on the thinner than heavy set patients.

There are three general methods by which manufacturers use in their dose reduction options [35, 36], each with their advantages and disadvantages. Implementation of the dose reduction option changes frequently in keeping with the state of technology, but the principles behind the methodology remain essentially the same. The three common dose modulation algorithms employed by manufacturers of CT scanners are AEC guided by image noise, AEC guided by reference image, and AEC guided by reference mAs. The dose modulation options are described in greater detail here because the operator has to make a selection when setting up a scan.

AEC Guided by Image Noise

Image noise can be described qualitatively as graininess of the image. Low noise images appear smooth with continuous shades of gray from the darkest to the lightest portions of the image. High noise images show characteristic salt and pepper grains interspersed through out the image. Resolution of low contrast objects can be greatly impaired by image noise. Image noise is influenced by a number of factors, but is most strongly influenced by the number of x-ray photons that contribute to the image. A simple way to quantify noise in an image is to calculate the percentage standard deviation. The standard deviation of an image is the square root of the total number of counts or dots that make up the image. The resulting standard deviation is then divided by the total counts in the image to arrive at the percentage standard deviation. The standard deviation of the number of counts in an image is a measure of noise in the image. The percentage standard deviation as computed by the ratio of the standard deviation to the total number of counts in the image indicates what fraction of the image is occupied by noise.

The number of counts in a given CT image is directly proportional to the number of x-ray photons available for image formation, which in turn depends on the intensity of the x-ray beam passing through the patient to strike the detectors, and the length of time the x-ray beam is on. The AEC modulates the beam intensity by varying the tube current. The exposure time is determined by the speed of the x-ray tube to make one rotation around the patient. The product of the tube current in mA and the rotation time in seconds is commonly called the mAs. The mAs selected for a CT scan determines the number of x-ray photons striking the patient. The higher the mAs, the greater the number of photons available to pass through the patient to reach the detectors, and lower is the noise in the reconstructed images. When all the other technical factors are held constant, the image noise is inversely proportional to the square root of the mAs, i.e.,

$$\text{Noise} \sim 1/\sqrt{\text{mAs}}$$

During CT scans, the tube rotation time is fixed. The image noise guided AEC continually adjusts the mAs by adjusting the mA to maintain the same number of photons reaching the detectors, and hence keeping the image noise at a pre-selected level. For example, the AEC can reduce the mA when the beam is passing through in the thinner anterior-posterior direction of the patient, and increases the mA when passing through laterally.

CT users have great flexibility in patient dose optimization by providing the AEC a target image noise appropriate for the particular CT procedure. The disadvantage is that the user may select a target noise level lower than necessary to obtain the diagnostic information, and results in giving unnecessary dose to the patient. A simple rule to remember is that reducing the mAs and hence the patient dose by a factor of 4, increases the image noise only by a factor of 2.

AEC Guided by Reference Image

This method of AEC is an extension of the constant image noise algorithm. Here, the target image noise is set on the AEC using a clinical image that is selected by the reader as of adequate quality for the given CT procedure. During scanning, the mA is adjusted at each tube position by the AEC to yield an image noise approximating the noise level in the reference image. The advantage of the reference image approach is that the target image noise is derived from a database of clinical images rather than some abstract percentage standard deviation. The major disadvantage of the reference image approach is the user inclination to select the a more aesthetic image as the reference image even though a less visually appealing image will suffice. This approach results in application more radiation to the patient than is necessary for diagnostic images.

AEC Guided by Reference mAs

This approach uses the mAs of a reference patient as a guide to modulate the mA for the actual patient. For a given CT procedure, a certain mAs that was found to produce images of acceptable quality on a reference patient is used as the standard of reference. From the attenuation profiles measured on a scout view of the patient being scanned, the AEC adjusts the tube current at each tube position to compensate for the difference in attenuation between the actual and reference patients. The image noise is not maintained for different patient size. The technique relies on the experience of the user to select the proper level of tube current modulation for a given patient and CT procedure.

Prospective Gating

The most dramatic reduction of dose was reported by using the prospective gating technique in combination with tube voltage reduction [27, 37, 38]. Prospective gating is a dose modulation technique guided by the patient's ECG. It is also known as the ECG guided step-and-shoot technique. The technique is based on the finding that the least amount of motion artifacts were found in the images reconstructed from data in the ventricular diastolic phase. The AEC raises the x-ray intensity to a high level during mid-diastole to acquire the image data, and reduces to a low level during the other phases of the cardiac cycle.

To implement the prospective gating technique, the x-ray tube current and consequently the x-ray beam intensity is modulated by the ECG tracings to synchronize with the patient's cardiac cycle. Signals from the ECG monitor trigger the tube current to increase for data acquisition during diastole, and drop down when data is not acquired during the systolic and early diastolic phases. During the quiescent period with no data acquisition, the table steps to the next position to prepare for scanning. The heart is thus scanned sequentially in a step-and-shoot fashion as shown in Fig. 3.4.

Immediately before the scan, a sample of the ECG traces is taken to measure the average R-R time interval. When the CT is set to scan, the computer sets the clock to zero upon receiving an R-wave from the ECG monitor. The R-wave simultaneously triggers the AEC system to reduce the tube current to a low value until, for example, after 70–80 % of

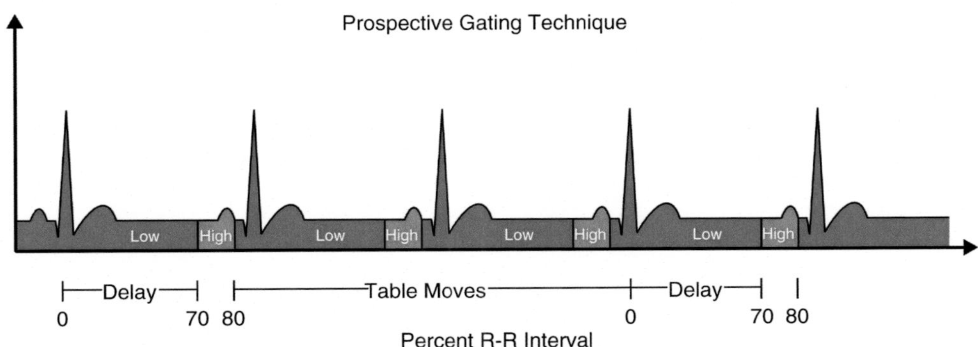

Fig. 3.4 In prospective gating, the ECG signals of the patient modulate the x-ray beam intensity to high levels only for a short duration in the R-R interval

the cardiac cycle has elapsed. After this initial delay, the tube current is raised to a high level and maintains the high output for the next 10–20 % of the cardiac cycle, corresponding to the time during which the heart is in the diastolic phase. At the 80–90 % mark that approximates the end of the diastolic phase, the system returns the tube current to the minimum and stops data acquisition. The time marker is reset to zero upon receiving the next R-wave. While the x-ray beam is at the low level, the table moves the patient to the next scanning position. This step-and-shoot cycle repeats until the scan length is completed. By turning the x-ray beam intensity to high during 10–20 % of the cardiac cycle for data acquisition, the patient dose was reported to reduce by 50–70 % in comparison with the retrospective gating which requires the x-ray beam on the high level continuously for the entire the scan length [39].

Slice Thickness and Patient Dose

Unlike single slice scanners in which the x-ray beam is completely intercepted by the detectors, multi-slice scanners extend the x-ray beam beyond the rows of detectors in the axial direction. The geometry in which the x-ray beam opens beyond the active rows of detectors is called over-beaming [38, 40]. Over-beaming is needed for multi-slice scanners to ensure each row of detectors is exposed to uniform intensity of x-rays to minimize helical artifacts. Unfortunately, the over-beam geometry exposes patients to x-rays not used for image formation. In general, the x-ray over beams the leading row of detectors by about 2 mm and the trailing row by 2 mm. Figure 3.5 shows how over-beam gives higher dose to the patient from thin than thick slice imaging. If the scanner is set to acquire 4 slices of 0.5 mm thickness (4 × 0.5), the x-ray beam over scans the first row of detectors by 2 mm and the last row by 2 mm. From a pure geometric consideration, only a 2 mm strip of the x-ray beam is used for imaging, while the other 4 mm exposed the patient without contributing information to the slice images. In other words, the acquisition protocol used only one third of the applied x-rays for imaging; whereas two thirds were wasted and contributed unnecessary radiation to the patient. If the protocol is set to acquire 4 slices of 1 mm wide (4 × 1) with the same 2 mm over-scan beyond the first and the fourth row of detectors. With the slice thickness increased to 1 mm, 56 % of the x-rays were used for imaging; therefore the amount of wasted x-rays was reduced to 44 %. This example shows that thick slice acquisition should be used whenever possible to make over-beaming a smaller proportion of the applied x-rays. Another reason for giving preference to thick slice acquisition is that the x-ray intensity or imaging time must be increased to provide a sufficient number of photons for reconstruction of thin slice images to keep image noise at acceptable levels. In the interest of reducing radiation to the patient, the slice thickness should be chosen consistent with the axial resolution required for diagnosis; therefore thinner slices are not always better.

Pitch and Patient Dose

The pitch has an inverse relationship with the patient dose, as a higher the pitch lowers the patient dose [38, 40, 41]. If scans were performed using a pitch greater than 1, x-rays sweep around the patient with gaps between successive loops of the beam. Because less tissue is exposed to x-rays, dose to the patient is lower. There are many advantages to using high pitch in order to lower patient dose. High pitch allows greater volume coverage in less time. Short scan time is obviously desirable for pediatric and trauma patients. High pitch is also desirable in CT angiography to ensure capture of the first pass of the contrast agent through the vessels. The disadvantages of high pitch are higher image noise, poorer image resolution, and appearance of helical artifacts due to fewer photons in the images. Conversely, for scans performed with a pitch less than 1, the table moves the patient slowly

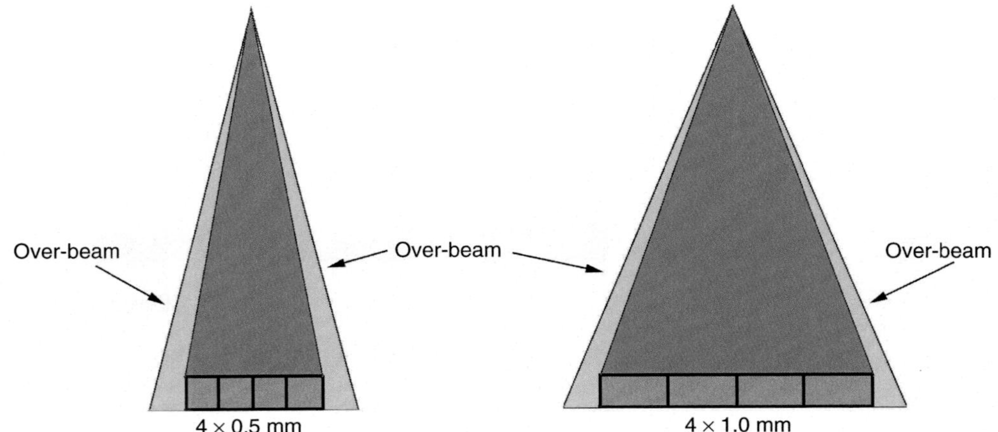

Fig. 3.5 For thin slice acquisition with narrow collimation, over-beaming causes a greater fraction of the x-ray beam to irradiate the patient without contributing to the image

through the gantry. Dose to the patient is higher due to redundant exposure from the x-ray beam overlapping in successive rotations around the patient. Coronary angiography requires low pitch for high image resolution and low noise. In this case, the patient table traverses slowly through the gantry at incremental distances less than the width of the x-ray beam in each gantry rotation. Redundant exposure reduces image noise and increases the low contrast resolution but gives higher dose to the patient. Recent advances in CT technology mitigate some of the issues with patient dose in coronary CT angiography.

Recent Advances in Cardiac CT

Expanding Rows of Detectors

Development of MSCT scanners beyond 64 rows of detectors to 128, 256 and 320 rows brought drastic changes to cardiovascular imaging techniques and lowering radiation dose to the patient. Of particular interest to cardiologists is the introduction of 320-detector row CT. When using a traditional 64-row scanner for coronary CT angiography, about 4 cm is covered with each tube rotation. A complete scan of the heart would require a minimum of 4 gantry rotations. The 320-slice CT with a 16 cm axial view could scan the entire heart in one rotation. It obviates helical scans, table indexing, and artifacts in images reconstructed from data acquired over several cardiac cycles. Dose savings are realized due to no overlapping helical scans and less over-beam dose. When used in combination with kV reduction, prospective gating, elimination of scan overlaps, and minimization of overbeaming, the patient dose can be reduced up to 90 % compared to a 64-row scanner without compromising image quality [42–44].

Dual Source Scanners

Another development in CT technology leading to an increase in temporal resolution and reduction in patient dose is the dual source CT scanner. A dual source CT scanner has two sets of x-ray tube and detectors mounted at 90° angles. For reconstruction of CT images, the algorithm requires projection profiles acquired at least over 180° plus the arc angle of the detectors, translating to approximately 240° of gantry rotation. This scan mode is called half scan. For a dual source scanner, the two sets of detectors only need to perform a quarter scan. The two sets of quarter scan data sets are joined together by software to satisfy the 180° angular requirement. Because sufficient data can be acquired in only one fourth of a gantry rotation, temporal resolution as short as 80 ms is achievable for a gantry rotation time of 330 ms. In addition, the pitch may be increased from 0.2 to 0.46 for higher heart rates to effect dose reduction of as much as 50 %, because the dose is inversely proportional to the pitch [45, 46].

Iterative Reconstruction

CT image reconstruction by iterative algorithm is not new. Until recently, though, filtered backprojection was the algorithm of choice. The advantage of filtered backprojection is the rapidity with which images can be reconstructed without elaborate computers. The reconstructed images suffer, however, from problems such as amplification of noise, beam hardening, scatter, streaks, and ring artifacts. Noise imbedded in the data amplifies by the backprojection algorithm during reconstruction and becomes a limiting factor on patient dose reduction by methods described above. As the number of photons, the amount of x-rays used to make up the image, decreases, image noise increases. Dose reduction becomes limited when noise begins to interfere with visualization of the image details. Iterative reconstruction algorithms overcome many of the shortcomings of the filtered backprojection methods [47, 48]. Iterative reconstruction starts with a filtered backprojection image. The projection profiles of the backprojection image are next computed and compared with the actual projection profiles measured during the CT scan. Various correction methods are then applied to correct discrepancies between the computed and the measured projection profiles. The corrected projection profiles are placed back to reconstruct a new image. The comparison, correction, and reconstruction processes repeat in loops until errors between the acquired and the computed projection profiles converge to a prescribed level. The number of iterations required to reconcile the differences between the computed and measured profiles is substantial. Long computation times previously precluded its use clinically. With the advent of computers in recent years with vastly improved speed, time is no longer a deterrent for implementing iterative reconstruction algorithms.

One reason why iterative reconstruction is superior to filtered backprojection for patient dose reduction is that the reconstructed images present much lower levels of noise. Lower image noise permits the user to apply less radiation to the patient to obtain the same quality images. Studies found that for images reconstructed with the same noise level as filtered backprojection, the iterative algorithms enabled use of lower beam current and therefore reduced the patient dose by up to 65 % [29]. However, for many of the CT systems in use today, implementation of iterative reconstruction requires major upgrading of their computing equipment.

Conclusion

High speed multi-slice CT with its high temporal and spatial resolution is increasingly applied for a wide spectrum of cardiac studies. Because of the high radiation dose associated with cardiac CT examinations, it is necessary for the clinicians to become familiar with the dosimetric principles, and to adopt dose reduction techniques in their clinical practice. This chapter reviewed the basic dosimetry parameters necessary to understand the terms and concepts invariably brought up in any discussion of radiation dose optimization methods. The abstract concept of effect dose should be well understood in order to explain to the patients the relative risks of different medical procedures that involve the use of radiation, such as the comparative risks of coronary CT angiography, chest x-rays, and radionuclide perfusion studies.

Patient dose reduction can be obtained on all CT systems by judiciously selecting the proper tube voltage, current-time product, and scan length. The numerous trade-names of dose modulation techniques offered by CT manufacturers can be confusing. However, the guiding principle of all techniques involves reducing the tube voltage, tube current, beam-on time, and scan volume to produce acceptable quality image with the less radiation to the patient. New systems on the market have incorporated many of the dose reduction principles and technologies into their systems, but users without the benefits of the new technologies can still minimize their patient dose by matching patient's size and weight with the dose reduction parameters discussed in this chapter.

References

1. NCRP Report No. 160. Ionizing radiation exposure of the population of the United States; 2009.
2. Brinjikji W, Kallmes D, Cloft H. Rising utilization of CT in adult fall patients. Am J Roentgenol. 2015;204:558–62.
3. ConsumerReport.org, "Consumer reports warns against the risks of radiation overexposure from unnecessary CT scans". Release Date: 27 Jan 2015. Last accessed 16 May 2015.
4. Watson SJ, Jones AL, Oatway WB, Hughes JS. Ionizing radiation exposure of the UK population: 2005 review. Health Protection Agency, Report HPA-RPD-001; 2005.
5. United Nations Scientific Committee on the Effects of Atomic Radiation. Sources and effects of atomic radiation: ionizing radiation, Publication n. E.00.IX4. New York: United Nations; 2000.
6. BEIR VII. Health risks from exposure to low levels of ionizing radiation: BEIR VII-Phase 2. Washington DC: National Academies Press; 2006.
7. Parker MS, Hui FK, Camacho MA, et al. Female breast radiation exposure during CT pulmonary angiography. Am J Roentgenol. 2005;185(5):1228–33.
8. NCRP Report No. 82. SI units in radiation protection and measurements; 1985.
9. ICRP. ICRP publication 92: relative biological effectiveness (RBE), quality factor (Q), and radiation weighting factor (wR). Oxford, UK: Elsevier Science Ltd; 2003. ISBN 0-08-044311-7.
10. 2007 report on occupational radiation exposures in Canada. Health Canada. http://www.hc-sc.gc.ca/ewh-semt/alt_formats/hecs-sesc/pdf/pubs/occup-travail/2007-report-rapport-eng.pdf.
11. Feng YJ, et al. Estimated cosmic radiation doses for flight personnel. Space Med Med Eng. 2002;15(4):265–9.
12. Department of Transportation Report – DOT/FAA/AM-03/16. What aircrews should know about their occupational exposure to ionizing radiation; 2003.
13. NCRP Report No. 101. Exposure of the U.S. population from occupational radiation; 1989.
14. ICRP. The 2007 recommendations of the International Commission on Radiological Protection. ICRP Publication 103. Ann ICRP. 2007;37(2–4):1–332.
15. Huda W, Ogden KM, Khorasani MR. Converting dose-length product to effective dose at CT. Radiology. 2008;248(3):995–1003.
16. NcNitt-Gray MF. AAPM/RSNA physics tutorial for residents: topics in CT, radiation dose in CT. Radiographics. 2002;22:1541–53.
17. Goldman LW. Principles of CT: radiation dose and image quality. J Nucl Med Technol. 2007;35:213–25.
18. Bauhs JA, Vriezze TJ, Primak AN, Bruesewitz MR, McCollough CH. CT dosimetry: comparison of measurement techniques and devices. Radiographics. 2008;28:245–53.
19. Christner JA, Kofler JM, McCollough CH. Estimating effective dose for CT using dose-length product compared with using organ doses: consequences of adopting international commission on radiological protection publication 103 or dual-energy scanning. Am J Roentgenol. 2010;194:881–9.
20. European Commission Study Group. European guidelines on quality criteria for computed tomography. Publication no. EUR 16262 EN. Brussels: Office for Official Publications of European Communities; 2000.
21. Radiation Exposure From Medical Exams and Procedures. https://hps.org/documents/Medical_Exposures_Fact_Sheet.pdf. Last accessed 25 July 2015.
22. Einstein AJ, Moser KW, Thompson RC, Cerqueira MD, Henzlova MJ. Radiation dose to patients from cardiac diagnostic imaging. Circulation. 2007;116:1290–305.
23. McCollough CH, Leng S, Yu L, Cody DD, Boone JM, McNitt-Gray MF. CT dose index and patient dose: they are not the same thing. Radiology. 2011;259(2):311–6.
24. Report No. 204. Size-Specific dose Estimates (SSDE) in pediatric and adult body CT examinations, 2011. College Park: American Association of Physicists in Medicine. https://www.aapm.org/pubs/reports/RPT_204.pdf. Last accessed 25 July 2015.
25. Dixon RL, Anderson JA, Bakalyar DM, et al. Comprehensive methodology for the evaluation of radiation dose in X-ray computed tomography. AAPM Report No. 111, College Park; 2010.
26. IAEA Human Health Reports 5. Status of computed tomography dosimetry for wide cone beam scanners, 2011, Vienna.
27. Budoff MJ, et al. Substantial radiation dose reduction in 64-multi-detector cardiac computed tomography by using lower X-ray energy during scanning. J Am Coll Cardiol. 2008;51:A148.
28. Budoff MJ. Maximizing dose reductions with cardiac CT. Int J Cardiovasc Imaging. 2009;25:279–87.
29. Maldjian PD, Goldman AR. Reducing radiation dose in body CT: a primer on dose metrics and Key CT technical parameters. Am J Roentgenol. 2013;200:741–7.
30. Raff GL, et al. radiation dose from cardiac computed tomography before and after implementation of radiation dose reduction techniques. JAMA. 2009;301:2340–8.
31. McCollough CH, Primak AN, Braun N, Kofler J, Yu L, Christner J. Strategies for reducing radiation dose in CT. Radiol Clin North Am. 2009;47(1):27–40.

32. Gopal A, Budoff MJ. A new method to reduce radiation exposure during multi-row detector cardiac computed tomographic angiography. Int J Cardiol. 2009;132:435–6.
33. Pflederer T, et al. Image quality in a Low radiation exposure protocol for retrospective ECG-gated coronary CT angiography. Am J Roentgenol. 2009;192:1045–50.
34. Gopal A, et al. Radiation reduction with prospective ECG-triggering acquisition using 64-multidetector computed tomographic angiography. Int J Cardiovasc Imaging. 2009;25:405–16.
35. Goodman TR, Brink JA. Adult CT: controlling dose and image quality. In: From invisible to visible – the science and practice of X-ray imaging and radiation dose optimization; 2006. Categorical course syllabus, Radiological Society of North America, Oak Brook, IL.
36. Lee CH, et al. Radiation dose modulation techniques in the multidetector CT era: from basics to practice. Radiographics. 2008;28:1451–9.
37. Sun Z. Coronary CT angiography with prospective ECG-triggering: an effective alternative to invasive coronary angiography. Cardiovasc Diagn Ther. 2012;2(1):28–37.
38. Mahesh M, Cody DD. Physics of cardiac imaging with multiple-row detector CT. Radiographics. 2007;27:1495–509.
39. Takakuwa KM, et al. Radiation dose in a "triple rule-Out" coronary CT angiography protocol of emergency department patients using 64-MDCT: the impact of ECG-based tube current modulation on age, sex, and body mass index. Am J Roentgenol. 2009;192:866–72.
40. Lewis M. Radiation dose issues in multi-slice CT scanning. ImPACT technology update no. 3, Jan 2005. http://www.impactscan.org/download/msctdose.pdf. Last accessed 25 July 2015.
41. Primak AN, McCollough CH, Bruesewitz MR, Zhang J, Fletcher JG. Relationship between noise, dose, and pitch in cardiac multi-detector row CT. Radiographics. 2006;26:1785–94.
42. Wong DTL, et al. Superior CT coronary angiography image quality at lower radiation exposure with second generation 320-detector row CT in patients with elevated heart rate: a comparison with first generation 320-detector row CT. Cardiovasc Diagn Ther. 2014;4(4):299–306.
43. Chen MY, Shanbhag SM, Arai AE. Submillisievert median radiation dose for coronary angiography with a second-generation 320-detector row CT scanner in 107 consecutive patients. Radiology. 2013;267(1):76–85.
44. Steigner ML, et al. Narrowing the phase window width in prospectively ECG-gated single heart beat 320-detector row coronary CT angiography. Int J Cardiovasc Imaging. 2009;25:85–90.
45. Yu L, Liu X, et al. Radiation dose reduction in computed tomography: techniques and future perspective. Imaging Med. 2009;1(1):65–84.
46. McCollough CH, et al. Dose performance of a 64-channel dual-source CT scanner. Radiology. 2007;243:775–84.
47. Tomizawa N, et al. Adaptive iterative dose reduction in coronary CT angiography using 320-row CT: assessment of radiation dose reduction and image quality. J Cardiovasc Comput Tomogr. 2012;6:318–24.
48. Kalendar W. Computed tomography: fundamentals, system technology, image quality, applications. Erlangen: Publicis Corporate Publishing; 2005.

Orientation and Approach to Cardiovascular Images

4

Jerold S. Shinbane and Antreas Hindoyan

Abstract

Mastery of conventional anatomy and physiology is essential as a template for understanding of cardiovascular variation and pathology. A multitude of analysis and reconstruction tools including orthogonal, double oblique, and curved multiplanar reformatted 2-D, and volume-rendered 3-D views can be utilized for comprehensive diagnosis of cardiovascular pathology. The goal of this chapter is orientation to review and analysis of cardiovascular structure from CCTA image sets using a systematic approach.

Keywords

Cardiovascular Computed Tomographic Angiography • Computed Tomography • Curved Multiplanar Reformatted • Double-Oblique • Orientation • Orthogonal Views • Volume-Rendered

Abbreviations

AAO	Ascending Aorta
DAO	Descending Aorta
AV	Aortic Valve
CS	Coronary Sinus
GCV	Great Cardiac Vein
IVC	Inferior Vena Cava
LA	Left Atrium
LAA	Left Atrial Appendage
LAD	Left Anterior Descending Coronary Artery
LV	Left Ventricle
LCx	Left Circumflex Coronary Artery
LIMA	Left Internal Mammary Artery
LM	Left Main Coronary Artery
LS	Left Sinus of Valsalva
MV	Mitral Valve
PA	Pulmonary Artery
PDA	Posterior Descending Coronary Artery
PV	Pulmonary Vein
RA	Right Atrium
RAA	Right Atrial Appendage
RCA	Right Coronary Artery
RIMA	Right Internal Mammary Artery
RV	Right Ventricle
TV	Tricuspid Valve

Electronic supplementary material The online version of this chapter (doi:10.1007/978-3-319-28219-0_4) contains supplementary material, which is available to authorized users.

J.S. Shinbane, MD, FACC, FHRS, FSCCT (✉) • A. Hindoyan, MD
Division of Cardiovascular Medicine, Department of Internal Medicine, Keck School of Medicine of the University of Southern California, 1520 San Pablo Suite 300, Los Angeles, CA 90033, USA
e-mail: shinbane@usc.edu

Introduction

A systematic and comprehensive approach to analysis of visualized structures is essential to interpretation of CCTA utilizing the multitude of analysis and reconstruction tools. The underpinning of this approach is an understanding of the 3-D anatomy and physiology of structures and their

M.J. Budoff, J.S. Shinbane (eds.), *Cardiac CT Imaging: Diagnosis of Cardiovascular Disease*, DOI 10.1007/978-3-319-28219-0_4

interrelation in the acquired tomographic data cube. Imagers will ultimately find their own individualized algorithm for image analysis, but this approach ultimately needs to be complete, methodical, and efficient. The goal of this chapter is orientation to viewing and analyzing cardiovascular structure from CCTA image sets, with mastery of conventional anatomy and physiology serving as a template for understanding of cardiovascular variation and pathology.

An important factor prior to image analysis is review of relevant clinical history and questions to be answered by the study. Before evaluation of individual structures, the image set needs to be assessed for limitations to analysis due to the field of view, percentage of the cardiac cycle imaged, and image quality based on degree of target region of interest contrast opacification and artifacts. Analysis should be systematic rather than focused on the most prominent findings. One systematic approach to analysis involves comprehensive evaluation through serial assessment of: (1) Non-coronary artery cardiovascular structure cranial to caudal with axial scrolling followed by additional 2- and 3-D analysis, (2) Coronary artery cardiovascular structure cranial to caudal with axial scrolling as an anchor followed by additional 2- and 3-D analysis, and (3) Non-cardiovascular structures in the available field of view by physicians with expertise in evaluation of these structures.

Image Views

Orthogonal Views: Axial, Sagittal and Coronal Planes (Figs. 4.1–4.134 shown at the end of the chapter; Videos 1, 2, and 3)

Even with the advent of a multitude of imaging software options, the axial images remain an anchor for analysis with additional information obtained from 2-D coronal sagittal, double oblique, curved multi-planar, and 3-D reconstructions useful for confirmation and specialized analysis of specific structures. In addition to structure, tissue characteristics related to the radiodensity of the tissue can be assessed through measurement of HUs (Fig. 4.135). The Hounsfield unit (HU) is based on an attenuation scale in which the radiodensity of water is 0 HU and air 1000 HU. Tissues have a spectrum of HU ranges depending on their radiodensity with approximate values for fat of −50 to −100 HU, muscle 10–40 HU, and wide spectrum for bone of 400–3000 HU based on architecture.

Analysis of CCTA relies significantly on evaluation of the axial plane images. In the axial plane, the thorax is viewed in serial cranial to caudal slices, with visualization of thinner slices enabling evaluation with greater resolution than thicker slices. If the CT system used does not provide true isotropic voxels due to limited Z axis resolution, the axial plane provides resolution superior to other planes. This is not the case for scanners providing imaging with isotropic voxels, as the voxels possess uniform resolution in all axes. The reader should visualize the patient in the supine position with the patient's feet coming out towards the reader. The sternum (anterior) and spine (posterior) can also be used to orient the reader in the axial plane (Fig. 4.136). The reader should never try to analyze a structure using one axial slice. Assessment of adjacent axial slices to establish anatomic continuity should be performed for comprehensive identification of a structure and its connections.

Non-coronary artery cardiovascular structure analysis includes: the size and architecture of the aorta and branch vessels at all visualized levels, the size and architecture of the main pulmonary artery and pulmonary artery branches, the 3-D relationships between the aorta and the pulmonary arteries, presence of anomalous thoracic vascular anatomy, location, number, and course of the pulmonary veins, atrioventricular and ventriculo-arterial concordance, continuity of the atrial septum, continuity of the ventricular septum, the presence of filling defects or masses in the left atrial appendage, atria and ventricles, valvular structure, myocardial thickness and tissue attenuation, and pericardial thickness and presence of effusion.

The thorax is viewed from anterior to posterior by scrolling through serial coronal images (Fig. 4.137) and from right to left on sagittal images (Fig. 4.138). In these reconstructions, multiple stacks of images are viewed at once, and therefore thin collimation lines can be seen. If the data sets are not aligned properly due to motion, step artifacts can occur. These artifacts would not be present using scanners which have an acquisition volume imaging the field of view in one gantry rotation, allowing single beat imaging. Respiratory motion artifacts are well seen on sagittal views.

In the sagittal and coronal views, assessment of contrast opacification of the descending aorta can be used as a marker of the adequacy of timing for contrast opacification of the distal coronary arteries. Measurement of contrast density and homogeneity measured by HU at serial levels of the descending aorta can be performed. If the HUs decrease significantly as the aorta descends, the distal coronary arteries may be poorly opacified and more difficult to analyze (Fig. 4.139).

The sagittal and coronal views display certain structures well in their natural planes. Sagittal images are helpful for viewing the right ventricular outflow tract, aorta in a "candy cane" view, and origins of venous coronary artery bypass grafts off of the aorta (Fig. 4.140). Coronal images facilitate display of the sternum, course of the left and right internal mammary arteries, mid-segment of the right coronary artery, left ventricular outflow tract, pulmonary veins and atrial appendage entering the left atrium, and descending aorta (Fig. 4.141).

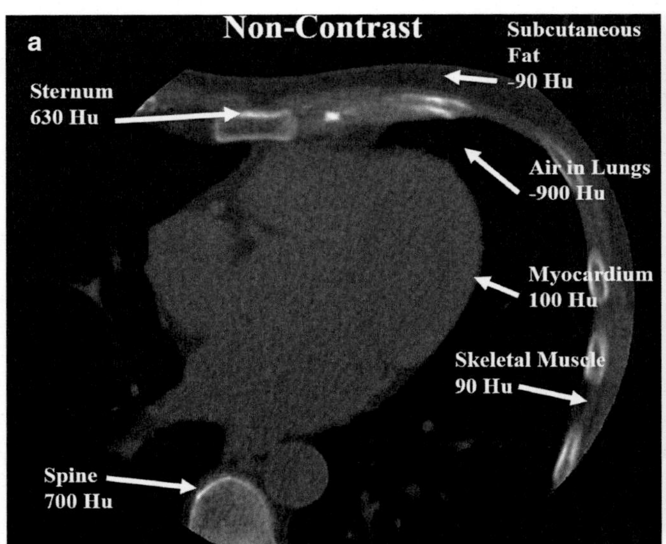

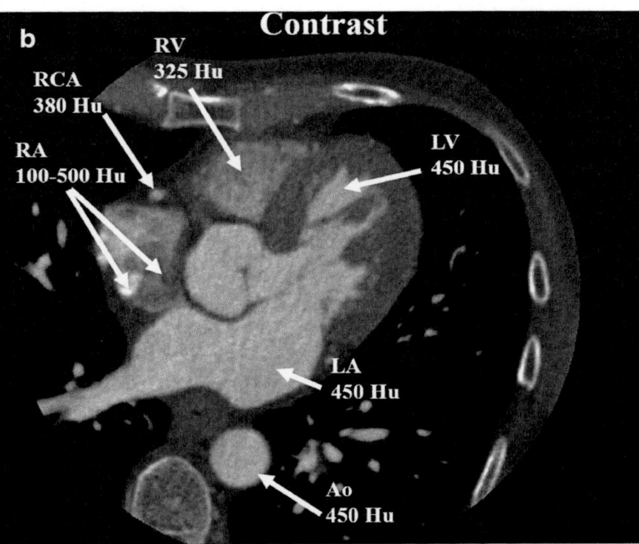

Fig. 4.135 Panel (**a**): A 2-D non-contrast axial view showing the Hounsfield Units of various tissues including subcutaneous fat, air in the lungs, bone, skeletal muscle and left ventricular myocardium. Panel (**b**): A 2-D contrast-enhanced axial view showing the Hounsfield Units of various tissues including subcutaneous fat, air in the lungs, bone, skeletal muscle, and left ventricular myocardium, and contrast enhanced right atrium (with inhomogeneity due to mixing of contrast enhanced and non-contrast enhanced blood), right ventricle, left atrium, left ventricle, and aorta. *Ao* aorta, *HU* Hounsfield units, *LA* left atrium, *LV* left ventricle, *RA* right atrium, *RCA* right coronary artery, *RV* right ventricle

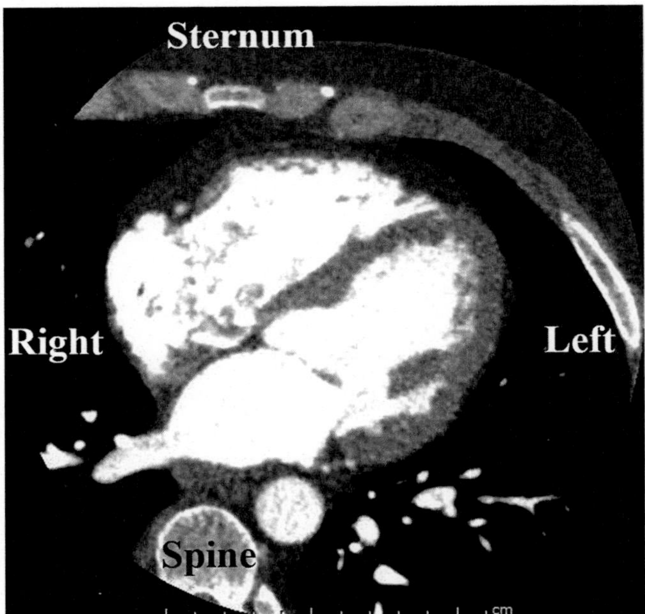

Fig. 4.136 A 2-D axial view showing anterior (sternum), posterior (spine), right and left orientation

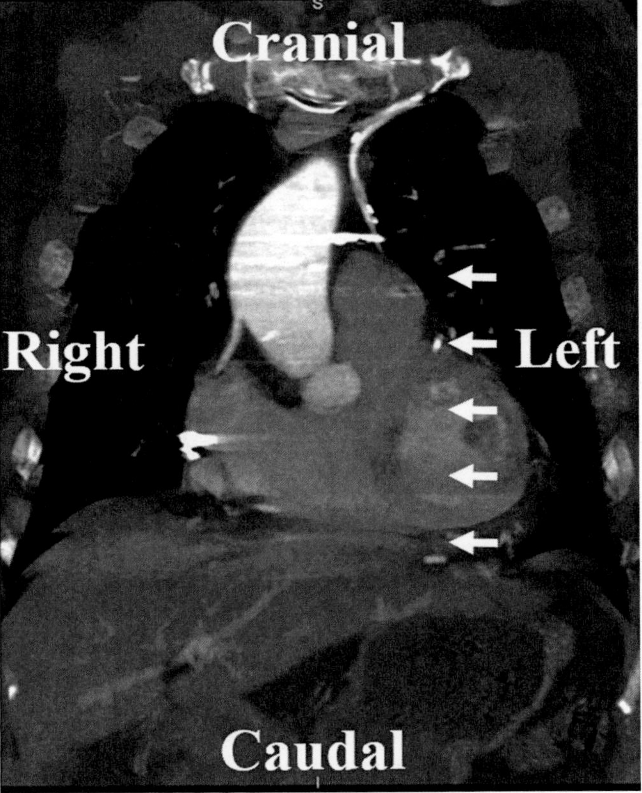

Fig. 4.137 2-D coronal view showing cranial, caudal, left and right orientation. Motion artifacts are seen as thin collimation lines (*arrows*)

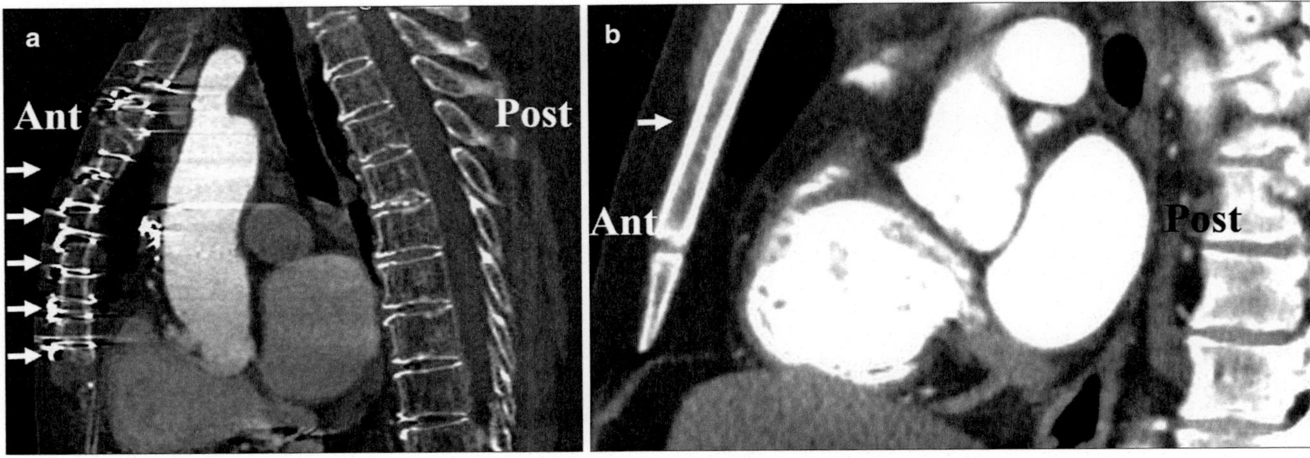

Fig. 4.138 2-D sagittal views showing anterior (sternum) and posterior (spine) orientation. Panel (**a**) Respiratory motion artifacts are seen as discontinuity of the sternum with thin collimation lines (*arrows*). Panel (**b**) Sternum with no evidence of respiratory motion (*arrow*)

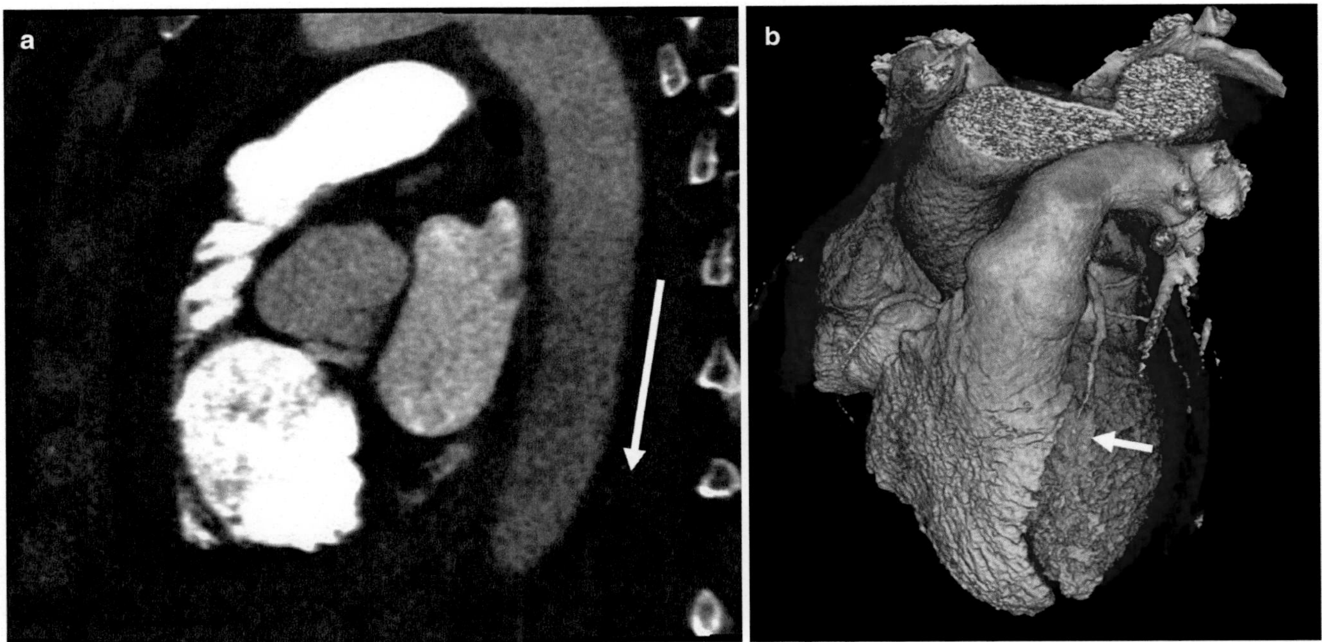

Fig. 4.139 Panel (**a**): A 2-D contrast-enhanced sagittal view showing decreased contrast density and homogeneity at serial levels of the descending aorta (*arrow*) as a marker of inadequate timing and contrast dose to visualize the distal segments coronary arteries. Panel (**b**): A 3-D contrast-enhanced reconstruction with lack of visualization of the mid to distal left anterior descending coronary artery (*arrow*)

Double Oblique 2-D Views

The axial, coronal, or sagittal views can be used as a starting point for rotation into planes providing coaxial long and short axis views of specific vascular structures (Fig. 4.142). "En face" measurements at various levels of the aorta (aortic annulus, sinus of Valsalva, sinotubular junction, ascending, arch, and descending aorta), pulmonary arteries, pulmonary vein ostia, and atrial or ventricular septal defects are important, as these structures often have ovoid rather than circular shapes, allowing the maximum and minimum diameters as well as the area of these structure to be quantified.

Curved Multiplanar Reformatted Views

Curved MPR images can evaluate an entire vascular structure in one view (Fig. 4.143). The plane of a specific artery can be chosen and displayed as a "curved surface" from

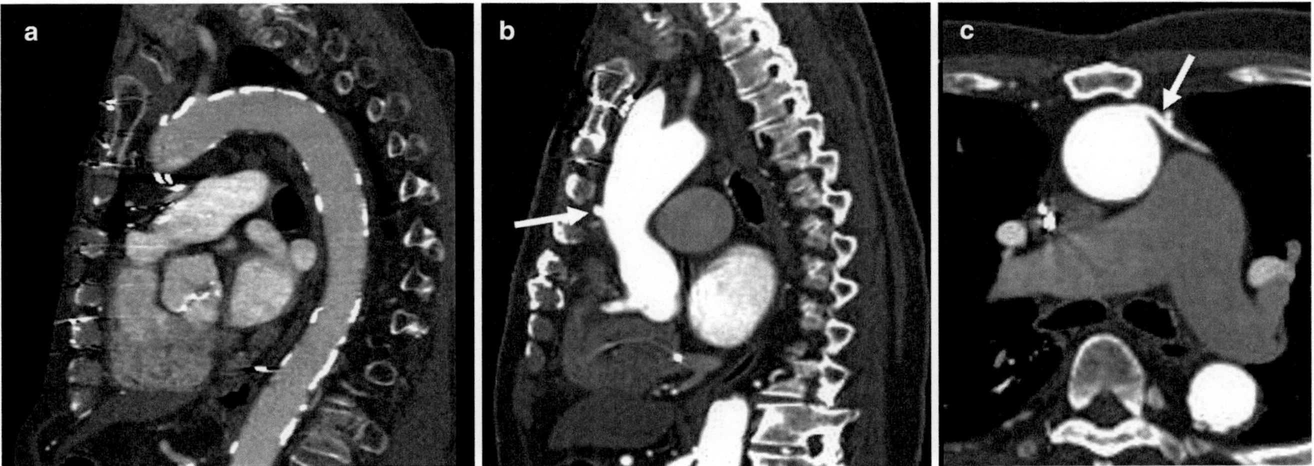

Fig. 4.140 Panel (**a**): A 2-D sagittal view displaying aorta in a "candy cane" view in a patient with atherosclerotic disease of the aorta. Panel (**b**): A 2-D sagittal view showing the origin of a saphenous venous coronary artery bypass graft off of the aorta in a patient with coronary artery bypass graft surgery (*arrow*). Panel (**c**): Axial view demonstrating the same saphenous vein graft (*arrow*)

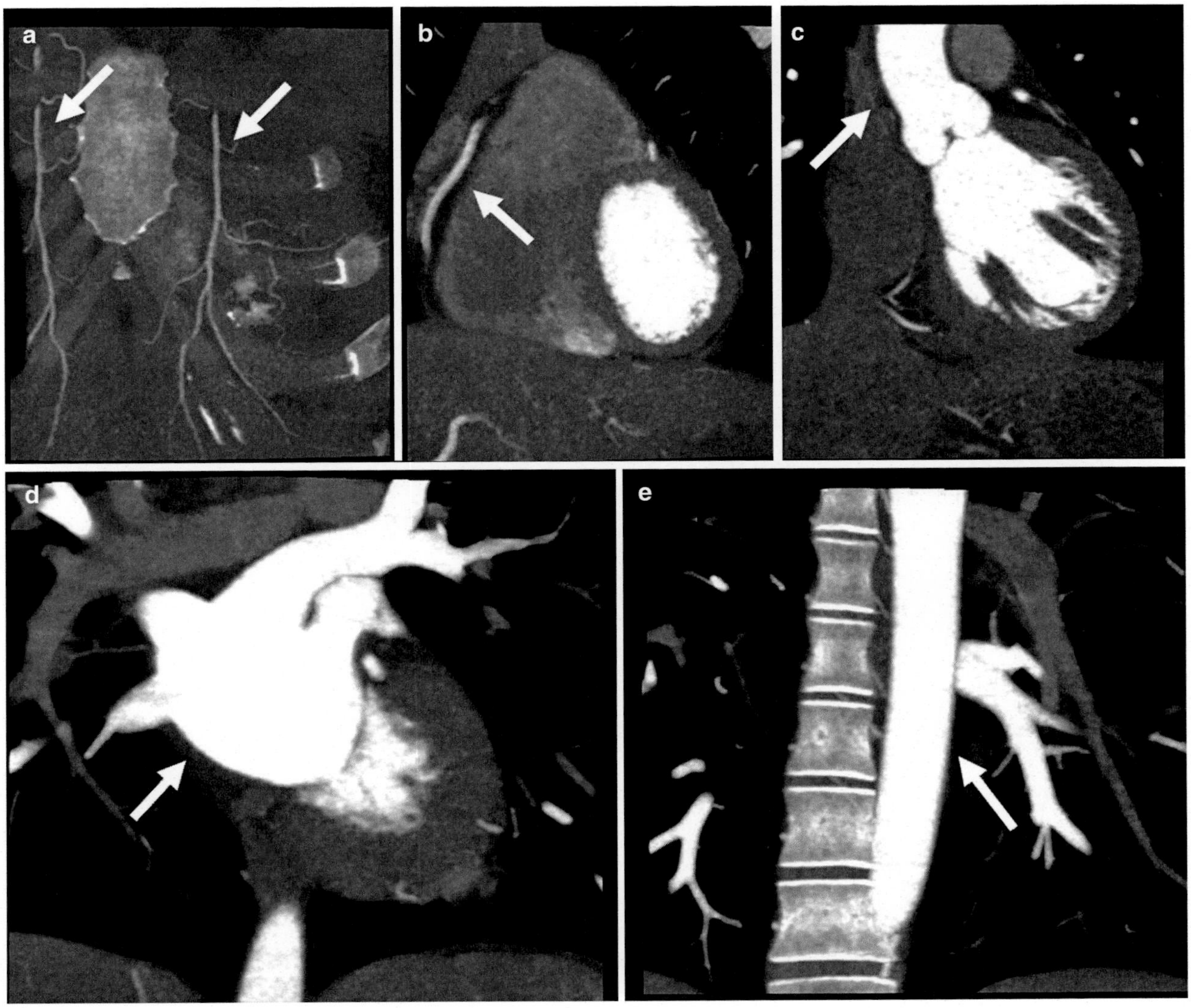

Fig. 4.141 Serial 2-D coronal images. Panel (**a**): Sternum with left and right internal mammary arteries (*arrow*). Panel (**b**): Mid-segment of the right coronary artery (*arrow*). Panel (**c**): Left ventricular outflow tract (*arrow*). Panel (**d**): Left atrium (*arrow*), pulmonary veins and left atrial appendage. Panel (**e**): Descending aorta (*arrow*)

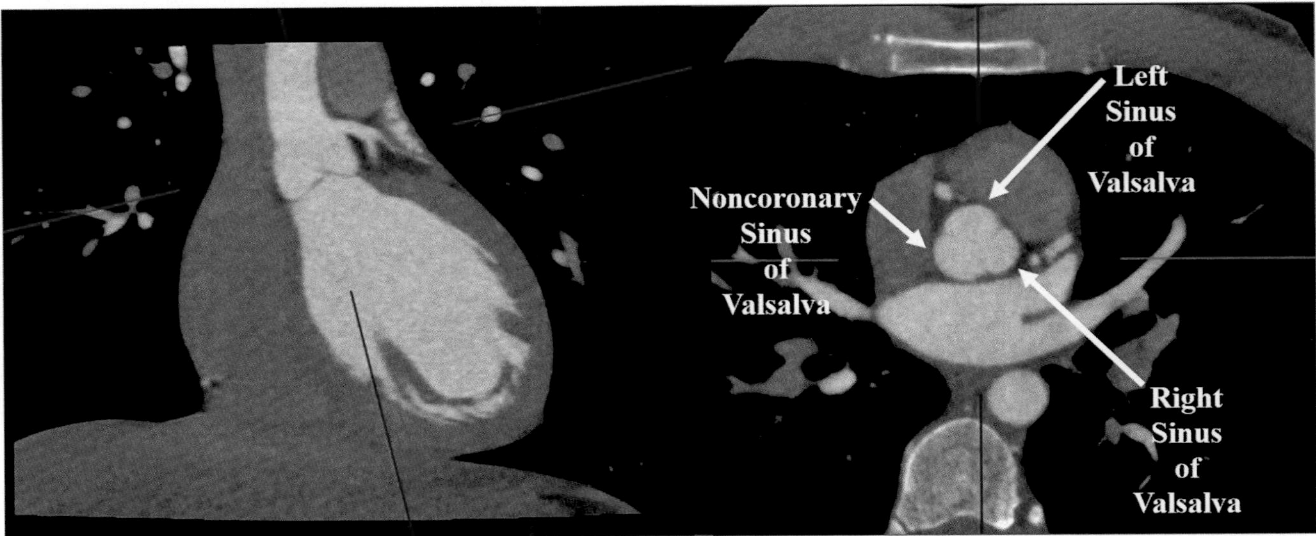

Fig. 4.142 Long (**a**) and short axis (**b**) 2-D double oblique views for coaxial assessment of the aorta at the sinuses of Valsalva (*arrows*)

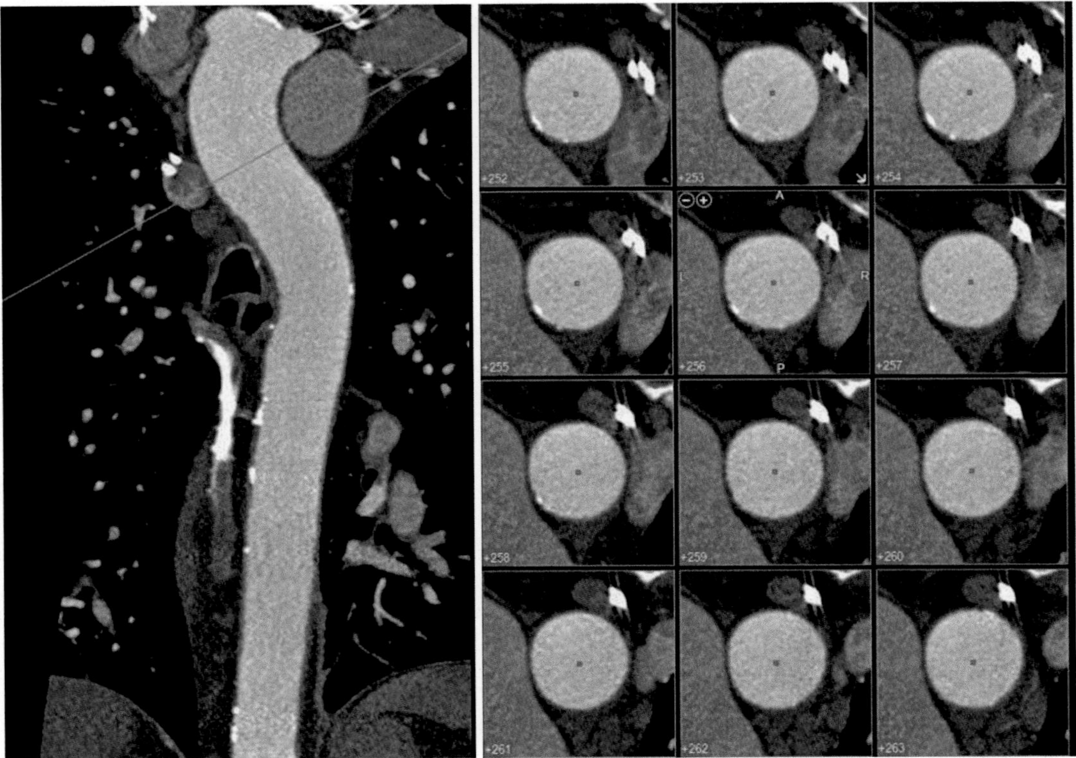

Fig. 4.143 Curved multiplanar reformatted views of the aorta with long axis (**a**) and serial coaxial cross sectional views (**b**)

within the 3D volume. This view also creates cross sectional cuts of each vascular segment. The thickness of the cross sectional cuts can be adjusted using workstation software. All other structures are automatically eliminated, including the side branches, and separate reconstructions can be rendered for each side-branch.

Volume-Rendered 3-D Views

The volume rendered technique relies on identification of all pixels within a specified attenuation range. The 3-D views may be helpful to obtain an overall sense of 3-D cardiovascular anatomy, but measurements related to structure should be performed using

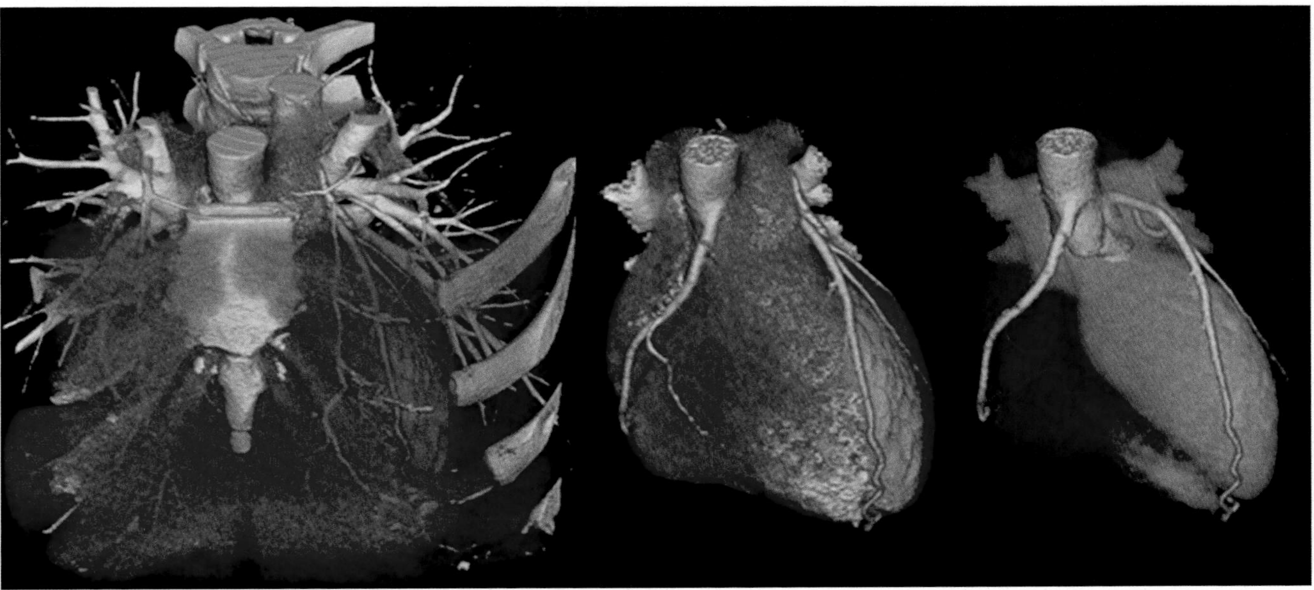

Fig. 4.144 Volume rendered 3-D reconstructions of the thorax with serial editing from thorax to cardiovascular structures to coronary arteries

2-D images in the appropriate plane. A variety of automatic and manual editing softwares allow visualization of specific structures and relationships in the 3-D data cube, but require care in utilization in order to avoid over or under editing of structures (Fig. 4.144).

Orientation to Analysis of Cardiovascular Structure

Orientation of the Great Vessels

Review of the spatial relationship between the aorta and main pulmonary artery is essential for analysis of rotational abnormalities of the great vessels. In the normal relationship of the aorta and main pulmonary artery, these vessels are perpendicular with the aorta rightward and posterior to the main pulmonary artery (Fig. 4.145). In D-transposition of the great arteries, the aorta is usually anterior to the main pulmonary artery, while in L-transposition, the aorta is usually anterior and rightward to the main pulmonary artery. In the setting of transposition of the great arteries, these vessels can be parallel with coaxial visualization in the same plane leading to a "double barrel shotgun" appearance.

Aorta

The aorta can be followed in the axial plane from the aortic root through the ascending aorta, arch and descending portions for morphology, atherosclerotic and non-atherosclerotic plaque, mural thrombus, penetrating ulcer, dissection, aneurysm and pseudoaneurysm. After review of the aorta in the axial position, double oblique views can be created so that coaxial measurements can be made at multiple levels including: the aortic annulus, sinuses of Valsalva, sinotubular junction, ascending aorta, arch, descending thoracic aorta, and potentially the upper abdominal aorta (Fig. 4.146). Due to limitation of the field of view for radiation dose reduction, portions of the aorta may not visualized. Recognition of the segments of the aorta not visualized is therefore important for analysis and reporting of findings.

Pulmonary Arteries

The initial axial assessment of the aortic to pulmonary artery relationship will bring the main pulmonary artery into view. The main pulmonary artery as well as proximal right and left pulmonary arteries can subsequently be assessed for morphology and measured coaxially using double oblique views, assessing for evidence of pulmonary arterial hypertension or aneurysm (Fig. 4.147). The pulmonary arterial tree is then assessed on the available full field of view on serial slices for vessel caliber and any evidence of filling defects, recognizing limitations if the contrast bolus has been focused on left-sided structures. Again, due to limited field of view for radiation dose reduction in studies performed for purposes such as coronary artery analysis, portions of the pulmonary arterial tree may not be visualized or

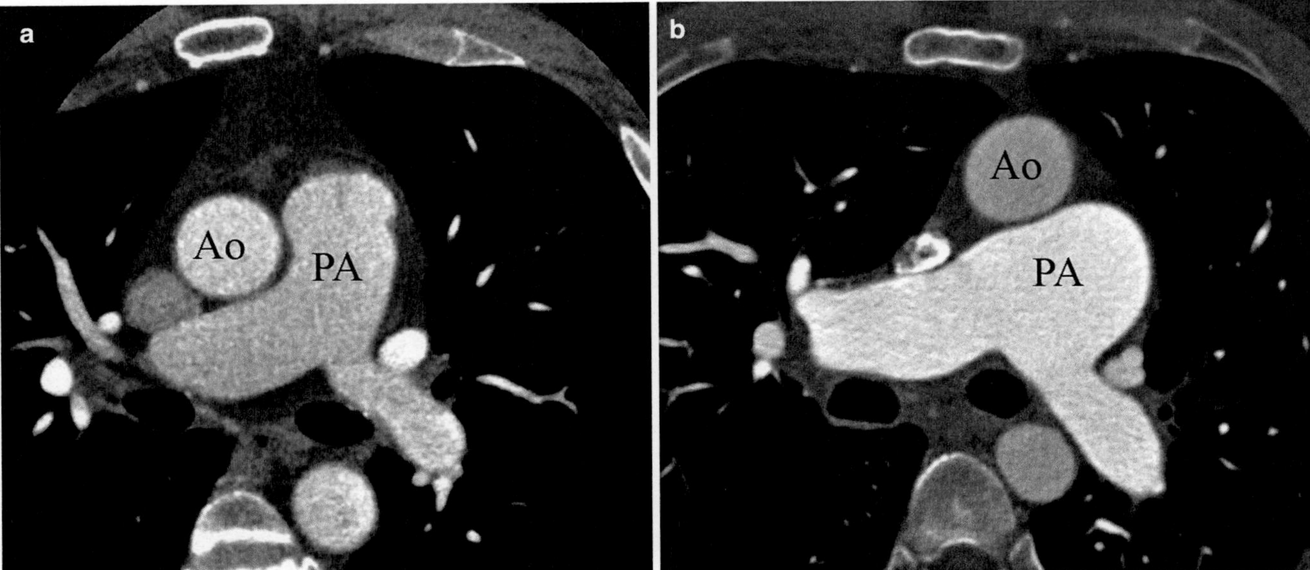

Fig. 4.145 2-D axial views demonstrating the spatial relationship between the aorta and main pulmonary artery for assessment of rotational abnormalities of the great arteries. Panel (**a**): Normal relationship of the aorta and main pulmonary artery with the aorta rightward and posterior to the main pulmonary artery. Panel (**b**): D-transposition of the great arteries, with parallel relationship of the great arteries with the aorta anterior and rightward to the main pulmonary artery. *Ao* aorta, *PA* pulmonary artery

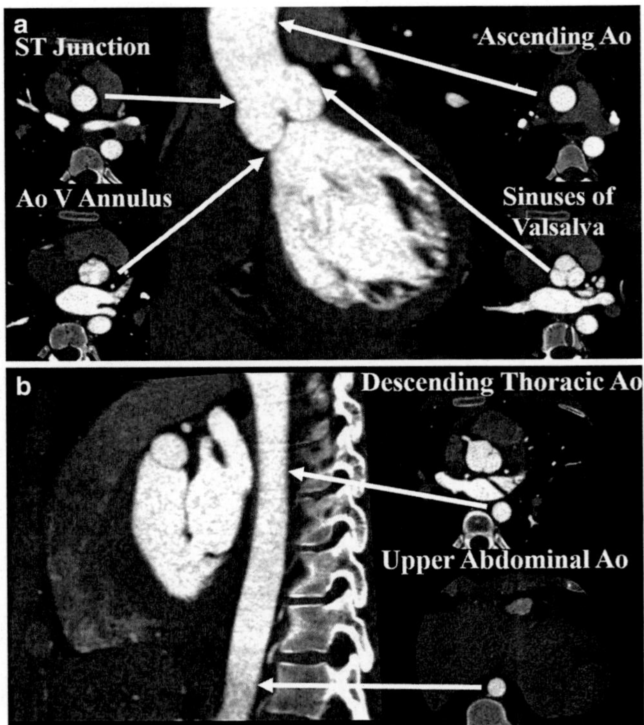

Fig. 4.146 2-D double oblique views demonstrating coaxial display of the aorta at multiple levels. Panel (**a**): The aortic annulus, sinuses of Valsalva, sinotubular junction, ascending aorta, Panel (**b**): Descending thoracic aorta and upper abdominal aorta. *Ao* aorta, *Ao V* aortic valve, *ST* sinotubular

adequately contrast opacified and therefore analysis is limited. Recognition of the portions of the pulmonary arterial tree not visualized is therefore important to analysis and reporting of findings.

Cardiac Chambers

Axial images should be reviewed for the spatial relationship between the heart and the thorax (Fig. 4.148). With normal anatomy, the heart is in the left hemithorax (levocardia), as opposed anomalous location in the right hemithorax (dextrocardia), or midline (mesocardia). The ventricles are normally D-looped, with the right ventricle rightward and anterior to the left ventricle, whereas in L-looped ventricles the relationship is inverted.

Right Atrium/SVC/IVC/Coronary Venous System

Visualization of the right atrium is dependent on the injection protocol. Even in circumstances where there is significant contrast bolus in the right atrium, there is still non-contrast enhanced blood flow from the contralateral arm venous drainage as well as the inferior vena cava. The presence of contrast and non-contrast enhanced blood causes Hounsfield Unit heterogeneity in the right atrium making endocardial assessment more challenging. The right atrium has a triangular shaped appendage as opposed to the

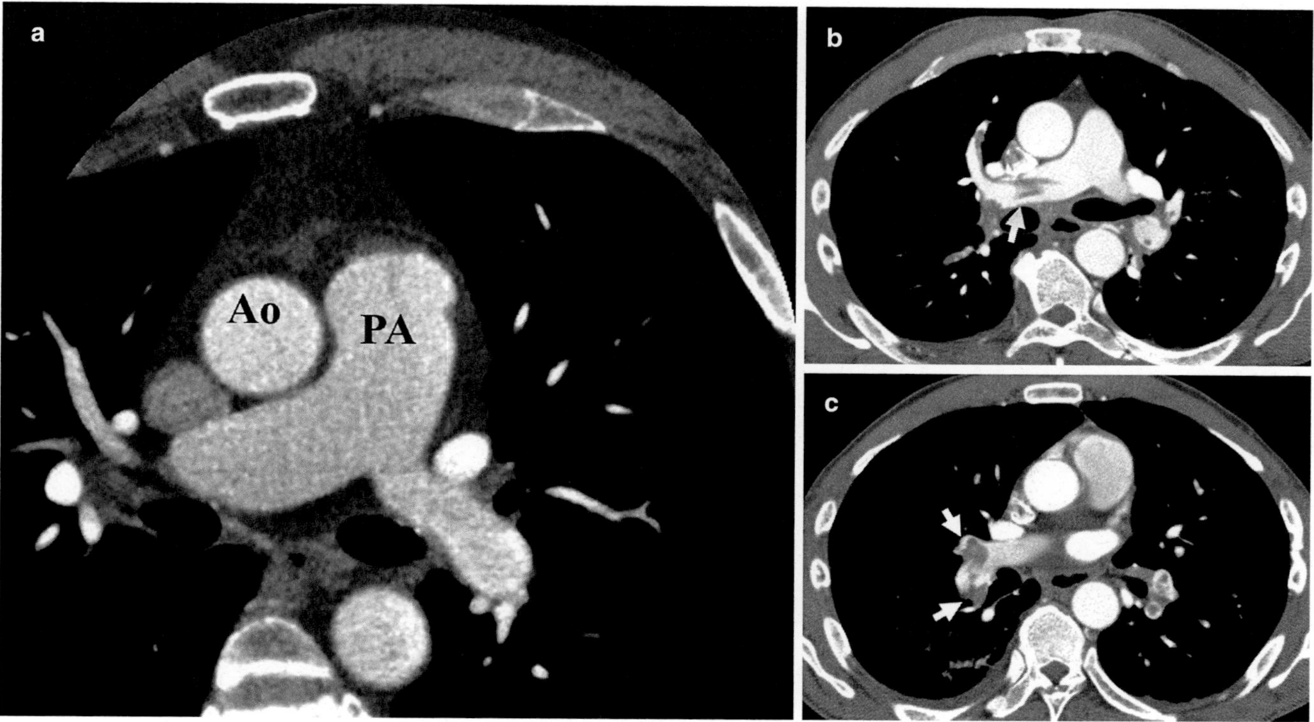

Fig. 4.147 2-D axial view of the main pulmonary artery. Panel (**a**): Pulmonary artery enlargement associated with pulmonary arterial hypertension. Panels (**b**, **c**): Large pulmonary artery emboli (*arrows*). *Ao* aorta, *PA* pulmonary artery

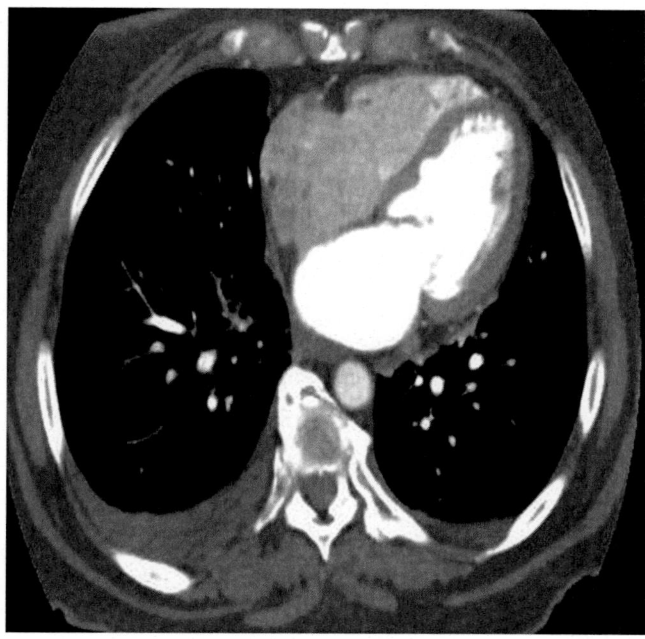

Fig. 4.148 2-D axial views of the normal orientation of the heart in the thorax (levocardia).

vermicular, "worm like", morphology of the left atrial appendage (Fig. 4.149). Familiarity with the division of the right atrium into a trabeculated lateral portion separated by the crista terminalis from a smooth walled septum is essential to avoid misinterpretation of structures as masses. Characteristics of the septum such as lipomatous hypertrophy (Fig. 4.150), atrial septal aneurysm, patent foramen ovale, and atrial septal defect require analysis of the entire septum. The size, shape and morphology of atrial septal defects including the surrounding rim require detailed assessment in double oblique views. Analysis for the presence, morphology and patency of the superior and inferior vena cavae should also include a search for any anomalous connections from the pulmonary veins as well as for the presence of other venous connection to the right atrium. The coronary sinus ostium is usually seen in the inferoposterior right atrium. The coronary sinus/great cardiac vein should be evaluated for continuity throughout course as well as for evidence of enlargement due to either right-sided pressure and volume overload or a left-sided superior vena cava with aneurysmal coronary sinus connection. The coronary sinus ostium may have a variable degree of presence of a remnant

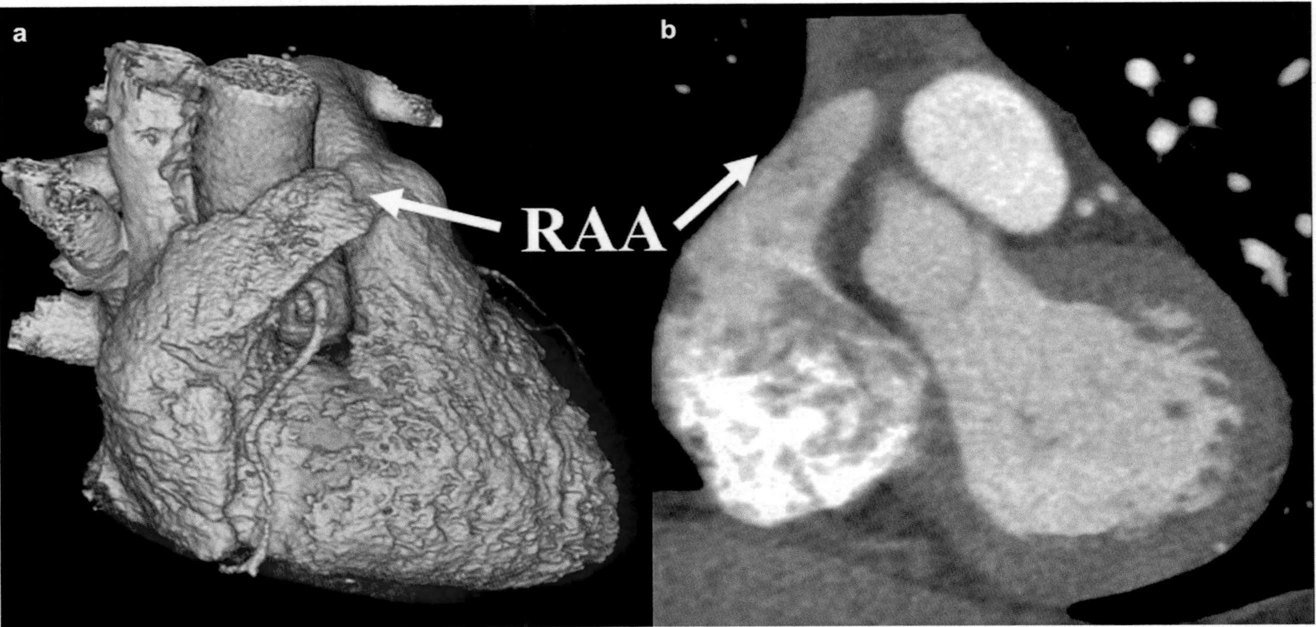

Fig. 4.149 Views of the triangular shaped, wide based right atrial appendage. Panel (**a**): 3-D reconstruction. Panel (**b**): 2-D double oblique image. *RAA* right atrial appendage

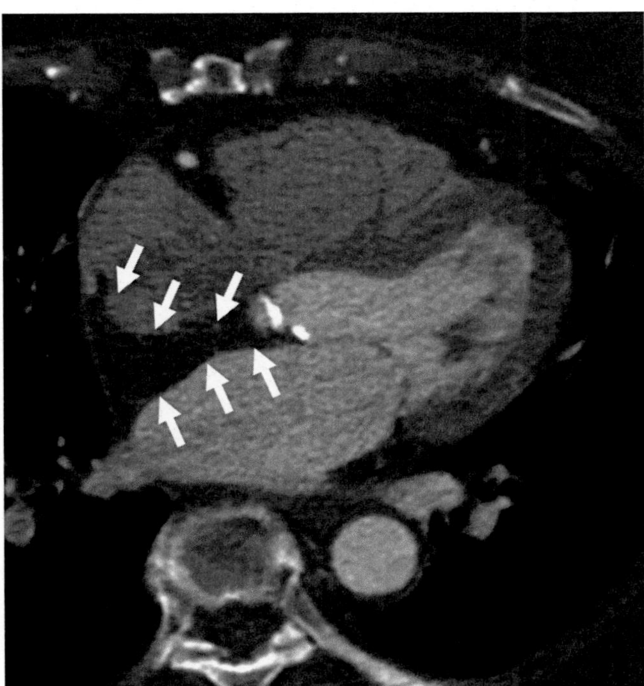

Fig. 4.150 2-D axial view of the atrial septum demonstrating lipomatous hypertrophy (*arrows*)

Thebesian valve. Evaluation of the entire coronary venous system necessitates a delay in timing of image acquisition from contrast injection as contrast-enhanced blood must flow back from the myocardium through the coronary venous branches, great cardiac vein and then to the coronary sinus. Adequate opacification of a left-sided superior vena cava requires images obtained with a left arm venous contrast injection.

Left Atrium/Pulmonary Veins

The left atrium and its relationship to the pulmonary veins and other thoracic structures can be characterized with multiple CCTA reconstruction modalities (Figs. 4.151 and 4.152). The left atrium is often trapezoidal in shape and becomes progressively more spherical when enlarged. The complex shape makes single plane assessment challenging and therefore volumetric assessment more completely characterizes size. The left atrial volume can be quantitated at end systole and end-diastole. The left atrial appendage is a complex structure, with variation in shape, size, lobulation, and the presence of pectinate muscles. Characterization of the left atrial appendage ostial characteristics, length of the main body, and number and morphology of lobes can be important to procedures such as left atrial appendage occlusion devices. Assessment should be made for filling defects in the left atrial appendage. Filling defects can be due to thrombus, mass, or inadequate opacification due to decreased left atrial appendage velocity. The left atrium should be assessed for masses as well as other anomalies

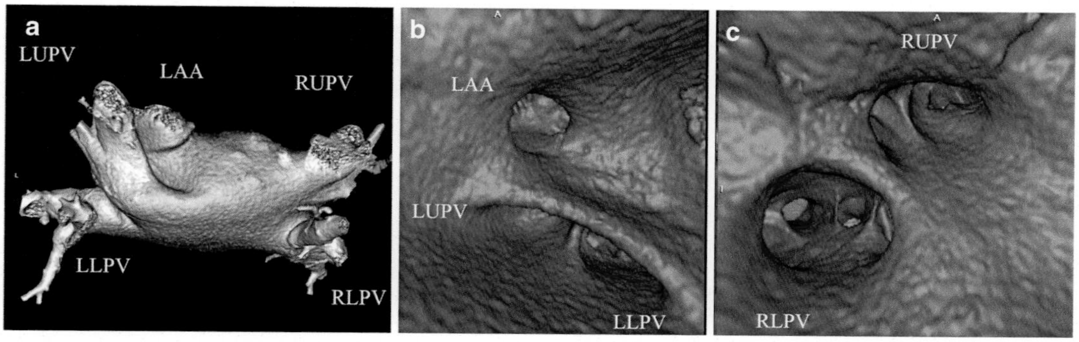

Fig. 4.151 Multimodal views of the left atrium. Panel (**a**): 3-D posterior view of the left atrium. Panel (**b**): Endovascular view of the left upper and lower pulmonary veins and the left atrial appendage. Panel (**c**): Endovascular view of the right upper and lower pulmonary veins. *LAA* left atrial appendage, *LLPV* left lower pulmonary vein, *LUPV* left upper pulmonary vein, *RLPV* right lower pulmonary vein, *RUPV* right upper pulmonary vein

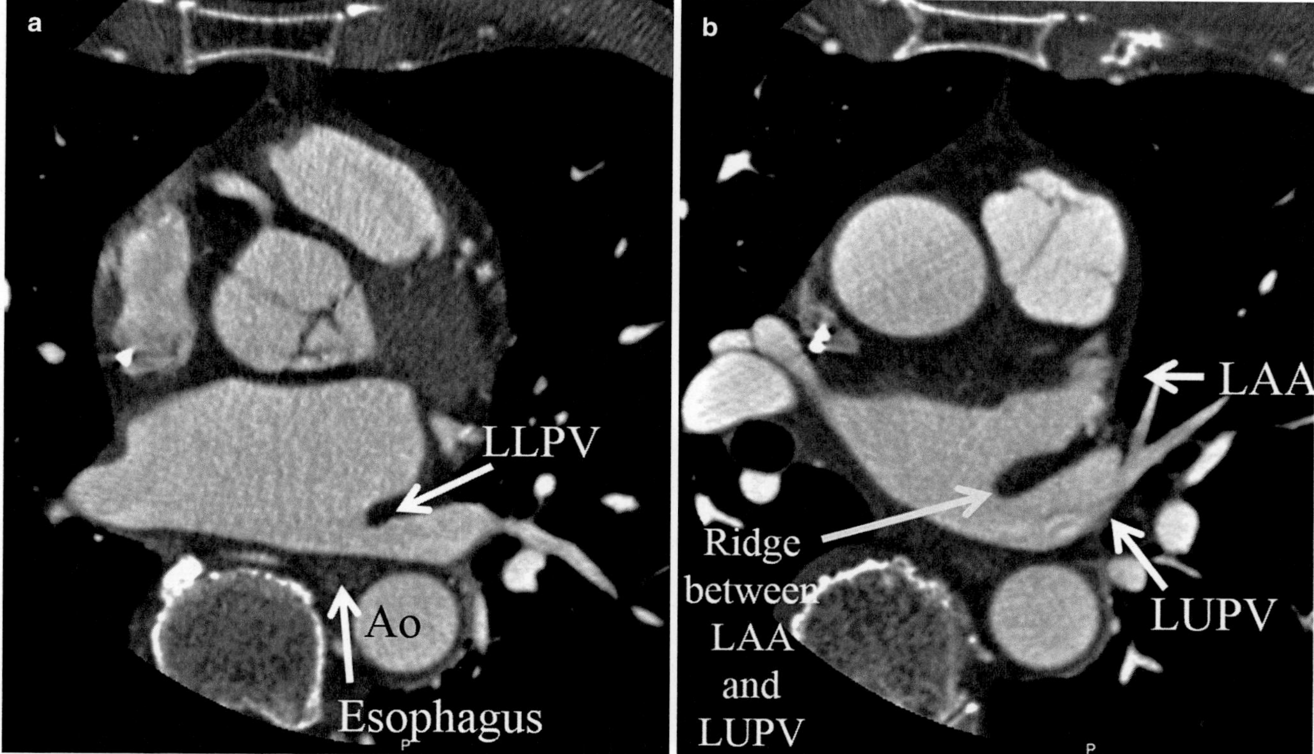

Fig. 4.152 2-D double oblique views of the left atrium. Panel (**a**): Relationship of the esophagus, left lower pulmonary vein and aorta. Panel (**b**): Relationship between the left atrial appendage, left upper pulmonary vein, and the ridge between these structures. In contradistinction to the right atrial appendage, the left atrial appendage is veriniform or "wormlike" with a narrow ostium. The ridge between the left atrial appendage and left upper pulmonary vein can be prominent and misdiagnosed as an atrial mass. *Ao* aorta, *LAA* left atrial appendage, *LLPV* left lower pulmonary vein, *LUPV* left upper pulmonary vein

such as accessory atrial appendages and diverticulae. The ridge between the left atrial appendage and left atrium, sometimes referred to as the "Coumadin ridge" can be prominent and misdiagnosed as an atrial mass.

The pulmonary veins can be assessed as they course to the left atrium on the coronal and axial views, with subsequent measurement of the pulmonary vein orifices made coaxially at the interface of the left atrium and pulmonary vein using a double oblique approach. Multiple variations in pulmonary venous anatomy occur, commonly with three right and two left pulmonary veins. Pulmonary veins can coalesce into a single trunk at the atrial interface. Each vein should be followed from its origin in the lungs and assessment should be made for any evidence of anomalous pulmonary venous return.

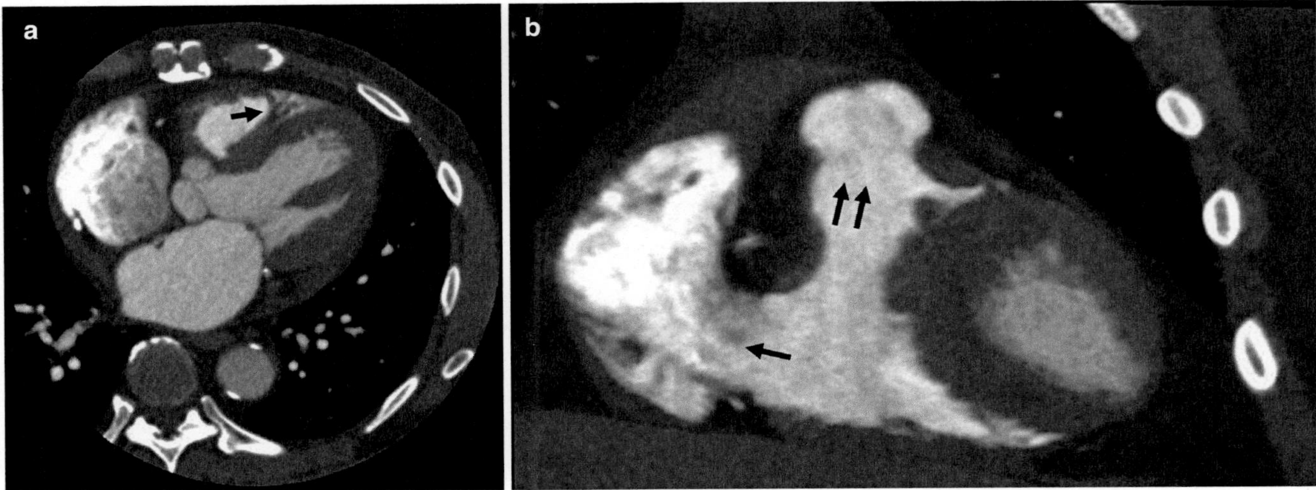

Fig. 4.153 2-D double oblique views of the right ventricle. Panel (**a**): Trabeculation of the septum and a moderator band (*black arrow*). Panel (**b**): Non-adjacent location of the tricuspid annulus (*single black arrow*) and pulmonic valve annulus (*double black arrows*), separated by the conus, creating divisions into an inflow, body, and outflow

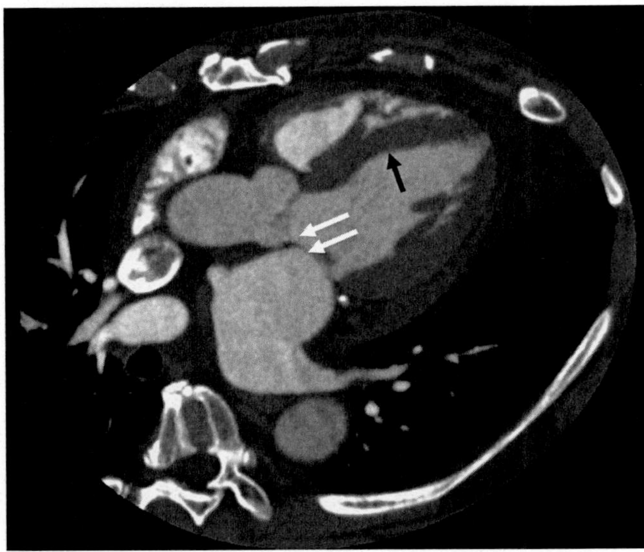

Fig. 4.154 2-D double oblique view of the left ventricle with the anatomic features of a smooth-walled septum (*black arrow*) and continuity between the aortic and mitral valve annuli (*white arrows*)

Right Ventricle

Similar to the right atrium, heterogeneous opacification of the contrast can occur in the right ventricle. Morphologic features of the right ventricle include trabeculation of the septum, moderator band, and non-adjacent location of the tricuspid valve and pulmonary valve annuli as they are separated by the conus arteriosus, therefore creating right ventricular divisions into an inflow, body, and outflow (Fig. 4.153). When retrospectively-gated images are acquired on an adequately opacified right ventricle, volumetric assessment of size and function can be measured. The right ventricle though is ovoid in shape and therefore can be more challenging to quantitate than the left ventricle.

Left Ventricle

Morphologic features of the left ventricle include a smooth-walled septum, adjacent location of the mitral valve and aortic valve annuli, and prominent papillary muscles (Fig. 4.154). Assessment can be made for wall thinning as well as lipomatous metaplasia associated with myocardial infarction. The ventricular septum can be assessed for continuity versus presence of a ventricular septal defect with characterization of location, shape, and size. The ventricle can be assessed for thrombi and masses. For retrospectively gated studies, functional views can be reformatted for assessment of left ventricular volumes, wall thicknesses and thickening, myocardial mass, regional wall motion and global ventricular function (Fig. 4.155, Video 4).

Valvular Structure and Function

On retrospectively-gated studies, aortic and mitral valve anatomy and motion including annular dimensions, valve leaflet number, morphology, degree of calcification, valve excursion, apposition, prolapse, valve area, and regurgitant orifice can be assessed (Figs. 4.156 and 4.157). Additionally, large vegetations or other masses, can be visualized. Functional image sets can be formatted following the traditional echocardiographic views, with the ability to view motion

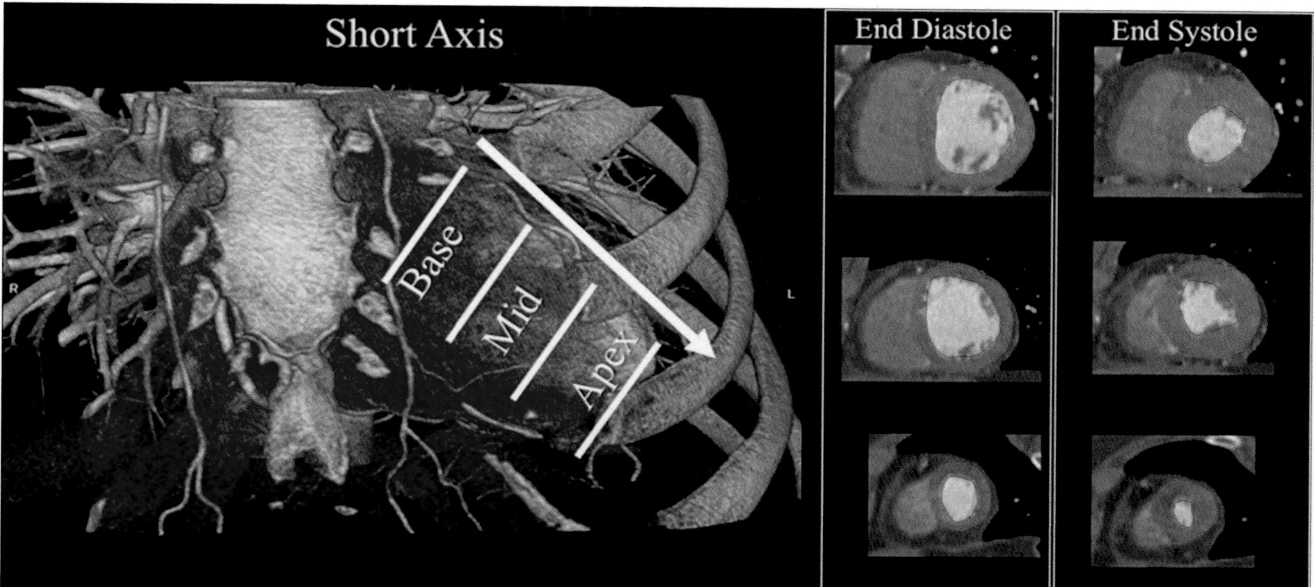

Fig. 4.155 2-D retrospectively-gated end-diastolic and end-systolic short axis ventricular views used for assessment of wall thickness, volumes, and ejection fraction

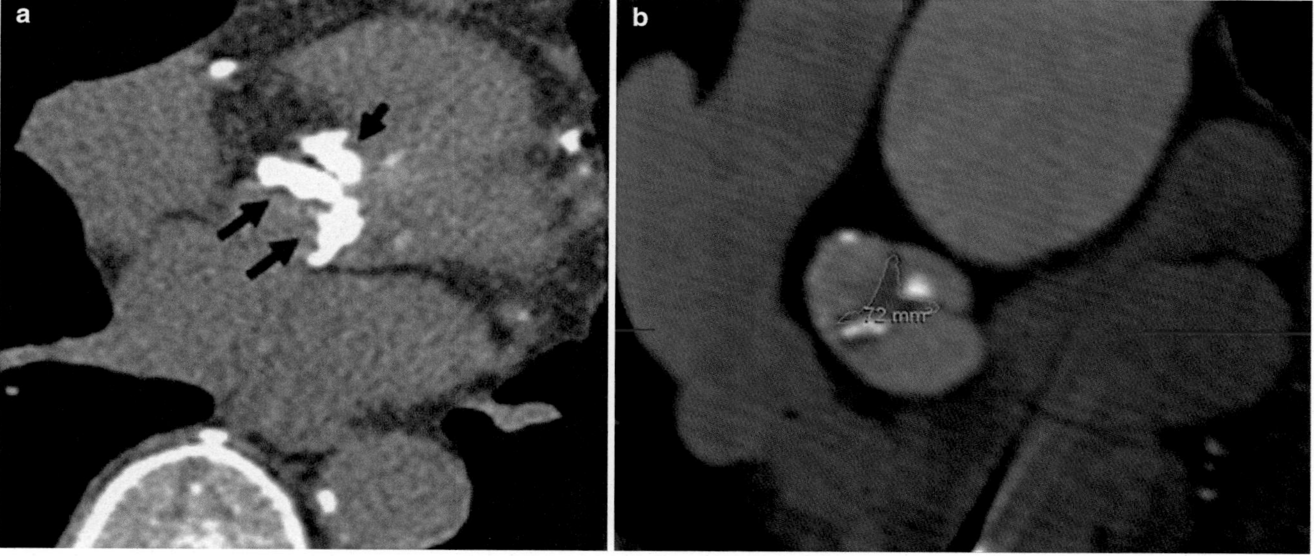

Fig. 4.156 2-D contrast-enhanced double oblique aortic valve images. Panel (**a**): Trileaflet calcific aortic stenosis. Panel (**b**): Planimetry of aortic valve area demonstrating severe aortic stenosis

through the entire cardiac volume in these views. Functional views can also be viewed in oblique planes for dynamic analysis of specific structures. Tricuspid and pulmonic valve assessment requires adequate contrast opacification of the right heart for analysis. With prospectively gated images more limited data related to valve morphology can be obtained (Fig. 4.158).

Pericardium

The pericardium should be assessed for evidence of regional or global thickening, calcification, pericardial effusion, and pericardial masses. This may be particularly helpful in scenarios of posterior pericardial effusions, where echocardiographic imaging may be more challeng-

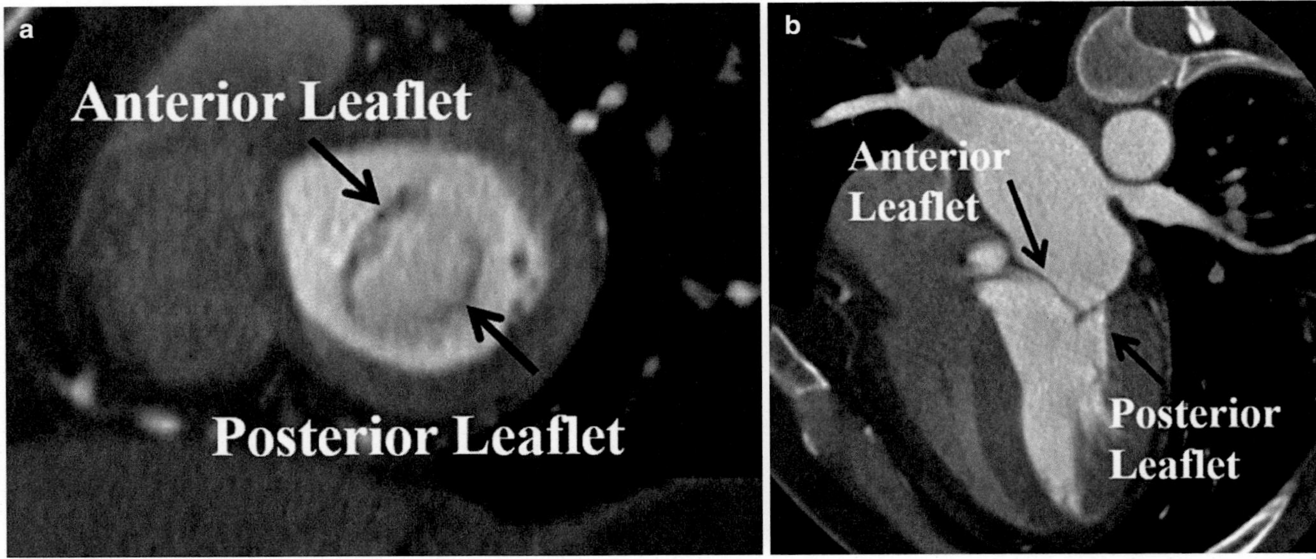

Fig. 4.157 2-D double oblique mitral valve images. Panel (**a**): Short axis view. Panel (**b**): 4 chamber view

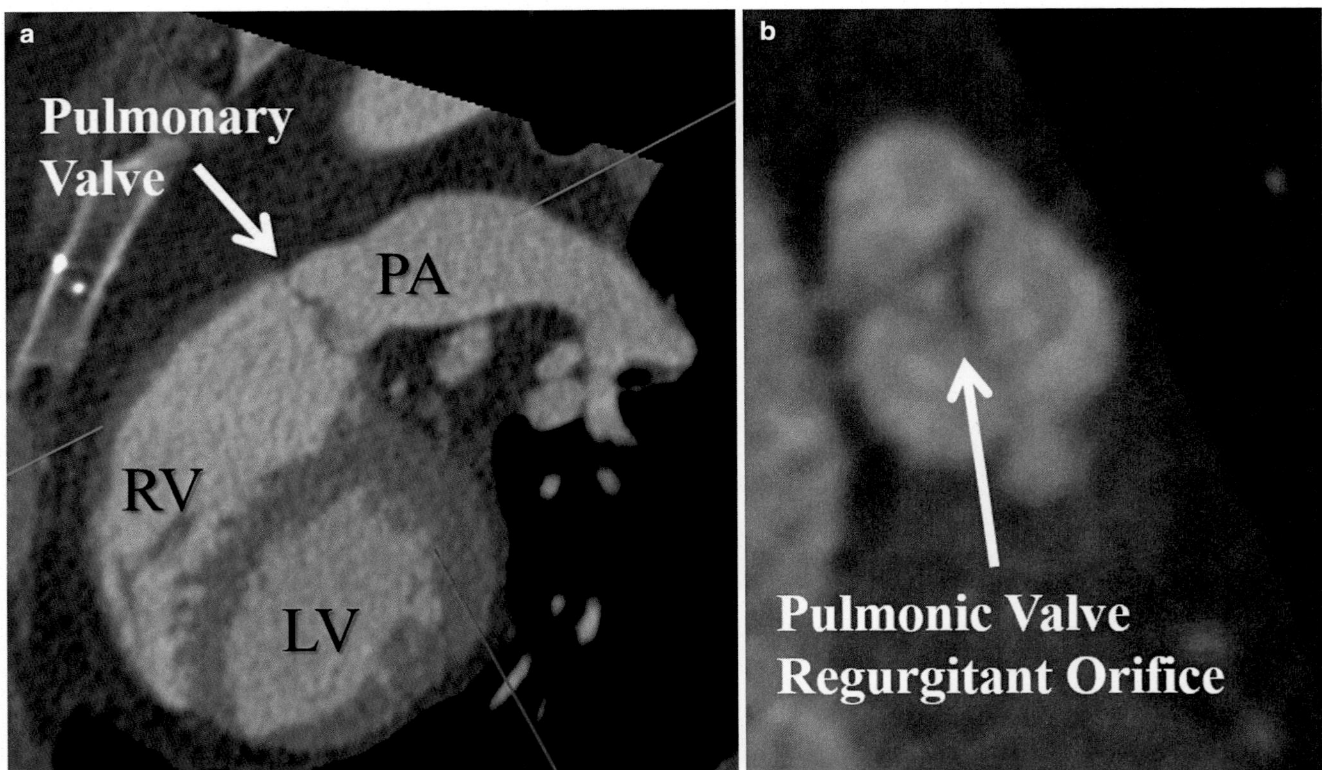

Fig. 4.158 2-D double oblique pulmonary valve images. Panel (**a**): Long axis view of right ventricular outflow tract. Panel (**b**): Coaxial view showing the pulmonary valve regurgitant orifice. *LV* left ventricle, *PA* pulmonary artery, *RA* right atrium

ing. Small pericardial effusion can be appreciated on coronal images with the fluid layering in the pericardial space just above the diaphragm. The HU cursor, if placed on the effusion, can confirm that the attenuation of the fluid is near water attenuation (0 HU).

Coronary Artery Assessment

Assessment of the coronary arteries requires a multimodal approach to reconstruction and analysis. Prior to assessment for coronary arterial atherosclerotic disease, the origin, course and termination of each coronary artery should be analyzed for coronary artery dominance and for anomalies. Viewing the aortic root in the axial plane as a clock face, the right coronary artery arises from the right sinus of Valsalva at approximately 11:30 on the clock face and the left main coronary artery arises off of the left sinus of Valsalva at approximately 3:30 on the clock face (Fig. 4.159)." The right coronary artery should be followed in the right AV groove, the left anterior descending coronary artery in the anterior interventricular groove and the left circumflex coronary artery in the left AV groove with branches of each artery coursing out of their respective grooves. The posterior

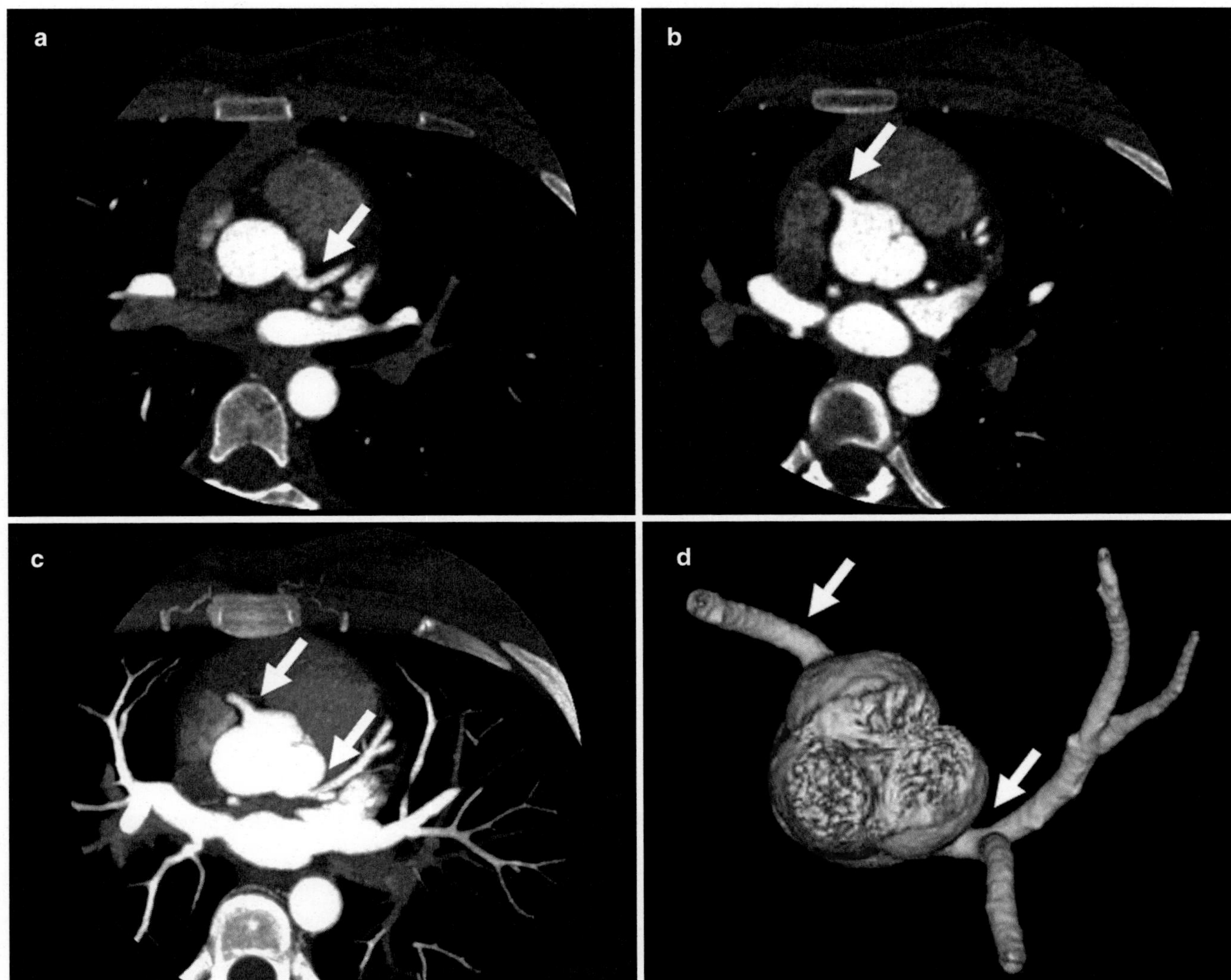

Fig. 4.159 Axial Images demonstrating the normal location of the origins of the coronary arteries. Viewing the aortic root in the axial plane as a "clock face," the right coronary artery arises from the right coronary sinus at approximately 11:30 on the "clock face" and the left main coronary artery arises off of the left coronary sinus at approximately 3:30 on the "clock face." Panel (**a**): 2-D axial view showing the origin of the left main coronary artery (*arrow*). Panel (**b**): 2-D axial view showing the origin of the right coronary artery (*arrow*). Panel (**c**): Thick maximal intensity projection showing the origin of the left main and right coronary arteries (*arrows*). Panel (**d**): Thick maximal intensity projection showing the origin of the left main and right coronary arteries (*arrows*)

descending artery can be visualized either from the right coronary artery or circumflex in the posterior interventricular groove, defining vessel dominance.

Anomalous coronary arteries can be characterized by ostial location and morphology, course and termination. An anomalous coronary artery can arise off of a shared ostium with another coronary artery, as its own separate ostium, off of another coronary artery, or off of another vascular structure such as the pulmonary artery. For a coronary artery off of the contralateral aortic sinus, the course can be pre-pulmonic, inter-arterial, intra-septal, or retro-aortic. Termination can occur in an anomalous myocardial vascular distribution or into another arterial or venous vascular structure.

Beginning at the most cranial slices, maximum intensity projections can be viewed at 5 mm slice thickness. These thicker slices facilitate visualization of the longitudinal course of the vessels, with one limitation being that the brightest pixel dominates the image. Therefore, in the presence of heavily calcified segments, one might miss a non-calcified plaque causing a significant narrowing of the coronary vessel. Adjusting the slice thickness back to 0.5 mm, each coronary artery segment can subsequently be followed, assessing for the presence of calcified, mixed, and non-calcified plaque in the vessels of mild, moderate, or severe grades. The coronary artery calcium images should also be referenced, as they demonstrate the presence and location of calcium without contrast in the coronary arteries.

In the axial view, the vessels are visualized in the plane of image acquisition. As previously mentioned, if the CT system used does not provide true isotropic voxels due to limited Z axis resolution, the axial view provides greater resolution than other reconstructed planes. Each individual artery should be followed through the cranial to caudal axial slices rather than attempting to view multiple arteries on one axial slice. The left main coronary artery, left anterior descending artery, circumflex coronary artery, and right coronary artery are analyzed individually along with their branches. A coronary arterial segment coaxial to the axial plane will appear as a circle, while an artery coursing perpendicular to the axial plane will appear linear. The limitation is that an arterial segment coursing in any other direction will be out of plane and therefore challenging to review. Therefore, other modalities including 2-D double oblique and curved multiplanar reconstructions are employed to follow the course of the arterial segment being analyzed.

Double oblique views allow each coronary artery to be followed in plane coaxially throughout its course (Fig. 4.160). Use of double oblique views allows the reader to follow the course of each coronary artery, which is especially useful for tortuous segments. The optimal assessment plane for the most proximal segment of a coronary artery can be identified in its long and short axis and then rotated 360 degrees. The oblique plane is then moved at small increments for serial assessment of segments and branches from proximal to distal artery.

Curved multiplanar reformatted images are extremely useful to evaluate an entire coronary artery in one view. The reader can choose the plane of a specific artery which is displayed as a "curved surface" from within the 3-D volume (Fig. 4.161). With curved multiplanar reformatted views, a centerline is created and the artery "straightened out" and viewed as a cylinder. The software also creates cross sectional cuts of each coronary arterial segment of the cylinder, with the ability to adjust the thickness of the cross sections. The arterial segment of interest (coronary artery stenosis) can be compared to the segments above and below it as a reference. All other structures are automatically eliminated, including the side branches, and separate reconstructions can be rendered for every side branch. The long axis luminal view can be rotated 360° around its central axis in order to assess eccentric plaques and stenoses. With curved multiplanar reformatted images, the computer software could create the appearance of a stenosis by following an area of dense calcium rather than the center of the vessel lumen. Additionally, the centerline can jump from the coronary artery to follow an adjacent cardiac vein. The centerline should therefore be viewed in order to ensure that it remains within the center of the vessel of analysis.

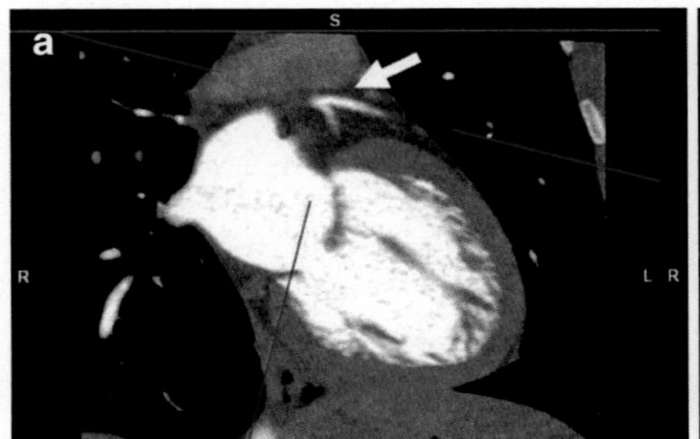

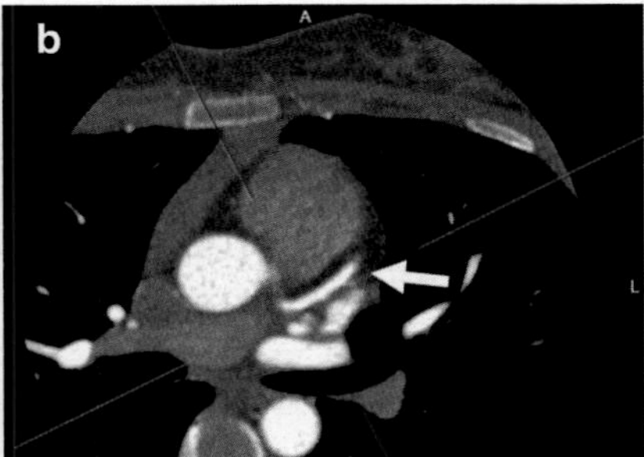

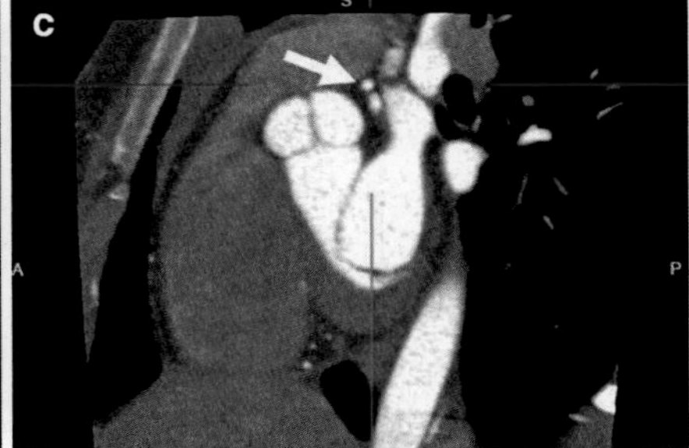

Fig. 4.160 2-D double oblique identification of a segment of the left anterior descending coronary artery with long (**a**, **b**) and short axis (**c**) views of the arterial segment

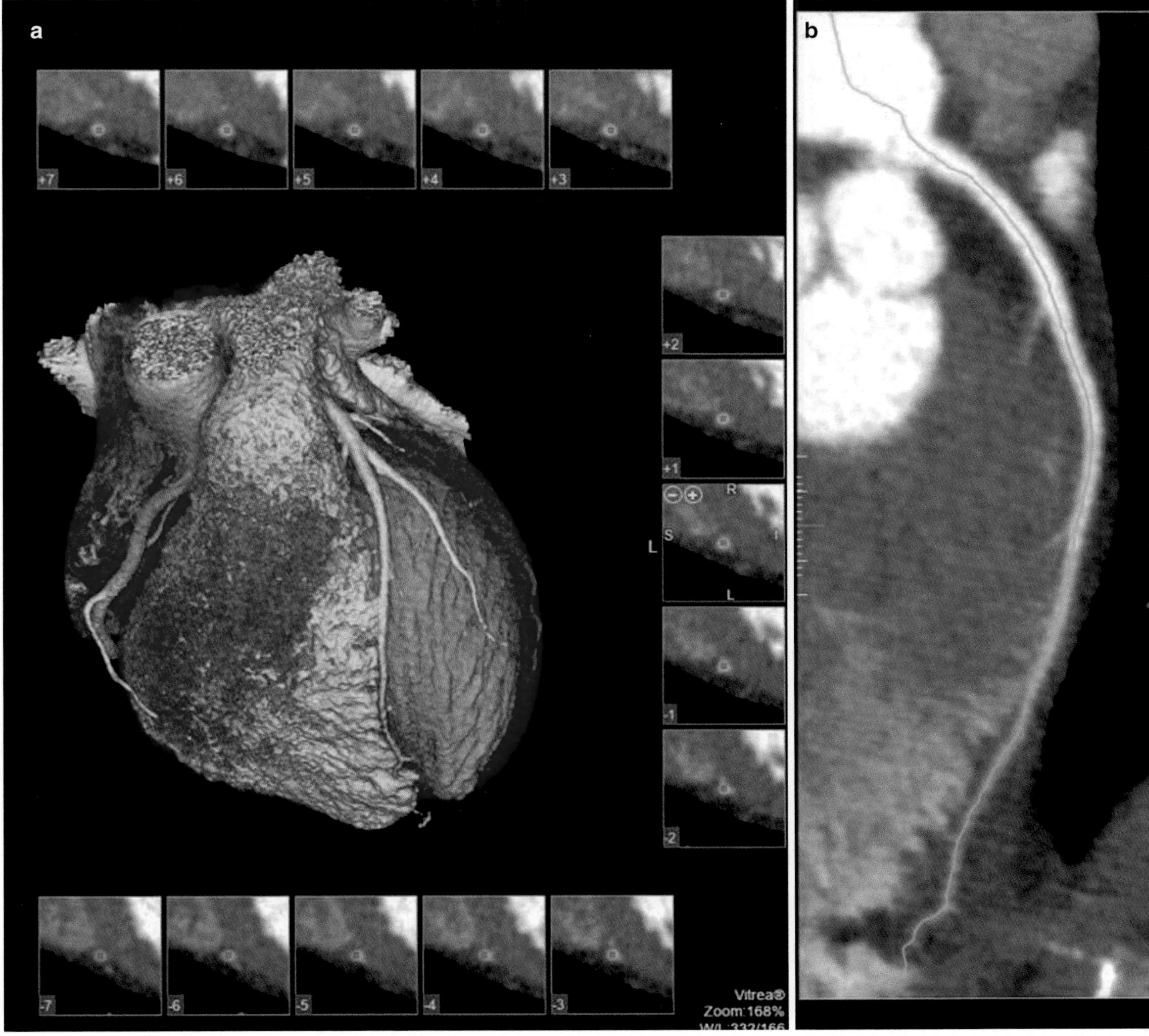

Fig. 4.161 Curved multiplanar reformatted view of a left anterior descending coronary artery. (**a**) The left anterior descending coronary artery is viewed as serial coaxial cross sections. (**b**) The centerline (*yellow line*) is used to determine the center of each arterial segment

The volume rendered technique relies on identifying all pixels above a certain threshold with various degrees of attenuation. The results are most similar in orientation to invasive coronary angiography images (Figs. 4.162 and 4.163, Videos 5 and 6). The coronary arteries are seen as relatively smooth structures with other cardiovascular landmarks present. The image can be rotated, allowing the interpreter some flexibility in visualizing the segment from multiple angles. A stenotic coronary artery segment will appear darker as well as narrowed on volume rendered images. The 3-D volume rendered images in CCTA help in identification of coronary anomalies as well as to assess the dominance of the coronary arterial tree. In patients with previous coronary artery bypass graft surgery, the origin of grafts from the aorta can be counted and the courses followed to the native vessels. Stumps of occluded grafts can also be easily identified. As there are potential artifacts with all these additional techniques, the thin axial slices should always be used to confirm or exclude any potential lesions that might be seen with other reconstructions.

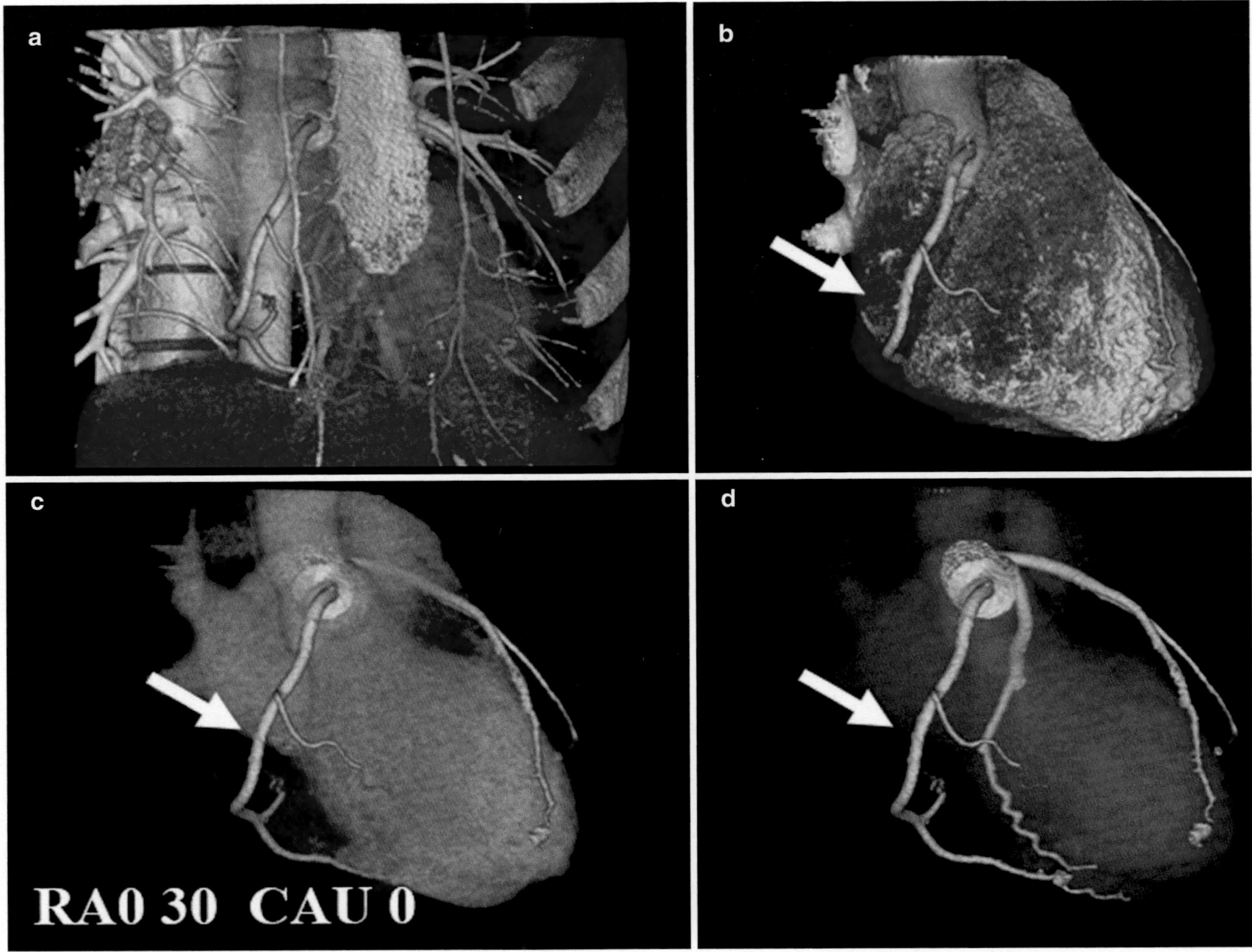

Fig. 4.162 3-D images of the right coronary artery (*arrows*) in the right anterior oblique 30 degree/ caudal 0 degree view. Panel (**a**): Image with skeletal structures. Panel (**b**): Image of heart and coronary arteries. Panels (**c**, **d**): Images of coronary arteries with varying degree of transparency of the heart. As opposed to invasive angiography, the left coronary artery is also visualized. *CAU* caudal, *RAO* right anterior oblique

Artifacts Affecting Assessment of The Coronary Arteries

A spectrum of artifacts may limit interpretation of the coronary arteries. Recognition of artifacts related to acquisition and reconstruction is important in order to avoid misinterpretation of coronary artery findings.

Coronary Artery Artifacts Due to Contrast Dose and Timing Relative to Image Acquisition

In the setting of right heart greater than left heart enhancement, the images may have been acquired too early after contrast administration. This early acquisition of images can also lead to the distal segments of the coronary arteries not being opacified, which can be misinterpreted as significant stenosis or occlusion. Measurement of contrast density and homogeneity at serial levels of the descending aorta can be performed. If the HUs decrease significantly as the aorta descends, the distal coronary arteries may be poorly opacified and more difficult to analyze. Additionally, inadequate flushing of contrast out of the superior vena cava can cause "streak artifact" potentially obscuring the mid right coronary artery.

Artifacts Due to Overlap of HU Attenuation Between Coronary Artery Lumen and Other Structures

Blooming artifacts can occur due to coronary artery or cardiac calcification, stents, clips, wires, pacemakers, implantable cardiac defibrillators and other radiopaque implanted materials. The non- contrast coronary artery calcium images can be used to assess for coronary artery segments which may be problematic prior to analysis of the CCTA images. Changing contrast level can diminish

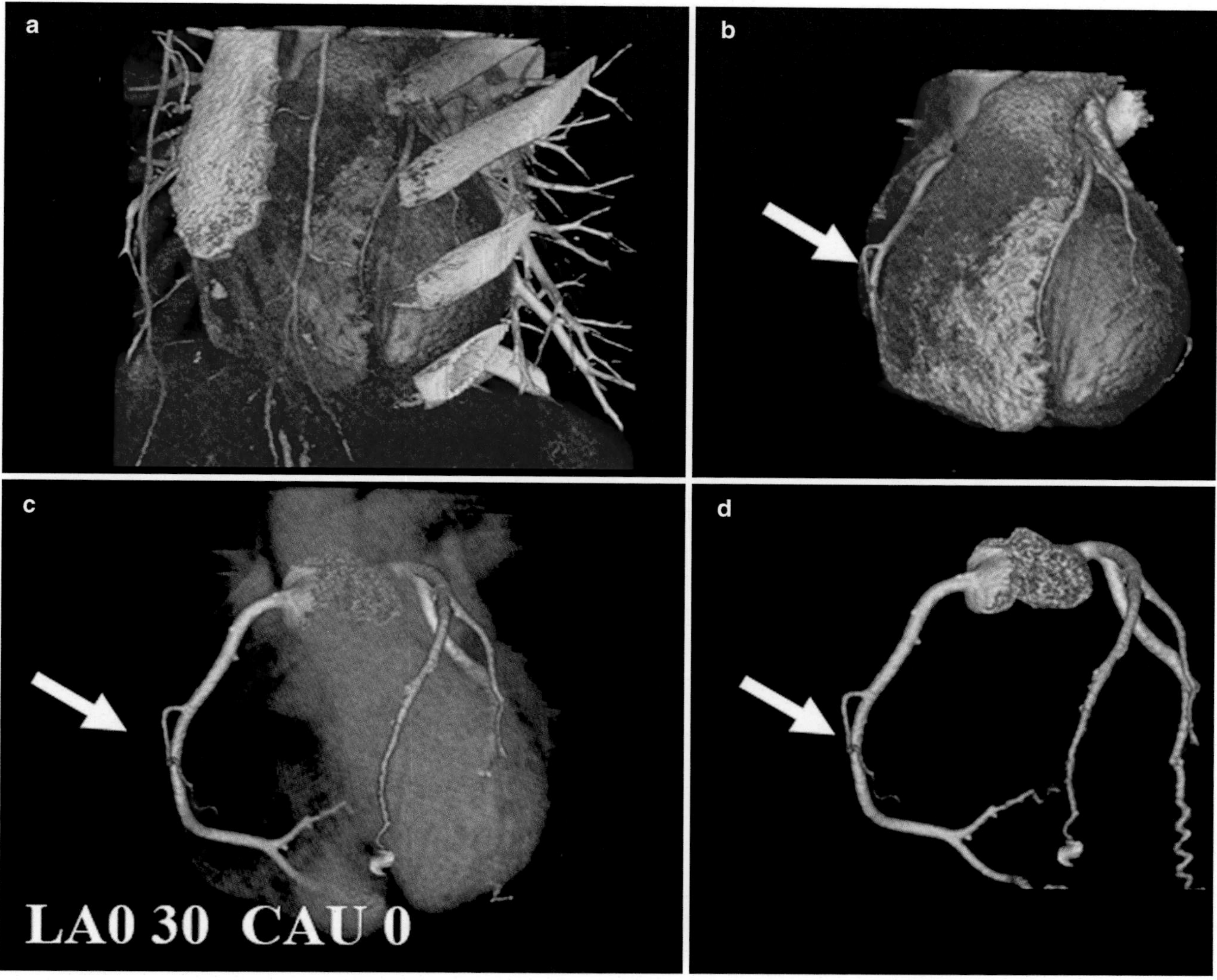

Fig. 4.163 3-D images of the right coronary artery (*arrows*) in the left anterior oblique 30°/ caudal 0° view. Panel (**a**): Image with skeletal structures. Panel (**b**): Image of heart and coronary arteries. Panels (**c**, **d**): Images of coronary arteries with varying degree of transparency of the heart. As opposed to invasive angiography, the left coronary artery is also visualized. *CAU* caudal, *LAO* left anterior oblique

these artifacts, and viewing of thin slices can decrease volume averaging artifact, but some arterial segment evaluation may be non-diagnostic.

Coronary Artery Artifacts Due to Motion

Artifacts can occur due to patient motion, respiratory motion, motion due to ectopic atrial and ventricular beats and other arrhythmias, and cardiac/coronary artery motion (Fig. 4.164). Respiratory and patient motion artifacts are well seen on sagittal views by viewing the sternum and other skeletal structures. In coronal images and sagittal reconstructions, multiple stacks of images are viewed simultaneously, and therefore thin collimation lines can be seen. If the data sets are not aligned properly due to motion, step artifact can occur.

Cardiac motion is complex, with contraction from apex to base as well as rotational movement of the heart during contraction. The motion of the right coronary artery is particularly complex and therefore images may appear blurred, appear as a "cashew nut" like shape or appear as a complete double image, depending on the phase of the R-R interval chosen to view. All available phases of the R-R interval should be assessed for each coronary artery segment with motion artifact in order to choose the most optimal images for analysis.

Coronary Artery Artifacts Due to 3-D Reconstruction

Although the 3-D images are intuitive regarding the gross location, orientation and relationships of the coronary arteries to cardiovascular structures, reconstruction can lead to the artifactual appearance of coronary artery stenosis or obstruction. The automated editing

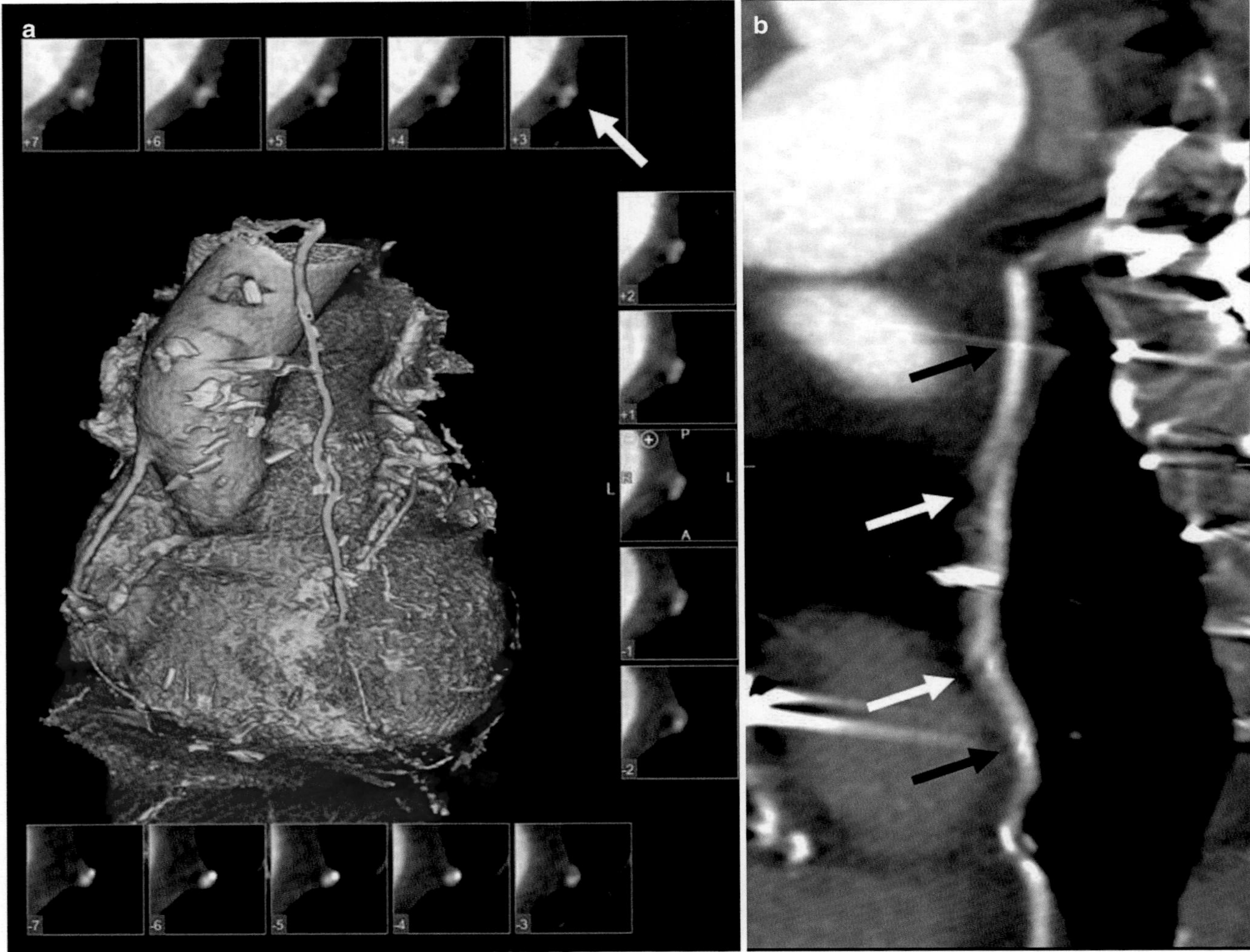

Fig. 4.164 Coronary artery artifacts due to curved multiplanar reformats of a left anterior mammary artery graft to the left anterior descending coronary artery. Panel (**a**): Double image of the LIMA graft due to motion (*arrow*). Panel (**b**): Areas of coronary artery discontinuity due to motion (*white arrows*). Additional blooming artifacts due to surgical clips are present (*black arrow*)

software may have edited out too much of the artery or left in overlying tissue obstructing view of the coronary artery (Fig. 4.165). The variety of motion artifacts mentioned above can lead to the discontinuous appearance of the artery. Intra-myocardial bridging can also appear as coronary artery occlusion as the artery courses internal to the epicardium. Due to these issues related to 3-D reconstruction, the volume rendered images are not used as the primary modality to document the presence of coronary artery stenoses.

Non-cardiovascular Structure

Additional assessment of appropriately windowed full field of view images need to be performed to assess: visceral situs, skeletal structure, lung parenchyma, presence of thoracic masses, and assessment of abdominal structures which may be in the field of view. Assessment of the non-cardiovascular structures in the field of view should be performed by physicians with expertise in analysis of these structures.

Conclusion

CCTA workstations and software provide multiple modalities to assess cardiovascular structure and function. Although axial images are most commonly relied on for final interpretation, other planes and reconstruction modalities, if used with a thorough knowledge of their strengths and limitations, are important to analysis. The employment of these modalities in an organized approach coupled with an understanding of the spatial relationships between cardiovascular structures allow for comprehensive diagnosis of cardiovascular pathology.

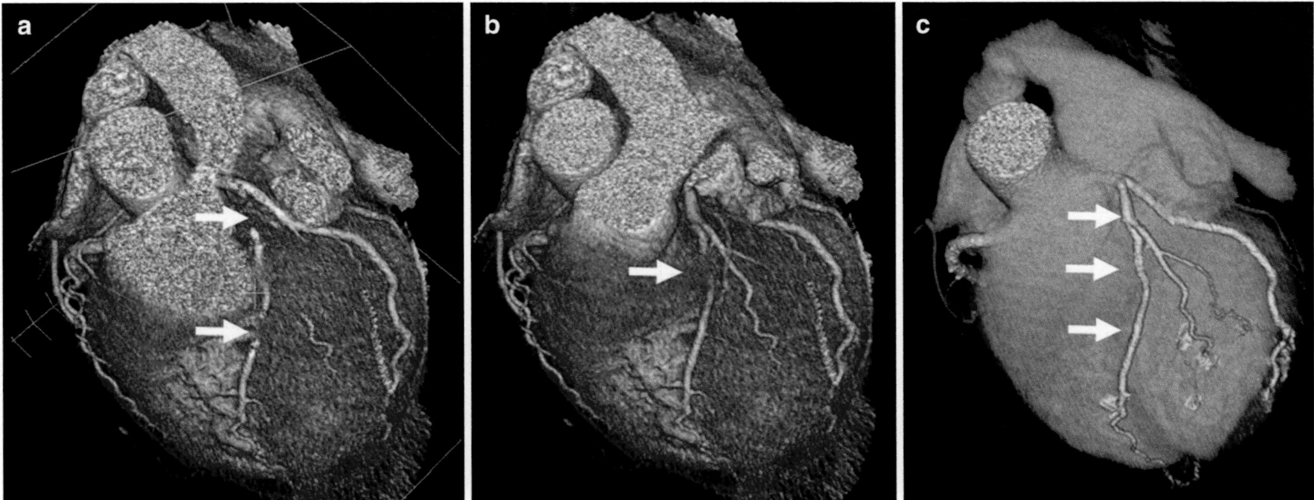

Fig. 4.165 Coronary artery artifacts due to 3-D reconstruction. Panel (**a**): Over editing of a portion of the left anterior descending coronary artery (*arrows*). Panel (**b**): Under editing with overlying tissue obstructing view of the coronary artery (*arrow*). Panel (**c**): 3-D view of the left anterior descending coronary artery without overlying tissue demonstrating a patent left anterior descending coronary artery (*arrows*)

Orientation to Axial Images

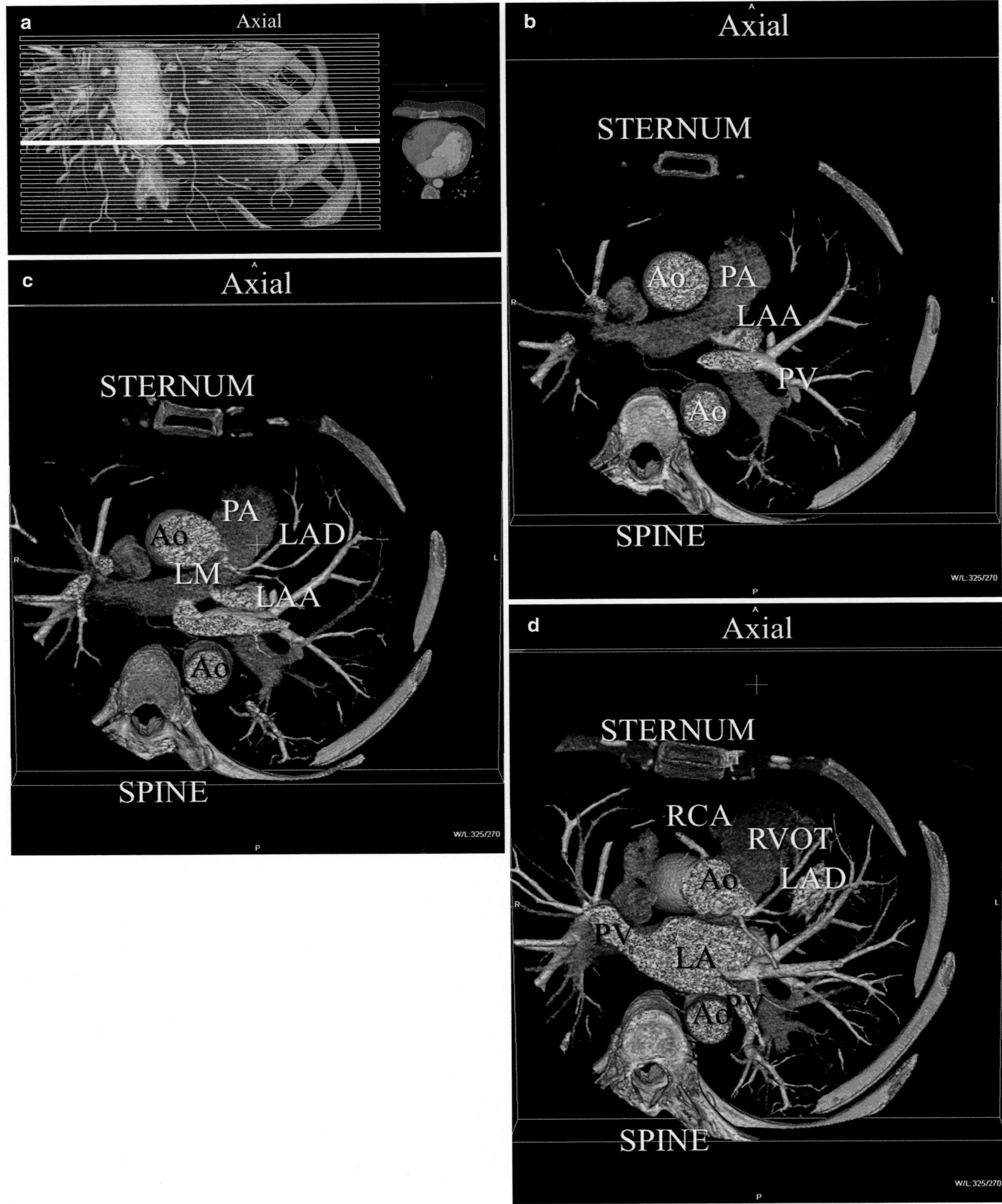

Fig. 4.1 (**a–m**) Serial axial 3-D CCTA images beginning at the level of the pulmonary artery with slices proceeding in a cranial to caudal direction

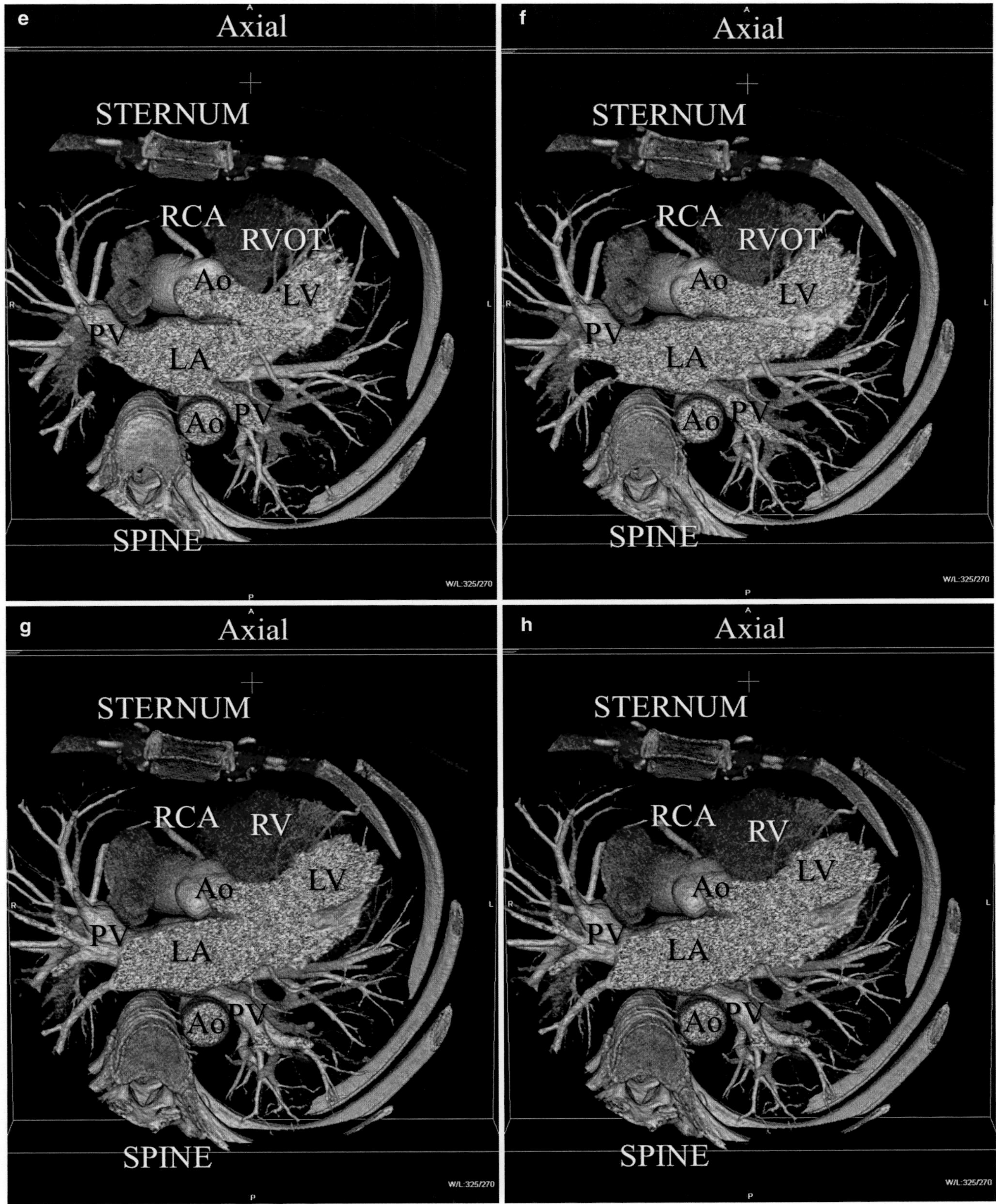

Fig. 4.1 (continued)

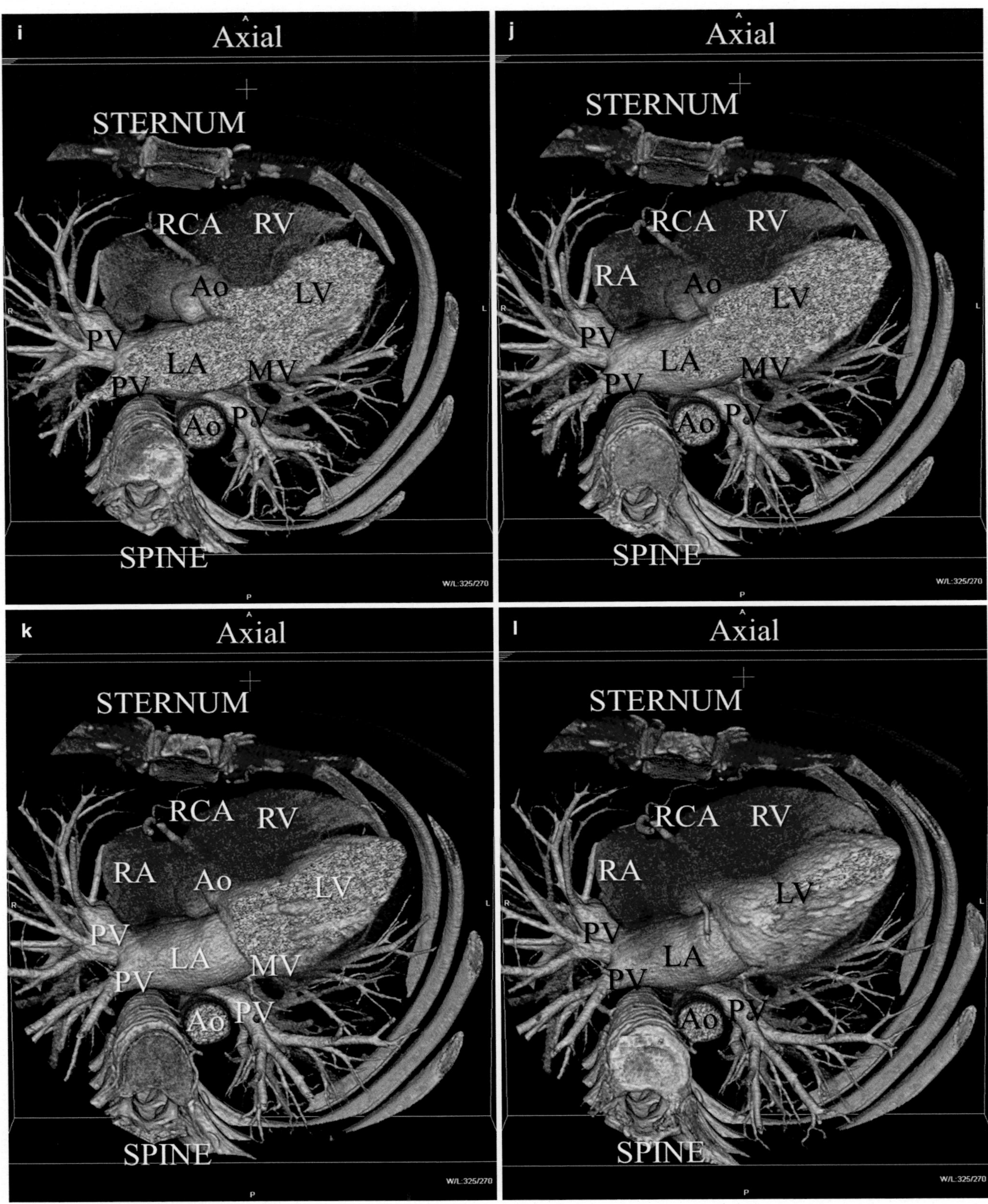

Fig. 4.1 (continued)

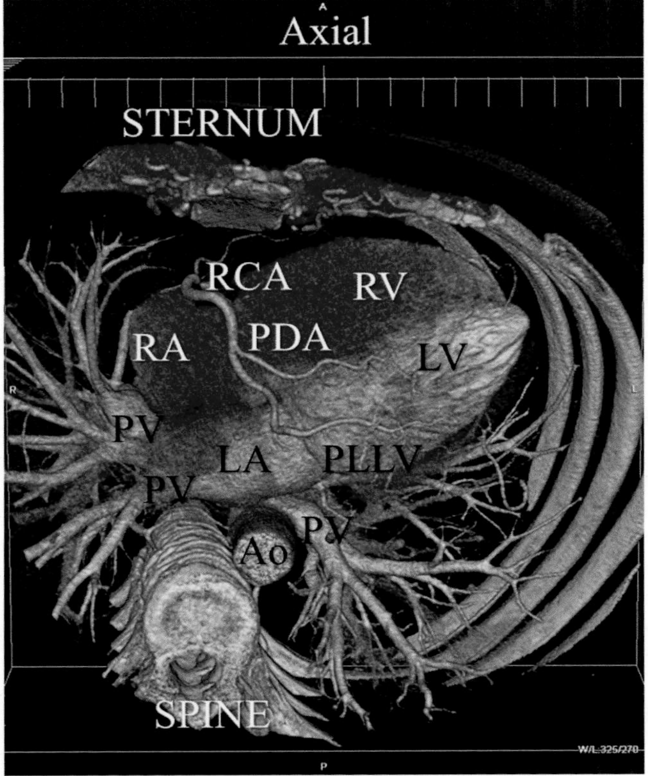

Fig. 4.1 (continued)

Orientation to Sagittal Images

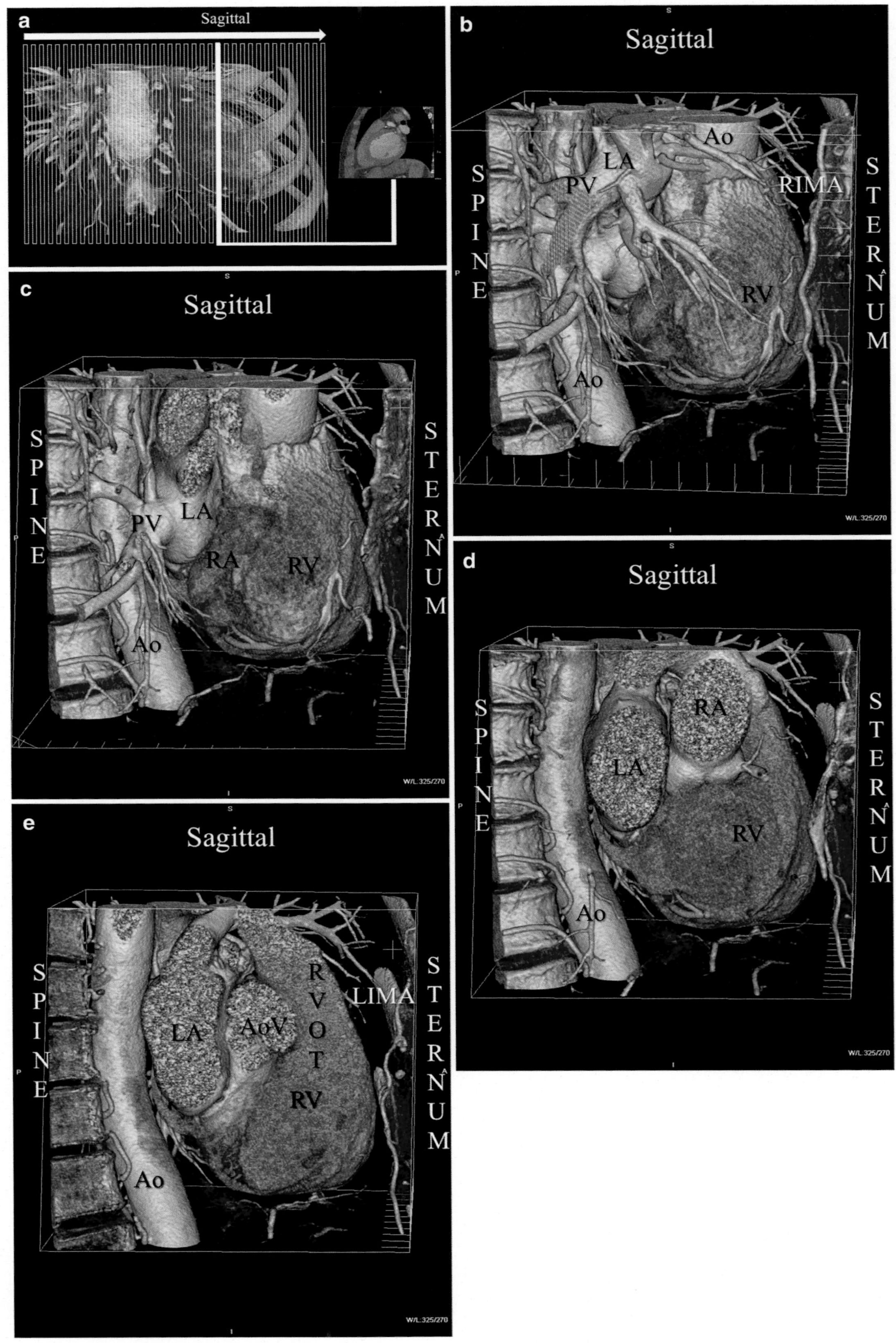

Fig. 4.2 (a–j) Serial sagittal 3-D CCTA images beginning Serial sagittal CT angiography images beginning at the sternum and proceeding leftward

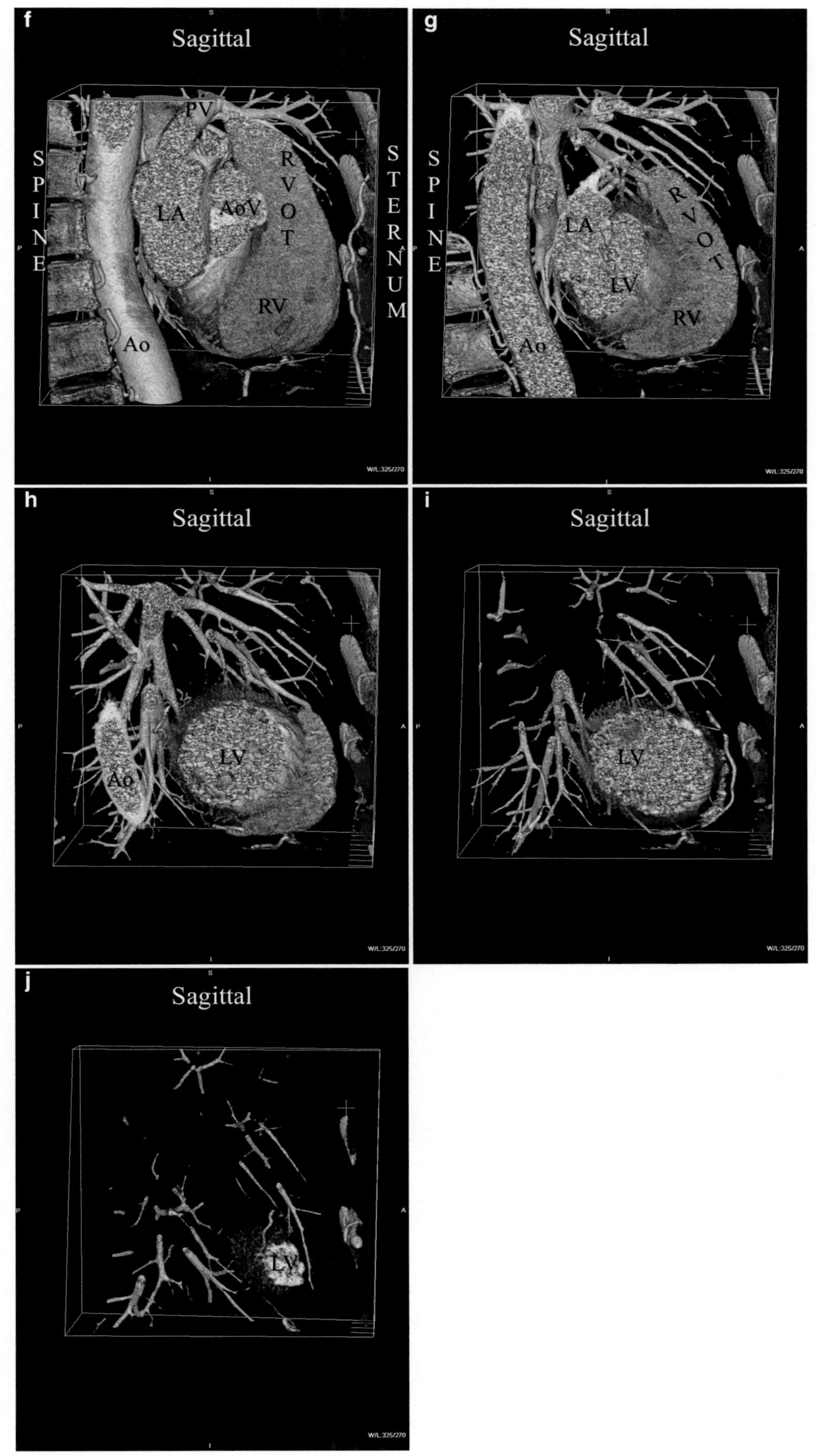

Fig. 4.2 (continued)

Orientation to Coronal Images

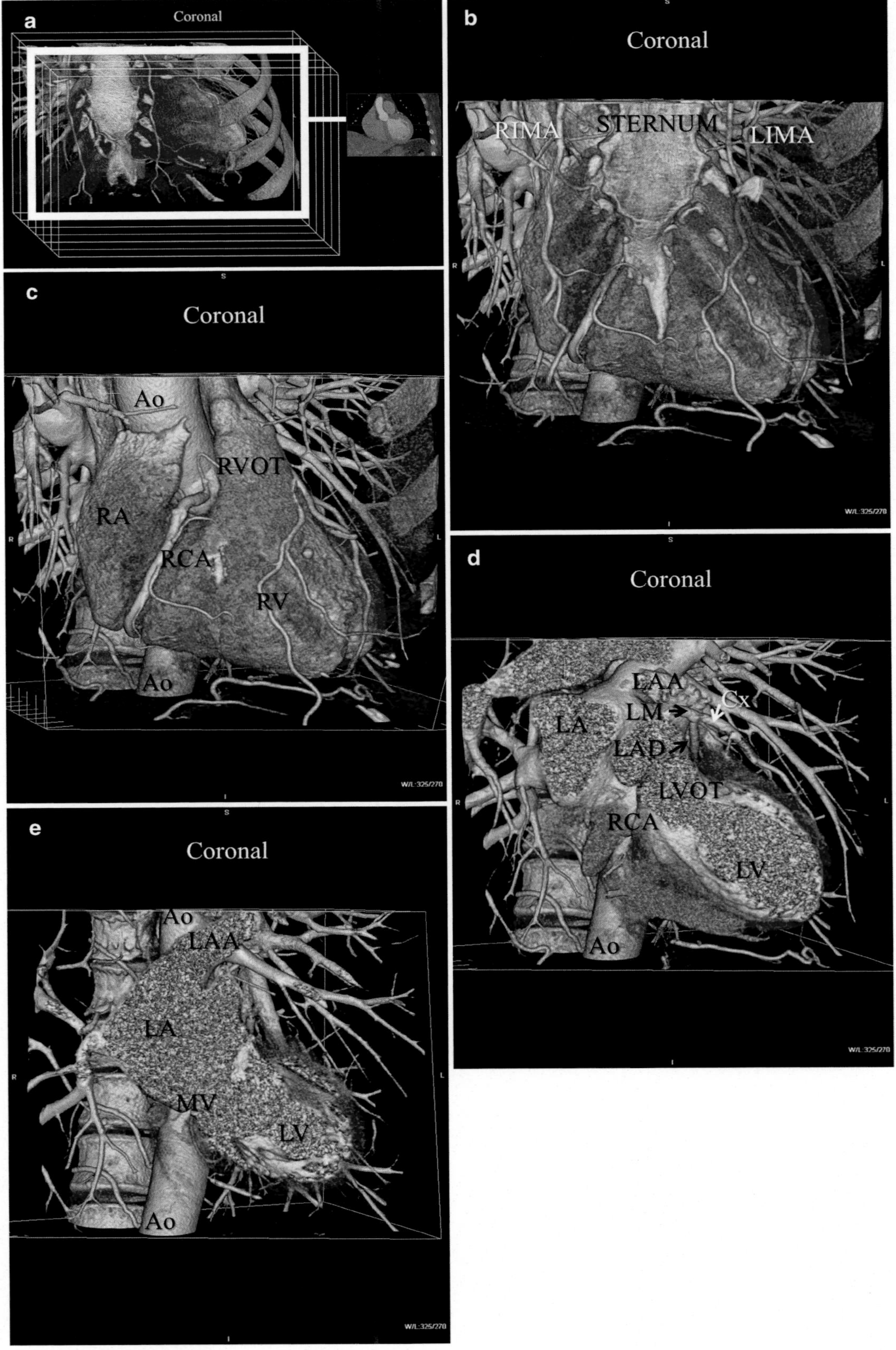

Fig. 4.3 (**a–g**) Serial coronal CCTA angiography images beginning at the sternum and proceeding posteriorly

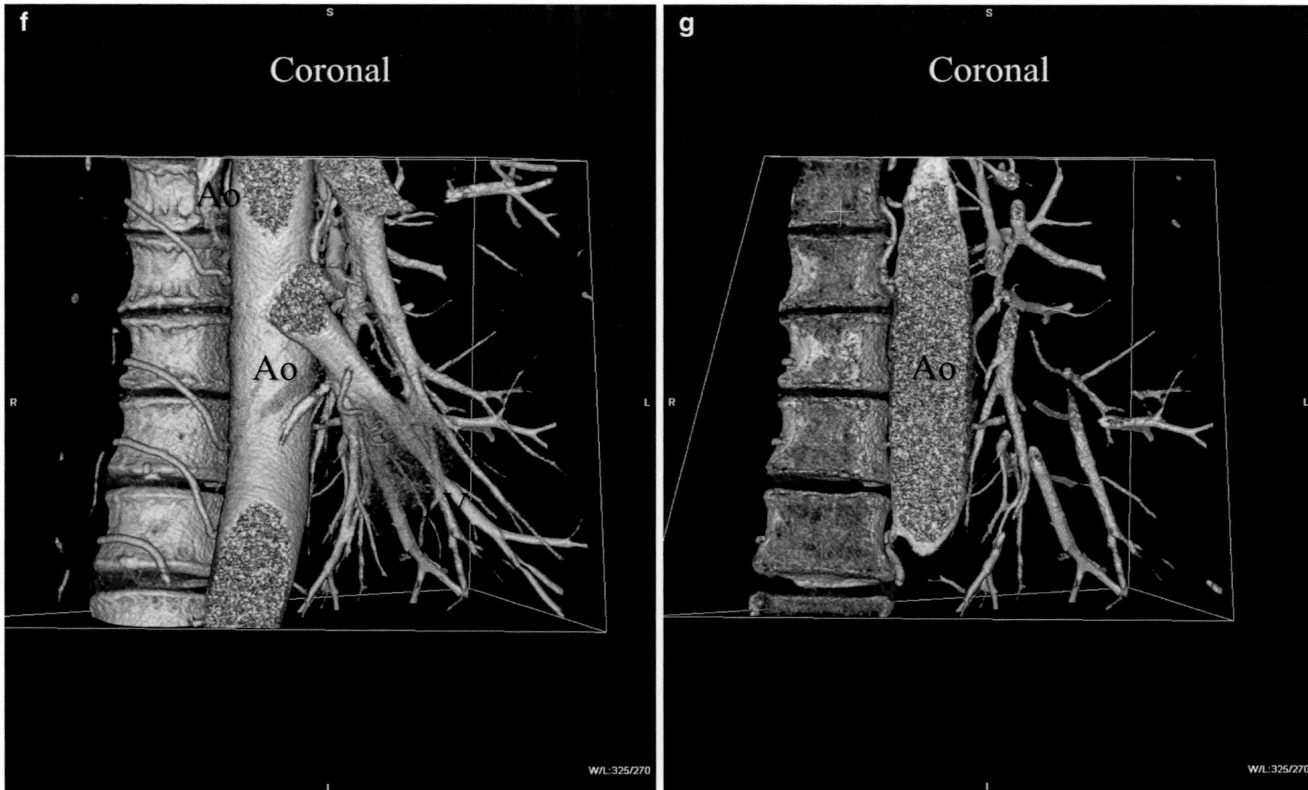

Fig. 4.3 (continued)

Serial 2-D Axial, Coronal, and Sagittal Images

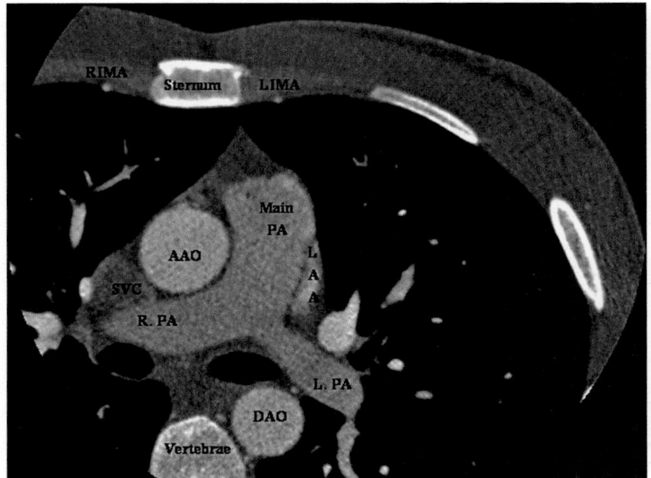

Fig. 4.4

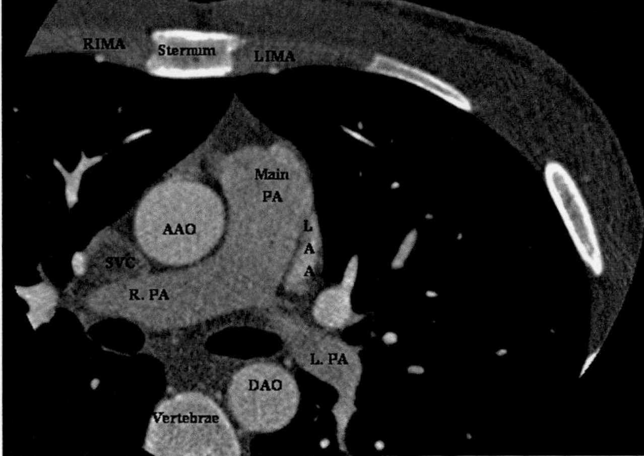

Fig. 4.5

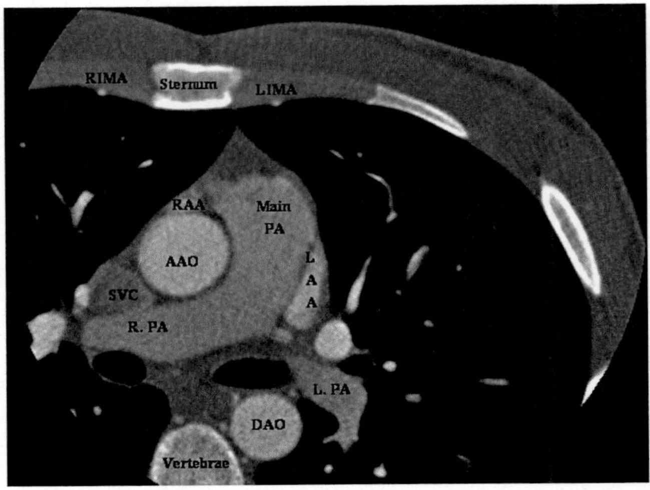

Fig. 4.6

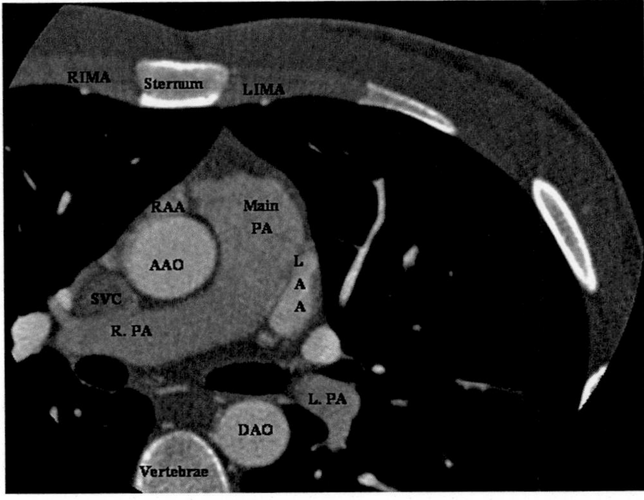

Fig. 4.7

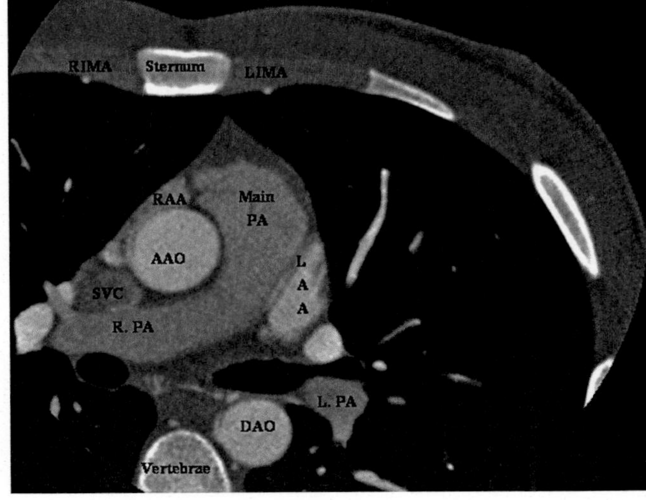

Fig. 4.8

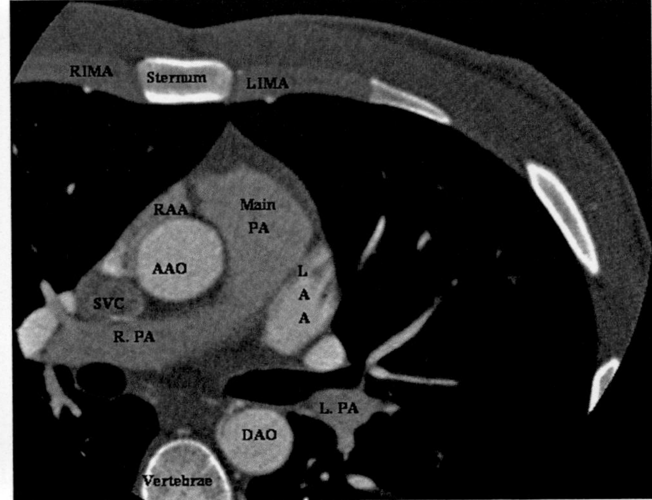

Fig. 4.9

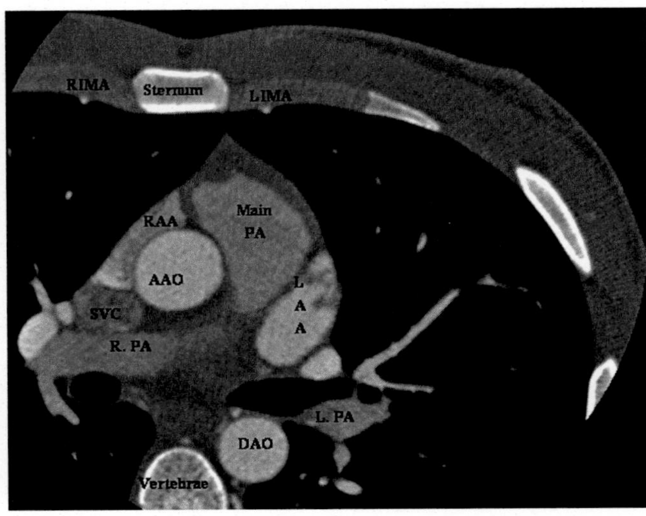

Fig. 4.10

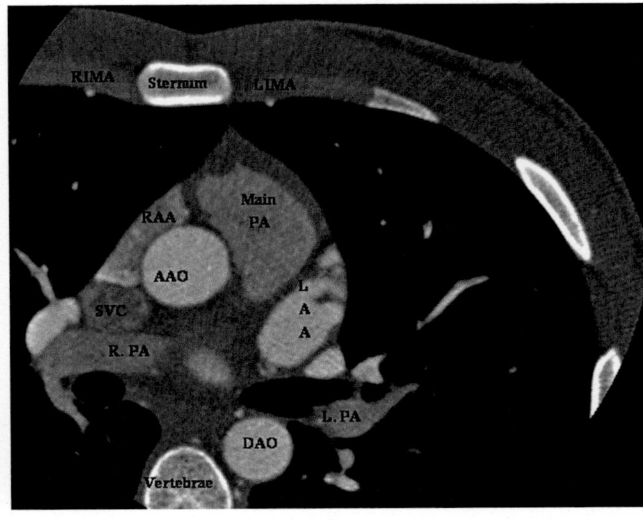

Fig. 4.11

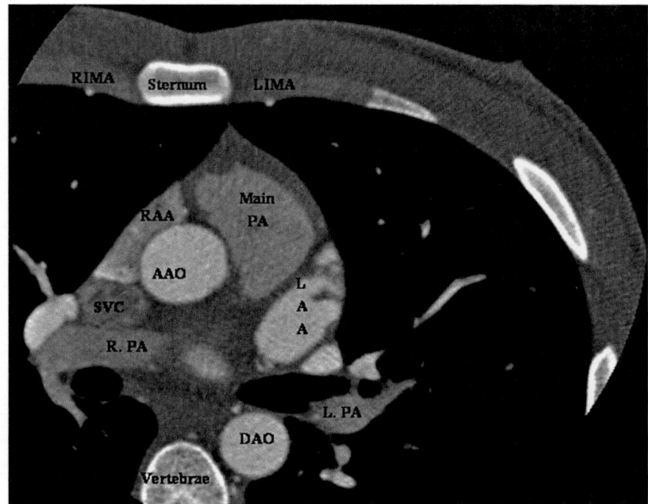

Fig. 4.12

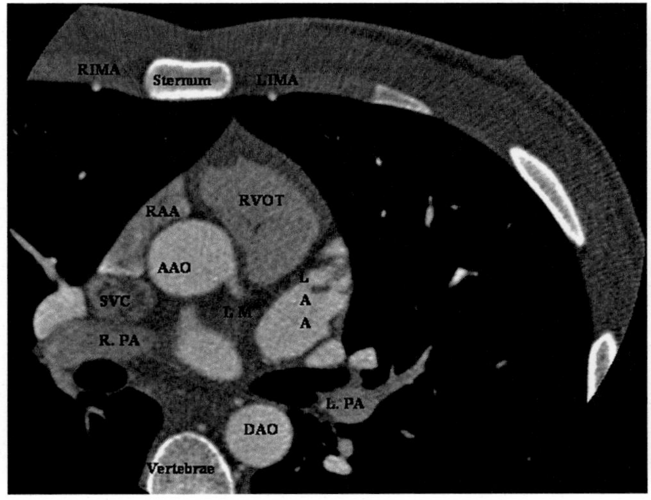

Fig. 4.13

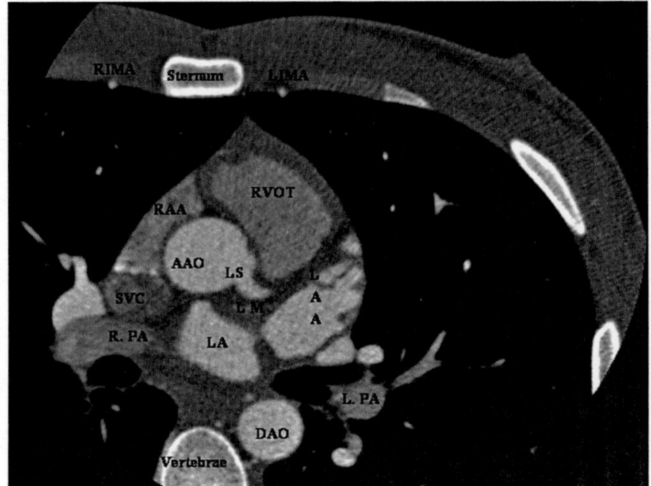

Fig. 4.14

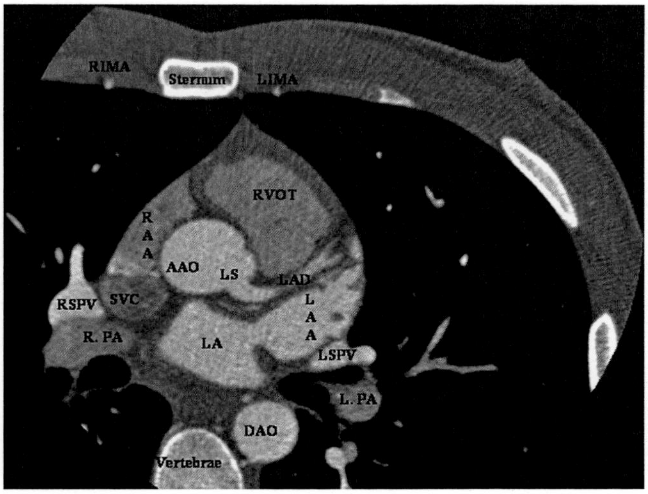

Fig. 4.15

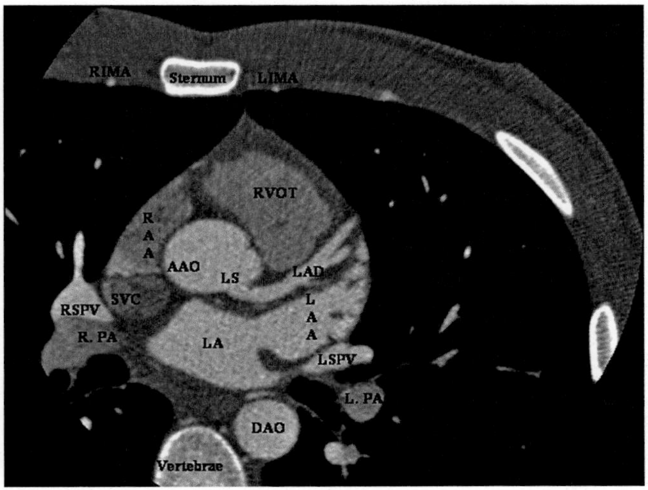

Fig. 4.16

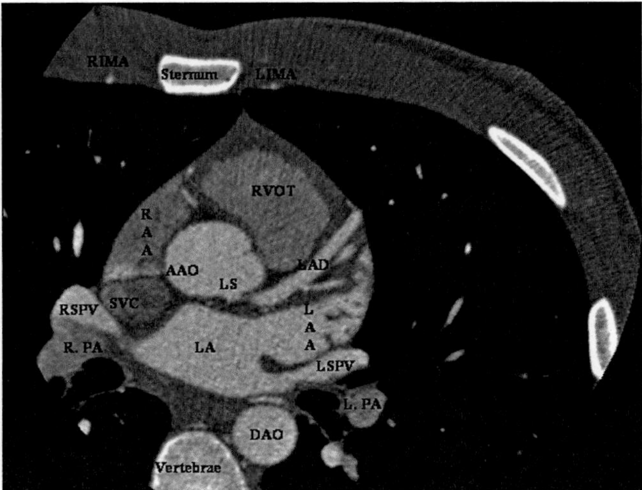

Fig. 4.17

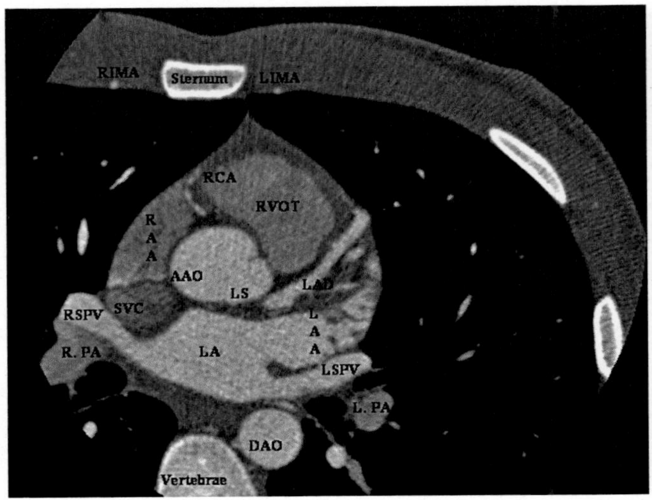

Fig. 4.18

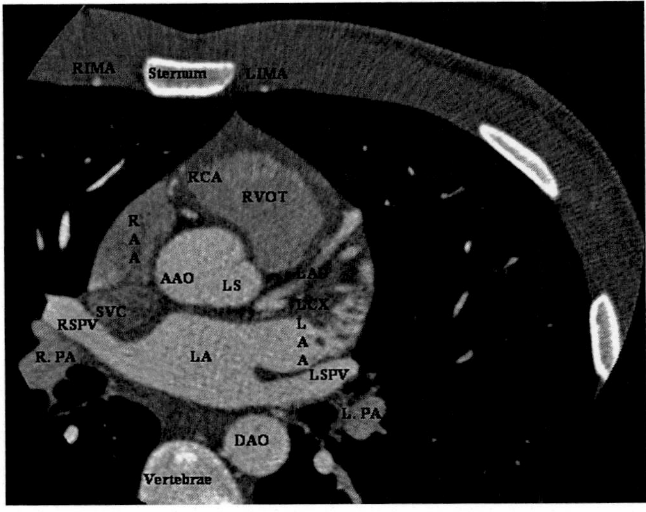

Fig. 4.19

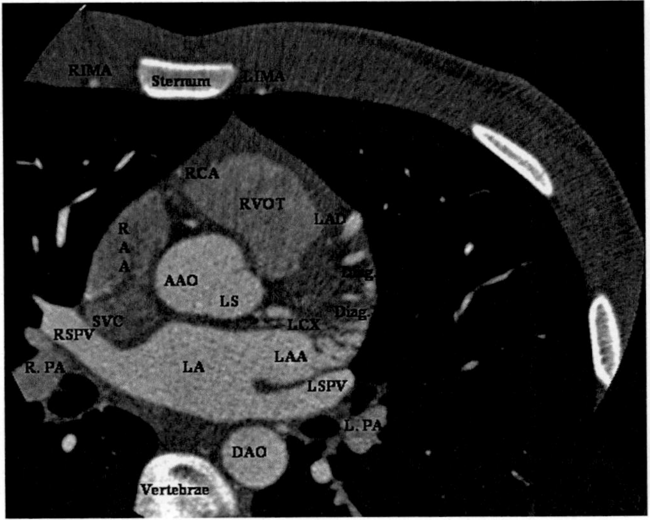

Fig. 4.20

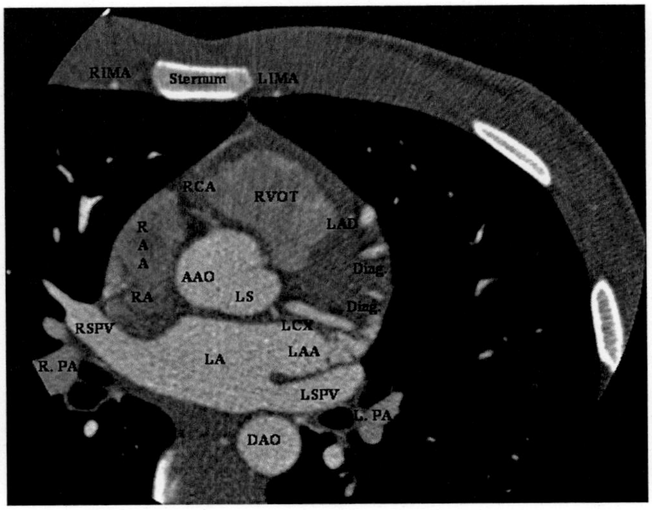

Fig. 4.21

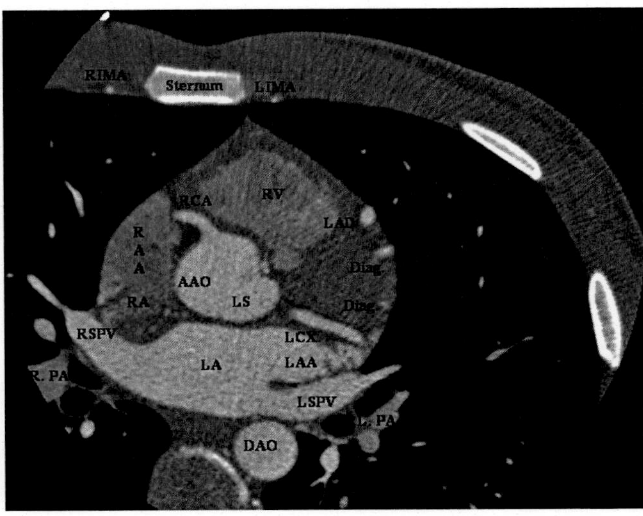

Fig. 4.22

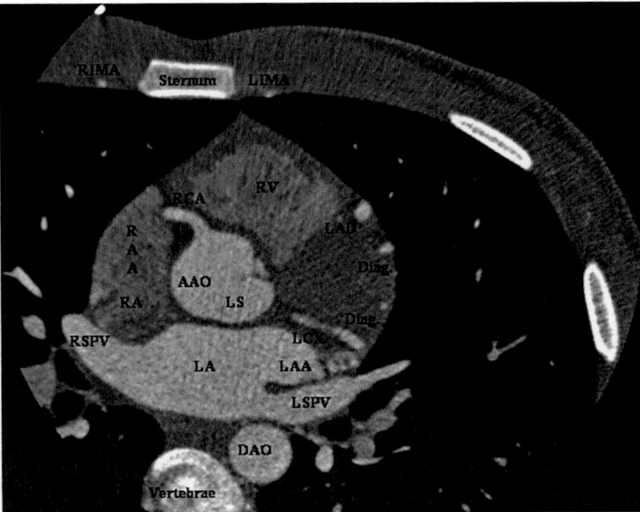

Fig. 4.23

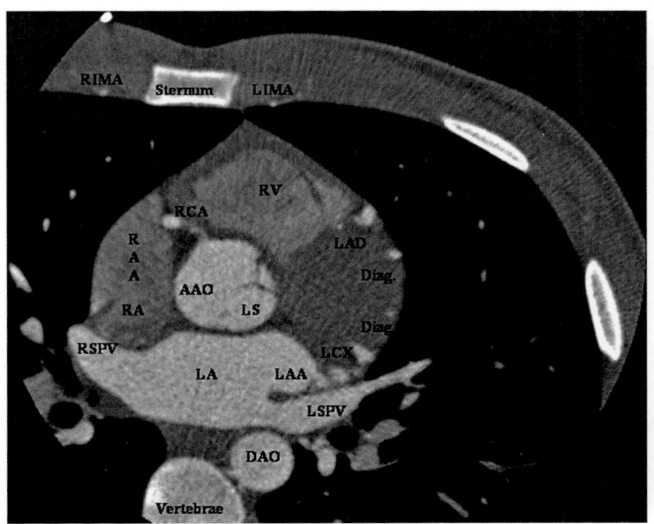

Fig. 4.24

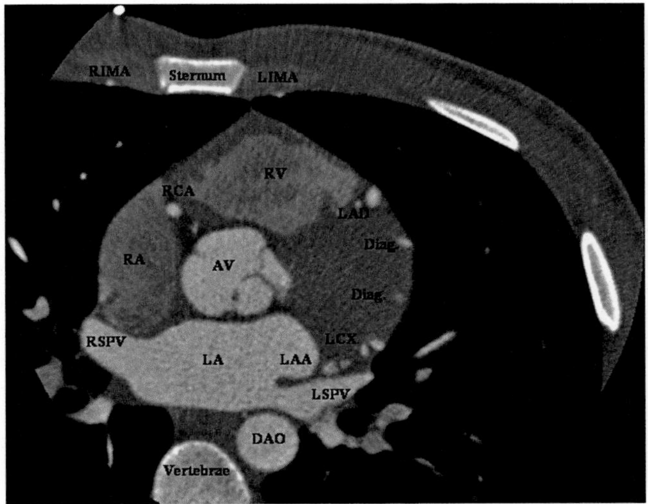

Fig. 4.25

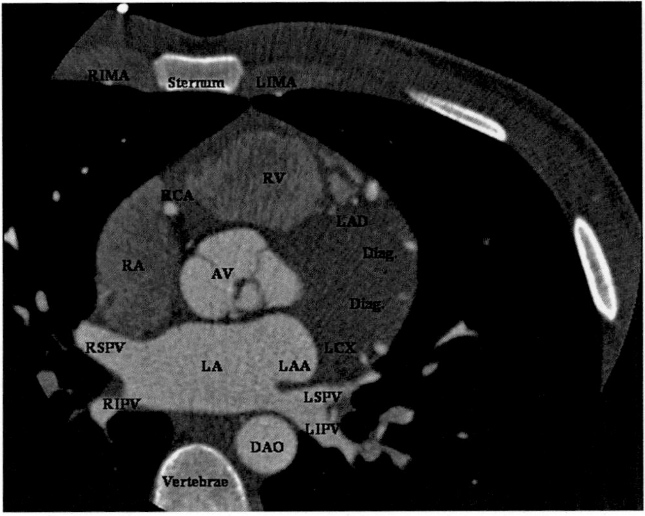

Fig. 4.26

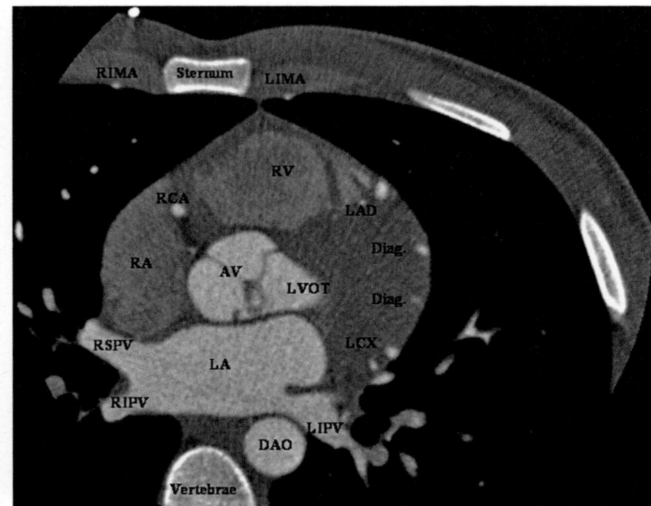

Fig. 4.27

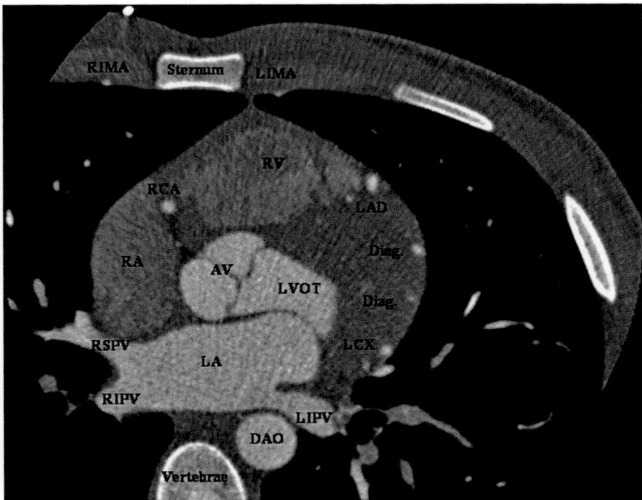

Fig. 4.28

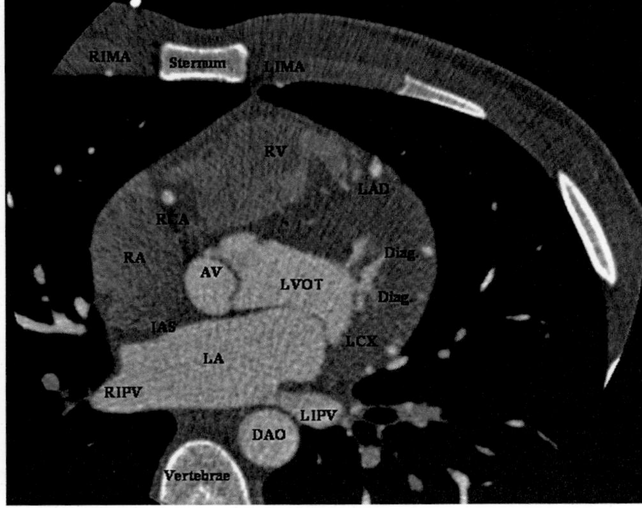

Fig. 4.29

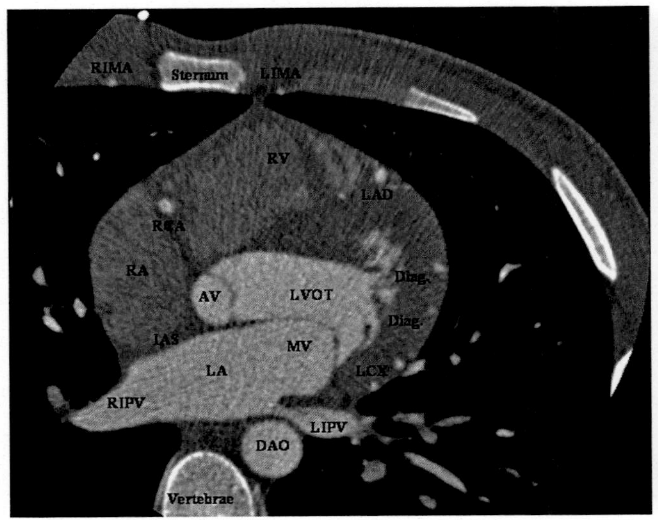

Fig. 4.30

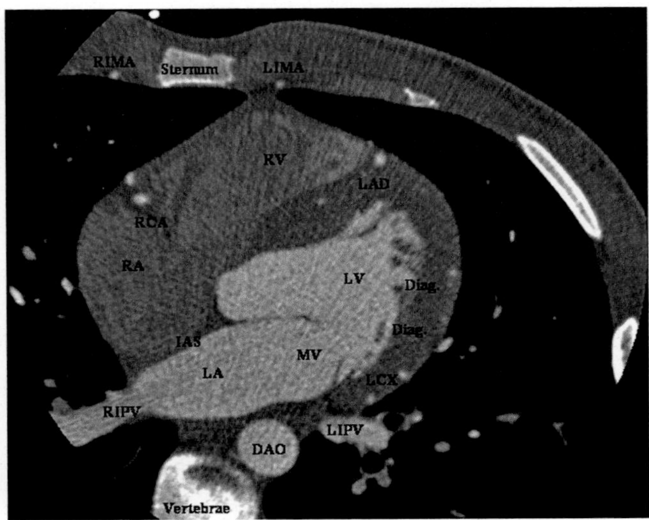

Fig. 4.33

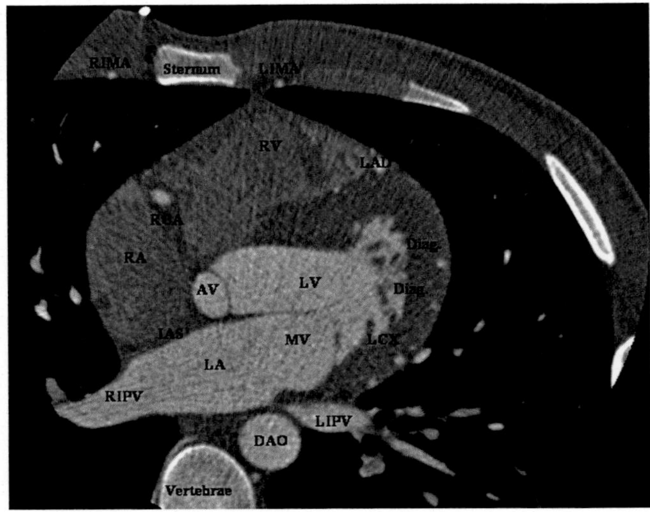

Fig. 4.31

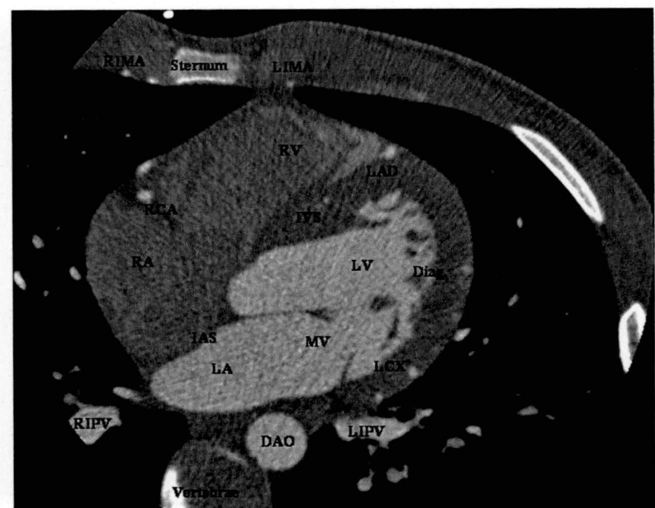

Fig. 4.34

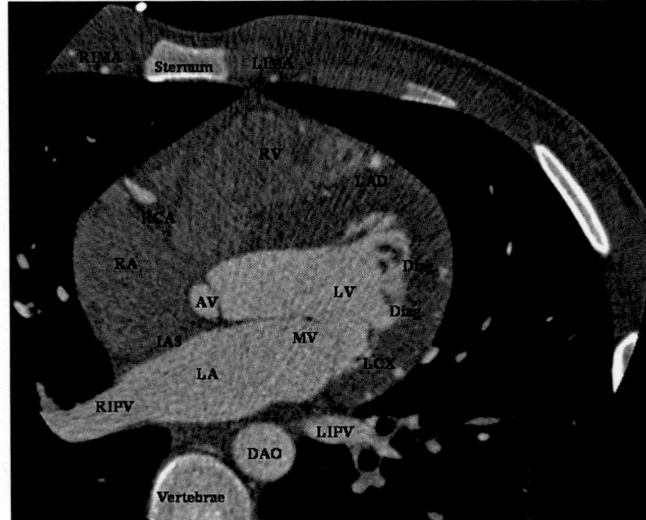

Fig. 4.32

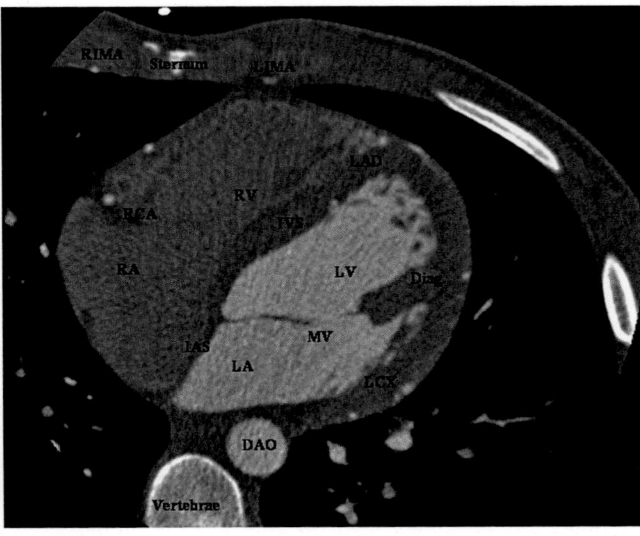

Fig. 4.35

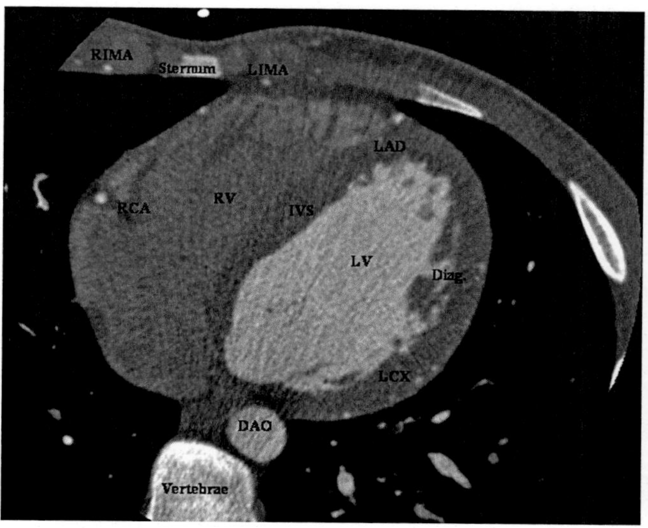

Fig. 4.36

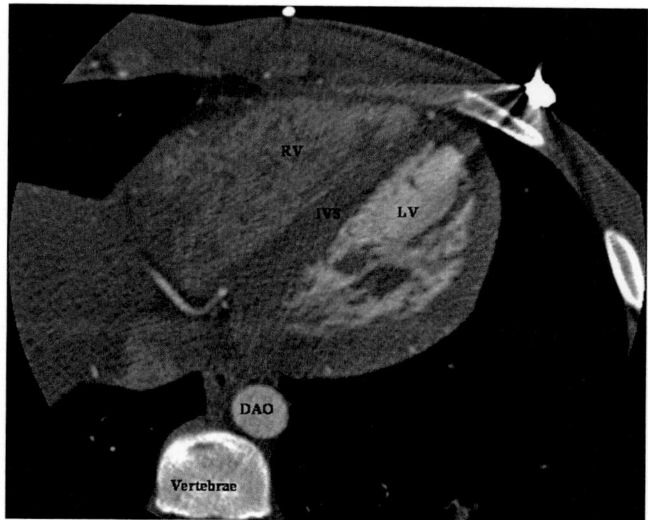

Fig. 4.37

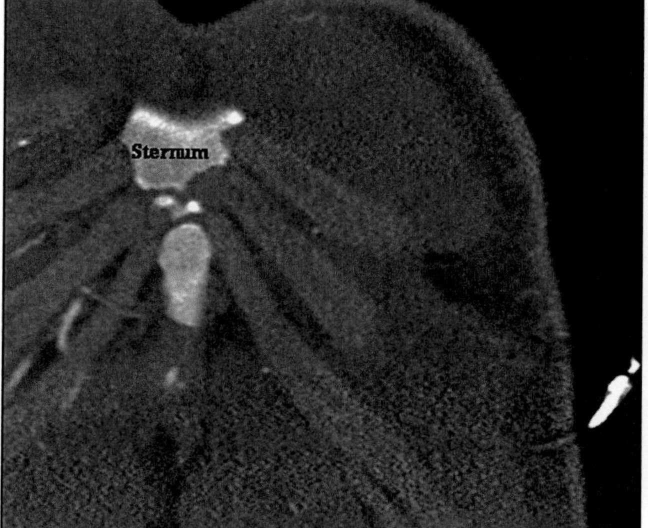

Fig. 4.38

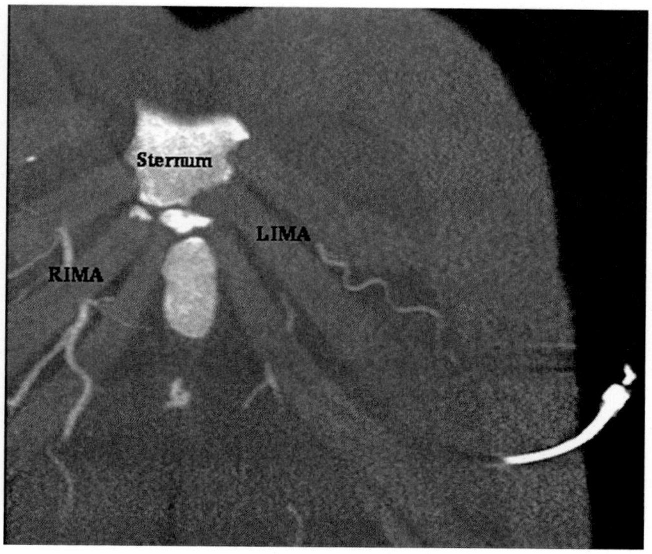

Fig. 4.39

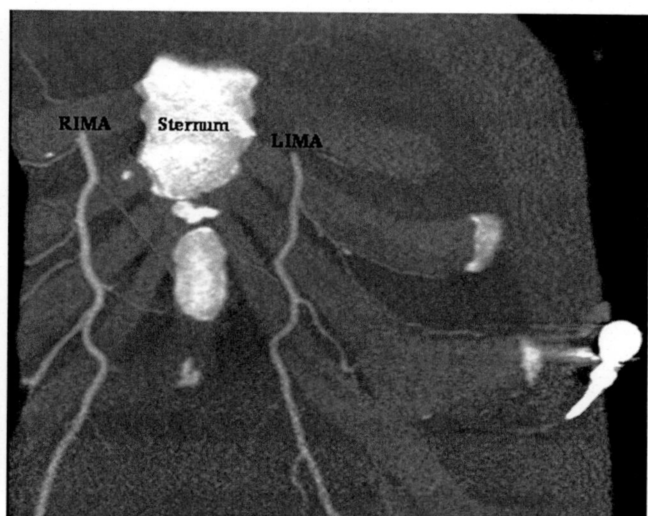

Fig. 4.40

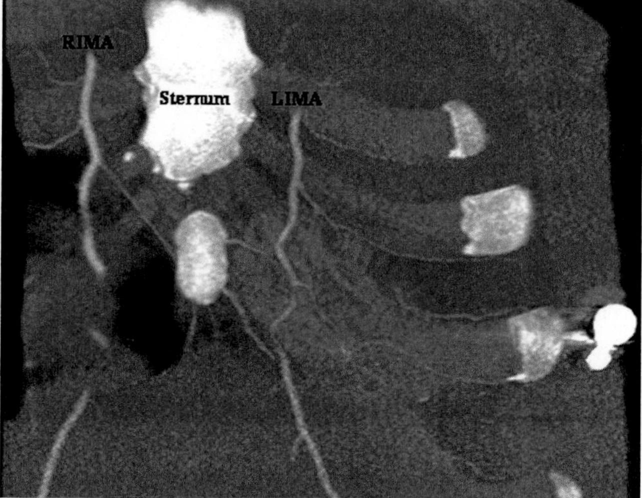

Fig. 4.41

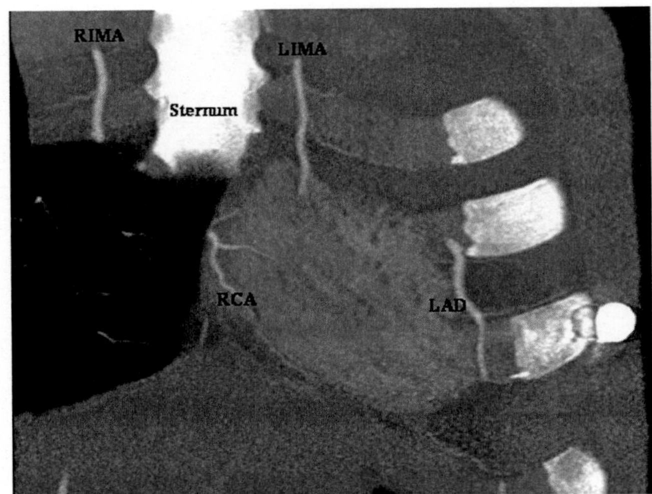

Fig. 4.42

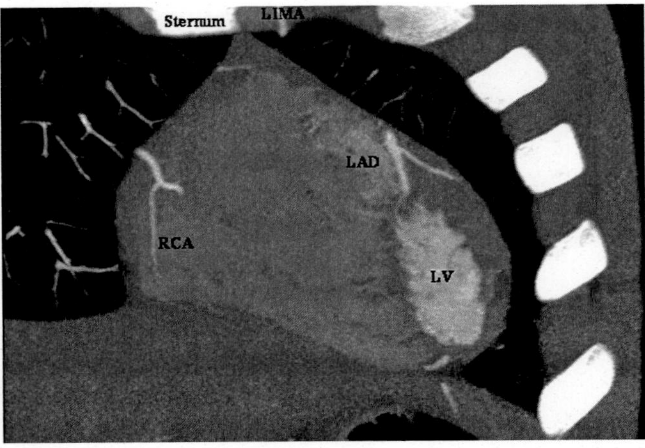

Fig. 4.45

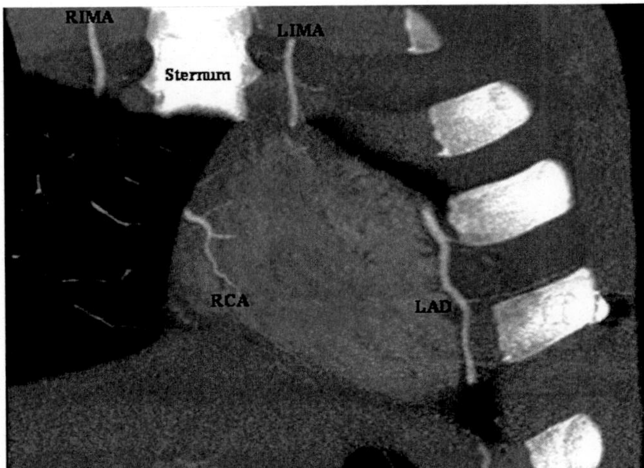

Fig. 4.43

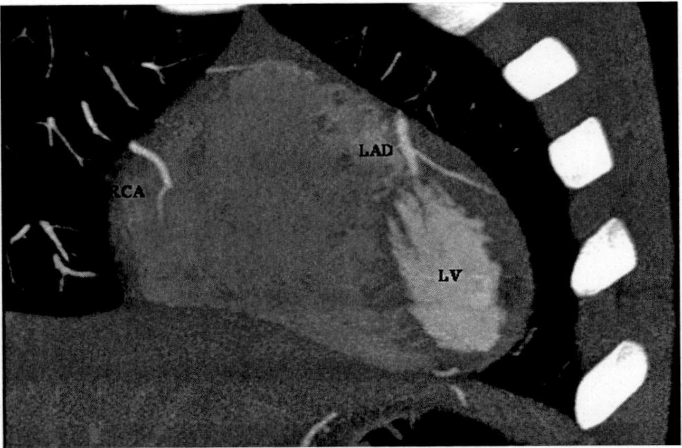

Fig. 4.46

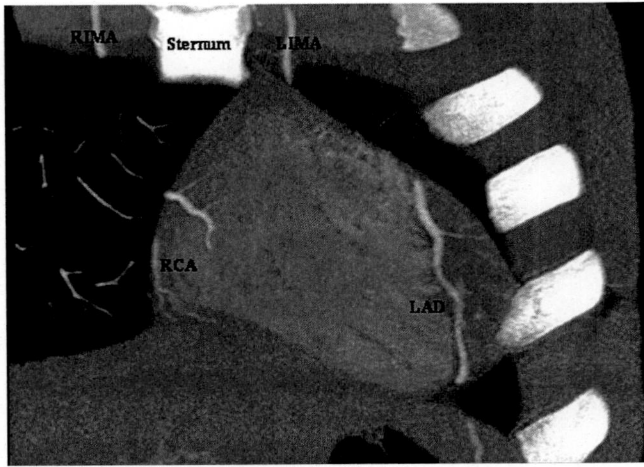

Fig. 4.44

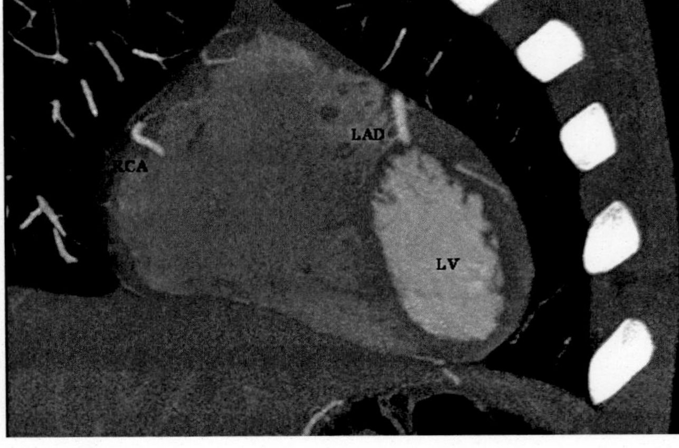

Fig. 4.47

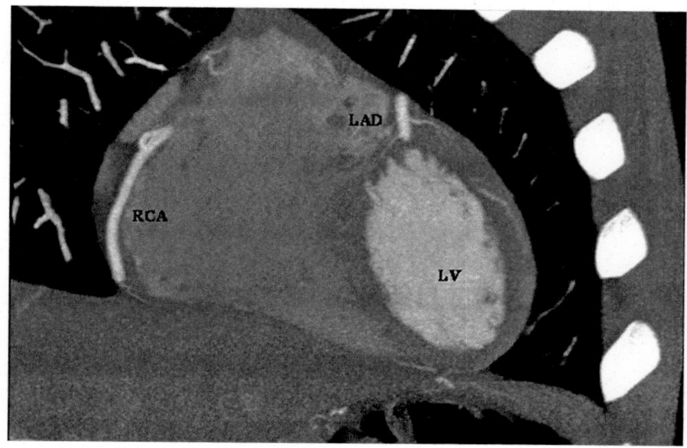

Fig. 4.48

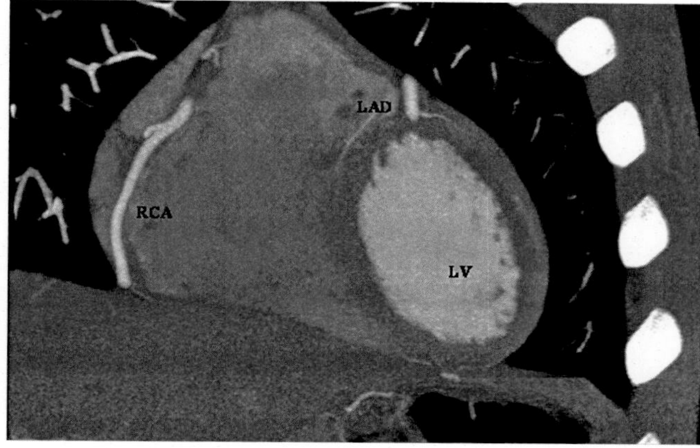

Fig. 4.49

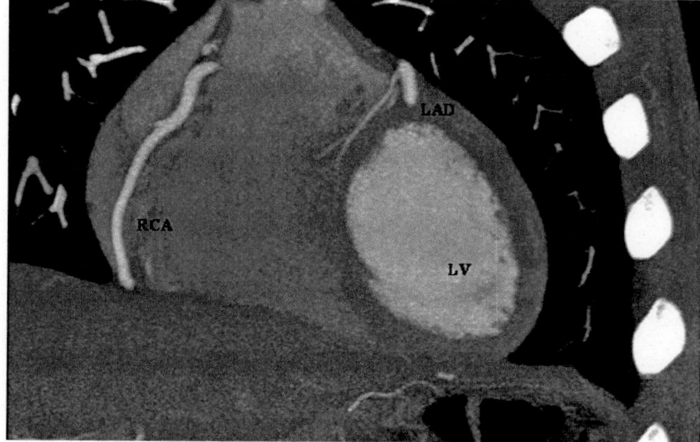

Fig. 4.50

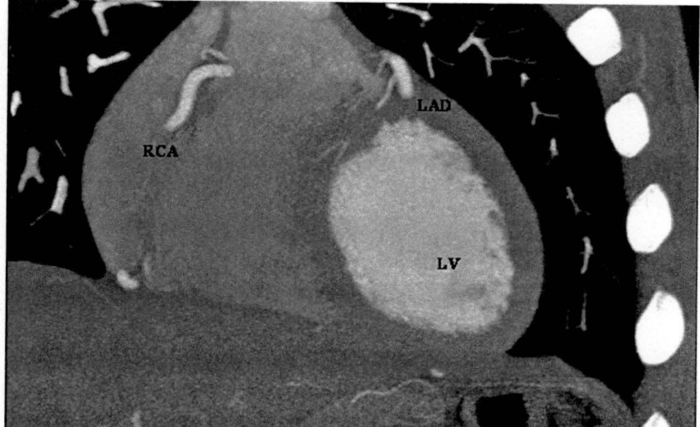

Fig. 4.51

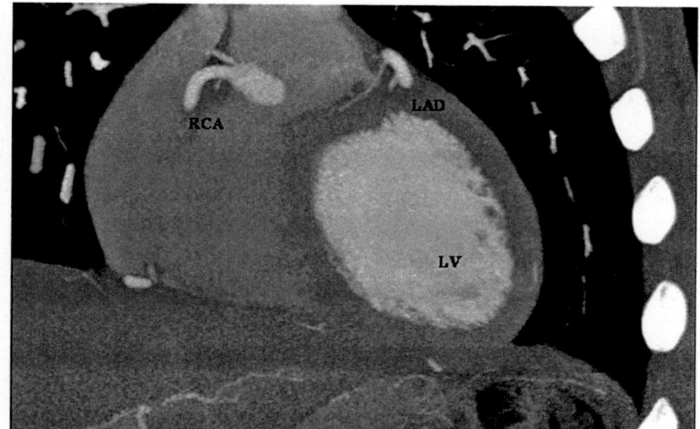

Fig. 4.52

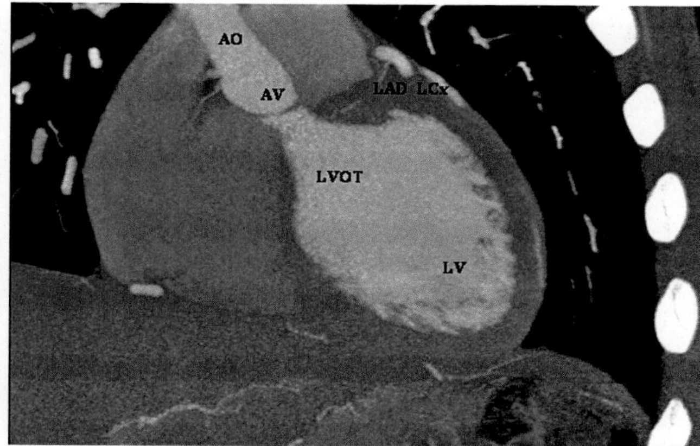

Fig. 4.53

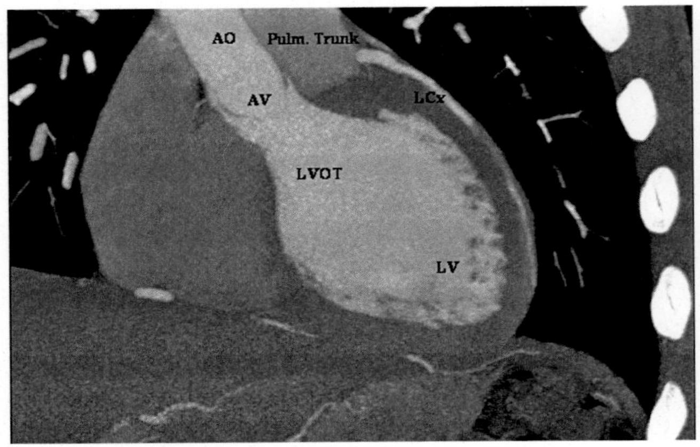

Fig. 4.54

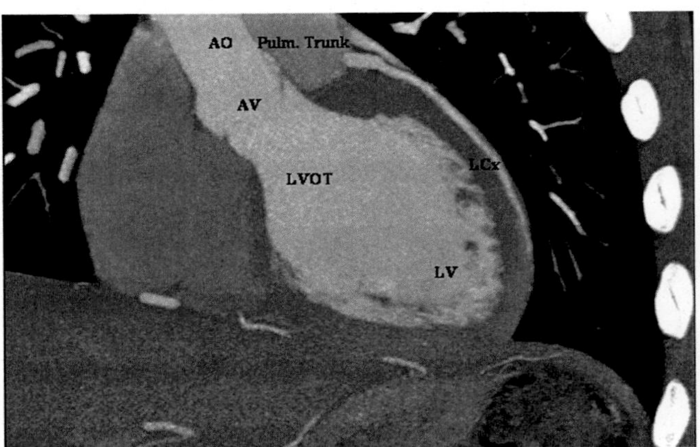

Fig. 4.55

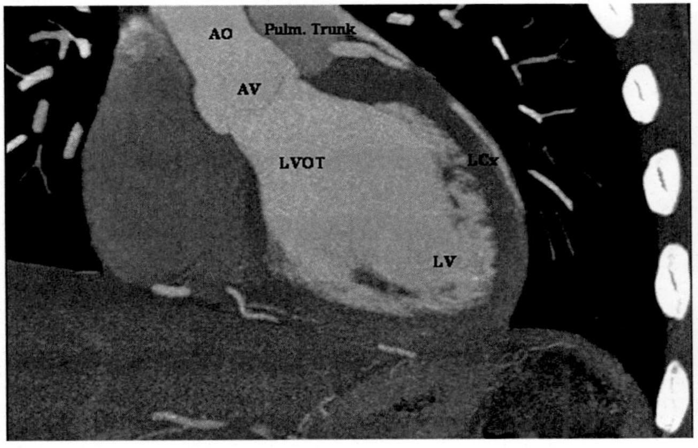

Fig. 4.56

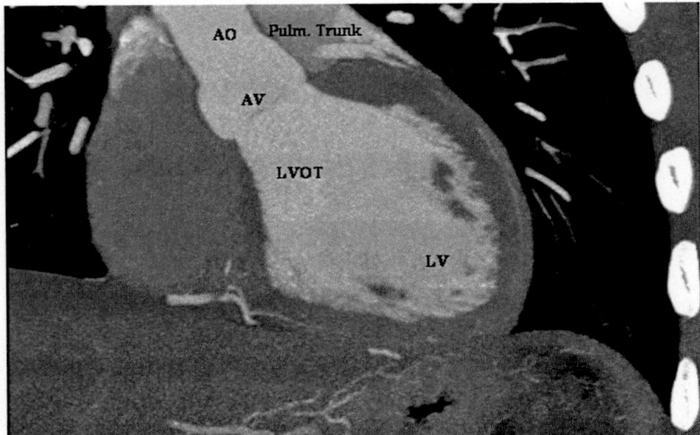

Fig. 4.57

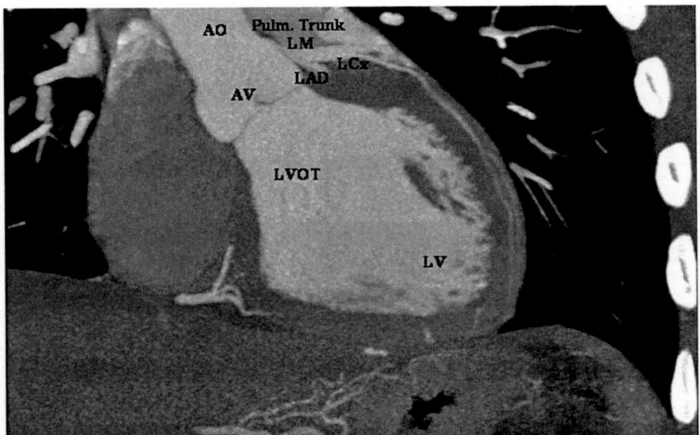

Fig. 4.58

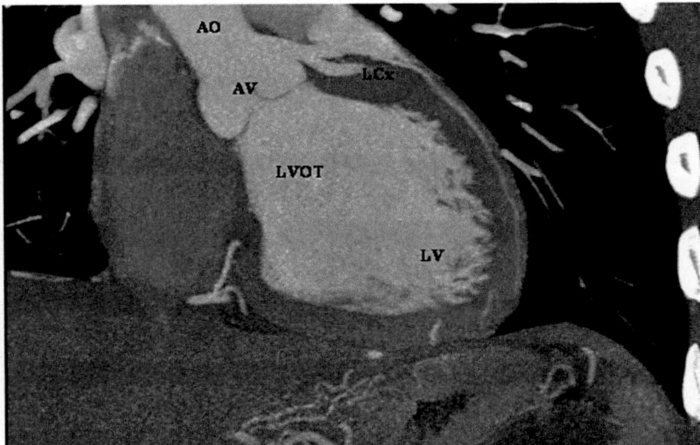

Fig. 4.59

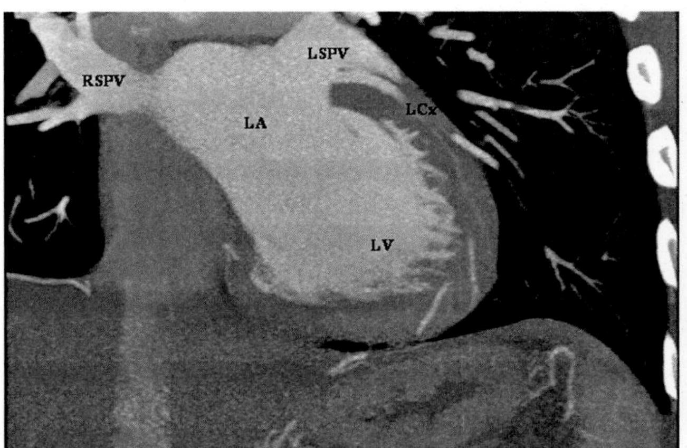

Fig. 4.60

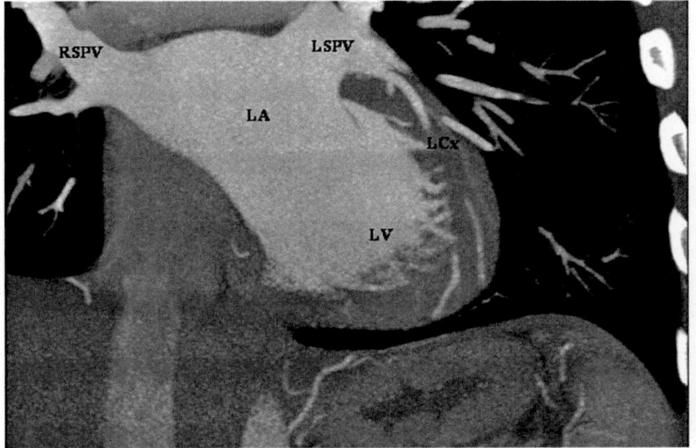

Fig. 4.61

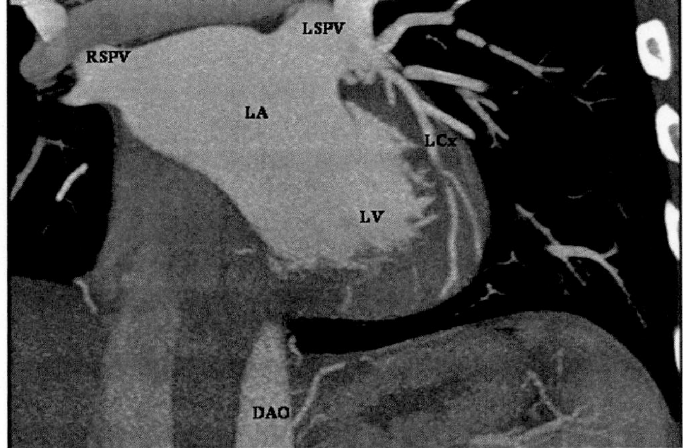

Fig. 4.62

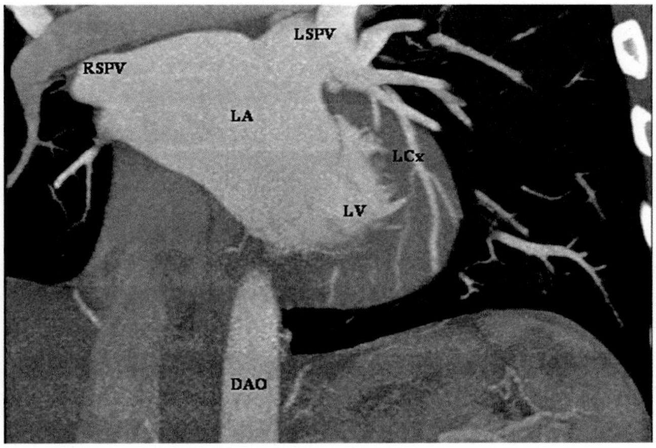

Fig. 4.63

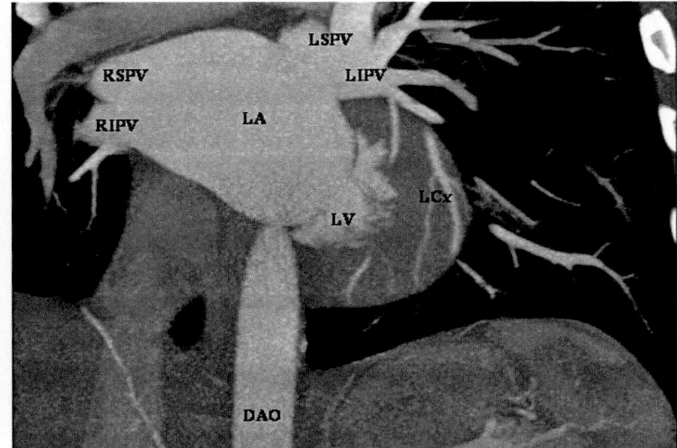

Fig. 4.64

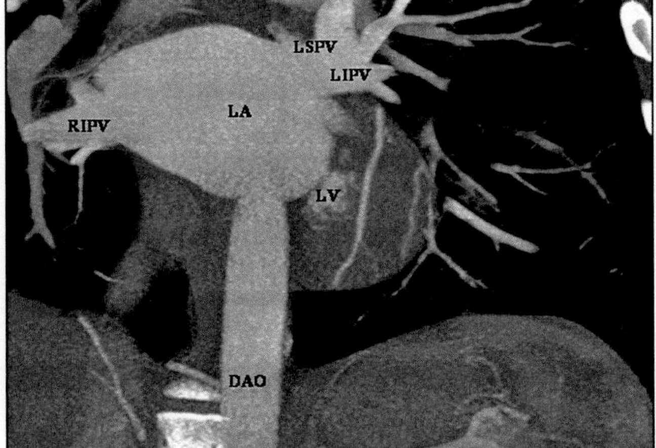

Fig. 4.65

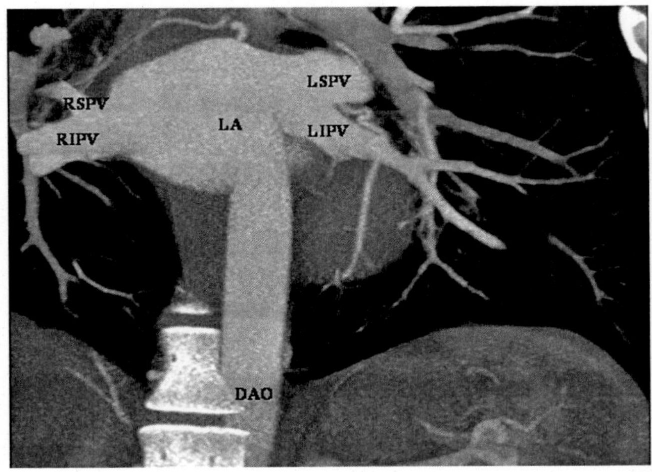

Fig. 4.66

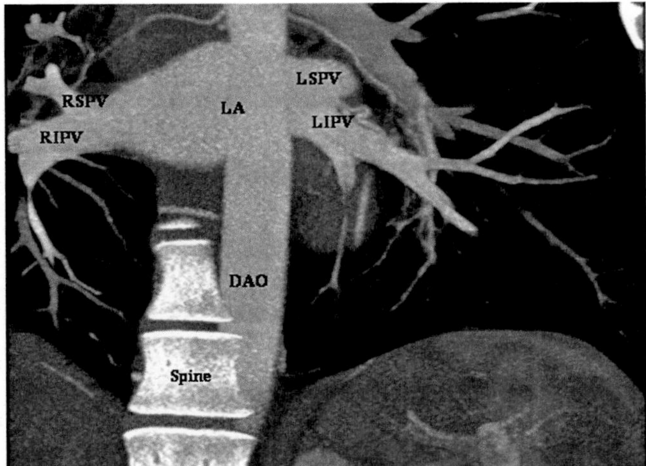

Fig. 4.67

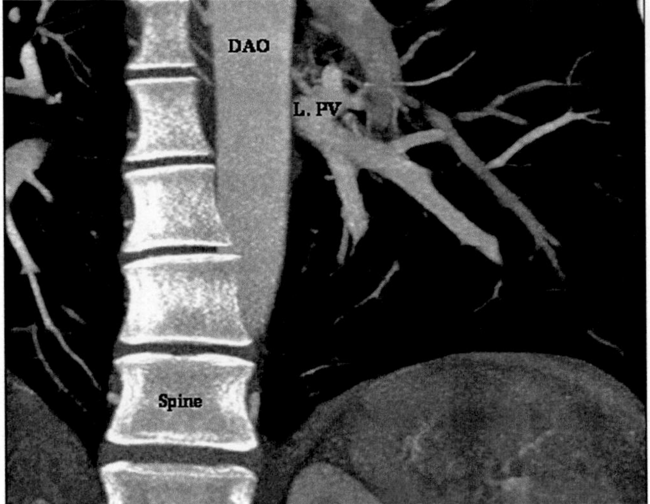

Fig. 4.68

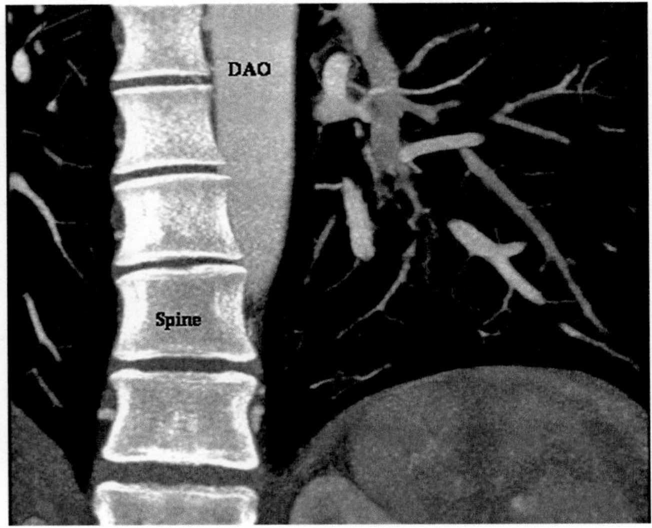

Fig. 4.69

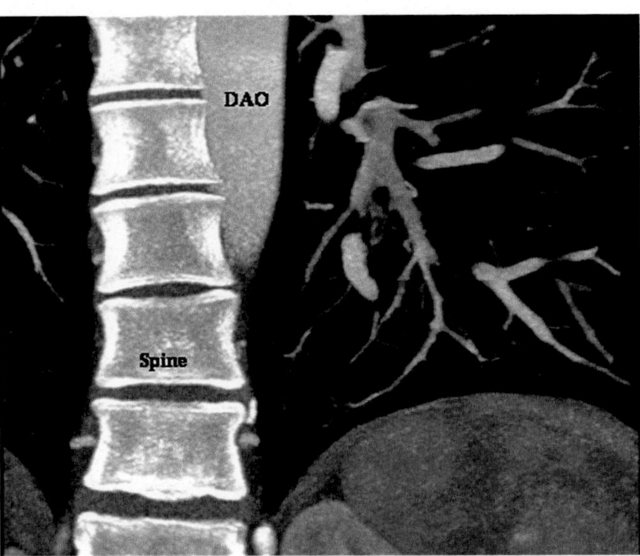

Fig. 4.70

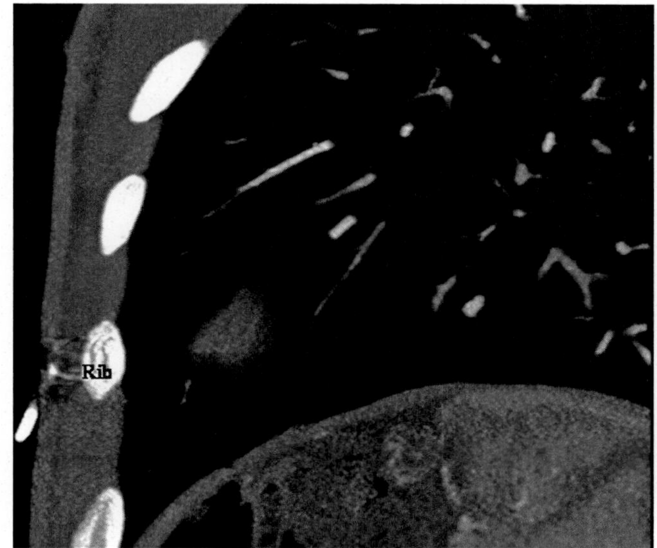

Fig. 4.71

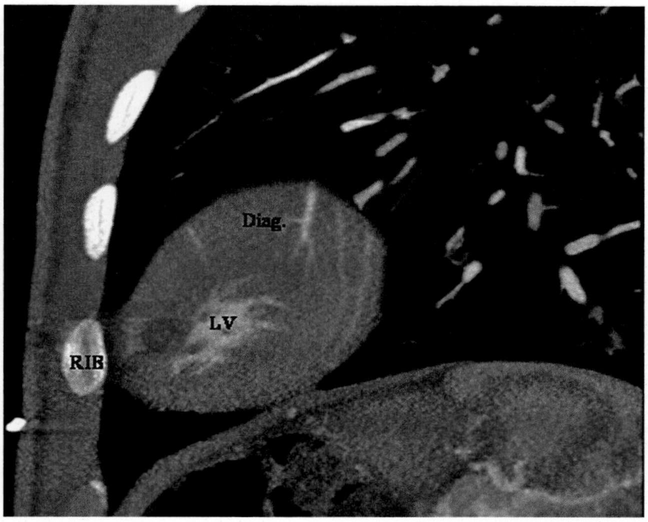

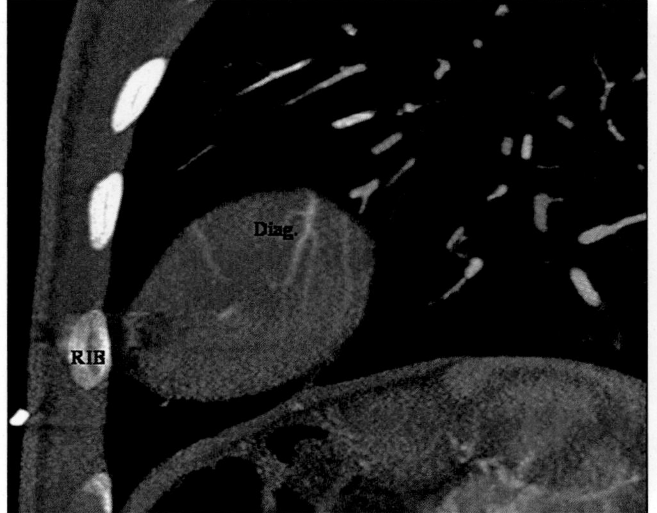

Fig. 4.72

Fig. 4.73

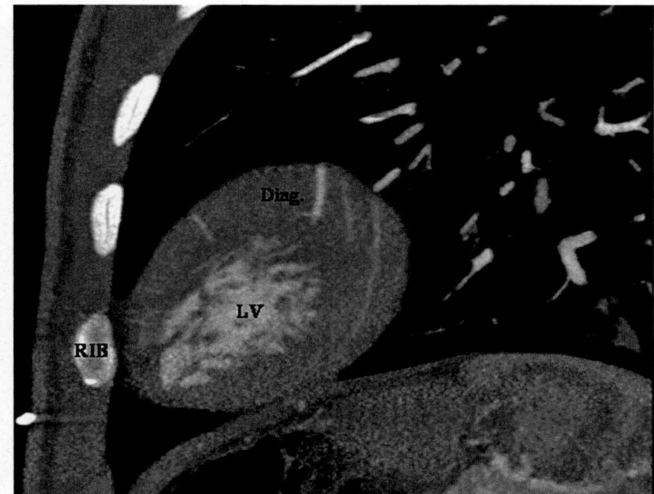

Fig. 4.74

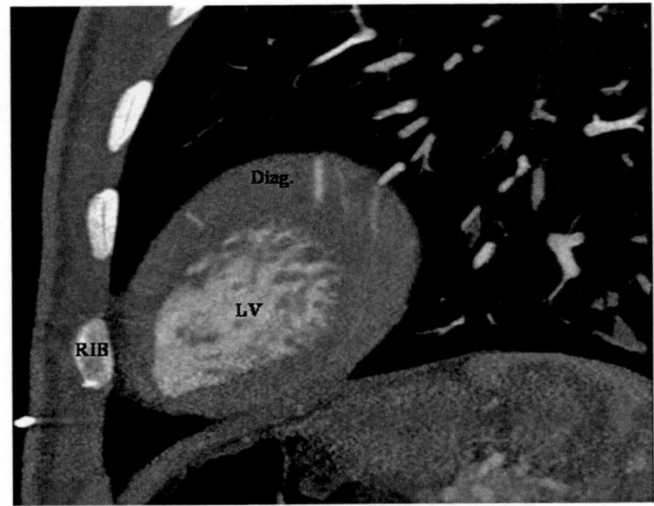

Fig. 4.75

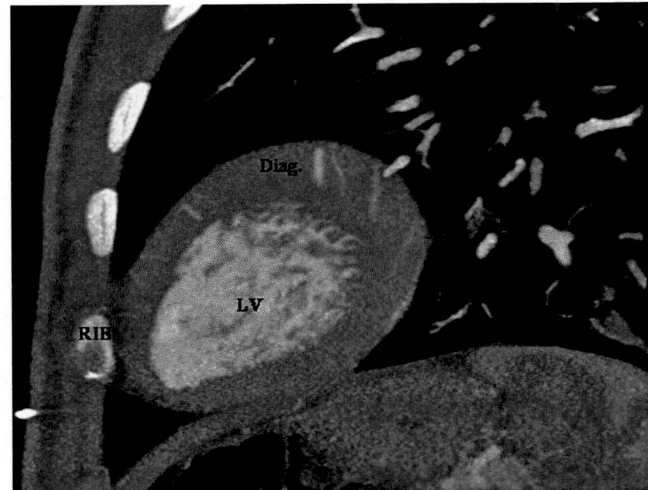

Fig. 4.76

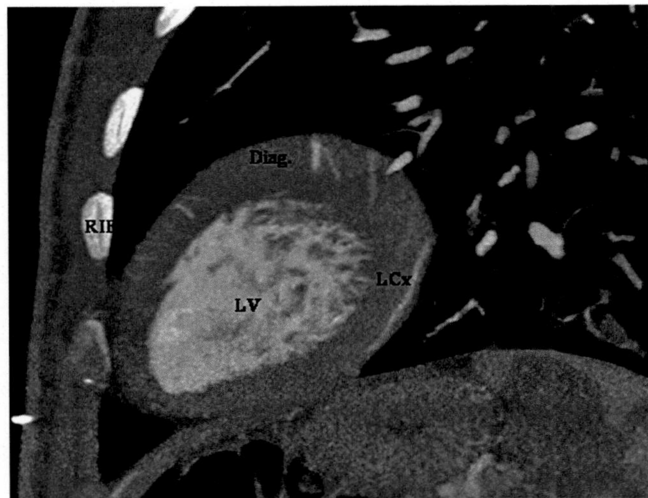

Fig. 4.77

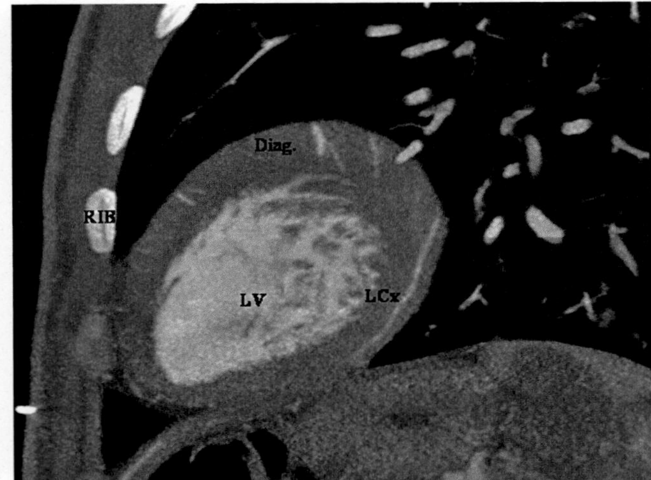

Fig. 4.78

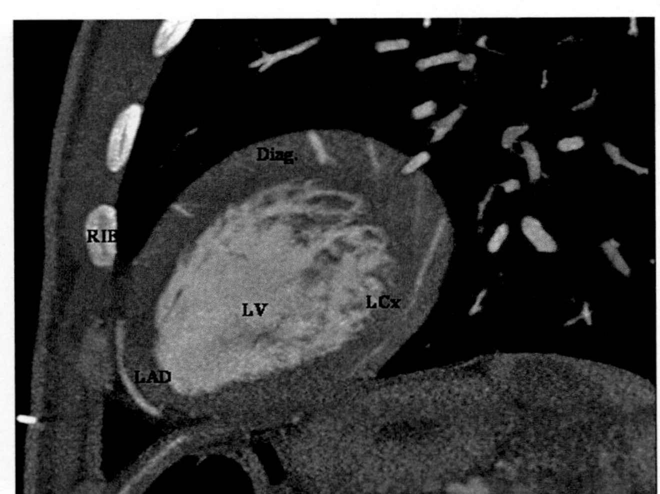

Fig. 4.79

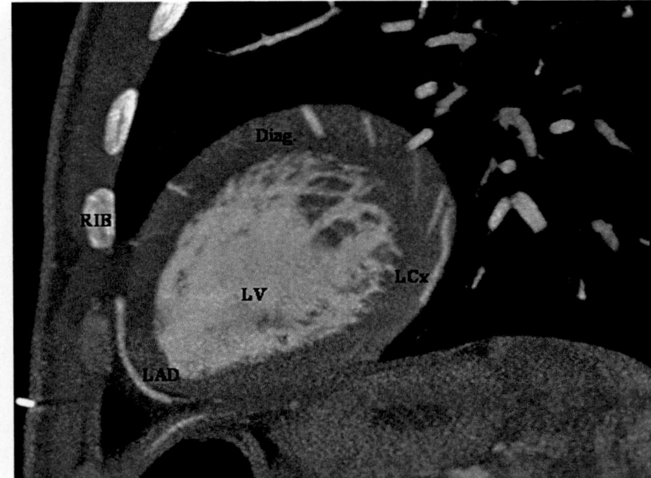

Fig. 4.80

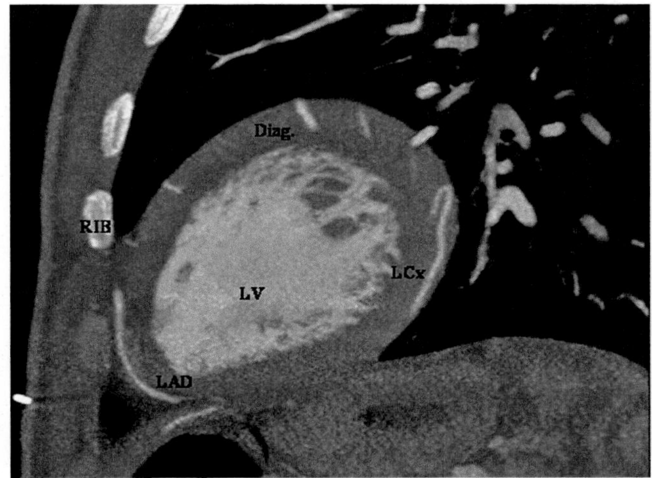

Fig. 4.81

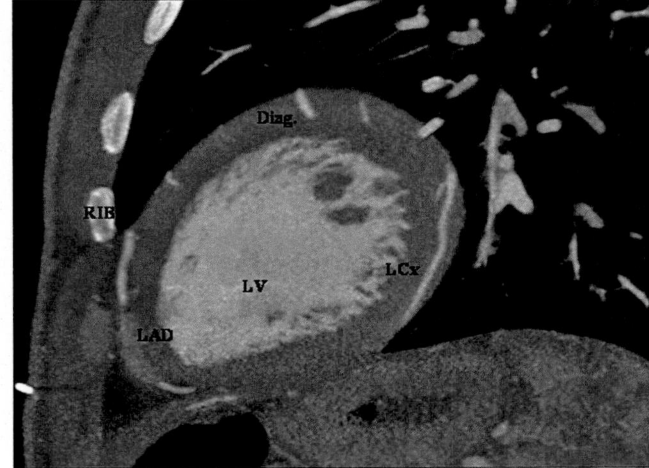

Fig. 4.82

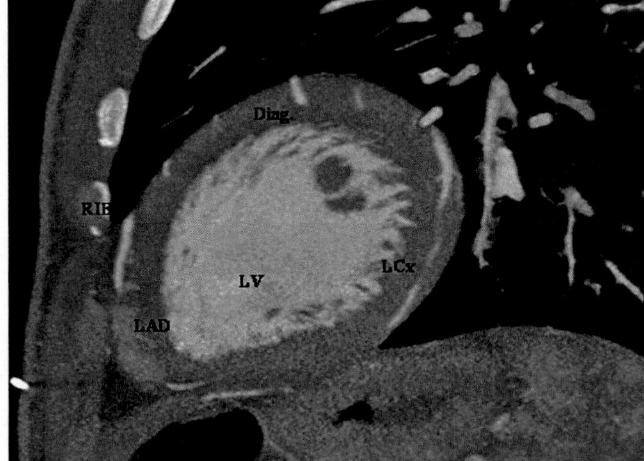

Fig. 4.83

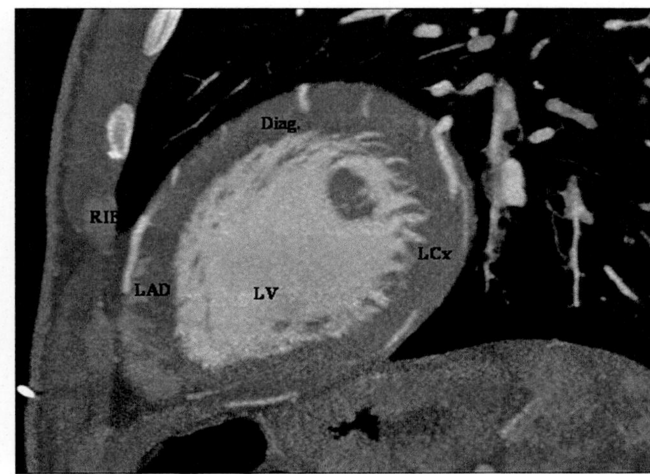

Fig. 4.84

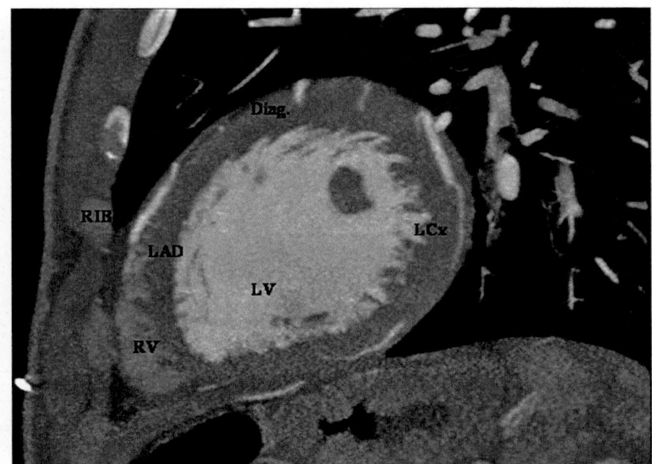

Fig. 4.85

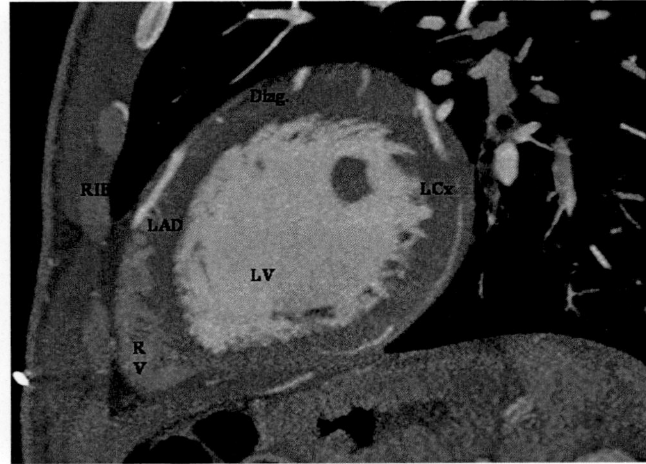

Fig. 4.86

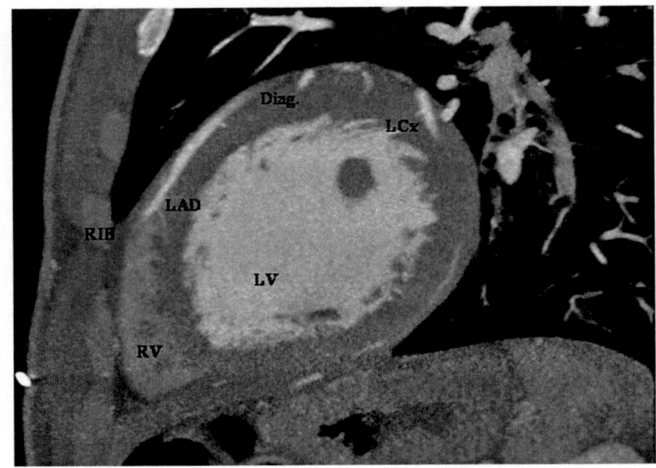

Fig. 4.87

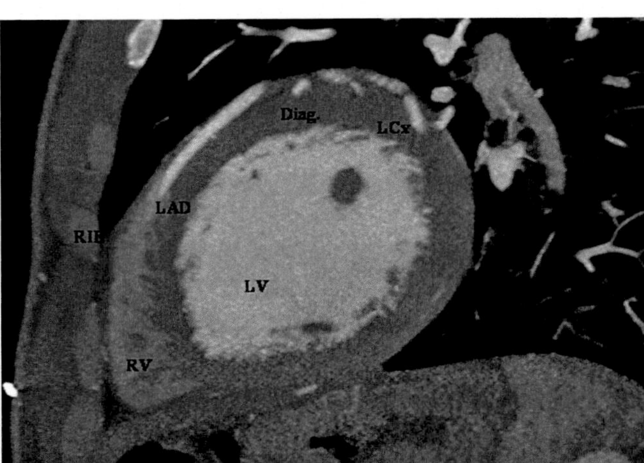

Fig. 4.88

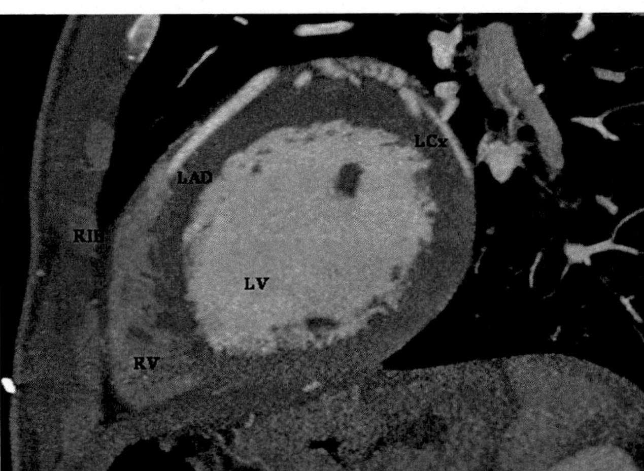

Fig. 4.89

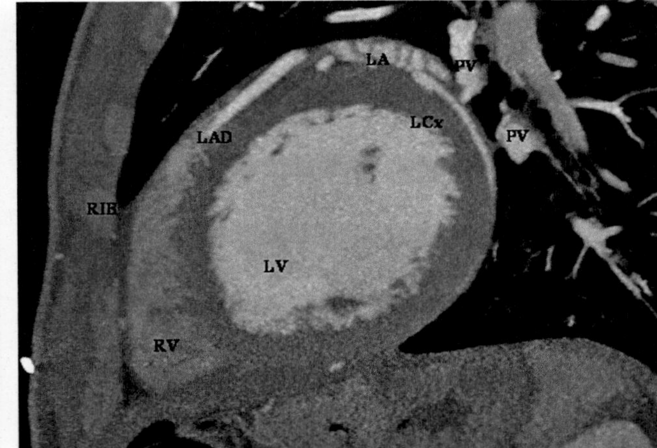

Fig. 4.90

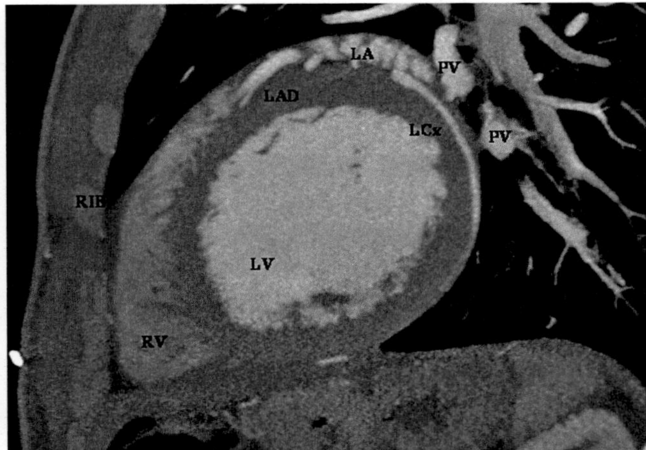

Fig. 4.91

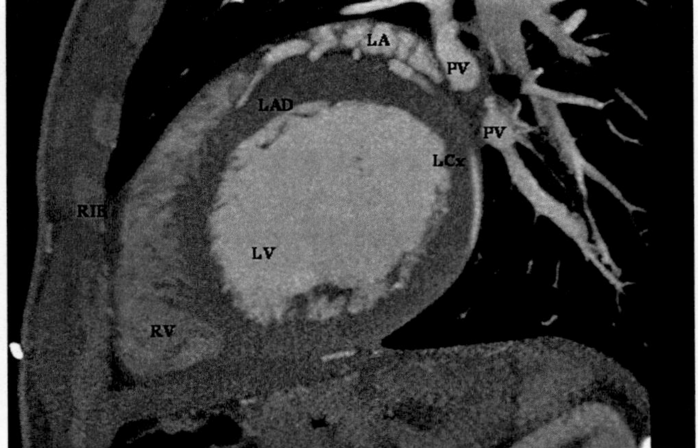

Fig. 4.92

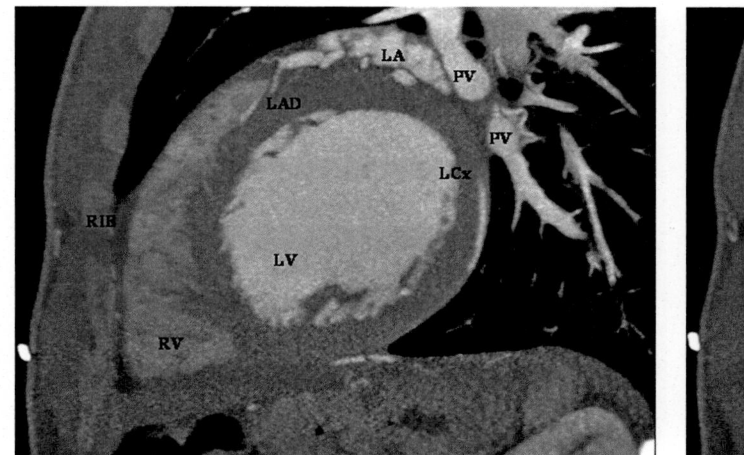

Fig. 4.93

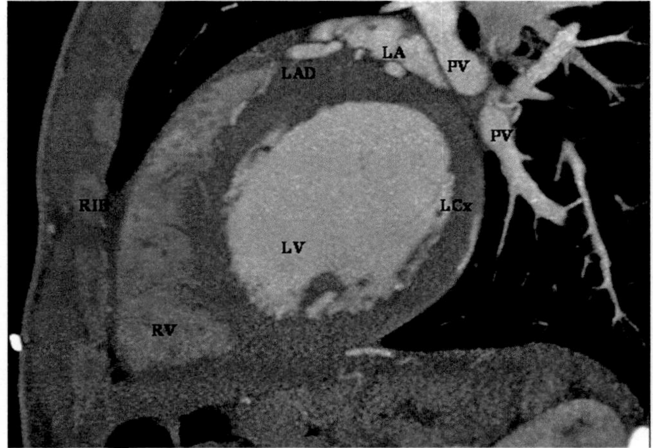

Fig. 4.94

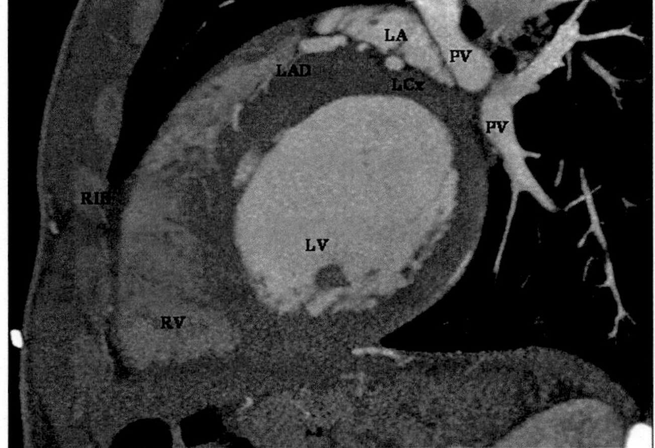

Fig. 4.95

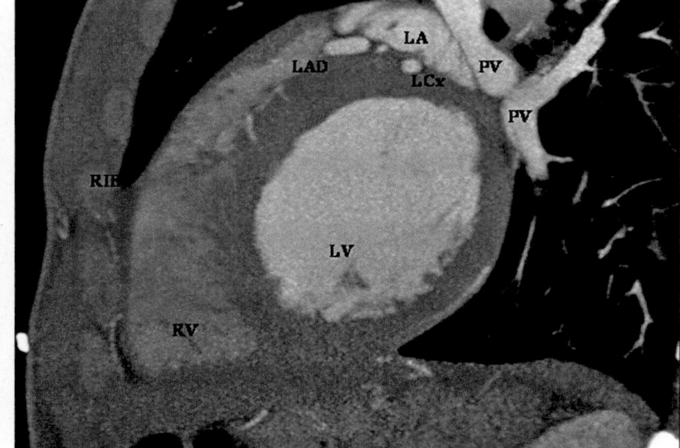

Fig. 4.96

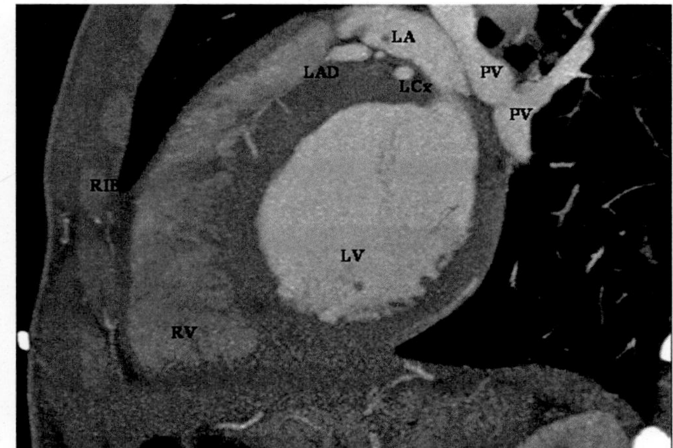

Fig. 4.97

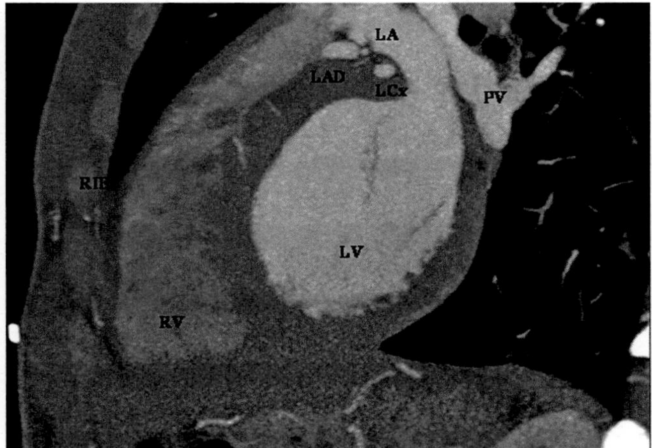

Fig. 4.98

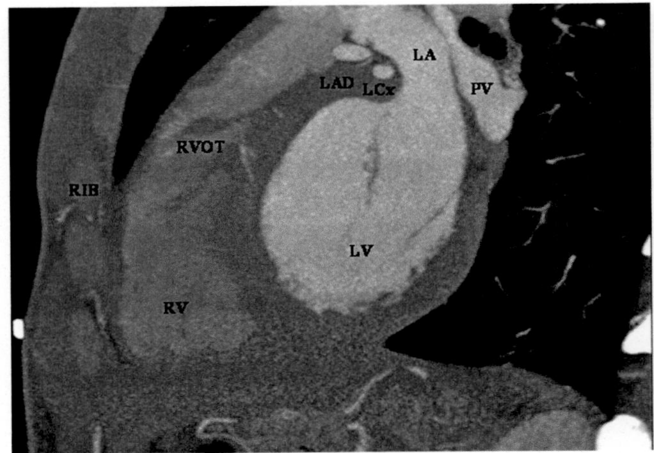

Fig. 4.99

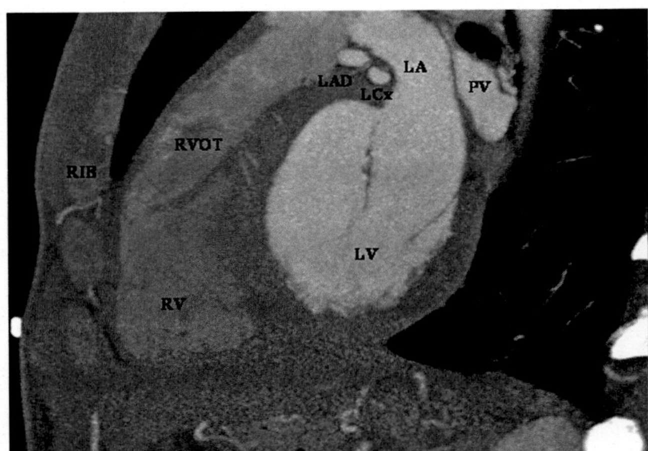

Fig. 4.100

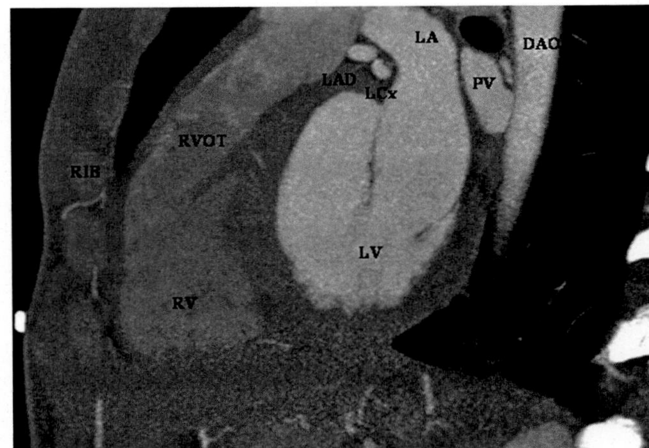

Fig. 4.101

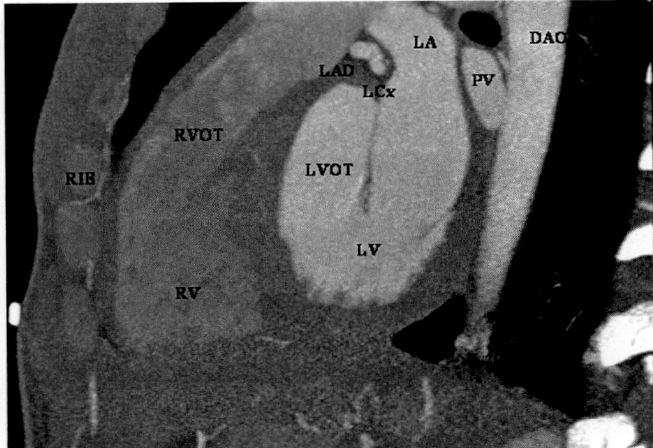

Fig. 4.102

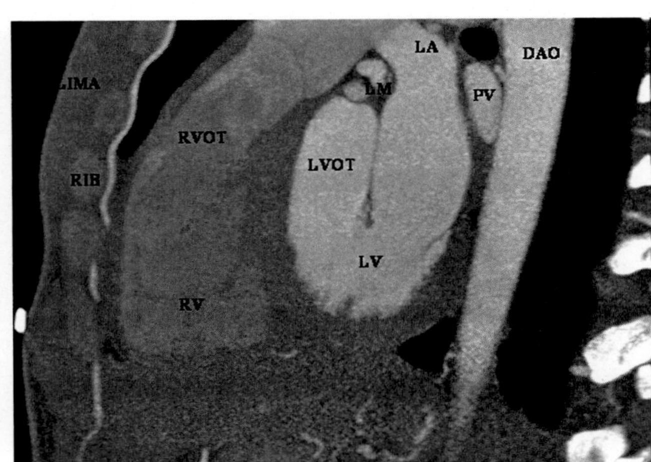

Fig. 4.103

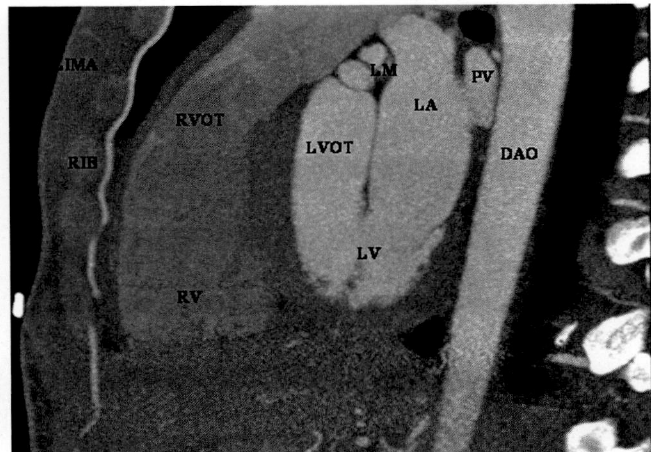

Fig. 4.104

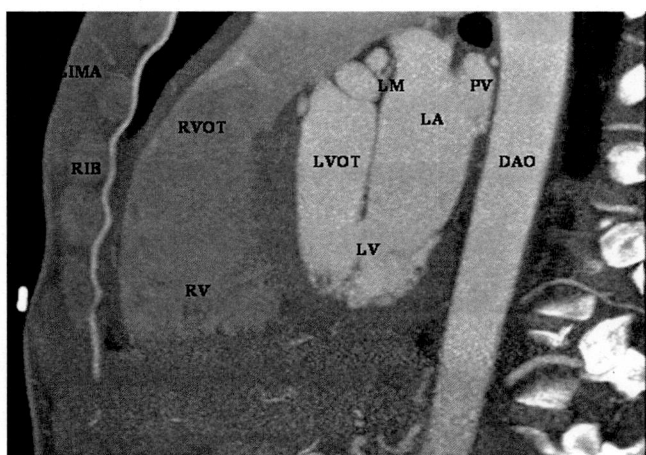

Fig. 4.105

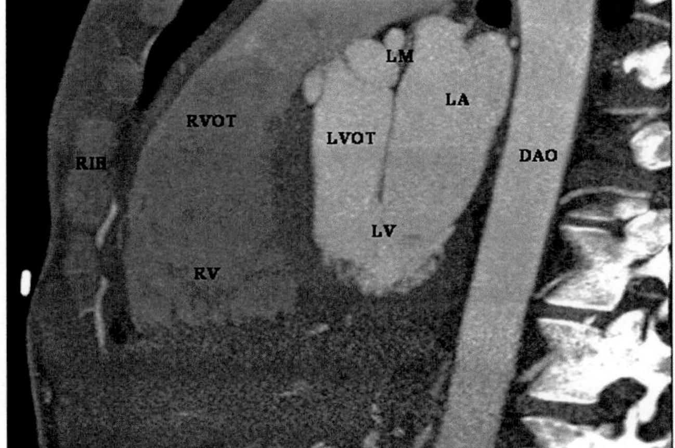

Fig. 4.106

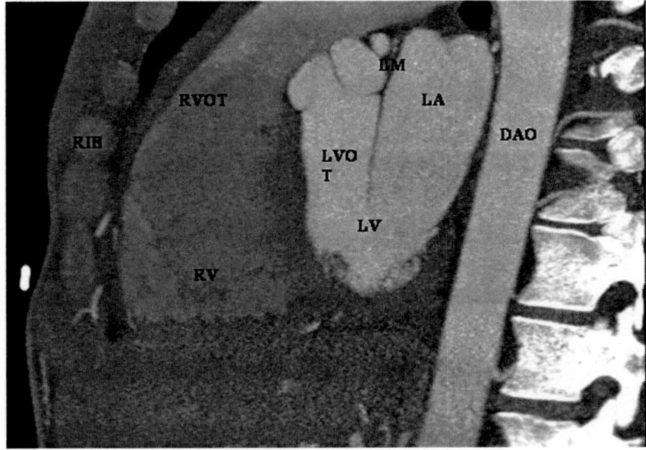

Fig. 4.107

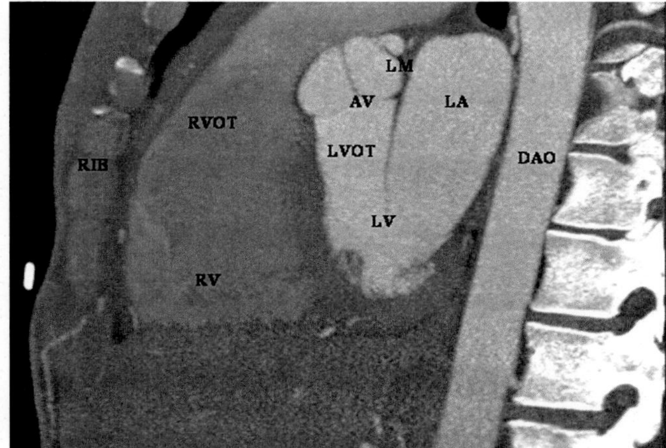

Fig. 4.108

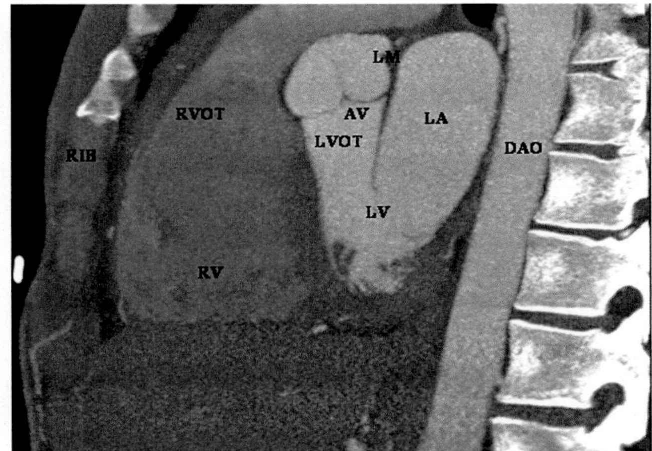

Fig. 4.109

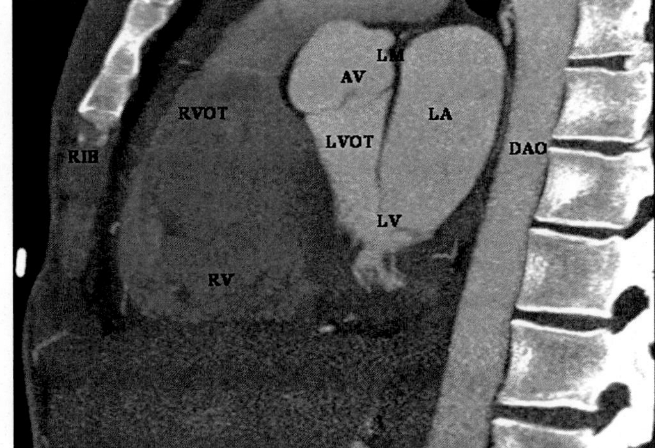

Fig. 4.110

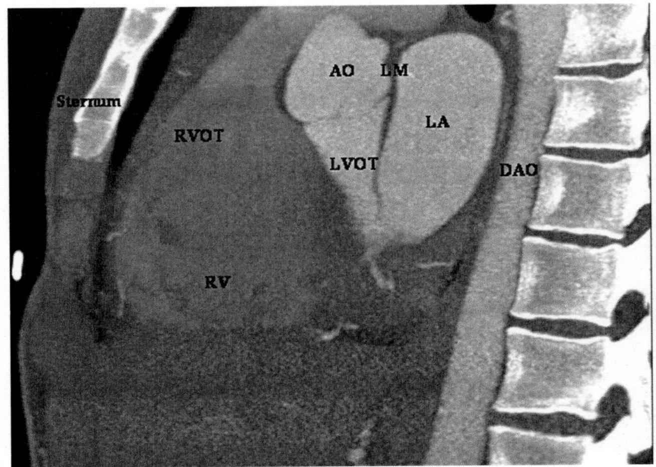

Fig. 4.111

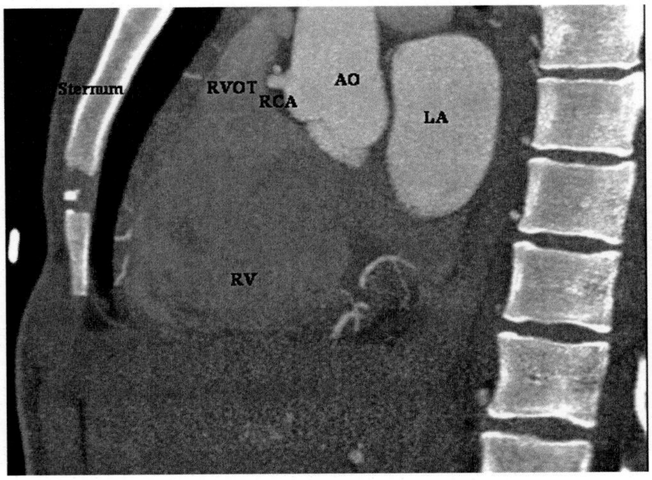

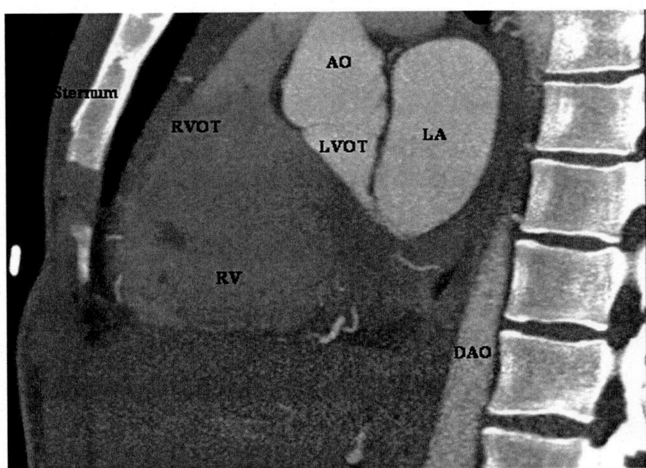

Fig. 4.112

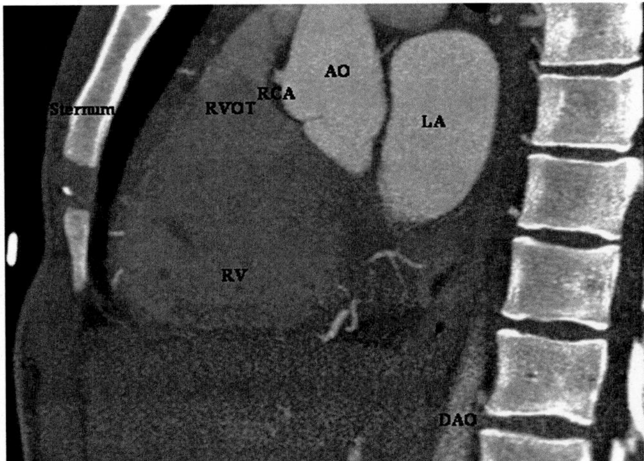

Fig. 4.113

Fig. 4.114

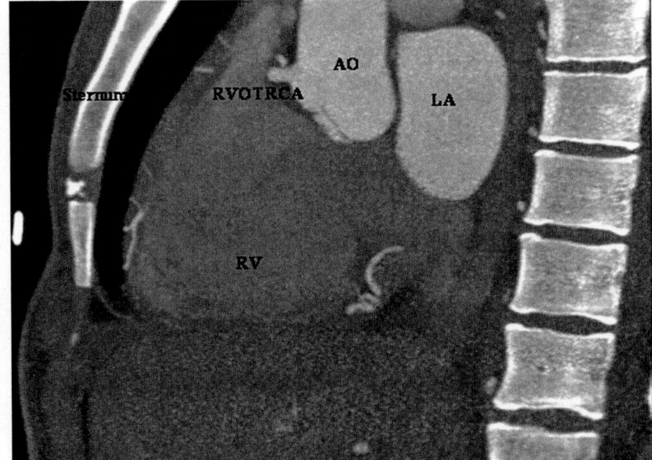

Fig. 4.115

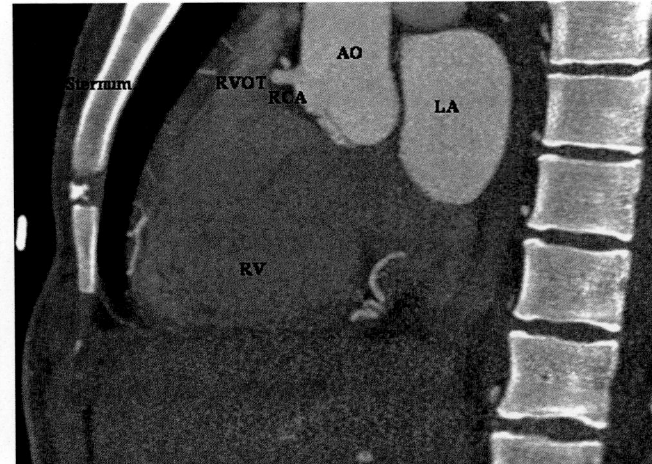

Fig. 4.116

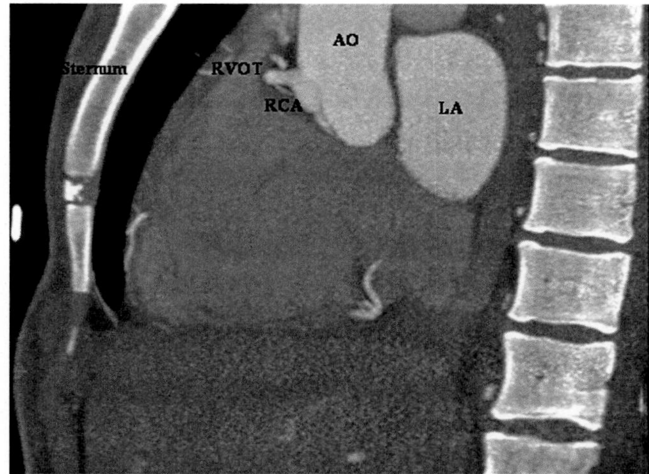

Fig. 4.117

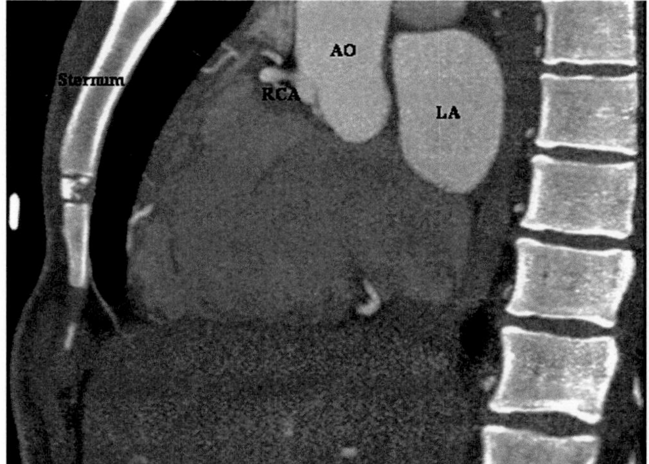

Fig. 4.118

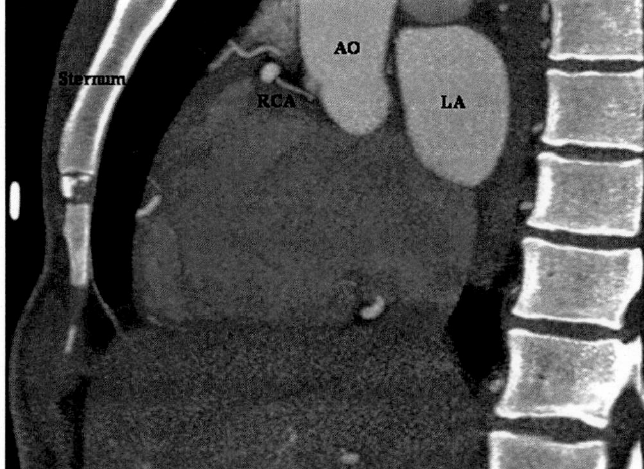

Fig. 4.119

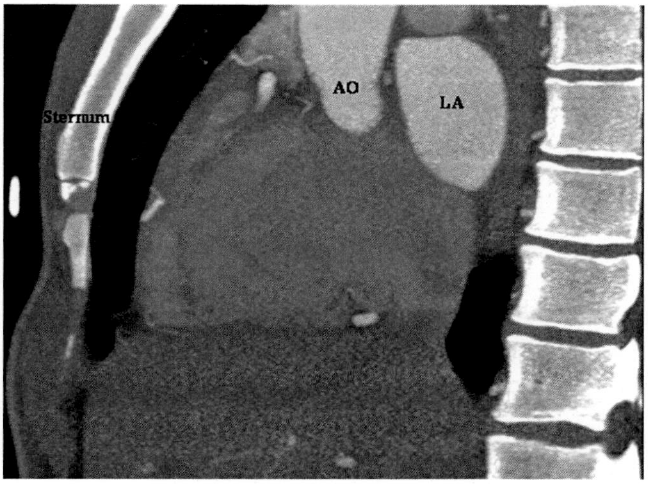

Fig. 4.120

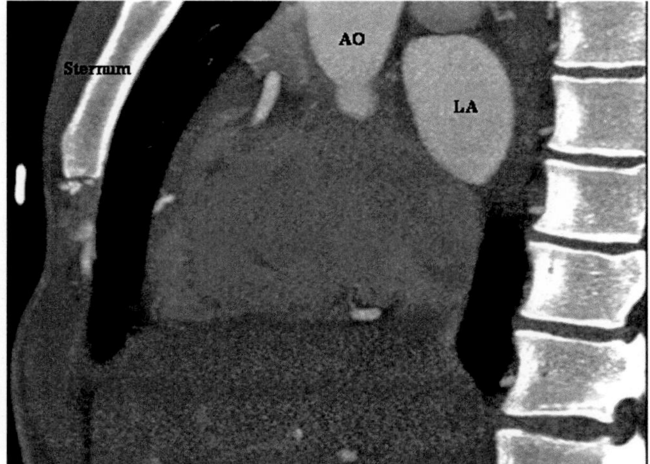

Fig. 4.121

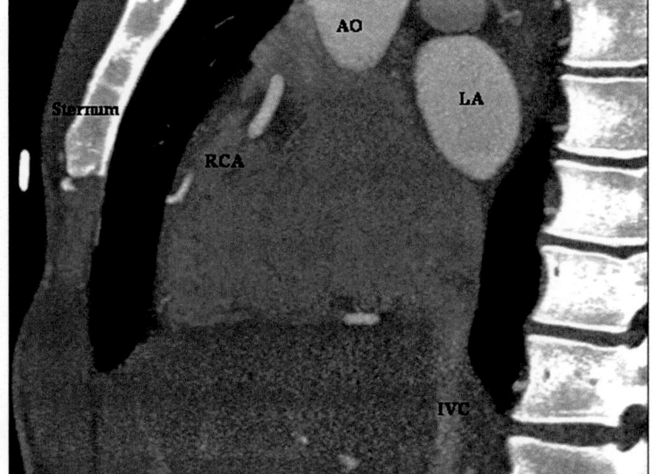

Fig. 4.122

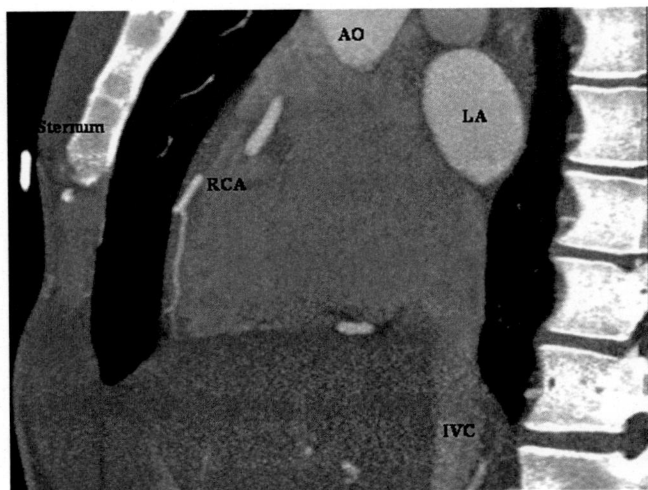

Fig. 4.123

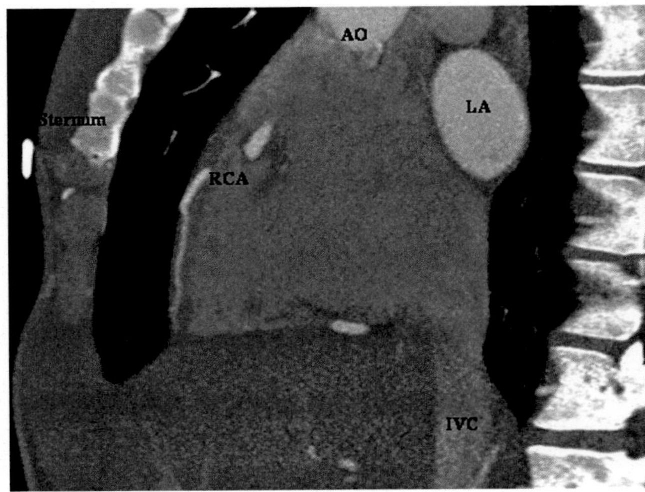

Fig. 4.124

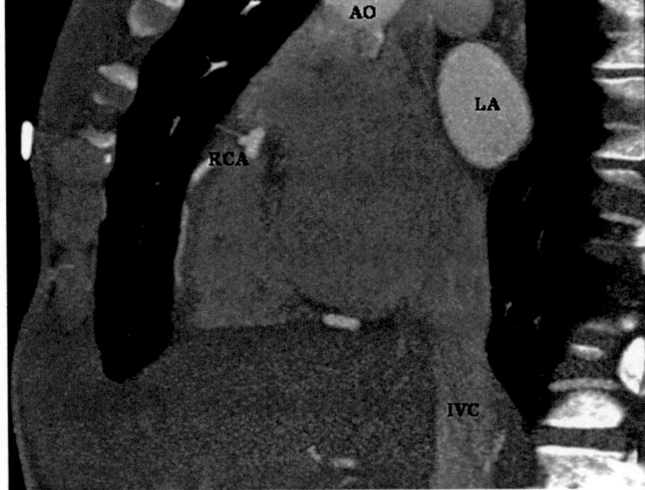

Fig. 4.125

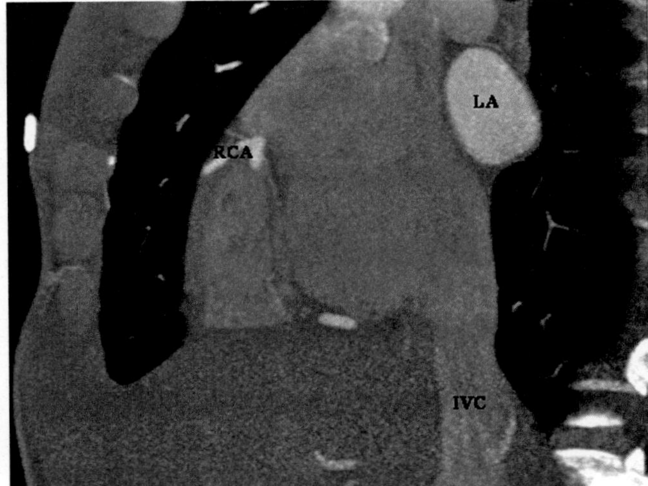

Fig. 4.126

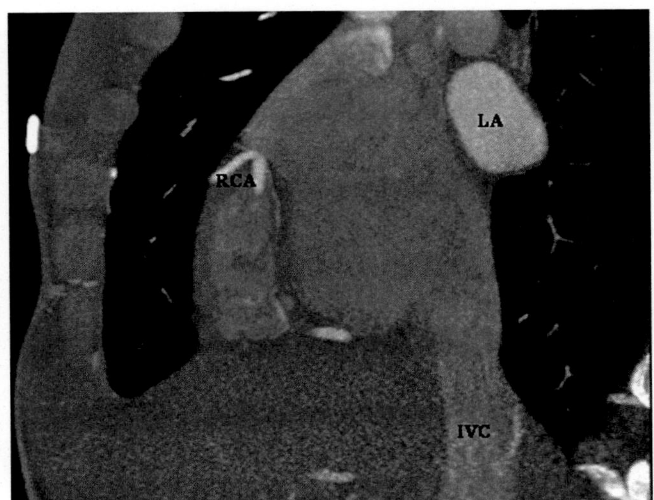

Fig. 4.127

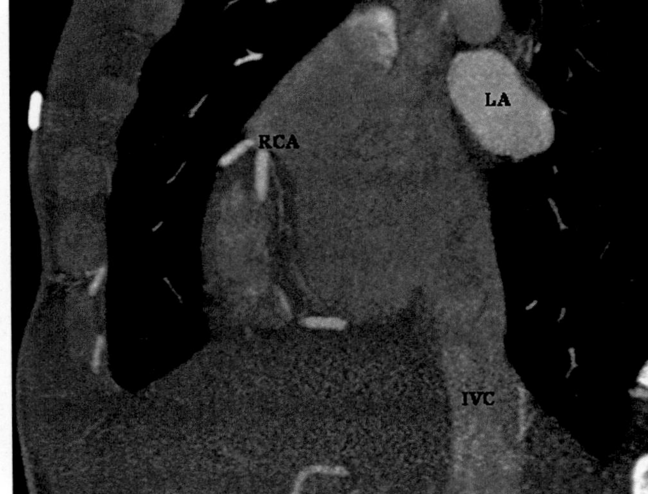

Fig. 4.128

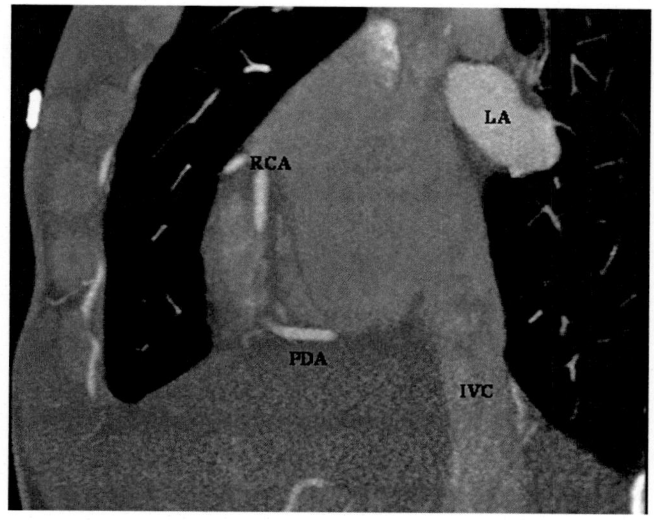

Fig. 4.129

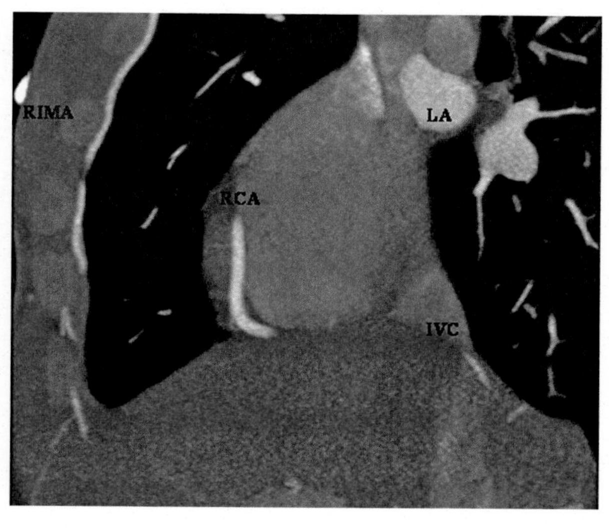

Fig. 4.132

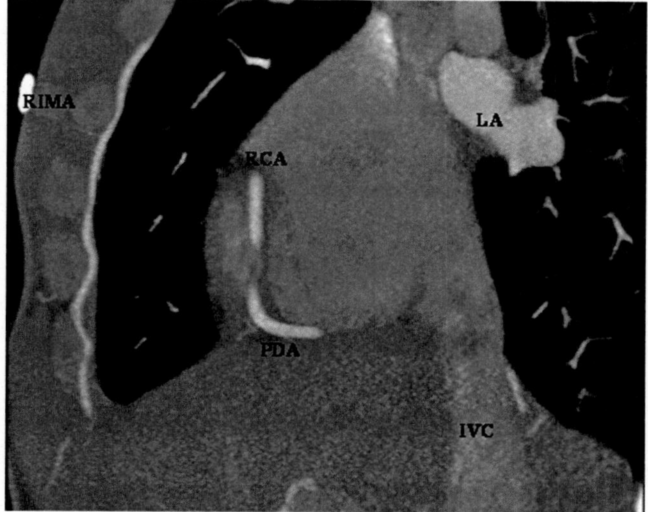

Fig. 4.130

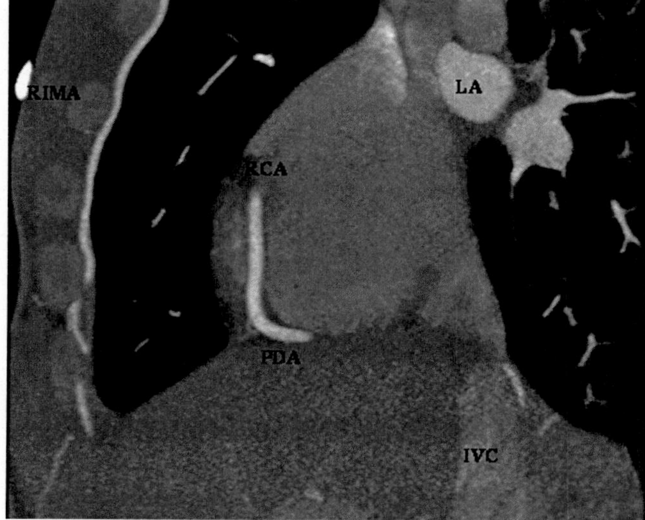

Fig. 4.131

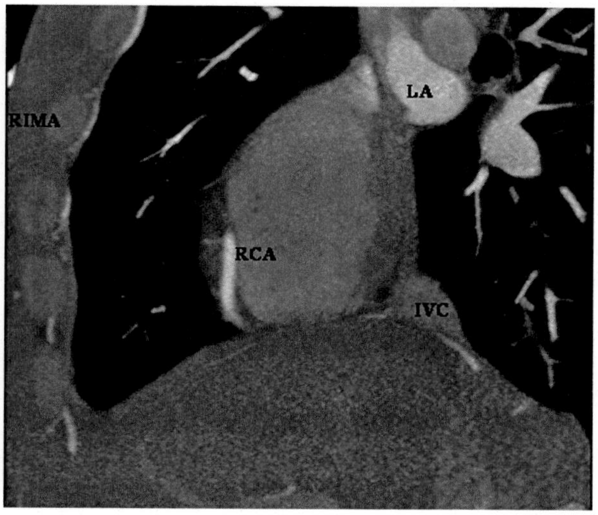

Fig. 4.133

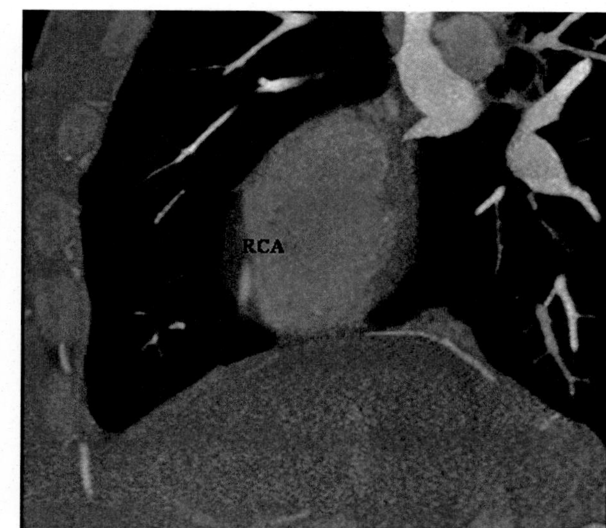

Fig. 4.134

Part II

Cardiac CT

Assessment of Cardiovascular Calcium: Interpretation, Prognostic Value, and Relationship to Lipids and Other Cardiovascular Risk Factors

5

Harvey S. Hecht

Abstract

Coronary artery calcium scanning has proven to be the most powerful predictor of cardiac risk in the primary prevention population, far exceeding conventional risk factors in prognostic value. It has also proven superior to all markers of inflammation, ankle brachial index, carotid intima-media thickness and flow mediated vasodilation. Its most accepted application is in the intermediate risk cohort, with an outcome based net reclassification index of the Framingham Risk Score exceeding 50 %. Application to young patients with a family history of premature coronary disease and to all diabetics older than 40 years of age is also appropriate.

Keywords

Coronary artery calcium • Primary prevention • Coronary artery disease • Risk factors • Risk prediction • Atherosclerosis

Cardiac risk assessment has traditionally been based on conventional risk factors; the shortcomings of this approach are all too often highlighted by major cardiac events occurring in presumably low-risk people. The annual presentation of 650,000 previously asymptomatic patients with an acute coronary event as the initial manifestation of coronary artery disease (CAD) [1] is a testimony to the failure of our current risk assessment model. Consequently, there has been a focus on markers of subclinical atherosclerosis that may be utilized for risk assessment of individuals, rather than extrapolating from risk factors that reflect trends in large groups of patients in epidemiologic studies. The most powerful of these subclinical markers is coronary artery calcium (CAC).

H.S. Hecht, MD, FACC, FSSCT
Department of Medicine, Icahn School of Medicine at Mount Sinai, New York, NY, USA

Mount Sinai Medical Center,
One Gustave L. Levy Place, Box 1030,
New York, NY 10029-6574, USA
e-mail: hhecht@aol.com

Background

CAC is pathognomonic for atherosclerosis [2–4]. Mönckeberg's calcific medial sclerosis does not occur in the coronary arteries [5]; atherosclerosis is the only vascular disease known to be associated with coronary calcification. Calcium phosphate (in the hydroxyapatite form) and cholesterol accumulate in atherosclerotic lesions. Circulating proteins that are normally associated with bone remodeling play an important role in coronary calcification, and arterial calcium in atherosclerosis is a regulated active process similar to bone formation, rather than a passive precipitation of calcium phosphate crystals [6–9]. Rumberger et al. [10] demonstrated that the total area of coronary artery calcification is highly correlated ($r=0.9$) in a linear fashion with the total area of coronary artery plaque on a segmental, individual, and whole coronary artery system basis (Fig. 5.1), and the areas of coronary calcification comprise approximately one fifth that of the associated coronary plaque. Additionally, there were plaque areas without associated coronary calcium, suggesting that there may be a coronary plaque size

M.J. Budoff, J.S. Shinbane (eds.), *Cardiac CT Imaging: Diagnosis of Cardiovascular Disease*,
DOI 10.1007/978-3-319-28219-0_5

most commonly associated with coronary calcium but, in the smaller plaques, the calcium is either not present or is undetectable.

Intravascular ultrasound [11, 12] measures of combined calcified and non-calcified plaque confirm the strong relationship (Fig. 5.2).

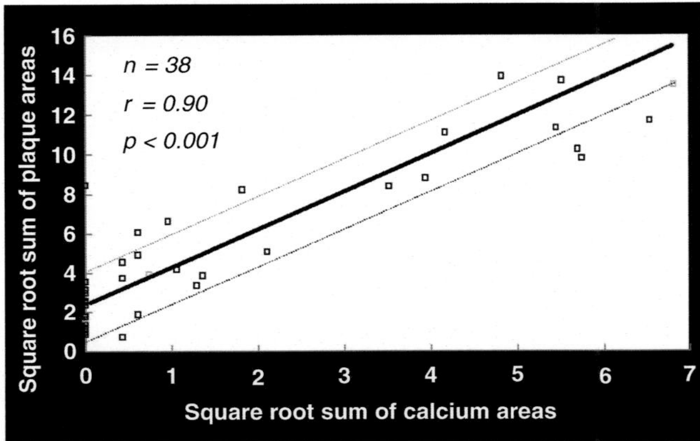

Fig. 5.1 Correlation between calcified and total plaque burden in histopathologic coronary artery specimens (Reproduced from Rumberger et al. [10], with permission from Wolters Kluwer Health)

Methodology

Technical

In the beginning, the data substantiating the importance of CAC were derived through the use of electron beam tomography (EBT), utilizing a rotating electron beam to acquire prospectively triggered, tomographic 100-ms X-ray images at 3 mm intervals in the space of a 30- to 40-s breathhold. The multidetector computed tomography (MDCT) technology has replaced EBT and employs a rotating gantry with a special X-ray tube and variable number of detectors (from 4 to 320), with 75–375-ms images at 0.5,1.5, 2.0, or 3.0 mm intervals, depending on the protocol and manufacturer.

Scoring

The presence of CAC is sequentially quantified through the entire epicardial coronary system. Coronary calcium is defined as a lesion above a threshold of 130 Hounsfield units (which range from −1000 (air), through 0 (water), and up to +1000 (dense cortical bone)), with an area of three or more adjacent pixels (at least 1 mm^2). The original calcium score

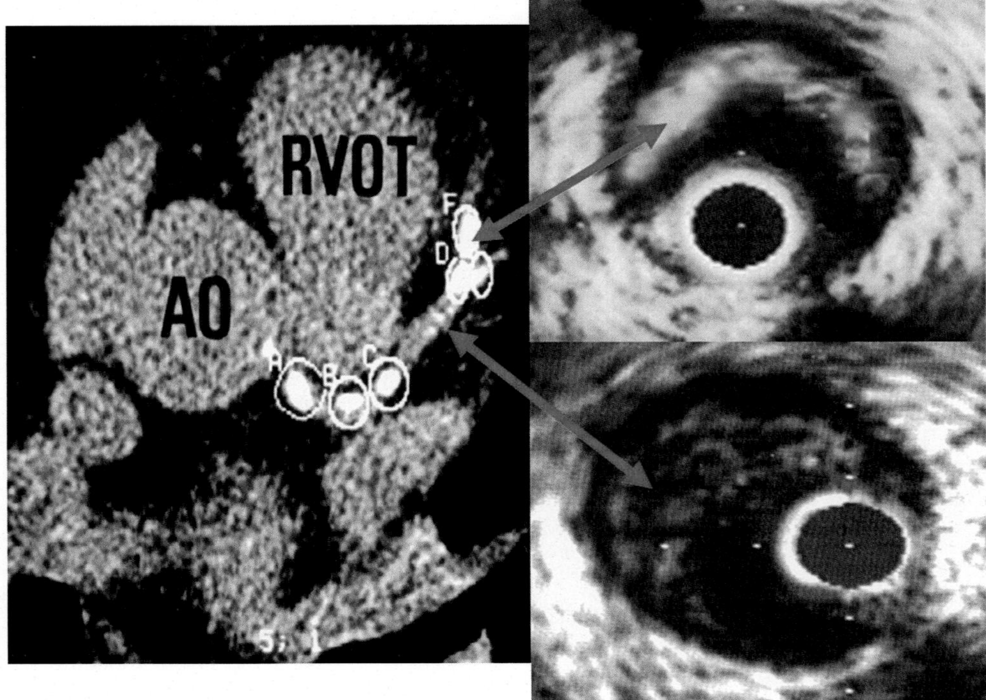

Fig. 5.2 Coronary artery calcium scan (*left*) demonstrating areas of extensive calcification corresponding to heavily calcified plaque on intravascular ultrasound (*upper right*), and less extensive calcification corresponding to less heavily calcified plaque on intravascular ultrasound (*lower right*), *AO* aorta, *RVOT* right ventricular outflow tract

developed by Agatston et al. [13] is determined by the product of the calcified plaque area and maximum calcium lesion density (from 1 to 4 based upon Hounsfield units). Standardized categories for the calcium score have been developed with scores of 0 indicating absence of calcified plaque, 1–10 considered minimal, 11–100 mild, 101–400 moderate, and >400 severe. Examples are shown in Fig. 5.1. The calcium volume score [14] is a more reproducible parameter that is independent of calcium density and may be the parameter of choice for serial studies to track progression or regression of atherosclerosis, but is rarely used. Phantom-based calcium mass scores are applicable to any CT scanner [15], but are never clinically used. Examples of CAC scans are shown in Fig. 5.3.

Epidemiology

By comparing a person's calcium score to others of the same age and gender through the use of large databases of asymptomatic subjects, a *calcium percentile* is generated [16]. This is an index of the prematurity of atherosclerosis; for example, a 50-year-old man in the 76th percentile has more plaque than 75 % but less plaque than 24 % of asymptomatic 50-year-old men. Although there is an increasing incidence of coronary calcification with increasing age, this simply parallels the development of coronary atherosclerosis.

Table 5.1 shows coronary calcification incidence in an unselected patient population of men and women [17]. The amount of CAC in women is similar to that in men a decade

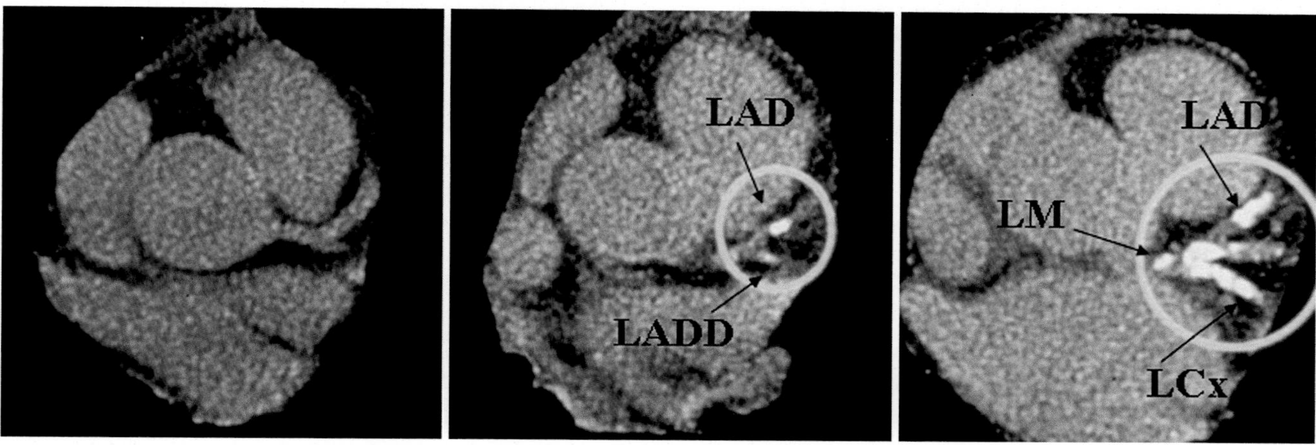

Fig. 5.3 Examples of coronary artery calcium scans. *Left* normal without CAC. *Center* moderate CAC involving the left anterior descending (*LAD*) and circumflex (*LCx*) coronary arteries. *Right* extensive CAC involving the left main (*LM*), anterior descending, and circumflex coronary arteries, *LADD* left anterior descending diagonal branch

Table 5.1 Calcium percentile database for asymptomatic men and women: coronary calcium scores as a function of patient age at the time of examination

Percentiles	40–45 years	46–50 years	51–55 years	56–60 years	61–65 years	66–70 years	71–75 years
Men (n = 28,250)							
10	0	0	0	1	1	3	3
25	0	1	2	5	12	30	69
50	2	3	15	54	117	166	350
75	11	36	110	229	386	538	844
90	69	151	346	588	933	1151	1650
Women (n = 14,540)							
10	0	0	0	0	0	0	0
25	0	0	0	0	0	1	4
50	0	0	1	1	3	25	51
75	1	2	6	22	68	148	231
90	4	21	61	127	208	327	698

younger, paralleling the 10-year lag in women of the development of clinical atherosclerosis.

Useful though these current nomograms are, variations according to ethnicity have been described, and data regarding these variations are still being collected and separated. In earlier studies, Blacks were noted to have either lower [18, 19] or similar [20, 21] amounts of CAC as Caucasians of the same age; Hispanics had less CAC than Caucasians [18]. In the more recent Multi-Ethnic Study of Atherosclerosis (MESA) of 6110 asymptomatic patients with 53 % female and an average age of 62 years, men had greater calcium levels than women, and calcium amount and prevalence continually increased with increasing age [22]. In men, Caucasians and Hispanics were the first and second highest respectively; Blacks were lowest at the younger ages, and Chinese were lowest at the older ages. In women, whites were highest, Chinese and Black were intermediate, and Hispanics were the lowest except for Chinese in the oldest age group. Thus, predictive indices should be extrapolated to non-whites with caution. However, MESA demonstrated very strong CAC predictive for all groups [23].

Younger patients with a family history of premature CAD have significantly higher CAC scores than similar aged individuals without this risk factor, particularly if there is a sibling history of premature CAD [24]. In MESA, the odds ratios for the presence of CAC independent of all risk factors in those with compared to those without a family history of premature CAD were 2.74 with premature CAD in both a parent and a sibling, 2.06 in a sibling alone, and 1.52 in a parent alone [25].

Radiation

The vast majority of CAC scanning is performed on MDCT scanners. The radiation exposure should not exceed 1.0 mSv [26]. Iterative reconstruction techniques that decrease noise will lead to even lower radiation exposure. Appropriate perspective is obtained by comparing this exposure to the 0.75 mSv of the annual mammographic examination recommended for women 45 years and older.

Coronary Artery Calcium and Obstructive Disease

Incidence

The relationship of CAC to obstructive disease has been extensively investigated, and was misunderstood by the 2000 ACC/AHA Consensus Document on EBT [27], which focused on the low specificity as a critical flaw. While the presence of CAC is nearly 100 % specific for atherosclerosis, it is not specific for obstructive disease since both obstructive and non-obstructive lesions have calcification present in the intima. Comparisons with pathology specimens have shown that the degree of luminal narrowing is weakly correlated with the amount of calcification on a site-by-site basis [28–30], whereas the likelihood of significant obstruction increases with the total CAC score [4, 31, 32]. Shavelle et al. [33] reported a 96 % sensitivity and 47 % specificity for a calcium score >0, with a relative risk for obstructive disease of 4.5, compared to a 76 % sensitivity and 60 % specificity for treadmill testing, with a relative risk of 1.7. Bielak et al. [34] noted a sensitivity and specificity of 99.1 % and 38.6 % for a calcium score >0. However, when corrected for verification bias, the specificity improved to 72.4 %, without loss of sensitivity (97 %). The likelihood ratio for obstruction ranged from 0.03–0.07 in men and women ≥50 years of age for 0 scores to 12.85 for scores >200. In the <50 years cohort, the likelihood ratios ranged from 0.1–0.29 for 0 scores to 54–189 for scores >100.

Rumberger et al. [35] demonstrated that higher calcium scores are associated with a greater specificity for obstructive disease at the expense of sensitivity; for example, a threshold score of 368 was 95 % specific for the presence of obstructive CAD. In 1764 persons undergoing angiography, the sensitivity and negative predictive value in men and women were >99 % [36]; a score of 0 virtually excluded patients with obstructive CAD. In a separate study of 1851 patients undergoing CAC scanning and angiography [37], CAC scanning by EBT in conjunction with pretest probability of disease derived by a combination of age, gender, and risk factors, facilitated prediction of the severity and extent of angiographically significant CAD in symptomatic patients.

In a recent meta-analysis of 10,355 symptomatic patients who underwent cardiac catheterization and CAC, 0 CAC was noted in 1941. Significant obstructive disease, defined as >50 % diameter stenosis, was noted in 5805 (56 %). For CAC >0 and the presence of >50 % diameter stenosis, the following were reported: sensitivity 98 %, specificity 40 %, positive predictive value 68 %, and negative predictive value 93 % [38].

Prognostic Studies in Symptomatic Patients

The prognostic value of extensive CAC (>1000) in symptomatic males with established advanced CAD was demonstrated in a 5-year follow-up study of 150 patients [39]. More recently, in a meta-analysis of 3924 symptomatic patients with a 3.5 year follow up, the cardiac event rate was

2.6 %/year in those with CAC >0 and 0.5 %/year in 0 CAC patients [38]. However, in this era of coronary computed tomographic angiography (CCTA), CAC alone is not justified in the symptomatic population; CCTA will identify the noncalcified plaque and obstructive disease that may be noted in these patients, even with 0 CAC.

Clarification

Despite the apparently reasonable specificities, which are similar to those of stress testing, it must be understood that the purpose of CAC scanning is not to detect obstructive disease and, therefore, it is inappropriate to even use "specificity" in the context of obstruction. Rather, its purpose is to detect subclinical atherosclerosis in its early stages, for which it is virtually 100 % specific.

CAC in Asymptomatic Patients

Key Prognostic Studies in Primary Prevention and Comparisons with Standard Risk Factor Paradigms

The utility of CAC for risk evaluation in the asymptomatic primary prevention population is dependent on prognostic studies documenting the relative risk conferred by calcified plaque quantitation compared to conventional risk factors. Raggi et al. [40] demonstrated, in 632 asymptomatic patients followed for 32 months, an annualized event rate of 0.1 %/year in patients with 0 scores, compared to 2.1 %/year with scores of 1–99, 4.1 %/year with scores of 100–400, and 4.8 %/year with scores >400. Thus, the annualized event rates associated with coronary calcium were in the range considered to warrant secondary prevention classification by the Framingham Risk Score (Fig. 5.4).

The odds ratio conferred by a calcium percentile >75 % was 21.5 times greater than for the lowest 25 %, compared to an odds ratio of 7 for the highest versus lowest quartiles of National Cholesterol Education Program (NCEP) risk factors (Fig. 5.5).

Wong et al. [41], in 926 asymptomatic patients followed for 3.3 years, noted a relative risk of 8 for scores >270, after adjusting for age, gender, hypertension, high cholesterol, smoking, and diabetes. Arad et al. [42], in 1132 subjects followed for 3.6 years, reported odds ratios of 14.3–20.2 for scores ranging from >80 to >600; these were 3–7 times greater than for the NCEP risk factors. In a retrospective analysis of 5635 asymptomatic, predominantly low to moderate risk, largely middle-aged patients followed for 37 ± 12 months, Kondos et al. [43] found that the presence of any CAC by EBT was associated with a relative risk for events of 10.5, compared to 1.98 and 1.4 for diabetes and smoking, respectively. In women, only CAC was linked to events, with a relative risk of 2.6; risk factors were not related. The presence of CAC provided prognostic information incremental to age and other risk factors.

Shaw et al. [44] retrospectively analyzed 10,377 asymptomatic patients with a 5-year follow-up after an initial EBT evaluation. All-cause mortality increased proportional to CAC, which was an independent predictor of risk after adjusting for all of the Framingham risk factors ($p<0.001$). Superiority of CAC to conventional Framingham risk factor assessment was demonstrated by a significantly greater area under the ROC curves (0.73 versus 0.67, $p<0.001$).

Greenland et al. [45] analyzed a population-based study of 1461 prospectively followed, asymptomatic subjects who

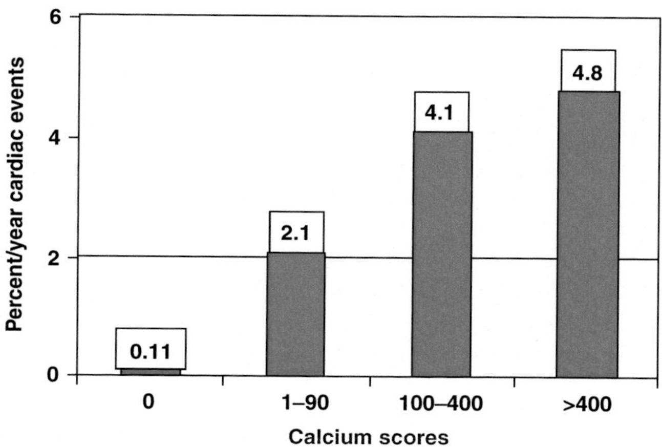

Fig. 5.4 Relationship of coronary artery calcium score to annual hard cardiac event rates in 632 asymptomatic patients undergoing EBT calcified plaque imaging. The solid line indicates the 2 %/year event rate consistent with secondary prevention risk

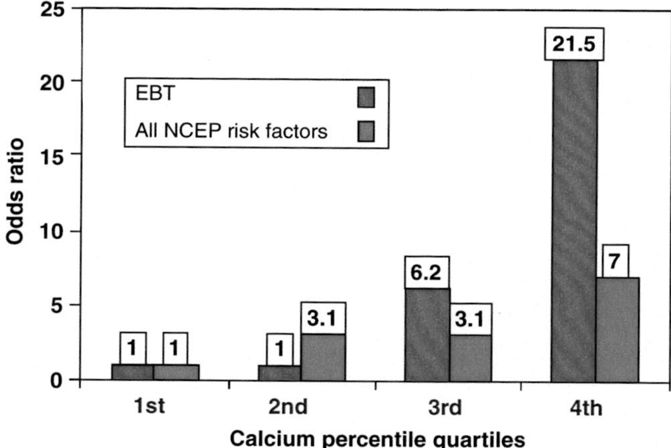

Fig. 5.5 Odds ratios of coronary artery calcium and NCEP risk factor quartiles for annual hard cardiac event rates in asymptomatic patients undergoing coronary artery calcium imaging

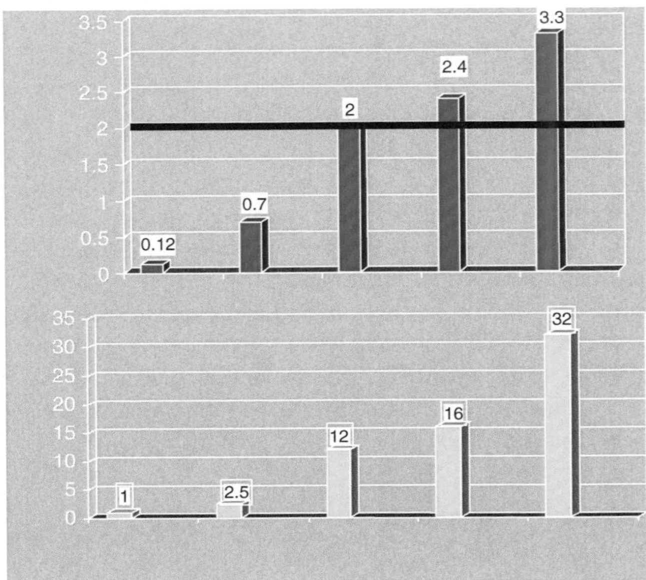

Fig. 5.6 Annual event rates and relative risks for cardiac events in 5585 asymptomatic patients at different levels of coronary artery calcium (St. Francis Heart Study). The solid line indicates the 2 %/year event rate consistent with secondary prevention risk

Table 5.2 Risk of coronary events associated with increasing coronary artery calcium after adjusting for standard risk factors in MESA

CAC	Annual rate	Events/no at risk	HR	P
0	0.11 %	15/3409	1.0	<0.001
1–100	0.59 %	39/1728	3.61	<0.001
101–300	1.43 %	41/752	7.73	<0.001
>300	2.87 %	67/833	9.67	<0.001
Doubling			1.26	<0.001

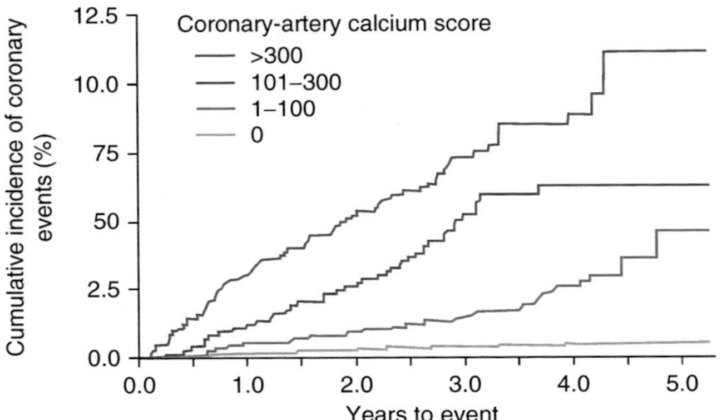

Fig. 5.7 Coronary events at different CAC levels in MESA

were predominantly moderate to high risk, and found that CAC scores >300 significantly added prognostic information to Framingham risk analysis in the 10–20 % Framingham risk category. The results of the St Francis Heart Study by Arad et al. [46] in a prospective, population-based study of 5585 asymptomatic, predominantly moderate- to moderately-high-risk men and women, mirrored previous retrospective studies [7, 18–20], and confirmed the higher event rates associated with increasing CAC scores. CAC scores >100 were associated with relative risks of from 12 to 32, and were secondary prevention equivalent, with event rates >2 %/year (Fig. 5.6). Incremental information over Framingham scores was documented with areas under the ROC curves of 0.81 for CAC and 0.71 for Framingham ($p<0.01$).

The prognostic significance of very high calcium scores was provided in a study of 98 asymptomatic patients with a CAC score >1000 who were followed for 17 months [47] during which 35 patients (36 %) suffered a hard cardiac event (myocardial infarction or cardiac death). The annualized event rate of 25 % refuted the erroneous concept that extensive calcified plaque may confer protection against plaque rupture and events.

In a younger cohort of 2000 asymptomatic Army personnel, Taylor et al. [48] demonstrated the powerful predictive value of CAC. There was a relative risk of 11.8 in patients with CAC >44 compared to those with 0 CAC, after correcting for the Framingham Risk Score. In a much more elderly population (71 years), Vliegenthart et al. found a hazard ratio of 4.6 for CAC 400–1000 compared to <100 after 3.3 years of follow up [49].

Subsequently, even more powerful data have emerged. Budoff et al. [50] in another all cause mortality study, with retrospective analysis of 25,203 asymptomatic patients after 6.8 years, found that CAC >400 was associated with a hazard ratio of 9.2. In the largest study using coronary calcium percentile rather than absolute scores, Becker et al. [51] in 1724 patients followed prospectively for 3.4 years, reported hazard ratios for CAC percentile >75 % versus 0 % of 6.8 for men and 7.9 for women. The area under the ROC curve for CAC percentile (0.81) was significantly superior to the Framingham (0.66), European Society of Cardiology (0.65), and PROCAM risk scores (0.63). Eighty two percent of patients who developed myocardial infarction or cardiac death were correctly classified as high risk by CAC percentile, compared to only 30 % by Framingham, 36 % by the European Society of Cardiology, and 32 % by PROCAM.

Perhaps the most important study is the Multiethnic Study of Atherosclerosis, an NHLBI sponsored prospective evaluation of 6814 patients followed for 3.8 years [23]. Compared to patients with 0 CAC, the hazard ratios for a coronary event were 7.73 for those with CAC 101–300, and 9.67 among participants for CAC >300 ($P<0.001$) (Table 5.2; Fig. 5.7).

Table 5.3 Characteristics and risk ratio for follow-up studies using coronary artery calcium in asymptomatic persons

Author	N	Mean age (years)	Follow-up duration (years)	Calcium score cutoff	Comparator group for RR calculation	Relative risk ratio
Arad [42]	1173	53	3.6	CAC >160	CAC <160	20.2
Park [108]	967	67	6.4	CAC >142.1	CAC <3.7	4.9
Raggi [40]	632	52	2.7	Top quartile	Lowest quartile	13
Wong [41]	926	54	3.3	Top quartile (>270)	First quartile	8.8
Kondos [43]	5635	51	3.1	CAC	No CAC	10.5
Greenland [45]	1312	66	7.0	CAC >300	No CAC	3.9
Shaw [44]	10,377	53	5	CAC ≥400	CAC ≤10	8.4
Arad [46]	5585	59	4.3	CAC ≥100	CAC <100	10.7
Taylor [48]	2000	40–50	3.0	CAC >44	CAC = 0	11.8
Vliegenthart [49]	1795	71	3.3	CAC >1000	CAC < 100	8.3
Budoff [50]	25,503	56	6.8	CAC >400	CAC 0	9.2
Lagoski [53]	3601	45–84	3.75	CAC >0	CAC 0	6.5
Becker [51]	1726	57.7	3.4	CAC >400	CAC 0	6.8 men 7.9 women
Detrano [23]	6814	62.2	3.8	CAC >300	CAC 0	14.1
Erbel [55]	4487	45–75	5	>75th %	<25th %	11.1 men 3.2 women

CAC coronary artery calcium score

Among the four racial and ethnic groups (Caucasian, Chinese, Hispanic, Black), doubling the CAC increased risk of any coronary event by 18–39 %. The ROC curve areas were significantly higher ($p<0.001$) with the addition of CAC to standard risk factors. CAC was more predictive of coronary disease than carotid intima-media thickness; the hazard ratios per 1-SD increment increased 2.5-fold (95 % CI, 2.1–3.1) for CAC and 1.2-fold (95 % CI, 1.0–1.4) for IMT [52].

In the 2684 patients in the female component of MESA [53], Lagoski et al. reported a 6.5 hazard ratio for the 32 % with a CAC >0 versus the 68 % with 0 CAC, even though 90 % were low risk by Framingham. In an analysis of all cause mortality in 44,052 asymptomatic patients followed for 5.6 years [54], the deaths/1000 patient years were 7.48 for CAC >10, compared to 1.92 for CAC 1–10, and 0.87 for 0 CAC. Finally, in a meta-analysis of 64,873 patients followed for 4.2 years, the coronary event rate was 1 %/year for the 42,283 with CAC >0, compared to 0.13 %/year in the 25,903 patients with 0 CAC [38].

Finally, in the Heinz Nixdorf Recall Study [55], 4487 subjects without CAD were followed for 5 years. Low ATP III risk was noted in 51.5 %, while 28.8 % and 19.7 % were at intermediate and high risk, respectively. The prevalence of low (<100), intermediate (100–399) and high (≥400) CAC scores was 72.9 %, 16.8 % and 10.3 %, respectively ($p<0.0001$). The relative risk of CAC >75th vs ≤25th percentile was 11.1 ($p<0.0001$) for men and 3.2 ($p=0.006$) for women. Adding CAC to the ATP III categories improved the AUC from 0.602 to 0.727 in men and from 0.660 to 0.723 in women, and led to a reclassification of 77.1 % of intermediate risk individuals (62.9 % into low risk, and 14.1 % into high risk group). The relative risk associated with doubling of the CAC score was 1.32 (95 % CI: 1.20–1.45, $p<0.001$) in men and 1.25 (95 % CI: 1.11–1.42, $p<0.0001$) in women.

Table 5.4 Summary of CAC absolute event rates from 14,856 patients in five prospective studies

CAC	FRS risk	Ten years event rate
0	Very low	1.1–1.7 %
1–100	Low	2.3–5.9 %
100–400	Intermediate	12.8–16.4 %
>400	High	22.5–28.6 %
>1000	Very high	37 %

Abbreviations: *CAC* coronary artery calcium, *FRS* Framingham risk score

In all of these studies, receiver operator characteristic curves for CAC were superior to the Framingham Risk Score and the annual event rate for CAC >100–400 exceeded the coronary artery disease equivalent of >2 %/year. Table 5.3 summarizes the relative risk results of the largest published outcome studies.

Amalgamation of data from five large prospective randomized studies [23, 46, 49, 51, 55] yields 10 year event rates that can be translated into Framingham Risk Score equivalents (Table 5.4). CAC >400 is a CAD equivalent,

Table 5.5 Reclassification of FRS risk by CAC primary prevention outcome studies

Study	% reclassified	N	Age	Follow up (years)
MESA		5878	62.2	5.8
FRS 0–6 %	11.6 %			
FRS 6–20 %	54.4 %			
FRS >20 %	35.8 %			
NRI	25 %			
Heinz Nixdorf		4487	45–75	5.0
FRS <10 %	15.0 %			
FRS 10–20 %	65.6 %			
FRS >20 %	34.2 %			
Rotterdam		2028	69.6	9.2
FRS <10 %	12 %			
FRS 10–20 %	52 %			
FRS >20 %	34 %			
NRI	19 %			

Abbreviations: *CAC* coronary artery calcium, *FRS* Framingham risk score, *MESA* multiethnic study of atherosclerosis

with 10 year event rates exceeding 20 % in asymptomatic patients. The absence of calcified plaque conveys an extraordinarily low 10 year risk (1.1–1.7 %), irrespective of the number of risk factors [56].

Of critical importance is the net reclassification index (NRI) conferred by CAC in the asymptomatic population by three major prospective population based studies [23, 49, 55] (Table 5.5). The percentage of patients with FRS risk estimate correctly reclassified by CAC based on outcomes ranged from 52 to 65.6 % in the intermediate risk population, 34–35.8 % in the high risk group and 11.6–15 % in the low risk cohort, with NRI's for the entire study population from 19 to 25 %.

Zero Coronary Artery Calcium Scores

Individuals with zero CAC scores have not yet developed detectable, calcified coronary plaque but they may have fatty streaking and early stages of plaque. Non-calcified plaques are present in many young adults. Nonetheless, the event rate in patients with CAC score 0 is very low [40, 45, 46]. Raggi et al. [40] demonstrated an annual event rate of 0.11 % in asymptomatic subjects with 0 scores (amounting to a 10-year risk of only 1.1 %), and in the St Francis Heart Study [46], scores of 0 were associated with a 0.12 % annual event rate over the ensuing 4.3 years. Greenland et al. [45], in a higher-risk asymptomatic cohort, noted a higher annual event rate (0.62 %) with 0 CAC scores; a less sensitive CAC detection technique and marked ethnic heterogeneity may have contributed to their findings. In the definitive MESA study [23], 0 CAC was associated with a 0.11 % annual event rate. In a meta-analysis of 64,873 patients followed for 4.2 years [54], the coronary event rate was 0.13 %/year in the 25,903 patients with 0 CAC compared to 1 %/year for the 42,283 with CAC >0. In an analysis of all cause mortality in 44,052 asymptomatic patients followed for 5.6 years [54], the deaths/1000 patient years for the 19,898 with 0 CAC was 0.87, compared to 1.92 for CAC 1–10, and 7.48 for CAC >10.

While non-calcified, potentially "vulnerable" plaque is by definition not detected by CAC testing, CAC can identify the pool of higher-risk asymptomatic patients out of which will emerge approximately 95 % of the patients presenting each year with sudden death or an acute myocardial infarction (MI). While the culprit lesion contains calcified plaque in only 80 % of the acute events [57], of greater importance is the observation that exclusively soft, non-calcified plaque has been seen in only 5 % of acute ischemic syndromes in both younger and older populations [12, 58]. In a more recent meta-analysis [38], only 2 of 183 (1.1 %) 0 CAC patients were ultimately diagnosed with an acute coronary syndrome after presenting with acute chest pain, normal troponin, and equivocal EKG findings. CAC >0 had 99 % sensitivity, 57 % specificity, 24 % positive predictive value, and 99 % negative predictive value for ACS. Thus, while it is uncommon that a patient with an imminent acute ischemic syndrome would have had a 0 CAC score, further evaluation, particularly with CCTA, is mandatory.

Adherence to Therapeutic Interventions

With the exception of a single study flawed by insufficient power [59], CAC has been shown to have a positive effect on initiation of and adherence to medication and life style changes. In 505 asymptomatic patients, statin adherence 3.6 years after visualizing their CAC scan was 90 % in those with CAC >400 compared to 75 % for 100–399, 63 % for 1–99, and 44 % for 0 CAC ($p<0.0001$) [60]. Similarly, in 980 asymptomatic subjects followed for 3 years, ASA initiation, dietary changes, and exercise increased significantly from those with 0 CAC (29 %, 33 %, 44 %, respectively) and was lowest (29 %) in those with CAC >400 (61 %, 67 %, 56 %, respectively [61]. Finally, after a 6 year follow up in 1640 asymptomatic subjects, the odds ratios for those with CAC >0 compared to 0 CAC for usage of statins, ASA, and statin+ASA were 3.53, 3.05 and 6.97, respectively [62]. In the Eisner (Early Identification of Subclinical Atherosclerosis by Noninvasive Imaging Research) trial, 2137 asymptomatic patients were randomized to using CAC to guide treatment or employing usual care [63]. CAC directed care produced significant improvement in systolic blood pressure, LDL-C, weight and waist size compared to usual care, without an increase in downstream testing. Patients with CAC >400

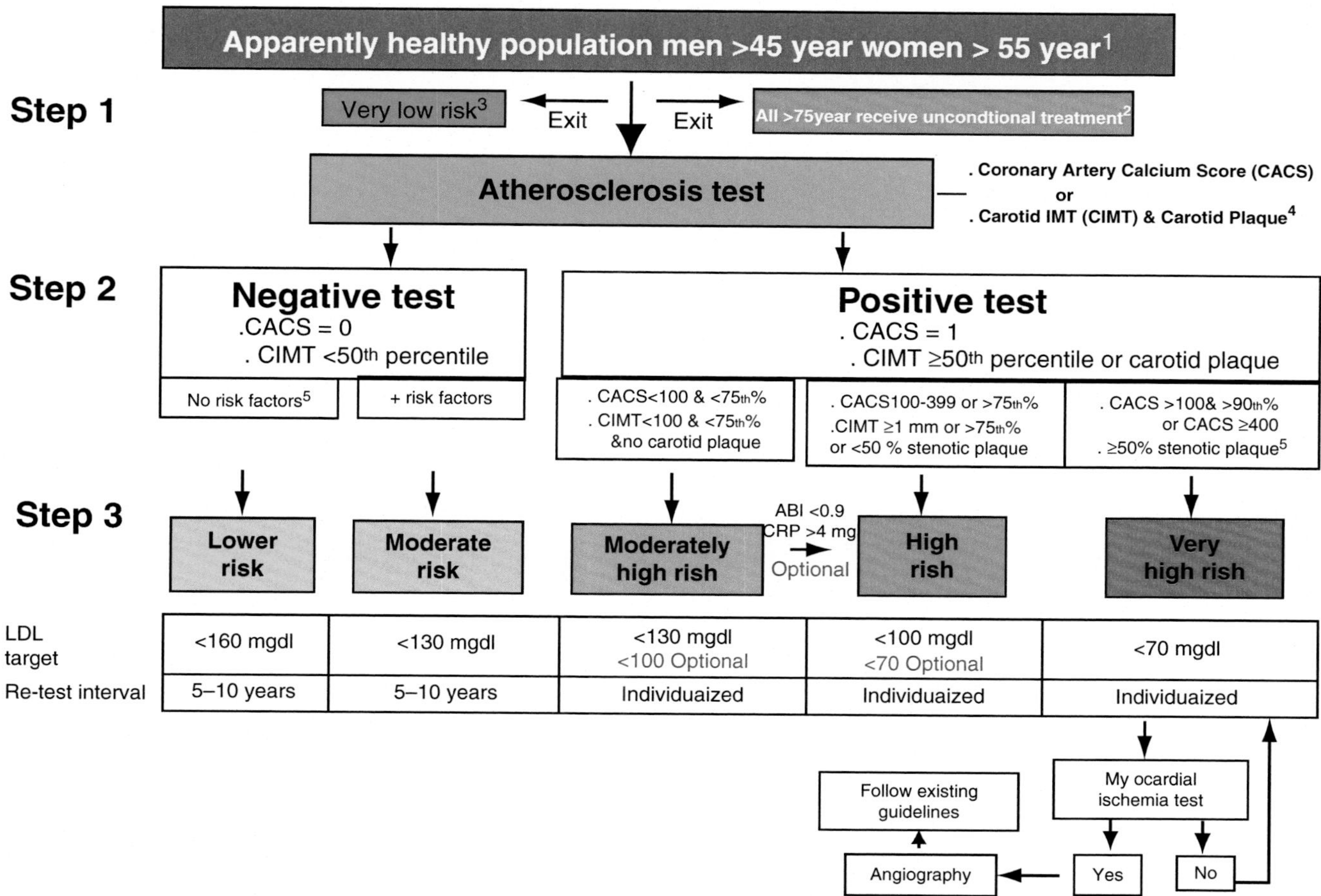

Fig. 5.8 The SHAPE guideline (Towards the National Screening for Heart Attack Prevention and Education Program)

had significantly greater improvement in all parameters than those with 0 CAC.

Coronary Artery Calcium and Guidelines

In 2006, the SHAPE guidelines (Fig. 5.8) recommended CAC or carotid intima-media thickening for all but the lowest risk asymptomatic men >45 years and women >55 years, with subsequent treatment based upon the amount of CAC [64].

The 2010 ACCF/AHA Guideline for Assessment of Cardiovascular Risk in Asymptomatic Adults appropriately assigned a class IIa recommendation to CAC for evaluation of the asymptomatic intermediate-risk population and for all patients older than 40 with diabetes mellitus [65]. On the basis of flawed assumptions, the 2013 American College of Cardiology (ACC)/AHA Guideline on the Treatment of Blood Cholesterol to Reduce Atherosclerotic Cardiovascular Risk in Adults [66] and the 2013 ACC/AHA Guideline on the Assessment of Cardiovascular Risk [67] assigned CAC to a class IIb recommendation for low intermediate risk (<7.5 %), similar to the 2010 guidelines for low-intermediate risk (6–10 %, class IIb). CAC is now recommended when clinical decision making is unclear (by physician or patient), for those with risk <7.5 % and they state "assessing CAC is likely to be the most useful of the current approaches to improving risk assessment among individuals found to be at intermediate risk after formal risk assessment." This however does essentially exclude the intermediate risk population for which the NRI by CAC in three major population-based prospective outcome studies [23, 49, 55] has ranged from 52 to 66 % (see Table 5.3). The outcomes on which the 2013 guidelines were based were changed by the addition of stroke, for which the investigators believed there was not sufficient CAC data, even though the Heinz Nixdorf Recall Study of 4180 patients demonstrated hazard ratios of CAC for stroke to be similar to age, hypertension, and smoking (Table 5.6) [68]. Further, the MESA data shows CVD (including stroke) performs as well as CAD [69]. Erroneous cost and radiation exposure concerns were also used to justify the classification, despite the $100 CAC cost and the decrease in radiation to <1 mSv.

Table 5.6 Relationship between coronary artery calcium and events in asymptomatic diabetic patients

Study	n	Prevalence	Hazard ratio	AUC	Event rates/year
Wong [85]	1823	Any CAC			
		No DM: 53 %			
		DM: 73.5 %			
Becker [86]	716 DM	0 CAC: 15 %		CAC: 0.77 0	CAC: 0.2 %
		CAC >400: 42 %		FRS: 0.68	CAC >400:5.6 %
				UKPDS: 0.71	
				P<0.01	
Eikeles [87]	589 DM		Compared to CAC 0–10	CAC: 0.73	CAC <10: 0 %
			CAC >1000: 13.8	UKPDS: 0.63	
			CAC 401–1000: 8.4	P<0.03	
			CAC 101–400: 7.1		
			CAC 11–100: 4.0		
Anand [88]	510 DM	CAC <10: 53.7 %	Compared with CAC <100	CAC: 0.92	
			CAC >1000: 58	UKPDS: 0.74	
			CAC 401–1000: 41	FRS: 0.60	
			CAC 101–400: 10	P<0.001	
			CAC 0–100: 1		
Malik [89]	881 DM		Inc. CAC: 2.9–6.5	CAC+RF: 0.78–0.80	1.5 %
	4036 No DM		Inc. CAC: 2.6–9.5	RF: 0.72–0.73	0.5 %
				P<0.001	

Source: Wiley from Hecht and Narula [107]

AUC area under curve, *CAC* coronary artery calcium, *DM* diabetes mellitu, *FRS* Framingham risk score, *Inc.* increasing, *MetS* metabolic syndrome, *RF* risk factors, *UKPDS* UK prospective diabetes study

Correlation with Risk Factors

Correlation in Individual Patients with Conventional Risk Factors

Conventional risk factors do correlate with CAC [70–72], even though CAC is superior to conventional risk factors in predicting outcomes. There is a clear association of CAC with a premature family history of CAD, diabetes, and lipid values in large groups of patients. However, the difficulty equating risk factors with CAC in individual patients has been highlighted by the work of Hecht et al. in 930 consecutive primary prevention subjects undergoing EBT [71]. They found increasing likelihoods of CAC with increasing levels of low-density lipoprotein cholesterol (LDL-C) and decreasing levels of high-density lipoprotein cholesterol (HDL-C) in the population as a whole, but found no differences in the amount of plaque between groups and demonstrated a total lack of correlation in *individual* patients between the EBT calcium percentile and the levels of total, LDL- and HDL-cholesterol, total/HDL-cholesterol, triglycerides, lipoprotein(a) (Lp(a)), homocysteine, and LDL particle size.

Postmenopausal women presented a striking example of the inability of conventional risk analysis to predict the presence or absence of subclinical atherosclerosis [73]. There were no differences in any lipid parameters or in the Framingham Risk Scores between postmenopausal women with and without calcified plaque, rendering therapeutic decisions that are not plaque- imaging-based extremely problematic.

The very limited value of individual risk factors for risk prediction was illustrated by Nasir et al. [56] in 44,952 primary prevention patients followed for 5.6 years. The decrease in survival in 0 CAC subjects with increasing numbers of risk factors was trivial, declining from 99.7 % with no risk factors to 99.0 % with ≥3 risk factors. Patients with a CAC >400 and no risk factors had 7× the risk of 0 CAC patients with ≥3 risk factors (16.9 vs 2.7 events per 1000 patients years.

Correlation with Novel Risk Factors

MESA extended the risk factor inferiority to more novel risk factors, including hs-CRP, carotid IMT, ankle bracial index, flow mediated vasodilation and family history of premature CAD, (Table 5.7). In 1330 intermediate risk patients followed for 7.6 years in the Multiethnic Study of Atherosclerosis, CAC had the highest HR and correctly reclassified 66 % of FRS predicted outcomes [69]. Similarly, in 1286 asymptomatic patients with a 4.1 year follow up, a combination of five blood biomarker risk factors, including hs-CRP, interleuk-6, myeloperoxidase, beta natriuretic protein and plasminogen activator-1, did not significantly increase the FRS c-statistic. CAC, on the other hand, increased it from 0.73 to 0.84 ($p<0.003$) [74].

The poor risk prediction performance of hs-CRP and its lack of correlation with CAC do not challenge the inflammatory aspects of the disease process. Rather, it emphasizes the greater value of evidence of the disease itself, namely CAC, compared to a risk marker, such as hs-CRP. Moreover, inflammation is the central commonality for a host of diseases characterized by higher incidences of both subclinical and clinical atherosclerosis (Fig. 5.9).

There is much less data regarding lipoprotein-associated phospholipase A2 (Lp-PLA2). In a nested case–control study among 266 CARDIA participants [75], Lp-PLA2 mass was significantly higher in subjects with CAC compared to those without CAC (OR 1.28). The numbers are too small to provide meaningful conclusions.

Table 5.7 Comparison of novel risk markers for improvement in cardiovascular risk assessment in 1330 intermediate-risk individuals

Marker	Multivariate HR	p	NRI vs FRS
ABI	0.79	.01	.036
Brachial FMD	0.82	.52	.024
CAC	2.60	<.001	.659
Carotid IMT	1.33	.13	.102
Family history	2.18	.001	.160
hs-CRP	1.26	.05	.079

Genetics

The lack of clear relationship between lipid levels and subclinical plaque in individual patients does not negate the atherogenic effect of these metabolic disorders. Rather, it highlights the variations in individual susceptibility to the atherogenic effects at a given plasma level, very likely mediated by as yet undetermined genetic factors. O'Donnell et al. [76], in an analysis of abdominal aortic calcium in 2151 patients in 1159 families in the Framingham Study, noted a heritability component accounting for up to 49 % of the variability in calcified plaque, and concluded that "AAC deposits are heritable atherosclerotic traits. A substantial portion of the variation is due to the additive effects of genes, which have yet to be characterized." Peyser et al. [77], analyzing coronary calcium in 698 patients in 302 families, found a variance of up to 48 % associated with additive polygenes after adjustment for covariates. They concluded that there is a: substantial genetic component for subclinical CAD variation . . . even after accounting for effects of genes acting through measured risk factors. These genes may act through other measurable risk factors or through novel pathways that have not or cannot be measured in vivo. Identification of such genes will provide a better basis for prevention and treatment of subclinical CAD.

Unfortunately, the single nucleotide polymorphism arena has not yet delivered any clinically concrete options.

The inevitable conclusion of the consistent lack of relationship between risk factors and disease and the superiority

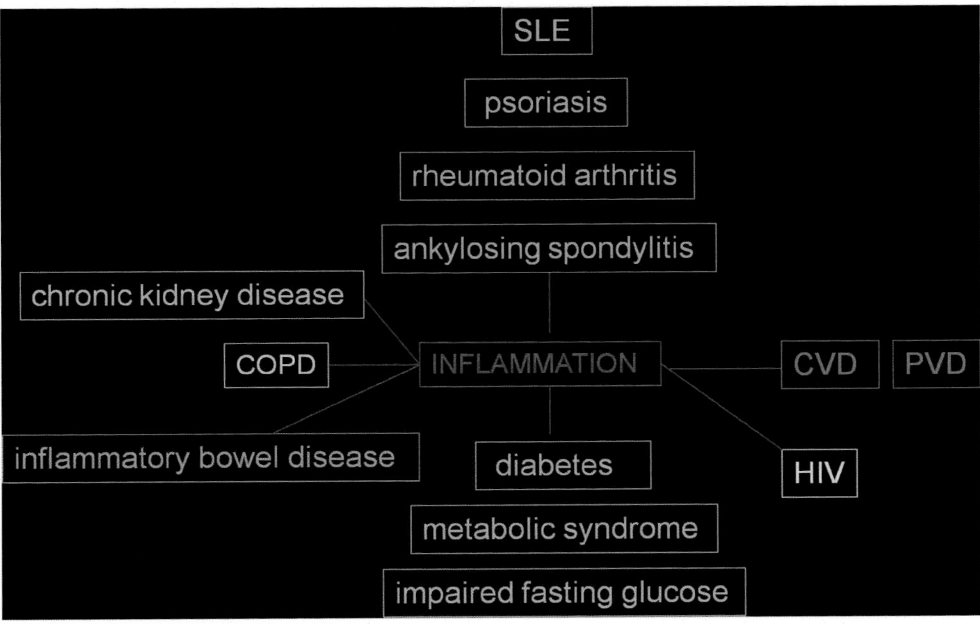

Fig. 5.9 Inflammatory diseases associated with a higher risk of coronary artery disease. *Abbreviations*: *COPD* chronic obstructive pulmonary disease, *CVD* cardiovascular disease, *HIV* human immunodeficiency virus, *PVD* peripheral vascular disease, *SLE* systemic lupus erythematosus

of CAC in individual patients was summarized by Hecht [78]: "*The most important role of risk factors may be to identify the modifiable targets of risk reduction in patients with risk already established by clinical events or significant CAC.*"

Clinical Applications

Patient Selection

Intermediate Risk

Hecht et al. [79] proposed recommendations for the application of CAC scanning (Table 5.8). The Framingham Risk Score [80], incorporating both age and gender, was recommended as the initial step in selecting the appropriate test populations. Asymptomatic patients in the National Cholesterol Education Adult Treatment Program III [81] classified 10–20 % Framingham 10-year risk category (intermediate risk) comprise the group that presents the greatest challenge to the treating physician, and are those in whom the application of CAC scoring is most appropriate; the CAC score can assist the physician in decisions regarding the initiation of statin therapy and lifestyle modifications. As previously noted, the NRI for this group ranges from 52 % to 66 %, with subsequent appropriate downgrading or upgrading of medical therapy for this majority of the intermediate risk group.

Lower Risk

Patients with less than 10 % Framingham risk may also benefit from CAC scoring to guide management decisions. For instance, most young patients with a family history of premature CAD will not have sufficient risk factors to even warrant Framingham scoring (lower NCEP risk) or will be in the moderate (1–10 % 10-year Framingham risk group), since family history, while an NCEP risk factor, does not contribute points to the Framingham score. In 222 young patients presenting with an MI as the first sign of CAD (mean age 50 years), Akosah et al. [82] demonstrated that 70 % were in these lesser risk categories and would not have been started on a statin using NCEP guidelines. Data from Schmermund et al. [12] and Pohle et al. [58] indicate that 95 % of acute MI patients would have been identified by CAC plaque imaging irrespective of age. On the basis of these observations, the use of CAC scoring should be considered in patients with a family history of premature CAD, irrespective of the FRS, as recommended by the 2009 CAC Appropriate Use Criteria [83]. Irrespective of family history, the NRI in the low risk population ranges from 11.6 to 16 %; approximately one of every eight low risk patients will miss the opportunity for recognition of their increased risk and upgrading of therapy in the absence of CAC scanning.

Higher Risk

With an NRI of 35 % for the FRS >20 % group, scanning of this cohort appears appropriate, with treatment and goals to be determined by the CAC level. Whether or not clinicians will consider downgrading intensity of treatment is quite problematic, since it is not guideline based.

Examples of risk transformation are shown in Figs. 5.10, 5.11, and 5.12. A 57-year old man with hypertension, total cholesterol 235 mg/dL, LDL-C 150 mg/dL, HDL-C 75 mg/dL, and a 10-year Framingham risk of 12 %, was referred for CAC scanning. The CAC score was 1872, in the >99th % for his age, placing him in the highest risk category with LDL-C treatment goal of <70 mg/dL (Fig. 5.10).

Figure 5.11a displays the CAC scan of a 41-year-old woman whose mother experienced a myocardial infarction at age 55. The total cholesterol was 188 mg/dL, LDL-C 112 mg/dL, HDL-C 50 mg/dL and triglycerides 132 mg/dL. She was in the 0–1 risk factor group in which a

Table 5.8 Recommendations for treatment in asymptomatic, NCEP classified moderately high-risk patients based upon CAC score

CAC score/percentile	Framingham risk group equivalent	LDL goal (mg/dL)	Drug therapy (mg/dL)
0	Lower risk; 0–1 risk factors; Framingham risk assessment not required	<160	≥190
			160–189: drug optional
1–10 and ≤75th %	Moderate risk; 2+risk factors (<10 % Framingham 10-year risk)	<130	≥160
11–100 and ≤75th %	Moderately high risk; 2+risk factors (10–20 % Framingham 10-year risk)	<130	≥130
			100–129: consider drug
101–400 or >75th %	High risk; CAD risk equivalent (>20 % Framingham 10-year risk)	<100 Optional goal <70	≥100
			<100: consider drug
>400 or >90th %	Highest risk[a]	<100 Optional goal <70	Any LDL level

[a]Based on CAC score; consider beta blockers

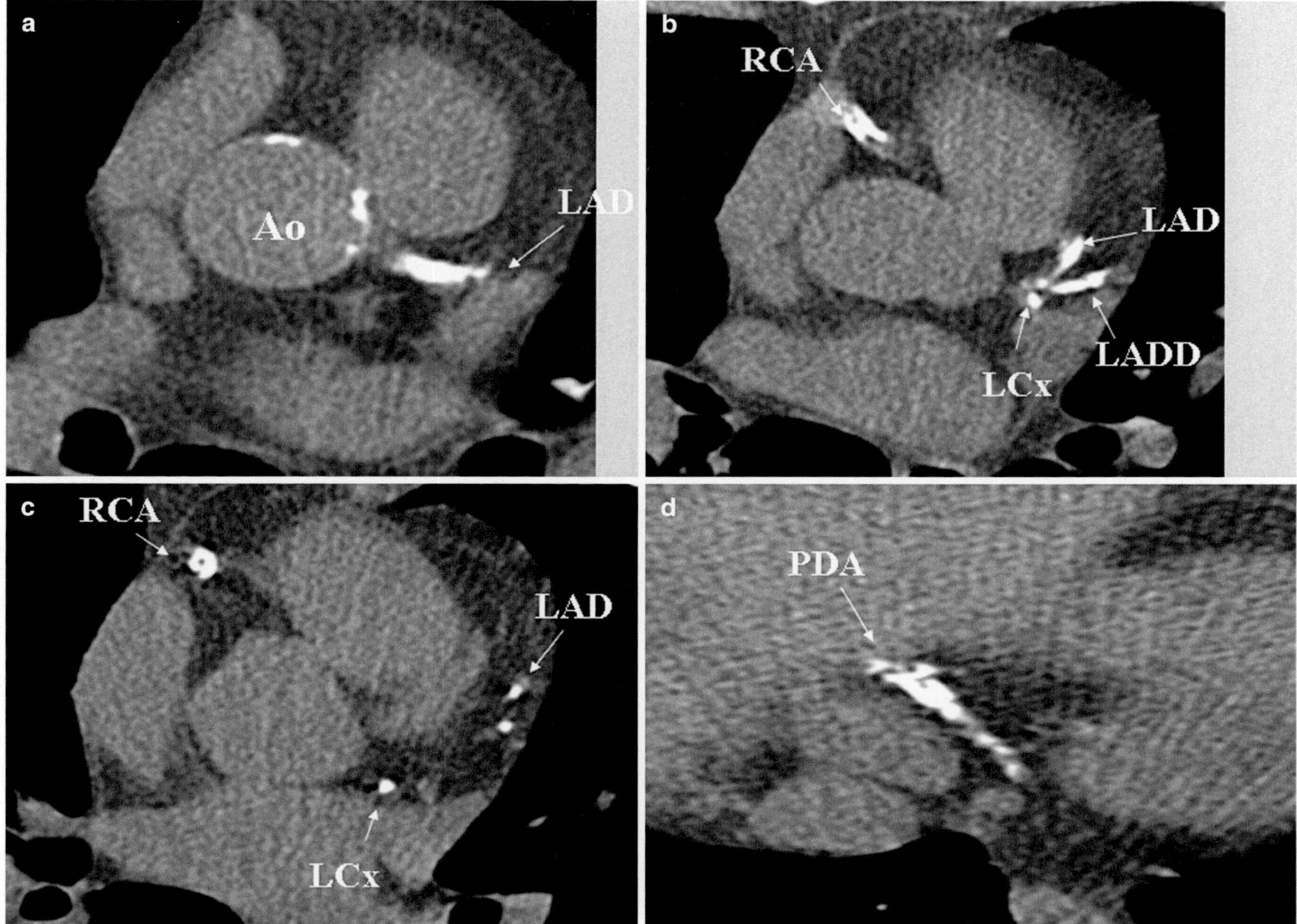

Fig. 5.10 A 57-year-old man with hypertension, total cholesterol 235 mg/dL, LDL-C 150 mg/dL, HDL-C 75 mg/dL, and a 10-year Framingham risk of 12 % referred for CAC scanning; CAC score was 1872, in the >99th percentile. Slices from base (**a**) through apex (**d**) reveal significant CAC in all coronary arteries and the ascending aorta. *Ao* aorta, *LAD* left anterior descending coronary artery, *LADD* diagonal branch of left anterior descending coronary artery, *LCx* left circumflex coronary artery, *PDA* posterior descending branch of right coronary artery, *RCA* right coronary artery

Framingham Risk Score need not be calculated. The CAC score was 110, in the left anterior descending (LAD) and diagonal branch, in the >99th percentile for her age, placing her in a high-risk category. She developed symptoms, underwent dual isotope nuclear stress testing (Fig. 5.11b), which revealed severe anteroseptal ischemia, followed by angiography and placement of a stent to treat a 95 % ostial LAD stenosis (Fig. 5.11c). Statin therapy was implemented to reduce the LDL-C to <70 mg/dL.

A 65- year-old male hypertensive smoker, with an LDL-C of 140 mg/dL and a 10-year Framingham risk of 25 %, was very reluctant to take a statin prescribed for his LDL-C. A CAC scan was performed (Fig. 5.12), which demonstrated total absence of calcified plaque, despite the presumed high risk. Therapeutic life changes, rather than statins, were recommended.

Other Applications

Diabetes

The 2010 ACC Guideline for Assessment of Risk in Asymptomatic Adults awarded CAC a Class IIa recommendation for all adults older than 40 with diabetes [65]. While the initial reasoning was to identify the high risk patients with CAC >400 for further evaluation to rule out obstructive disease, CAC prognostic data have challenged the ingrained concept of diabetes mellitus as a CAD disease equivalent. Patients with diabetes and CAC have higher risks than those without diabetes and similar CAC, but the absence of CAC conveys a similar low risk in both groups [84–90]. Therefore, the more appropriate rationale is for straightforward risk classification as with any other risk factor, allowing for the possibility of downgrading risk.

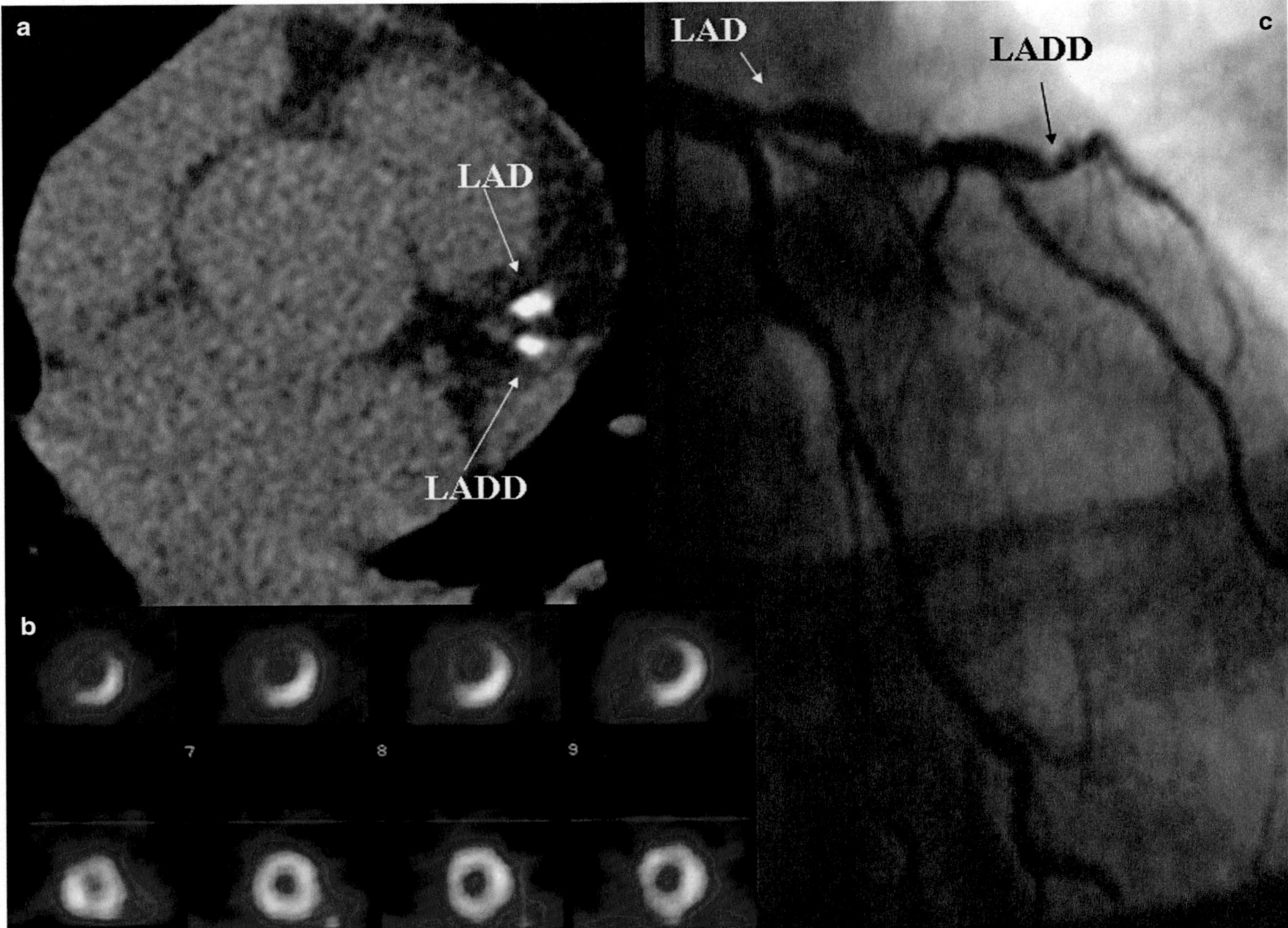

Fig. 5.11 A 41-year-old woman with a premature family history of CAD, total cholesterol 188 mg/dL, LDL-C 112 mg/dL, HDL-C 50 mg/dL, and triglycerides 132 mg/dL, in the lowest Framingham risk group. (**a**) CAC score of 110, in the left anterior descending and diagonal branch, in the >99th percentile. (**b**) Dual isotope nuclear stress testing revealing severe anteroseptal ischemia. (**c**) Angiography demonstrating 95 % ostial LAD stenosis and severe LADD disease. *LAD* left anterior descending coronary artery, *LADD* diagonal branch of left anterior descending coronary artery

Repeat Scanning

The use of serial CAC scanning to evaluate the progression of disease and the effects of therapy is a powerful emerging indication that will be covered in greater detail in Chap. 6. Asymptomatic patients with a 0 CAC score should not undergo repeat scanning for at least 4 years. The average time to conversion to a >0 CAC was 4.1 ± 0.9 years and the average score at the time of conversion was 19 ± 19 [91]. The repeat scanning interval in patients with >0 CAC is not data determined. Rather, logic dictates that the greater the concern, the shorter should be the interval. The low radiation dose makes repeat scanning less problematic.

Stress Testing

Since stress testing should only be performed in symptomatic patients, in whom CAC is not indicated, the interplay between the two is limited. Nonetheless, a combination of CAC and stress EKG has been advocated in symptomatic patients. However, coronary CTA is clearly the CT modality of choice, and will very likely replace stress testing as the first test in the evaluation of symptomatic patients [92].

In asymptomatic patients, post CAC stress testing is an issue, and the appropriateness of stress testing after CAC scanning is directly related to the CAC score. The data indicate that the incidence of abnormal nuclear stress testing is 1.3 %, 11.3 % and 35.2 % for CAC scores of <100,100–400

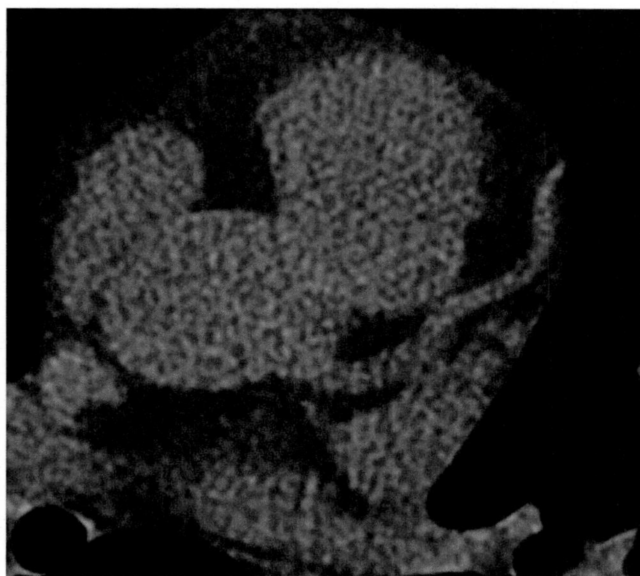

Fig. 5.12 A 65-year-old male hypertensive smoker, LDL-C of 140 mg/dL and a 10-year Framingham risk of 25 %. CAC scan demonstrated total absence of calcified plaque

and >400, respectively [93–97]. It is only in the >400 group that the pretest likelihood is sufficiently high to warrant further evaluation with functional testing. Coronary computed tomographic angiography is appropriate in patients with CAC <1000; higher CAC scores may preclude accurate evaluation. It is never appropriate to proceed directly to the catheterization laboratory from a CAC scan in asymptomatic patients.

Evaluation of incidental findings, particularly lung nodules, should follow standard radiology guidelines [98].

Cardiomyopathy

CAC may be used to differentiate ischemic from nonischemic cardiomyopathies. Budoff et al. [99] demonstrated in 120 patients with heart failure of unknown etiology that the presence of CAC was associated with a 99 % sensitivity for ischemic cardiomyopathy. Nonetheless, coronary CTA has replaced CAC for this indication.

Emergency Department Chest Pain Evaluation

Emergency department triage of chest pain patients by CAC has been totally supplanted by CCTA. Several early studies demonstrated potential application of CAC to the ED. Laudon et al. [100] reported on 105 patients. Of the 46 with positive scores (>0), 14 had abnormal follow-up inpatient testing. Of the 59 with 0 calcium scores, stress evaluation and/or coronary arteriography were normal in the 54 who underwent further testing and all were free of cardiac events 4 months later (100 % negative predictive value). Georgiou et al. [101] noted 41 cardiac events in 192 emergency room patients followed for 37 months; all but four were associated with calcium scores ≥4. However, CCTA data have clearly demonstrated a small (5 %) but finite incidence of obstructive disease in 0 CAC patients with chest pain [102], mandating performance of CCTA rather than CAC alone in this setting

Limitations

Frequently cited limitations of CAC are assuming much less importance. Radiation is no longer a significant issue as the absorbed radiation dose falls to the level of mammography. Unfortunately, irresponsible scare tactics have magnified public concern; education is needed to counter these negative effects. Cost has also become less of a concern as the price of CAC scanning has plummeted to ~ $100. "Incidentalomas" and their subsequent evaluation have generated negative sentiments. The frequency of clinically significant findings is 1.2 %, with indeterminate findings at 7.0 % [103]. The associated costs do not negatively impact the cost effectiveness of CAC [104]. Standard guidelines on how to handle these findings may reassure patients and physicians [98]. Patient anxiety related to CAC findings has also been cited as a negative. Anxiety is not an intended consequence but a certain amount is appropriate and inevitable when informed of increased cardiac risk, and may motivate increased adherence. On the other hand, for those with high anxiety of early ASCVD based on a severe family history or a high calculated ASCVD risk score, concern can often be calmed when reclassified toward significantly less risk by CAC. The most persistent criticism is the lack of randomized controlled trials that demonstrate improved patient outcomes through the use of CAC. The appropriate response notes that there "... is a double standard that demands randomized controlled (outcome) trials for CAC screening while ignoring their necessity for every other technology.... It is incumbent on the cardiology community to temper the inflexible need for randomized trials with the reality of 565,000 patients presenting with myocardial infarctions annually as their first symptoms, 95 % of whom could be identified as at high risk by CAC screening and aggressively treated to significantly reduce events [105]."

Conclusions

The validation of CAC scanning as a risk assessment tool may well represent one of the most significant advances in the history of preventive medicine. It offers the possibility of accurately identifying the vast majority of patients destined to suffer acute cardiac events, and, in so doing, should allow for substantial reduction of cardiovascular mortality and morbidity by increasingly effective pharmacologic and lifestyle therapy of the underlying disease process.

It is appropriate to conclude by quoting Dr. Scott Grundy [106]:

The power of imaging for detecting subclinical atherosclerosis to predict future ASCVD events is increasingly being recognized. Imaging has at least three virtues. It individualizes risk assessment beyond use of age, which is a less reliable surrogate for atherosclerosis burden; it provides an integrated assessment of the lifetime exposure to risk factors; and it identifies individuals who are susceptible to developing atherosclerosis beyond established risk factors. Also of importance, in the absence of detectable atherosclerosis, short-term risk appears to be very low. Thus, for primary prevention, a recommendation could be established that detection of significant plaque burden is a preferred strategy for initiation of LDL-lowering drugs. With such a recommendation, major risk factors and emerging risk factors could be used as a guide for selecting subjects for imaging more than as a primary guide for therapy. Once subclinical atherosclerosis is detected, intensity of drug therapy could be adjusted for plaque burden. This 2-step approach to risk assessment could provide a solution to the dilemma of patient selection for cholesterol-lowering drugs in primary prevention. In addition, it could be applied to all population subgroups. It could also be useful as a guide to low-dose aspirin prophylaxis and cholesterol-lowering therapy.

References

1. Heart and stoke statistical update. Dallas: American Heart Association; 2001.
2. Blankenhorn DH, Stern D. Calcification of the coronary arteries. Am J Roentgenol. 1959;81:772–7.
3. Frink RJ, Achor RW, Brown AL, et al. Significance of calcification of the coronary arteries. Am J Cardiol. 1970;26:241–7.
4. Wexler L, Brundage B, Crouse J, et al. Coronary artery calcification: pathophysiology, epidemiology, image methods and clinical implications. A scientific statement from the American Heart Association. Circulation. 1996;94:1175–92.
5. Faber A. Die Arteriosklerose, from Pathologische Anatomie, from Pathogenese Und Actiologie. G. Fischer; 1912.
6. Bostrom K, Watson KE, Horn S, et al. Bone morphogenetic protein expression in human atherosclerotic lesions. J Clin Invest. 1993;91:1800–9.
7. Ideda T, Shirasawa T, Esaki Y, et al. Osteopontin mRNA is expressed by smooth muscle-derived foam cells in human atherosclerotic lesions of the aorta. J Clin Invest. 1993;92:2814–20.
8. Hirota S, Imakita M, Kohri K, et al. Expression of osteopontin messenger RNA by macrophages in atherosclerotic plaques. A possible association with calcification. Am J Pathol. 1993;143:1003–8.
9. Shanahan CM, Cary NR, Metcalfe JC, Weissberg PL. High expression of genes for calcification-regulating proteins in human atherosclerotic plaque. J Clin Invest. 1994;93:2393–402.
10. Rumberger JA, Simons DB, Fitzpatrick LA, et al. Coronary artery calcium areas by electron beam computed tomography and coronary atherosclerotic plaque area: a histopathologic correlative study. Circulation. 1995;92:2157–62.
11. Baumgart D, Schmermund A, Goerge G, et al. Comparison of electron beam computed tomography with intracoronary ultrasound and coronary angiography for detection of coronary atherosclerosis. J Am Coll Cardiol. 1997;30:57–64.
12. Schmermund A, Baumgart D, Gorge G, et al. Coronary artery calcium in acute coronary syndromes: a comparative study of electron beam CT, coronary angiography, and intracoronary ultrasound in survivors of acute myocardial infarction and unstable angina. Circulation. 1997;96:1461–9.
13. Agatston AS, Janowitz WR, Hildner FJ, et al. Quantification of coronary artery calcium using ultrafast computed tomography. J Am Coll Cardiol. 1990;15:827–32.
14. Callister TQ, Cooil B, Raya SP, et al. Coronary artery disease: improved reproducibility of calcium scoring with an electron-beam CT volumetric method. Radiology. 1998;208:807–14.
15. Becker CR, Kleffel T, Crispin A, et al. Coronary artery calcium measurement. Agreement of multirow detector and electron beam CT. Am J Roentgenol. 2001;176:1295–8.
16. Janowitz WR, Agatston AS, Kaplan G, Viamonte M. Differences in prevalence and extent of coronary artery calcium detected by ultrafast computed tomography in asymptomatic men and women. Am J Cardiol. 1993;72:247–54.
17. Hoff JA, Chomka EV, Krainik AJ, et al. Age and gender distributions of coronary artery calcium detected by electron beam tomography in 35,246 adults. Am J Cardiol. 2001;87:1335–9.
18. Budoff MJ, Yang TP, Shavelle RM. Ethnic differences in coronary atherosclerosis. J Am Coll Cardiol. 2002;39:408–12.
19. Newman AB, Naydeck BL, Whittle J, et al. Racial differences in coronary artery calcification in adults. Arterioscler Thromb Vasc Biol. 2002;22:424–30.
20. Khuran C, Rosenbaum CG, Howard BV, et al. Coronary artery calcification in black women and white women. Am Heart J. 2003;145:724–9.
21. Jain T, Peshock R, Darren K, McGuire DK. African Americans and Caucasians have a similar prevalence of coronary calcium in the Dallas Heart Study. J Am Coll Cardiol. 2004;44:1011–7.
22. McClelland RL, Chung H, Detrano R, et al. Distribution of coronary artery calcium by race, gender, and age. Results from the Multi-Ethnic Study of Atherosclerosis (MESA). Circulation. 2006;113:30–7.
23. Detrano R, Guerci AD, Carr JJ, et al. Coronary calcium as a predictor of coronary events in four racial or ethnic groups. N Engl J Med. 2008;358:1336–45.
24. Nasir K, Michos ED, Rumberger JA, et al. Coronary artery calcification and family history of premature coronary heart disease: sibling history is more strongly associated than parental history. Circulation. 2004;110:2150–6.
25. Khurram Nasir K, Budoff MJ, Wong ND, et al. Family history of premature coronary heart disease and coronary artery calcification. Multi-Ethnic Study of Atherosclerosis (MESA). Circulation. 2007;116:619–62.
26. Gerber TC, Carr JJ, Arai AE, et al. Ionizing radiation in cardiac imaging: a science advisory from the American Heart Association

Committee on Cardiac Imaging of the Council on Clinical Cardiology and Committee on Cardiovascular Imaging and Intervention of the Council on Cardiovascular Radiology and Intervention. Circulation. 2009;119:1056–196526.
27. O'Rourke RA, Brundage BH, Froelicher VF, et al. American College of Cardiology/American Heart Association expert consensus document on electron beam computed tomography for the diagnosis and prognosis of coronary artery disease. Circulation. 2000;102:126–40.
28. Simons DB, Schwartz RS, Edwards WD, et al. Noninvasive definition of anatomic coronary disease by ultrafast computed tomographic scanning: a quantitative pathologic comparison study. J Am Coll Cardiol. 1992;20:1118–26.
29. Detrano R, Tang W, Kang X, et al. Accurate coronary calcium phosphate mass measurements from electron beam computed tomograms. Am J Card Imaging. 1995;9:167–73.
30. Mautner GC, Mautner SL, Froelich J, et al. Coronary artery calcification: assessment with electron beam CT and histomorphometric correlation. Radiology. 1994;192:619–23.
31. Budoff MJ, Georgiou D, Brody A, et al. Ultrafast computed tomography as a diagnostic modality in the detection of coronary artery disease-a multicenter study. Circulation. 1996;93:898–904.
32. Guerci AD, Spadaro LA, Popma JJ, et al. Electron Beam tomography of the coronary arteries: relationship of coronary calcium score to arteriographic findings in asymptomatic and symptomatic adults. Am J Cardiol. 1997;79:128–33.
33. Shavelle DM, Budoff MJ, LaMont DH, et al. Exercise testing and electron beam computed tomography in the evaluation of coronary artery disease. J Am Coll Cardiol. 2000;36:32–8.
34. Bielak LF, Rumberger JA, Sheedy PF, et al. Probabilistic model for prediction of agiographically defined obstructive coronary artery disease using electron beam computed tomography calcium score strata. Circulation. 2000;102:380–5.
35. Rumberger JA, Sheedy PF, Breen FJ, et al. Electron beam CT coronary calcium score cutpoints and severity of associated angiography luminal stenosis. J Am Coll Cardiol. 1997;29:1542–8.
36. Haberl R, Becker A, Leber A, et al. Correlation of coronary calcification and angiographically documented stenoses in patients with suspected coronary artery disease: results of 1,764 patients. J Am Coll Cardiol. 2001;37:451–7.
37. Budoff MJ, Raggi P, Berman D, et al. Continuous probabilistic prediction of angiographically significant coronary artery disease using electron beam tomography. Circulation. 2002;105(15):1791–6.
38. Sarwar A, Shaw LJ, Shapiro MD, et al. Diagnostic and prognostic value of absence of coronary artery calcification. J Am Coll Cardiol Img. 2009;2:675–88.
39. Mohlenkamp S, Lehmann N, Schmermund A, et al. Prognostic value of extensive coronary calcium quantities in symptomatic males – a 5-year follow-up study. Eur Heart J. 2003;24:845–54.
40. Raggi P, Callister TQ, Cooil B, et al. Identification of patients at increased risk of first unheralded acute myocardial infarction by electron beam computed tomography. Circulation. 2000;101:850–5.
41. Wong ND, Hsu JC, Detrano RC, et al. Coronary artery calcium evaluation by electron beam compute tomography and its relation to new cardiovascular events. Am J Cardiol. 2000;86:495–8.
42. Arad Y, Spadaro LA, Goodman K, et al. Prediction of coronary events with electron beam computed tomography. J Am Coll Cardiol. 2000;36:1253–60.
43. Kondos GT, Hoff JA, Sevrukov A, et al. Electron-beam tomography coronary artery calcium and cardiac events: a 37-month follow-up of 5,635 initially asymptomatic low to intermediate risk adults. Circulation. 2003;107:2571–6.
44. Shaw LJ, Raggi P, Schisterman E, et al. Prognostic value of cardiac risk factors and coronary artery calcium screening for all-cause mortality. Radiology. 2003;28:826–33.
45. Greenland P, LaBree L, Azen SP, et al. Coronary artery calcium score combined with Framingham score for risk prediction in asymptomatic individuals. JAMA. 2004;291:210–5.
46. Arad Y, Goodman KJ, Roth M, et al. Coronary calcification, coronary risk factors, and atherosclerotic cardiovascular disease events. The St Francis Heart Study. J Am Coll Cardiol. 2005;46(1):158–65.
47. Wayhs R, Zelinger A, Raggi P. High coronary artery calcium scores pose an extremely elevated risk for hard events. J Am Coll Cardiol. 2002;39:225–30.
48. Taylor AJ, Bindeman J, Feuerstein I, et al. Coronary calcium independently predicts incident premature coronary heart disease over measured cardiovascular risk factors mean three-year outcomes in the prospective army C\coronary C\calcium (PACC) project. J Am Coll Cardiol. 2005;46:807–14.
49. Vliegenthart R, Oudkerk M, Song B, et al. Coronary calcification detected by electron-beam computed tomography and myocardial infarction. The Rotterdam Coronary Calcification Study. Eur Heart J. 2002;23:1596–603.
50. Budoff MJ, Shaw LJ, Liu ST, et al. Long-term prognosis associated with coronary calcification. Observations from a registry of 25,253 patients. J Am Coll Cardiol. 2007;49:1860–70.
51. Becker A, Leber A, Becker C, Knez A. Predictive value of coronary calcifications for future cardiac events in asymptomatic individuals. Am Heart J. 2008;155:154–60.
52. Folsom AR, Kronmal RA, Detrano RC, et al. Coronary artery calcification compared with carotid intima-media thickness in the prediction of cardiovascular disease incidence the Multi-Ethnic Study of Atherosclerosis (MESA). Arch Intern Med. 2008;168:1333–9.
53. Lakoski SG, Greenland P, Wong ND, et al. Coronary artery calcium scores and risk for cardiovascular events in women classified as "Low Risk" based on Framingham risk score. The Multi-Ethnic Study of Atherosclerosis (MESA). Arch Intern Med. 2007;167(22):2437–42.
54. Blaha M, Budoff MJ, Shaw LJ, et al. Absence of coronary artery calcification and all-cause mortality. J Am Coll Cardiol Img. 2009;2:692–700.
55. Erbel R, Möhlenkamp S, Moebus S, et al. Signs of subclinical coronary atherosclerosis measured as coronary artery calcification improve risk prediction of hard events beyond traditional risk factors in an unselected general population – The Heinz Nixdorf Recall Study five-year outcome data. J Am Coll Cardiol 2009;56:1397–406. In press.
56. Nasir K, Rubin J, Blaha MJ, Shaw LJ, et al. Interplay of coronary artery calcification and traditional risk factors for the prediction of all-cause mortality in asymptomatic individuals. Circ Cardiovasc Imaging. 2012;5:467–73.
57. Mascola A, Ko J, Bakhsheshi H, et al. Electron beam tomography comparison of culprit and non-culprit coronary arteries in patients with acute myocardial infarction. Am J Cardiol. 2000;85:1357–9.
58. Pohle K, Ropers D, Mäffert R, et al. Coronary calcifications in young patients with first, unheralded myocardial infarction: a risk factor matched analysis by electron beam tomography. Heart. 2003;89:625–8.
59. O'Malley PG, Feuerstein IM, Taylor AJ. Impact of electron beam tomography, with or without case management, on motivation, behavioral change, and cardiovascular risk profile: a randomized controlled trial. JAMA. 2003;289:2215–23.
60. Kalia NK, Miller LG, Nasir K, Blumenthal RS, et al. Visualizing coronary calcium is associated with improvements in adherence to statin therapy. Atherosclerosis. 2006;185:394–9.
61. Orakzai RH, Nasir K, Orakzai SH, et al. Effect of patient visualization of coronary calcium by electron beam computed tomography on changes in beneficial lifestyle behaviors. Am J Cardiol. 2008;101:999–1002.

62. Taylor AJ, Bindeman J, Feuerstein I, et al. Community-based provision of statin and aspirin after the detection of coronary artery calcium within a community-based screening cohort. J Am Coll Cardiol. 2008;51:1337–41.
63. Rozanski A, Gransar H, Shaw LJ, et al. Impact of coronary artery calcium scanning on coronary risk factors and downstream testing: The EISNER (Early Identification of Subclinical Atherosclerosis by Noninvasive Imaging Research) prospective randomized trial. J Am Coll Cardiol. 2011;57:1622–32.
64. Naghavi M, Falk E, Hecht HS, et al. From vulnerable plaque to vulnerable patient—Part III: executive summary of the Screening for Heart Attack Prevention and Education (SHAPE) task force report. Am J Cardiol. 2006;98(Suppl 2A):2H–15.
65. Greenland P, Alpert JS, Beller GA, et al. 2010 ACCF/AHA guideline for assessment of cardiovascular risk in adults. A report of the American College of Cardiology Foundation/American Heart Association Task Force on Practice Guidelines. J Am Coll Cardiol. 2010;56:e50–103.
66. Stone NJ, Robinson J, Lichtenstein AH, et al. 2013 ACC/AHA guideline on the treatment of blood cholesterol to reduce atherosclerotic cardiovascular risk in adults. J Am Coll Cardiol. 2013. doi:10.1016/j.jacc.2013.11.002.
67. Goff Jr DC, Lloyd-Jones DM, Bennett G, et al. 2013 ACC/AHA guideline on the assessment of cardiovascular risk. J Am Coll Cardiol. 2013. doi:10.1016/j.jacc.2013.11.005.
68. Hermann DM, Gronewold J, Lehmann N, et al. Heinz Nixdorf Recall Study Investigative Group. Coronary artery calcification is an independent stroke predictor in the general population. Stroke 2013;44:1008–13.
69. Yeboah J, McClelland RL, Polonsky TS, et al. Comparison of novel risk markers for improvement in cardiovascular risk assessment in intermediate-risk individuals. JAMA. 2012;308:788–95.
70. Kuller LH, Matthews KA, Sutton-Tyrrell K, et al. Coronary and aortic calcification among women 8 years after menopause and their premenopausal risk factors: the Healthy Women Study. Arterioscler Thromb Vasc Biol. 1999;19:2189–98.
71. Hecht HS, Superko HR, Smith LK, et al. Relation of coronary artery calcium identified by electron beam tomography to serum lipoprotein levels and implications for treatment. Am J Cardiol. 2001;87:406–12.
72. Daviglus ML, Pirzada A, Liu K, et al. Comparison of low risk and higher risk profiles in middle age to frequency and quantity of coronary artery calcium years later. Am J Cardiol. 2004;94:367–9.
73. Hecht HS, Superko HR. Electron beam tomography and national cholesterol education program guidelines in asymptomatic women. J Am Coll Cardiol. 2001;37:1506–11.
74. Rana JS, Gransar H, Wong ND, et al. Comparative value of coronary artery calcium and multiple blood biomarkers for prognostication of cardiovascular events. Am J Cardiol. 2012;109:1449–53.
75. Iribarren C, Gross MD, Darbinian JA, et al. Association of lipoprotein-associated phospholipase A2 mass and activity with calcified coronary plaque in young adults. The CARDIA Study. Arterioscler Thromb Vasc Biol. 2005;25:216–21.
76. O'Donnell CJ, Chazaro I, Wilson PW, et al. Evidence for heritability of abdominal aortic calcific deposits in the Framingham Heart Study. Circulation. 2002;106:337–41.
77. Peyser PA, Bielak LF, Chu J, et al. Heritability of coronary artery calcium quantity measured by electron beam computed tomography in asymptomatic adults. Circulation. 2002;106:304–8.
78. Hecht HS. Risk factors revisited. Am J Cardiol. 2003;93:73–5.
79. Hecht HS, Budoff M, Ehrlich J, Rumberger J. Coronary artery calcium scanning: clinical recommendations for cardiac risk assessment and treatment. Am Heart J. 2006;151:1139–46.
80. Wilson PW, D'Agostino B, Levy D, et al. Prediction of coronary heart disease using risk factor categories. Circulation. 1998;97: 1837–47.
81. Grundy SM, Cleeman JI, Merz CN, et al. Implications of recent clinical trials for the National Cholesterol Education Program Adult Treatment Panel III guidelines. Circulation. 2004;110: 227–39.
82. Akosah K, Schaper A, Cogbill C, Schoenfeld P. Preventing myocardial infarction in the young adult in the first place: how do the National Cholesterol Education Panel III guidelines perform? J Am Coll Cardiol. 2003;41:1475–9.
83. Taylor A, Cerqueira M, Hodgson JM, et al. Appropriate use criteria for cardiac computed tomography. J Am Coll Cardiol. 2010;56: 1864–94.
84. Raggi P, Shaw LJ, Berman DS, Callister TQ. Prognostic value of coronary artery calcium screening in subjects with and without diabetes. J Am Coll Cardiol. 2004;43:1663–9.
85. Wong ND, Sciammarella MG, Polk D, et al. The metabolic syndrome, diabetes, and subclinical atherosclerosis assessed by coronary calcium. J Am Coll Cardiol. 2003;41:1547–53.
86. Becker A, Leber A, Becker B, et al. Predictive value of coronary calcifications for future cardiac events in asymptomatic patients with diabetes mellitus: prospective study in 716 patients over 8 years. BMC Cardiovasc Disord. 2008;27:1–8.
87. Elkeles R, Godsland IF, Feher MD, et al. Coronary cal- cium measurement improves prediction of cardiovascular events in asymptomatic patients with type 2 diabetes: the PREDICT study. Eur Heart J. 2008;29:2244–51.
88. Anand DV, Lim E, Hopkins D, Corder R, et al. Risk stratification in uncomplicated type 2 diabetes: prospective evaluation of the combined use of coronary artery calcium imaging and selective myocardial perfusion scintigraphy. Eur Heart J. 2006;27:713–21.
89. Malik S, Budoff M, Katz R. Impact of subclinical atherosclerosis on cardiovascular disease events in individuals with metabolic syndrome and diabetes: the Multi-Ethnic Study of Atherosclerosis. Diabetes Care. 2011;34:2285–90.
90. Kuller LH, Velentgas P, Barzilay J, et al. Diabetes mellitus, subclinical cardiovascular disease and risk of incident cardiovascular disease and all-cause mortality. Arterioscler Thromb Vasc Biol. 2000;20:823–9.
91. Min JK, Lin FY, Gidseg DS, et al. Determinants of coronary calcium conversion among patients with a normal coronary calcium scan. What is the "Warranty Period" for remaining normal? J Am Coll Cardiol. 2010;55:1110–7.
92. Hecht HS. A paradigm shift: coronary computed tomographic angiography before stress testing. Am J Cardiol. 2009;104(4):613–8.
93. He ZX, Hedrick TD, Pratt CM, et al. Severity of coronary artery calcification by electron beam computed tomography predicts silent myocardial ischemia. Circulation. 2000;101:244–51.
94. Moser KW, O'Keefe JH, Bateman TM, et al. Coronary calcium screening in asymptomatic patients as a guide to risk factor modification and stress myocardial perfusion imaging. J Nucl Cardiol. 2003;10:590–8.
95. Berman DS, Wong ND, Gransar H, et al. Relationship between stress-induced myocardial ischemia and atherosclerosis measured by coronary calcium tomography. J Am Coll Cardiol. 2004;44: 923–30.
96. Anand DJ, Lim E, Raval U, et al. Prevalence of silent myocardial ischemia in asymptomatic individuals with subclinical atherosclerosis detected by electron beam tomography. J Nucl Cardiol. 2004;11:450–7.
97. Chang SM, Nabi F, Xu J, et al. The coronary artery calcium score and stress myocardial perfusion imaging provide independent and complementary prediction of cardiac risk. J Am Coll Cardiol. 2009;54:1872–82.
98. MacMahon H, Austin JH, Gamsu G, et al. Guidelines for management of small pulmonary nodules detected on CT scans: a statement from the Fleischner Society. Radiology. 2005;237: 395–4002101.

99. Budoff MJ, Shavelle DM, Lamont DH, et al. Usefulness of electron beam computed tomography scanning for distinguishing ischemic from non-ischemic cardiomyopathy. J Am Coll Cardiol. 1998;32:1173–8.
100. Laudon DA, Vukov LF, Breen JF, et al. Use of electron-beam computed tomography in the evaluation of chest pain patients in the emergency department. Ann Emerg Med. 1999;33:15–21.
101. Georgiou D, Budoff MJ, Kaufer E, et al. Screening patients with chest pain in the emergency department using electron beam tomography: a follow-up study. J Am Coll Cardiol. 2001;38:105–10.
102. Rosen BD, Fernandes V, McClelland RL, et al. The prevalence of flow limiting stenoses in coronary arteries with previously documented zero calcium score: the Multi-Ethnic Study of Atherosclerosis (MESA). J Am Coll Cardiol Img. 2009;2:1175–83.
103. MacHaalany J, Yeung Y, Ruddy TD, et al. Potential clinical and economic consequences of noncardiac incidental findings on cardiac computed tomography. J Am Coll Cardiol. 2009;54:1533–4.
104. Pletcher MJ, Pignone M, Earnshaw S, et al. Using the coronary artery calcium score to guide statin therapy: a cost-effectiveness analysis. Circ Cardiovasc Qual Outcomes. 2014;7:276–84.
105. Hecht HS. The Deadly double standard: the saga of screening for subclinical atherosclerosis. Am J Cardiol. 2008;101:1085–7.
106. Grundy SM. Is lowering low-density lipoprotein an effective strategy to reduce cardiac risk? Promise of low-density lipoprotein–lowering therapy for primary and secondary prevention. Circulation. 2008;117:569–73.
107. Hecht HS, Narula J. Coronary calcium in diabetes mellitus. J Diabetes. 2012;4:342–50.
108. Park R, Robert Detrano R, Xiang M et al. Combined use of computed tomography coronary calcium scores and C-reactive protein levels in predicting cardiovascular events in non-diabetic individuals. Circulation. 2002.

Natural History and Impact of Interventions on CAC

6

Paolo Raggi

Abstract

Coronary artery calcium is a marker of sub-clinical atherosclerosis and it is deposited via an active process similar to bone formation. Sequential non-contrast CT has been proposed as a method to accurately quantify and monitor progression of calcification. While interventions have generally failed to slow progression of calcification, it has become apparent that continued progression of CAC is associated with an increased risk of myocardial infarction and cardiac death. As a consequence, researchers have implemented sequential cardiac CT to follow the progression of coronary artery calcium in a variety of clinical settings and in some cases have reported encouraging results.

Keywords

Coronary artery calcium • Progression • Statins • Serial CT imaging • Atherosclerosis • All-cause mortality • Epicardial adipose tissue • Chronic kidney disease • Human immunodeficiency virus

Preface

Coronary artery calcium has long been known to be associated with atherosclerotic plaque and its development is due to an active process resembling bone formation. Similarly, aortic valve degeneration and calcification appear to follow a pathophysiologic process very similar to atherosclerosis. With non-contrast CT it is possible to detect and accurately quantify the extent of calcification of vessels and cardiac valves offering an opportunity to monitor progression of disease. While interventions have generally failed to slow progression of calcification, it has become apparent that continued progression of coronary artery calcium (CAC) is associated with an increased risk of myocardial infarction and cardiac death, suggesting that there might be some utility for sequential imaging. Therefore, researchers have investigated the utilization of cardiac CT imaging to follow the progression of cardiovascular calcification in a variety of clinical settings, as will be discussed in this chapter.

P. Raggi, MD
Department of Medicine, Mazankowski Alberta
Heart Institute, University of Alberta,
4A7.050, 8440 – 112 Street, Edmonton, AB T6G 2B7, Canada
e-mail: raggi@ualberta.ca

Natural History of Plaque Calcification

In Western societies pre-atherosclerotic changes in the arterial wall begin very early in life. Necropsy data from 2876 subjects between the ages of 15 and 34 revealed intimal lesions in the aortas of all patients and in the right coronary artery of more than half of the youngest patients (15–19 year old). The prevalence and extent of disease increased with advancing age [1]. CAC has long been known to be associated with atherosclerosis and it is now clearly established that plaque calcification may be dependent upon an active process of mineralization resembling bone formation [2–5]. Several enzymes necessary for the assembly of normal bone have been found in the context of human atherosclerotic plaques [2–4] and cells normally found in the vessel wall,

M.J. Budoff, J.S. Shinbane (eds.), *Cardiac CT Imaging: Diagnosis of Cardiovascular Disease*,
DOI 10.1007/978-3-319-28219-0_6

such as smooth muscle cells [5], macrophages and pericytes [6] can transform into osteoblast-like cells with bone generating potential. Pericytes are of particular interest given the modern view that atherosclerosis is a process partially driven from the outside of the arterial lumen. Pericytes are interspersed with endothelial cells in the vasa vasorum penetrating through the adventitia of vessels developing atherosclerosis and have been shown to be able to undergo osteoblastic differentiation [6]. As vasa vasorum proliferate and expand in the vessel wall, bringing more pericytes in its context, they cause a series of intramural hemorrhages [7]. The cellular membrane of erythrocytes is rich in cholesterol and cell death in the context of the vessel wall causes accumulation of large amounts of lipids promoting inflammation and possibly inducing osteoblasic changes in the pericytes. As a result of a complex cascade of events, in advanced stages of atherosclerosis true ossification can be observed in pathological specimen. It is currently unknown if arterial calcification is part of the ongoing inflammatory phenomena in the plaque or an attempt at repairing the damage brought to the vascular wall by noxious stimuli. Some investigators have suggested that calcium deposition simply results from recurrent hemorrhage and thrombosis with deposition of minerals in the context of the plaque [8].

Numerous researchers have investigated what factors are associated with CAC appearance (conversion of calcium score from 0 to >0) and progression. In an analysis of racial differences in disease progression, the Multi Ethnic Study of Atherosclerosis (MESA) investigators reported that all traditional risk factors correlated with calcium progression in Whites, Asians, Hispanics and African Americans alike [9]. However, Whites showed the greatest progression and diabetes mellitus had a stronger impact on Blacks than other races. The European Heinz Nixdorf Recall (HNR) population study confirmed that all traditional risk factors impact inception and progression of CAC [10]. However, the MESA investigators further stressed the importance of family history of premature coronary artery disease [11], diabetes mellitus and the metabolic syndrome [12], while the HNR researchers highlighted the importance of smoking [13] in promoting conversion from nil to positive calcium.

As the process of calcification of a plaque appears to be dependent upon active phenomena of mineralization, it is plausible that the formation and degradation of calcification may be a dynamic phenomenon in the atherosclerotic plaque similar to what happens in bone, and that these processes may be activated or inhibited by external interventions. Numerous studies have addressed atherosclerosis regression in animal models. In one experiment, 59 Rhesus monkeys were fed a high cholesterol diet for several years and then exposed to a cholesterol restricted diet for three more years [14]. The animals were progressively sacrificed along the experimental period and histology revealed development of typical plaques with a lipid-rich core and scattered calcific granules. As plaques expanded the calcific deposits grew. After exposing the animals to a diet severely restricted in cholesterol, the plaques became more fibrotic, with a lower cholesterol content and the calcium deposits stopped growing [14]. In another experiment Williams et al. [15] used a monkey model of atherosclerosis to study the effect of medical therapy in addition to diet on atherosclerosis progression and regression. Thirty-two adult (7–10 years of age) male cynomolgus monkeys were fed an atherogenic diet for 2 years (progression phase). During the subsequent 2-year a low cholesterol diet was begun (treatment phase). Additionally, 14 monkeys received pravastatin (20 mg/kg body weight per day), while the diet of the other 18 monkeys was adjusted to maintain equal plasma LDL levels between groups over time. At the end of the treatment phase the total, low density and high-density lipoprotein cholesterol levels were similar in the two animal groups. However, histological analysis of the coronary, carotid and iliac arteries revealed important differences between treatment groups. While the lumen area was not different, pravastatin treated animals showed a reduction in intimal neovascularization, plaque macrophage infiltration and a decrease in calcification of early as well as advanced plaques. These findings suggested that statins might benefit the arterial wall in ways that differ from simple lipoprotein lowering. However, Stary [16], Daoud [17] and Clarkson [18] did not find any reduction in calcium deposition in the atherosclerotic plaque with interventions in experiments conducted in swine and monkeys. Hence, although attractive, the histological proof that arterial calcification may regress remains very controversial.

Technical Considerations

The severity of calcification is assessed by means of quantitative calcium-scores. The first score was developed by Agatston et al. [19]; this score holds a good correlation with the underlying atherosclerotic plaque burden [20] and has been used widely in research and clinical trials. The Agatston score is derived by multiplying the area of a calcified plaque by a density coefficient rated 1 through 4. This scoring method was shown to have a limited inter-scan reproducibility, especially when used with the older EBCT technology, and new scoring methods were therefore introduced for the purpose of performing reliable sequential studies [21–23]. The calcium volume score (measured in picoliters) is derived using an isotropic interpolation principle and it represents the volume of matter denser than 130 Hounsfield units (i.e. calcium) contained in an atherosclerotic plaque. The inter-scan reproducibility of this score is significantly higher than that of the Agatston method [21].

The mass score was the third and last score to be introduced [22, 23]. Though reportedly more reliable and reproducible than the other two scores, to date this measurement has not yet been employed extensively. Another important technical consideration is the method used to report change and the numerous imaging platforms currently available with the various brands and models of CT scanners present on the market. The change in absolute score tends to minimize while a change in percent score exaggerates the difference at follow-up in the presence of small baseline scores (the reverse is true for large baseline scores). A novel method was therefore introduced by Hokanson based on the difference between the square root of the follow-up and the square root of the baseline calcium volume score [24]. This score is not affected by the baseline score and an increase ≥2.5 is considered a reliable indication of true change. A final word of caution should be reserved for the type of scanner and imaging protocol utilized for sequential imaging; it is unlikely that an Agatston score measured with an original EBCT scanner can be compared with a follow-up scan obtained years later with a high-resolution MDCT. If possible, a patient should be re-scanned with the same equipment and with the same parameters (slice thickness, voltage, electrocardiographic gating etc.)

Effect of Statins on Progression of CAC

Initial human studies of atherosclerosis progression and regression were conducted by means of quantitative coronary angiography [25, 26]. The cardiovascular event reduction associated with luminal stenosis improvements seen on quantitative coronary angiography far outweighed the magnitude of the regression recorded over long-term follow-up periods [27]. This observation became germane to the concept that induction of plaque regression is an important surrogate marker worth achieving since it may translate in substantial cardiovascular risk reduction. Nonetheless, the invasive nature of coronary angiography greatly limits the utility of this tool for sequential studies, especially in asymptomatic people. More modernly atherosclerosis imaging to gauge the effect of treatment has been assessed with sequential measurements of CAC and carotid artery intimal medial thickness [28–32]. This approach presumes that limiting the progression or inducing the regression of atherosclerosis in asymptomatic individuals will provide the same benefit observed in symptomatic patients who underwent sequential invasive studies. This is an obvious limitation as symptomatic patients may have a very different substrate for their on-going atherosclerotic disease compared to asymptomatic subjects harboring sub-clinical disease.

Callister et al. [28] published the first report of sequential EBCT scanning to measure progression of CAC in asymptomatic patients. They conducted an observational study on 149 patients referred by primary care physicians for calcium screening. Treatment with HMG-CoA reductase inhibitors (statins) was recommended for all patients, but the initiation of such therapy was left to the discretion of the referring physician. Baseline and follow-up EBCT scan at a minimum of 12-month interval (range 12–15 months) and serial LDL-cholesterol measurements were obtained in all patients. Of the 149 patients, 105 received treatment with statins and 44 did not. Progression of CAC was seen in all untreated patients (mean LDL ± SD: 147 ± 22 mg/dl) and averaged 52 ± 36 %/year (Fig. 6.1). In contrast, the mean yearly calcium volume score change for all treated patients (mean LDL: 114 ± 23 mg/dl) was 5 ± 28 % ($p<0.001$ vs. untreated patients). Budoff et al. [29] reported the results of an observational study of 299 asymptomatic patients followed for 1–6.5 years after an initial EBCT scan. All patients underwent a second scan at a minimum of 12 months. The follow-up scans showed an increase in CAC in all untreated patients while patients treated with statins showed significant slowing of progression (15 ± 8 %/year on treatment vs. 39 ± 12 %/year without treatment). Two more

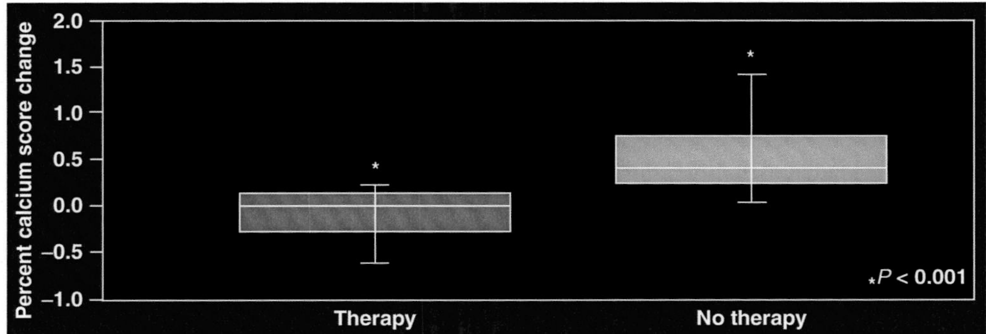

Fig. 6.1 Progression of calcium volume score in 105 patients treated for a year with statins and 44 untreated patients. There was a significant difference in progression between the two groups. The box plots indicate median (line in the middle of the box), confidence intervals (*vertical lines*) as well as 25th and 75th percentile (lower and top border of the box) [28]

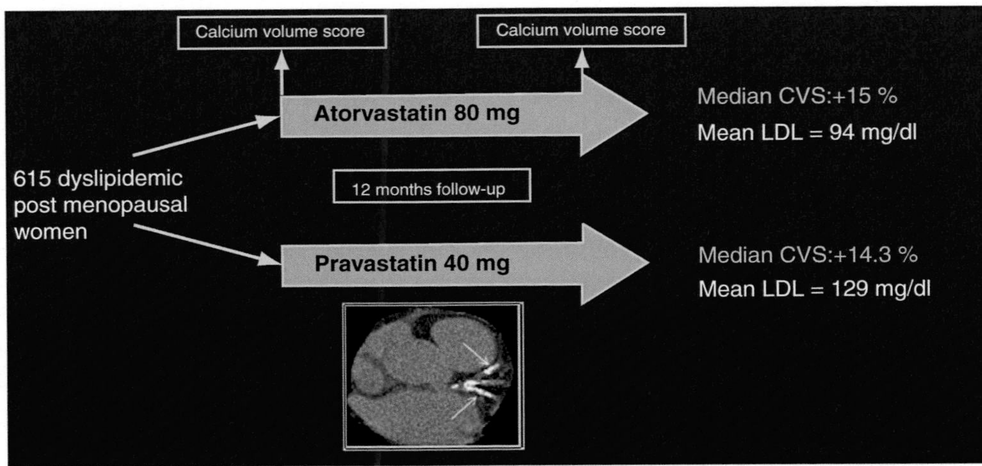

Fig. 6.2 Design of the BELLES trial and main study results. Aggressive lipid lowering therapy with atorvastatin did not slow progression of CAC more than moderate treatment with pravastatin [37]

small studies, in 66 men treated with cerivastatin [30] and eight patients with familial hypercholesterolemia receiving LDL apheresis [31], contributed to the growing evidence that statin therapy may retard the progression of CAC. Finally, in a subanalysis of the Women's Health Initiative Observational Study, Hsia et al. [33] evaluated prospectively the rate of progression of CAC in healthy postmenopausal women. Of 914 postmenopausal women enrolled in the main study, 305 women with a baseline calcium score ≥10 were invited for a repeat scan and 94 agreed to undergo a second scan. In multivariable analyses, statin use at baseline was a negative predictor ($p = 0.015$), whereas the baseline calcium score was a strong positive predictor ($p < 0.0001$) of progression of CAC.

Despite these encouraging results, other observational studies [34–36] and several randomized trials [37–39] failed to confirm an association between LDL lowering and progression of CAC. The BELLES trial (Beyond Endorsed Lipid Lowering With EBT Scanning) was a prospective, randomized study of post-menopausal and dyslipidemic women with a minimal calcium volume score of 30 at baseline [37]. After the initial EBCT scan, the 615 women enrolled were randomized to treatment with atorvastatin 80 mg/day or pravastatin 40 mg/day; a follow-up scan was performed 12 months after randomization (Fig. 6.2). The mean LDL cholesterol level was significantly lower with atorvastatin (94 mg/dl) than pravastatin (129 mg/dl). Nonetheless, the median percent change of the calcium volume score was not different between the two treatment arms (15.1 % and 14.3 % for atorvastatin and pravastatin respectively, P = NS). The St. Francis Heart Study [38] was a prospective, randomized study of 1005 healthy individuals with a CAC score above the 80th percentile for age and sex at screening. The study compared the effect of 20 mg/daily of atorvastatin along with vitamin C and E versus placebo on progression of CAC. At the end of a mean follow-up of 4.3 years the progression was similar among treatment arms (~20 %/year). Schmermund et al. [39] randomized 366 patients with no known cardiovascular disease to 10 mg vs 80 mg of atorvastatin daily for 1 year. The mean LDL levels on treatment were 109 ± 28 and 87 ± 33 mg/dl, respectively. Again the mean calcium volume score progression was not different at the end of 12 months of follow-up (25 % vs 27 %). Finally, Houslay et al. [40] randomized 48 patients to atorvastatin 80 mg/daily and 54 patients to placebo. After a median follow-up of 24 months the atorvastatin group had progressed by 26 %/year from baseline and the placebo group by 18 %/year (P = NS).

In conclusion, the results of randomized trials failed to confirm that lipid lowering therapy may slow progression of CAC; indeed there was a trend for statin therapy to attain the opposite effect.

Effect of Non-lipid Lowering Interventions on Progression of CAC

Besides medical therapy for dyslipidemia, other treatment modalities have been studied to slow the progression of CAC. An example of therapy of critical importance is represented by the effect of tight diabetic control on atherosclerosis progression. Snell-Bergeon et al. [41] assessed the effect of glycemic control in type 1 diabetes patients on progression of CAC. In 109 type 1 diabetic patients (22–50 year old), sequential EBCT scans were performed at an interval of 2.7 years. Progression of CAC was noted in 21 patients and it was associated with baseline hyperglycemia (odds ratio 7.11, 95 % CI 1.38–36.6, P = 0.02), after adjustment for baseline CAC, duration of diabetes, age and sex. There was also a significant interaction between higher insulin dose and higher body mass index (P = 0.03), suggesting that glycemic control and insulin resistance affected progression of CAC. Similarly, Anand et al. followed 392 type-2 diabetic patients. Progression of CAC was noted in 56 % of those with CAC at baseline; the best predictors of progression were the baseline CAC score, statins use and hemoglobin A1c >7 % during follow-up [42].

In the Women's Health Initiative (WHI), menopausal women between the ages of 50–59 years were randomized to treatment with conjugated estrogens or placebo [43]. In a sub-study of the WHI, 1064 women were submitted to CAC screening after 8.7 years from trial initiation. Women who had received estrogens showed a lower CAC score at follow-up compared to those who had received placebo (83.1 vs 123.1, P=0.02). Similarly, in a prospective observational study, combined hormone replacement therapy (progestin plus estrogens) and placebo were associated with a significantly greater progression of CAC (22–24 %/year) then treatment with unopposed estrogens alone (9 %/year) [44].

Several other approaches have been attempted to slow CAC progression. In a small, randomized study, Rath et al. [45] assessed the progression rate of CAC in subjects treated with a combination of vitamins, minerals and coenzymes. Untreated patients showed an average annual score increase of 44 % as assessed by the Agatston method. The rate of progression was slowed to 15 % yearly when patients were given nutritional supplements.

Budoff et al. [46] used aged garlic extract (AGE) to inhibit CAC progression. AGE was employed because it was previously shown to reduce multiple cardiovascular risk factors, including blood pressure, serum cholesterol levels, platelet aggregation and adhesion, while stimulating nitric oxide generation in endothelial cells. In a placebo-controlled, double-blind, randomized pilot study 23 patients were treated with 4 ml of oral AGE or the equivalent amount of placebo per day. Nineteen patients completed the 1-year protocol. At the end of follow-up the mean change in calcium volume score for the AGE group (n=9) was significantly smaller (7.5±9.4 %) than for the placebo group (n=10) that demonstrated an average increase of 22±18.5 % (P=0.046). Throughout the study there were no significant differences in individual cholesterol parameters or CRP between treatment group.

For a long time microscopic organisms called nanobacteria were thought to be implicated in the process of atherosclerosis where they operated as nucleating factors for CAC. More recently what was once believed to be an infectious agent has been described as a core of phosphate and calcium crystals with adherent molecules of fetuin-A; these complexes have been shown to act as nucleating factors for fast growth of calcification [47]. Nonetheless, before such knowledge was acquired tetracyclines – as treatment for nanobacteria – were combined with ethylenediaminetetraacetic acid disodium salt (EDTA) – as a chelating agent, as well as vitamins and CoQ10 and administered to 77 volunteers with stable coronary artery disease [48]. EBT scans were performed at baseline and after a short follow-up of 4 months. Of the 77 patients, 44 (57 %) showed CAC score regression (average −14 %), while the remaining 33 showed either no change or an increase in score. Of interest, serum lipid levels were reduced in a large proportion of patients despite the fact that most patients were already receiving statins prior to enrollment. No liver, renal or hematological side effects were recorded.

Obviously, these studies were very small and mainly exploratory in nature and the utility of such interventions will need to be confirmed in larger prospective studies.

Cardiovascular Calcification in End Stage Renal Disease and the Effect of Therapies on Its Progression

The cardiovascular disease rates of patients suffering from end-stage chronic kidney disease receiving dialysis (CKD stage 5D) are 30–50 fold higher than in the general population [49]. However, the cardiovascular mortality and morbidity of this patient group is only partially explained by traditional risk factors [50], and disorders of mineral metabolism may contribute substantially to the high incidence of events [51–56]. Hyperphosphatemia and its traditional management with calcium-based phosphate binders has been implicated in the development and progression of cardiovascular calcification, and the dose of oral calcium has been correlated with the severity of calcification [51, 57]. Vascular and valvular calcifications are very extensive in CKD-5D (Fig. 6.3) and progress rapidly. In an attempt to curb the rapid progression of calcification, the Treat-to-Goal Study—a randomized, multicenter clinical trial—compared the calcium-free, non-absorbable polymer sevelamer with traditional calcium-based phosphate binders [58]. Study outcomes included serum levels of phosphorus, calcium, intact parathyroid hormone (PTH), and lipids, as well as change in calcification of the coronary arteries and thoracic aorta quantified by EBCT. Two hundred adult patients who had received hemodialysis for a median of 3 years prior to study entry, were enrolled at 15 medical centers in Europe and the United States. During the study period, phosphate binders were adjusted to maintain serum phosphorus levels between 3.0 and 5.0 mg/dL, serum calcium levels between 8.5 and 10.5 mg/dL and serum PTH levels between 150 and 300 pg/mL. EBCT was performed at the start of the study, and after 6 and 12 months of treatment. In spite of a similar control of serum phosphorus and calcium, coronary and aortic calcification progressed significantly in the calcium-treated patients while there was no statistically significant change from baseline in the sevelamer group. At 1 year (Fig. 6.4), the median percent change in coronary and aorta scores were 25 % and 28 % and 6 % and 5 % in the calcium and sevelamer group, respectively (p=0.02 for all intergroup comparisons). Of note, the mean LDL cholesterol was significantly lower in the sevelamer group, than in patients treated with calcium salts, despite the fact that the latter

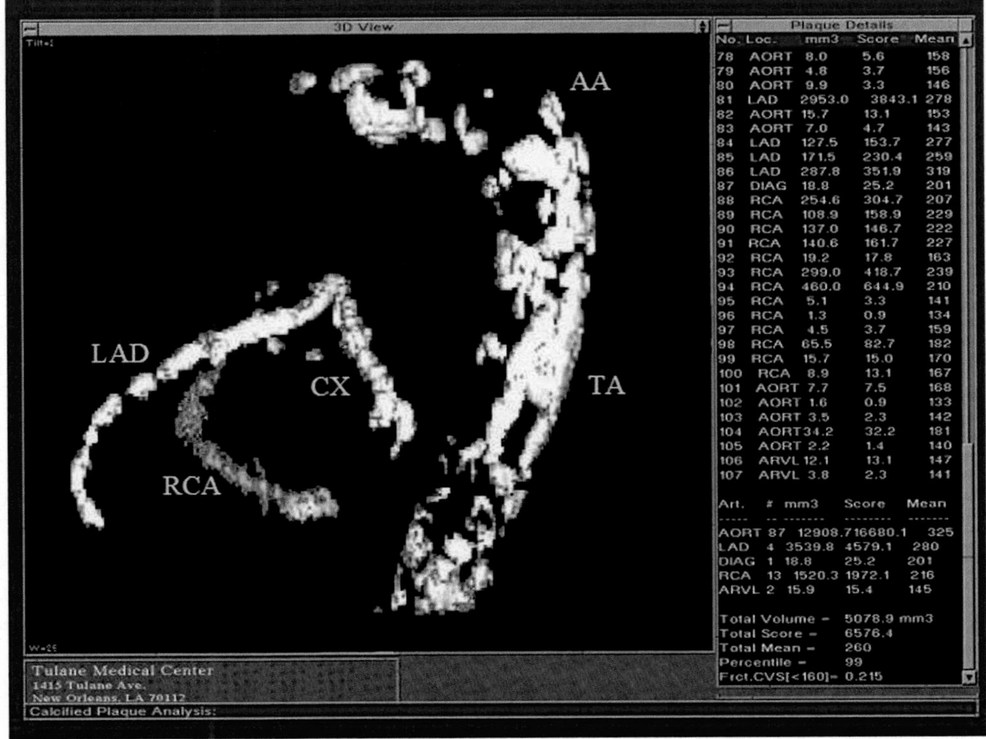

Fig. 6.3 Extensive cardiovascular calcification in a patient suffering from end-stage renal disease. The soft tissues have been removed and only the calcified portion of the aorta and coronary arteries are shown. *AA* aortic arch, *LAD* left anterior descending coronary artery, *CX* circumflex coronary artery, *RCA* right coronary artery, *TA* thoracic aorta

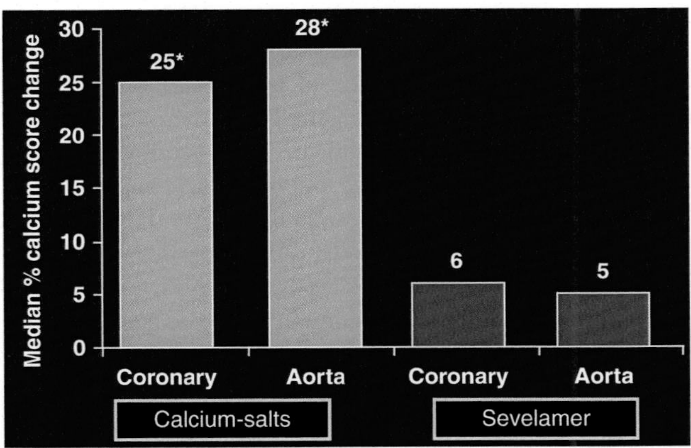

Fig. 6.4 Median percentage calcium score change for coronary arteries and aorta in end-stage renal disease patients randomized to 1-year treatment with sevelamer or calcium-based salts. The progression was significant for both coronary arteries and aorta only in the calcium salt treated patients [58]

received statins more often. However, the changes in calcium score severity seen at 52 weeks were independent of the levels of LDL cholesterol, HDL cholesterol and C-reactive protein. Additionally, sevelamer therapy was accompanied by a simultaneous improvement in bone mineral density [59]. Interestingly, an inverse relationship between CAC and bone mineral density has also been observed in non-uremic individuals [60, 61] and suggests an interaction between bone and vascular health.

A second randomized study was performed with the same primary end-point of CAC progression in patients randomized to sevelamer or calcium-based phosphate binders within a few weeks of beginning hemodialysis [62]. At the end of 18 months of follow-up calcium treated patients again showed a significant 11-fold greater progression of CAC than sevelamer treated patients ($p<0.002$). The secondary end point of this study was long-term mortality; at the end of 4.5 years of follow-up the mortality of calcium treated patients was double that of sevelamer treated subjects (hazard ratio: 3.2; $p<0.02$) [63]. In contrast with these 2 studies, the investigators of the CARE-2 study were unable to confirm that sevelamer and calcium-acetate phosphate binders affect CAC progression differently and showed an approximate 30 % progression at the end of 1 year for both treatment arms [64]. In this protocol the investigators meant to ascertain whether the effect of sevelamer on CAC progression is due to its lipid lowering ability; therefore they planned to randomize patients to sevelamer or a combination of calcium salts and statins. However, 80 % of the sevelamer treated patients also received statins and this may have caused CAC progression in both arms as shown in the general population (see above). Furthermore, the PTH level of sevelamer treated patients was double that of prior studies [58, 62], suggesting a very poor control of mineral metabolism. In a more recent trial cinacalcet and vitamin D, both used to reduce the PTH levels in secondary hyperparathyroidism, were compared as far as their ability to slow CAC progression [65]. At the end of 1 year of follow-up cinacalcet showed a non-significant but clear trend toward slowing of calcification of the cardiac valves, coronary arteries and aorta. Due to the numerous protocol violations committed by the participating physicians, a subanalysis was performed to assess the effect of protocol adherence [66]. Patients who were treated with cinacalcet in close adherence with the protocol showed a very significant slowing of CAC and aortic valve calcification compared to controls. Although this was an unplanned sub-analysis it highlighted the importance of protocol adherence and the possibility that many unsuccessful randomized studies may be marred by poor compliance with the protocol design by the participating physicians rather than the patients.

Coronary Atherosclerosis in Human Immunodeficiency Virus Infected Patients

With the advent of highly effective anti-retroviral therapy (HART), the mortality due to AIDS related diseases has dropped dramatically. However, other diseases have surfaced and are now affecting these patients in premature age. Among the most prominent is atherosclerosis and coronary artery disease [67, 68]. Initially believed to be a consequence of the dyslipidemia induced by several HART drugs, the concept has now evolved to include a more complex interaction of traditional risk factors and HIV-specific risk factors, such as chronic inflammation, proliferation of pro-inflammatory lymphocytes, endothelial damage and dysfunction and global activation of the immune system. HIV infected patients have been demonstrated to have a higher prevalence and larger than expected deposits of CAC [69–71] and CAC seems to progress rapidly in HIV infected patients [72, 73]. In addition to traditional risk factors, immunological factors have been associated with the prevalence and progression of CAC such as nadir CD4 count [69], HIV infection per se [72], volume of epicardial fat [73], and circulating CD16+ monocytes [74].

Visceral Adipose Tissue and Coronary Artery Calcium

The current epidemic of obesity, insulin resistance and diabetes mellitus in western countries, has generated a strong interest in the potential role of visceral adipose tissue in the development of atherosclerosis and its complications. The intra-abdominal and epicardial adipose tissues (EAT) (Fig. 6.5) are highly inflamed in obese patients, patients with the metabolic syndrome and in those with established coronary artery disease; large quantities of pro-inflammatory

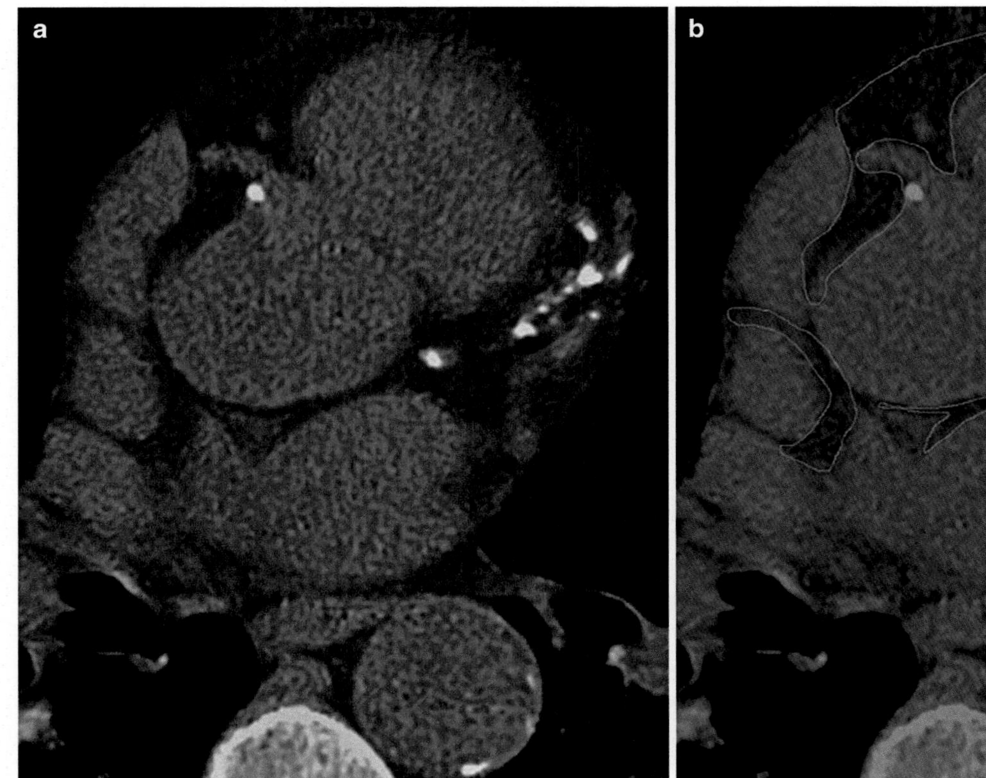

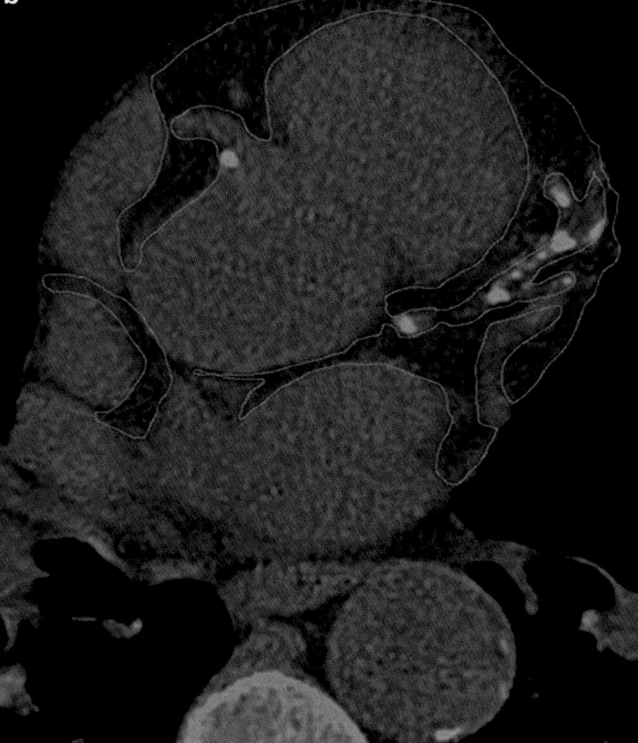

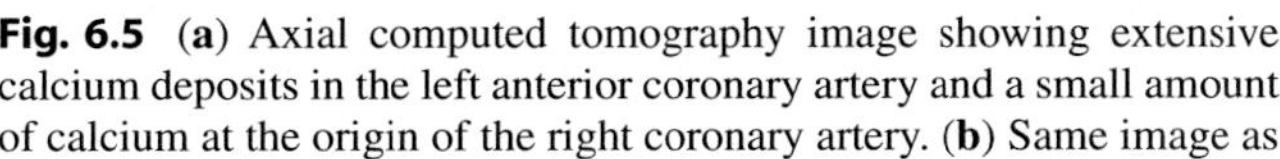

Fig. 6.5 (**a**) Axial computed tomography image showing extensive calcium deposits in the left anterior coronary artery and a small amount of calcium at the origin of the right coronary artery. (**b**) Same image as in (**a**); the epicardial adipose tissue is encased between the visceral and parietal pericardium highlighted by the orange line

cytokines and free fatty acids are released by these fat compartments [75]. The exact mechanisms by which EAT may predispose to atherosclerosis development are unknown, although several plausible mechanisms may be involved in this process. The adventitia of the coronary arteries comes in direct contact with EAT without the interposition of a fascia. EAT may thus exert a paracrin effect with direct exposure of the adventitia to humoral and cellular inflammatory mediators; this in turn may promote proliferation of vasa vasorum and growth of subendothelial atherosclerotic lesions [75]. Adipocytes are capable of secreting numerous cytokines that affect metabolic, inflammatory and vascular pathways; some of them are specifically secreted by adipocytes (such as adiponectin, leptin, and resistin), while others are also produced by other tissues (plasminogen activator inhibitor type-1 (PAI-1), tumor necrosis factor-α, interleukin 1 and 6, monocyte chemo-attractant protein 1 (MCP-1), angiotensin II, and cholesteryl ester transfer protein) [75]. Several studies showed an association of EAT with CAC, while others have shown an association of EAT with plaques showing characteristics of vulnerability [75]. In 3 studies in the general population [76–78] and one study of HIV infected patients [73] there was a significant association between EAT and CAC progression. In the Heinz Nixdorf Recall study [78], the association of EAT and CAC progression was significant in patients with a small burden of atherosclerosis at baseline (defined as a CAC score less than 100) but not in patients with more advanced disease. Additionally, the association was stronger in younger subjects and patients with lower body mass index. The authors hypothesized that these seemingly paradoxical results suggest that EAT acts as an initial promoter of atherosclerosis but that it may not have a prolonged long-term effect on CAC.

Clinical Implications of CAC Progression

The clinical significance of progression of CAC has been addressed in several observational studies and one randomized trial to date. Raggi et al. [79] followed 817 asymptomatic individuals referred by primary care physicians for sequential EBCT imaging at an average interval of 2.2 ± 1.3 years. Telephone interviews and chart reviews were conducted to ascertain the occurrence of myocardial infarction after the second CT scan. The mean yearly CAC volume score change for the individuals who suffered a myocardial infarction was 47 ± 50 % while it averaged 26 ± 32 % in those free of events (P<0.001). Treatment of hyperlipidemia (a probable marker of greater baseline risk) and CAC score change were independent predictors of myocardial infarction.

In a second observation [80], the occurrence of myocardial infarction was estimated in a cohort of 495 asymptomatic individuals submitted to sequential EBCT scanning while undergoing treatment with statins. The mean follow-up was 3 years, men and women were enrolled in equal proportions and the mean age of the enrolled subjects was 57 ± 8 years. In spite of an identical average LDL level on treatment (~120 mg/dl in each group), the 41 patients who suffered a myocardial infarction showed a much greater yearly CAC score progression than the 454 event-free survivors (42 ± 23 % vs 17 ± 25 %, P<0.001, Fig. 6.6). The investigators further applied a threshold of 15 %/year increase in CAC score to differentiate a true score change from a measurement reproducibility error [21]. Independent of the baseline CAC score patients with an increase smaller than 15 %/year (i.e no progression from baseline) suffered very few events (N = 5) and the events occurred late during follow-up. On the contrary, the majority of events (N = 36) occurred in patients showing a CAC score progression >15 %/year and the events occurred early during follow-up. Figure 6.7 shows an example of rapid progression of CAC and the occurrence of an acute coronary event in a 64 year old man. In the MESA study [81] 5862 patients had a baseline and follow-up CAC scan at approximately 2.5 year interval while the median clinical follow-up time was 7.5 years. Progression of CAC was a predictor of incident cardiovascular events both in patients without and those with CAC at baseline. An increase of ≥300 Agatston score units in patients with CAC at baseline was associated with a hazard ratio of 6.3 of developing hard cardiovascular events. In an observational study of 4609 asymptomatic patients, Budoff et al. [82] performed sequential CT scans an average of 3.5 years from baseline. The intent was to test whether CAC progression measured by three different methods (absolute change, increase >15 %/year and square root) predicted mortality and which method was the most predictive. During follow-up there were 288 all-cause deaths and CAC progression measured by any of the three methods was predictive of an event, although the square root method was the best model. Finally, three

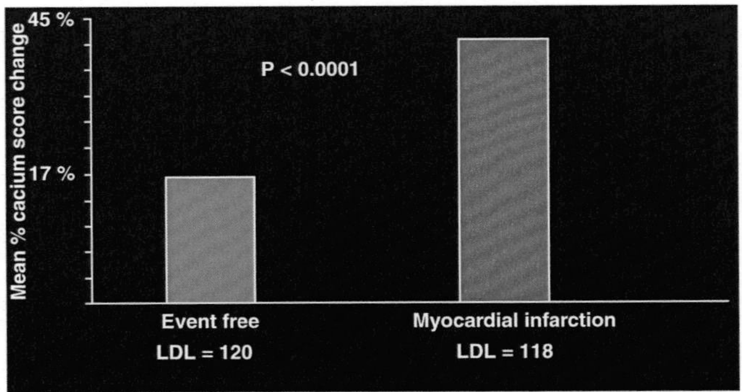

Fig. 6.6 Mean CAC volume score in patients treated with statins who suffered a myocardial infarction during follow-up and event-free subjects. Despite attaining a similar mean LDL level with treatment, the calcium score progression was significantly different between groups [80]

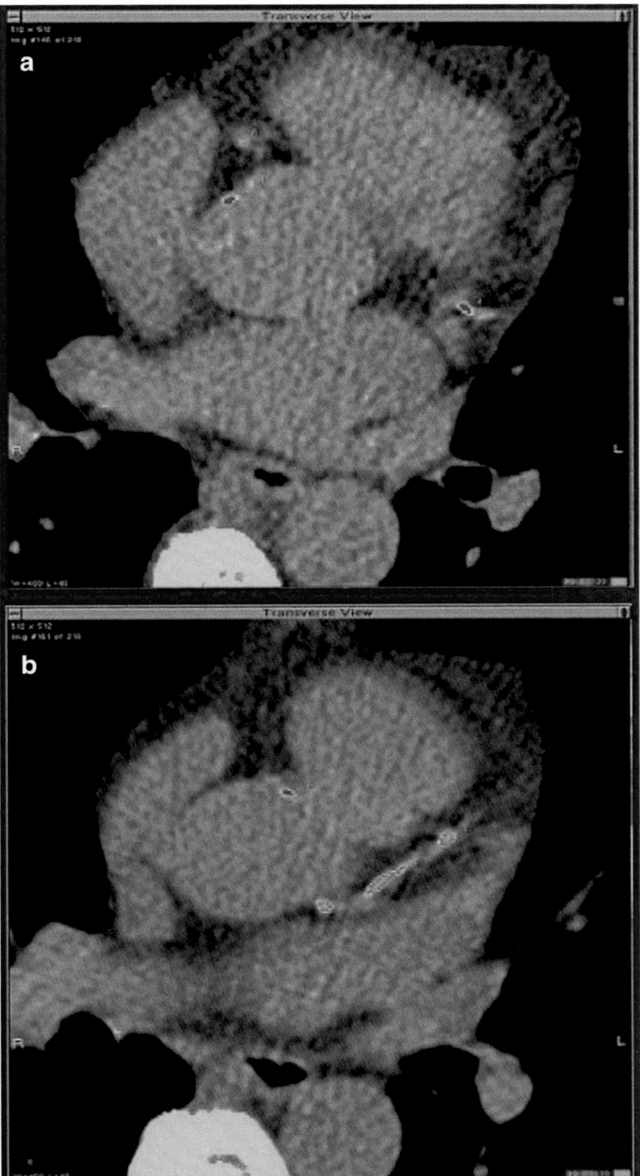

Fig. 6.7 (**a**) This 64 year old man at intermediate risk of cardiovascular events by Framingham categories had a baseline CAC score of 106. (**b**) After 18 months from the first CT his score increased to 296. Within 3 months of the second CT scan he suffered a non-ST elevation myocardial infarction

independent groups of researchers made the observation that progression of CAC is faster in patients with the metabolic syndrome and diabetes mellitus and it is linked with increased risk of cardiovascular events [12, 83, 84].

The only prospective randomized trial that tested the hypothesis of CAC progression as a predictor of an adverse event was the St. Francis Heart Study [85]. In the natural history arm of the study 4903 patients (age 50–70) were submitted to a baseline and repeat CT scan 2 years after enrollment. After approximately 4 years of follow-up 119 incident cardiovascular events were recorded of which 49 occurred after the second CT scan; the median absolute CAC score increase was 4 units in event-free survivors and 247 units in those who suffered events ($P<0.0001$). In multiple logistic regression analyses, age ($p=0.03$), male gender ($p=0.04$), LDL cholesterol ($p=0.01$), HDL cholesterol ($p=0.04$), and 2-year change in CAC score ($p=0.0001$) were significantly associated with risk of events.

The studies reviewed above clearly indicate that CAC progression poses a serious threat for the occurrence of future events. Nonetheless, whether sequential CAC screening should be recommended in clinical practice remains controversial since available therapies are not effective in slowing calcium accrual.

Conclusion

Despite a basic science construct, there has been no validation of the clinical utility of sequential CAC imaging to monitor the effectiveness of lipid lowering therapy. On the other hand, the benefit of non-calcium based therapies for phosphate-binding purposes in end-stage renal disease has been clearly shown with this technique. A number of small and preliminary studies have shown that CT can be of potential use in monitoring the outcome of various therapies. Nonetheless, there is an urgent need to standardize the scoring methods and assess the equivalence of the existing CT equipment [23, 86]. Additionally, the rigid application of a density threshold of 130 HU to define the presence of tissue calcification in all patients limits our ability to identify more recent and less densely calcified plaques and may be incorrectly applied to all the different CT brands and models available on the market. Although there is a need for further prospective studies, the most interesting finding that has emerged so far is that progression of CAC is associated with a greater risk of adverse events.

Future directions of research may include studying the effect of novel therapies such as HDL raising drugs, new LDL lowering therapies (i.e. – PCSK-9 inhibitors), new treatments for HIV that do not affect lipid metabolism, etc. If sequential CT imaging were confirmed to be useful in assessing the effectiveness of anti-atherosclerotic therapies, it would greatly facilitate the conduction of prevention trials by allowing a reduction in the number of patients needed to treat. Furthermore, a physician's effort to implement preventive measures might be facilitated by sharing information with his patients about the course of their disease.

With continued improvements in CT technology and further reduction in radiation exposure, it is hoped that the role of sequential CT imaging may become better defined either for follow-up of CAC or non-calcified plaque changes by CT angiography [87].

References

1. Strong JP, Malcom GT, McMahan A, Tracy RE, Newman III WP, Herderick EE, Cornhill F. Prevalence and extent of atherosclerosis in adolescents and young adults. The Pathobiological Determinants of Atherosclerosis in Youth Study. JAMA. 1999;281:727–35.
2. Bostrom K, Watson KE, Horn S, Wortham C, Herman IM, Demer LL. Bone morphogenic protein expression in human atherosclerotic lesions. J Clin Invest. 1993;91:1800–9.
3. Fitzpatrick LA, Severson A, Edwards WD, Ingram RT. Diffuse calcification in human coronary arteries: association of osteopontin with atherosclerosis. J Clin Invest. 1994;94:1597–604.
4. Shanahan CM, Cary NR, Metcalfe JC, Weissberg PL. High expression of genes for calcification-regulating proteins in human atherosclerotic plaques. J Clin Invest. 1994;93:2393–402.
5. Proudfoot D, Davies JD, Skepper JN, Weissberg PL, Shanahan CM. Acetylated low-density lipoprotein stimulates human vascular smooth muscle cell calcification by promoting osteoblastic differentiation and inhibiting phagocytosis. Circulation. 2002;106:3044–50.
6. Collett GD, Canfield AE. Angiogenesis and pericytes in the initiation of ectopic calcification. Circ Res. 2005;96:930–8.
7. Subbotin V. Neovascularization of coronary tunica intima (DIT) is the cause of coronary atherosclerosis. Lipoproteins invade coronary intima via neovascularization from adventitial vasa vasorum, but not from the arterial lumen: a hypothesis. Theor Biol Med Model. 2012;9:11.
8. Bini A, Mann KG, Kudryk BJ, Schen FJ. Noncollagenous bone matrix proteins, calcification and thrombosis in carotid artery atherosclerosis. Arterioscler Thromb Vasc Biol. 1999;19:1852–61.
9. Kronmal RA, McClelland RL, Detrano R, Shea S, Lima JA, Cushman M, Bild DE, Burke GL. Risk factors for the progression of coronary artery calcification in asymptomatic subjects: results from the Multi-Ethnic Study of Atherosclerosis (MESA). Circulation. 2007;115(21):2722–30.
10. Erbel R, Lehmann N, Churzidse S, Rauwolf M, Mahabadi AA, Möhlenkamp S, Moebus S, Bauer M, Kälsch H, Budde T, Montag M, Schmermund A, Stang A, Führer-Sakel D, Weimar C, Roggenbuck U, Dragano N, Jöckel KH; on behalf of the Heinz Nixdorf Recall Study Investigators. Progression of coronary artery calcification seems to be inevitable, but predictable – results of the Heinz Nixdorf Recall (HNR) study. Eur Heart J. 2014;pii:ehu288. [Epub ahead of print].
11. Pandey AK, Blaha MJ, Sharma K, Rivera J, Budoff MJ, Blankstein R, AlMallah M, Wong ND, Shaw L, Carr J, O'Leary D, Lima JA, Szklo M, Blumenthal RS, Nasir K. Family history of coronary heart disease and the incidence and progression of coronary artery calcification: Multi-Ethnic Study of Atherosclerosis (MESA). Atherosclerosis. 2014;232:369–76.
12. Wong ND, Nelson JC, Granston T, Bertoni AG, Blumenthal RS, Carr JJ, Guerci A, Jacobs Jr DR, Kronmal R, Liu K, Saad M, Selvin E, Tracy R, Detrano R. Metabolic syndrome, diabetes, and incidence and progression of coronary calcium: the Multiethnic Study of Atherosclerosis study. JACC Cardiovasc Imaging. 2012;5:358–66.
13. Lehmann N, Möhlenkamp S, Mahabadi AA, Schmermund A, Roggenbuck U, Seibel R, Grönemeyer D, Budde T, Dragano N, Stang A, Mann K, Moebus S, Erbel R, Jöckel KH. Effect of smoking and other traditional risk factors on the onset of coronary artery calcification: results of the Heinz Nixdorf recall study. Atherosclerosis. 2014;232:339–45.
14. Stary HC. Natural history of calcium deposits in atherosclerosis progression and regression. Z Kardiol. 2000;89 Suppl 2:28–35.
15. Williams JK, Sukhova GK, Herrington DM, Libby P. Pravastatin has cholesterol-lowering independent effects on the artery wall of atherosclerotic monkeys. J Am Coll Cardiol. 1998;31:684–91.
16. Stary HC. The development of calcium deposits in atherosclerotic lesions and their persistence after lipid regression. Am J Cardiol. 2001;88(2A):16E–9.
17. Daoud AS, Jarmolych J, Augustyn JM, Fritz KE. Sequential morphologic studies of regression of advanced atherosclerosis. Arch Pathol. 1981;105:233–9.
18. Clarkson TB, Bond MG, Bullock BC, Marzetta CA. A study of atherosclerosis regression in Macaca mulatta. IV. Changes in coronary arteries from animals with atherosclerosis induced for 19 months and then regressed for 24 months or 48 months at plasma cholesterol concentrations of 300 or 200 mg/dl. Exp Mol Pathol. 1981;34:345–68.
19. Agatston AS, Janowitz WR, Hildner JR, Zusmer NR, Viamonte Jr M, Detrano R. Quantification of CAC using ultrafast computed tomography scanning. J Am Coll Cardiol. 1990;15: 827–32.
20. Sangiorgi G, Rumberger JA, Severson A, Edwards WD, Gregoire J, Fitzpatrick LA, Schwartz RS. Arterial calcification and not lumen stenosis is highly correlated with atherosclerotic plaque burden in humans: a histologic study of 723 coronary artery segements using non-decalcifying methodology. Electron beam computed tomography and coronary artery disease: scanning for coronary artery calcification. J Am Coll Cardiol. 1998;31:126–33.
21. Callister TQ, Cooil B, Raya S, Lippolis NJ, Russo DJ, Raggi P. Coronary artery disease: improved reproducibility of calcium scoring with electron-beam CT volumetric method. Radiology. 1998;208:807–14.
22. Rumberger JA, Kaufman L. A rosetta stone for CAC risk stratification: agatston, volume, and mass scores in 11,490 individuals. AJR Am J Roentgenol. 2003;181:743–8.
23. McCollough CH, Ulzheimer S, Halliburton SS, Shanneik K, White RD, Kalender WA. CAC: a multi-institutional, multimanufacturer international standard for quantification at cardiac CT. Radiology. 2007;243:527–38.
24. Hokanson JE, MacKenzie T, Kinney G, Snell-Bergeon JK, Dabelea D, Ehrlich J, Eckel RH, Rewers M. Evaluating changes in coronary artery calcium: an analytic method that accounts for interscan variability. AJR Am J Roentgenol. 2004;182:1327–32.
25. Jukema JW, Bruschke AV, van Boven AJ, Reiber JH, Bal ET, Zwinderman AH, Jansen H, Boerma GJ, van Rappard FM, Lie KI. Effects of lipid lowering by pravastatin on progression and regression of coronary artery disease in symptomatic men with normal to moderately elevated serum cholesterol levels. The Regression Growth Evaluation Statin Study (REGRESS). Circulation. 1995;91:2528–40.
26. Brown G, Albers JJ, Fisher LD, Schaefer SM, Lin JT, Kaplan C, Zhao XQ, Bisson BD, Fitzpatrick VF, Dodge HT. Regression of coronary artery disease as a result of intensive lipid-lowering therapy in men with high levels of apolipoprotein B. N Engl J Med. 1990;323:1289–98.
27. Levine GN, Keaney Jr JF, Vita JA. Cholesterol reduction in cardiovascular disease: clinical benefits and possible mechanisms. N Engl J Med. 1995;332:512–21.
28. Callister TQ, Raggi P, Cooil B. Effects of HMG-CoA reductase inhibitors on coronary artery disease. N Engl J Med. 1998;339: 1972–7.
29. Budoff MJ, Lane KL, Bakhsheshi H, Mao S, Grassmann BO, Friedman BC, Brundage BH. Rates of progression of CAC by electron beam tomography. Am J Cardiol. 2000;86:8–11.
30. Achenbach S, Dieter R, Pohle K, Leber A, Thilo C, Knez A, Menendez T, Maeffert R, Kusus M, Regenfus M, Bickel A, Haberl R, Stienbeck G, Moshage W, Daniel WG. Influence of lipid-lowering therapy on the progression of coronary artery calcification. Circulation. 2002;106:1077–82.
31. Hoffmann U, Derfler K, Haas M, Stadler A, Brady TJ, Kostner K. Effects of combined low density lipoprotein apheresis and

aggressive statin therapy on coronary calcified plaque as measured by computed tomography. Am J Cardiol. 2003;91:461–4.
32. Taylor AJ, Kent SM, Flaherty PJ, Coyle LC, Markwood TT, Vernalis MN. ARBITER: Arterial Biology for the Investigation of the Treatment Effects of Reducing Cholesterol: a randomized trial comparing the effects of atorvastatin and pravastatin on carotid intima medial thickness. Circulation. 2002;106:2055–60.
33. Hsia J, Klouj A, Prasad A, Burt J, Adams-Campbell LL, Howard BV. Progression of coronary calcification in healthy postmenopausal women. BMC Cardiovasc Disord. 2004;4:21.
34. Hecht HS, Harman SM. Comparison of the effects of atorvastatin versus simvastatin on subclinical atherosclerosis in primary prevention as determined by electron beam tomography. Am J Cardiol. 2003;91:42–5.
35. Hecht HS, Harman SM. Relation of aggressiveness of lipid-lowering treatment to changes in calcified plaque burden by electron beam tomography. Am J Cardiol. 2003;92:334–6.
36. Wong ND, Kawakubo M, LaBree L, Azen SP, Xiang M, Detrano R. Relation of CAC progression and control of lipids according to the National Cholesterol Education Program guidelines. Am J Cardiol. 2004;94:431–6.
37. Raggi P, Davidson M, Callister TQ, Welty FK, Bachmann GA, Hecht H, Rumberger JA. Aggressive versus moderate lipid-lowering therapy in hypercholesterolemic post-menopausal women: Beyond Endorsed Lipid Lowering with EBT Scanning (BELLES). Circulation. 2005;112(4):563–71. (In press).
38. Arad Y, Spadaro LA, Roth M, Newstein D, Guerci A. Treatment of asymptomatic adults with elevated calcium scores with atorvastatin, vitamin C and vitamin E. The St. Francis Heart Study randomized clinical trial. J Am Coll Cardiol. 2005;46:166–72.
39. Schmermund A, Achenbach S, Budde T, Buziashvili Y, Förster A, Friedrich G, et al. Effect of intensive versus standard lipid-lowering treatment with atorvastatin on the progression of calcified coronary atherosclerosis over 12 months: a multicenter, randomized, double-blind trial. Circulation. 2006;113:427–37.
40. Houslay ES, Cowell SJ, Prescott RJ, Reid J, Burton J, Northridge DB, Boon NA, Newby DE, Scottish Aortic Stenosis and Lipid Lowering Therapy, Impact on Regression trial Investigators. Progressive coronary calcification despite intensive lipid-lowering treatment: a randomised controlled trial. Heart. 2006;92:1207–12.
41. Snell-Bergeon JK, Hokanson JE, Jensen L, MacKenzie T, Kinney G, Dabelea D, Eckel RH, Ehrlich J, Garg S, Rewers M. Progression of coronary artery calcification in type 1 diabetes: the importance of glycemic control. Diabetes Care. 2003;26:2923–8.
42. Anand DV, Lim E, Darko D, Bassett P, Hopkins D, Lipkin D, Corder R, Lahiri A. Determinants of progression of coronary artery calcification in type 2 diabetes role of glycemic control and inflammatory/vascular calcification markers. J Am Coll Cardiol. 2007;50(23):2218–25.
43. Manson JE, Allison MA, Rossouw JE, Carr JJ, Langer RD, Hsia J, et al. Estrogen therapy and coronary-artery calcification. N Engl J Med. 2007;356:2591–602.
44. Budoff MJ, Chen GP, Hunter CJ, Takasu J, Agrawal N, Sorochinsky B, Mao S. Effects of hormone replacement on progression of coronary calcium as measured by electron beam tomography. J Womens Health (Larchmt). 2005;14:410–7.
45. Rath M, Niedzwiecki A. Nutritional supplement program halts progression of early coronary atherosclerosis documented by ultrafast computed tomography. J Appl Nutr. 1996;48:67–78.
46. Budoff MJ, Takasu J, Flores FR, Niihara Y, Lu B, Lau BH, Rosen RT, Amagase H. Inhibiting progression of coronary calcification using Aged Garlic Extract in patients receiving statin therapy: a preliminary study. Prev Med. 2004;39:985–91.
47. Kuro-O M. A phosphate-centric paradigm for pathophysiology and therapy of chronic kidney disease. Kidney Int Suppl (2011). 2013;3:420–6.
48. Maniscalco BS, Taylor KA. Calcification in coronary artery disease can be reversed by EDTA-tetracycline long-term chemotherapy. Pathophysiology. 2004;11:95–101.
49. Renal Data System US. USRDS 2004 Annual Data Report: Atlas of End-Stage Renal Disease in the United States. Bethesda: National Institutes of Health, National Institute of Diabetes and Digestive and Kidney Diseases; 2004.
50. Longenecker JC, Coresh J, Powe NR, Levey AS, Fink NE, Martin A, et al. Traditional cardiovascular disease risk factors in dialysis patients compared with the general population: the CHOICE Study. J Am Soc Nephrol. 2002;13:1918–27.
51. Guérin AP, London GM, Marchais SJ, Metivier F. Arterial stiffening and vascular calcifications in end-stage renal disease. Nephrol Dial Transplant. 2000;15:1014–21.
52. Blacher J, Guerin AP, Pannier B, Marchais SJ, London GM. Arterial calcifications, arterial stiffness, and cardiovascular risk in end-stage renal disease. Hypertension. 2001;38:938–42.
53. Raggi P, Boulay A, Chasan-Taber S, Amin N, Dillon M, Burke SK, et al. Cardiac calcification in adult hemodialysis patients. A link between end-stage renal disease and cardiovascular disease? J Am Coll Cardiol. 2002;39:695–701.
54. London GM, Guérin AP, Marchais SJ, Métivier F, Pannier B, Adda H. Arterial media calcification in end-stage renal disease: impact on all-cause and cardiovascular mortality. Nephrol Dial Transplant. 2003;18:1731–40.
55. London GM. Cardiovascular calcifications in uremic patients: clinical impact on cardiovascular function. J Am Soc Nephrol. 2003;14:S305–9.
56. Block GA, Klassen PS, Lazarus JM, Ofsthun N, Lowrie EG, Chertow GM. Mineral metabolism, mortality, and morbidity in maintenance hemodialysis. J Am Soc Nephrol. 2004;15:2208–18.
57. Goodman WG, Goldin J, Kuizon BD, Yoon C, Gales B, Sider D, et al. Coronary-artery calcification in young adults with end-stage renal disease who are undergoing dialysis. N Engl J Med. 2000;342:1478–83.
58. Chertow GM, Burke SK, Raggi P. Sevelamer attenuates the progression of coronary and aortic calcification in hemodialysis patients. Kidney Int. 2002;62:245–52.
59. Raggi P, James G, Burke S, Bommer J, Taber SC, Holzer H, Braun J, Chertow GM. Paradoxical decrease in vertebral bone density with calcium-based phosphate binders in hemodialysis. J Bone Miner Res. 2005;20:764–72.
60. Barengolts EI, Berman M, Kukreja SC, Kouznetsova T, Lin C, Chomka EV. Osteoporosis and coronary atherosclerosis in asymptomatic postmenopausal women. Calcif Tissue Int. 1998;62:209–13.
61. Sirola J, Sirola J, Honkanen R, Kroger H, Jurvelin JS, Maenpaa P, Saarikoski S. Relation of statin use and bone loss: a prospective population-based cohort study in early postmenopausal women. Osteoporos Int. 2002;13:537–41.
62. Block GA, Spiegel DM, Ehrlich J, Mehta R, Lindbergh J, Dreisbach A, et al. Effects of sevelamer and calcium on coronary artery calcification in patients new to hemodialysis. Kidney Int. 2005;68(4):1815–24.
63. Block GA, Raggi P, Bellasi A, Kooienga L, Spiegel DM. Mortality effect of coronary calcification and phosphate binder choice in incident hemodialysis patients. Kidney Int. 2007;7:438–41.
64. Qunibi W, Moustafa M, Muenz LR, He DY, Kessler PD, Diaz-Buxo JA, et al. A 1-year randomized trial of calcium acetate versus sevelamer on progression of coronary artery calcification in hemodialysis patients with comparable lipid control: the Calcium Acetate Renagel Evaluation-2 (CARE-2) study. Am J Kidney Dis. 2008;5:952–65.
65. Raggi P, Chertow GM, Torres PU, Csiky B, Naso A, Nossuli K, Moustafa M, Goodman WG, Lopez N, Downey G, Dehmel B, Floege J, on behalf of the ADVANCE Study Group. The ADVANCE

Study: a randomized study to evaluate the effects of cinacalcet plus low dose vitamin D on vascular calcification in patients on hemodialysis. Nephrol Dial Transplant. 2011;26(4):1327–39.
66. Ureña-Torres PA, Floege J, Hawley CM, Pedagogos E, Goodman WG, Pétavy F, Reiner M, Raggi P. Protocol adherence and the progression of cardiovascular calcification in the ADVANCE study. Nephrol Dial Transplant. 2013;28:146–52.
67. Triant VA, Lee H, Hadigan C, Grinspoon SK. Increased acute myocardial infarction rates and cardiovascular risk factors among patients with human immunodeficiency virus disease. J Clin Endocrinol Metab. 2007;92:2506–12.
68. Freiberg MS, Chang CC, Kuller LH, Skanderson M, Lowy E, Kraemer KL, Butt AA, Bidwell Goetz M, Leaf D, Oursler KA, Rimland D, Rodriguez Barradas M, Brown S, Gibert C, McGinnis K, Crothers K, Sico J, Crane H, Warner A, Gottlieb S, Gottdiener J, Tracy RP, Budoff M, Watson C, Armah KA, Doebler D, Bryant K, Justice AC. HIV infection and the risk of acute myocardial infarction. JAMA Int Med. 2013;173(8):614–22.
69. Post WS, Budoff M, Kingsley L, Palella Jr FJ, Witt MD, Li X, George RT, Brown TT, Jacobson LP. Associations between HIV infection and subclinical coronary atherosclerosis. Ann Intern Med. 2014;160:458–67.
70. Mangili A, Gerrior J, Tang AM, O'Leary DH, Polak JK, Schaefer EJ, Gorbach SL, Wanke CA. Risk of cardiovascular disease in a cohort of HIV-infected adults: a study using carotid intima-media thickness and coronary artery calcium score. Clin Infect Dis. 2006;43:1482–9.
71. Kingsley LA, Cuervo-Rojas J, Munoz A, Palella FJ, Post W, Witt MD, et al. Subclinical coronary atherosclerosis, HIV infection and antiretroviral therapy: multicenter AIDS Cohort Study. Aids. 2008;22:1589–99.
72. Guaraldi G, Zona S, Orlando G, Carli F, Ligabue G, Fiocchi F, Menozzi M, Rossi R, Modena MG, Raggi P. Human immunodeficiency virus infection is associated with accelerated atherosclerosis. J Antimicrob Chemother. 2011;66(8):1857–60.
73. Zona S, Raggi P, Bagni P, Orlando G, Carli F, Ligabue G, Scaglioni R, Rossi R, Guaraldi MG. Parallel increase of subclinical atherosclerosis and epicardial adipose tissue in patients with HIV. Am Heart J. 2012;163:1024–30.
74. Baker JV, Hullsiek KH, Singh A, Wilson E, Henry K, Lichtenstein K, Onen N, Kojic E, Patel P, Brooks JT, Hodis HN, Budoff M, Sereti I, CDC SUN Study Investigators. Immunologic predictors of coronary artery calcium progression in a contemporary HIV cohort. AIDS. 2014;28(6):831–40.
75. Alexopoulos N, Katritsis D, Raggi P. Visceral adipose tissue as a source of inflammation and promoter of atherosclerosis. Atherosclerosis. 2014;233:104–12.
76. Nakanishi R, Rajani R, Cheng VY, Gransar H, Nakazato R, Shmilovich H, Otaki Y, Hayes SW, Thomson LE, Friedman JD, Slomka PJ, Berman DS, Dey D. Increase in epicardial fat volume is associated with greater coronary artery calcification progression in subjects at intermediate risk by coronary calcium score: a serial study using non-contrast cardiac CT. Atherosclerosis. 2011;218: 363–8.
77. Yerramasu A, Dey D, Venuraju S, Anand DV, Atwal S, Corder R, Berman DS, Lahiri A. Increased volume of epicardial fat is an independent risk factor for accelerated progression of sub-clinical coronary atherosclerosis. Atherosclerosis. 2012;220: 223–30.
78. Mahabadi AA, Lehmann N, Kälsch H, Robens Y, Bauer M, Dykun I, Budde T, Moebus S, Jöckel KH, Erbel R, Möhlenkamp S. Association of epicardial adipose tissue with progression of coronary artery calcification is more pronounced in the early phase of atherosclerosis – results from the Heinz Nixdorf Recall study. JACC Cardiovasc Imaging. 2014;7(9):909–16.
79. Raggi P, Cooil B, Shaw LJ, Aboulhson J, Takasu J, Budoff MJ, Callister TQ. Progression of coronary calcification on serial electron beam tomography scanning is greater in patients with future myocardial infarction. Am J Cardiol. 2003;92:827–9.
80. Raggi P, Callister T, Budoff M, Shaw L. Progression of CAC and risk of first myocardial infarction in patients receiving cholesterol-lowering therapy. Arterioscler Thromb Vasc Biol. 2004;24: 1272–7.
81. Budoff MJ, Young R, Lopez VA, Kronmal RA, Nasir K, Blumenthal RS, Detrano RC, Bild DE, Guerci AD, Liu K, Shea S, Szklo M, Post W, Lima J, Bertoni A, Wong ND. Progression of coronary calcium and incident coronary heart disease events: MESA (Multi-Ethnic Study of Atherosclerosis). J Am Coll Cardiol. 2013;61: 1231–9.
82. Budoff MJ, Hokanson JE, Nasir K, Shaw LJ, Kinney GL, Chow D, Demoss D, Nuguri V, Nabavi V, Ratakonda R, Berman DS, Raggi P. Progression of coronary artery calcium predicts all-cause mortality. JACC Cardiovasc Imaging. 2010;3:1229–36.
83. Raggi P, Cooil B, Ratti C, Callister TQ, Budoff M. Progression of coronary calcification and occurrence of myocardial infarction in patients with and without diabetes mellitus. Hypertension. 2005;45:1–6.
84. Kiramijyan S, Ahmadi N, Isma'eel H, Flores F, Shaw LJ, Raggi P, Budoff MJ. Impact of coronary artery calcium progression and statin therapy on clinical outcome in subjects with and without diabetes mellitus. Am J Cardiol. 2013;111:356–61.
85. Arad Y, Goodman KJ, Roth M, Newstein D, Guerci AD. Coronary calcification, coronary risk factors, and atherosclerotic cardiovascular disease events. The St. Francis Heart Study. J Am Coll Cardiol. 2005;46:158–65.
86. Oudkerk M, Stillman AE, Halliburton SS, Kalender WA, Mohlenkamp S, McCollough CH, et al. CAC screening: current status and recommendations from the European Society of Cardiac Radiology and North American Society for Cardiovascular Imaging. Int J Cardiovasc Imaging. 2008;24(6):645–71.
87. Zeb I, Li D, Nasir K, Malpeso J, Batool A, Flores F, Dailing C, Karlsberg RP, Budoff M. Effect of statin treatment on coronary plaque progression – a serial coronary CT angiography study. Atherosclerosis. 2013;23:198–204.

Methodology for CCTA Image Acquisition

7

Mathew J. Budoff, Jerold S. Shinbane, and Songshao Mao

Abstract

Cardiovascular computed tomographic angiography (CCTA) can assess cardiovascular pathology through visualization of gross anatomic abnormalities, characterization of tissue attenuation, and cardiac functional analysis. As cardiac structures are in constant motion, special attention to the methodology of image acquisition is essential to capturing high quality images during the most quiescent stage of cardiac and coronary artery motion. Successful imaging requires an understanding of the interplay of multiple motions, including the complexities of cardiac motion, motion related to variation in heart rate and rhythm, potential respiratory motion, potential patient movement, table motion, gantry rotation, and timing and movement of the intravenous contrast bolus through the structures of interest (Fig. 7.1).

Optimization of image acquisition is achieved through localization of target structures, timing of scanning for capture of images during the segment of the R-R interval with relatively slow cardiac motion, and injection of contrast media to enhance opacification of structures throughout all slice levels. These techniques help to avoid or minimize motion artifacts and suboptimal opacification of structures of interest, which would make subsequent image reconstruction and diagnostic analysis a challenge. Imaging methodology must also focus on minimizing the exposure to radiation and the amount of intravenous contrast. This chapter will focus on methods essential to acquisition of diagnostic images for the assessment of cardiovascular pathology.

Keywords

Cardiac computed tomography • Image Acquisition • Methodology • Non-invasive angiography • Radiation • Contrast • Calcium scoring • Scan protocols

Introduction

Cardiovascular computed tomographic angiography (CCTA) can assess cardiovascular pathology through visualization of gross anatomic abnormalities, characterization of tissue attenuation, and cardiac functional analysis. As cardiac structures are in constant motion, special attention to the methodology of image acquisition is essential to capturing high quality images during the most quiescent stage of cardiac and coronary artery motion. Successful imaging requires an understanding of the interplay of multiple motions, including the complexities of cardiac motion, motion related

M.J. Budoff, MD (✉)
David Geffen School of Medicine at UCLA, Los Angeles Biomedical Research Institute, Torrance, CA, USA
e-mail: mbudoff@labiomed.org

J.S. Shinbane, MD, FACC FHRS FSCCT
Division of Cardiovascular Medicine, Department of Internal Medicine, University of Southern California, Keck School of Medicine, Los Angeles, CA, USA

S. Mao, MD
Department of Medicine, Division of CardiologyLos Angeles Biomedical Research Institute, Los Angeles, CA 90713, USA

M.J. Budoff, J.S. Shinbane (eds.), *Cardiac CT Imaging: Diagnosis of Cardiovascular Disease*, DOI 10.1007/978-3-319-28219-0_7

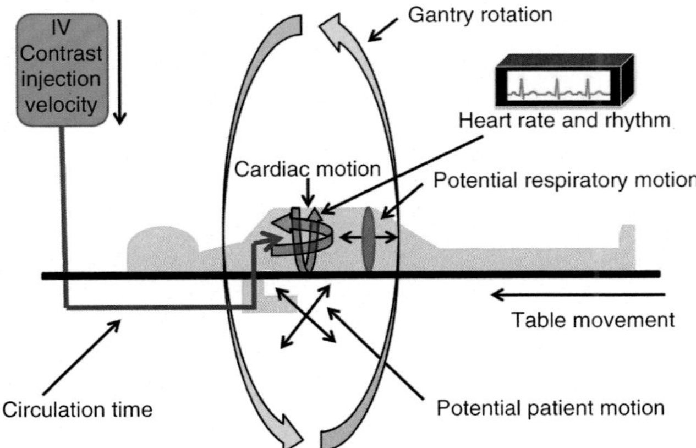

Fig. 7.1 Schematic demonstrating multiple motion factors which must be accounted for during imaging, including the complexities of cardiac motion, motion related to variation in heart rate and rhythm, potential respiratory motion, potential patient movement, table motion, gantry rotation, and the movement of the intravenous contrast bolus to the structures of interest

to variation in heart rate and rhythm, potential respiratory motion, potential patient movement, table motion, gantry rotation, and timing and movement of the intravenous contrast bolus through the structures of interest (Fig. 7.1).

Optimization of image acquisition is achieved through localization of target structures, timing of scanning for capture of images during the segment of the R-R interval with relatively slow cardiac motion, and injection of contrast media to enhance opacification of structures throughout all slice levels. These techniques help to avoid or minimize motion artifacts and suboptimal opacification of structures of interest, which would make subsequent image reconstruction and diagnostic analysis a challenge. Imaging methodology must also focus on minimizing the exposure to radiation and the amount of intravenous contrast. This chapter will focus on methods essential to acquisition of diagnostic images for the assessment of cardiovascular pathology.

Image Acquisition Concepts

The ability to visualize the coronary vasculature is due to advances in spatial and temporal resolution of scanning technology. There are multiple factors that affect spatial and temporal resolution, many of which are interdependent. The goal of image acquisition is to visualize the target structures in their entirety while limiting the field of view to exclude additional structures, as a larger field of view will increase radiation exposure and may diminish image quality. The field of view defines the imaging boundaries important to ensuring visualization of structures of interest. As the 512 by 512 voxel matrix is assigned to a particular field of view, a smaller field of view leads to greater spatial resolution. For example, if a field of view is set at 20 cm, the voxel size is 20 cm divided by 512 voxels, or 0.4 mm. If the field of view is set a 50 cm to include evaluation of axilla, breast and lungs, the voxel size is approximately 1 mm, or 2.5 fold worse resolution. Structures are delineated by their attenuation, as measured in Hounsfield units (HU), named after Sir Godfrey Hounsfield, the inventor of computed tomography. Each voxel is assigned a unit of attenuation based on a scale, with the attenuation values of different substances represented by a different HU value [1]. Representative HU values include: air −1000, fat −50 to −100, water 0, muscle 10–40, contrast 80–300, calcium 130–1500.

Scanner

Conceptually, multidetector computed tomography (MDCT) systems work using similar principles, but vary in regard to specific components and features. A MDCT system has an x-ray tube/collimator and detector/collimator housed in a gantry capable of extremely rapid rotation. The x-ray tube provides radiation energy quantified through tube current (mAs) and tube voltage (kVP). Multidetector scanners have multiple rows of detectors arranged in a variety of arrays with the goal of covering a specified volume during each gantry rotation. Advances in detector number and arrangement have lead to increases in the volume of coverage per rotation, with imaging of the entire heart now achievable within one cardiac cycle [2].

The relationship between table movement, gantry rotation speed and beam collimation defines the degree volume coverage per rotation, as well as the degree of overlap between rotations. The concept of "pitch" quantifies this relationship, as pitch relates to coverage obtained by the x-ray beam, through beam width and table movement, during one rotation of the gantry. The pitch therefore defines the amount of overlap of the acquired data and the speed at which the study is complete. Overlapping images allow for oversampling, permitting multisector image reconstruction, but also lead to greater radiation exposure. With a pitch value of less than 1, there is overlap between volumes of coverage. The definition of pitch has evolved with advancement of scanner technologies, and various equations have been proposed depending on the specific type of scanner [3]. Using conventional ECG-gated helical data acquisition, the pitch values for coronary CT angiography are typically considerably less than 1 (e.g., 0.22), which indicates that the table is advanced by much less than one detector row width during one rotation of the scanner. Thus, the same region within the heart is exposed during several consecutive rotations, which increases radiation dose. Newer systems enable thinner slice thickness and collimation, allowing for an even lower pitch resulting in more images, thinner reconstruction intervals, and better visualization of the coronary anatomy. Systems which provide enough Z axis coverage for whole heart imaging in one gantry rotation eliminate the variable of pitch, by allowing for imaging without table movement [2]. In contrast, the latest generation dual-source CT technology permits ECG-triggered helical scanning at very high pitch values. By inter-weaving data measured from two detector systems separated by approximately 90°, pitch can be increased up to 3.4 [4]. Helical scanning with such high pitch values reduces the amount of redundant data collected, thus substantially decreasing radiation exposure. This dual-source CT configuration allows prospectively ECG-triggered high-pitch helical scan mode, first introduced in 2009. With single-source CT systems, this pitch is limited to a maximum value of 1.5 for gapless data acquisition in the z-axis. At higher pitch values, data gaps occur, which may result in image artifacts and errors in image reconstruction. However, with second-generation dual-source CT, the second tube/detector system is used to fill the data gaps; accordingly, the pitch can be increased to values above 3. This results in very short CT data acquisition and radiation exposure times.

ECG Triggering

ECG triggering is essential to minimize the effects of cardiac motion on image acquisition. Cardiac and coronary motion during a single cardiac cycle is extremely complex and can be analyzed in the context of the X, Y, and Z axis planes. Left ventricular contraction and relaxation are the main source of cardiac motion. Multiple types of cardiac motion have been noted including: inward or outward motion of the endocardium with systole and diastole; rotation; torsion or wringing; translocation; and "accordion-like" base to apex motion [3]. There is greater X-Y direction motion at the mid-portion of the left ventricle and greater Z direction motion at the base of the heart [5]. Left ventricular endocardial maximal motion speed has been reported at 41–100 mm/s [6, 7].

Specific motion issues also relate to individual coronary arteries. Since the right coronary artery is further from the center of the left ventricle than the left coronary artery, this artery exhibits faster motion, especially in its mid-section [8]. Atrial systole and diastole are important factors causing motion of the right coronary artery and the left circumflex coronary artery [9]. The right coronary artery has 50 mm/s motion speed by angiography [10]. The left main and proximal portion of left anterior descending coronary artery have greater Z plane motion, and therefore Z axis motion can induce left main motion abnormalities [5, 7].

Given the imaging challenges caused by cardiac motion, appropriate collimation size and acquisition speed are factors important to minimizing CCTA motion artifact. Since the acquisition speed is insufficient to completely freeze heart motion, cardiac triggering is essential in order to capture and process images at times of minimal cardiac and coronary artery motion speed to avoid blurring of images.

Based on ventricular and atrial contraction and relaxation, there are six phases in a cardiac cycle (R-R interval). These include: isovolumic contraction time, ejection time, isovolumic relaxation time, left ventricular rapid filling, diatasis, and atrial contraction time. During ventricular systole, the motion of right coronary artery and left circumflex mid-segment are in an anterior and inner direction, which reverses in diastole. At end isovolemic contraction and relaxation, the motion speed is close zero, but the time interval for imaging is very short.

There are three relatively low speed motion segments: isovolumic contraction, isovolumic relaxation, and diastasis. The isovolumic contraction time (after the R wave) and relaxation time (after the T wave) are approximately 50–140 ms. Diastasis is the other slower motion segment, but the length is more variable following heart rate changes. In patient with heart rates of greater than 100–110 bpm, diastasis is minimal [11]. The diatasis segment is the optimal scan time in patient with a lower heart rate, and is the most common time period for assessment in patients with regular and controlled heart rates.

With image acquisition, an ECG signal is simultaneously recorded with the raw data set. Two ECG gating techniques are used for CCTA imaging, retrospective and prospective triggering. With retrospective ECG gating, images are acquired throughout the cardiac cycle (Figs. 7.2 and 7.3) [12]. The strength of this approach is that images can be reconstructed using the most optimal timing for each coronary artery or arterial segment after image acquisition has occurred. Additionally, acquisition of images throughout the cardiac cycle allows for volumetric assessment of cardiac function. The major drawback of this approach is that radiation exposure is significantly greater than with a prospective ECG gated approach. Retrospective gating with current tube modulation leads to a significant decrease in radiation by decreasing radiation exposure during the systolic phase of the cardiac cycle [13].

With prospective triggering, images are obtained at a set percentage of the R-R interval. The advantage of this technique is the limitation to radiation exposure [14]. The disadvantage relates to the limited dataset obtained. If the images obtained demonstrate significant motion artifact, there are no other images to reconstruct. Given the variability of heart rate with arrhythmias, prospective gating can be problematic with significant atrial or ventricular ectopy or atrial fibrillation.

In regard to variability of heart rate or rhythm, any change in heart rate or rhythm can alter chamber size, and therefore change of the spatial location of target structure in axial or

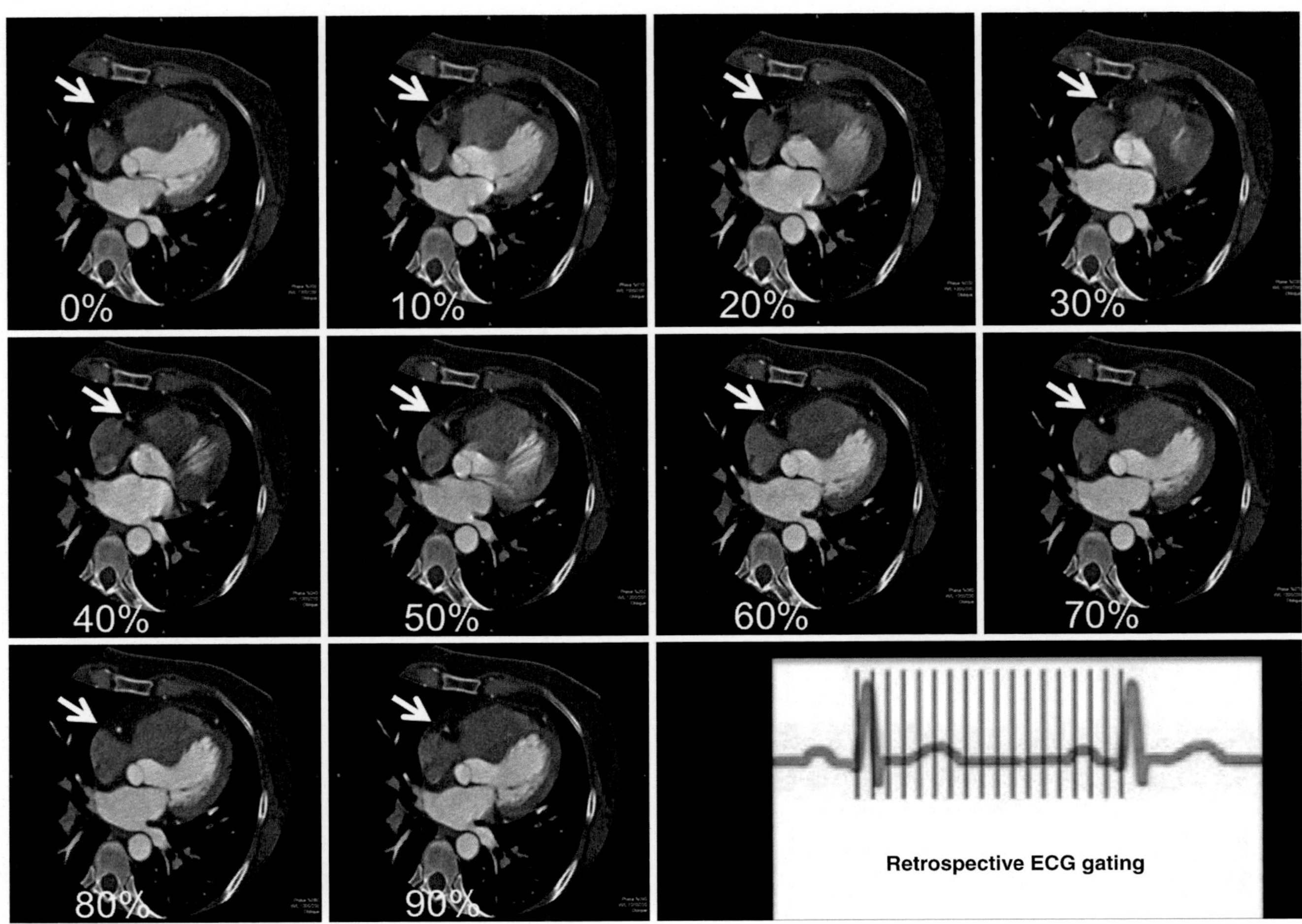

Fig. 7.2 Demonstration of motion of the right coronary artery at serial decile percentages of the R-R interval during retrospective gating. The most optimal R-R percentage is 70 %, as blurring of the right coronary artery is seen at other phases. The *arrow* depicts the right coronary artery, which should be a round structure, but with motion, appears as a 'cashew-nut' shape

3-D images, even if the individual axial image is not blurred. All patients have some variability in heart rate, even those without atrial or ventricular ectopy. Scanning protocols exist which can withhold imaging during short R-R intervals during image acquisition [15]. Post processing analysis includes editing and deletion of images from ectopic beats and analysis of mid-diastolic phases of the R-R interval with an absolute rather than relative time from the preceding R wave when the R-R interval is variable.

Heart rate control is essential for image optimization. Premedication with beta blockers, or calcium channel blockers when beta blockers are contra-indicated, is used to achieve sinus rates of 60 beats/min using most standard MDCT systems. With dual source MDCT systems, imaging can be performed with heart rates in a higher range (although radiation doses will still go up with faster heart rates, so good justification for beta blockade with this system still exists) [16, 17].

High quality images on CCTA depend on a low and steady heart rate (below 70 bpm, and preferably below 60 bpm in most cases), as a consistently wide diastolic time interval is needed with techniques such as ECG-based tube current modulation, prospectively ECG-triggered axial scanning, and prospectively ECG-triggered high-pitch helical scanning. Without adequate patient preparation (generally, beta-blocker drugs), it is rare that this goal is achieved. Calcium channel blockers with good chronotropic effects (verapamil, diltiazem) can be used as an alternative, or in conjunction with, beta blockade in patients with high resting heart rates undergoing CCTA.

Nitroglycerin is given sublingually prior to scanning to maximally dilate coronary arteries. Since there may be catecholamine stimulation with breath hold, the sound of the scanner, nitroglycerin administration, and the sensation of contrast administration, a resting sinus rate that appears to be controlled without medications prior to scanning may still increase during scanning. Special attention to monitoring of heart rate and blood pressure is important, as in some circumstances patients may not be able to tolerate medications for heart rate control and dilation of coronary arteries.

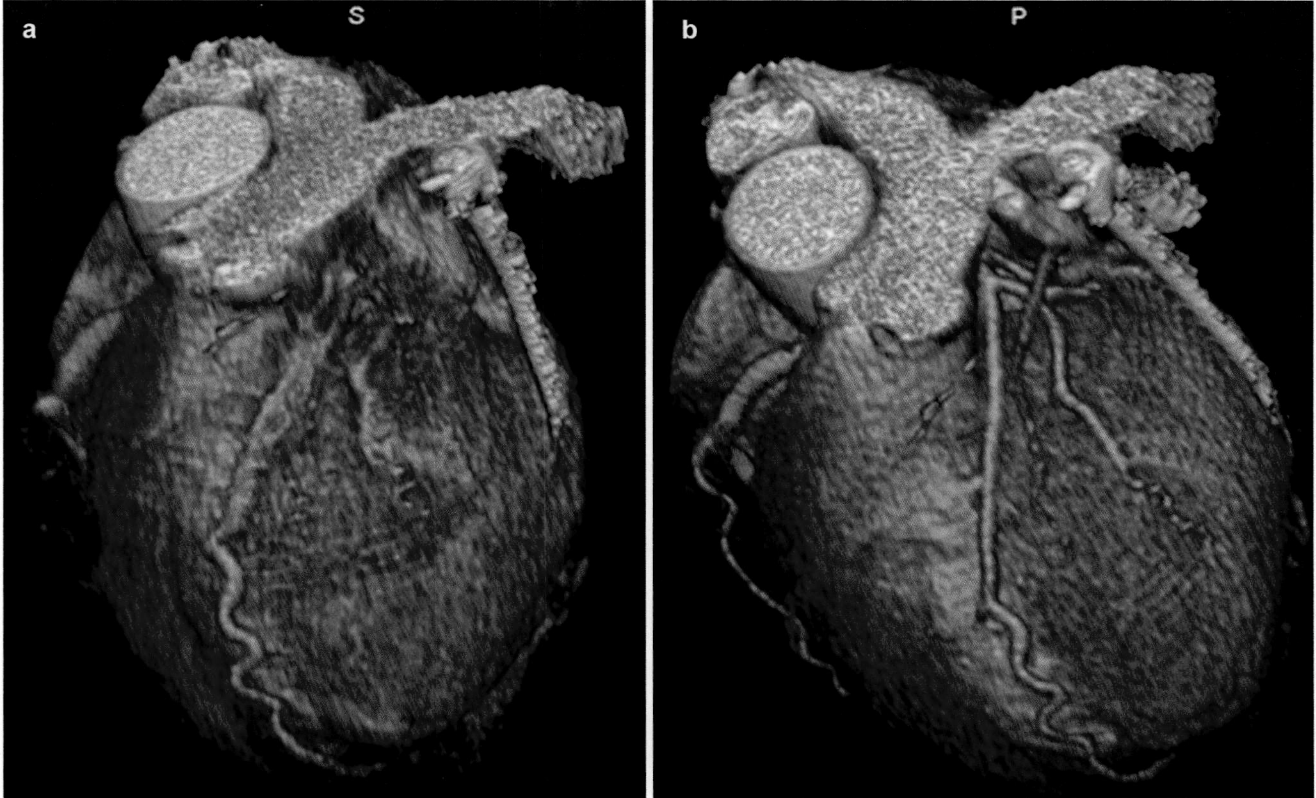

Fig. 7.3 3-D reconstructions of the LAD at different phases of the R-R interval, demonstrating reconstruction at a suboptimal phase and an optimal phase for artery visualization. (**a**) Reconstruction at 30 % of the R-R interval. (**b**) Reconstruction at 70 % of the R-R interval

Breath hold is essential to limit motion of structures due to respiration during image acquisition. Breath hold times have decreased significantly with advances in technology and allow for cardiac imaging to be completed during a single breath hold. There is some controversy as to the optimal phase of respiration for breath hold. Regardless of the phase chosen in an individual lab, it is important to practice breath hold commands and exercises prior to the scan. The technologist, by assessing whether breath holding was optimal during the scout film, calcium score and/or contrast timing run, can further educate the patient prior to the CTA scan acquisition. As an end-inspiratory breath hold will move thoracic structures more caudally than an end-expiratory breath hold, consistent breath hold instructions need to be given for preview images and actual scans, and critical for the CTA for diagnostic images.

Contrast Media Injection

The aim of contrast media injection is to enhance the contrast differentiation between target structure and surrounding tissues, by increasing the CT Hounsfield Units (CT HU) of the interest structure. Ideally, an injection protocol will achieve optimal enhancement with uniformity of contrast enhancement at all slice levels using as small a dose of contrast medium as possible. Important factors to consider in regard to contrast media injection are circulation time and injection methodology.

Assessment of the circulation time is important to timing the acquisition of images, and is defined as the time from contrast injection to the optimal enhancement of target structures. This sequence typically consists of repetitively imaging a single slice using a low radiation serial scanning of the same slice to obtain the peak enhancement time through time density curve analysis (Figs. 7.4 and 7.5). With CCTA, scans are obtained at the level of the takeoff of the left main coronary artery or descending aorta, to create a time–density curve to assess the time to peak opacification. The measured transit time is then used as the delay time from the start of the contrast injection to imaging start for the CCTA. It is important to use the same injection rate for the circulation time as for the subsequent CCTA study.

Another contrast timing method utilizes an automatic bolus-triggering technique. With this method, angiography imaging is automatically activated when the CT HU reaches a pre-specified HU value [18]. Circulation times vary based on the cardiac output. Patients with low output states having increased times and high output states with decreased times. Many factors influence circulation time, including venous

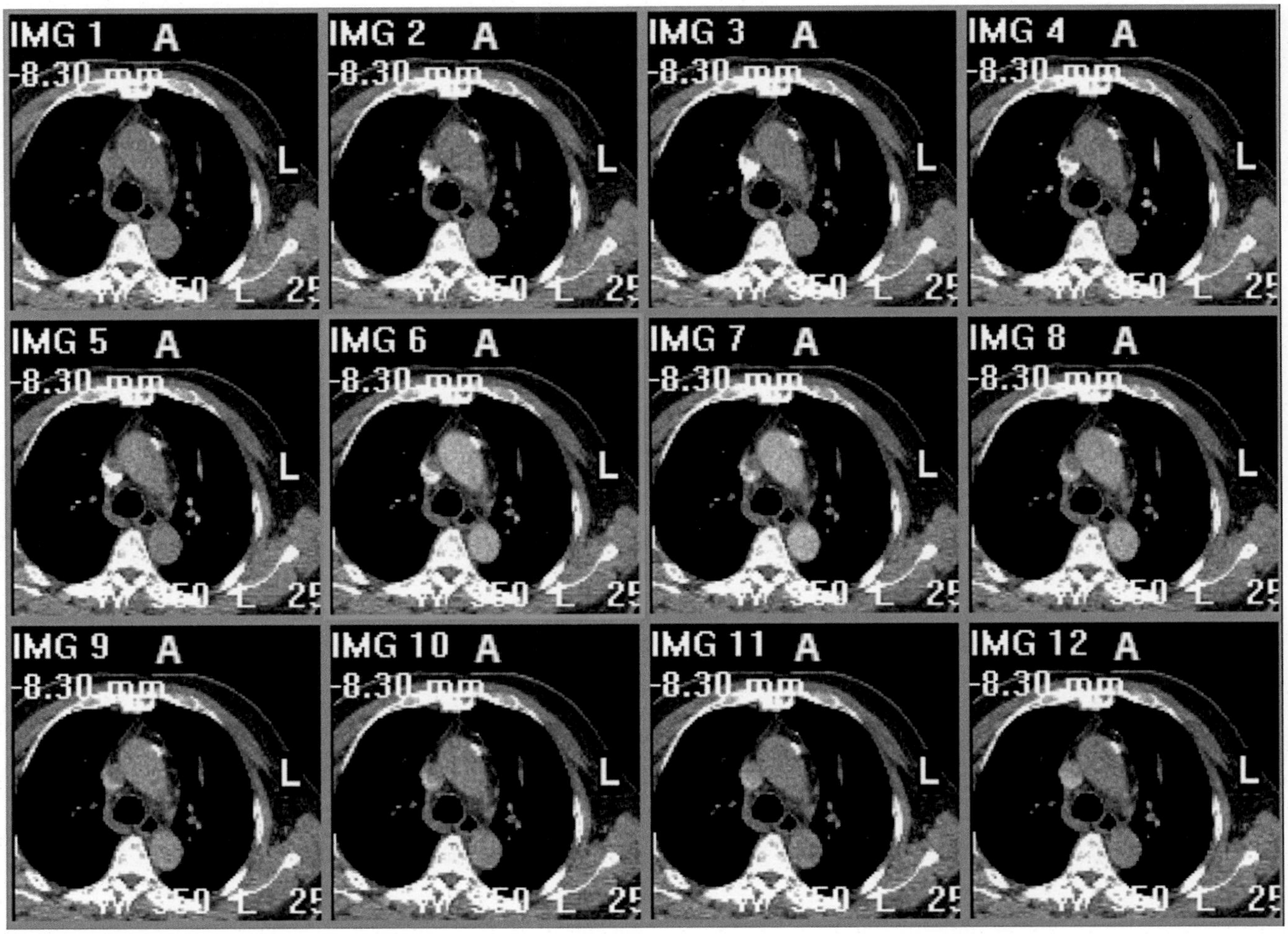

Fig. 7.4 Serial axial images of the target slice demonstrating opacification for determination of the circulation time

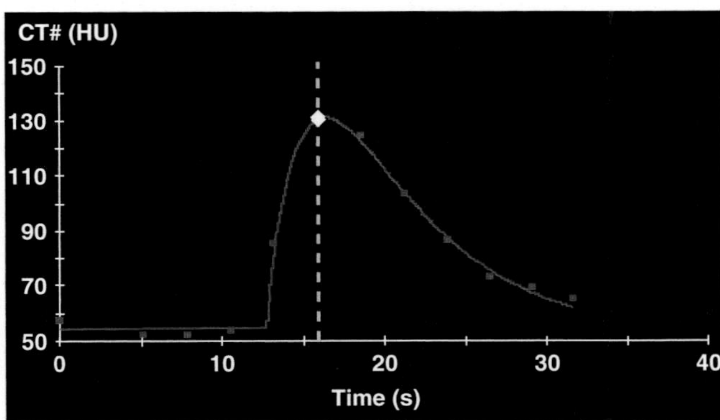

Fig. 7.5 Graph of CT Hounsfield Units versus time, demonstrating the time to maximal opacification of the region of interest

anatomy, cardiac output, and underlying cardiac and valvular function and therefore must be individually determined.

Low osmolar nonionic contrast media contrast medium is usually administered via an 20-gauge needle in the antecubital vein. Optimal enhancement depends on the contrast media dose and injection rate. The goal is to maintain the same level of vascular enhancement throughout image acquisition. The dose of contrast media is dependent on multiple factors, such as patient size, scan time, and desired enhancement level (CT HU). Multiphase contrast injectors with preset volumes and injection velocities are used to maintain uniformity of contrast enhancement throughout the study. A first injection stage with a high velocity, often 5 ml/s, is followed by saline injection to flush the remaining contrast out of the intravenous line and antecubital vein using a multiphase injector. The use of a saline bolus after contrast injection moves the residual contrast in the intravenous tubing and arm veins into the heart and coronary vasculature. The timing of the saline bolus is important, as in some studies clearance of the venous circulation and right heart structures can help with visualization of arterial structures, while in other studies, these structures are important to analysis. A middle phase with diluted contrast can also be utilized for some opacification of right heart and venous structures.

Specific injection protocols may be necessary for certain specialized indications including congenital heart disease. Since image quality on CT is based upon contrast to noise ratios (CNR), maintaining good contrast opacification is important. In larger patients or more obese subjects, the noise will be greater, so to ensure good image quality, faster rates of contrast injection are preferable to maintain the CNR. Thus, for patients who are very obese, increasing the rate of contrast to 6 ml/s is often necessary. A larger IV access may be necessary to ensure good flow at higher injection rates.

Preview, Calcium, and Contrast Scans

CCTA is performed in the following sequence: planar scout images, a non-contrast coronary artery calcium scan, a timing scan for assessment of the circulation time, and a contrast scan. Planar scout images are obtained in order to define the most cranial and caudal scanning levels (Z-axis) of the structures of interest. The scout images are obtained in anteroposterior and lateral views and aligned to the patient by a laser system. The scan volume is selected with the structures of interest placed within the center of the scanning volume. Important landmarks can be identified including the left atrial appendage, which is usually the most cranial structure of the heart, and the ventricular apex, which is the most caudal structure. Although the carina had served as a marker to localize the most cranial aspect of the heart, the distance from carina to left main coronary artery is extremely variable [19]. Also, the left anterior descending coronary artery can course cranial to the left main coronary artery (Fig. 7.6). For coronary artery imaging, scanning 10 mm cranial to the left main coronary artery and 10 mm caudal to the apex is subsequently performed with CCTA. In patients with coronary artery bypass grafts, the starting point is the top of the aortic arch or 10 mm higher than the surgical metal clips. The mid level of the right pulmonary artery can also be used as the beginning of the scan level, if it can be defined in preview images.

After the scout images, a calcium scan is performed (Fig. 7.7). This is a high resolution non-contrast cardiac-gated study which provides important prognostic information regarding future cardiovascular risk. For the calcium scan, the 2-D axial images are analyzed with the identification of calcium either using manual or automated methods, with quantification of calcium score based on identification of HU units with an attenuation of at least 130 HU in the areas of identified calcium. There are two major methods of quantifying coronary artery calcium, the Agatston score and volumetric analysis. The Agatston score is based on the plaque number, and plaque area times a coefficient based on the peak HU units in the plaque [20]. Calcium volume score describes a volumetric analysis of calcium with calculation based on volumetric reconstruction and is more reproducible on serial study [21]. The calcium score is a marker of plaque burden and is an independent risk factor for coronary artery disease beyond traditional risk factors [22, 23].

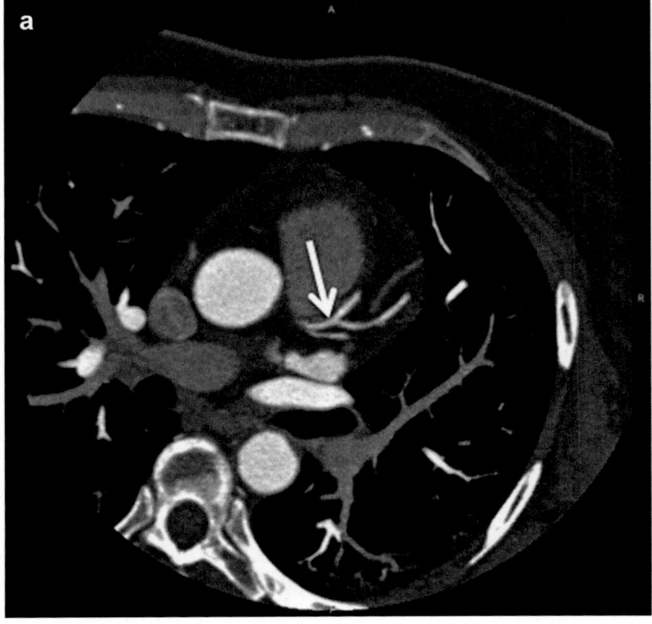

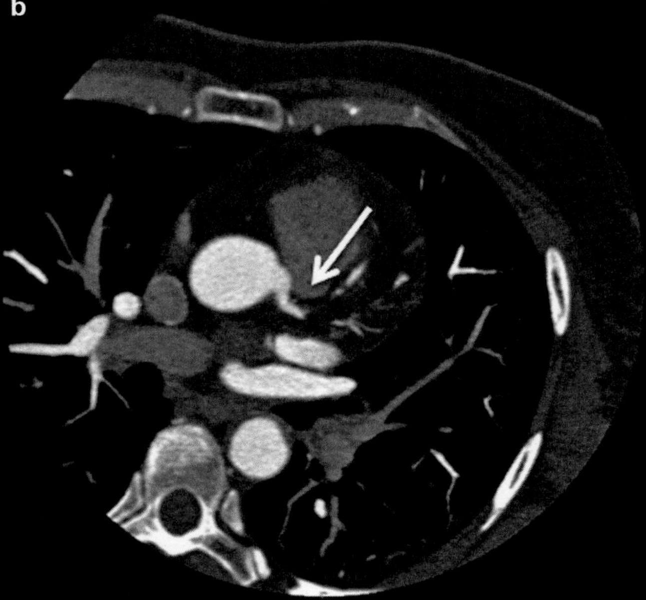

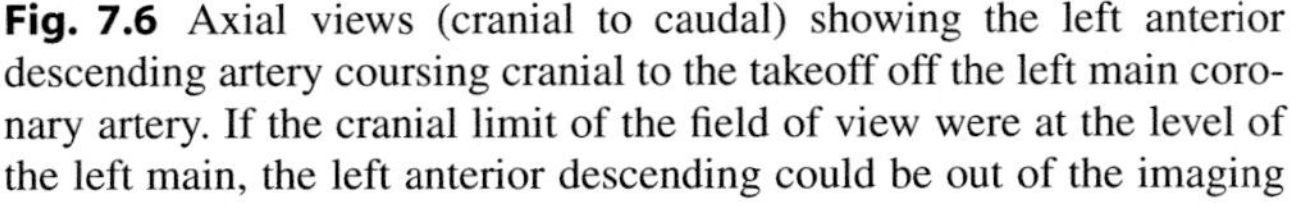

Fig. 7.6 Axial views (cranial to caudal) showing the left anterior descending artery coursing cranial to the takeoff off the left main coronary artery. If the cranial limit of the field of view were at the level of the left main, the left anterior descending could be out of the imaging field. (**a**) The cranial slice, showing the left anterior descending (*arrow*). (**b**) A more caudal slice, demonstrating the left main artery (*arrow*) is visualized inferiorly to the left anterior descending artery

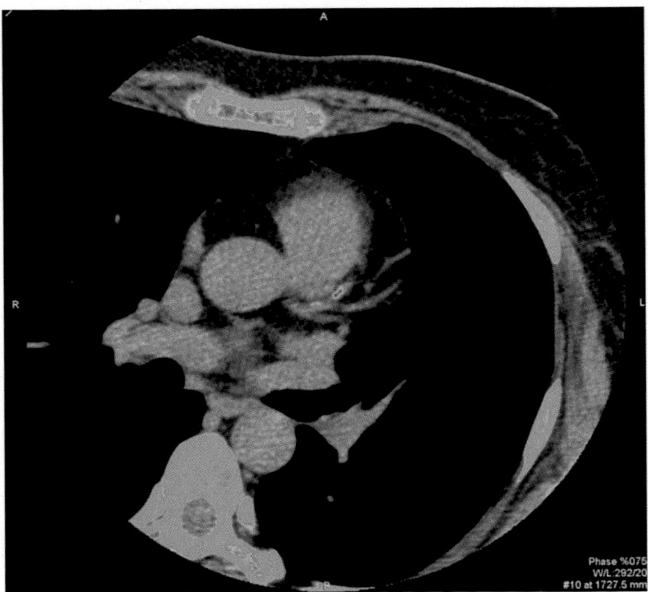

Fig. 7.7 Coronary artery calcium score axial image showing a calcification of the left anterior descending coronary artery

The calcium scan is useful to the planning, performance, and interpretation of the CCTA. Assessment of the images can be used to ensure that there is complete coverage of the coronary anatomy in the image set prior to contrast angiography, as well as to determine the minimum volume to be covered to minimize radiation exposure [24]. The degree of coronary calcification may prohibit the accurate assessment of coronary artery stenoses.

The calcium score as well as the calcium distribution should be assessed prior to the performance of the CCTA to determine whether the contrast study should be performed. Different imaging centers use various cutoffs for the performance of CCTA in the setting of a significantly elevated calcium score, with some center using >500 or >1000. It is important though to have an understanding of the specific goal of an individual study, as depending on the question asked and the location of calcium, some studies may still be performed in settings of an elevated calcium score. For example, in cases where the location and patency of coronary artery bypass grafts are the clinical questions, calcium in the native coronary arteries may still not necessarily prohibit the study from being performed. In addition to traditional cardiac risk factors, knowledge of the calcium score is helpful in assessing the pretest probability of coronary artery disease when interpreting the contrast angiography images.

After performance of the calcium scan, a contrast angiography study is performed, requiring the administration of iodinated contrast timed to enhance the structures of interest. This may vary by the type of study, with some studies performed specifically for assessment of coronary artery anatomy, while others are performed for additional assessment of thoracic vasculature, such as in the case of congenital heart disease.

Relation of Image Acquisition to Image Analysis

Image reconstruction is dependent on image acquisition, as the reconstructed images are only as good as the acquired data. The raw datasets are imported to workstations with software allowing the analysis of images in multiple 2-D and 3-D formats. Prior to reconstruction, the 2-D axial dataset must be reviewed to ensure that the structures of interest were scanned in their entirety and that there is uniformity of contrast throughout the study. A decrease in contrast in the distal vessels can appear as stenoses. Adequate and uniform enhancement of the distal aorta can be helpful in ensuring that distal coronary arteries have been adequately opacified.

Interpretation of CT coronary angiography requires reconstruction and analysis of multiple 2-D and 3-D analyses so that findings can be confirmed on multiple views and artifacts related to image acquisition can be identified. Image reconstruction allows a 3-D understanding of cardiovascular anatomy from large vessel to small vessel. The serial axial 2-D images are reconstructed into a 3-D data cube with subsequent use of software to edit out and analyze cardiovascular structure. Workstation software has dramatically reduced the time for image editing and reconstruction. Systematic reconstruction, serial automated editing, and analysis of this data cube allows one to glean information important to characterization of the structure and relationship between structures essential to clinical diagnosis and planning and facilitation of cardiovascular procedures. These reconstructions include: assessment of thoracic structures in relation to skeletal structures, relation of large vessel vasculature and structures, cardiac chambers, valves, and coronary vasculature (Fig. 7.8).

Reconstruction of coronary artery anatomy requires assessment of the phase of the cardiac cycle during which an artery or arterial segment is most quiescent. Retrospectively gated axial images can be reconstructed at different diastolic phases of the cardiac cycle and assessed for the most optimal images regarding minimizing cardiac motion (Figs. 7.2 and 7.3). As the optimal phase of the cardiac cycle may vary by artery and arterial segment, different arteries or segments may need to be analyzed using multiple modalities. Once the correct phase or phases have been chosen, 2-D images can be rapidly formatted in axial, sagittal, and coronal planes.

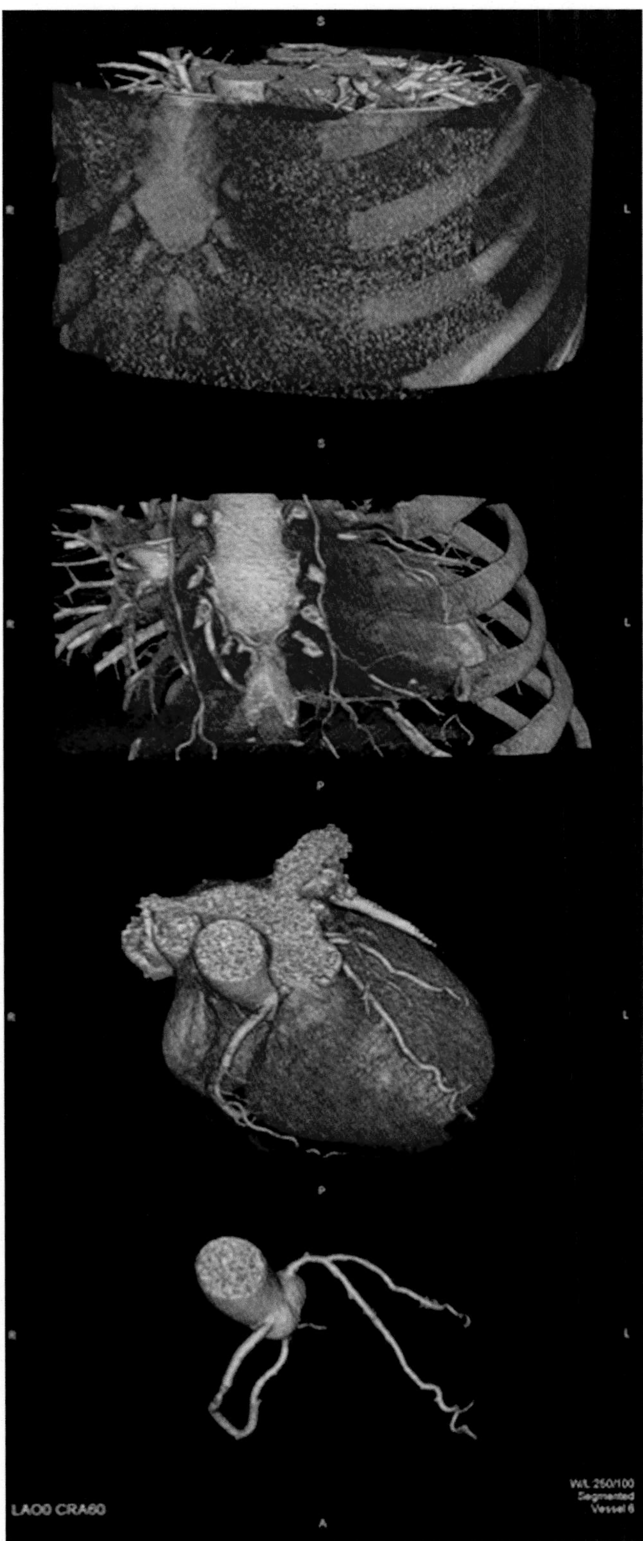

Fig. 7.8 Reconstructions of thoracic structures in relation to skeletal structures, relation of large vessel vasculature and structures, cardiac chambers, valves, and coronary vasculature

Subsequent analysis is performed primarily from axial images with additional analysis with multiple modalities of image reconstruction (Fig. 7.9a–g). Functional analysis for retrospectively gated scans can be formatted and assessed in standard echo views (Fig. 7.10).

Although the 3-D reconstructed images are both aesthetic and intuitive regarding orientation, it is essential to recognize that the process of reconstruction has limitations. It is essential to remember that the 2-D views provide an entire dataset whereas the 3-D techniques lead to loss of data and potential artifacts that adversely affect interpretation of images. Given the limitations of reconstruction techniques, it is essential to continually reference back to the 2-D images and view potential findings using multiple types of reconstructions before making a diagnosis.

There are many factors related to image acquisition that may affect image reconstruction and analysis. With volume rendering, pixels are assigned HU depending on their attenuation. With automated editing, pixels below a certain HU cutoff (lower threshold 80–100 HU) are edited out. Volume rendering and editing software allows creation of 3-D image with structures removed to adequately visualize structures of interest, but involves potential loss of data through over-editing of structures. If over-edited, the coronary arteries can appear as though stenoses are present.

Construction of 3-D images from 2-D image sets with cardiac respiratory or patient motion between slices can lead to artifactually discontinuous arterial segments that could be misinterpreted as stenoses. Lack of uniformity of contrast enhancement on serial slices may also result in the artifactual appearance of stenoses. If only viewed on 3-D images, myocardial bridging can be misinterpreted as obstructive coronary artery disease. Misalignment artifacts (formed from movement between the large acquisitions of the 64–160 detector arrays or collimation), can also form regions of pseudo-stenosis. Misalignment artifacts have been previously known as mis-registration, stair step, collimation or a multitude of prior names. The Society of Cardiovascular Computed Tomography has developed a nomenclature document to standardize these names [25].

Partial volume effects may limit reconstruction and analysis. The goal of scanning is to acquire isotropic data, where the spatial resolution is equal in the X, Y, and Z axes, allowing for accurate images with multiplane reconstructions [26]. As spatial resolution in the Z axis may not be truly isotropic, some volume averaging of data may occur. Therefore, volumes averaging may occur with only a portion of the depth of the image being represented as present throughout the dataset.

Calcified plaques may also limit reconstruction and analysis of images. The purpose of contrast enhanced studies

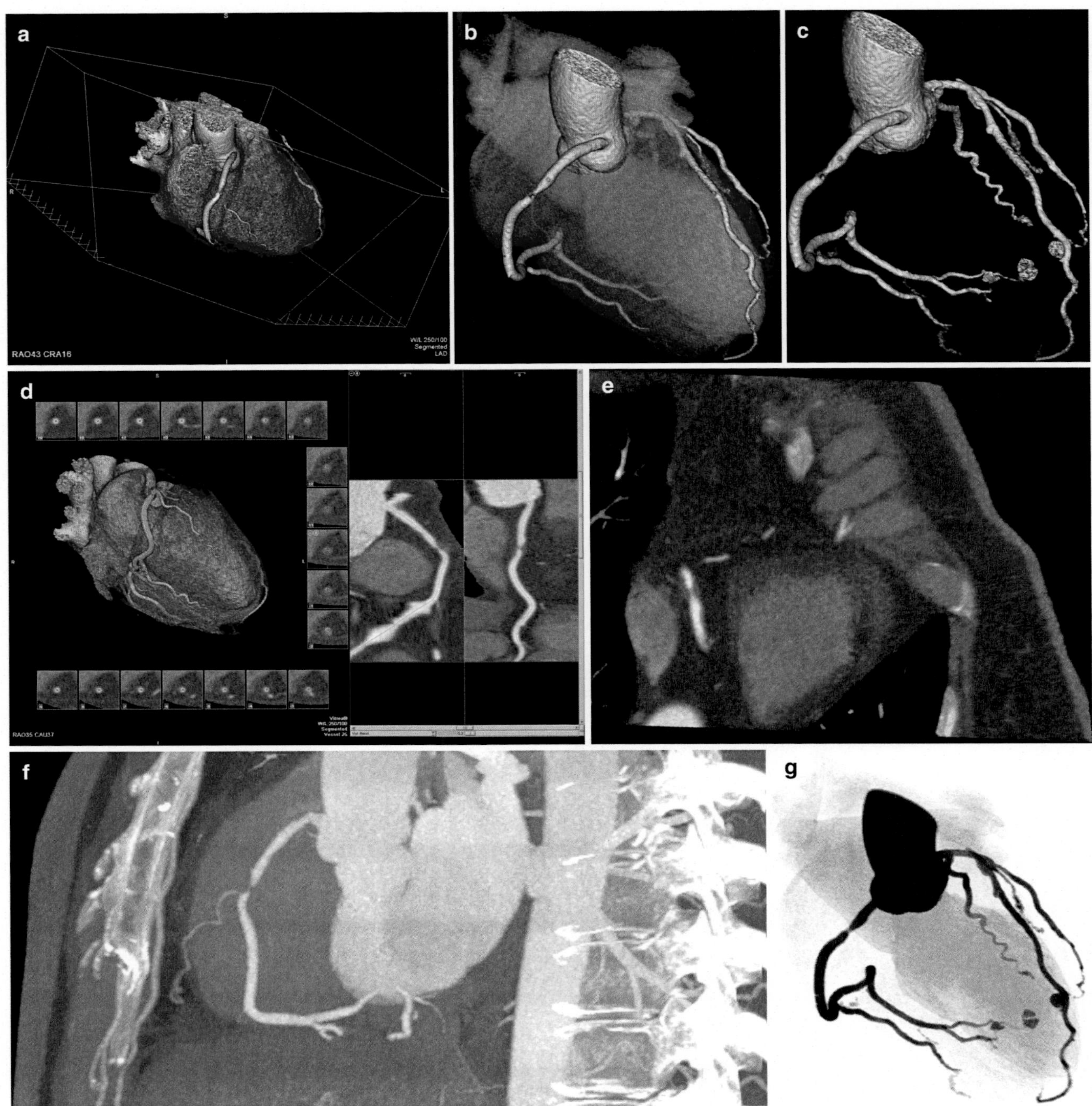

Fig. 7.9 A significant right coronary artery non-calcified stenosis is shown using multiple reconstruction modalities. Multiple CCTA angiography views are demonstrated including; (**a**) 3-D volume rendered view of the heart and coronary arteries; (**b**) 3-D volume rendered view of the heart and coronary arteries; (**c**) 3-D volume rendered view of only the coronary arteries; (**d**) Curved multiplanar reformatted view; (**e**) Double oblique reformat; (**f**) Sagittal view with a thick maximum intensity projection; (**g**) Cardiac catheterization angiography emulation

is to increase contrast between coronary vessel lumen and surrounding tissues. Greater lumen enhancement (represented by increased CT HU) will create greater contrast between the vessel lumen and non-calcified vessel wall, which is especially important for visualization of small vessels. Luminal enhancement though, will decrease the contrast between enhanced vessel lumen and calcified plaques. This can make assessment of the coronary arterial wall challenging for assessment of different tissue components of the plaque wall.

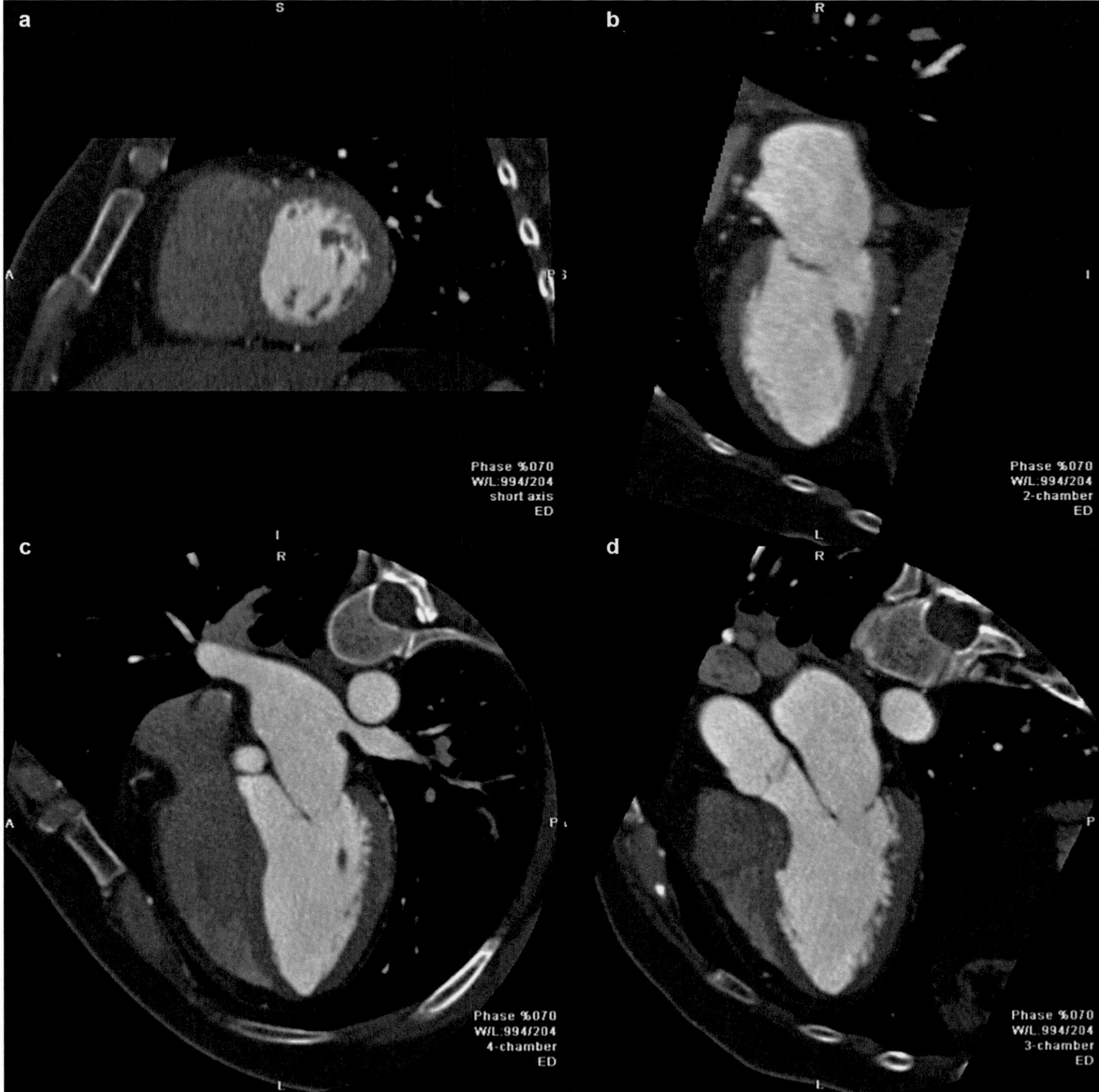

Fig. 7.10 Functional views in standard echo planes. (**a**) Short axis view; (**b**) 2 chamber view; Panel; (**c**) 4 chamber view; (**d**) 3 chamber view

Other reconstruction and viewing modalites can are useful for analysis of images that are problematic due to issues related to image acquisition [27]. Maximal intensity projections demonstrate the maximal density point at each point in a 3-D volume. Conceptually, this provides the ability to move through the 3-D data cube with a thick slab focused on the maximum intensity of the images in the slab. The modality provides for assessment of small and distal vessels and is helpful for differentiating calcium, contrast, and metal in the coronary arteries and avoids issues of volume averaging of structures. As editing is not involved with this modality, there will be overlap of structures as one moves through the dataset.

Multiplanar curved reformatting allows for in plane analysis of an individual vessel (Fig. 7.11) [28]. A reconstruction is performed orthogonal to vessel centerline

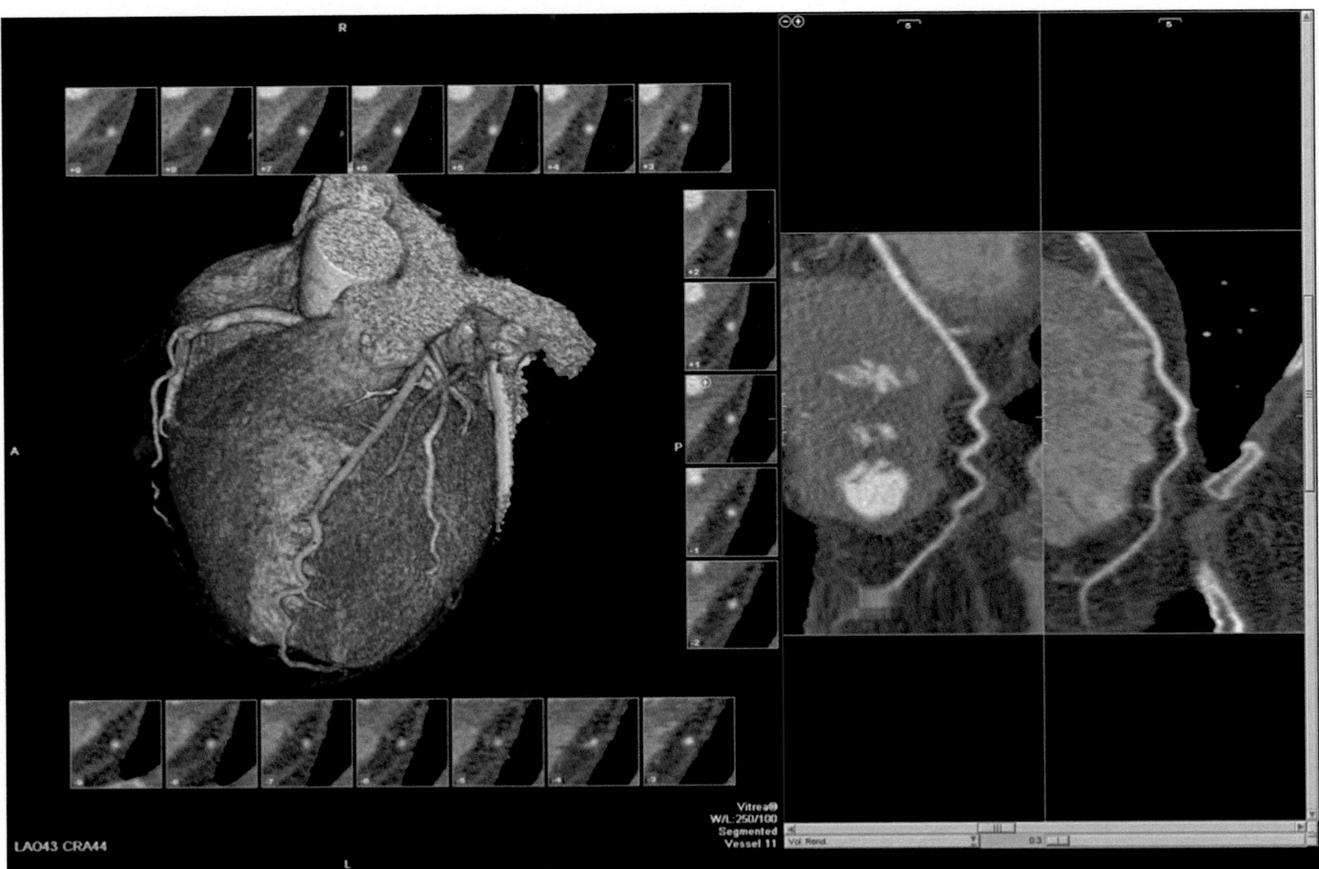

Fig. 7.11 Curved multiplanar reformation of the left anterior descending coronary artery, allowing in plane analysis of the vessel

and does not require editing. Vessels can be analyzed in a 360° rotation allowing for assessment of eccentricity of plaque in relation to the vessel lumen. The technique requires accurate vessel tracking and determination of the centerline of the vessel. Interactive display methods may provide greater diagnostic accuracy than pre-rendered images [27]. Virtual endoscopic views, which provide a perspective from inside a vessel or chamber have been developed, but are very dependent on filtering and smoothing techniques. Fluoroscopic views are helpful for assessment of metallic structures such as pacemaker leads.

The evolution of CT scanners and workstations allow for rapid acquisition and reconstructions of images for the characterization of cardiovascular disease processes. CCTA imaging poses challenges due to the complex motion of the heart, variation in heart rate and rhythm, and tissue characteristics of cardiovascular structures. An understanding of these factors and meticulous attention to triggering techniques, contrast injection methods, and preview methods can lead to images visualizing anatomy and function critical to the diagnosis and treatment of patients with cardiovascular disease.

References

1. Brooks RA. A quantitative theory of the Hounsfield unit and its application to dual energy scanning. J Comput Assist Tomogr. 1977;1(4):487–93.
2. Dewey M, Zimmermann E, Deissenrieder F, et al. Noninvasive coronary angiography by 320-row computed tomography with lower radiation exposure and maintained diagnostic accuracy: comparison of results with cardiac catheterization in a head-to-head pilot investigation. Circulation. 2009;120(10):867–75.
3. Silverman PM, Kalender WA, Hazle JD. Common terminology for single and multislice helical CT. AJR Am J Roentgenol. 2001;176(5):1135–6.
4. Hausleiter J, Bischoff B, Hein F, Meyer T, Hadamitzky M, Thierfelder C, Allmendinger T, Flohr TG, Schomig A, Martinoff S. Feasibility of dual-source cardiac CT angiography with high-pitch scan protocols. J Cardiovasc Comput Tomogr. 2009;3: 236–42.
5. Mao S, Budoff MJ, Bin L, Liu SC. Optimal ECG trigger point in electron-beam CT studies: three methods for minimizing motion artifacts. Acad Radiol. 2001;8(11):1107–15.
6. Ritchie CJ, Godwin JD, Crawford CR, Stanford W, Anno H, Kim Y. Minimum scan speeds for suppression of motion artifacts in CT. Radiology. 1992;185(1):37–42.
7. Rogers Jr WJ, Shapiro EP, Weiss JL, et al. Quantification of and correction for left ventricular systolic long-axis shortening by

magnetic resonance tissue tagging and slice isolation. Circulation. 1991;84(2):721–31.

8. Mao S, Lu B, Oudiz RJ, Bakhsheshi H, Liu SC, Budoff MJ. Coronary artery motion in electron beam tomography. J Comput Assist Tomogr. 2000;24(2):253–8.
9. Achenbach S, Ropers D, Holle J, Muschiol G, Daniel WG, Moshage W. In-plane coronary arterial motion velocity: measurement with electron-beam CT. Radiology. 2000;216(2):457–63.
10. Topol EJ, Nissen SE. Our preoccupation with coronary luminology. The dissociation between clinical and angiographic findings in ischemic heart disease. Circulation. 1995;92(8):2333–42.
11. Weyman AE. Principles and practice of echocardiography. 2nd ed. Philadelphia: Lea and Febiger; 1994. p. 721–41.
12. Becker CR, Knez A, Ohnesorge B, Schoepf UJ, Reiser MF. Imaging of noncalcified coronary plaques using helical CT with retrospective ECG gating. AJR Am J Roentgenol. 2000;175(2):423–4.
13. Abada HT, Larchez C, Daoud B, Sigal-Cinqualbre A, Paul JF. MDCT of the coronary arteries: feasibility of low-dose CT with ECG-pulsed tube current modulation to reduce radiation dose. AJR Am J Roentgenol. 2006;186(6 Suppl 2):S387–90.
14. Husmann L, Valenta I, Gaemperli O, et al. Feasibility of low-dose coronary CT angiography: first experience with prospective ECG-gating. Eur Heart J. 2008;29(2):191–7.
15. Matsutani H, Sano T, Kondo T, et al. ECG-edit function in multidetector-row computed tomography coronary arteriography for patients with arrhythmias. Circ J. 2008;72(7):1071–8.
16. Brodoefel H, Burgstahler C, Tsiflikas I, et al. Dual-source CT: effect of heart rate, heart rate variability, and calcification on image quality and diagnostic accuracy. Radiology. 2008;247(2):346–55.
17. Ropers U, Ropers D, Pflederer T, et al. Influence of heart rate on the diagnostic accuracy of dual-source computed tomography coronary angiography. J Am Coll Cardiol. 2007;50(25):2393–8.
18. Cademartiri F, Nieman K, van der Lugt A, et al. Intravenous contrast material administration at 16-detector row helical CT coronary angiography: test bolus versus bolus-tracking technique. Radiology. 2004;233(3):817–23.
19. Bakhsheshi H, Mao S, Budoff MJ, Bin L, Brundage BH. Preview method for electron-beam CT scanning of the coronary arteries. Acad Radiol. 2000;7(8):620–6.
20. Agatston AS, Janowitz WR, Hildner FJ, Zusmer NR, Viamonte Jr M, Detrano R. Quantification of coronary artery calcium using ultrafast computed tomography. J Am Coll Cardiol. 1990;15(4): 827–32.
21. Callister TQ, Cooil B, Raya SP, Lippolis NJ, Russo DJ, Raggi P. Coronary artery disease: improved reproducibility of calcium scoring with an electron-beam CT volumetric method. Radiology. 1998;208(3):807–14.
22. Greenland P, LaBree L, Azen SP, Doherty TM, Detrano RC. Coronary artery calcium score combined with Framingham score for risk prediction in asymptomatic individuals. JAMA. 2004; 291(2):210–5.
23. Greenland P, Bonow RO, Brundage BH, et al. ACCF/AHA 2007 clinical expert consensus document on coronary artery calcium scoring by computed tomography in global cardiovascular risk assessment and in evaluation of patients with chest pain: a report of the American College of Cardiology Foundation Clinical Expert Consensus Task Force (ACCF/AHA Writing Committee to Update the 2000 Expert Consensus Document on Electron Beam Computed Tomography) developed in collaboration with the Society of Atherosclerosis Imaging and Prevention and the Society of Cardiovascular Computed Tomography. J Am Coll Cardiol. 2007;49(3):378–402.
24. Gopal A, Budoff MJ. A new method to reduce radiation exposure during multi-row detector cardiac computed tomographic angiography. Int J Cardiol. 2009;132(3):435–6.
25. Weigold WG, Abbara S, Achenbach S, et al. Consensus document on standardized nomenclature for cardiac computed tomography a report of the society of cardiovascular computed tomography writing committee. J Cardiovasc Comput Tomogr. 2011;5(3):136–44. doi:10.1016/j.jcct.2011.04.004.
26. Tsukagoshi S, Ota T, Fujii M, Kazama M, Okumura M, Johkoh T. Improvement of spatial resolution in the longitudinal direction for isotropic imaging in helical CT. Phys Med Biol. 2007;52(3): 791–801.
27. Ferencik M, Ropers D, Abbara S, et al. Diagnostic accuracy of image postprocessing methods for the detection of coronary artery stenoses by using multidetector CT. Radiology. 2007;243(3): 696–702.
28. Achenbach S, Moshage W, Ropers D, Bachmann K. Curved multiplanar reconstructions for the evaluation of contrast-enhanced electron beam CT of the coronary arteries. AJR Am J Roentgenol. 1998;170(4):895–9.

Post-processing and Reconstruction Techniques for the Coronary Arteries

8

Swaminatha V. Gurudevan

Abstract

Proper post-processing of cardiac CT images is crucial to obtain high-quality diagnostic images of the coronary arteries. The design of acquisition protocols take into account scan-related factors such as the temporal and spatial resolution of the scanner as well as patient-relate factors such as the patient weight and ECG tracing. ECG gating can be performed with either prospective or retrospective gating, with each method having distinct advantages. The next phase of post-processing involves the layout of images on the cardiac CT workstation. These reconstruction techniques enable the interpreting physician to reliably identify the anatomy and course of the coronary arteries and interpret coronary artery plaque and luminal obstruction.

Keywords

Reconstruction • Temporal resolution • Spatial resolution • Maximum intensity projection • Convolution kernel • Pitch • Retrospective and prospective ECG gating

Introduction

With the advent of multidetector computed tomography, noninvasive imaging of the coronary arteries is now possible. Attention to detail in the post-processing aspects of coronary artery imaging is crucial to obtain high-quality, clinically diagnostic images. This chapter will review the scan-related and post-scan related post-processing parameters that with careful adjustment can greatly aid the reader in accurately interpreting cardiovascular CT images.

S.V. Gurudevan, MD, FACC
Department of Medicine, Healthcare Partners Medical Group, 401 S. Fair Oaks Ave., Pasadena, CA 91105, USA
e-mail: SGurudevan@healthcarepartners.com

Scan-Related Post-processing Parameters

Temporal and Spatial Resolution

Two important parameters to understand when evaluating an imaging modality are temporal and spatial resolution. **Temporal resolution** refers to the ability of an imaging modality to detect two distinct events in time as separate events, and is expressed in units of time. It can be likened to the shutter speed on a camera. Fast shutter speeds have superior temporal resolution to slow shutter speeds and produce superior images of rapidly moving subjects in action shots. Slow shutter speeds, on the other hand, will produce blurring artifacts when subjects move. The intrinsic temporal resolution of single source multidetector CT systems (using half-scan reconstruction) ranges from 160 to 225 ms, while dual source CT systems have a temporal resolution as low as 83 ms. Two approaches to optimize temporal resolution in cardiac CT include improving the imaging speed with ultrafast

M.J. Budoff, J.S. Shinbane (eds.), *Cardiac CT Imaging: Diagnosis of Cardiovascular Disease*,
DOI 10.1007/978-3-319-28219-0_8

gantry rotation speeds and slowing the motion of the heart during the examination through effective beta blockade. Each technique is essential to produce motion-free images.

Spatial resolution, on the other hand, refers to the ability of an imaging modality to detect two distinct objects in space as separate objects, and is expressed in units of distance. Smaller objects such as coronary arteries require submillimeter spatial resolution to clearly define the vessel wall, lumen, coronary plaque. The spatial resolution of multidetector CT ranges from 0.5 to 0.625 mm, and is most directly related to the width of the collimated beam.

Cardiac CT Gating

Coronary artery motion that occurs during the cardiac cycle remains the greatest challenge to effective imaging of the coronary arteries with cardiovascular CT [1, 2]. Reconstruction algorithms target phases of the cardiac cycle where the coronary arteries move the least. Coronary artery motion occurs predictably in specific phases of the cardiac cycle. The two phases of the cardiac cycle in which the coronary arteries move the least are *mid-diastole*, during the diastasis period between early rapid ventricular filling (the E wave) and atrial contraction (the A wave) and *end-systole*, immediately prior to the E wave [3]. At slow heart rates (Fig. 8.1), the diastasis period (between 70 and 80 % of the R-R interval) is the most optimal imaging period. At faster heart rates (Fig. 8.2), the diastasis period shrinks, making the end-systolic period (between 30 and 50 % of the R-R interval) the period of least coronary motion [4].

Due to the motion of the beating heart, ECG gating is necessary to achieve consistent images of the heart that are free of motion artifacts. **Prospective ECG gating** relies on the scanner initiating imaging only during a pre-specified interval of the cardiac cycle (Fig. 8.3), usually the mid-diastolic interval. Systolic images are not obtained, and a slow, steady heart rate is necessary to avoid motion artifacts.

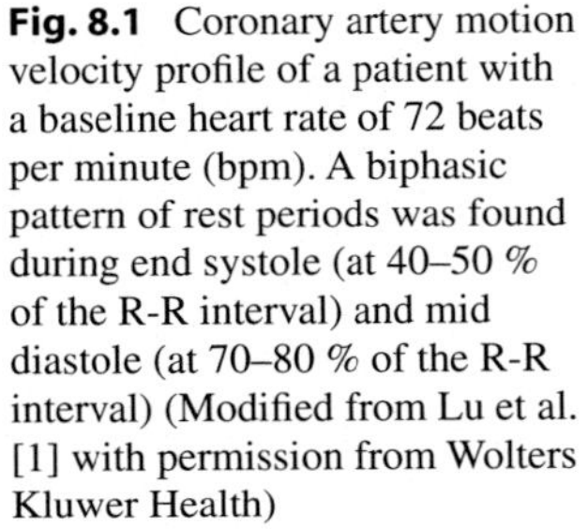

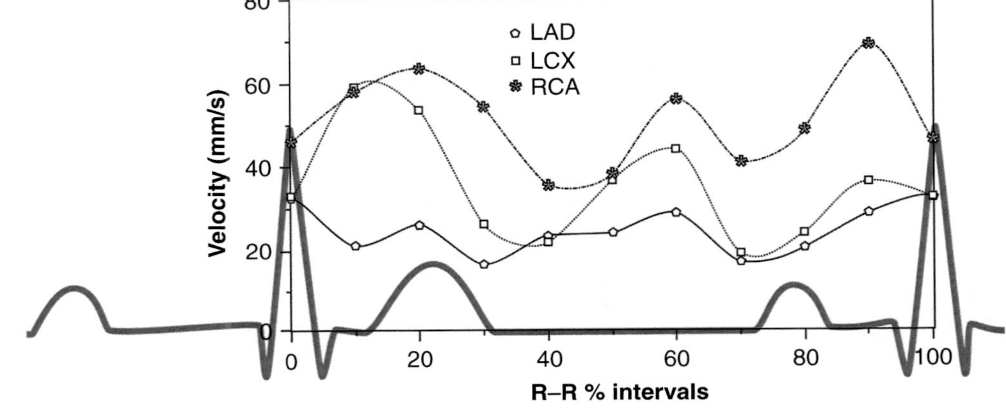

Fig. 8.1 Coronary artery motion velocity profile of a patient with a baseline heart rate of 72 beats per minute (bpm). A biphasic pattern of rest periods was found during end systole (at 40–50 % of the R-R interval) and mid diastole (at 70–80 % of the R-R interval) (Modified from Lu et al. [1] with permission from Wolters Kluwer Health)

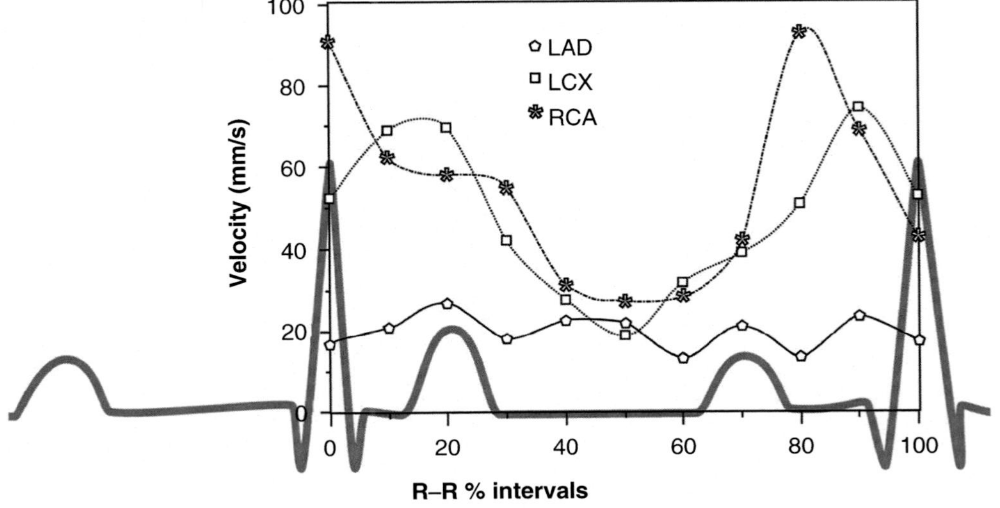

Fig. 8.2 Coronary artery motion velocity profile of a patient with a baseline heart rate of 89 bpm. A monophasic rest period pattern was found near end systole (at 40–60 % of the R-R interval) (Modified from Lu et al. [1] with permission from Wolters Kluwer Health)

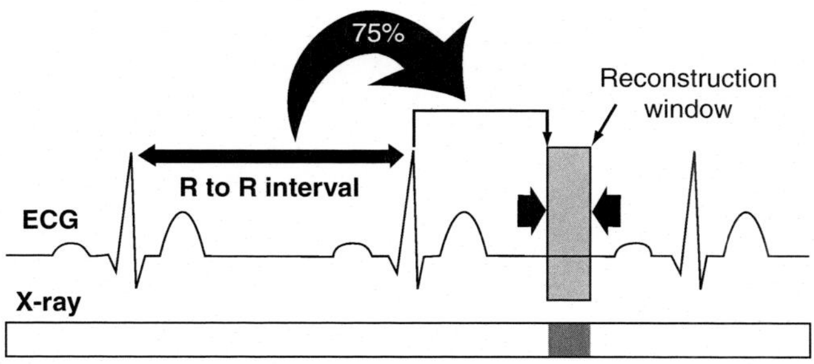

Fig. 8.3 Prospective ECG-gating

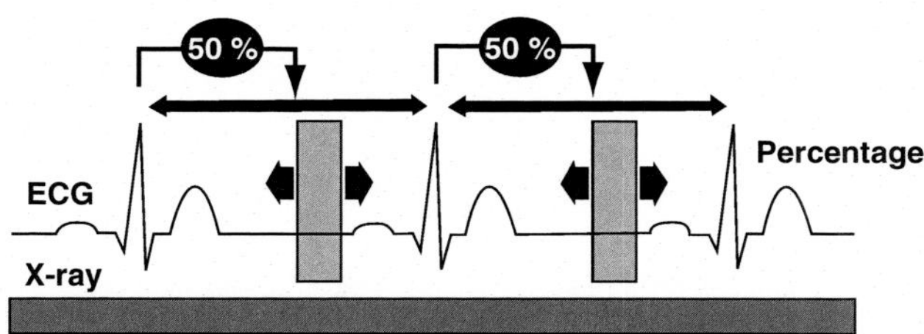

Fig. 8.4 Retrospective ECG-gating

The greatest advantage of prospective ECG gating is the use of a low radiation dose (as low as 1 mSv) [5].

Retrospective ECG gating involves a continuous spiral feed and scan wherein the entire heart volume is covered continuously. Data acquisition occurs from all phases of the cardiac cycle (Fig. 8.4). The patient's ECG is recorded simultaneously with the CT data acquisition and from the raw scan data, specific phases of the cardiac cycle are reconstructed to create multiple data sets [6]. Data overlap is necessary to capture each table position at more than one cardiac cycle. Retrospective gating enables imaging at more rapid heart rates by employing multi-segment reconstruction to increase the effective temporal resolution of the scanner. In addition, by overlapping data acquisition, errant reconstruction from premature heartbeats and variations in heart rate can be corrected through ecg-editing programs (Fig. 8.5) [7].

Field of View

While the **scanned field of view** represents the entire object scanned within the gantry, the **displayed field of view** is defined as the angular size of the displayed scan on the 3 dimensional matrix. For a given CT application, the size of the matrix is 512×512, which limits the number of voxels that can be displayed within a particular field of view. For general thoracic CT applications, the entire chest is included in the field of view. However, with cardiac imaging applications, it is necessary to reduce the displayed field of to maximize X-axis and Y-axis spatial resolution. Typically a field of view that encompasses the heart, pericardium and great vessels (20 cm or less) is selected so that the X-axis and Y-axis spatial resolution matches the Z-axis resolution, which is related only to the collimated beam width. This resolution ranges from 0.5 to 0.625 mm for most CT systems. Figure 8.6 demonstrates representative axial images from a gated thoracic CT exam with a larger field of view and a more refined field of view.

Convolution Kernel

The generation of interpretable cardiac CT images involves the application of a variety of reconstruction filters, the goal of which are to maximize signal to noise ratio and improve visualization of the object of interest. This image processing occurs on the CT scanner console and can be employed following acquisition of the raw CT data. **The convolution kernel** is defined as the image processing filter applied to the raw data to yield a final scan image. The sharpness of the final image is most directly influenced by the type of filter employed.

A *soft convolution kernel* will tend to smooth edges and reduce the amount of image noise. It can be advantageous to employ this kernel in obese patients where signal-to-noise ratio can be diminished secondary to attenuation from adipose tissue. *Sharp convolution kernels* tend to enhance edges at the cost of increased overall image noise. These sharp kernels can be used in patients with stents or heavily calcified vessels [8–10] to reduce blooming artifacts that can occur, as shown in Fig. 8.7. For the majority of coronary CT imaging applications, a neutral convolution kernel is employed that balances image noise and edge detection.

Spiral Pitch

An important parameter for characterizing a spiral CT is the pitch. The pitch is defined as the table feed per gantry rotation divided by the width of the collimated beam. A pitch of greater than 1 implies there are gaps in data acquisition, while a pitch of less than 1 implies that there is overlap in data acquisition (Fig. 8.8). Retrospectively gated multidetector cardiac CT data acquisitions are performed with a pitch of approximately 0.2, as cardiac gating is always necessary for motion-free images and it is necessary to image an entire cardiac cycle at least once at each table position. Modern 64-slice CT scanners automatically determine pitch based on the scan length and heart rate. The major advantages of using a slower pitch is an improved temporal resolution due to increased data overlap while the major disadvantage is an increased radiation exposure. Multisegment reconstruction (discussed below) requires a decreased pitch compared to half-scan reconstruction [6].

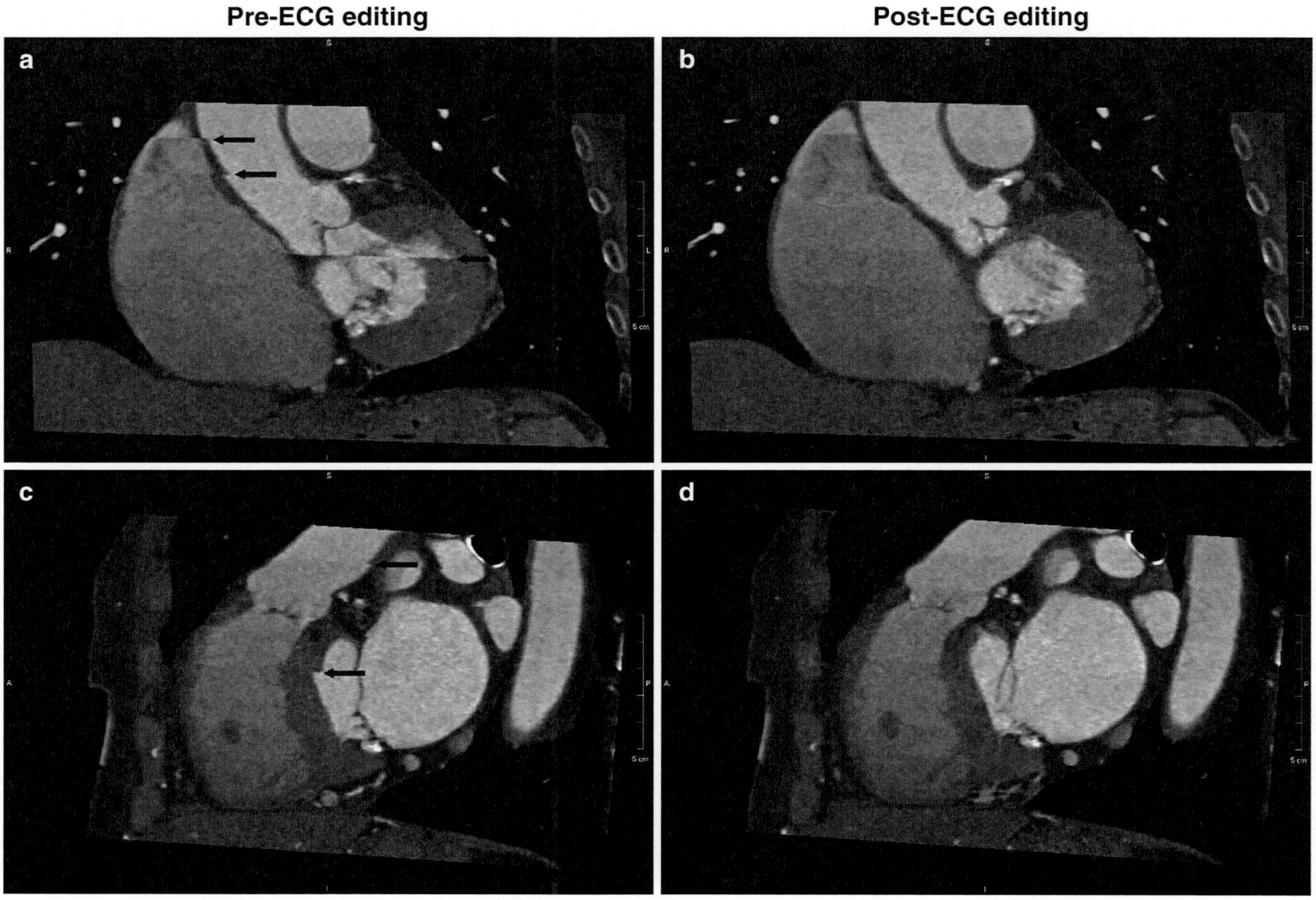

Pre-ECG editing

Post-ECG editing

Fig. 8.5 ECG editing to eliminate misregistration artifacts can be employed on retrospectively gated CT acquisitions. (**a**) Is an oblique coronal section taken at 40 % of the R-R interval demonstrating stairstep-like misregistration artifacts (*arrows*) in a patient with atrial fibrillation undergoing a retrospectively gated 64-slice cardiac CT examination, in whom the R-R interval was notably irregular. (**c**) Is an oblique sagittal section at the same reconstruction interval demonstrating similar misregistration artifacts (*arrows*). (**b** and **d**) Demonstrate successful elimination of the artifacts in the same oblique coronal and sagittal planes using ECG editing to perform precise reconstruction at the end of the T wave (end systole)

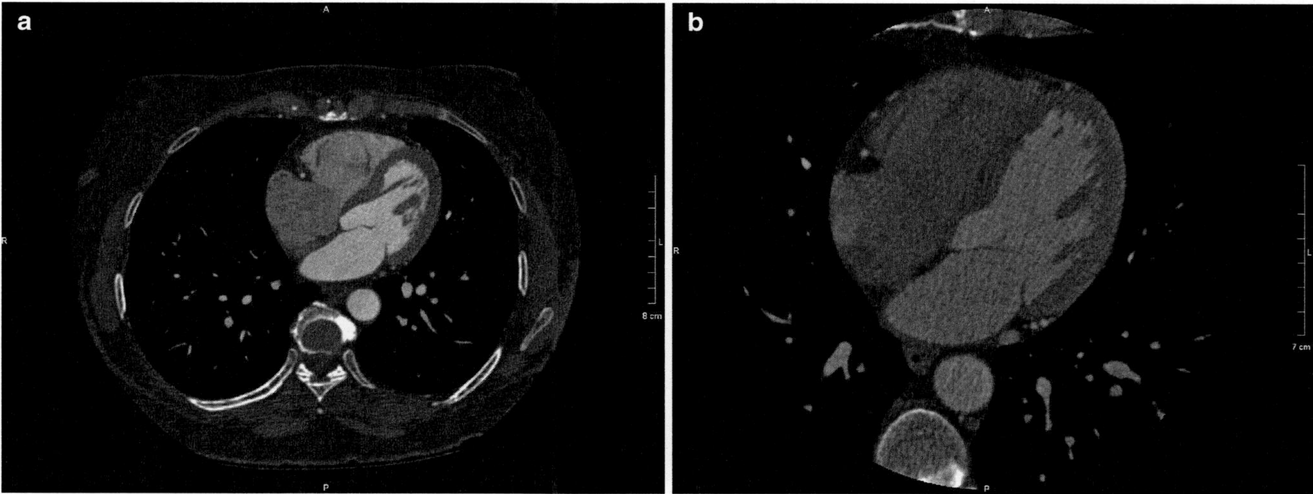

Fig. 8.6 Axial projections of two gated cardiac CT examinations at different displayed fields of view. (**a**) Demonstrates a displayed field of view encompassing the entire chest. This will tend to limit image resolution in the X and Y axes. (**b**) Demonstrates an appropriately limited field of view for a cardiac CT examination

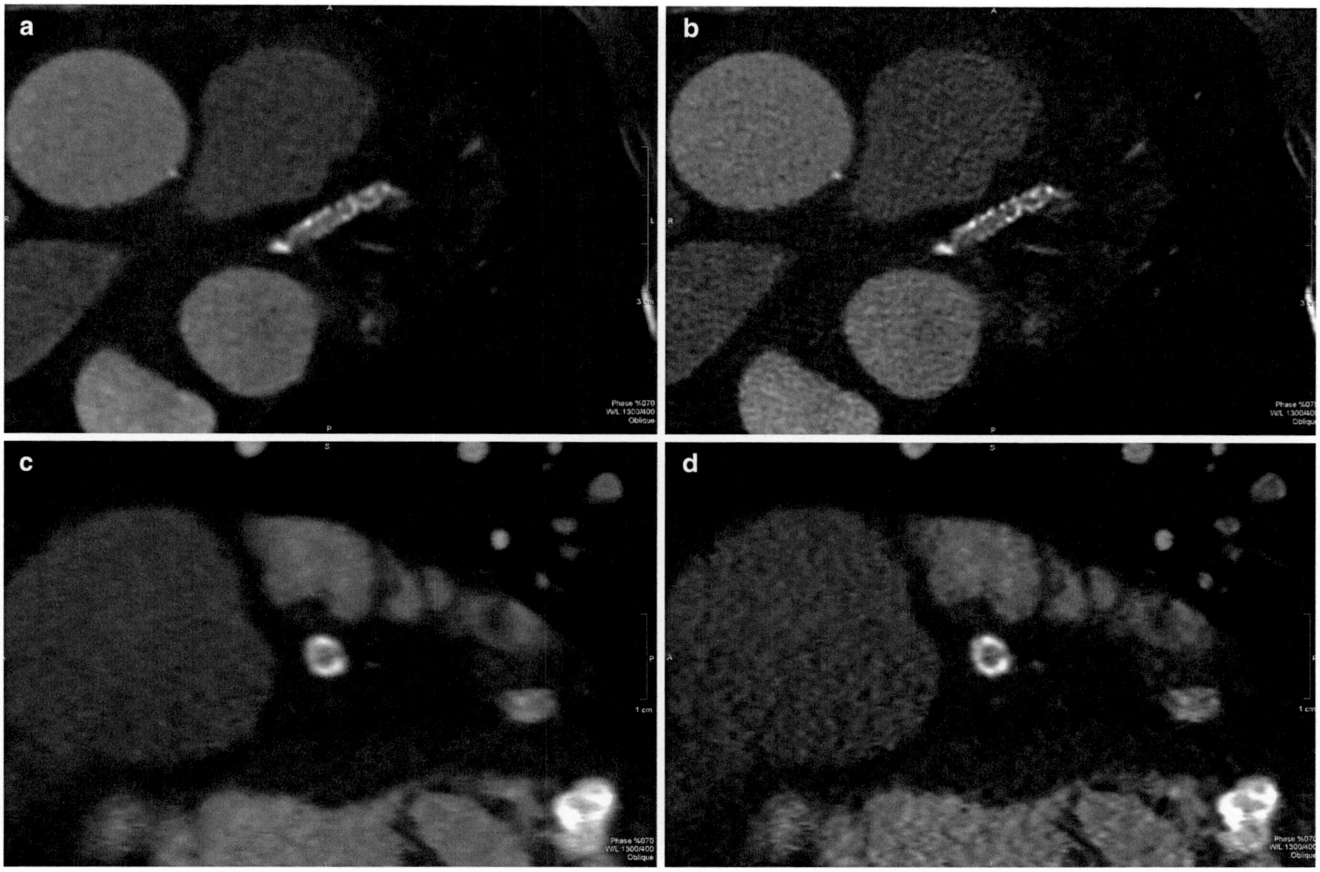

Fig. 8.7 Sharp and smooth convolution kernels are employed to improve visualization of stents and calcified vessels while reducing blooming artifacts. (**a** and **c**) Depict long axis and short axis oblique thin-slice projections of an LAD stent using a standard smooth (B26f) kernel. (**b** and **d**) are similar projections using a sharp (B46f) convolution kernel. Blooming artifacts are reduced, and the edge of the stent is more clearly delineated at the expense of increased noise in the remainder of the image

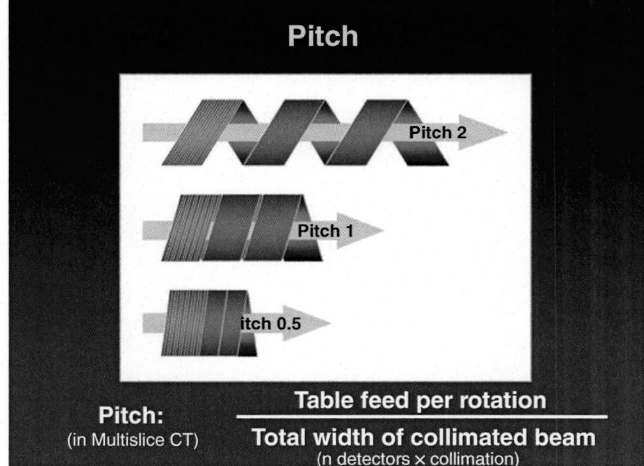

Fig. 8.8 Pitch refers to the table feed per gantry rotation during a spiral acquisition divided by the width of the collimated beam. A pitch of exactly 1 (*central diagram*) implies that there are no data gaps and there is no overlap of data. When pitch is greater than 1 (*top diagram*), there are gaps in data acquisition, whereas when pitch is less than 1 (*bottom diagram*), there is data overlap. Retrospectively gated cardiac CT examinations are performed with a pitch of approximately 0.2

Reconstruction of CT Data in 64-Detector CT Systems

With 64-detector CT systems, each revolution of the gantry enables imaging of 3.2–4.0 cm of the heart (64 detectors times the width of each detector). To cover the entire heart, the required length of most cardiac scans is 9–10 cm; this necessitates combining data from multiple table positions to yield a final volume of data. The greatest challenge in the reconstruction of this volumetric cardiac CT data is the maintenance of temporal uniformity: that is, one should be able to provide cardiac images at each table position from the same part of each cardiac cycle. A breakdown of temporal uniformity can lead to characteristic "stairstep" artifacts.

The most commonly used reconstruction algorithm in spiral cardiac CT is **the half-scan reconstruction method**, which involves the use of scan data from a single gantry rotation to generate an axial CT image. Half-scan reconstruction excludes the fan beam width (approximately 30°), so that approximately 210° of rotation are necessary to generate a single axial image. Using the half-scan method, the temporal resolution is approximately 60 % of the rotational speed of the scanner (due to the fan beam width exclusion). For modern single source 64-slice CT scanners which have gantry rotation times ranging from 330 to 375 ms, the temporal resolution using the half-scan reconstruction method is approximately 200–225 ms. In patients with heart rates of 60 beats per minute or less, the mid-diastolic diastasis period of minimal coronary motion is long enough to allow effective reconstructions in mid diastole in the majority of patients.

In patients with heart rates faster than 80 beats per minute, the duration of the diastasis period decreases considerably and may be only 100–200 ms. This makes it nearly impossible to reconstruct motion-free images using the half-scan reconstruction method. In these cases, **multi-segment reconstruction** may be utilized to improve the effective temporal resolution of the CT scanner. Multisegment reconstruction relies on additional data overlap with slower table movement and decreased pitch during CT acquisition [11, 12]. This overlap results in the same table position being available for imaging at multiple heart beats from multiple detectors (Fig. 8.9). By combining views at a single table position from different subsequent gantry rotations, one simulated half-scan rotation is generated. This results in improved image quality with fewer motion artifacts. By combining images from 3 cardiac cycles, the effective temporal resolution can be improved to as much as 65 ms. Multi-segment reconstruction relies heavily on a consistent R-R interval on the consecutive beats used to generate the final axial image. Irregularities from atrial fibrillation or sinus arrhythmia during breath holding may cause misregistration artifacts.

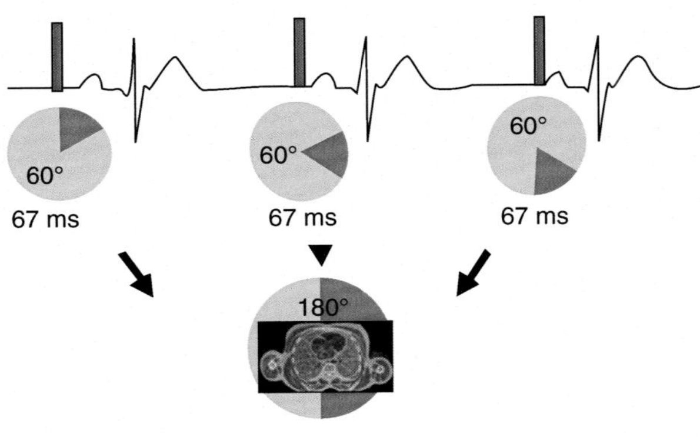

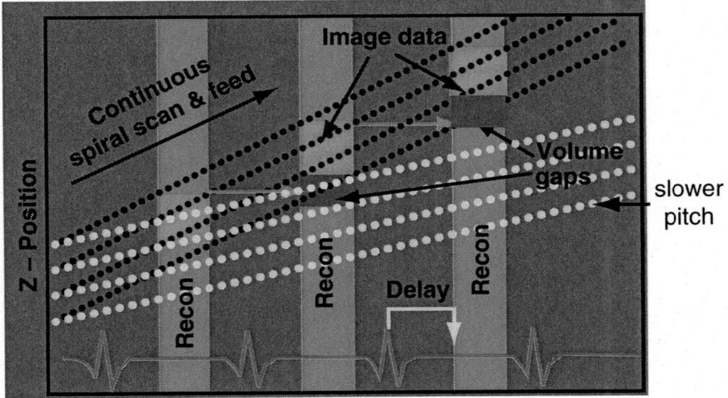

Fig. 8.9 (**a** and **b**) Multisegment reconstruction of a CT acquisition involves the acquisition of data at a single table position over several cardiac cycles. The volumetric data are combined to yield a final summed volume. The major requirement for multisegment reconstruction is data overlap, which results in a slower pitch and higher radiation dose during the CT acquisition. Using this technique, effective temporal resolution can be improved to 67 ms for a scanner with a half-scan acquisition time of 200 ms

Reconstruction of CT Data in 320-Detector CT Systems

With 320-detector CT systems, one axial rotation can cover up to 16 cm of tissue, although typically all 320 detectors cannot be employed simultaneously to image the heart. To accomplish this, the use of a wide X-ray beam and a wide cone angle is required. Figures 8.10 and 8.11 demonstrate the concept of the fan angle and the cone angle. The cone angle determines the coverage of the X-ray beam in the longitudinal, or z-axis while the fan angle determines the coverage in the x/y plane. The use of a wide cone angle gives the 320-detector scanner the ability to cover up to 16 cm of tissue

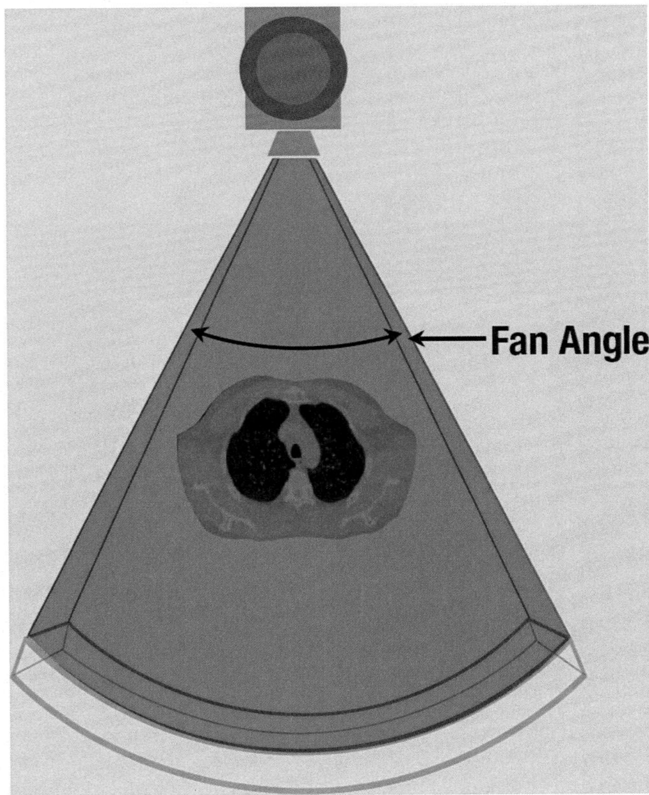

Fig. 8.10 The fan angle represents the spread of the X-ray beam in the x/y plane and is a factor in determining the diameter of the field of view (Reproduced with permission from Toshiba America Medical Systems)

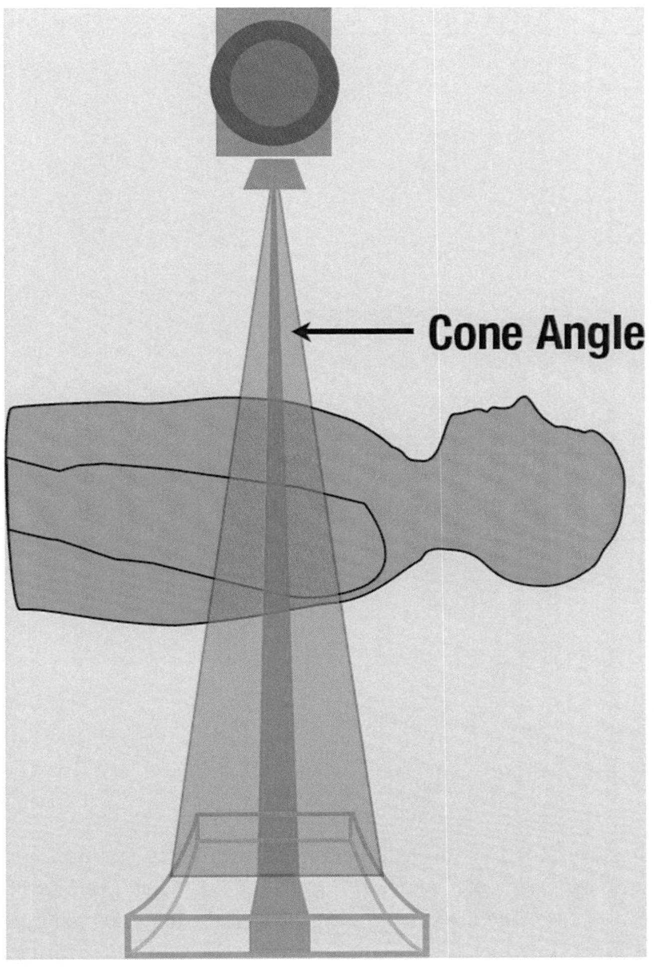

Fig. 8.11 The cone angle quantifies the spread of the X-ray beam in the z-direction, along the length of the patient (Reproduced with permission from Toshiba America Medical Systems)

in one axial rotation [13]. As a result, it is not necessary to move the patient through a spiral scan line. Instead, the patient can remain stationary and the entire heart to be imaged in a single gantry revolution. This has the potential to substantially improve image clarity by eliminating stairstep and misregistration artifacts that are sometimes seen with 64-detector systems, but will have no impact on temporal resolution, based upon the gantry rotation speed (as described above).

While use of a wide cone angle offers the capability of whole organ coverage, it also presents a challenge to image reconstruction algorithms employed in 64-detector systems. Traditional reconstruction algorithms cannot successfully incorporate the highly tilted X-ray planes created by the cone angle trajectory. As a result, one can get cone-beam artifacts including shading, ghosting, and diminished resolution as shown in Fig. 8.12a. With more advanced reconstruction algorithms specifically designed for 320-detector systems that account for the cone angle, these artifacts can be eliminated, shown in Fig. 8.12b [14].

Post Scan Related Post-processing Parameters

After the scan has been completed and datasets have been generated, additional post-processing techniques on a cardiac CT workstation are essential to accurately interpreting cardiac morphology as well as coronary artery anatomy and disease burden. The presence of an isotropic data set in which the spatial resolution is identical across all planes of examination facilitates manipulation of the data on a workstation.

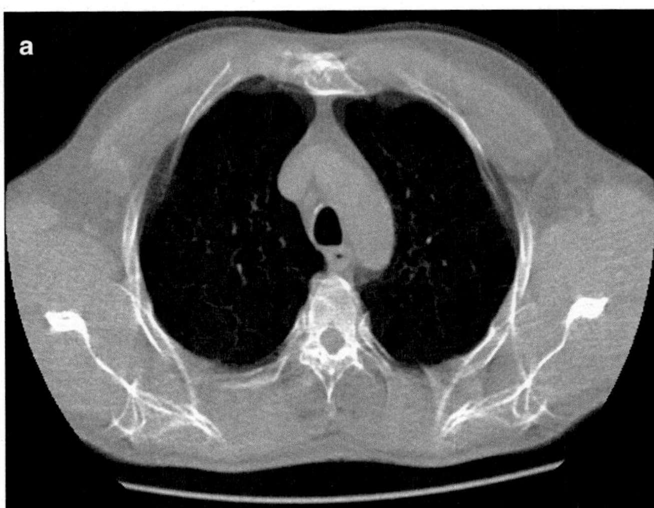

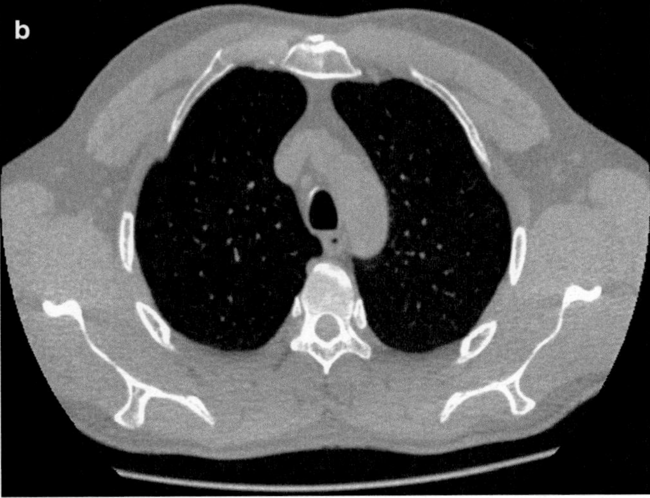

Fig. 8.12 Panel A (*top*) illustrates cone beam artifact. The image demonstrates shading, ghosting, and diminished resolution. This is a result of a reconstruction algorithm that does not properly take into account the wide cone angle. Panel B (*bottom*) shows an identical image reconstructed with a novel reconstruction algorithm that takes into account the wide cone angle, thereby eliminating the artifact (Reproduced with permission from Toshiba America Medical Systems)

The raw axial images are the most reliable for diagnosis, as they reflect the source data in the order the images were acquired. To assist the reader in processing large volumes of data and illustrating key findings, additional rendering techniques have been developed [15, 16]. These include the multiplanar reformatting, maximum intensity projection, the volume averaging and volume rendering techniques, and the curved multiplanar projection. All involve rendering data contained within a 3 dimensional slab (the thickness of which the user can change) of data as a single 2-dimensional projection.

Multiplanar Reformatting (MPR)

Multiplanar reformatting involves the selection of an arbitrary image plane in a cardiac CT volume. This technique requires an isotropic volumetric data set with equal spatial resolution in the X, Y, and Z axes. The plane may not conform to the conventional axial, coronal, and sagittal imaging planes and can be modified by the user, as shown in Fig. 8.13. MPR is the mainstay for analysis of cardiac CT data sets and is the most reliable method for the reader to arrive at the correct diagnosis. It can be performed using a single slice or with differing numbers of stacked slices. When more than one slice is selected, a rendering option must be selected to display a composite image of the multiple slices.

Maximum Intensity Projection

The maximum intensity projection (MIP) involves the projection of data in a 3-dimensional slab so that only the voxels of highest HU are displayed on a 2-dimensional image (Fig. 8.14). Initially developed by Rubin and colleagues [17, 18]. for use in peripheral CT angiography, the MIP is now used for nearly all CT angiography applications and is the mainstay of coronary artery interpretation. The MIP is ideal for the display of coronary artery images from a contrast CT examination as the maximum intensity in the coronary arteries is usually the intraluminal contrast. The coronary arteries

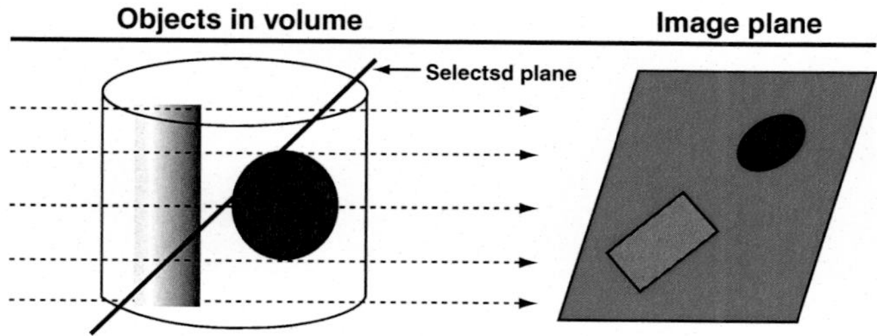

Fig. 8.13 Multiplanar Reformat Projection (MPR)

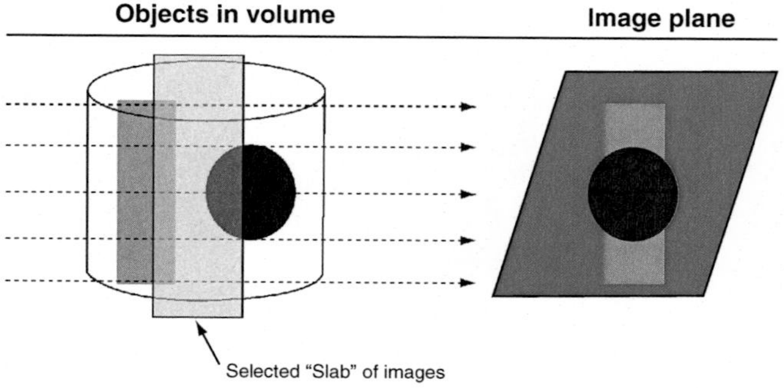

Fig. 8.14 Maximum Intensity Projection (MIP)

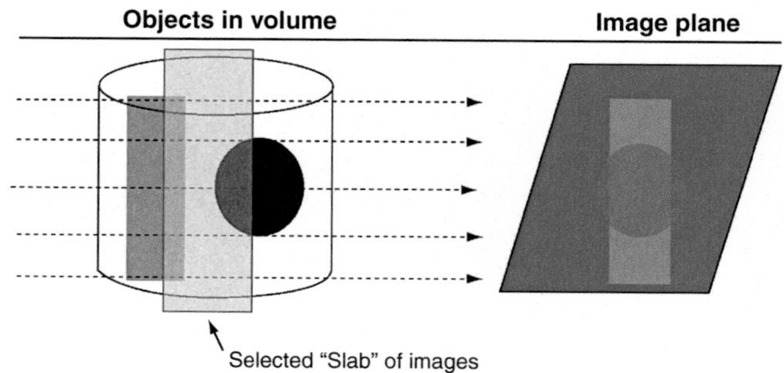

Fig. 8.15 Volume averaging

are surrounded by low-attenuation epicardial fat, resulting in an angiogram-like image with excellent edge definition (Fig. 8.14). Due the selection of the highest intensity voxels within a slab, the MIP tends to overestimate stenosis severity in calcified vessels and stented segments (bright objects like calcium and metal get further enhanced). Overreliance on MIPs can also lead the reader to overlook subtle findings in the coronary arteries, including motion and misalignment artifacts. In general, readers should always reconfirm findings on MIP with the source axial data.

Volume Averaging and Volume Rendering

Volume averaging (VA) involves the projection of data in a 3-dimensional slab so that the intensity of all the voxels in the slab is averaged on a final 2-dimensional image (Fig. 8.15). While edge definition is poorer than with MIP, VA enables the reader to "see through" a dense object in a slab and can be useful in interpreting stenoses in calcified vessels. When specific colors are assigned to specific ranges of HU in a 3-dimensional volumetric slab, this is termed volume rendering (VR); this is available on virtually every cardiac workstation. The relative position and 3-dimensional relationship of the coronary arteries, cardiac veins, and cardiac chambers is possible using 3-dimensional VR (Fig. 8.16). While especially helpful in evaluating coronary

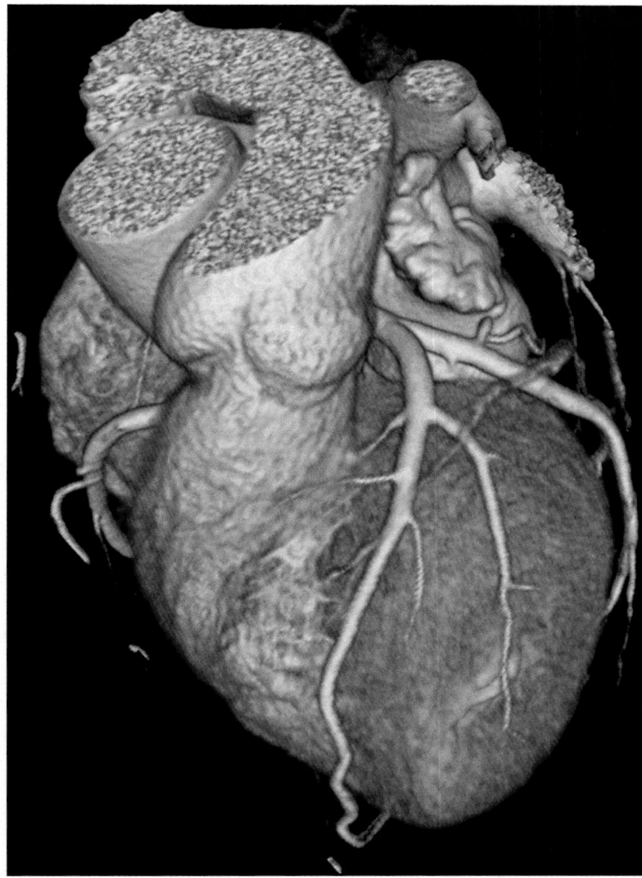

Fig. 8.16 3D volume rendering

anomalies and bypass grafts, the reader should never attempt to interpret stenoses purely on the basis of a 3D VR images: as calcium and intraluminal contrast have attenuation ranges that are near one another, significant coronary artery stenoses in calcified vessels can be misinterpreted.

Curved Multiplanar Projection

The curved multiplanar projection (CMP) is a centerline method for analysis of vessels whereby a virtual plane is created using the center of the column of contrast visualized on a series of consecutive axial slices (Fig. 8.17). A virtual plane in which the vessel is "stretched out" can then be displayed. CMP is useful for confirming and illustrating the appearance of stenoses identified using standard axial multiplanar projections. It is particularly useful for tortuous vessels and those vessels that cannot be easily tracked in a single plane or thin slab using MIP. The CMP is only as reliable as the accuracy of the centerline, and should not be used as a first-line assessment of coronary stenosis severity. Artifacts from inaccurate centerlines can lead to incorrect assessment of stenosis severity.

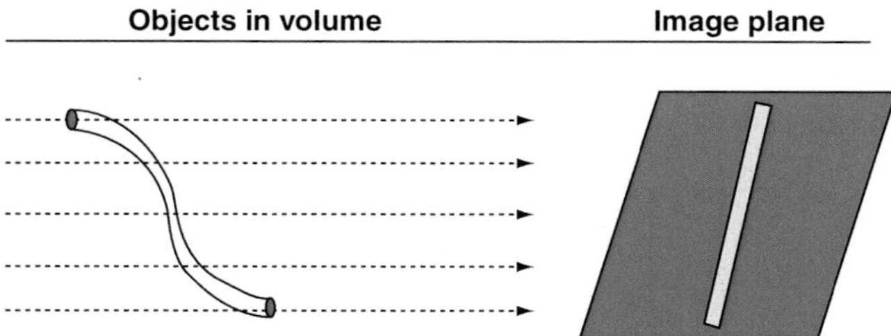

Fig. 8.17 Curved Planar Reformat (CPR)

References

1. Lu B, Mao SS, Zhuang N, et al. Coronary artery motion during the cardiac cycle and optimal ECG triggering for coronary artery imaging. Invest Radiol. 2001;36(5):250–6.
2. Mao S, Lu B, Oudiz RJ, Bakhsheshi H, Liu SC, Budoff MJ. Coronary artery motion in electron beam tomography. J Comput Assist Tomogr. 2000;24(2):253–8.
3. Kim WY, Stuber M, Kissinger KV, Andersen NT, Manning WJ, Botnar RM. Impact of bulk cardiac motion on right coronary MR angiography and vessel wall imaging. J Magn Reson Imaging. 2001;14(4):383–90.
4. Isma'eel H, Hamirani YS, Mehrinfar R, et al. Optimal phase for coronary interpretations and correlation of ejection fraction using late-diastole and end-diastole imaging in cardiac computed tomography angiography: implications for prospective triggering. Int J Cardiovasc Imaging. 2009;25(7):739–49.
5. Gurudevan SV, Narula J. Prospective electrocardiogram-gating: a new direction for CT coronary angiography? Nat Clin Pract Cardiovasc Med. 2008;5(7):366–7.
6. Flohr TG, Schaller S, Stierstorfer K, Bruder H, Ohnesorge BM, Schoepf UJ. Multi-detector row CT systems and image-reconstruction techniques. Radiology. 2005;235(3):756–73.
7. Cademartiri F, Mollet NR, Runza G, et al. Improving diagnostic accuracy of MDCT coronary angiography in patients with mild heart rhythm irregularities using ECG editing. AJR Am J Roentgenol. 2006;186(3):634–8.
8. Ehara M, Kawai M, Surmely JF, et al. Diagnostic accuracy of coronary in-stent restenosis using 64-slice computed tomography: comparison with invasive coronary angiography. J Am Coll Cardiol. 2007;49(9):951–9.
9. Nieman K, Cademartiri F, Raaijmakers R, Pattynama P, de Feyter P. Noninvasive angiographic evaluation of coronary stents with multi-slice spiral computed tomography. Herz. 2003;28(2):136–42.
10. Maintz D, Seifarth H, Flohr T, et al. Improved coronary artery stent visualization and in-stent stenosis detection using 16-slice computed-tomography and dedicated image reconstruction technique. Invest Radiol. 2003;38(12):790–5.
11. Kachelriess M, Ulzheimer S, Kalender WA. ECG-correlated image reconstruction from subsecond multi-slice spiral CT scans of the heart. Med Phys. 2000;27(8):1881–902.
12. Ohnesorge B, Flohr T, Becker C, et al. Cardiac imaging by means of electrocardiographically gated multisection spiral CT: initial experience. Radiology. 2000;217(2):564–71.
13. Tuy HK. An inverse formula for cone-beam reconstruction. SIAM J Appl Math. 1983;43:546–52.
14. Feldkamp LA, Davis LC, Kress JW. Practical cone beam algorithm. J Opt Soc Am. 1984;1:612–9.
15. Addis KA, Hopper KD, Iyriboz TA, et al. CT angiography: in vitro comparison of five reconstruction methods. AJR Am J Roentgenol. 2001;177(5):1171–6.

16. Pavone P, Luccichenti G, Cademartiri F. From maximum intensity projection to volume rendering. Semin Ultrasound CT MR. 2001;22(5):413–9.
17. Rubin GD, Dake MD, Napel S, et al. Spiral CT of renal artery stenosis: comparison of three-dimensional rendering techniques. Radiology. 1994;190(1):181–9.
18. Prokop M, Shin HO, Schanz A, Schaefer-Prokop CM. Use of maximum intensity projections in CT angiography: a basic review. Radiographics. 1997;17(2):433–51.

Coronary CT Angiography: Native Vessels

9

Stephan Achenbach

Abstract

Coronary CT Angiography has become increasingly stable and robust and accuracy to identify and rule out high-grade stenosis of the coronary arteries is high. The main clinical application is to rule out significant coronary artery disease in patients with a relatively low pre-test likelihood of disease. For this application, several guidelines in the US and Europe endorse the use of cardiac CT. Other applications of coronary CTA include the support of coronary interventions, especially in the context of chronic total coronary occlusion, the identification of coronary anomalies, and, to some extent, the assessment of non-obstructive coronary atherosclerosis. However, the use of coronary CTA for screening purposes is currently not supported by official recommendations.

Keywords

Coronary CT Angiography • Coronary CTA • Coronary Artery Disease • Computed Tomography • Stenosis • Atherosclerosis • Plaque

Introduction

Visualization of the coronary arteries has been the major focus of cardiac CT in the past years. Non-invasive "coronary CT angiography" has tremendous clinical potential for detecting or ruling out coronary artery stenoses in selected patients (see Figs. 9.1 and 9.2). As a consequence of continuous and substantial progress regarding image quality and robustness of the investigation, it is incorporated in several recent official guidelines and recommendations. In addition, imaging of coronary atherosclerotic plaque may play a potential role in risk stratification. However, spatial resolution and temporal resolution of CT imaging, even with the latest scanner generations, are not equal to those of invasive coronary angiography. Interpreters of coronary CT angiography data sets must therefore be aware that artefacts can occur and may lead to false-positive and, less frequently, to false-negative results. Diagnostic accuracy is impaired when image quality is reduced and image quality, in turn, is influenced by many factors such as the patient's heart rate, body weight, ability to cooperate, and extent of coronary calcification. Therefore, the clinical utility of coronary CT angiography significantly depends on the specific clinical situation and patient under investigation. The specific advantages and disadvantages of coronary CT angiography must be carefully considered before using this method in the workup of a patient with known or suspected coronary artery disease.

Imaging Protocol

Since the small dimensions and the rapid motion of the coronary vessels pose tremendous challenges for non-invasive imaging, high-end CT equipment and adequate imaging protocols must be used. Currently, 64-slice CT is considered the minimum requirement for coronary artery imaging, and newer

S. Achenbach, MD
Department of Cardiology, University of Erlangen, Ulmenweg 18, Erlangen 91054, Germany
e-mail: Stephan.Achenbach@uk-erlangen.de

M.J. Budoff, J.S. Shinbane (eds.), *Cardiac CT Imaging: Diagnosis of Cardiovascular Disease*,
DOI 10.1007/978-3-319-28219-0_9

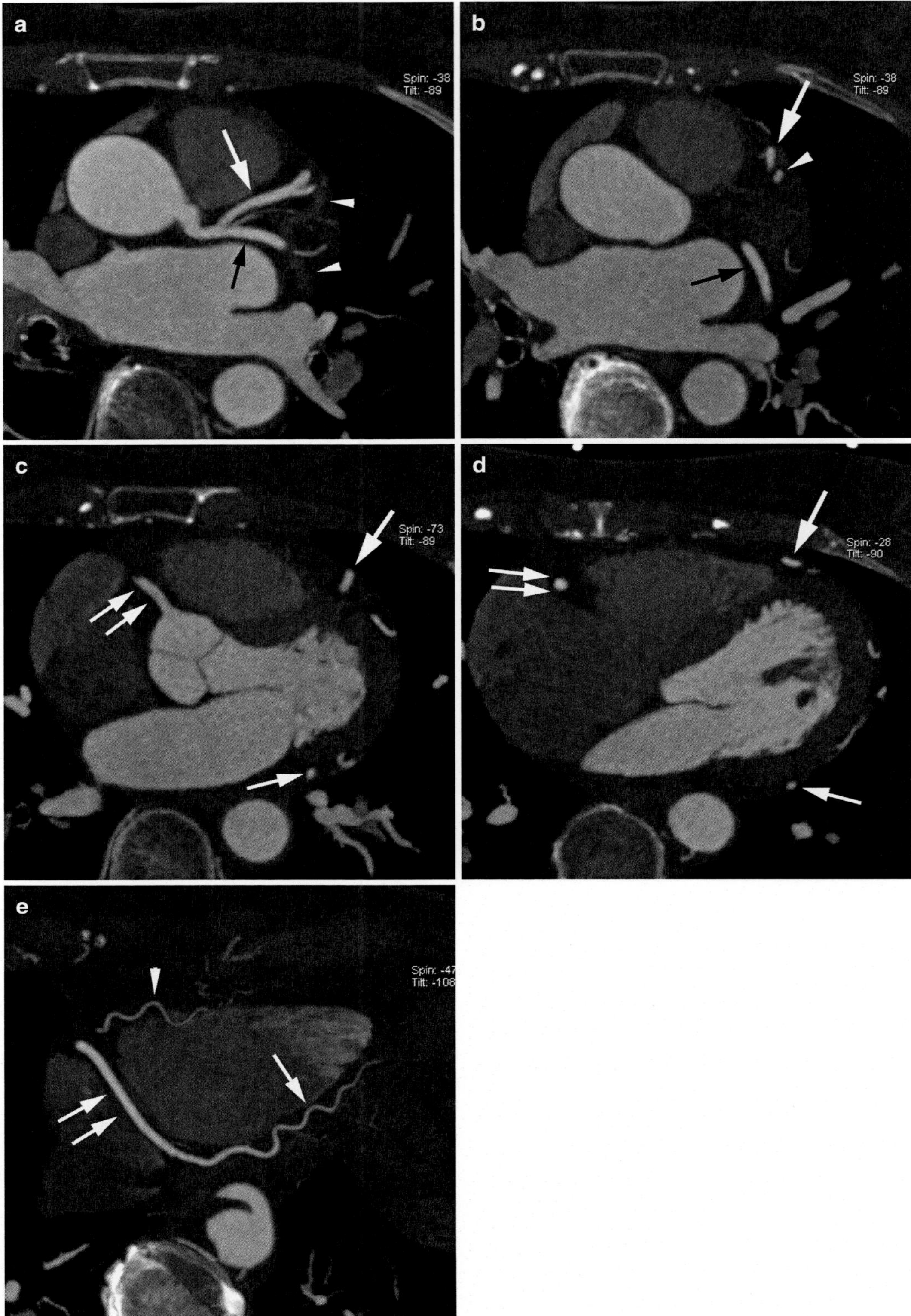

Fig. 9.1 Normal anatomy of the coronary arteries in transaxial images. (**a**) Level of the left main origin from the aortic root. The bifurcation of the left main into the left anterior descending (*large arrow*) and left circumflex coronary artery (*small arrow*) can be seen. The *arrowheads* point at a coronary vein. (**b**) A few mm further distal, the left anterior descending coronary artery (*large arrow*) has given rise to a diagonal branch (*arrowhead*). (**c**) Level of the right coronary ostium. A short section of the right coronary artery is visible (*double arrows*). *Large arrow*: Mid left anterior descending coronary artery, *small arrow*: left circumflex coronary artery. (**d**) Mid-ventricular level. The left anterior descending coronary artery (*large arrow*), left circumflex coronary artery (*small arrow*), and right coronary artery can be seen (*double arrows*). (**e**) Distal segment of the right coronary artery (*double arrow*), which ends in the posterior descending artery (*small arrow*). The *arrowhead* points at a right ventricular branch

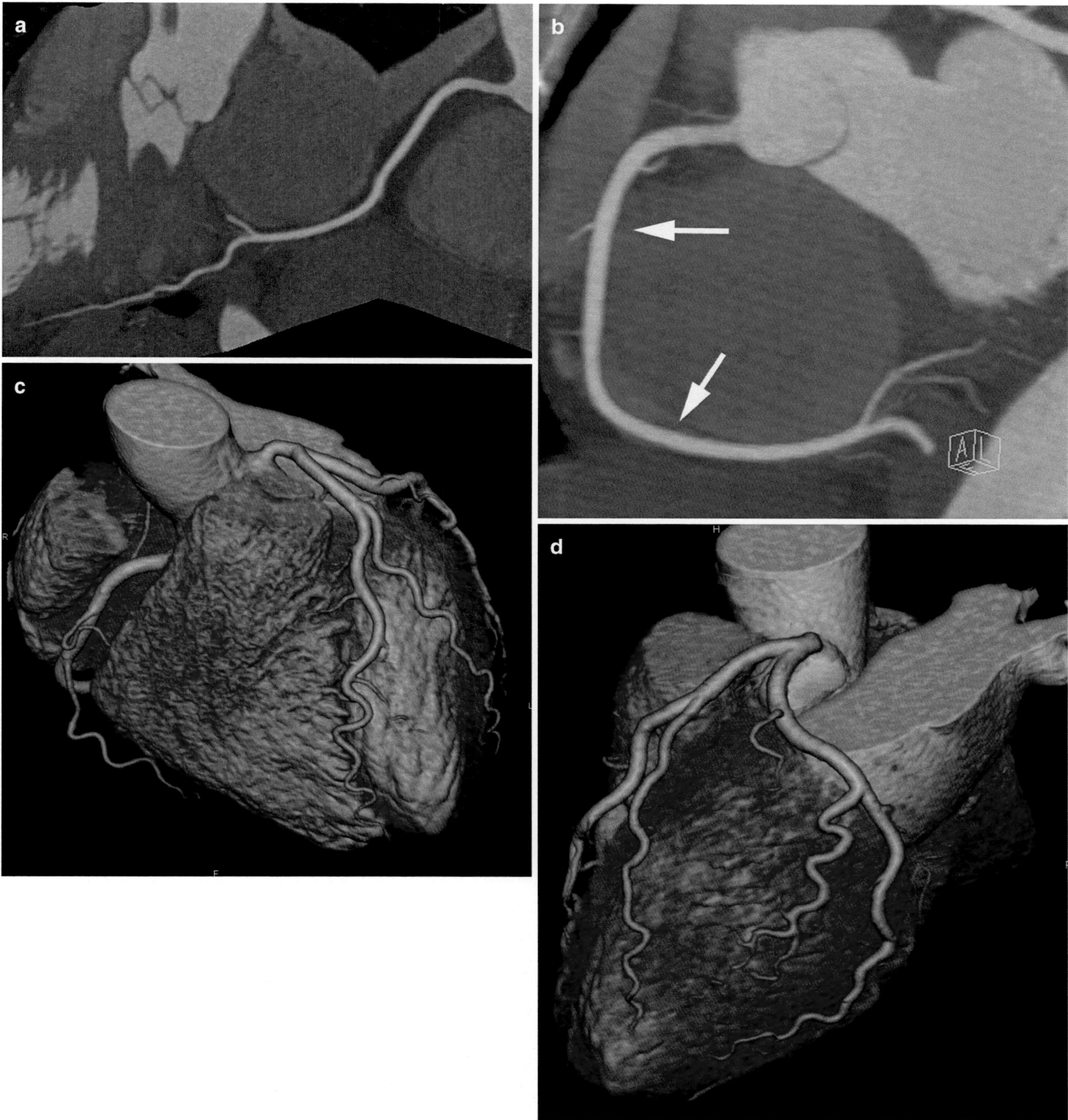

Fig. 9.2 Same patient as in Fig. 9.1. Various forms of post-processing have been used to visualize longer segments of the coronary arteries. (**a**) Curved multiplanar reconstruction (curved MPR) of the right coronary artery. (**b**) Maximum Intensity projection (MIP) of the right coronary artery (*arrows*) in a double-oblique plane. (**c**, **d**) 3-dimensional, surface-weighted Volume Rendering Technique (VRT) reconstructions in two different angulations

technology [1], such as Dual Source CT and scanners that allow simultaneous acquisition of 256 or 320 cross-sections, provide for more robust image quality and further improved image quality.

A basic prerequisite for CT imaging of the coronary arteries is the patient's ability to understand and follow breathhold commands. Even slight respiratory motion during data acquisition will cause substantial artefact and may render the coronary arteries (or parts of them) unevaluable. Therefore, patients should be able to reliably hold their breath for approximately 10 s. Otherwise, coronary CT angiography should not be performed. Heart rate should be regular and preferably low (optimally below 60/min, even though this is not as strictly required for Dual Source CT)

[1, 2]. It is usually recommended that patients receive premedication with short acting beta blockers to lower the heart rate. Beta blockers can be administered orally approximately 1 hr prior to scanning, or intravenously immediately before the scan. Sometimes, a combination of both is necessary. Nitrates should be given to all patients who have no contraindications in order to achieve coronary dilatation, which substantially improves image quality [1].

Intravenous contrast enhancement is necessary for coronary CT angiography and typically, 50–100 ml of iodine-based, high concentration contrast agent are injected. High flow rates are recommended, injection should be between 4 and 7 ml/s. Synchronization of contrast injection and data acquisition can be achieved either through a "bolus tracking" method or by using a separate "test bolus" acquisition to measure the contrast transit time.

Subsequent data acquisition can follow various principles. The obtained data need to be synchronized with the heart beat, and this can either be achieved through retrospective ECG gating or prospective ECG triggering [1].

Retrospectively gated scans are acquired in spiral mode and usually provide for robust and high image quality, flexibility to choose the cardiac phase during which images are reconstructed, as well as the ability to reconstruct "functional" data sets throughout the cardiac cycle in order to analyse left ventricular function and regional wall motion. In order to limit radiation exposure, the output of the x-ray tube can be "modulated" during the acquisition, with lower output in systole, and higher output in diastole, when the most relevant image reconstructions are usually performed.

Prospectively triggered scans are associated with substantially lower radiation exposure. Images are acquired in axial mode without table movement and the patient table is advanced by one detector width following the acquisition, with subsequent images acquired in the next or second to next cardiac cycle. Less flexibility to reconstruct data at different time instants in the cardiac cycle as well as greater susceptibility to artefacts caused by arrhythmia are trade-offs for the advantage of lower dose. Especially in young patients – in whom radiation dose may be of major concern – prospectively triggered scans should be strongly considered [2–5]. Heart rate must be low so that artefact-free images can be guaranteed at the time instant of radiation exposure. The lowest radiation dose is achieved when the x-ray exposure window in each cardiac cycle is only as long as one-half rotation of the gantry requires (just long enough to reconstruct one set of transaxial slices), but "padding" (x-ray exposure over a longer time period in each cardiac cycle) may be used to provide some flexibility regarding the time instant of image reconstruction [6, 7].

A combination of spiral acquisition and prospective triggering is the so-called "Flash Mode" (*prospectively ECG triggered high pitch spiral acquisition*). It is only available with a limited number of scanners that have either two detectors or a very wide detector. Images are acquired during continuous, very fast motion of the table, and the volume of the heart is typically covered within 150–250 ms. In the cranio-caudal direction, the data for each subsequent image are acquired with a very slight temporal offset as compared to the previous image (approximately 0.5 ms), so that the consecutive images represent ever so slightly different time instants within the cardiac cycle. Since the transition is smooth and image acquisition is typically performed in diastole with very little cardiac motion, this offset is not noticeable in the data set and in reconstructed images. This mode of data acquisition provides high image quality at very low doses, but requires stable heart rates below 60 beats/min to avoid artefact [8–11].

Radiation Exposure

Unless specific measures are taken to limit radiation dose, the exposure during coronary CTA can be high. A landmark study performed several years ago demonstrated that in individual centers, the average estimated effective radiation exposure was as high as 30 mSv (while in the same study, sites at the lower end of the spectrum performed coronary CTA with an average exposure of only 4–5 mSv) [12]. Since then, substantial progress has been achieved regarding radiation exposure (see Table 9.1). ECG-based tube current modulation in spiral acquisition and prospectively ECG-triggered image acquisition avoid x-ray exposure during the entire cardiac cycle and limit x-ray tube output to those phases of the heart beat which are likely to be used for image reconstruction. This limits the flexibility of reconstructing images during different parts of the R-R interval, which would be desirable to assess ventricular function (a question, however, that is rarely relevant in coronary CTA), and which is also advantageous when motion artefacts are present, to identify a phase with no or little artefact. Hence, low heart rates, which make it extremely likely that artefact-free images are obtained in diastole, facilitate the use of these techniques and in this way, reducing the heart rate by premedication contributes to lower radiation exposure [2]. While the tube voltage for coronary CTA used to uniformly be 120 kV, it has been observed that depending on patient size, it is possible to reduce tube voltage to 100 or 80 kV, or in very selected cases even 70 kV [13–17]. The increase in noise is tolerable depending on patient size, and to some extent is offset by higher iodine contrast. A "rule of thumb" is that tube voltage can be reduced to 100 kV for all patients with a body weight below 100 kg. Finally, there is a linear relationship between tube current and image noise, so that again, especially in patients with low body weight there is potential to reduce exposure.

Table 9.1 Measures to reduce radiation exposure in coronary CTA

Method	Downsides	Specifics	Prerequisites
Avoid x-ray exposure during the entire cardiac cycle	Loss of flexibility to reconstruct data during freely selectable time instants in the cardiac cycle	Spiral acquisition with ECG-based tube current modulation	Low and stable heart rate
		Prospectively ECG triggered axial acquisition	CT scanner with wide detector
Reduce tube voltage (as compared to standard 120 kV)	Increased image noise (to some degree offset by higher iodine contrast)	100 kV or 80 kV, with some scanners 70 kV	Low body weight
Reduce tube current	Increased image noise	Scanner specific	Low body weight
Iterative reconstruction	Altered image impression as compared to filtered back projection	Various algorithms, vendor-specific	None

Many of the measures that decrease radiation exposure do, on the other hand, increase image noise. Since "iterative reconstruction" can reduce noise as compared to the standard "filtered back projection" (at the cost of longer computation time), it can offset the downsides of reduced exposure to some extent and therefore allows to use lower exposure protocols [2, 18, 19].

The combination of various methods that limit exposure permit to perform coronary CTA with doses well below 1 mSv (see Fig. 9.3). This is clinically possible with high-end hardware in somewhat selected patients (low heart rate and reasonable body weight) [17]. There are published series that demonstrated high accuracy for stenosis detection using such protocols [20, 21]. In a very strictly selected patient cohort, it has even been reported that doses below 0.1 mSv are possible [10], but image quality at this extreme end of the spectrum is not good and robust enough for routine clinical practice.

Without going to the extreme and by using measures that are widely available, do not require special training and are straightforward to implement, Chinnayan et al. reported a mean effective dose of 6.4 mSv across 15 centers routinely performing coronary CTA [22]. In the most recent multicenter trial, the average effective dose for coronary CT angiography was 3.2 mSv (as compared to 9.75 mSv for SPECT and 12.0 mSv for invasive angiography) [23].

Image Reconstruction and Post-processing

Typical data sets for coronary artery visualization by CT consist of approximately 200–300 thin (0.5–0.75 mm) transaxial cross-sections (see Figs. 9.1, 9.2, and 9.3). In most cases, workstations are used for data interpretation. While many workstations provide pre-rendered reconstructions that are intended to show the coronary arteries over their entire course, readers should not rely on such atomatoed post-processing tools alone. In fact, official recommendations mandate that the reader manipulates the original data and does not rely on pre-rendered reconstructions [24]. The most useful post-processing tools are thin-slab maximum intensity projections (approximately 5 mm slice thickness) and multiplanar reconstructions (see Figs. 9.2 and 9.3) in oblique or curved planes that are adapted to the orientation of the coronary arteries. 3-dimensional renderings allow quite impressive visualization of the heart and coronary arteries, but they are not accurate for stenosis detection and play no role in data interpretation (see Fig. 9.3) [25].

Typical Findings

In most cases, coronary CT angiography is performed to detect or rule out significant coronary artery stenoses (See Fig. 9.4). In most cases, presence of a "significant" luminal stenosis is assumed when the diameter reduction of the coronary lumen appears to be more than 70 %. Stenosis severity is usually determined my visual estimation, since quantitative approaches are not exact – the spatial resolution of coronary CT angiography, approximately 0.5 mm, is not sufficient to allow for accurate, quantitative stenosis grading. In fact, visual estimation of stenosis degree has no downsides as compared to quantitative approaches [26–28]. Stenosis severity in CT can appear to be less or more than invasive angiography – the typical margin of agreement is approximately ±20 % [27]. Hence, stenoses that appear to be less than 50 % in CT can be expected to be less than 70 % in invasive angiography with a very high degree of certainty. In most cases, however, there is a tendency to *over*estimate, rather than underestimate, the degree of luminal stenosis in coronary CT angiography as compared to catheter-based invasive coronary angiography (Fig. 9.5). Often, high grade coronary artery stenoses appear as complete or near-complete interruptions of the coronary artery lumen in the CT data set (Fig. 9.6). Categories of stenosis severity that are recommended for use in coronary CT angiography reports care listed in Table 9.2 [24]. The differentiation between complete coronary artery occlusions and high-grade stenoses can be difficult in coronary CT angiography. Very long lesions typically correspond to complete occlusions (Fig. 9.7), while shorter lesions can either be secondary to high grade luminal

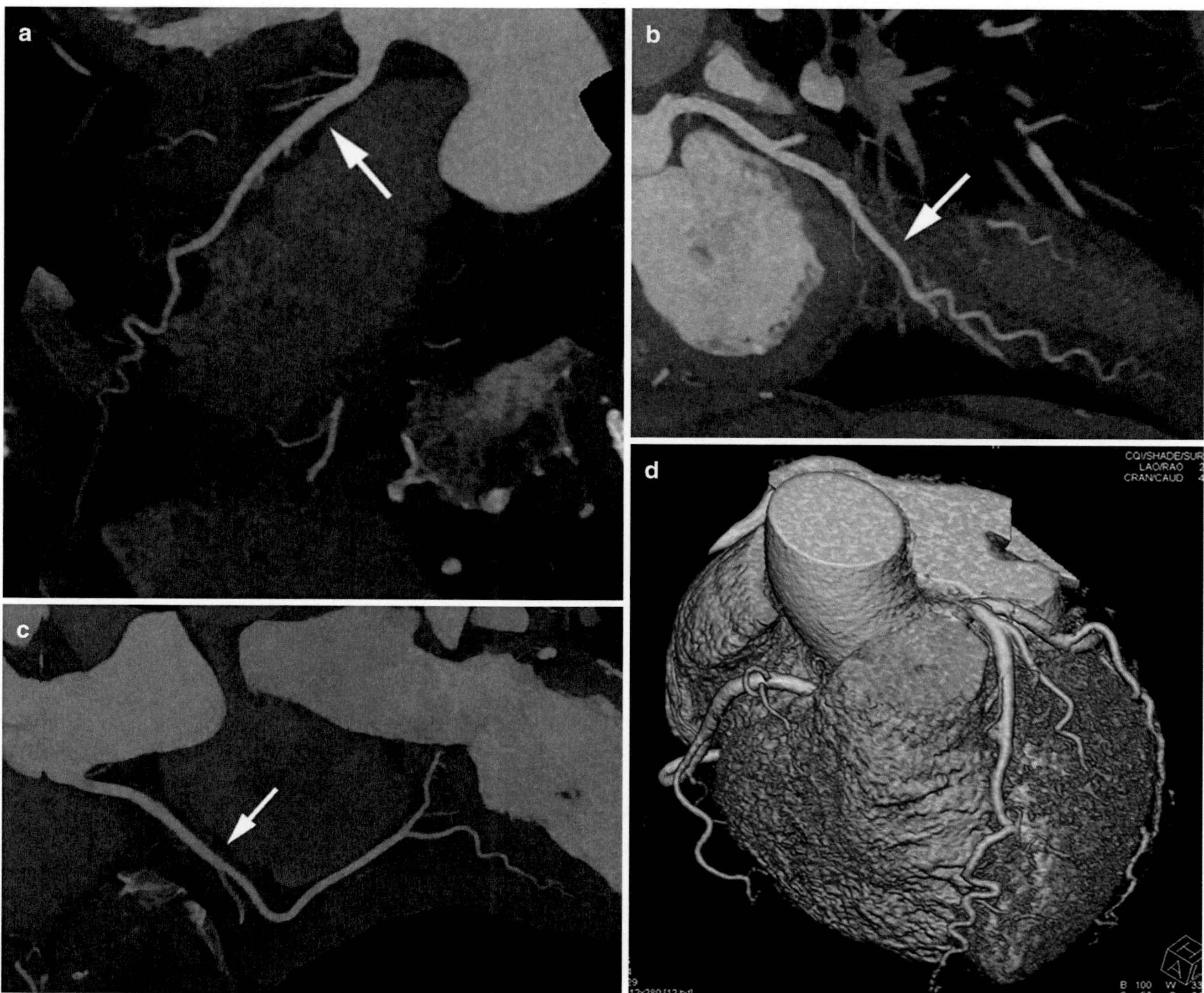

Fig. 9.3 Very low dose coronary CT angiography. Using a combination of a low-dose image acquisition mode (prospectively ECG-triggered high-pitch spiral acquisition), low tube voltage (70 kV), low tube current and iterative reconstruction, CT angiography was performed with an estimated effective dose of 0.35 mSv. Curved multiplanar reconstructions of the left anterior descending coronary artery (**a**, *arrow*), left circumflex coronary artery (**b**, *arrow*), and right coronary artery (**c**, *arrow*)) clearly demonstrate the absence of coronary artery stenosis. (**d**) 3-dimensional surface-weighted reconstruction

narrowing or to a complete occlusion with good distal filling via collateral flow [29]. Since CT only shows a static image and flow in the coronary arteries can not actually be seen, retrograde filling of a coronary artery segment can not be differentiated from antegrade flow (Fig. 9.8).

Insufficient image quality is most frequently the consequence of motion artefact (as a consequence of coronary movement or respiration), high image noise, or a combination of both. Additional problems can be caused by severe calcification, which causes partial volume effects (often referred to as "blooming") and aggravates motion artefacts (Fig. 9.9). In some cases, artefacts render the entire data set or some coronary segments unevaluable. This has become less frequent with more modern scanners but can still occur, especially if data acquisition is not carefully and expertly performed. If artefacts caused by motion, calcium, or a combination of both cause misinterpretation, it will in most cases be overestimation of stenosis degree or a false-positive reading of a stenosis [30, 31]. False-negative interpretations are less frequent.

Accuracy for Stenosis Detection

Coronary CT angiography has high accuracy for the detection of coronary artery stenoses (see Fig. 9.4). In addition to numerous small, single-center studies, four multi-center trials have investigated the accuracy of coronary CT angiography

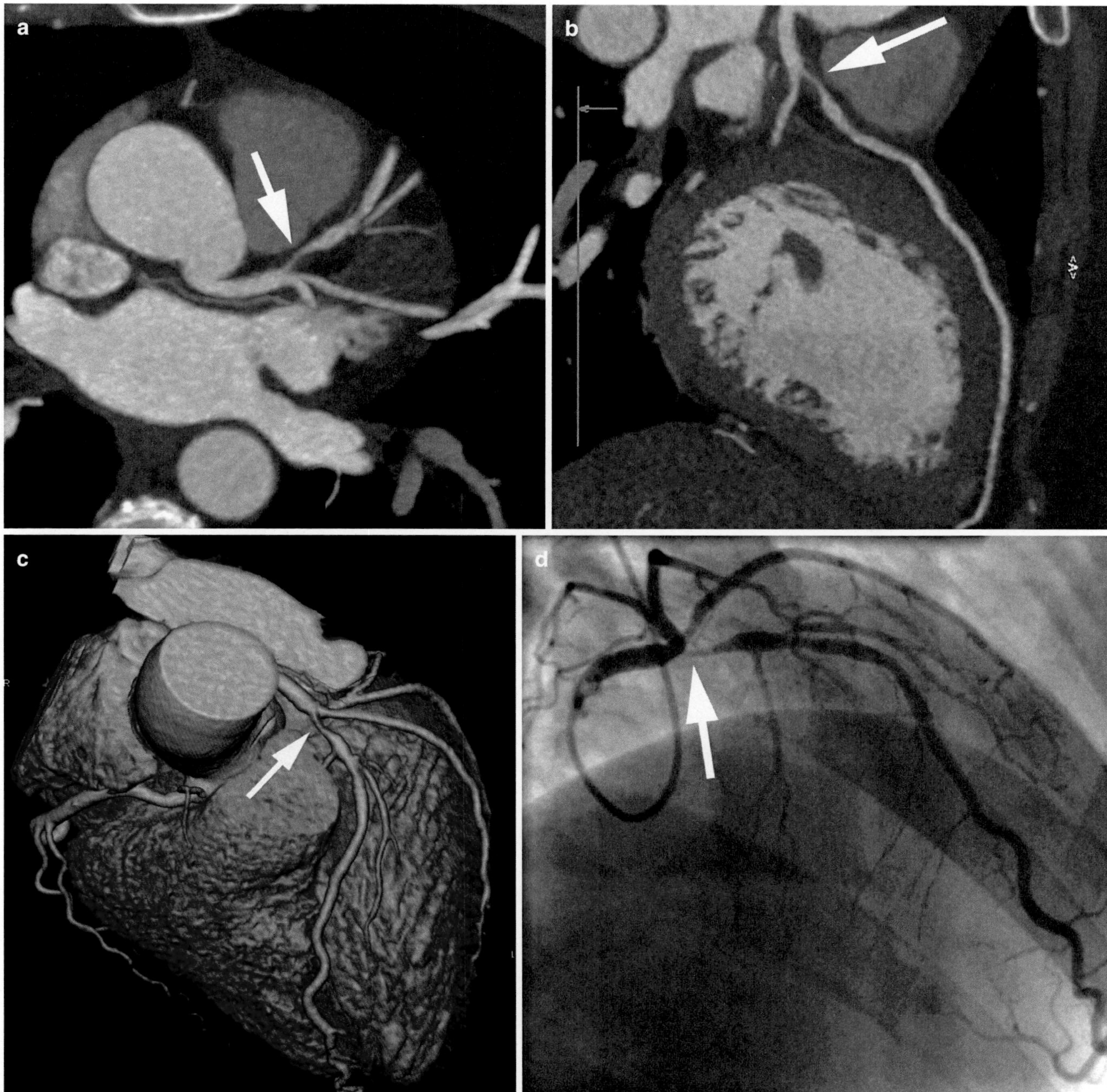

Fig. 9.4 Coronary CT angiography in a patient with a very proximal, high-grade stenosis of the left anterior descending coronary artery. (**a**) Maximum intensity projection in a transaxial orientation. The stenosis of the left anterior descending coronary artery, just distal to the left main trifurcation, can be seen (*arrow*). (**b**) Curved multiplanar reconstruction of the left main and left anterior descending coronary artery (*arrow*: stenosis). (**c**) 3-dimensional reconstruction (*arrow*: stenosis). (**d**) Invasive coronary angiogram (*arrow*: stenosis)

for the identification of coronary artery stenosis in comparison to invasive coronary angiography (see Table 9.3). Two trials performed in patients with suspected coronary artery disease using 64-slice CT have demonstrated sensitivities of 95–99 % and specificities of 64–83 % as well as negative predictive values of 97–99 % for the identification of individuals with at least one coronary artery stenosis [32, 33]. The positive predictive values were lower (64 and 86 % in the trials cited above), which is due to a tendency to overestimate stenosis degree in coronary CTA as well as the fact that image artefacts often result in false-positive interpretations. As in any diagnostic test, there is a trade-off between sensitivity and specificity in coronary CT angiography: Most studies – and most clinical users – will aim to keep sensitivity high, at the cost of specificity. If, on the other hand, a high specificity is desired, sensitivity will suffer. In a multicenter study of 291

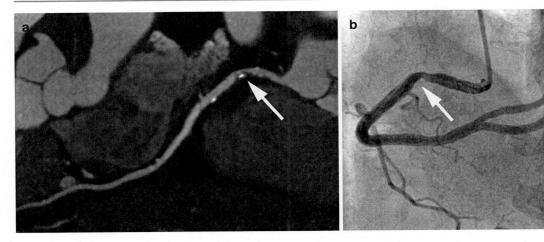

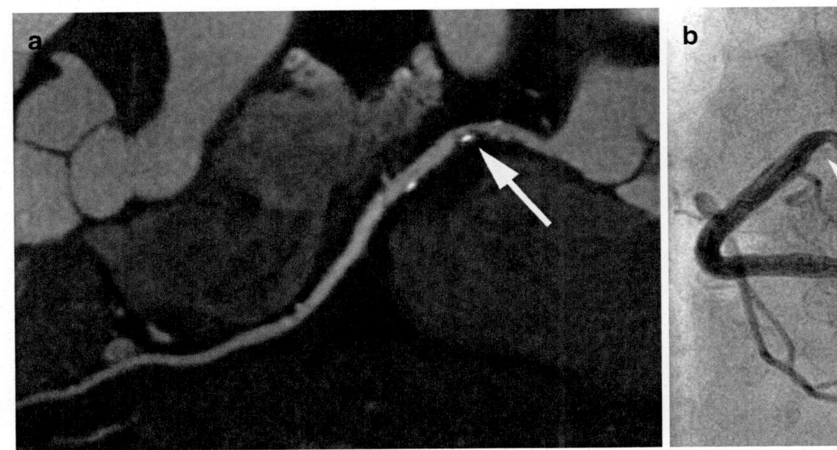

Fig. 9.5 Frequently, the degree of luminal narrowing appears more severe in coronary CT angiography than in the invasive, catheter-based coronary angiogram. (**a**) Curved multiplanar reconstruction showing a stenosis in the proximal right coronary artery (*arrow*). (**b**) In the corresponding invasive angiogram, the stenosis appears less severe (*arrow*)

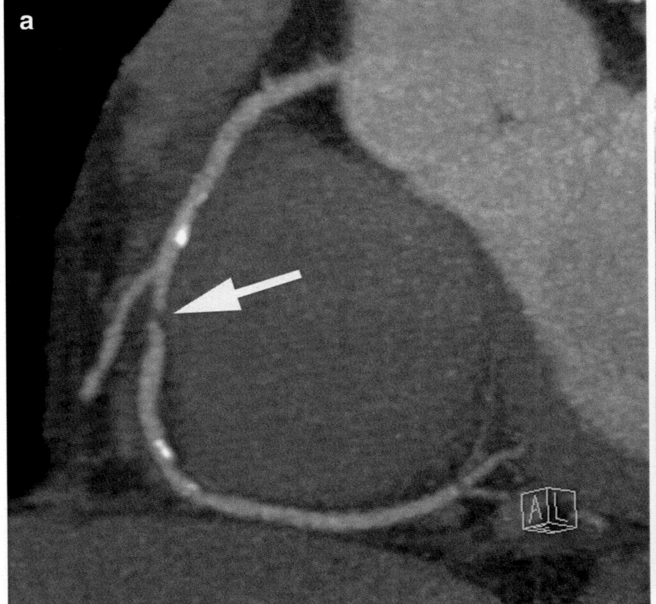

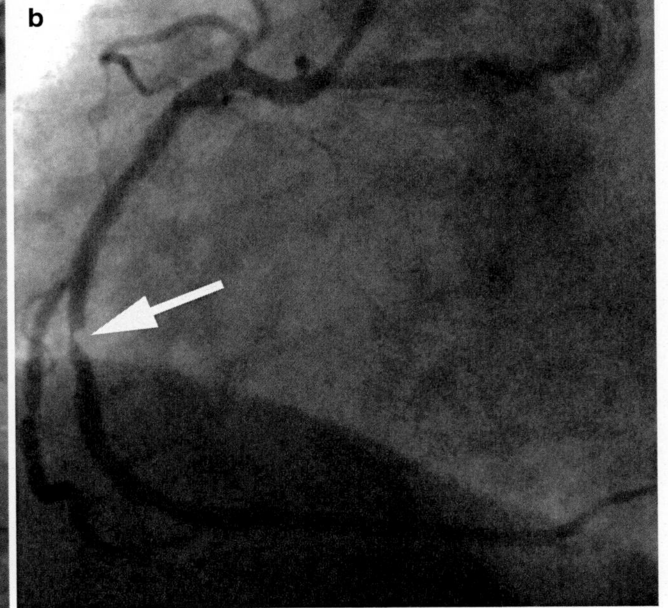

Fig. 9.6 High-grade luminal stenoses often appear as complete interruption of the coronary artery lumen in coronary CT angiography. (**a**) Maximum Intensity Projection in a patient with a high grade stenosis of the right coronary artery (*arrow*). At the site of the stenosis, the arterial lumen is completely interrupted. (**b**) Corresponding invasive coronary angiogram. A small residual lumen is present (*arrow*). The spatial resolution of CT is not sufficient to reliably visualize such small remaining lumina

Table 9.2 Recommended categories of luminal stenosis severity for reporting coronary CT angiography [24]

Recommended quantitative stenosis grading	
0 – Normal	Absence of plaque and no luminal stenosis
1 – Minimal	Plaque with <25 % stenosis
2 – Mild	25–49 % stenosis
3 – Moderate	50–69 % stenosis
4 – Severe	70–99% stenosis
5 – Occluded	

patients with 56 % prevalence of coronary artery stenoses, as well as 20 % of patients with previous myocardial infarction and 10 % with prior revascularization, specificity was high (90 %) and the positive predictive value was 91 % [34]. However, this came at the cost of decreased sensitivity (85 %) and negative predictive value (83 %, see Table 9.3) [23].

A large meta-analysis of trials that compared coronary CT angiography to invasive coronary angiography for stenosis detection in a total of 3764 patients yielded a patient-based sensitivity of 98 % and specificity of 82 % to identify

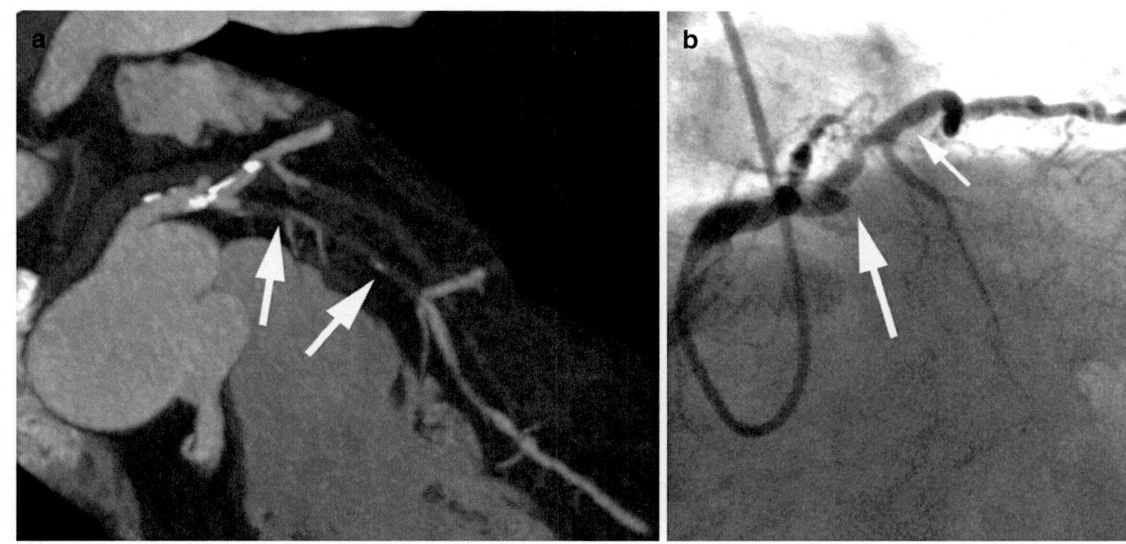

Fig. 9.7 Total occlusion of the left anterior descending coronary artery. (**a**) Coronary CT angiography displays interruption of the coronary artery lumen over a long distance (*arrows*). (**b**) The invasive angiogram confirms proximal occlusion of the left anterior descending coronary artery (*large arrow*). The *small arrow* points at the diagonal branch

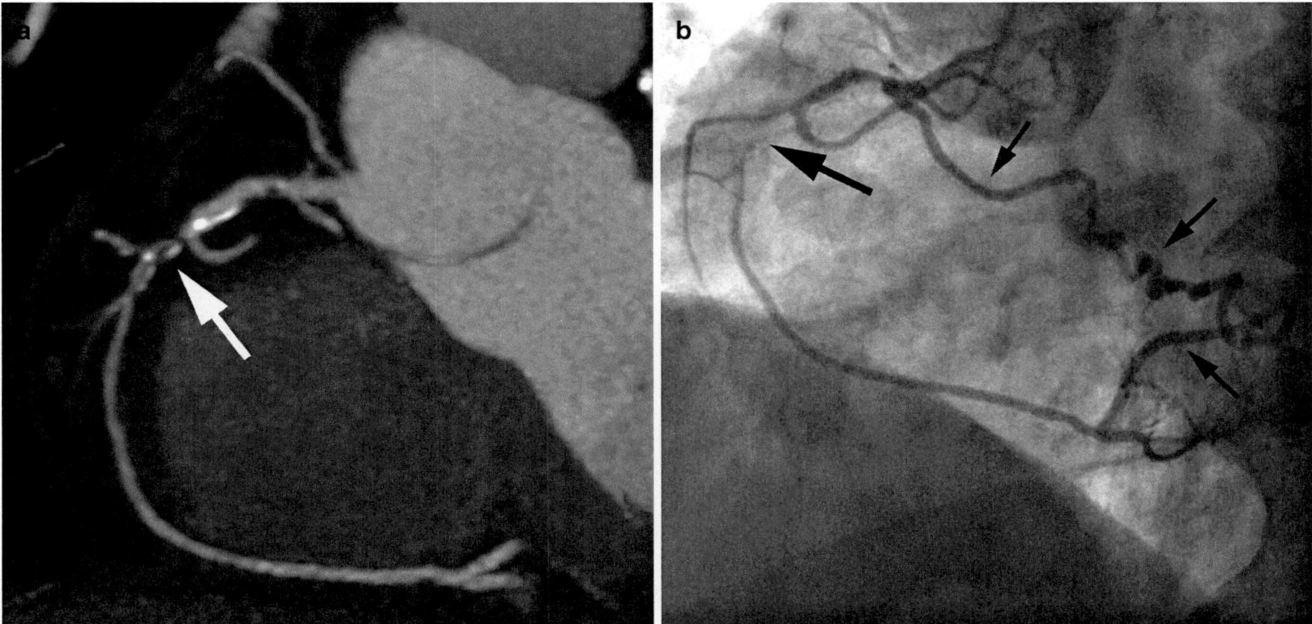

Fig. 9.8 Coronary CT angiography cannot identify retrograde filling of a coronary artery via collaterals. (**a**) Maximum Intensity Projection of the right coronary artery showing lesion with severe impairment of the lumen (*arrow*). The distal vessel segments are filled with contrast. (**b**) Invasive coronary angiography shows chronic total occlusion of the proximal right coronary artery (*arrow*) and retrograde filling of the mid and distal right coronary artery via a collateral vessel (Kugel's collateral)

individuals with at least one significant coronary artery stenosis. The negative predictive value was 99 % and the positive predictive value was 91 %. On an individual artery-based level, sensitivity was 95 %, specificity 90 %, negative predictive value 99 % and positive predictive value 75 % [35] (see Table 9.4)

Accuracy values are not uniform across all patients. Several trials have demonstrated that high heart rates, obesity, and extensive calcification negatively influence accuracy [36–40]. Usually, degraded image will lead to false-positive rather than false-negative findings. Specificity is therefore typically reduced when image quality is not very good (see Fig. 9.10).

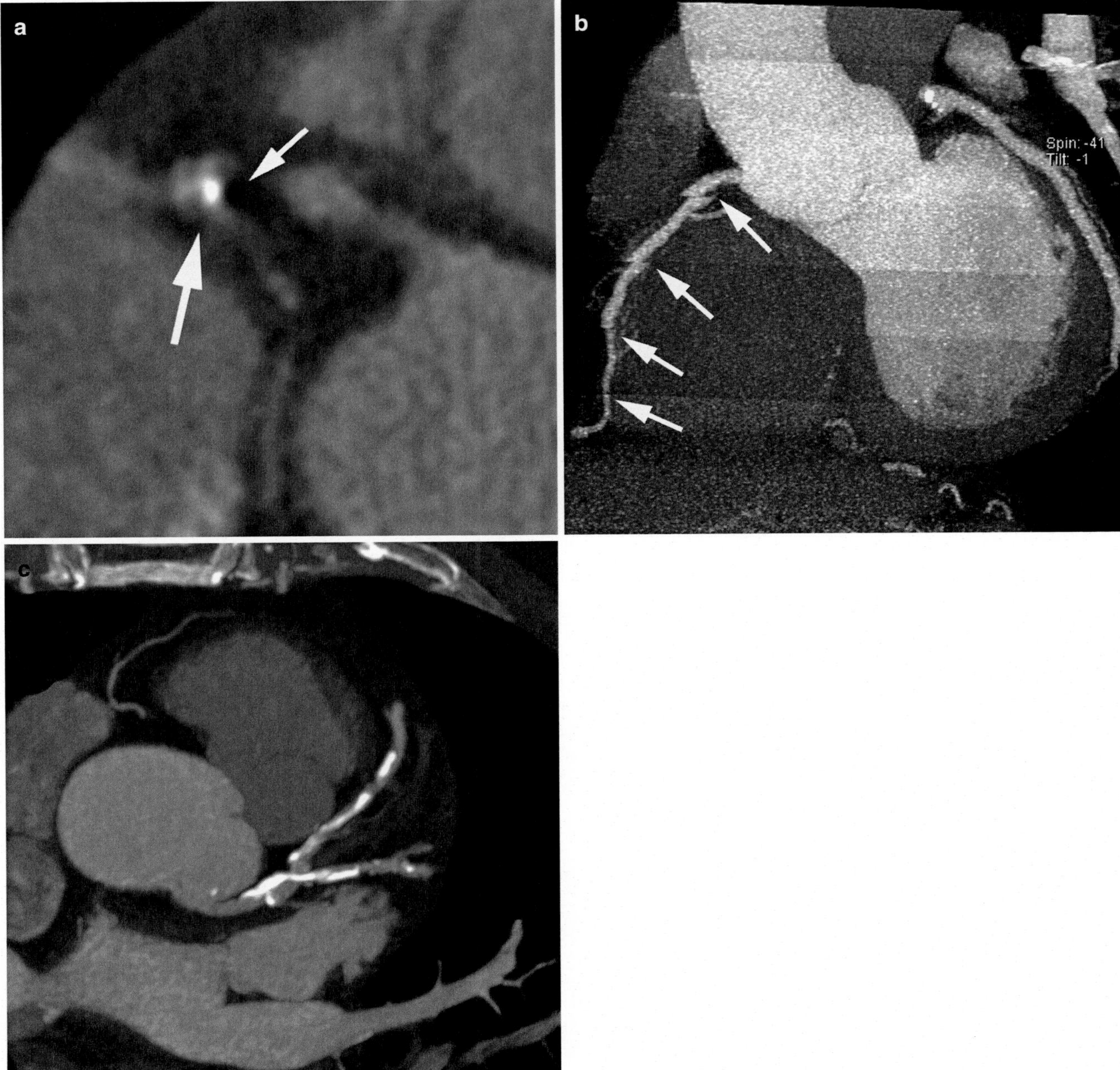

Fig. 9.9 Typical artifacts that can occur in coronary CT angiography. (**a**) Motion artifact due to rapid coronary artery movement. Here, the right coronary is affected. Motion causes blurring of the arterial contour (*large arrow*). It also causes low-density artifacts that, in this case, are outside the actual vessel cross-section (*small arrow*). Such artifacts are aggravated by the presence of calcium or other high-density material. (**b**) "Misaligment" or "Step" artifacts (*arrows*). Such artifacts can occur due to respiratory or other body motion or due to arrhythmias. (**c**) Severe calcification can render the coronary arteries uninterpretable regarding the presence of stenoses

Along with patient factors that influence image quality (such as body weight, heart rate, and the degree of calcification), the accuracy of coronary CT angiography depends on the pre-test likelihood of disease [39, 41]. In an analysis of 254 patients referred to invasive angiography and also studied by CT, it was demonstrated that coronary CT angiography performs best in patients with a low to intermediate clinical likelihood of coronary artery stenoses (negative predictive value: 100 % in both groups), while accuracy is substantially lower in high-risk patients (see Table 9.5) [41].

Overall, the good diagnostic performance of coronary CT angiography in patients who are not at high likelihood of having coronary artery stenoses, and especially the very high negative predictive value found for such patients make coronary CTA is a clinically useful tool in symptomatic patients who have a low or intermediate likelihood of coronary

Table 9.3 Multi-center studies that investigated the accuracy of coronary artery stenosis detection by contrast-enhanced 64-slice coronary CT angiography in comparison to invasive coronary angiography. The last of the cited studies (Rochitte et al.) used a combined reference standard of "At least 50 % stenosis in coronary angiography plus perfusion defect in SPECT". All values are based on per-patient analyses

Author	Number of sites	Number of patients	Prevalence of obstructive CAD[a]	Sensitivity (95 % CI)	Specificity (95 % CI)	Negative predictive value (95 % CI)	Positive predictive value (95 % CI)
Budoff [32]	16	230	25 %	95 (85–99 %)	83 % (76–88 %)	99 % (96–100 %)	64 % (53–75 %)
Meijboom [33]	3	360	68 %	99 % (98–100 %)	64 % (55–73 %)	97 % (94–100 %)	86 % (82–90 %)
Miller [34]	9	291[a]	56 %	85 % (79–90 %)	90 % (83–94 %)	83 % (75–89 %)	91 % (86–95 %)
Rochitte [23]	16	381[b]	38 %	92 %[c] (87–96 %)	51 %[c] (44–57 %)	92 %[c] (86–96 %)	53 %[c] (47–60 %)

[a]This trial included 58 patients with previous myocardial infarction and 28 patients with previously percutaneous coronary intervention
[b]This trial included 104 patients with previous myocardial infarction and 109 patients with previously placed coronary stents
[c]Combined reference standard of angiographic stenosis plus perfusion defect

Table 9.4 Results of a meta-analysis that investigated the accuracy of coronary artery stenosis detection by computed tomography angiography in comparison to invasive coronary angiography [35]

	Number of trials	Sensitivity (95 % CI)	Specificity (95 % CI)	Negative predictive value (range)	Positive predictive value (range)
Per patient analysis	18	98.2 % (97.4–98.8 %)	81.6 % (79.0–84.0 %)	99.0 % (88–100 %)	90.5 %(75–100 %)
Per-artery analysis	17	94.9 % (93.9–95.8 %)	89.5 % (88.8–90.2 %)	99.0 % (93–100 %)	75.0 % (53–95 %)
Per-segment analysis	17	91.3 % (90.2–92.2 %)	94 % (93.7–94.2 %)	99.0 % (98–100 %)	69.0 % (44–86 %)

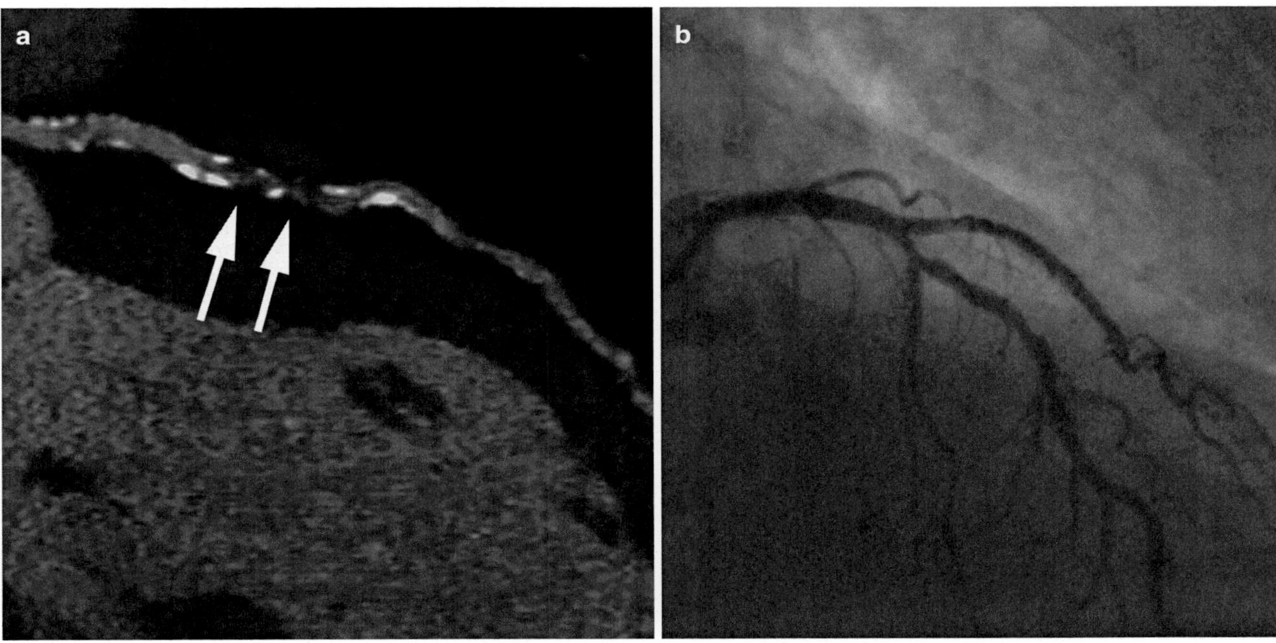

Fig. 9.10 Artifacts typically lead to false-positive results of coronary CT angiography. (**a**) Calcification, slight motion and somewhat high image noise lead to a false-positive interpretation of the mid left anterior descending coronary artery (*arrows*). (**b**) Invasive angiography shows that no relevant stenosis is present

disease, but for clinical reasons require further workup to rule out significant coronary stenoses. A negative coronary CT angiography will obviate the need for further testing. Indeed, several observational trials clearly demonstrated that symptomatic patients have an extremely favourable clinical outcome when coronary CT angiography is "negative" and hence do not require any further testing [42–46]. The large-scale, multi-center international CONFIRM registry

Table 9.5 Diagnostic performance of 64-slice CT depending on the clinical pre-test likelihood of coronary artery disease in 254 patients [41]

Pre-test probability	N	Sensitivity %	Specificity %	Pos. pred. value %	Neg. pred. value %
High	105	98	74	93	89
Intermediate	83	100	84	80	100
Low	66	100	93	75	100

supports the extremely good prognosis of symptomatic patients after a normal coronary CTA examination [47]. The registry collected data from 12 centers in 6 countries between 2005 and 2009 who underwent clinically indicated coronary CTA. Min et al. analyzed 24 775 of these patients, with follow-up obtained in 23 854, of which 5594 patients had obstructive coronary artery disease and 18 260 did not. Over a mean period of 2.3 years, 404 deaths were recorded. The mean annualized death rate in patients with a normal coronary CTA examination was only 0.28 % [48].

Based on the same registry, Shaw et al. analyzed the relationship between coronary CTA results, invasive coronary angiography, and subsequent mortality [49]. They found that in patients without any obstructive stenosis in coronary CTA, performing invasive coronary angiography was associated with a relative hazard for death of 2.2 ($p=0.011$), while in patients with obstructive stenosis in coronary CTA, invasive angiography was associated with a relative hazard for death of 0.61 ($p=0.047$). Min et al. reported that a benefit of revascularization was only present in patients with high-risk anatomy in coronary CTA (at least two-vessel coronary artery disease with involvement of the left anterior descending coronary artery, three-vessel coronary disease or left main stenosis) [50]. Revascularization was associated with a hazard ratio for death of 0.38 (95 % CI: 0.18–0.83) in patients with “high-risk CAD” in coronary CTA, but there was no survival difference in patients without “high-risk CAD” in coronary CTA (hazard ratio 3.24 with a 95 % CI between 0.76 and 13.89). Thus, sufficient data is available that coronary CTA is an excellent prognostic tool and that it is safe to avoid any further testing in chest pain patients if coronary CT angiography demonstrates the absence of coronary artery stenoses.

Acute Chest Pain

In the setting of acute chest pain, it is clinically very useful to reliably and quickly rule out – or identify – coronary artery stenosis (see Fig. 9.11). This is especially the case if the ECG is normal and myocardial enzymes are not elevated, the likelihood of coronary disease is low, but the possibility of myocardial infarction requires a rapid and definite diagnosis. Numerous trials have demonstrated that CT angiography is accurate and safe to stratify patients with acute chest pain and absence of ECG changes as well as myocardial enzyme elevation [51], and that outcome is excellent if CT demonstrates the absence of coronary stenosis in acute chest pain patients [52–59]. A cost advantage of incorporating CT angiography in the workup of low-likelihood acute chest pain patients as compared to the standard of care has been demonstrated [54]. Most trials of coronary CTA in acute chest pain patients can justifiably be criticized for including very low-risk patients [60], but their results can likely be extrapolated to patients with somewhat higher risk. In fact, both US [61] and European guidelines on acute coronary syndromes incorporate coronary CT angiography as a useful tool to rule out stenosis in patients with low-risk acute chest pain [62]. As for other applications, coronary CT angiography should be considered in acute chest pain patients only if patient characteristics promise full evaluability and high image quality [62].

Coronary CT Angiography and Ischemia

Coronary CTA, like invasive angiography, is a purely morphologic imaging modality and cannot demonstrate the functional relevance of stenoses (ischemia). The correlation of CT results with the presence of ischemia is poor [63–65]. Especially in the case of lesions with borderline degree of stenosis, this may be a limitation for the clinical application of CT angiography. Not surprisingly, coronary CT angiography a better predictor of angiographic findings than testing for ischemia [63–65]. A “negative” coronary CT angiography result is a reliable predictor to rule out the presence of coronary artery stenoses and the need for revascularization, and it may therefore be used as a “gatekeeper” to avoid invasive angiograms. On the other hand, coronary CTA – like invasive angiography – should not be performed in an unselected patient population and not for “screening” purposes. A positive coronary CTA scan taken by itself does not strongly predict the need for revascularization [66].

Several methods are under evaluation to improve the ability of coronary CT angiography to predict ischemia. They include the combination with CT-based myocardial perfusion [67, 68] assessment and specific analysis methods, such as the “transluminal attenuation gradient” or CT-based determination of the “fractional flow reserve” (FFR) [69, 70]. Especially the latter receives widespread interest. Based on the anatomic CT data set, computational

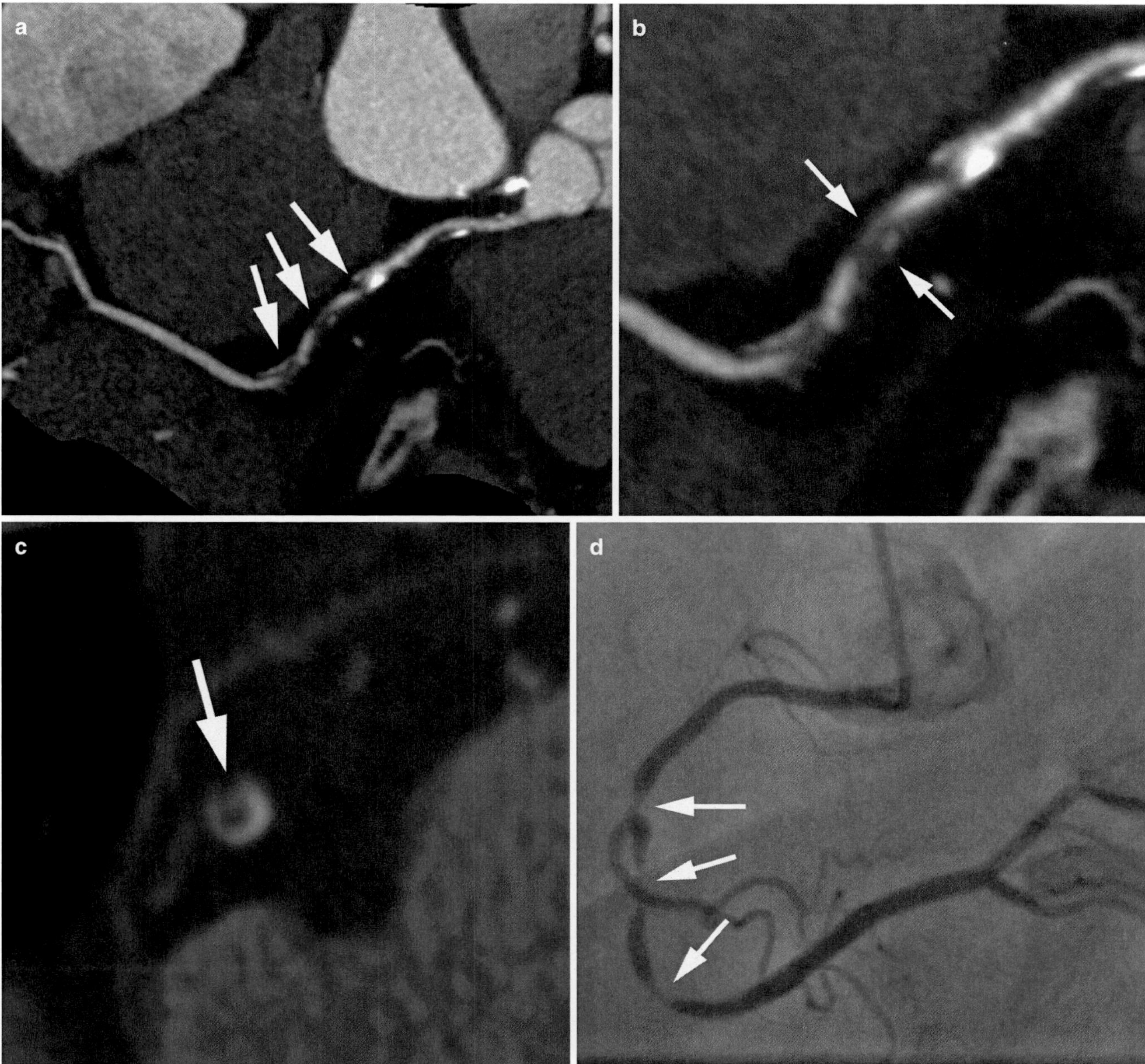

Fig. 9.11 Typical findings of coronary CT angiography in patients with an acute coronary syndrome. (**a**) Coronary CT angiography (curved multiplanar reconstruction) shows three high-grade stenoses of the right coronary artery (*arrows*). (**b**) As frequently seen in acute coronary lesions, there is pronounced "positive remodeling" of the of the lesion (*arrows*), a consequence of plaque rupture with subsequent thrombus formation inside the vessel. (**c**) A cross-sectional view of the right coronary artery at the site of the lesion shows ring-like enhancement with a central filling defect (*arrow*). Similar to the pronounced positive remodeling shown in Fig. 9.11b, this finding, when present, typically indicates an acute coronary lesion, but is not necessarily observed in all lesions associated with an acute coronary syndrome. (**d**) Invasive coronary angiogram (*arrows*: serial stenoses)

fluid dynamics are applied to model the flow and resistance pattern under adenosine stress and to obtain the FFR value for all segments of the coronary artery tree Initial publications show that this is feasible, and can improve the specificity of CT to identify ischemia causing lesions over a purely anatomic assessment alone. However, further validation will be necessary.

Imaging of Coronary Atherosclerotic Plaque

Coronary CT angiography allows to visualize non-stenotic coronary atherosclerotic plaque if image quality is good (see Fig. 9.12). Given the fact that the vast majority of cardiac events are caused by plaque rupture, the detection and

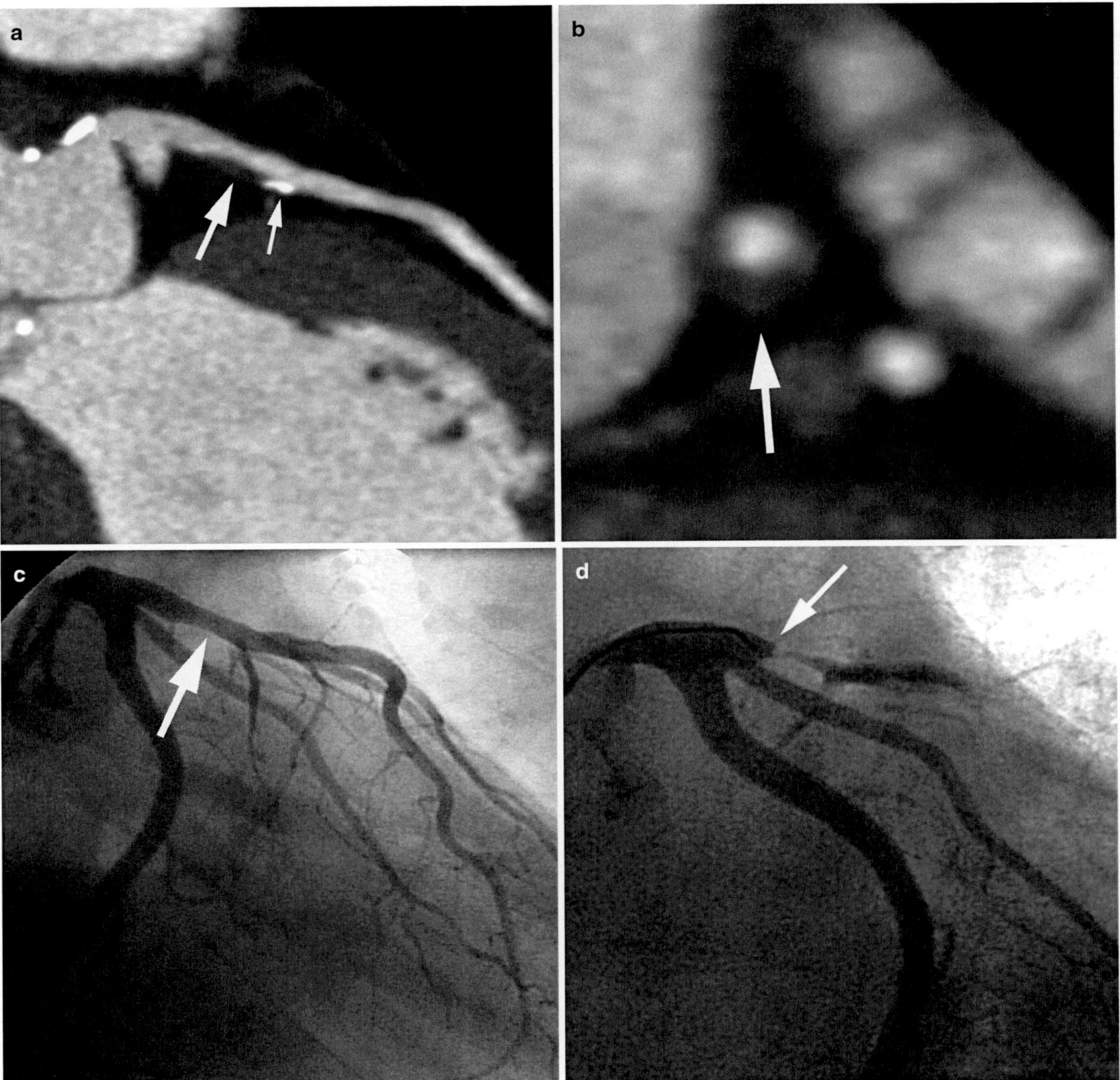

Fig. 9.12 Visualization of non-obstructive coronary atherosclerotic plaque by CT. (**a**) Multiplanar reconstruction of the left anterior descending coronary artery. In the proximal vessel segment, a non-obstructive plaque which is partly calcified (*small arrow*) and partly non-calcified (large arrow) can easily be detected by CT. (**b**) Cross-sectional view of the plaque (*arrow*) shows its eccentric position. (**c**) Invasive coronary angiogram. Only a very slight luminal stenosis is present at the site of the plaque (*arrow*). (**d**) 7 years after coronary CT angiography shown in panels **a** and **b** and after the invasive angiogram shown in panel **c**, the patient developed acute symptoms and presented with ST-elevation myocardial infarction of the anterior wall. The left anterior descending coronary artery was occluded at the site of the formerly non-obstructive, partly calcified atherosclerotic plaque

characterization not only of calcified, but also of non-calcified plaque components is a promising tool for improved risk stratification. In comparison to IVUS, accuracy for detecting non-calcified plaque has been found to be approximately 80–90 % [71–73] but these studies were performed in selected patients. With some limitations and again under the prerequisite of excellent image quality, plaque quantification and characterization is possible. On average, the CT attenuation within "fibrous" plaques is higher than within "lipid-rich" plaques (mean attenuation values of 91–116

HU versus 47–71 HU) [74–77] However, the variability of density measurements within plaque types is large and numerous factors, including the degree of intraluminal contrast attantuation as well as various image reconstruction parameters influence the density that is measured by CT within coronary plaques [78, 79]. Therefore, accurate classification of plaque composition by coronary CTA is not currently possible. On the other hand, some parameters that are more readily available from CT might also contribute to the detection of "vulnerable" plaques. They include a "spotty" pattern of calcification, and a large degree of positive remodelling [80–83].

Some characteristics of coronary atherosclerotic plaque that can determined by CT, such as positive remodeling (see Fig. 9.13) and low CT attenuation of the atherosclerotic material (below 30 HU), are associated with the occurrence of future acute coronary syndromes [83]. However, the presence and extent of coronary atherosclerotic plaque seems to be a more robust marker of risk than individual plaque characteristics. Several studies and data based on large registries have been able to demonstrate a prognostic value of atherosclerotic lesions detected by coronary CT angiography both in symptomatic and asymptomatic individuals. An analysis of the clinical CONFIRM registry, including more than 23,000 patients, confirmed the prognostic value of coronary CT angiography, where the presence of coronary stenoses, but also the presence of non-obstructive plaque was associated with an increased risk of mortality [48]. However, the hazard ratio for non-obstructive plaque was relatively low (HR 1.6; 95 % CI 1.2–2.2). Other trials and analyses confirm similar findings [84, 85]. The problematic issue is that while absence of plaque is clearly associated with an extremely good prognosis, the presence of some non-obstructive plaque is very frequent in the population and the positive predictive value regarding future cardiovascular events is very low [85]. Also, a relevant incremental prognostic value of contrast-enhanced coronary CT angiography over coronary calcium measurements has so far not convincingly been demonstrated [86]. Therefore, coronary CT angiography for the identification of coronary atherosclerotic plaque is currently not recommended for risk assessment purposes in asymptomatic individuals.

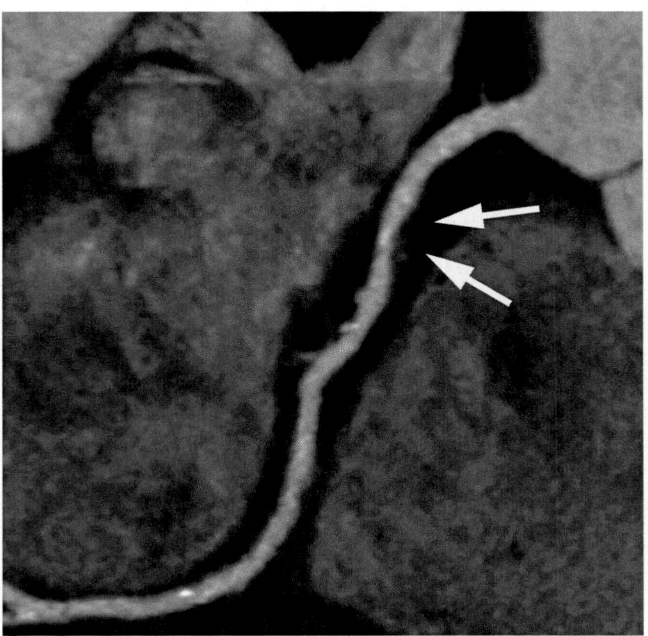

Fig. 9.13 Pronounced positive remodeling of a non-obstructive, non-calcified coronary atherosclerotic plaque of the right coronary artery (*arrows*)

Anomalous Coronary Arteries

Coronary CT angiography is an excellent tool to investigate patients with known or suspected congenital coronary artery anomalies (Figs. 9.14 and 9.15). Coronary CT angiography can classify both the origin and also the often complex course of anomalous coronary vessels [87–91]. While the necessity for contrast agent injection and radiation exposure are certain drawbacks of CT imaging as compared to MR, which is also a potential diagnostic tool in coronary artery anomalies, the ease of data acquisition and the predictability with which a high-resolution data set with optimal image quality for evaluation can be expected make coronary CT angiography a method of choice for the workup of known or suspected anomalous coronary vessels. Obviously, the use of low-dose image acquisition protocols is recommendable in the often young patients who undergo evaluation for anomalous coronary arteries.

Guidelines and Recommendations

A group of US-based professional societies (both cardiology and radiology) has jointly issued a statement of "Appropriateness Criteria" for cardiac CT in the year 2010 (see Table 9.6). The document lists clinical situations in which coronary CTA could be applied, and rates them as inappropriate, appropriate, or uncertain [92]. Such situations include the use of CT coronary angiography to rule out coronary artery stenoses in patients who are symptomatic, but who have a non-interpretable or equivocal stress test, who are unable to exercise, or who have a non-interpretable ECG. Furthermore, the document considers the use of coronary CT angiography appropriate for patients with new onset heart failure and for patients who present witch acute chest pain and an intermediate pre-test likelihood of coronary artery disease, but who have a normal ECG and absence of enzyme elevation (see Table 9.5) [92]. Finally, the use of CT

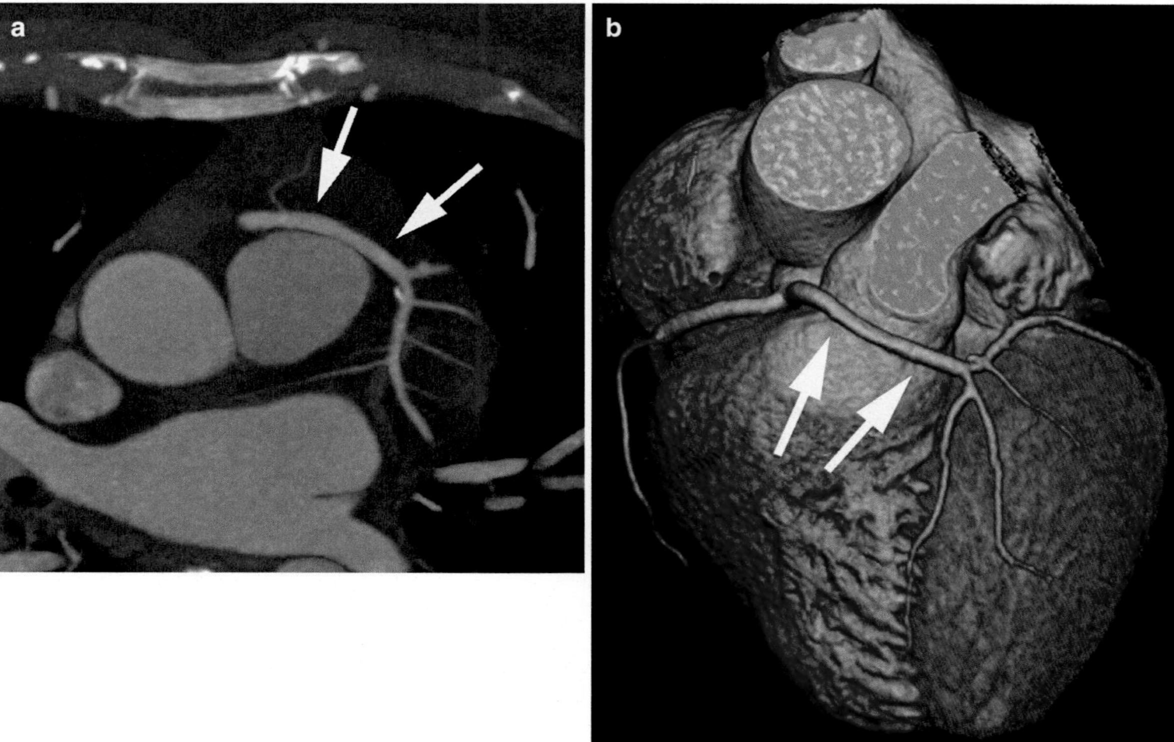

Fig. 9.14 Visualization of a coronary anomaly by CT. Due to its three-dimensional nature, coronary CT angiography allows excellent delineation of the origin and course of anomalous coronary arteries. This patient has an anomalous left main coronary artery arising from the right coronary sinus and travelling anterior to the pulmonary artery, with subsequent division into the left anterior descending and left circumflex coronary artery. This infrequent anomaly is clinically harmless. (**a**) Two-dimensional CT image in transaxial orientation which shows the position of the anomalous left main coronary artery anterior to the pulmonary artery (*arrows*). (**b**) Three-dimensional reconstruction. The *arrows* point at the anomalous left main coronary artery

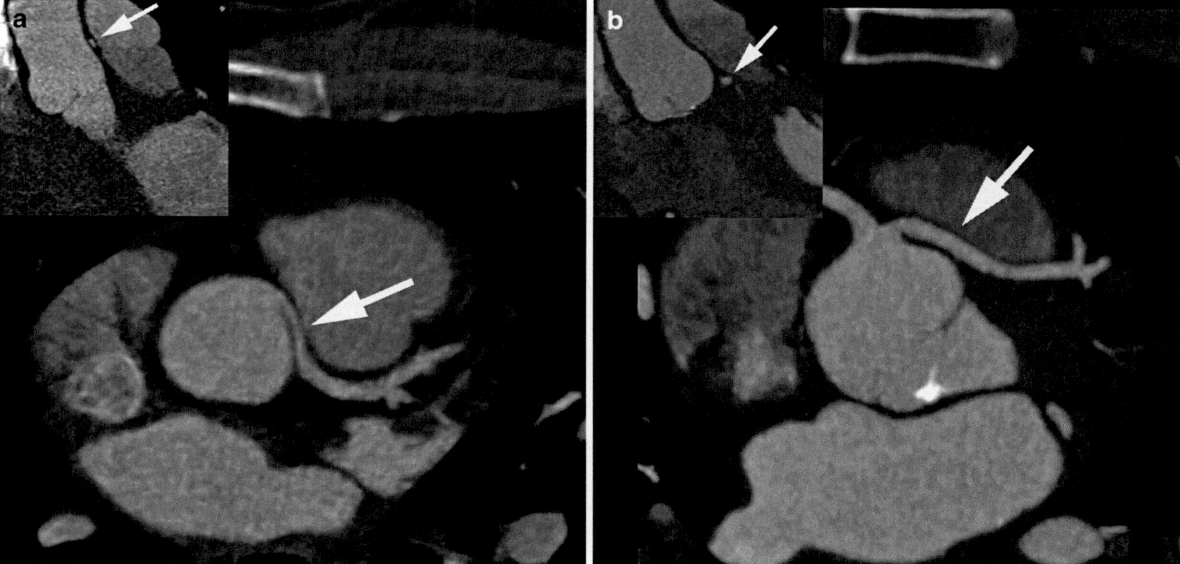

Fig. 9.15 "Interarterial" versus "sub-pulmonary" course of an anomalous left main coronary artery. (**a**) Patient with an anomalous left main coronary artery (*arrows*) that arises from the right coronary sinus and follows an "interarterial" course between the ascending aorta and right pulmonary artery. In this location (see *inset*), there is potential danger of ischemia due to kinking or compression of the left main coronary artery. Surgical correction, irrespective of symptoms, is frequently suggested. (**b**) Patient with an anomalous left main coronary which also arises from the right coronary sinus but then travels below the pulmonary artery, embedded in the septum ("subpulmonary" or "transseptal" course, see *arrows*). This anomaly is typically considered less harmful

Table 9.6 Appropriateness of coronary CT angiography in various clinical situations [92]

Non-acute symptoms possibly representing an ischemic equivalent – no stress test done	
ECG interpretable **and** able to exercise	
Low pre-test likelihood (<10 %)	Uncertain
Intermediate pre-test likelihood (10–90 %)	**Appropriate**
High pre-test likelihood (>90 %)	Inappropriate
ECG uninterpretable **or** unable to exercise	
Low or intermediate pre-test likelihood	**Appropriate**
High pre-test likelihood	Uncertain
Non-acute symptoms, prior ECG exercise test	
Normal but continued symptoms	**Appropriate**
Abnormal	
Intermediate duke treadmill score	**Appropriate**
Low or high duke treadmill score	Inappropriate
Non-acute symptoms, prior stress imaging procedure	
Equivocal	**Appropriate**
Mildly positive	Uncertain
Moderately or severely positive	Inappropriate
Discordant ECG exercise and stress imaging results	**Appropriate**
New or worsening symptoms with a past stress imaging study	
Past study normal	**Appropriate**
Past study abnormal	Uncertain
Acute symptoms with suspicion of ACS (urgent presentation)	
Definite MI	Inappropriate
"Triple Rule Out" for acute chest pain of uncertain cause (differential diagnosis includes pulmonary embolism, aortic dissection, and ACS)	Uncertain
Cardiac biomarkers normal or equivocal and ECG normal or uninterpretable	
Low or intermediate pre-test likelihood	**Appropriate**
Intermediate pre-test likelihood	**Appropriate**
Patient with previous revascularization by CABG and	
Symptoms, assessment of bypass patency required	**Appropriate**
No symptoms, surgery <5 years ago	Inappropriate
No symptoms, surgery ≥5 years ago	Uncertain
Patient with previous revascularization by PCI and	
Symptoms, stent <3 mm	Inappropriate
Symptoms,, stent ≥3 mm	Uncertain
No symptoms, left main stent ≥3 mm	**Appropriate**
No symptoms, other stents	Inappropriate

angiography is considered "appropriate" to evaluate patients with anomalous coronary arteries [92]. CT angiography for screening purposes is not endorsed.

Official guidelines issued by the European Society of Cardiology assign a "Class IIa" recommendation ("should be considered") to coronary CTA in patients with suspected stable coronary artery disease [93] and patients with acute chest pain but absence of ECG changed and enzyme elevation [62]. United States guidelines on non-ST-elevation acute coronary syndromes, jointly issued by the ACC and AHA [61], assign a "Class IIa" recommendation to coronary CTA and state that:

In patients with possible ACS and a normal ECG, normal cardiac troponins, and no history of CAD, it is reasonable to initially perform (without serial ECGs and troponins) coronary CT angiography to assess coronary artery anatomy (Level of Evidence: A) or rest myocardial perfusion imaging with a technetium-99 m radiopharmaceutical to exclude myocardial ischemia (Level of Evidence: B)

ACC/AHA guidelines on stable coronary disease, in their last version dated 2012, provide the following recommendations regarding the use of coronary CTA [94]:

Class IIa ("Should be considered")

Patients unable to exercise, with low to intermediate pretest probability of ischemic heart disease

Patients with intermediate pretest probability of ischemic heart disease and an inconclusive exercise test, ongoing symptoms in spite of a normal exercise test, as well as patients unable to undergo stress testing by myocardial perfusion imaging or stress echocardiography

Class IIb ("might be reasonable")

Patients able to exercise, with intermediate pretest probability of ischemic heart disease

Summary and Outlook

In spite of the impressive and continuously improving image quality, coronary CT angiography does not currently constitute a general replacement for invasive, catheter-based diagnostic coronary angiography. A somewhat lower spatial and temporal resolution as compared to invasive angiography, the requirement for regular and low heart rates, and the necessity for breathhold cooperation will preclude CT angiography in a relevant fraction of patients who require a workup for coronary artery disease. In addition, coronary CT angiography performs less well in patients with diffuse, severe disease, with substantial coronary calcification, or with small coronary arteries (as encountered, for example, in some individuals with diabetes). For these cases and all situations where the need for a revascularization procedure is expected based on clinical grounds, an invasive approach and catheter-based angiography will remain the best diagnostic option.

However, there are numerous patients with a lower pre-test likelihood of disease and with characteristics that promise high image quality and diagnostic accuracy. In these patients, coronary CTA, if performed expertly, is a superb test to rule out the presence of coronary artery stenosis and avoid the need for any further testing. Data on the prognostic value of coronary CTA will continue to accumulate and the continuous technical improvements of CT hardware will make coronary CTA ever more robust and accurate. It can therefore be expected that the role of coronary CTA in clinical cardiology will continue to expand. The challenges to meet will include the identification of the specific patient groups that benefit most from coronary CTA, assuring the widespread availability of high-end CT hardware, and the incorporation of training in coronary CTA into the curriculum of cardiology training.

References

1. Abbara S, Arbab-Zadeh A, Callister TQ, Desai MY, Mamuya W, Thomson L, Weigold WG. SCCT guidelines for performance of coronary computed tomographic angiography: a report of the Society of Cardiovascular Computed Tomography Guidelines Committee. J Cardiovasc Comput Tomogr. 2009;3:190–204.
2. Halliburton SS, Abbara S, Chen MY, Gentry R, Mahesh M, Raff GL, Shaw LJ, Hausleiter J. SCCT guidelines on radiation dose and dose-optimization strategies in cardiovascular CT. J Cardiovasc Comput Tomogr. 2011;5:198–224.
3. Bischoff B, Hein F, Meyer T, Krebs M, Hadamitzky M, Martinoff S, Schömig A, Hausleiter J. Comparison of sequential and helical scanning for radiation dose and image quality: results of the Prospective Multicenter Study on Radiation Dose Estimates of Cardiac CT Angiography (PROTECTION) I Study. AJR Am J Roentgenol. 2010;194(6):1495–9.
4. Hausleiter J, Meyer TS, Martuscelli E, Spagnolo P, Yamamoto H, Carrascosa P, Anger T, Lehmkuhl L, Alkadhi H, Martinoff S, Hadamitzky M, Hein F, Bischoff B, Kuse M, Schömig A, Achenbach S. Image quality and radiation exposure with prospectively ECG-triggered axial scanning for coronary CT angiography: the multicenter, multivendor, randomized PROTECTION-III study. JACC Cardiovasc Imaging. 2012;5(5):484–93.
5. Kim JS, Choo KS, Jeong DW, Chun KJ, Park YH, Song SG, Park JH, Kim JH, Kim J, Han D, Lim SJ. Step-and-shoot prospectively ECG-gated vs. retrospectively ECG-gated with tube current modulation coronary CT angiography using 128-slice MDCT patients with chest pain: diagnostic performance and radiation dose. Acta Radiol. 2011;52(8):860–5.
6. Labounty TM, Leipsic J, Min JK, Heilbron B, Mancini GB, Lin FY, Earls JP. Effect of padding duration on radiation dose and image interpretation in prospectively ECG-triggered coronary CT angiography. AJR Am J Roentgenol. 2010;194(4):933–7.
7. Leipsic J, LaBounty TM, Ajlan AM, Earls JP, Strovski E, Madden M, Wood DA, Hague CJ, Poulter R, Branch K, Cury RC, Heilbron B, Taylor C, Grunau G, Haiducu L, Min JK. A prospective randomized trial comparing image quality, study interpretability, and radiation dose of narrow acquisition window with widened acquisition window protocols in prospectively ECG-triggered coronary computed tomography angiography. J Cardiovasc Comput Tomogr. 2013;7:18–24.
8. Lell M, Marwan M, Schepis T, Pflederer T, Anders K, Flohr T, Allmendinger T, Kalender W, Ertel D, Thierfelder C, Kuettner A, Ropers D, Daniel WG, Achenbach S. Prospectively ECG-triggered high-pitch spiral acquisition for coronary CT angiography using dual source CT: technique and initial experience. Eur Radiol. 2009;19:2576–83.
9. Achenbach S, Goroll T, Seltmann M, Pflederer T, Anders K, Ropers D, Daniel WG, Uder M, Lell M, Marwan M. Detection of coronary artery stenoses by low-dose, prospectively ECG-triggered, high-pitch spiral coronary CT angiography. JACC Cardiovasc Imaging. 2011;4(4):328–37.
10. Schuhbaeck A, Achenbach S, Layritz C, Eisentopf J, Hecker F, Pflederer T, Gauss S, Rixe J, Kalender W, Daniel WG, Lell M, Ropers D. Image quality of ultra-low radiation exposure coronary CT angiography with an effective dose <0.1 mSv using high-pitch spiral acquisition and raw data-based iterative reconstruction. Eur Radiol. 2013;23(3):597–606.
11. Neefjes LA, Dharampal AS, Rossi A, Nieman K, Weustink AC, Dijkshoorn ML, Ten Kate GJ, Dedic A, Papadopoulou SL, van Straten M, Cademartiri F, Krestin GP, de Feyter PJ, Mollet NR. Image quality and radiation exposure using different low-dose scan protocols in dual-source CT coronary angiography: randomized study. Radiology. 2011;261:779–86.
12. Hausleiter J, Meyer T, Hermann F, Hadamitzky M, Krebs M, Gerber TC, McCollough C, Martinoff S, Kastrati A, Schömig A, Achenbach S. Estimated radiation dose associated with cardiac CT angiography. JAMA. 2009;301:500–7.
13. Bischoff B, Hein F, Meyer T, Hadamitzky M, Martinoff S, Schömig A, Hausleiter J. Impact of a reduced tube voltage on CT angiography and radiation dose: results of the PROTECTION I study. JACC Cardiovasc Imaging. 2009;2:940–6.
14. Jun BR, Yong HS, Kang EY, Woo OH, Choi EJ. 64-slice coronary computed tomography angiography using low tube voltage

of 80 kV in subjects with normal body mass indices: comparative study using 120 kV. Acta Radiol. 2012;53(10):1099–106.
15. Cao JX, Wang YM, Lu JG, Zhang Y, Wang P, Yang C. Radiation and contrast agent doses reductions by using 80-kV tube voltage in coronary computed tomographic angiography: a comparative study. Eur J Radiol. 2014;83(2):309–14.
16. LaBounty TM, Leipsic J, Poulter R, Wood D, Johnson M, Srichai MB, Cury RC, Heilbron B, Hague C, Lin FY, Taylor C, Mayo JR, Thakur Y, Earls JP, Mancini GB, Dunning A, Gomez MJ, Min JK. Coronary CT angiography of patients with a normal body mass index using 80 kVp versus 100 kVp: a prospective, multicenter, multivendor randomized trial. AJR Am J Roentgenol. 2011;197(5):W860–7.
17. Hell MM, Bittner D, Schuhbaeck A, Muschiol G, Brand M, Lell M, Uder M, Achenbach S, Marwan M. Prospectively ECG-triggered high-pitch coronary angiography with third-generation dual-source CT at 70 kVp tube voltage: Feasibility, image quality, radiation dose, and effect of iterative reconstruction. J Cardiovasc Comput Tomogr. 2014;8:418–25.
18. Yin WH, Lu B, Li N, Han L, Hou ZH, Wu RZ, Wu YJ, Niu HX, Jiang SL, Krazinski AW, Ebersberger U, Meinel FG, Schoepf UJ. Iterative reconstruction to preserve image quality and diagnostic accuracy at reduced radiation dose in coronary CT angiography: an intraindividual comparison. JACC Cardiovasc Imaging. 2013;6:1239–49.
19. Leipsic J, Nguyen G, Brown J, Sin D, Mayo JR. A prospective evaluation of dose reduction and image quality in chest CT using adaptive statistical iterative reconstruction. AJR Am J Roentgenol. 2010;195(5):1095–9.
20. Achenbach S, Marwan M, Ropers D, Schepis T, Pflederer T, Anders K, Kuettner A, Daniel WG, Uder M, Lell MM. Coronary computed tomography angiography with a consistent dose below 1 mSv using prospectively ECG-triggered high-pitch spiral acquisition. Eur Heart J. 2010;31:340–6.
21. Alkadhi H, Stolzmann P, Desbiolles L, Baumueller S, Goetti R, Plass A, Scheffel H, Feuchtner G, Falk V, Marincek B, Leschka S. Low-dose, 128-slice, dual-source CT coronary angiography: accuracy and radiation dose of the high-pitch and the step-and-shoot mode. Heart. 2010;96(12):933–8.
22. Chinnaiyan KM, Boura JA, DePetris A, Gentry R, Abidov A, Share DA, Raff GL, Advanced Cardiovascular Imaging Consortium Coinvestigators. Progressive radiation dose reduction from coronary computed tomography angiography in a statewide collaborative quality improvement program: results from the Advanced Cardiovascular Imaging Consortium. Circ Cardiovasc Imaging. 2013;6:646–54.
23. Rochitte CE, George RT, Chen MY, Arbab-Zadeh A, Dewey M, Miller JM, Niinuma H, Yoshioka K, Kitagawa K, Nakamori S, Laham R, Vavere AL, Cerci RJ, Mehra VC, Nomura C, Kofoed KF, Jinzaki M, Kuribayashi S, de Roos A, Laule M, Tan SY, Hoe J, Paul N, Rybicki FJ, Brinker JA, Arai AE, Cox C, Clouse ME, Di Carli MF, Lima JA. Computed tomography angiography and perfusion to assess coronary artery stenosis causing perfusion defects by single photon emission computed tomography: the CORE320 study. Eur Heart J. 2014;35:1120–30.
24. Leipsic J, Abbara S, Achenbach S, Cury R, Earls JP, Mancini GJ, Nieman K, Pontone G, Raff GL. SCCT guidelines for the interpretation and reporting of coronary CT angiography: a report of the Society of Cardiovascular Computed Tomography Guidelines Committee. J Cardiovasc Comput Tomogr. 2014;8(5):342–58.
25. Ferencik M, Ropers D, Abbara S, Cury RC, Hoffmann U, Nieman K, Brady TJ, Moselewski F, Daniel WG, Achenbach S. Diagnostic accuracy of image postprocessing methods for the detection of coronary artery stenoses by using multidetector CT. Radiology. 2007;243(3):696–702.
26. Cheng V, Gutstein A, Wolak S, Suzuki Y, Dey D, Gransar H, Thomson LE, Hayes SW, Friedman JD, Berman DS. Moving beyond binary grading of coronary arterial stenoses on coronary computed tomographic angiography: insights for the imager and referring clinician. JACC Cardiovasc Imaging. 2008;1:472–4.
27. Cury RC, Pomerantsev EV, Ferencik M, Hoffmann U, Nieman K, Moselewski F, Abbara S, Jang IK, Brady TJ, Achenbach S. Comparison of the degree of coronary stenoses by multidetector computed tomography versus by quantitative coronary angiography. Am J Cardiol. 2005;96(6):784–7.
28. Boogers MJ, Schuijf JD, Kitslaar PH, van Werkhoven JM, de Graaf FR, Boersma E, van Velzen JE, Dijkstra J, Adame IM, Kroft LJ, de Roos A, Schreur JH, Heijenbrok MW, Jukema JW, Reiber JH, Bax JJ. Automated quantification of stenosis severity on 64-slice CT: a comparison with quantitative coronary angiography. JACC Cardiovasc Imaging. 2010;3(7):699–709.
29. von Erffa J, Ropers D, Pflederer T, Schmid M, Marwan M, Daniel WG, Achenbach WG. Differentiation of total occlusion and high-grade stenosis in coronary CT angiography. Eur Radiol. 2008;18(12):2770–5.
30. Hoffmann U, Moselewski F, Cury RC, Ferencik M, Jang IK, Diaz LJ, Abbara S, Brady TJ, Achenbach S. Predictive value of 16-slice multidetector spiral computed tomography to detect significant obstructive coronary artery disease in patients at high risk for coronary artery disease: patient-versus segment-based analysis. Circulation. 2004;110:2638–43.
31. Yan RT, Miller JM, Rochitte CE, Dewey M, Niinuma H, Clouse ME, Vavere AL, Brinker J, Lima JA, Arbab-Zadeh A. Predictors of inaccurate coronary arterial stenosis assessment by CT angiography. JACC Cardiovasc Imaging. 2013;6(9):963–72.
32. Budoff MJ, Dowe D, Jollis JG, Gitter M, Sutherland J, Halamert E, Scherer M, Bellinger R, Martin A, Benton R, Delago A, Min JK. Diagnostic performance of 64-multidetector-row coronary computed tomographic angiography for evaluation of coronary artery stenosis in individuals without known coronary artery disease. J Am Coll Cardiol. 2008;52:1724–32.
33. Meijboom WB, Meijs MF, Schuijf JD, Cramer MJ, Mollet NR, van Mieghem CA, Nieman K, van Werkhoven JM, Pundziute G, Weustink AC, de Vos AM, Pugliese F, Rensing B, Jukema JW, Bax JJ, Prokop M, Doevendans PA, Hunink MG, Krestin GP, de Feyter PJ. Diagnostic accuracy of 64-slice computed tomography coronary angiography: a prospective, multicenter, multivendor study. J Am Coll Cardiol. 2008;52:2135–44.
34. Miller JM, Rochitte CE, Dewey M, Arbab-Zadeh A, Niinuma H, Gottlieb I, Paul N, Clouse ME, Shapiro EP, Hoe J, Lardo AC, Bush DE, de Roos A, Cox C, Brinker J, Lima JA. Diagnostic performance of coronary angiography by 64-row CT. N Engl J Med. 2008;359:2324–36.
35. Paech DC, Weston AR. A systematic review of the clinical effectiveness of 64-slice or higher computed tomography angiography as an alternative to invasive coronary angiography in the investigation of suspected coronary artery disease. BMC Cardiovasc Disord. 2011;11:32.
36. Vanhoenacker PK, Heijenbrok-Kal MH, Van Heste R, Decramer I, Van Hoe LR, Wijns W, Hunink MG. Diagnostic performance of multidetector CT angiography for assessment of coronary artery disease: meta-analysis. Radiology. 2007;244:419–28.
37. Westwood ME, Raatz HD, Misso K, Burgers L, Redekop K, Lhachimi SK, Armstrong N, Kleijnen J. Systematic review of the accuracy of dual-source cardiac CT for detection of arterial stenosis in difficult to image patient groups. Radiology. 2013;267(2):387–95.
38. Chen CC, Chen CC, Hsieh IC, Liu YC, Liu CY, Chan T, Wen MS, Wan YL. The effect of calcium score on the diagnostic accuracy of coronary computed tomography angiography. Int J Cardiovasc Imaging. 2011;27 Suppl 1:37–42.
39. Arbab-Zadeh A, Miller JM, Rochitte CE, Dewey M, Niinuma H, Gottlieb I, Paul N, Clouse ME, Shapiro EP, Hoe J, Lardo AC, Bush DE, de Roos A, Cox C, Brinker J, Lima JA. Diagnostic

accuracy of computed tomography coronary angiography according to pre-test probability of coronary artery disease and severity of coronary arterial calcification. The CORE-64 (Coronary Artery Evaluation Using 64-Row Multidetector Computed Tomography Angiography) International Multicenter Study. J Am Coll Cardiol. 2012;59(4):379–87.
40. Kruk M, Noll D, Achenbach S, Mintz GS, Pręgowski J, Kaczmarska E, Kryczka K, Pracoń R, Dzielińska Z, Sleszycka J, Witkowski A, Demkow M, Rużyłło W, Kępka C. Impact of coronary artery calcium characteristics on accuracy of CT angiography. JACC Cardiovasc Imaging. 2014;7(1):49–58.
41. Meijboom WB, van Mieghem CA, Mollet NR, Pugliese F, Weustink AC, van Pelt N, Cademartiri F, Nieman K, Boersma E, de Jaegere P, Krestin GP, de Feyter PJ. 64-slice computed tomography coronary angiography in patients with high, intermediate, or low pretest probability of significant coronary artery disease. J Am Coll Cardiol. 2007;50:1469–75.
42. Gilard M, Le Gal G, Cornily JC, Vinsonneau U, Joret C, Pennec PY, Mansourati J, Boschat J. Midterm prognosis of patients with suspected coronary artery disease and normal multislice computed tomography findings. A prospective management outcome study. Arch Intern Med. 2007;165:1686–9.
43. Lesser JR, Flygenring B, Knickelbine T, Hara H, Henry J, Kalil A, Pelak K, Lindberg J, Pelzel J, Schwartz RS. Clinical utility of coronary CT angiography: coronary stenosis detection and prognosis in ambulatory patients. Cath Cardiovasc Interv. 2007;69:64–72.
44. Hadamitzky M, Freissmuth B, Meyer T, Hein F, Kastrati A, Martinoff S, Schömig A, Hausleiter J. Prognostic value of coronary computed tomographic angiography for prediction of cardiac events in patients with suspected coronary artery disease. JACC Cardiovasc Imaging. 2009;2:404–11.
45. Ostrom MP, Gopal A, Ahmadi N, Nasir K, Yang E, Kakadiaris I, Flores F, Mao SS, Budoff MJ. Mortality incidence and the severity of coronary atherosclerosis assessed by computed tomography angiography. J Am Coll Cardiol. 2008;52:1335–43.
46. Abidov A, Gallagher MJ, Chinnayan KM, Mehta LS, Wegner JH, Raff GH. Clinical effectiveness of coronary computed tomographic angiography in the triage of patients to cardiac catheterization and revascularization. J Nucl Cardiol. 2009;16:701–13.
47. Otaki Y, Arsanjani R, Gransar H, Cheng VY, Dey D, Labounty T, Lin FY, Achenbach S, Al-Mallah M, Budoff MJ, Cademartiri F, Callister TQ, Chang HJ, Chinnaiyan K, Chow BJ, Delago A, Hadamitzky M, Hausleiter J, Kaufmann P, Maffei E, Raff G, Shaw LJ, Villines TC, Dunning A, Cury RC, Feuchtner G, Kim YJ, Leipsic J, Berman DS, Min JK. What have we learned from CONFIRM? Prognostic implications from a prospective multicenter international observational cohort study of consecutive patients undergoing coronary computed tomographic angiography. J Nucl Cardiol. 2012;19:787–95.
48. Min JK, Dunning A, Lin FY, Achenbach S, Al-Mallah M, Budoff MJ, Cademartiri F, Callister TQ, Chang HJ, Cheng V, Chinnaiyan K, Chow BJ, Delago A, Hadamitzky M, Hausleiter J, Kaufmann P, Maffei E, Raff G, Shaw LJ, Villines T, Berman DS, CONFIRM Investigators. Age- and sex-related differences in all-cause mortality risk based on coronary computed tomography angiography findings results from the International Multicenter CONFIRM (coronary CT angiography evaluation for clinical outcomes: an International Multicenter Registry) of 23,854 patients without known coronary artery disease. J Am Coll Cardiol. 2011;58(8):849–60.
49. Shaw LJ, Hausleiter J, Achenbach S, Al-Mallah M, Berman DS, Budoff MJ, Cademartiri F, Callister TQ, Chang HJ, Kim YJ, Cheng VY, Chow BJ, Cury RC, Delago AJ, Dunning AL, Feuchtner GM, Hadamitzky M, Karlsberg RP, Kaufmann PA, Leipsic J, Lin FY, Chinnaiyan KM, Maffei E, Raff GL, Villines TC, Labounty T, Gomez MJ, Min JK, CONFIRM Registry Investigators. Coronary computed tomographic angiography as a gatekeeper to invasive diagnostic and surgical procedures: results from the multicenter CONFIRM (coronary CT angiography evaluation for clinical outcomes: an International Multicenter) registry. J Am Coll Cardiol. 2012;60(20):2103–14.
50. Min JK, Berman DS, Dunning A, Achenbach S, Al-Mallah M, Budoff MJ, Cademartiri F, Callister TQ, Chang HJ, Cheng V, Chinnaiyan K, Chow BJ, Cury R, Delago A, Feuchtner G, Hadamitzky M, Hausleiter J, Kaufmann P, Karlsberg RP, Kim YJ, Leipsic J, Lin FY, Maffei E, Plank F, Raff G, Villines T, Labounty TM, Shaw LJ. All-cause mortality benefit of coronary revascularization vs. medical therapy in patients without known coronary artery disease undergoing coronary computed tomographic angiography: results from CONFIRM (COronary CT Angiography EvaluatioN For Clinical Outcomes: An InteRnational Multicenter Registry). Eur Heart J. 2012;33:3088–97.
51. Meijboom WB, Mollet NR, Van Mieghem CA, Weustink AC, Pugliese F, van Pelt N, Cademartiri F, Vourvouri E, de Jaegere P, Krestin GP, de Feyter PJ. 64-slice computed tomography coronary angiography in patients with non-ST elevation acute coronary syndrome. Heart. 2007;93:1386–92.
52. Hoffmann U, Nagurney JT, Moselewski F, Pena A, Ferencik M, Chae CU, Cury RC, Butler J, Abbara S, Brown DF, Manini A, Nichols JH, Achenbach S, Brady TJ. Coronary multidetector computed tomography in the assessment of patients with acute chest pain. Circulation. 2006;114:2251–60.
53. Gallagher MJ, Ross MA, Raff GL, Goldstein JA, O'Neill WW, O'Neil B. The diagnostic accuracy of 64-slice computed tomography coronary angiography compared with stress nuclear imaging in emergency department low-risk chest pain patients. Ann Emerg Med. 2007;49:125–36.
54. Goldstein JA, Gallagher MJ, O'Neill WW, Ross MA, O'Neil BJ, Raff GL. A randomized controlled trial of multi-slice coronary computed tomography for evaluation of acute chest pain. J Am Coll Cardiol. 2007;49:863–71.
55. Coles DR, Wilde P, Oberhoff M, Rogers CA, Karsch KR, Baumbach A. Multislice computed tomography coronary angiography in patients admitted with a suspected acute coronary syndrome. Int J Cardiovasc Imaging. 2007;23:603–14.
56. Litt HI, Gatsonis C, Snyder B, Singh H, Miller CD, Entrikin DW, Leaming JM, Gavin LJ, Pacella CB, Hollander JE. CT angiography for safe discharge of patients with possible acute coronary syndromes. N Engl J Med. 2012;366:1393–403.
57. Hoffmann U, Truong QA, Schoenfeld DA, Chou ET, Woodard PK, Nagurney JT, Pope JH, Hauser TH, White CS, Weiner SG, Kalanjian S, Mullins ME, Mikati I, Peacock WF, Zakroysky P, Hayden D, Goehler A, Lee H, Gazelle GS, Wiviott SD, Fleg JL, Udelson JE, ROMICAT-II Investigators. Coronary CT angiography versus standard evaluation in acute chest pain. N Engl J Med. 2012;367:299–308.
58. Jones RL, Thomas DM, Barnwell ML, Fentanes E, Young AN, Barnwell R, Foley AT, Hilliard M, Hulten EA, Villines TC, Cury RC, Slim AM. Safe and rapid disposition of low-to-intermediate risk patients presenting to the emergency department with chest pain: a 1-year high-volume single-center experience. J Cardiovasc Comput Tomogr. 2014;8(5):375–583.
59. Staniak HL, Bittencourt MS, Pickett C, Cahill M, Kassop D, Slim A, Blankstein R, Hulten E. Coronary CT angiography for acute chest pain in the emergency department. J Cardiovasc Comput Tomogr. 2014;8(5):359–67.
60. Redberg RF. Coronary CT, angiography for acute chest pain. N Engl J Med. 2012;367(4):375–6.
61. Amsterdam EA, Wenger NK, Brindis RG, Casey Jr DE, Ganiats TG, Holmes Jr DR, Jaffe AS, Jneid H, Kelly RF, Kontos MC, Levine GN, Liebson PR, Mukherjee D, Peterson ED, Sabatine MS, Smalling RW, Zieman SJ. 2014 AHA/ACC guideline for the management of patients with non-ST-elevation acute coronary

syndromes: a report of the American College of Cardiology/American Heart Association Task Force on Practice Guidelines. J Am Coll Cardiol. 2014;64(24):e139–228.

62. Hamm CW, Bassand JP, Agewall S, Bax J, Boersma E, Bueno H, Caso P, Dudek D, Gielen S, Huber K, Ohman M, Petrie MC, Sonntag F, Uva MS, Storey RF, Wijns W, Zahger D, ESC Committee for Practice Guidelines. ESC guidelines for the management of acute coronary syndromes in patients presenting without persistent ST-segment elevation: the Task Force for the management of acute coronary syndromes (ACS) in patients presenting without persistent ST-segment elevation of the European Society of Cardiology (ESC). Eur Heart J. 2011;32(23):2999–3054.
63. Schuijf JD, Wijns W, Jukema JW, Atsma DE, de Roos A, Lamb HJ, Stokkel MP, Dibbets-Schneider P, Decramer I, De Bondt P, van der Wall EE, Vanhoenacker PK, Bax JJ. Relationship between noninvasive coronary angiography with multi-slice computed tomography and myocardial perfusion imaging. J Am Coll Cardiol. 2006;48:2508–14.
64. Min JK, Shaw LJ, Berman DS. The present state of coronary computed tomography angiography – a process in evolution. J Am Coll Cardiol. 2010;55:957–65.
65. Hacker M, Jakobs T, Hack N, Nikolaou K, Becker C, von Ziegler F, Knez A, Konig A, Klauss V, Reiser M, Hahn K, Tiling R. Sixty-four slice spiral CT angiography does not predict the functional relevance of coronary artery stenoses in patients with stable angina. Eur J Nucl Med Mol Imaging. 2007;34:4–10.
66. Berman DS, Hachamovitch R, Shaw LJ, Friedman JD, Hayes SW, Thomson LE, Fieno DS, Germano G, Wong ND, Kang X, Rozanski A. Roles of nuclear cardiology, cardiac computed tomography, and cardiac magnetic resonance: noninvasive risk stratification and a conceptual framework for the selection of noninvasive imaging tests in patients with known or suspected coronary artery disease. J Nucl Med. 2006;47:1107–18.
67. Bamberg F, Becker A, Schwarz F, Marcus RP, Greif M, von Ziegler F, Blankstein R, Hoffmann U, Sommer WH, Hoffmann VS, Johnson TR, Becker HC, Wintersperger BJ, Reiser MF, Nikolaou K. Detection of hemodynamically significant coronary artery stenosis: incremental diagnostic value of dynamic CT-based myocardial perfusion imaging. Radiology. 2011;260:689–98.
68. Tashakkor AY, Nicolaou S, Leipsic J, Mancini GB. The emerging role of cardiac computed tomography for the assessment of coronary perfusion: a systematic review and meta-analysis. Can J Cardiol. 2012;28:413–22.
69. Taylor CA, Fonte TA, Min JK. Computational fluid dynamics applied to cardiac computed tomography for noninvasive quantification of fractional flow reserve: scientific basis. J Am Coll Cardiol. 2013;61:2233–41.
70. Nørgaard BL, Leipsic J, Gaur S, Seneviratne S, Ko BS, Ito H, Jensen JM, Mauri L, De Bruyne B, Bezerra H, Osawa K, Marwan M, Naber C, Erglis A, Park SJ, Christiansen EH, Kaltoft A, Lassen JF, Bøtker HE, Achenbach S, NXT Trial Study Group. Diagnostic performance of noninvasive fractional flow reserve derived from coronary computed tomography angiography in suspected coronary artery disease: the NXT trial (analysis of coronary blood flow using CT angiography: next steps). J Am Coll Cardiol. 2014;63(12):1145–55.
71. Achenbach S, Moselewski F, Ropers D, Ferencik M, Hoffmann U, MacNeill B, et al. Detection of calcified and noncalcified coronary atherosclerotic plaque by contrast-enhanced, submillimeter multidetector spiral computed tomography: a segment-based comparison with intravascular ultrasound. Circulation. 2004;109:14–7.
72. Leber AW, Knez A, Becker A, Becker C, von Ziegler F, Nikolaou K, et al. Accuracy of multidetector spiral computed tomography in identifying and differentiating the composition of coronary atherosclerotic plaques: a comparative study with intracoronary ultrasound. J Am Coll Cardiol. 2004;43:1241–7.
73. Leber AW, Becker A, Knez A, von Ziegler F, Sirol M, Nikolaou K, Ohnesorge B, Fayad ZA, Becker CR, Reiser M, Steinbeck G, Boekstegers P. Accuracy of 64-slice computed tomography to classify and quantify plaque volumes in the proximal coronary system: a comparative study using intravascular ultrasound. J Am Coll Cardiol. 2006;47:672–7.
74. Pohle K, Achenbach S, MacNeill B, Ropers D, Ferencik M, Moselewski F, Hoffmann U, Brady TJ, Jang IK, Daniel WG. Characterization of non-calcified coronary atherosclerotic plaque by multi-detector row CT: comparison to IVUS. Atherosclerosis. 2007;190:174–80.
75. Sun J, Zhang Z, Lu B, Yu W, Yang Y, Zhou Y, Wang Y, Fan Z. Identification and quantification of coronary atherosclerotic plaques: a comparison of 64-MDCT and intravascular ultrasound. AJR Am J Roentgenol. 2008;190(3):748–54.
76. Nakazato R, Shalev A, Doh JH, Koo BK, Dey D, Berman DS, Min JK. Quantification and characterisation of coronary artery plaque volume and adverse plaque features by coronary computed tomographic angiography: a direct comparison to intravascular ultrasound. Eur Radiol. 2013;23(8):2109–17.
77. Obaid DR, Calvert PA, Gopalan D, Parker RA, Hoole SP, West NE, Goddard M, Rudd JH, Bennett MR. Atherosclerotic plaque composition and classification identified by coronary computed tomography: assessment of computed tomography-generated plaque maps compared with virtual histology intravascular ultrasound and histology. Circ Cardiovasc Imaging. 2013;6(5):655–64.
78. Cademartiri F, Mollet NR, Runza G, Bruining N, Hamers R, Somers P, Knaapen M, Verheye S, Midiri M, Krestin GP, de Feyter PJ. Influence of intracoronary attenuation on coronary plaque measurements using multislice computed tomography: observations in an ex vivo model of coronary computed tomography angiography. Eur Radiol. 2005;15:1426–31.
79. Achenbach S, Boehmer K, Pflederer T, Ropers D, Seltmann M, Lell M, Anders K, Kuettner A, Uder M, Daniel WG, Marwan M. Influence of slice thickness and reconstruction kernel on the computed tomographic attenuation of coronary atherosclerotic plaque. J Cardiovasc Comput Tomogr. 2010;4(2):110–5.
80. Achenbach S, Ropers D, Hoffmann U, MacNeill B, Baum U, Pohle K, Brady TJ, Pomerantsev E, Ludwig J, Flachskampf FA, Wicky S, Jang IK, Daniel WG. Assessment of coronary remodeling in stenotic and nonstenotic coronary atherosclerotic lesions by multidetector spiral computed tomography. J Am Coll Cardiol. 2004;43:842–7.
81. Moselewski F, Ropers D, Pohle K, Hoffmann U, Ferencik M, Chan RC, Cury RC, Abbara S, Jang IK, Brady TJ, Daniel WG, Achenbach S. Comparison of measurement of cross-sectional coronary atherosclerotic plaque and vessel areas by 16-slice multidetector computed tomography versus intravascular ultrasound. Am J Cardiol. 2004;94:1294–7.
82. Gauss S, Achenbach S, Pflederer T, Schuhbäck A, Daniel WG, Marwan M. Assessment of coronary artery remodelling by dual-source CT: a head-to-head comparison with intravascular ultrasound. Heart. 2011;97(12):991–7.
83. Motoyama S, Sarai M, Harigaya H, Anno H, Inoue K, Hara T, Naruse H, Ishii J, Hishida H, Wong ND, Virmani R, Kondo T, Ozaki Y, Narula J. Computed tomographic angiography characteristics of atherosclerotic plaques subsequently resulting in acute coronary syndrome. J Am Coll Cardiol. 2009;54: 49–57.
84. Bittencourt MS, Hulten E, Ghoshhajra B, O'Leary D, Christman MP, Montana P, Truong QA, Steigner M, Murthy VL, Rybicki FJ, Nasir K, Gowdak LH, Hainer J, Brady TJ, Di Carli MF, Hoffmann U, Abbara S, Blankstein R. Prognostic value of nonobstructive and obstructive coronary artery disease detected by coronary computed tomography angiography to identify cardiovascular events. Circ Cardiovasc Imaging. 2014;7(2):282–91.

85. Hulten EA, Carbonaro S, Petrillo SP, Mitchell JD, Villines TC. Prognostic value of cardiac computed tomography angiography: a systematic review and meta-analysis. J Am Coll Cardiol. 2011;57(10):1237–47.
86. Cho I, Chang HJ, Sung JM, Pencina MJ, Lin FY, Dunning AM, Achenbach S, Al-Mallah M, Berman DS, Budoff MJ, Callister TQ, Chow BJ, Delago A, Hadamitzky M, Hausleiter J, Maffei E, Cademartiri F, Kaufmann P, Shaw LJ, Raff GL, Chinnaiyan KM, Villines TC, Cheng V, Nasir K, Gomez M, Min JK, CONFIRM Investigators. Coronary computed tomographic angiography and risk of all-cause mortality and nonfatal myocardial infarction in subjects without chest pain syndrome from the CONFIRM Registry (coronary CT angiography evaluation for clinical outcomes: an international multicenter registry). Circulation. 2012;126(3):304–13.
87. Ropers D, Moshage W, Daniel WG, et al. Visualization of coronary artery anomalies and their course by contrast-enhanced electron beam tomography and three-dimensional reconstruction. Am J Cardiol. 2001;87:193–7.
88. Datta J, White CS, Gilkeson RC, Meyer CA, Kansal S, Jani ML, Arildsen RC, Read K. Anomalous coronary arteries in adults: depiction at multi-detector row CT angiography. Radiology. 2005;235:812–8.
89. Kim SY, Seo JB, Do KJ, Heo JN, Lee JS, Song JW, Choe YH, Kim TH, Yong HS, Choi SI, Song KS, Lim TH. Coronary artery anomalies: classification and ECG-gated multi-detector row CT findings with angiographic correlation. Radiographics. 2006;26:317–33.
90. Duran C, Kantarci M, Durur Subais I, Gulbaran M, Sevimli S, Bayram E, Eren S, Karaman A, Fil F, Al O. Remarkable anatomic anomalies of coronary arteries and their clinical importance: a multidetector computed tomography angiographic study. J Comput Assist Tomogr. 2006;30:939–48.
91. Bozlar U, Uğurel MS, Sarı S, Akgün V, Ors F, Taşar M. Prevalence of dual left anterior descending artery variations in CT angiography. Diagn Interv Radiol. 2015;21:34–41.
92. Taylor AJ, Cerqueira M, Hodgson JM, Mark D, Min J, O'Gara P, Rubin GD, American College of Cardiology Foundation Appropriate Use Criteria Task Force; Society of Cardiovascular Computed Tomography; American College of Radiology; American Heart Association; American Society of Echocardiography; American Society of Nuclear Cardiology; North American Society for Cardiovascular Imaging; Society for Cardiovascular Angiography and Interventions; Society for Cardiovascular Magnetic Resonance. ACCF/SCCT/ACR/AHA/ASE/ASNC/NASCI/SCAI/SCMR 2010 appropriate use criteria for cardiac computed tomography. A report of the American College of Cardiology Foundation Appropriate Use Criteria Task Force, the Society of Cardiovascular Computed Tomography, the American College of Radiology, the American Heart Association, the American Society of Echocardiography, the American Society of Nuclear Cardiology, the North American Society for Cardiovascular Imaging, the Society for Cardiovascular Angiography and Interventions, and the Society for Cardiovascular Magnetic Resonance. J Am Coll Cardiol. 2010;56:1864–94.
93. Montalescot G, Sechtem U, Achenbach S, Andreotti F, Arden C, Budaj A, Bugiardini R, Crea F, Cuisset T, Di Mario C, Ferreira JR, Gersh BJ, Gitt AK, Hulot JS, Marx N, Opie LH, Pfisterer M, Prescott E, Ruschitzka F, Sabaté M, Senior R, Taggart DP, van der Wall EE, Vrints CJ. 2013 ESC guidelines on the management of stable coronary artery disease: the task force on the management of stable coronary artery disease of the European Society of Cardiology. Eur Heart J. 2013;34:2949–3003.
94. Fihn SD, Gardin JM, Abrams J, Berra K, Blankenship JC, Dallas AP, Douglas PS, Foody JM, Gerber TC, Hinderliter AL, King SB, Kligfield PD, Krumholz HM, Kwong RY, Lim MJ, Linderbaum JA, Mack MJ, Munger MA, Prager RL, Sabik JF, Shaw LJ, Sikkema JD, Smith Jr CR, Smith Jr SC, Spertus JA, Williams SV, Anderson JL, American College of Cardiology Foundation/American Heart Association Task Force. 2012 ACCF/AHA/ACP/AATS/PCNA/SCAI/STS guideline for the diagnosis and management of patients with stable ischemic heart disease: a report of the American College of Cardiology Foundation/American Heart Association task force on practice guidelines, and the American College of Physicians, American Association for Thoracic Surgery, Preventive Cardiovascular Nurses Association, Society for Cardiovascular Angiography and Interventions, and Society of Thoracic Surgeons. Circulation. 2012;126(25):e354–471.

10 Coronary CT Angiography After Revascularization

Joachim Eckert, Marco Schmidt, Thomas Voigtländer, and Axel Schmermund

Abstract

Because of the high number of coronary revascularizations clinicians frequently have to assess bypass or stent function in patients presenting with chest pain or other symptoms suggesting dysfunction. Predominantly, invasive coronary angiography is performed for this purpose. In the last decade innovations in CT scanners, protocols and reconstructions have led to a remarkable increase in diagnostic accuracy of coronary CT angiography for the assessment of coronary bypass grafts and stents whereas radiation exposure has significantly decreased. Occlusions of bypass grafts and occlusive in-stent stenoses can be ruled out with a high negative predictive value approaching 100 %.

Keywords

Coronary CT angiography • Stents • Bypass grafts

Background

Coronary artery revascularization is one of the most frequent medical procedures. In the year 2009 about 350,000 percutaneous coronary interventions (PCI) were performed and 200,000 patients underwent bypass surgery in the United States [1]. In clinical practice, patients after coronary revascularization frequently present with symptoms suggesting progression of coronary artery disease (CAD). Physicians have to reevaluate the patency of the coronary arteries, especially concerning an in-stent-stenosis or occluded bypass grafts. These patients often undergo invasive coronary angiography (ICA) even though there is no evidence of ischemia. As an alternative to ICA, coronary computed tomography angiography (CCTA) plays an increasing role for obtaining reliable information on coronary anatomy noninvasively.

J. Eckert, MD (✉) • M. Schmidt, MD • T. Voigtländer, MD
A. Schmermund, MD
Department of Cardiology, Cardioangiologisches Centrum Bethanien, Im Pruefling 23, Frankfurt, Hessen 60389, Germany
e-mail: j.eckert@ccb.de; m.schmidt@ccb.de; t.voigtlaender@ccb.de; a.schmermund@ccb.de

Bypass Grafts

Venous Grafts: Anatomy and Natural History

Venous bypass grafts still represent the majority of all grafts used for bypass surgery. Due to differences in anatomy and surgical techniques, their patency rates are inferior to internal mammary artery grafts [2, 3]. Three modes of venous bypass graft degeneration have been described which occur at different time points after surgery. Within hours to weeks after surgery, technical deficiencies and thrombotic activation lead to early thrombotic occlusion in approximately 5–10 % of the grafts [4]. Over the course of the following year, intimal hyperplasia and thrombosis appear to be the major mechanisms, accounting for an overall occlusion rate of 10–15 % within the first year [4, 5]. Finally, after the first year, mechanisms known from native coronary artery atherosclerosis predominate. Bypass attrition between postoperative years 1 and 5 appears to be minimal. After year 5, atherothrombotic occlusion of venous grafts accounts for a reduced patency rate. It has traditionally been estimated to range between 40 and 60 % at 10–12 years [4, 6]. However, data from the Veteran Affairs Cooperative Study indicate that venous grafts which

M.J. Budoff, J.S. Shinbane (eds.), *Cardiac CT Imaging: Diagnosis of Cardiovascular Disease*,
DOI 10.1007/978-3-319-28219-0_10

are open 1 week after surgery have a patency rate of 68 % after 10 years [2]. The presence of angiographic stenoses between 50 and 99 % of graft diameter appears to be 17–22 % at 10 years [2]. As opposed to native coronary arteries and arterial grafts, venous bypass grafts tend to develop an extensive thrombotic burden and occlude quite rapidly once a high-grade stenosis has formed.

Arterial Grafts: Anatomy and Natural History

The left internal mammary artery ("IMA") is most often used as arterial graft. Arterial vessels are by design much better adapted to systemic blood pressure values and shear stress than venous vessels, and this translates into improved patency rates [2, 3]. IMA grafts patent at 1 week after surgery had a 10 year patency rate of 88 % in the Veterans Affairs Cooperative Study [2]. As with venous grafts, recipient vessel location and status influence graft survival. Survival is best for grafts to the left anterior descending coronary artery and a native vessel diameter ≥ 2 mm [2]. Interestingly, IMA grafts sewed to a recipient vessel with < 50 % diameter stenosis may have a very high rate of occlusion, probably due to competing flow through the native vessel [7]. Regarding CT imaging, the smaller lumen diameter of arterial grafts and frequent use of metal clips represent a challenge for diagnostic image quality.

Non-invasive CT Examination

Venous bypass grafts are typically larger in diameter than the native large epicardial coronary arteries (approximately 4 – 10 mm versus 2 – 5 mm), and they are less subjected to cardiac motion. Accordingly, even with older-generation ("non-cardiac") CT machines, investigators examined contrast enhancement along the course of the graft to establish bypass patency [8, 9]. Due to the inherent limitations of non-gated scanning with relatively long acquisition times, overall diagnostic accuracy regarding bypass graft patency remained at approximately 90 %, with better results for (larger) vein grafts than for the arterial grafts. It was not possible to identify potential non-occlusive high-grade bypass body stenoses, the distal anastomosis of grafts, or the native coronary arterial run-off. The advent of electron-beam computed tomography (EBCT) as the first dedicated cardiac CT scanner and the development of non-invasive coronary angiography beginning in 1994 allowed for visualization of coronary bypass grafts and three-dimensional representation of the graft vessels [10]. Still, however, image quality was in part insufficient for detailed analysis of small diameter grafts or the complex anatomy of native vessels and the anastomosis region. Also, artifacts related to metal clips and breathing / arrhythmias hampered image quality. Despite these limitations, EBCT bypass angiography was used for some years for detecting venous bypass graft occlusion or stenosis

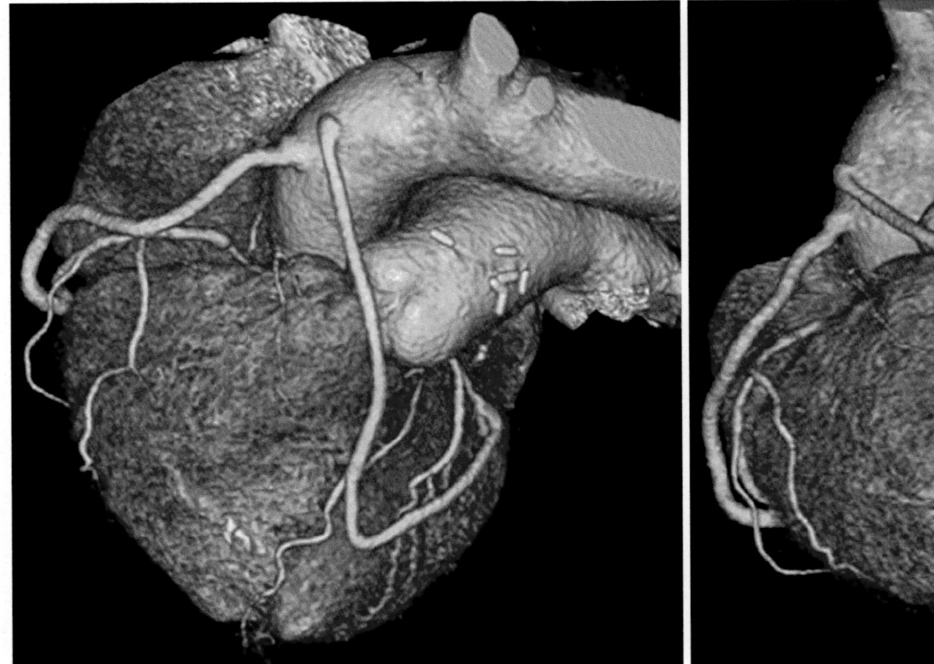

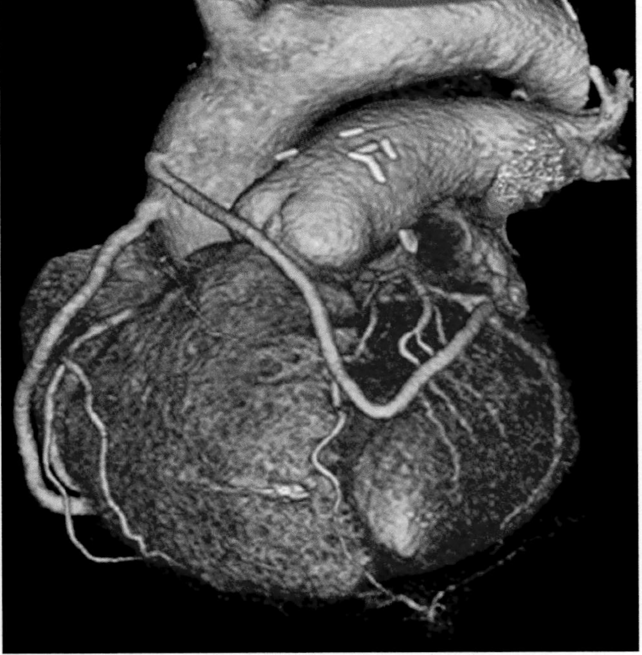

Fig. 10.1 64-row MDCT 3-dimensional image reconstruction shows two patent venous grafts coursing to a right coronary artery and an obtuse marginal branch (Courtesy of Dr. Dieter Ropers, University Clinic Erlangen-Nürnberg, Germany)

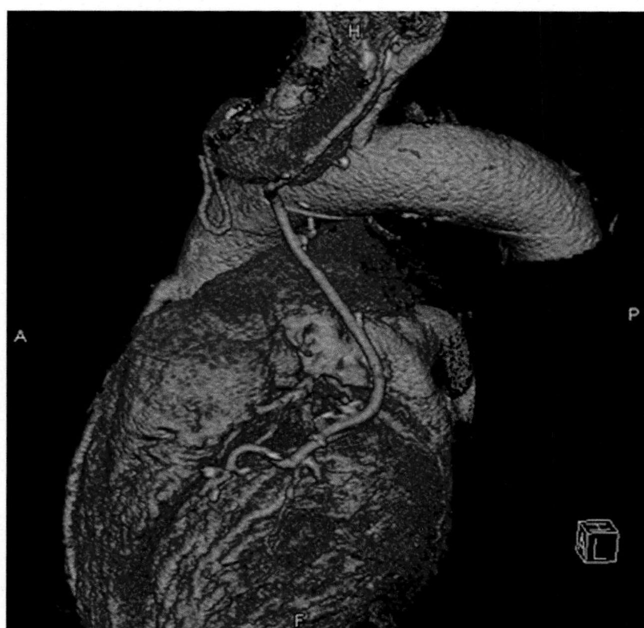

Fig. 10.2 64-row MDCT 3-dimensional image reconstruction shows a patent left internal mammary graft with two anostomoses to the first diagonal branch and left anterior descending coronary artery itself, respectively

within the shaft body and proved to be helpful in a subset of patients with unspecific symptoms after bypass surgery.

With later generations of multidetector CT systems and improvements in spatial and temporal resolution stenosis detection in more difficult situations such as the bypass anastomosis region or visualization of arterial grafts surrounded by metal clips was enhanced. Currently, arterial grafts and the anastomosis region of venous and arterial grafts can be analyzed with increased diagnostic yield [11–19] (Figs. 10.1 and 10.2). Even the analysis of native vessel disease progression became more accurate with multidetector CT scanners [15] (Fig. 10.3). Regarding the exclusion of high-grade stenoses, the negative predictive value was 100 % for bypass grafts and 96–98 % for the native coronary arteries (grafted or nongrafted). Only 9 % of the native coronary arteries were unevaluable due to severe calcifications or motion artifacts.

A meta-analysis by Hamon et al. comprised studies using 16- and 64-slice MDCT published up to May 2007 [11]. A total of 15 studies were included, six of which used 64-slice CT [12–17]. Table 10.1 gives an overview of the diagnostic performance of 64-slice MDCT in a total of 355 patients and 976 bypass grafts [11]. Between 87 and 100 % of the grafts were fully assessable regarding the detection / exclusion of angiographically significant stenoses. In particular, a high negative predictive value was obtained in the studies, indicating the ability to reliably rule out high-grade stenoses or obstruction of the bypass grafts using 64-slice MDCT. More recent studies have confirmed a negative predictive value for ruling out high-grade bypass graft stenoses ranging between 96 and 99 % [18–20]. However, depending on the anatomy, the distal anastomosis can still be challenging to examine, and the degree of stenosis tends to be overestimated [18]. The native coronary circulation can be assessed despite previous bypass surgery [19–21] (Fig. 10.4), however, as in a population with no previous bypass surgery, heavy coronary calcification or a small native vessel diameter can render the CT analysis difficult. Sensitivities for the detection of significant lesions range between 86–95 % for distal runoffs and 86–97 % for non grafted arteries.

A recent publication demonstrated the prognostic value of CCTA in coronary bypass patients [22]. Both bypass grafts and native coronary arteries were analyzed regarding the number of unprotected coronary territories (UCT). The incidence of myocardial infarction as well as the risk of death increased significantly with higher numbers of UCT. Hence, CCTA not only provides morphologic information on the coronary anatomy but also prognostic data.

Imaging Protocols

Most experts agree that consequential betablockade should be undertaken with the aim of reaching heart rates ≤ 60–65 bpm, which improves image quality due to less motion artifacts and may reduce radiation exposure. Although most recent scanner generations are less susceptible to motion artifacts, practical experience dictates that this approach yields superior visibility of coronary artery segments. The administration of oral or intravenous nitrates for vasodilatation immediately prior to the scan is recommended. A temporal window of 60 % of the RR-interval appears to be best suited [23]. Caudo-cranial scan direction seems to be superior in terms of image quality and radiation exposure [24]. The latest development in CT scanners led to a remarkable decrease in radiation exposure (prospective ECG-gating, reduced tube voltage, tube current modulation, higher acquisition speed) which is on average lower than in ICA.

Specific scanning protocols with the various scanners are detailed elsewhere in this book.

Conclusions to Bypass Grafts

CCTA is increasingly used as a modality for the non-invasive assessment of bypass graft patency and stenoses. As compared to ICA, a small proportion of grafts remains unassessable due to artifacts or anatomic complexity. However, this proportion has decreased with improvements in scanner technology. Bypass grafts as well as native coronary arteries can be evaluated with high diagnostic accuracy. ICA remains gold standard for defining coronary

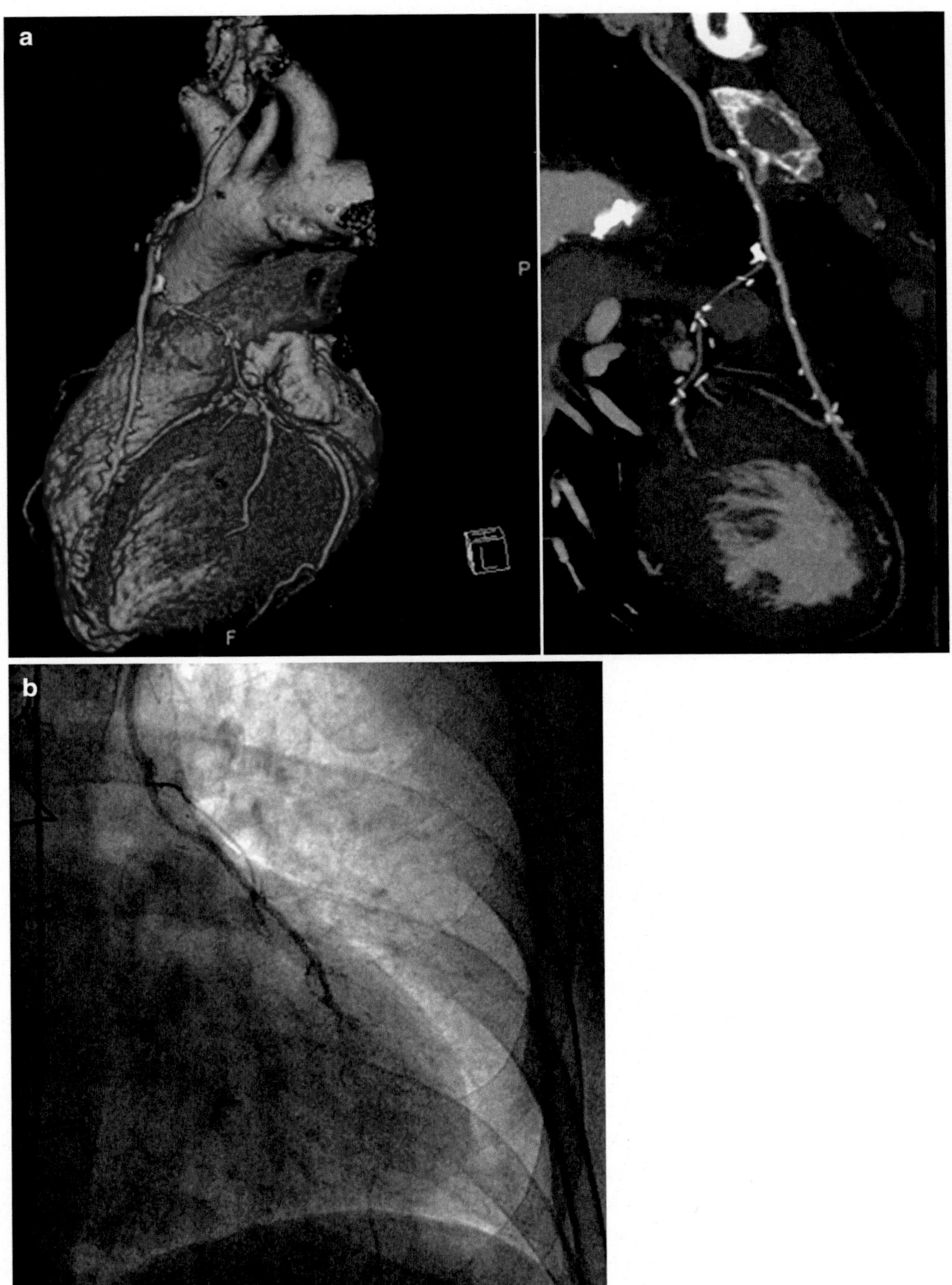

Fig. 10.3 64-row MDCT 3-dimensional image reconstruction (**a**) shows a patent left internal mammary graft to the left anterior descending coronary artery and the corresponding selective angiogram. Distal to the anastomosis, the left anterior descending coronary artery is occluded; see corresponding invasive angiographc image (**b**)

Table 10.1 Results of 64-slice MDCT examination of 976 bypass grafts as documented in a meta-analysis by Hamon et al.[a]

Sensitivity (%)	Specificity (%)	Positive predictive value (%)	Negative predictive value (%)	Positive likelihood ratio	Negative likelihood ratio
98.1 (96.0,99.3)	96.9 (95.3,98.1)	94.1 (91.0,96.3)	99.1 (98.0,99.7)	24.7 (12.5,47.7)	0.03 (0.01,0.06)

Numbers in parentheses = 95 % CI
[a]Data from Hamon et al. [11]

bypass anatomy, but especially in patients with non-specific complaints, CCTA is an excellent alternative and provides a nice roadmap to see the origin locations and number of patent grafts in those patients without prior recent angiography, including use of right and left internal mammaries non-invasively.

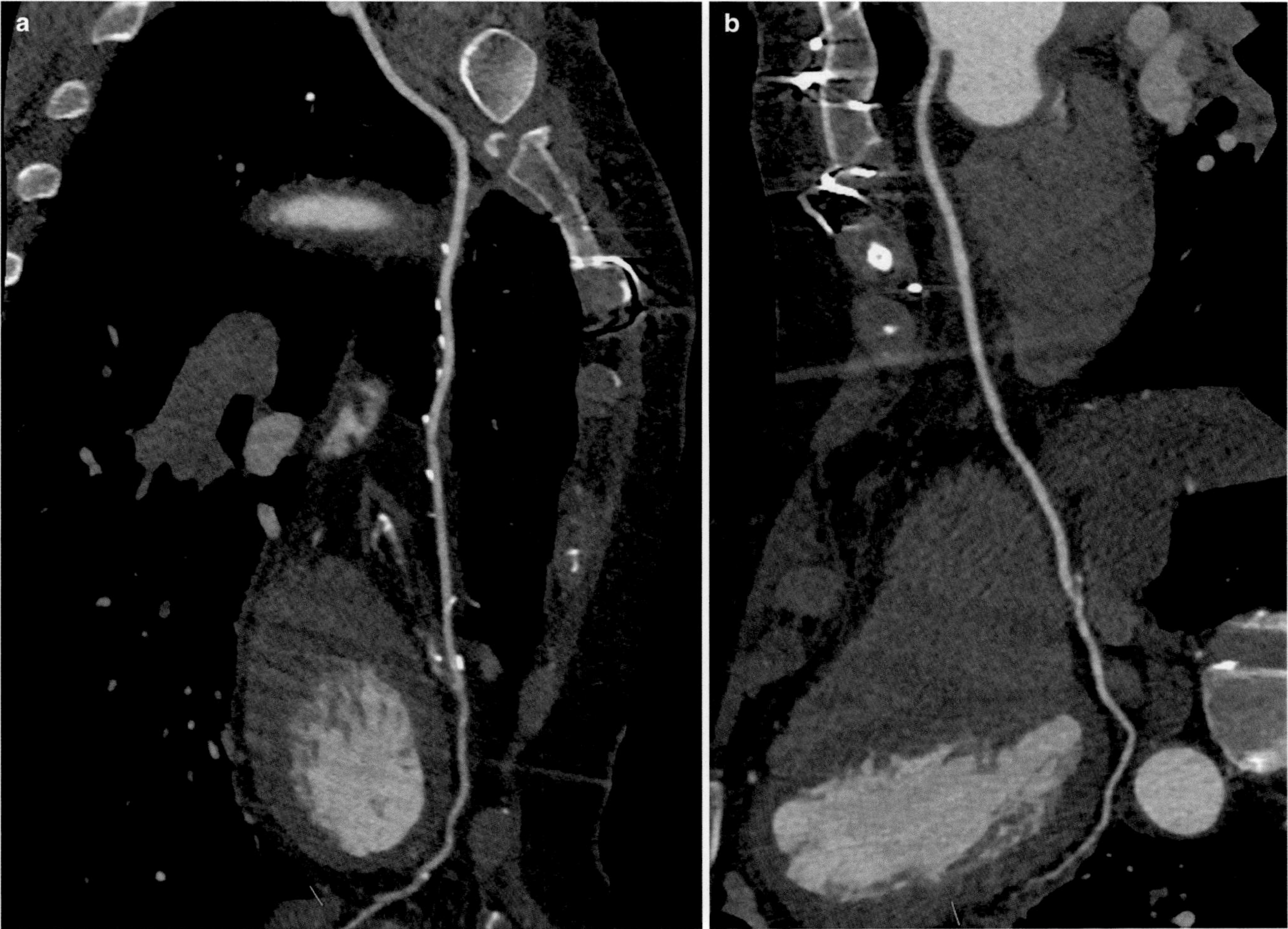

Fig. 10.4 Patent left internal mammary graft to the left anterior descending coronary artery with normal runoff (**a**). Patent single vein graft to the right coronary artery with normal runoff (**b**). Bypass grafts as well as the native coronary arteries can be evaluated with good image quality

Coronary Stents

Background

The majority of percutaneous coronary angioplasties are performed with placement of a stent in the vessel wall [25]. Most stents are made of stainless steel or cobalt-chromium, which can both be challenging to visualize using CCTA due to motion artifacts and "blooming". Usual stent diameters range between 2.5 and 4 mm. The widespread use of drug eluting stents has significantly reduced the risk of in-stent restenosis [26]. Vessel size, stented length, co morbidities, lesion morphology, and previous bypass surgery are predictors of higher rates of restenosis [26].

Depending on materials and size, stents can have a widely different appearance in CCTA. A closed cell design with a higher metal-to-surface ratio makes it more difficult to visualize the stent lumen than an open cell design. New generations of bioresorbable scaffolds (BRS), on the other hand, made of magnesium or polylactid polymer, are free of metal and may be visualized only by radioopaque markers at the extreme ends of the scaffold.

Non-invasive CT Examination

Early EBCT-studies used time-density curve analysis in a region of interest distal to the stent comparing it to the pattern in the aorta [27–29]. This led to a reliable detection of complete occlusions whereas high-grade and subtotal stenoses were frequently missed because of the fact that contrast flow may pass subtotal stenoses and collateral vessels may fill the vessel lumen retrogradely.

Apart from motion artifacts, in vitro studies revealed further stent-related problems — in CT imaging such as enhancement of the stent struts ("blooming"), apparent reduction of the stent lumen, attenuation of contrast values

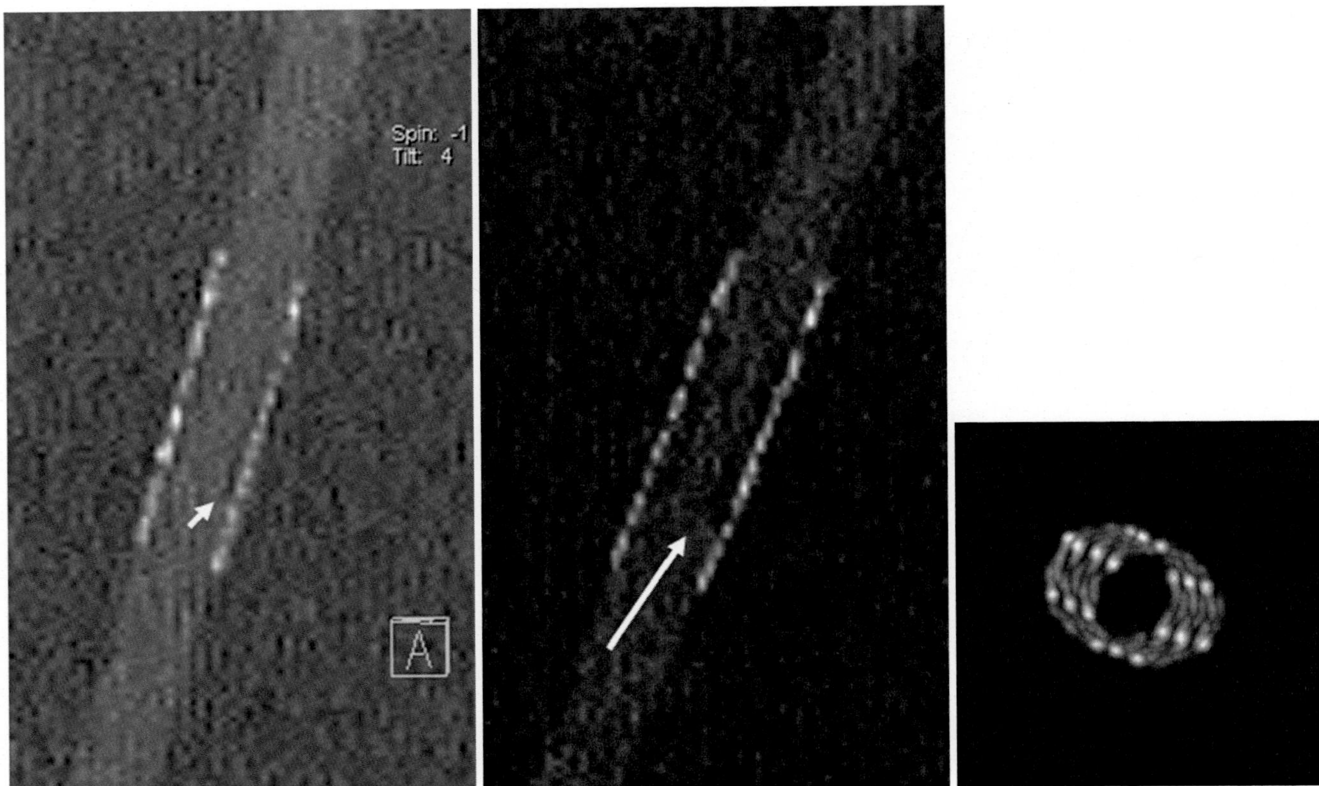

Fig. 10.5 Ultra-high resolution images of a coronary stent using 64-row MDCT. The two *left panel* pictures show the stent mounted on a vessel model placed in a phantom with realistic attenuation values. The *short arrow* marks an artificial 30 % in-stent restenosis (produced within the stented vessel model), the *longer arrow* a 50 % restenosis in the same setting. The *right panel* shows a three-dimensional reconstruction of the stent

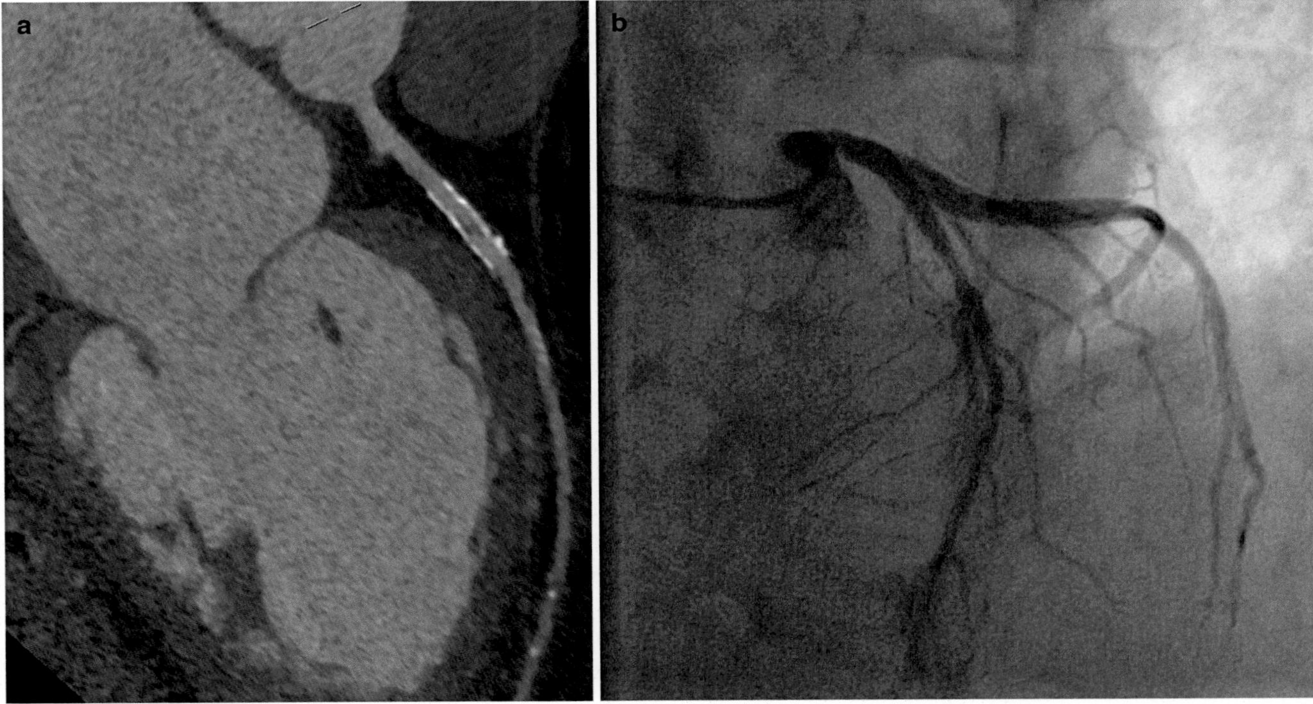

Fig. 10.6 Intermediate in-stent-stenosis of a 3.25 × 16 mm bare-metal-stent in the proximal left anterior descending artery (**a**). Corresponding invasive coronary angiogram of the left coronary artery (**b**)

inside the lumen and beamlike artifacts adjacent to the stent [30–33] (Fig. 10.5). Improvements in CT technology like multi slice and dual-source scanners in recent years have increased the accuracy of detection of in-stent stenoses (Fig. 10.6). Nevertheless, stent artifacts are still problematic, and they vary between different types of stents [34]. Several studies have evaluated the accuracy of multislice CCTA in diagnosing in-stent stenoses versus ICA (gold-standard) [35–40], partly combined with IVUS [38] or OCT [39]. Taking all segments into account, sensitivity was 50–100 %, specificity 57–98 %, and negative predictive value (NPV) 96–100 %. Looking only at the assessable stents (predominantly stents ≥ 3.0 mm), sensitivity was 86–100 %, specificity 93–97 %, and NPV 98–100 %.

Besides patient-related aspects that impede image quality, in particular heart rate, vessel calcifications, motion artifacts, and obesity, stent diameter has been identified as the most important stent-related factor. Stent diameters of 3.0 mm or more appear to have a significantly higher diagnostic accuracy on CCTA than smaller stents [38, 40] (Fig. 10.7). A good correlation between CCTA and IVUS can be observed in the analysis of left main coronary artery stents [41]. The type of stent plays an essential role. A strut thickness of less than 100 μm is associated with less artifacts und thus improves diagnostic accuracy [38]. Due to the artifacts mentioned above, CCTA tends to underestimate lumen area which may result in false positive findings. On the other hand, stent occlusions or high-grade in-stent stenoses can be ruled out with confidence (NPV 98–100 %). In 2010, a meta-analysis combined 14 studies assessing diagnostic accuracy of CCTA versus ICA [42]. In total, 89 % of all stents were assessable. Sensitivity for assessable stents was 90 %, specificity 91 %.

Rief et al. showed improved diagnostic precision in combining CCTA with myocardial CT perfusion (CTP) [43]. CTP can add functional information concerning an in-stent stenosis and the need for revascularization (93 % sensitivity). Fixed perfusion deficits due to previous myocardial infarctions result, however, in a sensitivity of 65 % and PPV of only 33 % for CTP alone.

Recent bioresorbable stents (BRS) are hardly visible in CCTA and, unlike metal stents, do not generate artifacts. So far, comparative studies with other DES concerning diagnostic yield exist only in vitro [34]. Onuma et al. demonstrated the feasibility of CCTA and fractional flow reserve (FFR) in patients after implantation of an ABSORB BRS [44].

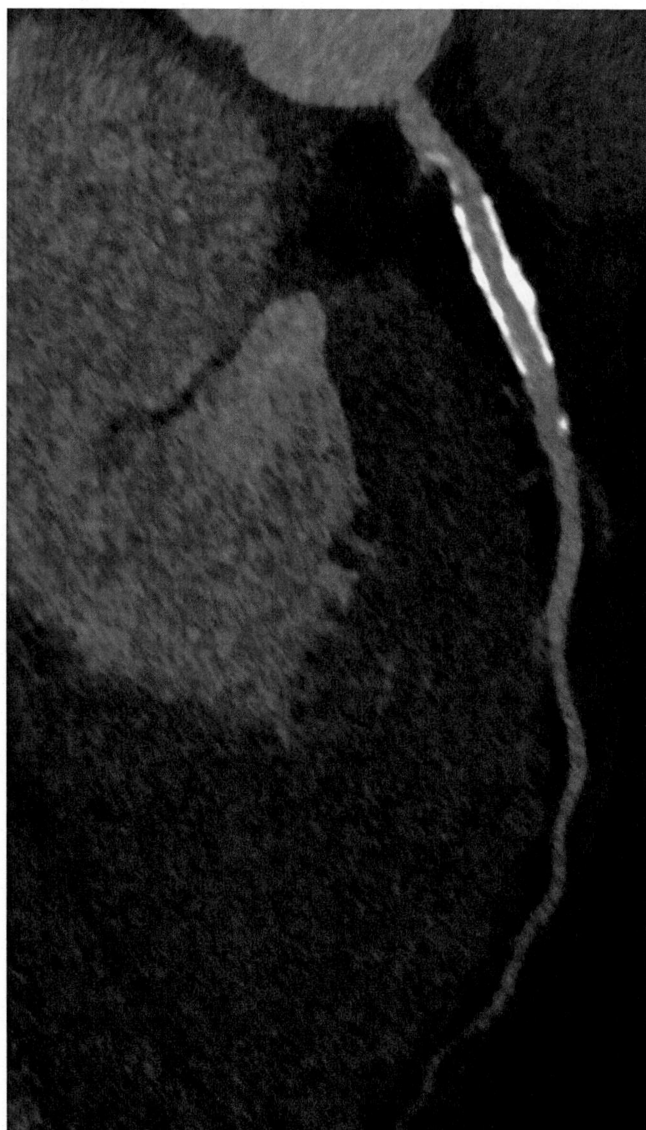

Fig. 10.7 Patent drug-eluting stent (3.0 × 18 mm) in the proximal left anterior descending artery

Imaging Protocols

Over the last decade there has been a dramatic reduction in radiation exposure with CCTA due to improvements in CT scanner technology and image reconstruction, e.g., iterative reconstruction [45, 46]. Image quality has improved due to the use of sharp, high-resolution kernels [47, 48]. Most patients can be scanned with prospective ECG-triggering, resulting in a significantly lower radiation exposure compared to the retrospective spiral mode. Xia et al. even examined patients after stent implantation with high-pitch spiral mode [49]. Diagnostic accuracy was equal to low-pitch spiral mode and sequential mode, effective dose was in the range of 1.0 mSv.

Preparations for CCTA are the same for stent imaging as for other CCTA indications and are described elsewhere in the book.

Conclusion

Using new dual-source CT systems, coronary stents can be visualized with high diagnostic accuracy. In stents with diameters of 3.0 mm or more, in-stent stenoses can be ruled out with reasonably high certainty. Importantly, strut thickness of the stents has an impact on image quality. Stents with a small strut thickness are better assessable by CCTA than those with thicker struts. A new quality has been introduced by bioresorbable stents, whose materials are partly not visible in CCTA. Such stents can only be identified by distinct radio-opaque markers at the extreme ends of the stent. ICA remains the gold-standard for the diagnosis of in-stent stenoses. For individual patients with prior implantation of relatively large coronary stents (≥3 mm), CCTA may offer an attractive alternative.

References

1. Riley RF, Don CW, Powell W, Maynard C, Dean LS. Trends in coronary revascularization in the United States from 2001 to 2009. Circ Cardiovasc Qual Outcomes. 2011;4:193–7.
2. Goldman S, Zadina K, Moritz T, VA Cooperative Study Group #207/297/364, et al. Long-term patency of saphenous vein and left internal mammary artery grafts after coronary artery bypass surgery: results from a Department of Veterans Affairs Cooperative Study. J Am Coll Cardiol. 2004;44:2149–56.
3. Schwartz L, Kip KE, Frye RL, Alderman EL, Schaff HV, Detre KM, Bypass Angioplasty Revascularization Investigation. Coronary bypass graft patency in patients with diabetes in the Bypass Angioplasty Revascularization Investigation (BARI). Circulation. 2002;106:2652–8.
4. Lytle BW, Loop FD, Cosgrove DM, Ratliff NB, Easley K, Taylor PC. Long-term (5 to 12 years) serial studies of internal mammary artery and saphenous vein coronary bypass grafts. J Thorac Cardiovasc Surg. 1985;89:248–58.
5. Shi Y, O'Brien Jr JE, Mannion JD, Morrison RC, Chung W, Fard A, Zalewski A. Remodeling of autologous saphenous vein grafts. The role of perivascular myofibroblasts. Circulation. 1997;95:2684–93.
6. Fitzgibbon GM, Kafka HP, Leach AJ, Keon WJ, Hooper GD, Burton JR. Coronary bypass graft fate and patient outcome: angiographic follow-up of 5,065 grafts related to survival and reoperation in 1,388 patients during 25 years. J Am Coll Cardiol. 1996;28:616–26.
7. Berger A, MacCarthy PA, Siebert U, Carlier S, Wijns W, Heyndrickx G, Bartunek J, Vanermen H, De Bruyne B. Long-term patency of internal mammary artery bypass grafts. Relationship with preoperative severity of the native coronary artery stenosis. Circulation. 2004;110(suppl II):II-36–40.
8. Brundage BH, Lipton MJ, Herfkens RJ, Berninger WH, Redington RW, Chatterjee K, Carlsson E. Detection of patent coronary bypass grafts by computed tomography. A preliminary report. Circulation. 1980;61:826–31.
9. Daniel WG, Dohring W, Stender HS, Lichtlen PR. Value and limitations of computed tomography in assessing aortocoronary bypass graft patency. Circulation. 1983;67:983–7.
10. Achenbach S, Moshage W, Ropers D, Nossen J, Bachmann K. Noninvasive, three-dimensional visualization of coronary artery bypass grafts by electron beam tomography. Am J Cardiol. 1997;79:856–61.
11. Hamon M, Lepage O, Malagutti P, et al. Diagnostic performance of 16- and 64-section spiral CT for coronary artery bypass graft assessment: meta-analysis. Radiology. 2008;247:679–86.
12. Malagutti P, Nieman K, Meijboom WB, et al. Use of 64-slice CT in symptomatic patients after coronary bypass surgery: evaluation of grafts and coronary arteries. Eur Heart J. 2007;28:1879–85.
13. Pache G, Saueressig U, Frydrychowicz A, et al. Initial experience with 64-slice cardiac CT: non-invasive visualization of coronary artery bypass grafts. Eur Heart J. 2006;27:976–80.
14. Dikkers R, Willems TP, Tio RA, Anthonio RL, Zijlstra F, Oudkerk M. The benefit of 64-MDCT prior to invasive coronary angiography in symptomatic post-CABG patients. Int J Cardiovasc Imaging. 2006;23:369–77.
15. Ropers D, Pohle FK, Kuettner A, et al. Diagnostic accuracy of noninvasive coronary angiography in patients after bypass surgery using 64-slice spiral computed tomography with 330-ms gantry rotation. Circulation. 2006;114:2334–41.
16. Meyer TS, Martinoff S, Hadamitzky M, et al. Improved noninvasive assessment of coronary artery bypass grafts with 64-slice computed tomographic angiography in an unselected patient population. J Am Coll Cardiol. 2007;49:946–50.
17. Jabara R, Chronos N, Klein L, et al. Comparison of multidetector 64-slice computed tomographic angiography to coronary angiography to assess the patency of coronary artery bypass grafts. Am J Cardiol. 2007;99:1529–34.
18. Feuchtner GM, Schachner T, Bonatti J, et al. Diagnostic performance of 64-slice computed tomography in evaluation of coronary artery bypass grafts. AJR Am J Roentgenol. 2007;189:574–80.
19. Nazeri I, Shahabi P, Tehrai M, Sharif-Kashani B, Nazeri A. Assessment of patients after coronary artery bypass grafting using 64-slice computed tomography. Am J Cardiol. 2009;103:667–73.
20. de Graaf FR, van Velzen JE, Witkowska AJ, et al. Diagnostic performance of 320-slice multidetector computed tomography coronary angiography in patients after coronary artery bypass grafting. Eur Radiol. 2011;21:2285–96.
21. Weustink AC, Nieman K, Pugliese F, et al. Diagnostic accuracy of computed tomography angiography in patients after bypass grafting: comparison with invasive coronary angiography. JACC Cardiovasc Imaging. 2009;2:816–24.
22. Mushtaq S, Andreini D, Pontone G, et al. Prognostic value of coronary CTA in coronary bypass patients: a long-term follow-up study. JACC Cardiovasc Imaging. 2014;7:580–9.
23. Desbiolles L, Leschka S, Plass A, et al. Evaluation of temporal windows for coronary artery bypass graft imaging with 64-slice CT. Eur Radiol. 2007;17:2819–28.
24. Lee SK, Jung JI, Ko JM, Lee HG. Image quality and radiation exposure of coronary CT angiography in patients after coronary artery bypass graft surgery: influence of imaging direction with 64-slice dual-source CT. J Cardiovasc Comput Tomogr. 2014;8:124–30.
25. Trikalinos TA, Alsheikh-Ali AA, Tatsioni A, Nallamothu BK, Kent DM. Percutaneous coronary interventions for non-acute coronary artery disease: a quantitative 20-year synopsis and a network meta-analysis. Lancet. 2009;373:911–8.
26. Cassese S, Byrne RA, Tada T, et al. Incidence and predictors of restenosis after coronary stenting in 10 004 patients with surveillance angiography. Heart. 2014;100:153–9.
27. Schmermund A, Haude M, Baumgart D, Görge G, Grönemeyer D, Seibel R, Sehnert C, Erbel R. Non-invasive assessment of coronary Palmaz-Schatz stents with contrast enhanced electron beam computed tomography. Eur Heart J. 1996;17:1546–53.
28. Möhlenkamp S, Pump H, Baumgart D, Haude M, Gronemeyer DH, Seibel RM, Schwartz RS, Erbel R. Minimally invasive evaluation of coronary stents with electron beam computed tomography: In

vivo and in vitro experience. Catheter Cardiovasc Interv. 1999;48:39–47.
29. Pump H, Möhlenkamp S, Sehnert CA, Schimpf SS, Schmidt A, Erbel R, Gronemeyer DH, Seibel RM. Coronary arterial stent patency: assessment with electron-beam CT. Radiology. 2000;214:447–52.
30. Maintz D, Juergens KU, Wichter T, Grude M, Heindel W, Fischbach R. Imaging of coronary artery stents using multislice computed tomography: in vitro evaluation. Eur Radiol. 2003;13:830–5.
31. Mahnken AH, Buecker A, Wildberger JE, Ruebben A, Stanzel S, Vogt F, Günther RW, Blindt R. Coronary artery stents in multislice computed tomography: in vitro artifact evaluation. Invest Radiol. 2004;39:27–33.
32. Schlosser T, Scheuermann T, Ulzheimer S, et al. In-vitro evaluation of coronary stents and 64-detector-row computed tomography using a newly developed model of coronary artery stenosis. Acta Radiol. 2008;49:56–64.
33. Schlosser T, Scheuermann T, Ulzheimer S, et al. In vitro evaluation of coronary stents and in-stent stenosis using a dynamic cardiac phantom and a 64-detector row CT scanner. Clin Res Cardiol. 2007;96:883–90.
34. Gassenmaier T, Petri N, Allmendinger T, et al. Next generation coronary CT angiography: in vitro evaluation of 27 coronary stents. Eur Radiol. 2014;24:2953–61.
35. Rixe J, Achenbach S, Ropers D, et al. Assessment of coronary artery stent restenosis by 64-slice multi-detector computed tomography. Eur Heart J. 2006;27:2567–72.
36. Ehara M, Kawai M, Surmely JF, et al. Diagnostic accuracy of coronary in-stent restenosis using 64-slice computed tomography: comparison with invasive coronary angiography. J Am Coll Cardiol. 2007;49:951–9.
37. Pugliese F, Weustink AC, Van Mieghem C, et al. Dual source coronary computed tomography angiography for detecting in-stent restenosis. Heart. 2008;94(7):848–54.
38. Andreini D, Pontone G, Bartorelli AL, et al. Comparison of feasibility and diagnostic accuracy of 64-slice multidetector computed tomographic coronary angiography versus invasive coronary angiography versus intravascular ultrasound for evaluation of in-stent restenosis. Am J Cardiol. 2009;103:1349–58.
39. Kubo T, Matsuo Y, Ino Y, et al. Diagnostic accuracy of CT angiography to assess coronary stent thrombosis as determined by intravascular OCT. JACC Cardiovasc Imaging. 2011;4:1040–3.
40. Zhang J, Li M, Lu Z, Hang J, Pan J, Sun L. In vivo evaluation of stent patency by 64-slice multidetector CT coronary angiography: shall we do it or not? Int J Cardiovasc Imaging. 2012;28:651–8.
41. Roura G, Gomez-Lara J, Ferreiro JL, et al. Multislice CT for assessing in-stent dimensions after left main coronary artery stenting: a comparison with three dimensional intravascular ultrasound. Heart. 2013;99:1106–12.
42. Sun Z, Almutairi AM. Diagnostic accuracy of 64 multislice CT angiography in the assessment of coronary in-stent restenosis: a meta-analysis. Eur J Radiol. 2010;73:266–73.
43. Rief M, Zimmermann E, Stenzel F, et al. Computed tomography angiography and myocardial computed tomography perfusion in patients with coronary stents: prospective intraindividual comparison with conventional coronary angiography. J Am Coll Cardiol. 2013;62:1476–85.
44. Onuma Y, Dudek D, Thuesen L, et al. Five-year clinical and functional multislice computed tomography angiographic results after coronary implantation of the fully resorbable polymeric everolimus-eluting scaffold in patients with de novo coronary artery disease: the ABSORB cohort A trial. JACC Cardiovasc Interv. 2013;6:999–1009.
45. Ebersberger U, Tricarico F, Schoepf UJ, et al. CT evaluation of coronary artery stents with iterative image reconstruction: improvements in image quality and potential for radiation dose reduction. Eur Radiol. 2013;23:125–32.
46. Eisentopf J, Achenbach S, Ulzheimer S, Layritz C, Wuest W, May M, Lell M, Ropers D, Klinghammer L, Daniel WG, Pflederer T. Low-dose dual-source CT angiography with iterative reconstruction for coronary artery stent evaluation. JACC Cardiovasc Imaging. 2013;6:458–65.
47. Oda S, Utsunomiya D, Funama Y, et al. Improved coronary in-stent visualization using a combined high-resolution kernel and a hybrid iterative reconstruction technique at 256-slice cardiac CT-Pilot study. Eur J Radiol. 2013;82:288–95.
48. Zhou Q, Jiang B, Dong F, et al. Computed tomography coronary stent imaging with iterative reconstruction: a trade-off study between medium kernel and sharp kernel. J Comput Assist Tomogr. 2014;38:604–12.
49. Xia Y, Junjie Y, Ying Z, et al. Accuracy of 128-slice dual-source CT using high-pitch spiral mode for the assessment of coronary stents: first in vivo experience. Eur J Radiol. 2013;82:617–22.

Part III

CT Angiography Assessment for Cardiac Pathology

Assessment of Cardiac Structure and Function by Computed Tomography Angiography

11

John A. Rumberger

Abstract

High-resolution multi-detector CT (MDCT) scanners capable of quantitative imaging of the heart were introduced around 2002. Initially 16-slice scanners were validated but the current state of the art is 64+-slice scanners. This chapter discusses the use of 64+-slice MDCT for quantitative assessment of cardiac structure and function.

Keywords

Left ventricle • Systolic function • Diastolic function • MDCT • Cardiac CT

Current State of the Art

CT has traditionally oriented and displayed images parallel or at 90° angles to the long axis of the body (i.e., transaxial, coronal, and sagittal image planes). Such presentations oriented about the long axis of the body do not satisfy prior established presentations of cardiac images as they do not cleanly transect the ventricles, atria, or myocardial regions as supplied by the major coronary arteries.

Knowledge of cardiac ejection fractions [1], absolute ventricular volumes [2, 3], and location and extent of regional wall motion abnormalities provides valuable diagnostic and prognostic information, and non-invasive cardiac imaging has become the reference standard in routine clinical practice.

The American Heart Association in 2002 [4] published standards of myocardial segmentation and nomenclature for tomographic imaging of the heart using non-invasive imaging modalities and divided the left ventricle (LV) into 17 segments. The nomenclature for image presentation for cardiac CT is: the short axis, horizontal long axis, and vertical long axis, as shown in Fig. 11.1. These cardiac axes are very familiar to practitioners performing SPECT or PET imaging; for those familiar with two-dimensional echocardiography, these correspond to the short axis, apical four-chamber, and apical two-chamber views, respectively. These cardiac imaging planes are oriented at 90°angles relative to each other [i.e. 3-orthogonal planes].

In order to employ CT to define the cardiac chambers and separate them from the surrounding myocardium, it is necessary to use intravenous contrast. In general, this can be accomplished with <100 mL of non-ionic contrast, and it is possible to perform complete imaging of the heart chambers, the coronary arteries, and the proximal great vessels (aorta and pulmonary artery) in a single setting with a single injection of contrast. Methods for contrast administration for MDCT scanning of the heart are found elsewhere.

Orthogonal (short and various long axes) cardiac CT images after intravenous contrast allow for identification of non-opacified intracardiac thrombi (Fig. 11.2a) and tumors (Fig. 11.2b) including excellent resolution of the left atrium and the left atrial appendage (Fig. 11.3), allowing localization of structures smaller than 1 mm [5, 6]. Cardiac CT can additionally be of assistance in defining thrombi or occult occlusion of the venae cavae and other right-sided structures. Cardiac CT can also be a primary method of defining intracardiac shunts such as those caused by inter-ventricular (Fig. 11.4a) and inter-atrial (Fig. 11.4b) congenital defects and other acquired defects post-infarction [7].

J.A. Rumberger, PhD, MD
Cardiac Imaging, The Princeton Longevity Center, Forestall Village, 136 Main Street, Princeton, NJ 08540, USA
e-mail: jrumberger@theplc.net

M.J. Budoff, J.S. Shinbane (eds.), *Cardiac CT Imaging: Diagnosis of Cardiovascular Disease*,
DOI 10.1007/978-3-319-28219-0_11

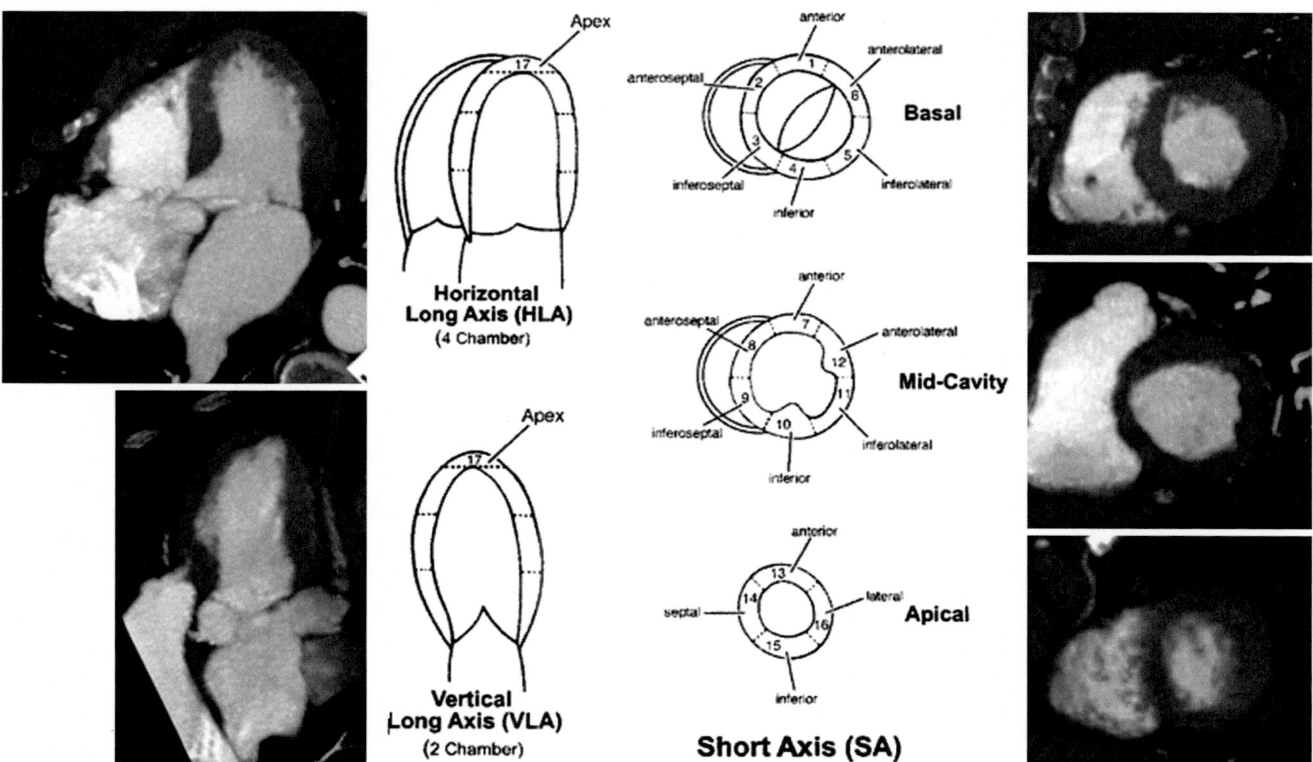

Fig. 11.1 Standardized presentation of the heart in cardiac CT. American Heart Association 17 segment model of the left ventricle (LV); the orthogonal imaging planes are the horizontal long axis, the vertical long axis, and the short axis (Reprinted from Cerqueira et al. [4], with permission of Wolters Kluwer Health, Copyright 2002, American Heart Association, Inc.)

Cardiac CT can be used to quantitate left and right ventricular volumes [8–10], left and right atrial volumes, left and right ventricular muscle mass [11–14], regional left ventricular function, wall thickening and contractility [15–17], rates of diastolic filling of the right and left ventricles [16, 18, 19], post-infarction left and right ventricular remodeling [20–24], cardiac remodeling following cardiac [25] and lung transplantation [26], and ejection fraction [27–30] in patients with no contraindication to the use of iodinated contrast medium. Additional applications include quantitation of uni-valvular regurgitation [31] and assessment of infarct size [32, 33]. The majority of these validation studies was performed in the 1980s and 1990s using EBT and has been adapted and/or re-validated in studies using MDCT. In most instances, these quantitative aspects can be performed or at least well-approximated in patients with generally normal sinus rhythm. Since the number of cardiac cycles imaged per scan is single (256- and 320-slice scanners) or generally limited to <5 (64-slice scanners), quantitation may be limited in those patients with significant dysrhythmias, such as non-regular atrial fibrillation.

All available post-processing workstations can provide quantitative and often non-interactive (i.e., automatic) measurements of the LV in particular. Shown in Fig. 11.5a–e, is the general outline of the procedure and subsequent display of the results. Table 11.1 shows validated norms for LV chamber size, wall thicknesses, ejection fraction, and ventricular volumes using cardiac CT. Reproducibility of CT in performing right and left ventricular volume and function measurements has also been established [34, 35].

Cardiac CT imaging using thin sections allows post-processing of images into end-diastolic and end-systolic short and "long" axis images at multiple ECG-phases to facilitate identification of structures and salient features of the ventricular anatomy (Fig. 11.6). Using short and long axis imaging also allows identification of infarct locations (Fig. 11.7). Demonstrated in this latter example is a common CT finding in contrast-enhanced images from patients with remote myocardial infarction. The "negative" contrast noted in Fig. 11.7 is actually due to lack of contrast opacification in the infarcted region causing "contrast rarefaction." Long axis (both vertical and horizontal) imaging of the left ventricle also allows for definition of basilar and apical infarcts, and true- and pseudo-apical aneurysms (Fig. 11.8). Two-dimensional and three-dimensional reconstruction methods, possible in nearly an infinite number of imaging planes, also allows for postoperative assessment of left ventricular aneurysectomy (Fig. 11.9). Global and regional details of the LV due to ischemic cardiomyopathy and hypertrophic cardiomyopathy using cardiac CT provide details commonly

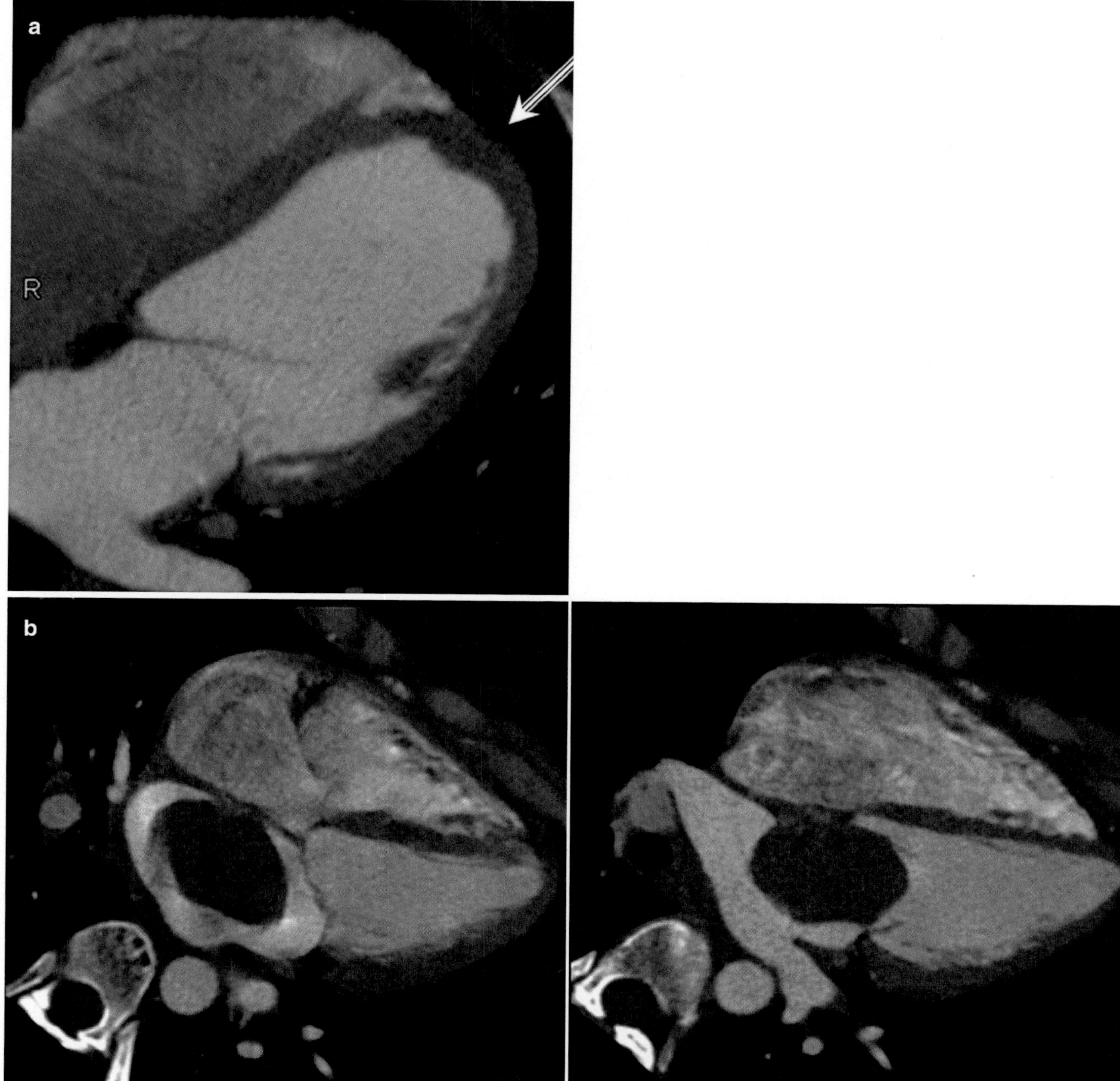

Fig. 11.2 Examples of non-opacified cardiac thrombus and tumor. (**a**) Modified vertical long axis tomogram of the left ventricle (LV); the area noted by the arrow is a non-opacified thrombus at the LV apex. (**b**) Modified horizontal long axis image of the left atrium (LA)/LV; the non-opacified area in the LA chamber is a left atrial myxoma shown at end-systole and end-diastole: note that, during diastole, the myxoma prolapses through the mitral valve

noted by other imaging methods. The right ventricle (RV) can also be imaged. Figure 11.10 shows a dilated RV in a patient with arrhythmogenic RV dysplasia, and Fig. 11.11 shows fatty infiltration of the RV; cardiac CT can often be an alternative or a confirmatory method to MRI in the evaluation of such patients [36]. Biventricular consequences to congenital (Fig. 11.12) and acquired heart disorders (Fig. 11.13) can also be imaged.

Three-dimensional calipers available on all CT workstations allow for quantitative measures of ventricular dimensions in any axis (Fig. 11.14a). Additionally, measures of ventricular muscle thicknesses can be done on all myocardial walls (Fig. 11.14b). Measures of the aorta and other chambers such as the left atrium (Fig. 11.14c) can also be helpful and augment data on ventricular volumes, muscle mass, and function by CT. Normal layers of fat on the epicardial surface of

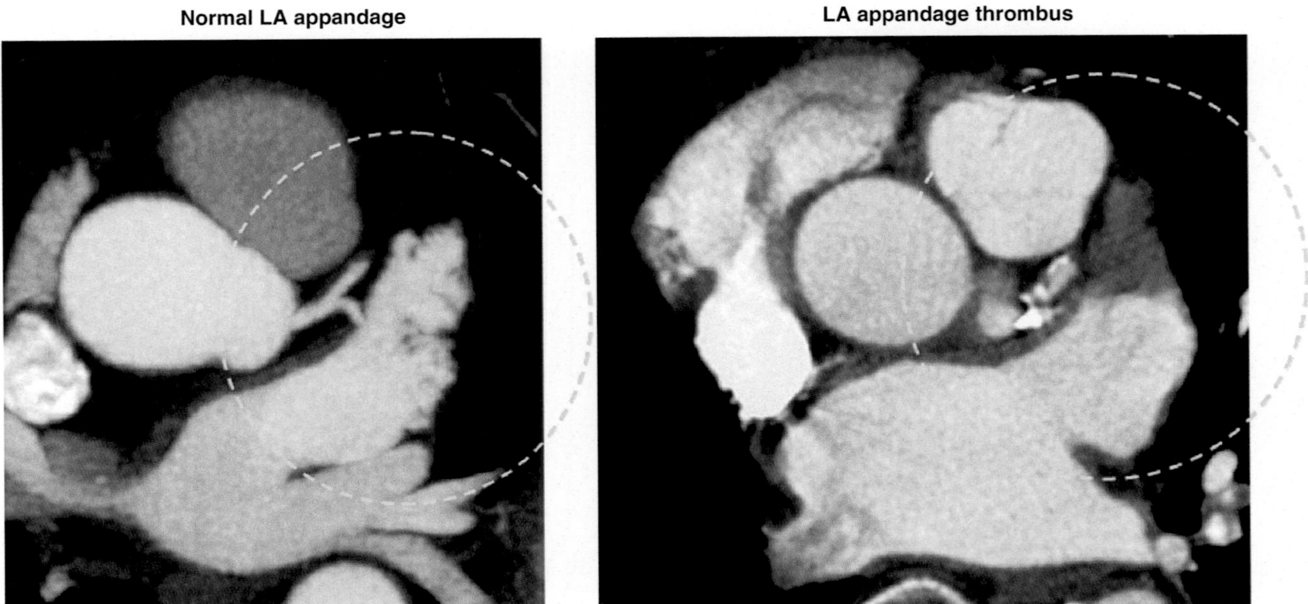

Fig. 11.3 Definition of the left atrial appendage by cardiac CT. *Left*: a normal LA (left atrial) appendage (*dotted circle*). *Right*: LA appendage with thrombus (*dotted circle*)

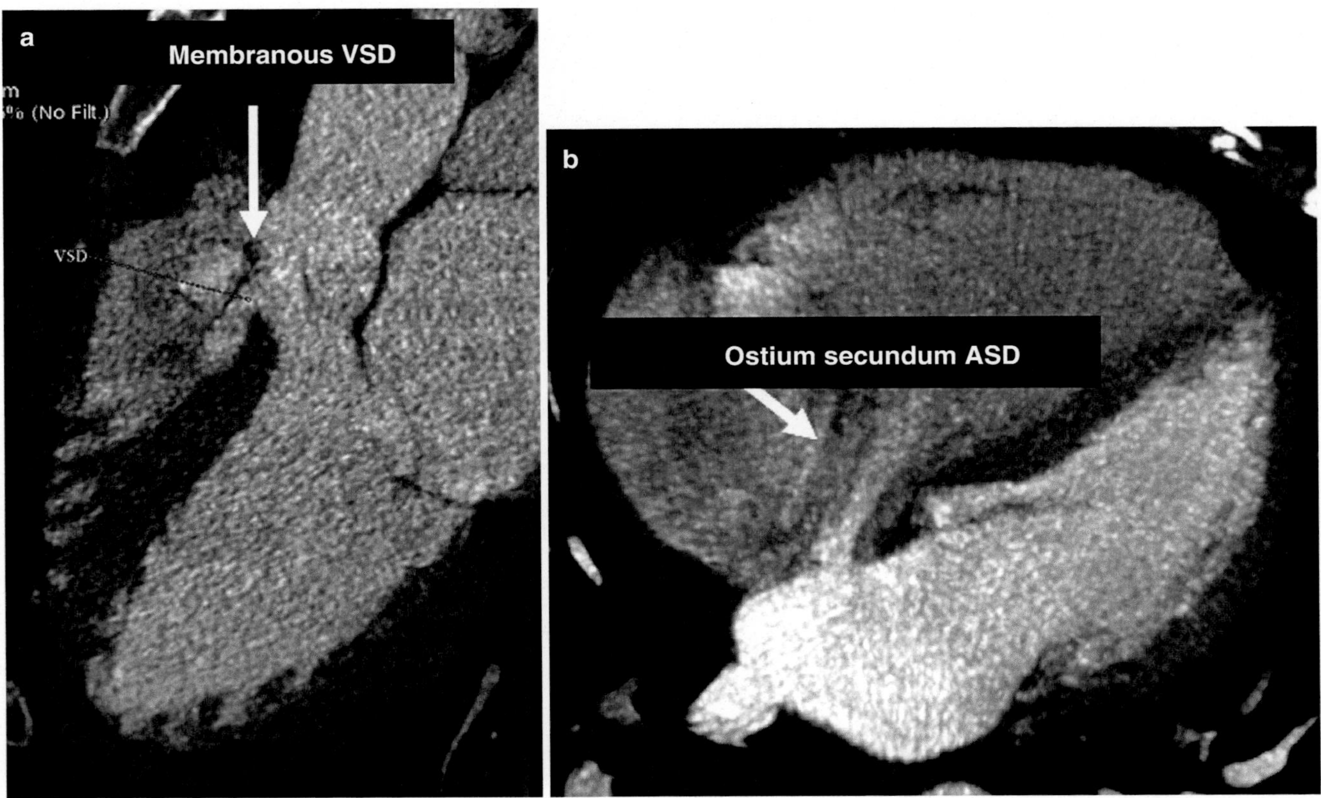

Fig. 11.4 Examples of congenital intra-cardiac shunts as shown by cardiac CT. (**a**) "Peri" membranous ventricular septal defect (VSD) as noted by the *arrow*. (**b**) Jet of contrast demonstrating a left to right shunt from an ostium secundum atrial septal defect (ASD) as noted by the *arrow*

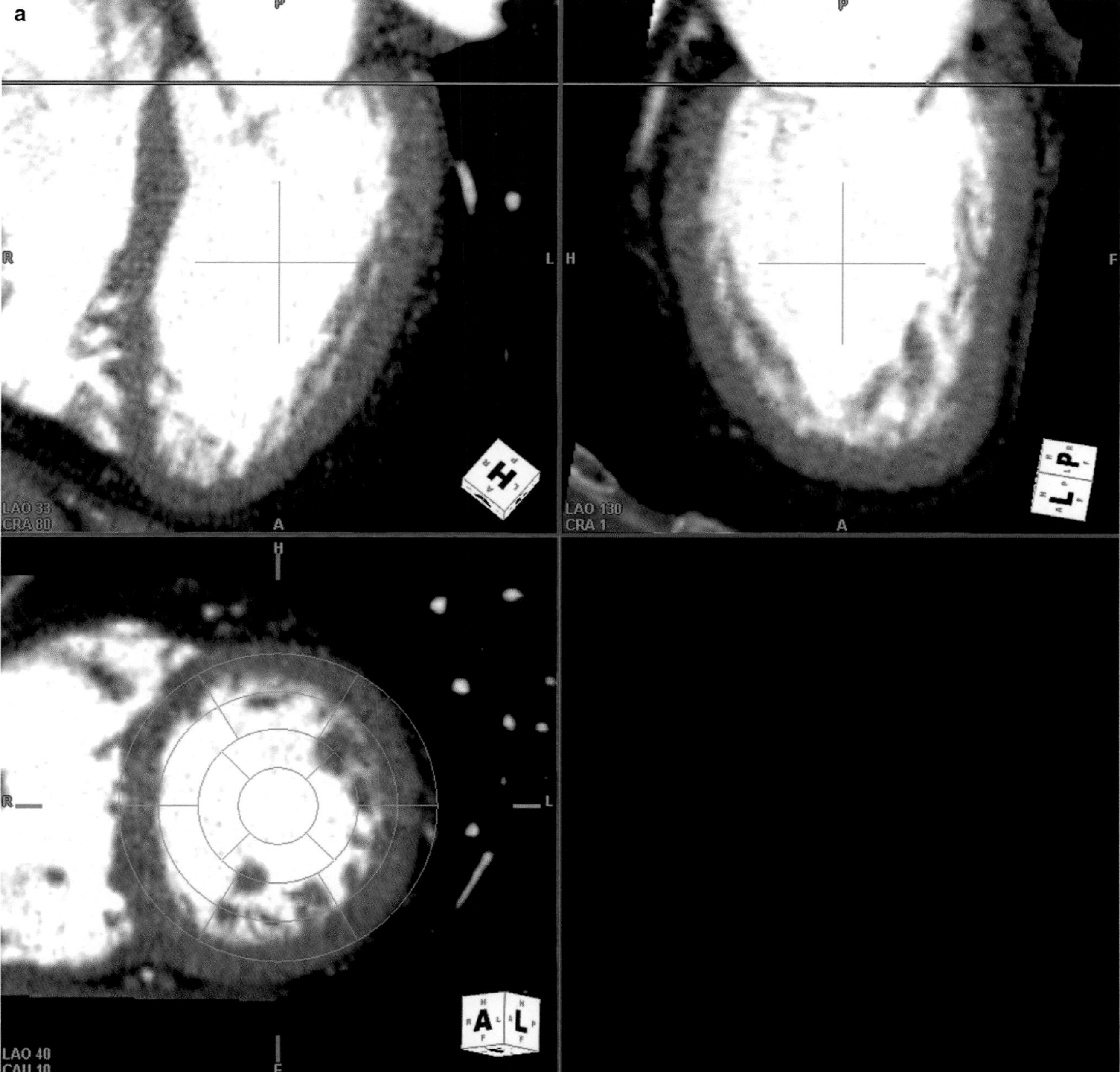

Fig. 11.5 Quantitation of LV (left ventricular) function by cardiac CT. (**a**) Horizontal long axis, vertical long axis, and short axis views of the left ventricle (LV); the line demonstrates the plane of the mitral valve: when performing quantitative analysis, it is necessary that the LV chamber be isolated. (**b**) Semi-quantitative edge definition of the cardiac endocardial surfaces using thresholding methods; from this information, the LV endocardial (chamber) volumes can be determined. (**c**) Semi-quantitative isolation of the LV myocardial epicardial and septal surfaces using thresholding methods; from this information the LV muscle mass and myocardial wall thicknesses can be determined. (**d**) Lower right of the figure: a color map of the myocardial surface systolic function is defined to provide definition of regional LV function. (**e**) LV chamber volume as a function of time during the cardiac cycle; from these data can be derived information on *EF* (ejection fraction), *EDV* (end-diastolic volume), *EDV* (end-systolic volume), *SV* (stroke volume), rates of systolic emptying (contractility), as well as rates of early and late diastolic filling (diastolic function)

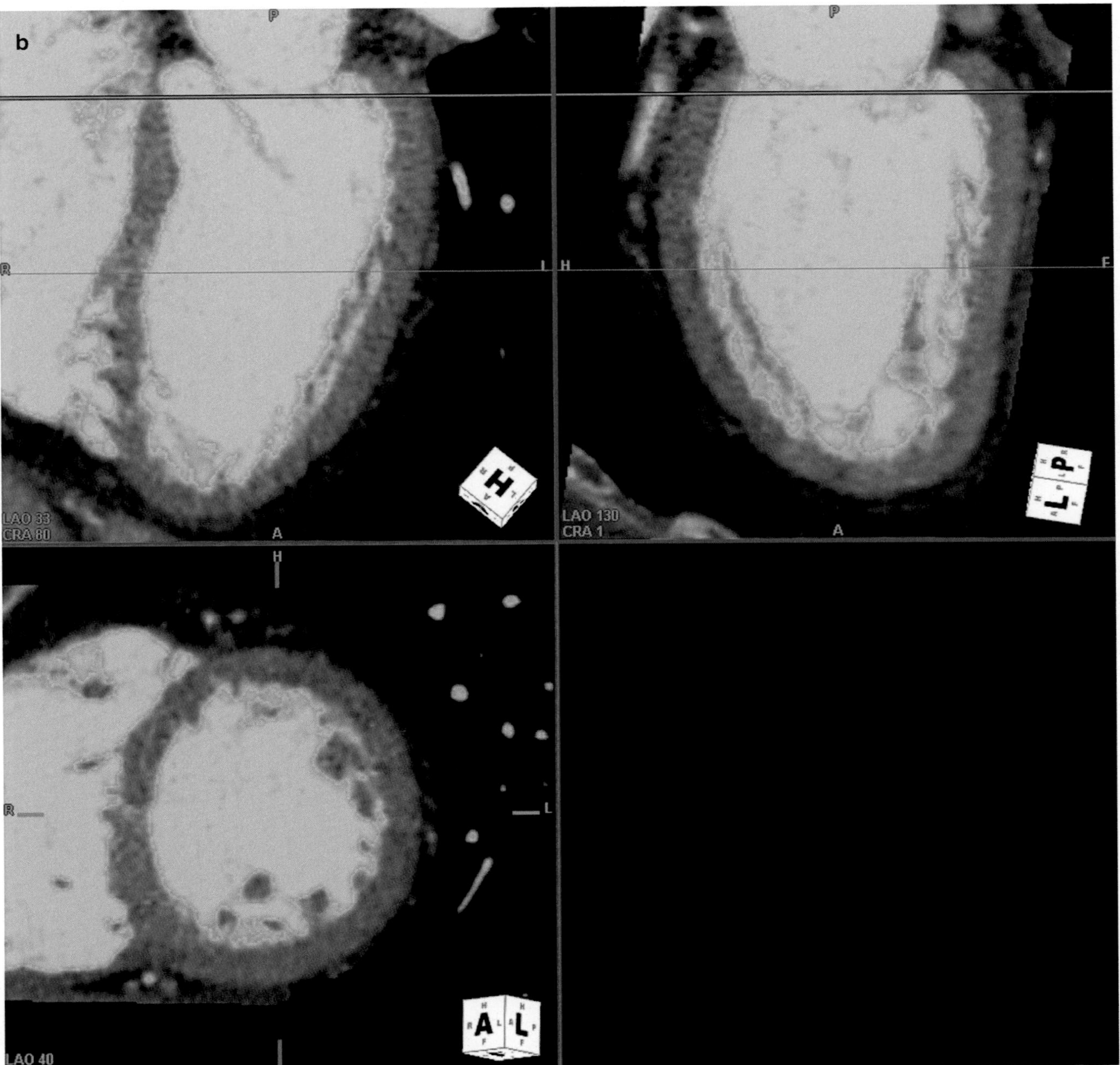

Fig. 11.5 (continued)

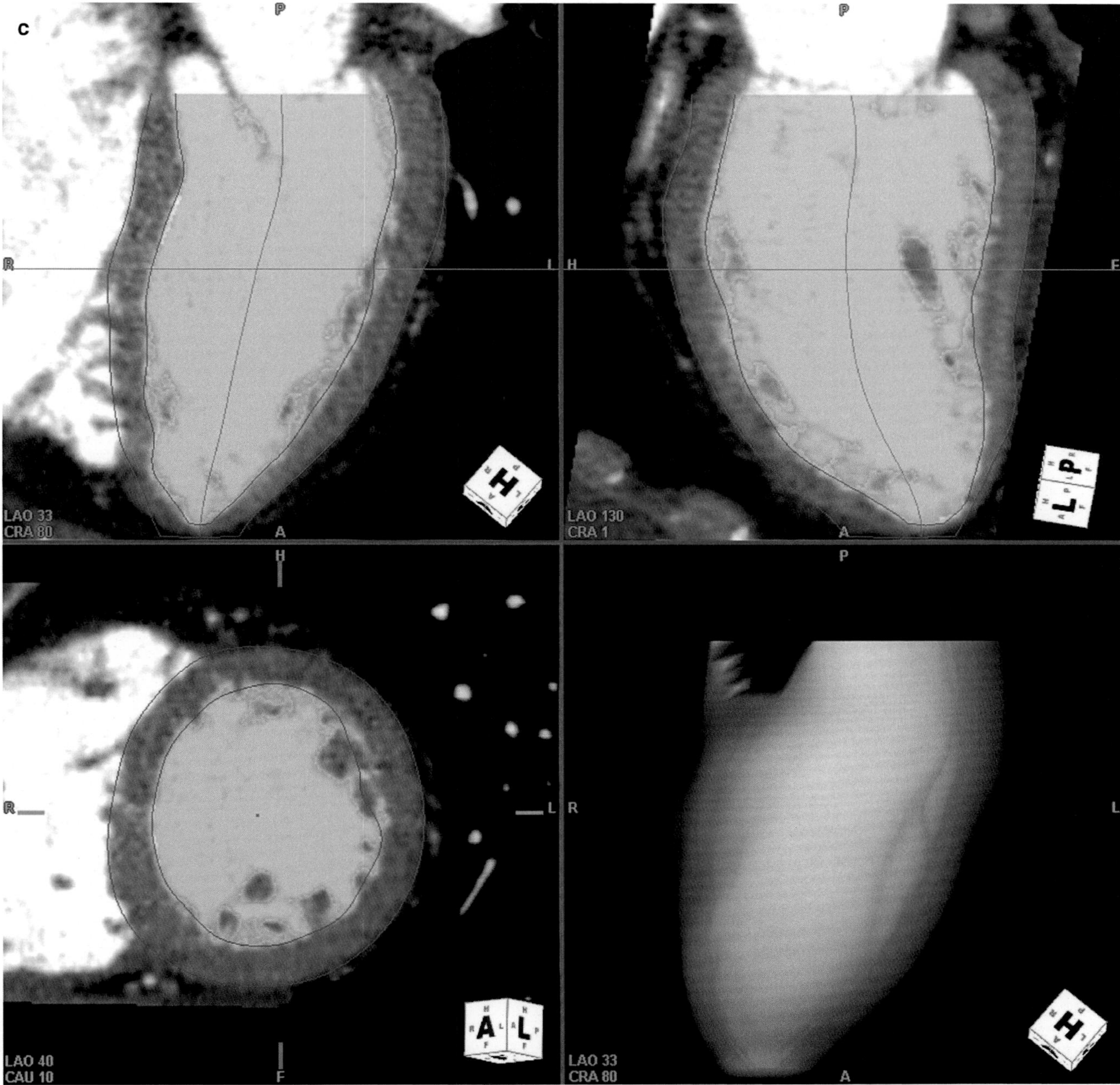

Fig. 11.5 (continued)

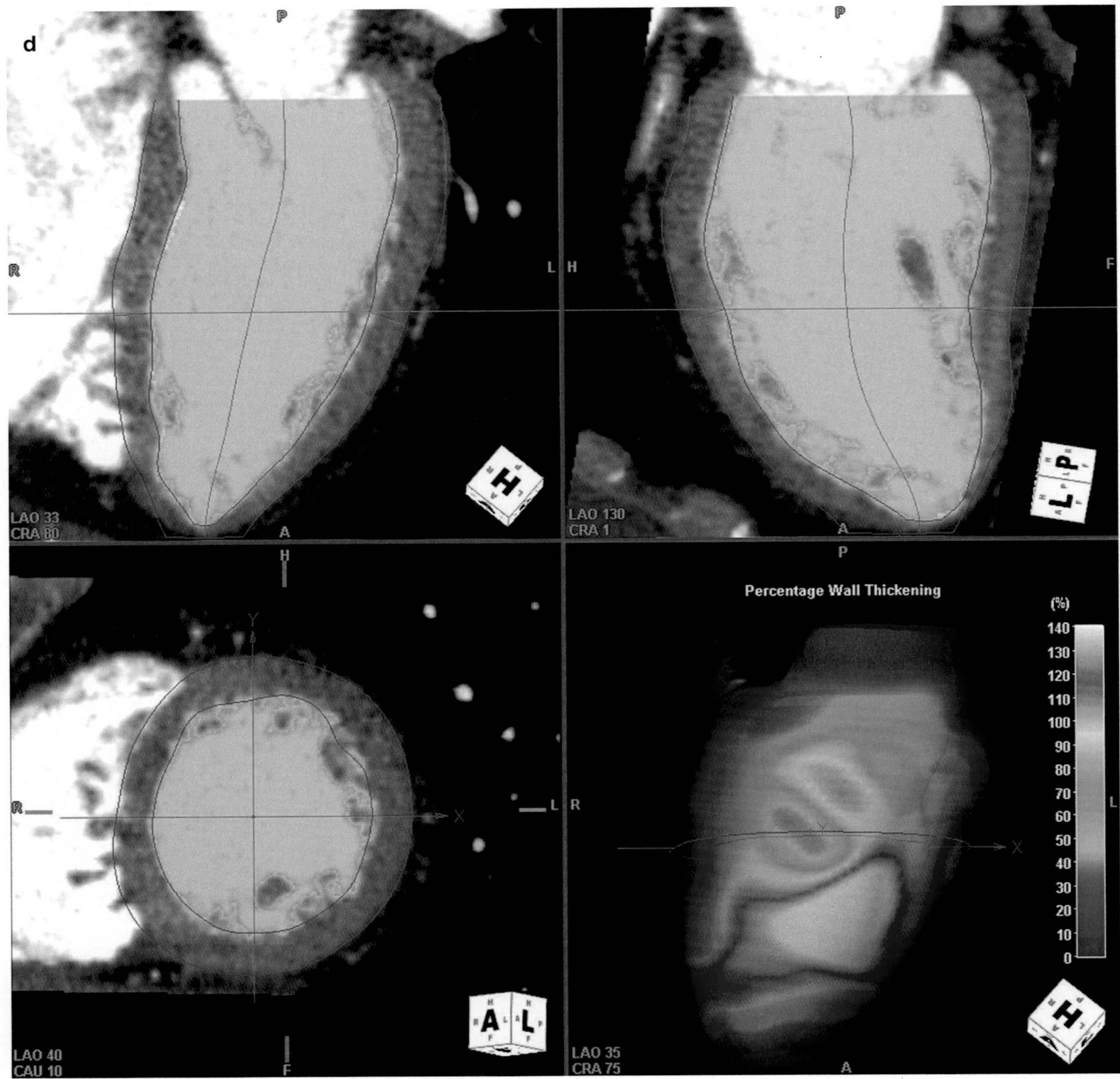

Fig. 11.5 (continued)

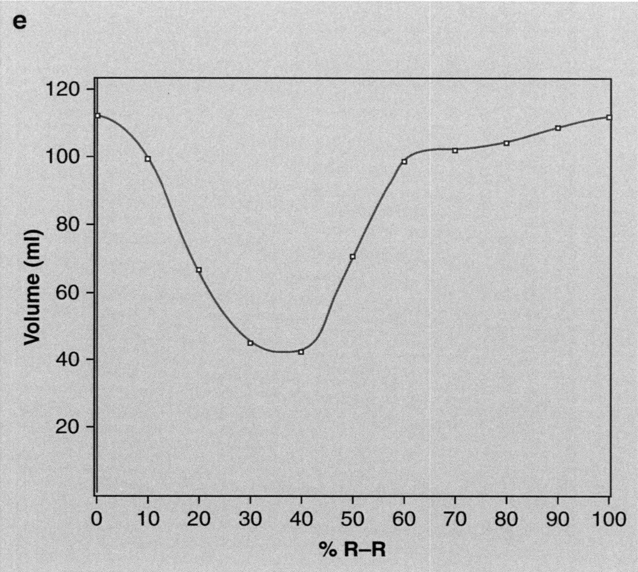

Fig. 11.5 (continued)

the heart and the outer surface of the pericardial sac provide natural contrast and permit the examiner to reliably identify the pericardium (Fig. 11.15). Contrast-enhanced CT often allows separating chronic effusive pericarditis from gross pericardial thickening since the parietal and epicardial layers of the pericardium have their own blood supply. CT can be used to define the entire anatomy of the pericardium and may be of greatest value in localization of loculated effusions such as those confined to the posterior areas of the heart (which are difficult to define using surface two-dimensional echocardiography). Tamponade can be identified with CT by right atrial or ventricular collapse or by indirect signs such as an inappropriately enlarged inferior vena cava or enlarged hepatic veins. High-resolution images can define the anatomic localization and extent of pericardial thickening. In the evaluation of a patient for constrictive pericarditis, CT can add considerably to the diagnosis. CT has an advantage over traditional echocardiography in that the entire cardiac volume is imaged very quickly, and then images of both two-dimensional and three-dimensional views can be rapidly generated. Contrast is usually not required to image the pericardium, as the natural delineation of the pericardial surface (usually 100 Hounsfield Units, HU) and adjacent air (<-700 HU) is dramatic. Calcified pericardial tissue is even easier to image, as the calcification is usually in the +300–400 HU range.

Indications

The mandate for a complete cardiac CT angiogram (CCTA) in routine clinical practice is to include quantitative cardiac structure and function as part of each evaluation performed for assessment of coronary plaque and lumen anatomy. However, quantitation of cardiac function using MDCT can only practically be performed using retrospective ECG-gating.

Prospective ECG-gating protocols provide static images of the heart and the coronary arteries and are appropriate if the indication for performing 64+-slice MDCT is solely assessment of coronary artery anatomy. Prospectively gated MDCT can also provide general information about cardiac chamber sizes, general cardiac anatomy, and some evaluations of the pericardium, but cannot be used to quantitate LV and RV systolic or diastolic function. In such instances, if LV function is also desired for overall clinical assessment, then alternative methods are widely available such a gated SPECT, MRI, and two-dimensional echocardiography. Although MRI and ultrasound provide no ionizing radiation exposure, SPECT imaging can result in radiation exposures up to 3–5 times that of cardiac CT.

Utilization of prospective ECG gating can significantly reduce the effective radiation dose to the patient using MDCT; however, if quantitation of LV function is also required, a retrospective gated cardiac CT can be performed with limited radiation by lowering the kV from 120–100 [and now even 80] and application of ECG-dose (mA) modulation. A properly planned retrospective 64+slice cardiac CT can be performed with effective patient radiation doses of 2–6 mSv versus a prospectively gated MDCT scan, which can be done generally with effective radiation doses of 1–3 mSv (or slightly higher using 256-slice and 320-slice scanners).

Contraindications

The contraindications to performing a retrospectively gated MDCT for assessment of cardiac structure and function are the same as those for performing any cardiac CT examination. Beta-blockers are almost universally applied to get resting heart rates in the range of 60 beats/min. Individuals with reactive airways disease (e.g., emphysema, asthma) should only be given beta-blockers under controlled conditions. Intravenous contrast is also required, thus reduced renal function (e.g., creatinine >1.9 mg/dl) might suggest that an alternative method of evaluating the LV/RV should be considered, but there is no absolute contraindication for MDCT cardiac imaging in the presence of abnormal renal function.

Issues of radiation exposure of the patient during diagnostic cardiac CT examinations and have been bandied about in the press for some time; it is of course important that this potential hazard be considered and risk versus benefit defined by the referring physician. But the American Association of Physicists in Medicine [AAPM] issued the following statement in 12/11 [37]:

Table 11.1 Reference values for left ventricular size, function, and muscle mass for cardiac CT in adult women and men[a]

	Women				Men			
Measurement	Reference range	Mildly abnormal	Moderately abnormal	Severely abnormal	Reference range	Mildly abnormal	Moderately abnormal	Severely abnormal
Septal wall thickness (mm)[a]	6–9	10–12	13–15	≥16	6–10	11–13	14–16	≥17
Posterior wall thickness (mm)[a]	6–9	10–12	13–15	≥16	6–10	11–13	14–16	≥17
LV muscle mass (gm)	66–155	156–176	177–187	>190	96–200	201–227	228–254	>260
LV diameter (mm)[a]	39–53	54–57	58–61	≥62	42–59	60–63	64–68	≥69
LV global EDV (ml)	60–110	111–122	123–136	≥140	70–160	161–190	191–210	≥210
LV global ESV (ml)	20–50	51–60	61–70	≥71	25–60	61–70	71–85	≥86
LV global EF (%)	≥55	45–54	30–44	<30	≥55	45–54	30–44	<30

Data from Rumberger et al. [32]; and Lang et al. [35]
EDV end-diastolic volume, *ESV* end-systolic volume, *EF* ejection fraction
[a]End-diastole, mid left ventricle

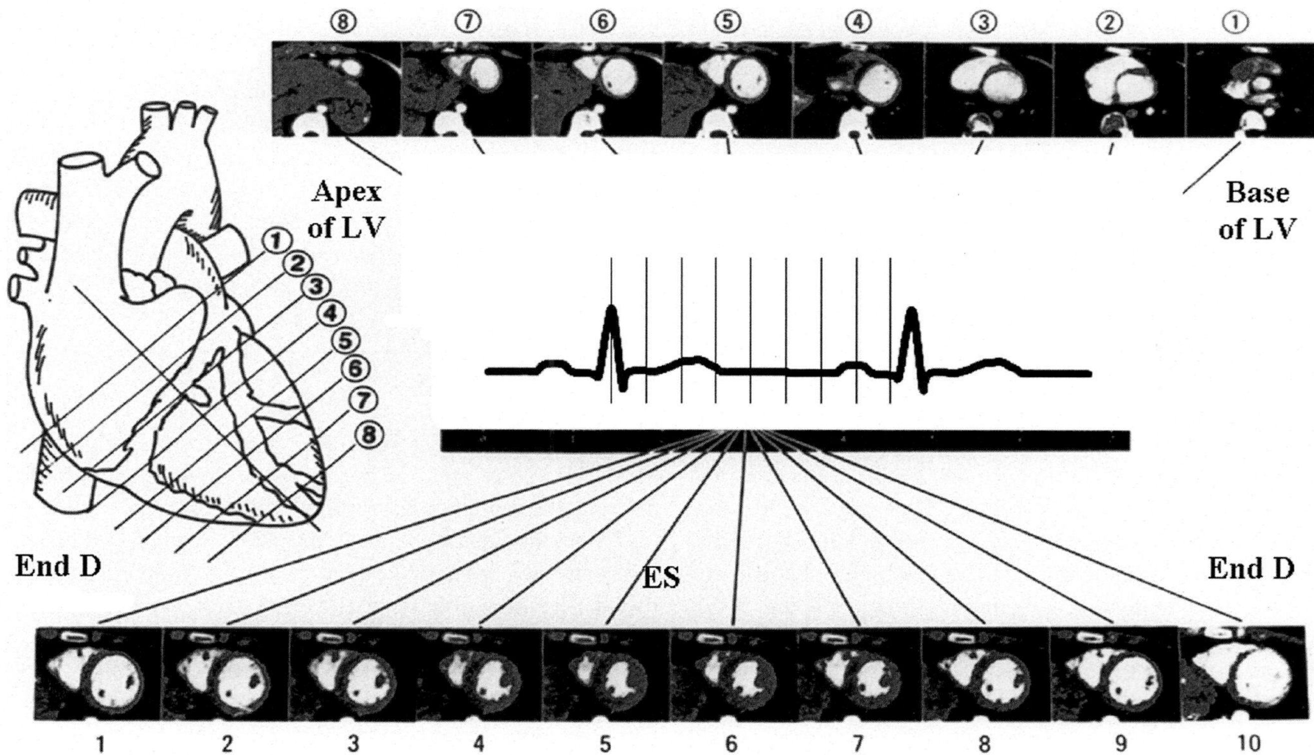

Fig. 11.6 Example of LV (left ventricle) short axis images from the apex to base of the heart and various ECG related phases defined from end-diastole (*End D*) to end-systole (*ES*) and back to end-diastole (end D) during a 10-phase ECG gated reconstruction of cardiac function using Cardiac CT

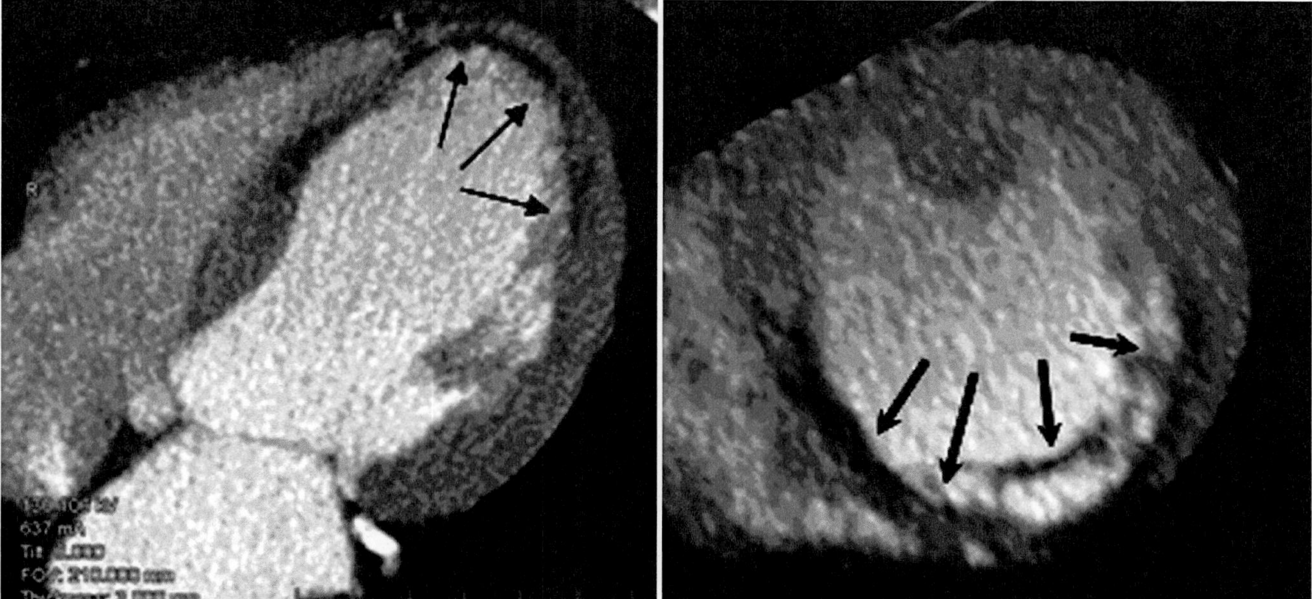

Fig. 11.7 Vertical long axis and mid-LV short axis images of a patient with remote myocardial infarction. *Left*: vertical long axis; the *arrows* point to regions of transmural infarction in the lower septal wall, apex, and lateral wall. *Right*: mid-LV short axis; the *arrows* point to regions of transmural infarction in the inferior septum, inferior (posterior) wall, and lateral wall; using such presentations, estimates of myocardial infarction size can be estimated

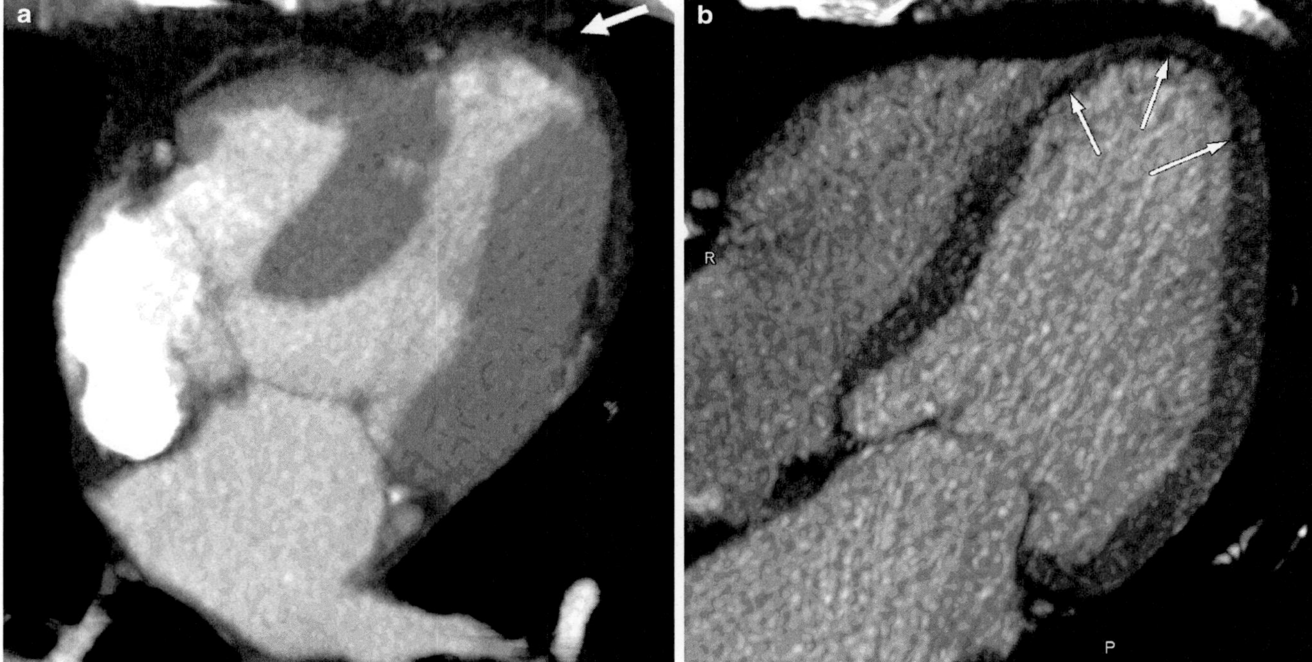

Fig. 11.8 Examples of left ventricular (LV) true aneurysm and "pseudo" aneurysm using Cardiac CT. (**a**) End-systolic long axis image of LV demonstrating LV apical aneurysm (*arrow*); (**b**) End-diastolic long axis image of LV demonstrating dilation of LV apex and thinning of myocardial with akinetic regional motion and "pseudo" aneurysm (*arrows*)

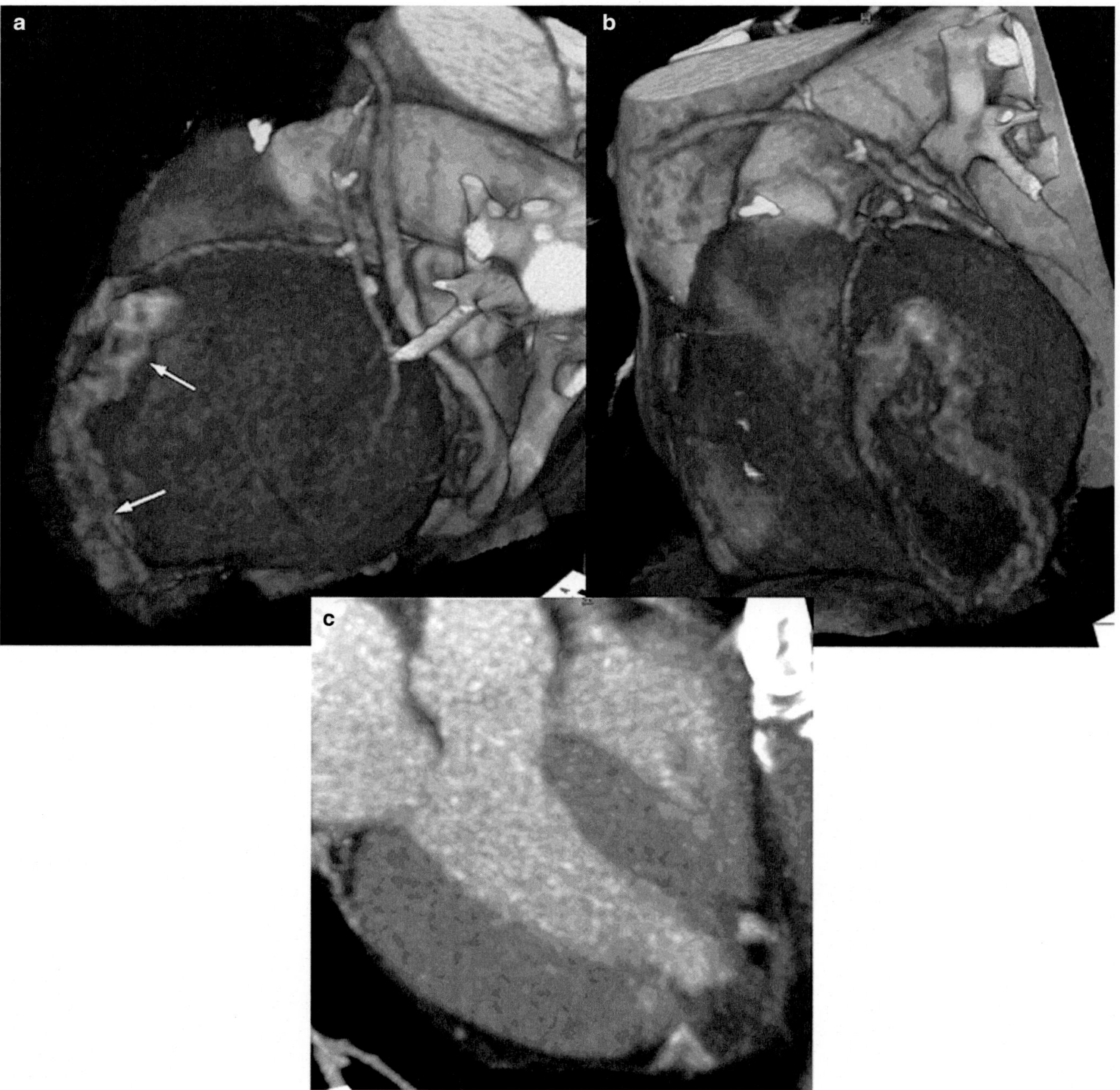

Fig. 11.9 Cardiac CT images of patient after left ventricular (LV) aneurysmectomy. (**a**, **b**) Volume rendering presentation from lateral and anterior views of the LV: the area of aneurysm repair is shown by the *arrows*. (**c**) A maximum intensity projection (2-dimensional) of the LV long axis showing the area of aneurysm repair: the two bright objects at the LV apex are surgical pledgets

> The American Association of Physicists in Medicine (AAPM) acknowledges that medical imaging procedures should be appropriate and conducted at the lowest radiation dose consistent with acquisition of the desired information. Discussion of risks related to radiation dose from medical imaging procedures should be accompanied by acknowledgement of the benefits of the procedures. Risks of medical imaging at effective doses below 50 mSv for single procedures or 100 mSv for multiple procedures over short time periods are too low to be detectable and may be nonexistent. Predictions of hypothetical cancer incidence and deaths in patient populations exposed to such low doses are highly speculative and should be discouraged. These predictions are harmful because they lead to sensationalistic articles in the public media that cause some patients and parents to refuse medical imaging procedures, placing them at substantial risk by not receiving the clinical benefits of the prescribed procedures.

Patients unable to hold their breath for 15 s or who are uncooperative should be avoided for cardiac CT. The presence of various dysrhythmias (frequent PACs/PVCs) can

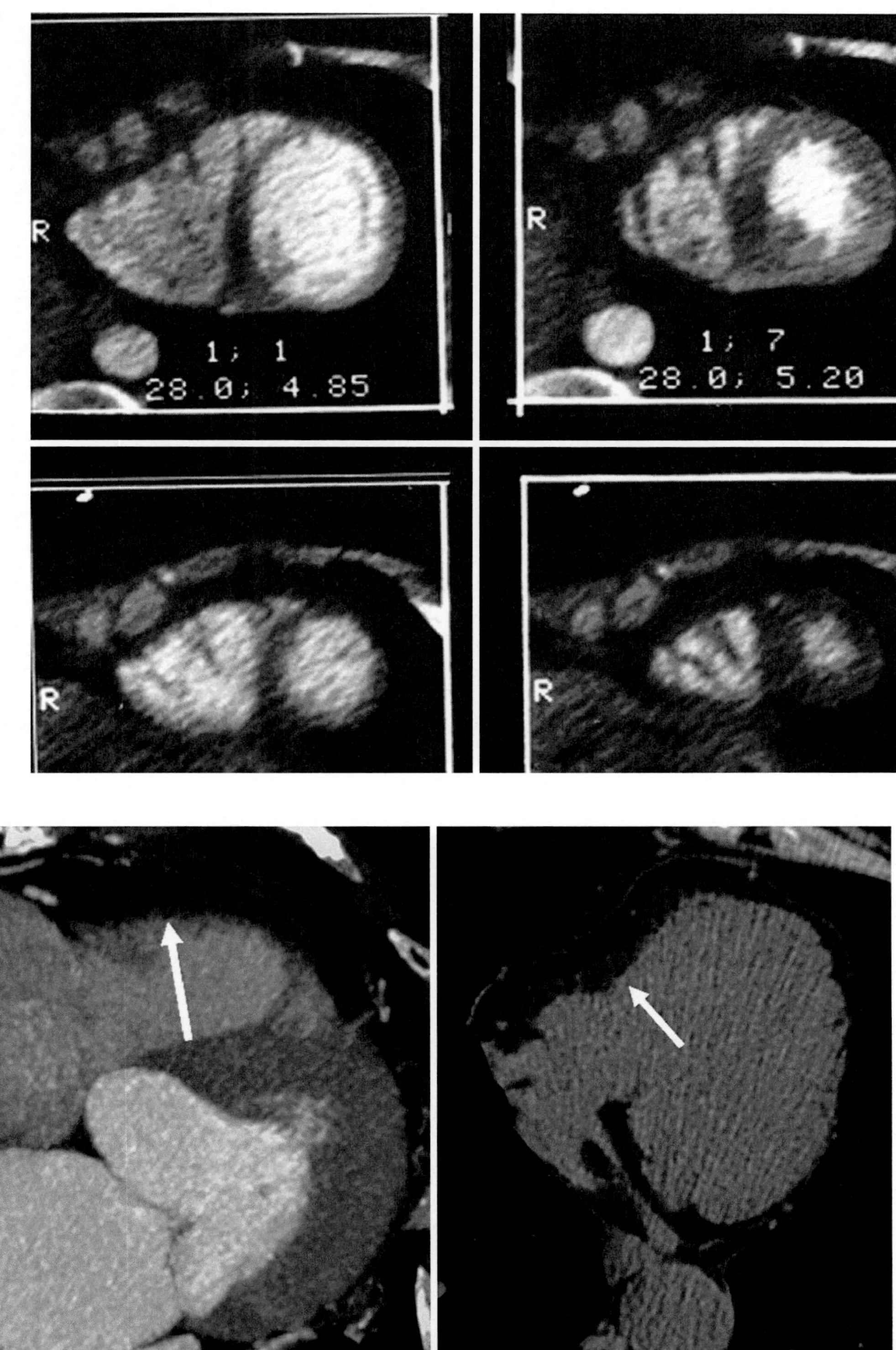

Fig. 11.10 Short axis images of the LV (*right*) and RV (right ventricle, *left*) from an 18 year old woman with syncope and ARVD (arrhythmogenic RV dysplasia). Note the enlargement of the RV compared to the LV and the presence of wide trabeculations in the RV, both major criteria for diagnosis of ARVD

Fig. 11.11 Cardiac CT Images of two patients with ARVD (arrhythmogenic right ventricular dysplasia). The *arrows* demonstrate "fatty infiltration" of the RV wall, a major diagnostic criteria for the diagnosis of ARVD

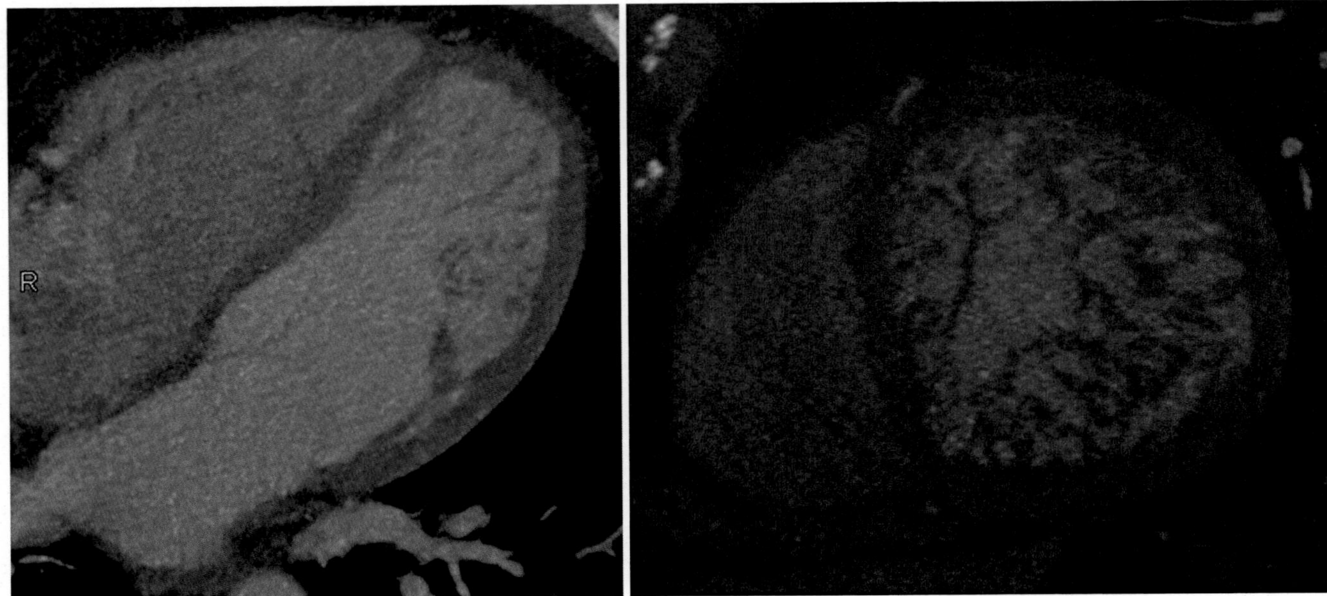

Fig. 11.12 Cardiac CT in a patient with "non-compaction" of the LV. *Left*: Long axis showing dilation of the lower (apical) one-half of the LV chamber. *Right*: a mid-LV short axis demonstrating dilation of the LV chamber and the presence of deep "sinusoids" (fenestrations) of the LV chamber

make quantitation of LV function with MDCT difficult, and individuals with pacemakers should have the ventricular rate set to 60 beats per minute. The presence of atrial fibrillation is not a contraindication, but, with uncontrollable rapid ventricular response, will likely result in sub-optimal data.

Strengths

A properly planned 64+slice, retrospectively ECG-gated, MDCT examination can provide quantitative data on LV/RV systolic (and diastolic function) both globally and regionally. It can also provide quantitative data on chamber sizes, valve (both natural (Fig. 11.16) and prosthetic) valve motion and cross-sectional areas, visualization of intra-cardiac shunts, definition of cardiac tumors and thrombi, quantitation of LV muscle mass, regional wall thicknesses and thickening, myocardial infarct size, and the gross physiologic consequences of pericardial effusions and pericardial constriction.

Limitations

Sub-optimal assessment of cardiac structures and function can occur due to cardiac dysrhythmias, inadequate heart rate control during imaging, and poor chamber contrast timing/administration. Definition of end-diastole is straight-forward by noting the timing of the R-wave on the ECG and the appropriate CT reconstructed phase. Definition of end-systole is more difficult. Although using a 10-phase retrospective reconstruction usually assigns end-systole to the smallest chamber volume, recent data suggest that at least a 15 phase reconstruction might be more appropriate for timing of this event [38]. The number of phases reconstructed from a 64+-slice MDCT retrospectively ECG gated cardiac CT is a choice made by the physician, and going from a 10-phase to a 20-phase reconstruction only results in more images to review for analysis and the subsequent increase in file size and image storage requirements. Also, many of the available image processing workstations have a limit to the number of images that can be placed into active memory for review.

Comparison to Other Imaging Modalities

EBT and by inference 64+slice MDCT has been validated for assessment of cardiac function in comparison to SPECT imaging, MRI, contrast-ventriculography, and two-dimensional echo.

Future Directions

The quantitation of cardiac structure and function by cardiac CT has been evolving for more than 25 years. Improvements in cardiac edge-detection methods have

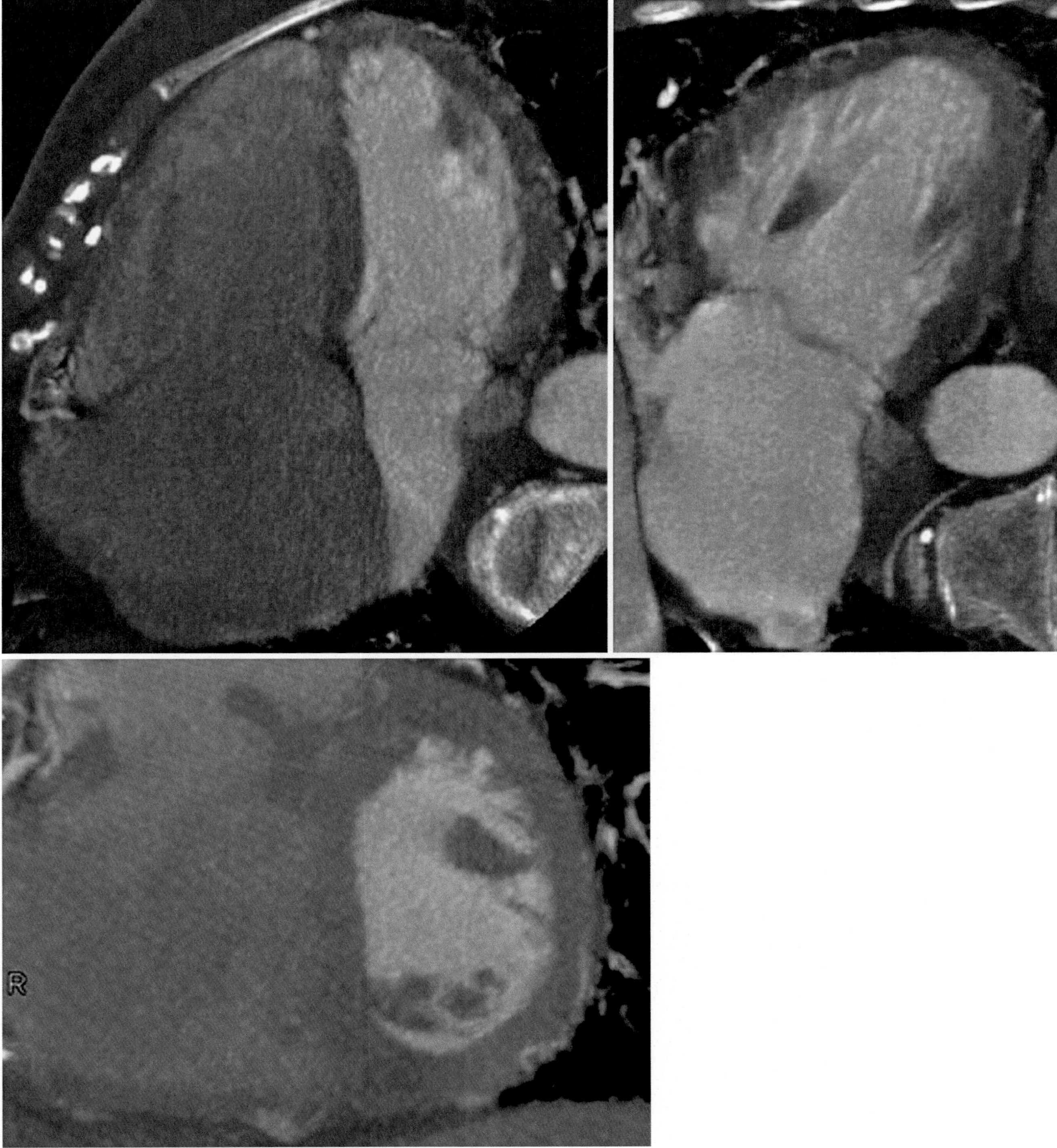

Fig. 11.13 Cardiac CT of a patient with severe pulmonary hypertension as a consequence to severe, chronic mitral valve regurgitation. The horizontal (*left*) and vertical (*middle*) long axis images demonstrate the dilation of the right ventricle (RV) and right atrium (RA)/left atrium; the short (*right*) axis image demonstrates a common characteristic of pulmonary hypertension and a "D" shaped interventricular septum (IVS)

essentially eliminated the need to laboriously trace images from each tomographic plane and apply a modified Simpson's (stack of coins) rule. All current workstations allow for straight-forward information on EF, regional wall thickening, regional wall motion, and LV volumes from 64+-slice MDCT cardiac examinations. Semi-quantitative information on left/right atrial volume/dimensions and RV volume/dimensions are also in development.

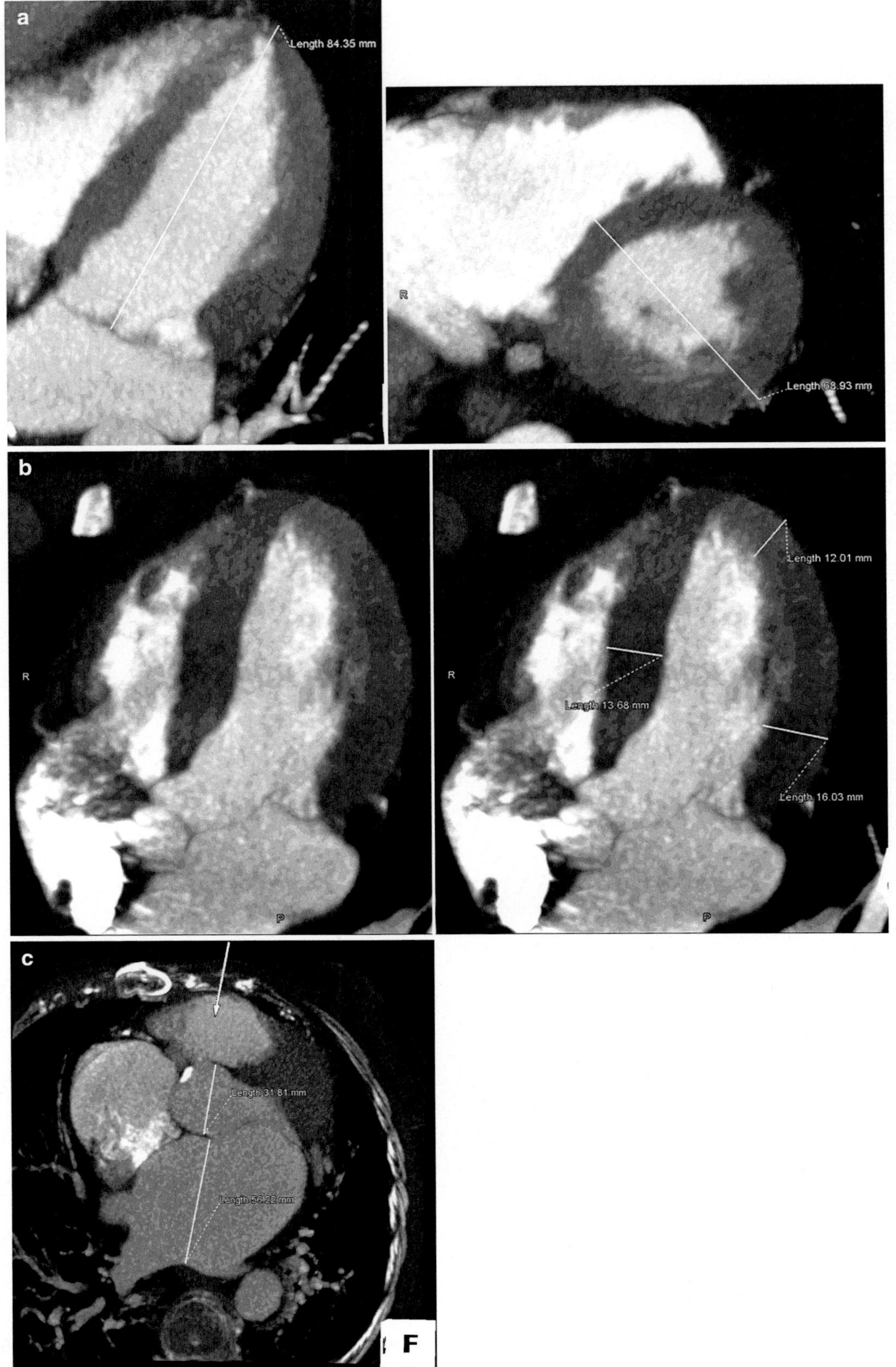

Fig. 11.14 Measurement of cardiac and chamber dimensions in cardiac CT. (**a**) Long axis and short axis dimensions of the left ventricular long axis and at mid ventricle short axis. (**b**) Measurements of septal, apical, and lateral wall thicknesses at end-diastole in a patient with severe cardiac hypertrophy. (**c**) Representative measurements of the aortic root and left atrium as measured mimicking a para-sternal measurement that might be done using two-dimensional echocardiography (direction indicated by *arrow*)

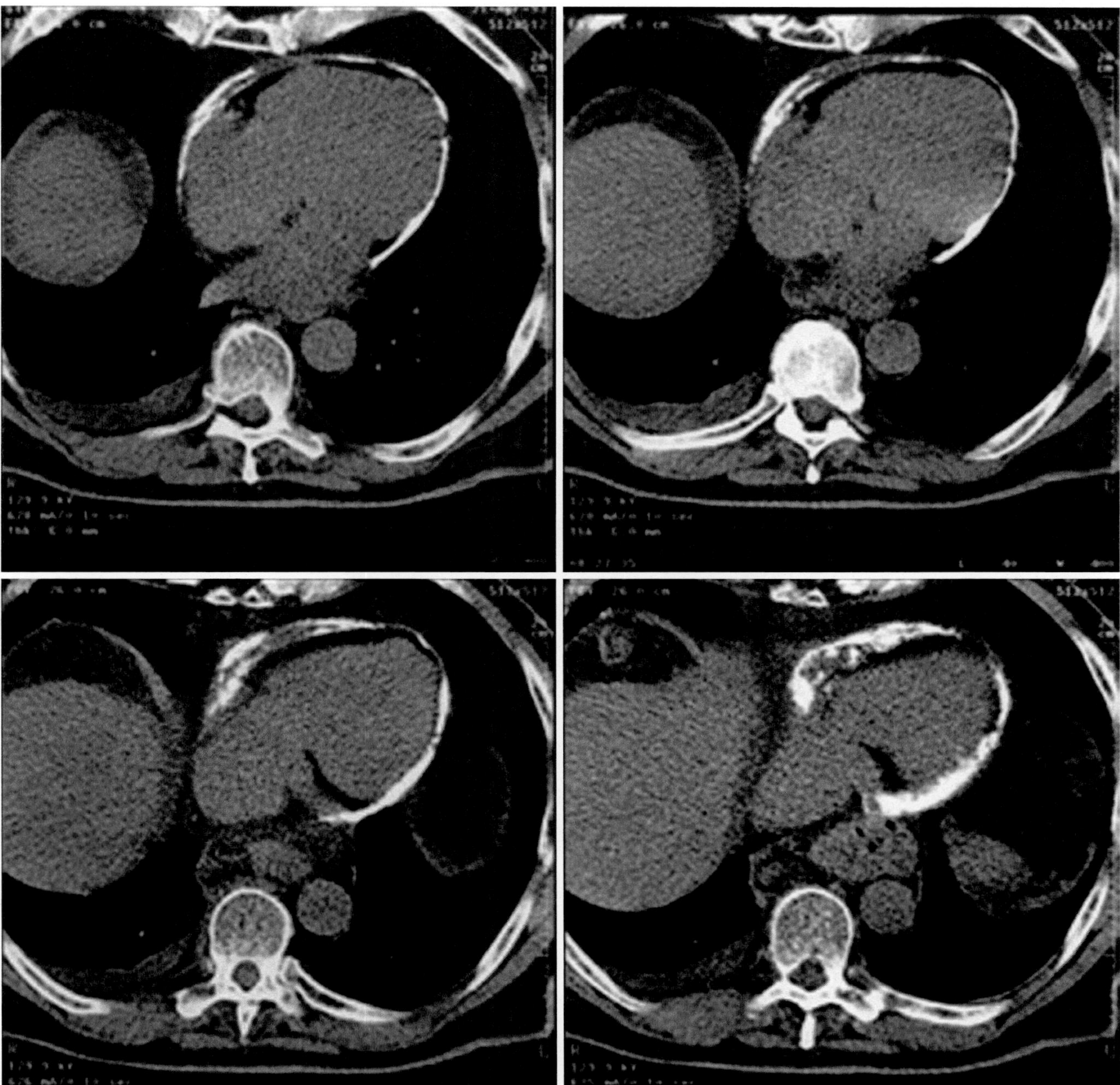

Fig. 11.15 Evaluation of the pericardium by cardiac CT. (**a**) *Left* – Concentric, densely calcified pericardium in a patient with constrictive pericarditis as a consequence to tuberculosis. *Right* – Images from a patient with pericardial tamponade from a concentric pericardial effusion. (**b**) *Top left* – Volume rendered image demonstrating entire cardiac volume; *Top right*: Volume rendered image demonstrating only the cardiac epicardial surface; this was performed by changing the CT display window and level settings on the image presented in **b**, *top left*; *Bottom*: a maximum intensity projection of the horizontal cardiac long axis demonstrating the opacified cardiac chambers and the surrounding low intensity circumferential pericardial effusion

Fig. 11.15 (continued)

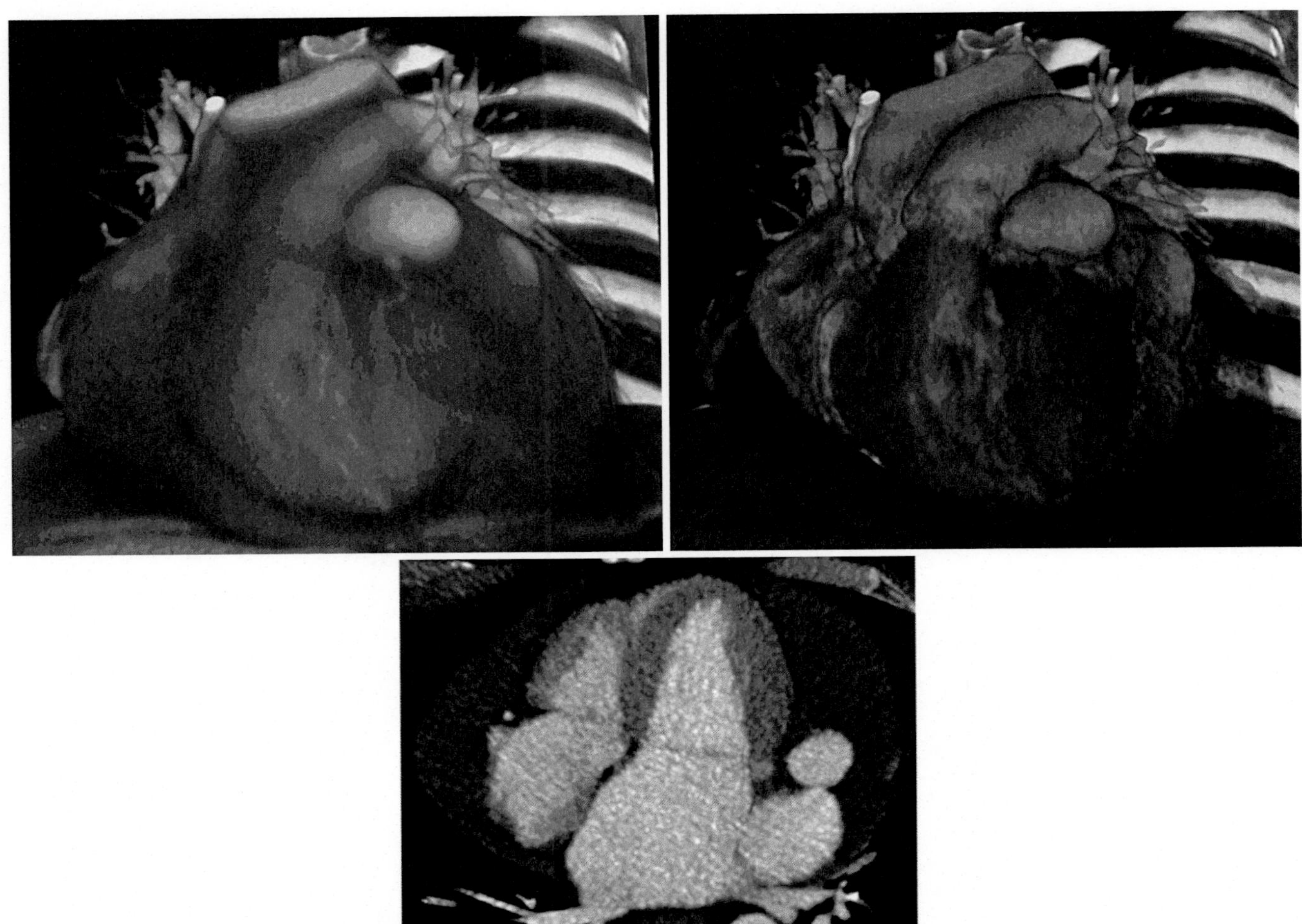

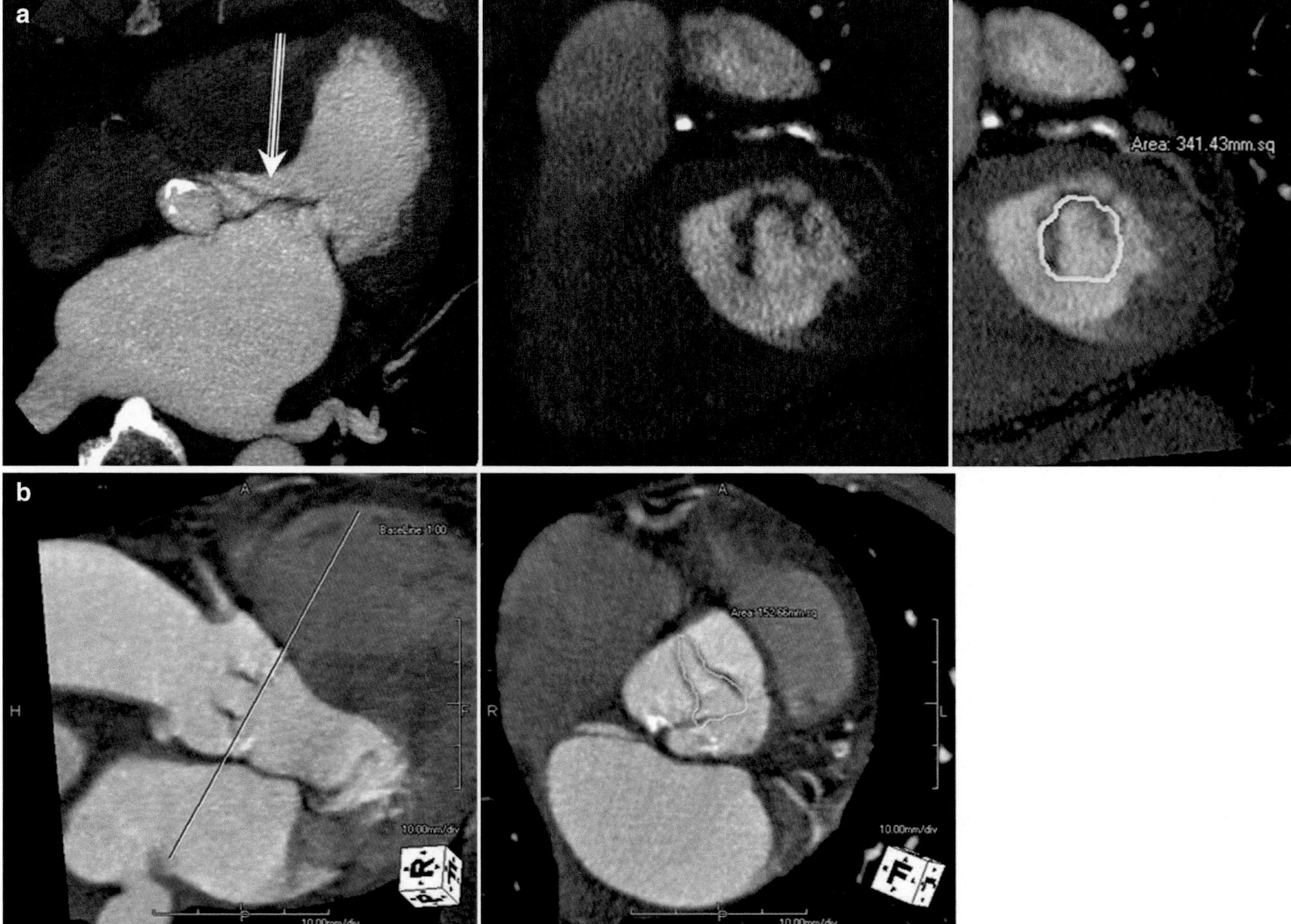

Fig. 11.16 Evaluation of cardiac valve stenosis using cardiac CT. (**a**) LV long axis and short axis images demonstrating thickened mitral valve leaflets (*arrow*) and dilated left atrium and measurement of mitral valve area in a patient with moderate mitral valve stenosis. (**b**) Representative orthogonal views of the aortic valve and measurement of aortic valve area in a patient with known mild aortic valve stenosis

References

1. Hammermeister KE, DeRouen TA, Dodge HT. Variables predictive of survival with coronary disease: selection by univariate and multivariate analyses from the clinical, electrocardiographic, exercise, arteriographic and quantitative angiographic evaluation. Circulation. 1979;59:421–50.
2. Norris RW, Barnaby PF, Brandt PWT. Prognosis after recovery from first acute myocardial infarction: determinant of reinfarction and sudden death. Am J Cardiol. 1984;53:408–13.
3. White HD, Norris RM, Brown MA, Brandt PWJ, Whitlock RML, Weld CJ. Left ventricular end-systolic volume as the major determinant of survival after recovery from myocardial infarction. Circulation. 1987;76:44–51.
4. Cerqueira MD, Weissman NJ, Dilsizian V, et al. Standardized myocardial segmentation and nomenclature for tomographic imaging of the heart – a statement for healthcare professions from the Cardiac Imaging Committee of the Council on Clinical Cardiology of the American Heart Association. Circulation. 2002;105:539–42.
5. Achenbach S, Sacher D, Ropers D, Pohle K, Nixdorff U, Hoffman U, Muschiol G, Flachskampf PA, Daniel WW. Electron beam computed tomography for the detection of left atrial thrombi in patients with atrial fibrillation. Heart. 2004;90(12):1477–8.
6. Meinel Jr JF, Wang G, Jiang M, Frei T, Vannier M, Hoffman E. Spatial variation of resolution and noise in multi-detector row spiral CT. Acad Radiol. 2003;10:607–10.
7. Paul JF, Macé L, Caussin C, Fsihi A, Berthaux X, Brenot P, et al. Multirow detector computed tomography assessment of intraseptal dissection and ventricular pseudo-aneurysm in postinfarction ventricular septal defect. Circulation. 2001;104:497–8.
8. Reiter SJ, Rumberger JA, Feiring AJ, Stanford W, Marcus ML. Precision of right and left ventricular stroke volume measurements by rapid acquisition cine computed tomography. Circulation. 1986;74:890–900.
9. Yamamuro M, Tadamura E, Kubo S, Toyoda H, Nishina T, Ohba M, et al. Cardiac functional analysis with multi-detector row CT and segmental reconstruction algorithm: comparison with echocardiography, SPECT, and MR imaging. Radiology. 2005;234:381–90.
10. Halliburton SS, Petersilka M, Schvartzman PR, Obuchowski N, White RD. Evaluation of left ventricular dysfunction using multiphasic reconstructions of coronary multi-slice computed tomography data in patients with chronic ischemic heart disease: validation

against cine magnetic resonance imaging. Int J Cardiovasc Imaging. 2003;19:73–83.
11. Feiring AJ, Rumberger JA, Reiter SJ, Skorton DJ, Collins SM, Lipton MJ, et al. Determination of left ventricular mass in the dog with rapid acquisition cardiac CT scanning. Circulation. 1985;72:1355–62.
12. Hajduczok Z, Weiss RM, Marcus ML, Stanford W. Determination of right ventricular mass in humans and dogs with ultrafast computed tomography. Circulation. 1990;82:202.
13. Kuroda T, Seward JB, Rumberger JA, Yanagi H, Tajik AJ. Left ventricular volume and mass: comparative study of 2-dimensional echocardiography and ultrafast computed tomography. Echocardiography. 1994;11:1–9.
14. Rumberger JA. Quantifying left ventricular regional and global systolic function using ultrafast computed tomography. Am J Card Imaging. 1991;5(1):29–37.
15. Feiring AJ, Rumberger JA, Reiter SJ, Collins SM, Skorton DJ, Rees M, et al. Sectional and segmental variability of left ventricular function: experimental and clinical studies using ultrafast computed tomography. J Am Coll Cardiol. 1988;12:415.
16. Lanzer P, Garrett J, Lipton MJ, Gould R, Sievers R, O'Connell W, et al. Quantitation of regional myocardial function by cine computed tomography: pharmacologic changes in wall thickness. J Am Coll Cardiol. 1986;8:682.
17. Feiring AJ, Rumberger JA. Ultrafast computed tomography analysis of regional radius-to-wall thickness ratios in normal and volume-overloaded human left ventricle. Circulation. 1992;85: 1423–32.
18. Rumberger JA, Weiss RM, Feiring AJ, Stanford W, Hajduczok ZD, Rezai K, et al. Patterns of regional diastolic function in the normal human left ventricle: an ultrafast-CT study. J Am Coll Cardiol. 1989;13:119–25.
19. Lipton MJ, Rumberger JA. The assessment of left ventricular systolic and diastolic function by ultrafast computed tomography. Am J Card Imaging. 1991;5:318–27.
20. Rumberger JA, Behrenbeck T, Breen JR, Reed JE, Gersh BJ. Nonparallel changes in global chamber volume and muscle mass during the first year following transmural myocardial infarction in man. J Am Coll Cardiol. 1993;21:673–82.
21. Hirose K, Reed JE, Rumberger JA. Serial changes in left and right ventricular systolic and diastolic mechanics during the first year after an initial left ventricular Q-wave myocardial infarction. J Am Coll Cardiol. 1995;25:1097–104.
22. Hirose K, Shu NH, Reed JE, Rumberger JA. Right ventricular dilatation and remodeling the first year after an initial transmural wall myocardial infarction. Am J Cardiol. 1993;72:1126.
23. Chareonthaitawee P, Christian TF, Hirose K, Gibbons RJA. Relation of initial infarct size with the extent of left ventricular remodeling in the year after acute myocardial infarction. J Am Coll Cardiol. 1995;25:567–73.
24. Sehgal M, Hirose K, Reed JE, Rumberger JA. Regional left ventricular systolic thickening and thicknesses during the first year after initial Q-wave myocardial infarction: serial effects of ventricular remodeling. Int J Cardiol. 1996;53:45–54.
25. Vigneswaran WT, Rumberger JA, Rodeheffer RJ, Breen JF, McGregor CGA. Ventricular remodeling following orthotopic cardiac trans-plantation. Mayo Clin Proc. 1996;71:735–42.
26. Rensing BJ, McDougall JC, Breen JR, Vigneswaran WT, McGregor CGA, Rumberger JA. Right and left ventricular remodeling after orthotopic single lung transplantation for end-stage emphysema. J Heart Lung Transplant. 1997;16:926–33.
27. Gerber T, Rumberger JA, Gibbons R, Behrenbeck T. Measurement of left ventricular ejection fraction by TC-99 M sestamibi first-pass angiography in patients with myocardial infarction: comparison with electron beam computed tomography. Am J Cardiol. 1999;83:1022–6.
28. Schuijf JD, Bax JJ, Jukema JW, Lamb HJ, Vliegen HW, Salm LP, et al. Noninvasive angiography and assessment of left ventricular function using multislice computed tomography in patients with type 2 diabetes. Diabetes Care. 2004;27:2905–10.
29. Dirksen MS, Bax JJ, de Roos A, Jukema JW, van der Geest RJ, Geleijns K, et al. Usefulness of dynamic multislice computed tomography of left ventricular function in unstable angina pectoris and comparison with echocardiography. Am J Cardiol. 2002;90:1157–60.
30. Rumberger JA, Sheedy PF, Breen JF. Use of ultrafast (cine) x-ray of right and left ventricular volume measurements by electron-beam computed tomography in cardiac and cardiovascular imaging. In: Guiliani ER, Gersh BJ, McGoon MD, Dayes DL, Shaff HF, editors. Mayo clinic practice of cardiology. 3rd ed. St. Louis: Mosby; 1996. p. 303–24.
31. Rumberger JA, Reed JE. Quantitative dynamics of left ventricular emptying and filling as a function of heart size and stroke volume in pure aortic regurgitation and in normal subjects. Am J Cardiol. 1992;70:1045–50.
32. Weiss RM, Stark CA, Rumberger JA, Marcus ML. Identification and quantitation of myocardial infarction or risk area size with cine-computed tomography. Am J Card Imaging. 1990;4:33–7.
33. Schmermund A, Gerber T, Behrenbeck T, Reed JE, Sheedy PF, Christian TF, et al. Myocardial infarct size by electron beam computed tomography: a comparison with ^{99m}Tc sestamibi. Invest Radiol. 1998;33:313–21.
34. Schmermund A, Breen JF, Sheedy PF, Rumberger JA. Reproducibility of right and left ventricular volume measurement by electron-beam CT in patients with congestive heart failure. Int J Card Imaging. 1998;14(3):201–9.
35. Lang RM, et al. Recommendations for chamber quantification: a report from the American Society of Echocardiography's Guidelines and Standards Committee and the Chamber Quantification Writing Group, Developed in Conjunction with the European Association of Echocardiography, A Branch of the Europena Society of Cardiology. J Am Soc Echocardiogr. 2005;18:1440–63.
36. Soh EK, villines TC, Feuerstein IM. Sixty-four-multislice computed tomography in a patient with arrhythmogenic right ventricular dysplasia. J Cardiovasc Comput Tomogr. 2008;2:191–2.
37. Policy number: PP25-A: AAPM position statement on radiations risks from medical imaging procedures. Policy Date 12/13/11; Sunset Date 12/31/16. http://www.aapm.org/org/policies/details.asp?id=318&type=PP¤t=true.
38. Bardo DME, Kachenoura N, Newby B, Lang RM, Mor-Avi V. Multidetector computed tomography evaluation of left ventricular volumes: sources of error and guidelines for their minimization. J Cardiovasc Comput Tomogr. 2008;2:222–30.

Cardiovascular CT for Perfusion and Delayed Contrast Enhancement Imaging

12

Ravi K. Sharma, Ilan Gottlieb, and João A.C. Lima

Abstract

Recent advancements in multi-detector computed tomography (MDCT) imaging have demonstrated the ability of MDCT to be a comprehensive imaging modality, which in a single scan setting could provide a wide array of complementary information. Advent of MDCT system with faster scan acquisition of entire myocardial volume has allowed assessment of stress myocardial perfusion that has shown to provide incremental diagnostic accuracy over coronary CT angiography (CTA) in assessing hemodynamically significant stenosis.

Detection of fibrosis by Delayed Enhanced MDCT (DE-MDCT) has been validated against gold standards such as histology and contrast enhanced MRI. DE-MDCT can accurately identify and characterize morphological features of acute and healed myocardial infarction, including infarct size, transmurality, and the presence of microvascular obstruction and collagenous scar. In addition, recent studies have also substantiated the utility of contrast enhanced MDCT in assessment of extracellular volume fraction (ECV) which corresponds to diffuse myocardial fibrosis. This has allowed comprehensive evaluation of myocardial tissue characteristics with significant bearing on the management, prognosis and follow-up of a myocardial disease process.

Keywords

Computed tomography perfusion • Stress CT perfusion • Delayed enhanced MDCT • MDCT myocardial viability • Myocardial fibrosis

Electronic supplementary material The online version of this chapter (doi:10.1007/978-3-319-28219-0_12) contains supplementary material, which is available to authorized users.

R.K. Sharma, MD • J.A.C. Lima, MD (✉)
Division of Cardiology, Johns Hopkins Hospital,
Blalock 524D, 600 N. Wolfe St, Baltimore, MD 21287, USA
e-mail: rsharm25@jhmi.edu; jlima@jhmi.edu

I. Gottlieb, MD Msc, PhD
Casa de Saúde São José – Radiologia,
R. Macedo Sobrinho, 21 – Humaitá, Rio de Janeiro,
RJ 22271-080, Brazil
e-mail: ilangottlieb@gmail.com

Abbreviations

CAD	Coronary Artery Disease
CTA	Coronary CT Angiography
DE-MDCT	Delayed enhanced MDCT
ECV	Extracellular Volume Fraction
LAD	Left Anterior Descending
LV	Left Ventricle
MDCT	Multi-Detector Computed Tomography
MRI	Magnetic Resonance Imaging
PET	Positron Emission Tomography
SPECT	Single Photon Emission Computed Tomography

M.J. Budoff, J.S. Shinbane (eds.), *Cardiac CT Imaging: Diagnosis of Cardiovascular Disease*,
DOI 10.1007/978-3-319-28219-0_12

Subject Overview

A 54 year old male with diabetes and family history of coronary artery disease (CAD) comes to a cardiologist for the first time for atypical chest pain. The patient reports "having to grasp for air" while in chest pain. A rest electrocardiogram (ECG) is done at the office, in which non-specific T wave changes were the only abnormality. Besides blood tests, the cardiologist orders an echocardiogram that shows reduced left ventricle (LV) function and akinesis of the mid and apical anterior-septal walls and a stress single photon emission computed tomography (SPECT) study that shows a perfusion defect in the same regions, with little reversibility on the rest images. Thinking this is most likely ischemic coronary disease, the cardiologist orders a cardiac magnetic resonance imaging (MRI) for viability evaluation prior to the invasive coronary angiography, which showed an occluded mid left anterior descending (LAD) artery with distal filling via collaterals. Given the presence of viability on the MRI scan, the patient successfully underwent percutaneous coronary intervention of the mid-LAD lesion and two months later LV function shows improvement and the patient is asymptomatic.

Cardiologists are familiar with relying on a number of different imaging modalities for a thorough assessment of cardiovascular diseases and further decision making. Coronary anatomy evaluation is usually performed using invasive catheterization or more recently by non-invasive MDCT scans. Global and regional myocardial function as well as structural abnormalities can be assessed with echocardiography, MRI and MDCT. Subclinical atherosclerosis is usually assessed via detection of coronary calcium using MDCT or electron beam CT scanners or via measuring carotid intima-media thickness with ultrasound; while ischemia detection and quantification at stress are usually performed with nuclear SPECT or positron emission tomography (PET), echo or MRI imaging. Finally myocardial fibrosis for viability and prognosis assessment is usually detected and quantified by MRI and nuclear techniques.

Recent advancements in MDCT imaging have demonstrated the feasibility of MDCT to be a comprehensive imaging modality, which in a single scan setting could provide a wide array of complementary information. Ideally, using one imaging modality to perform all these assessments during a single scan setting could have substantial economic implications, may serve to reduce patient anxiety, and improve workflow.

Ischemia Detection by MDCT

The notion that CT could provide information on myocardial perfusion has been documented in the past by investigators using electron beam CT [1]. However, the combination of a reliable coronary angiogram with stress-induced myocardial perfusion assessment had to wait until spiral CT technology progressed sufficiently to enable the acquisition of 64 slices simultaneously [2]. Advent of wide array single source (256 or 320) and dual source detector scanning system with faster gantry rotation time has allowed rapid acquisition of entire cardiac volume with low radiation exposure, making MDCT perfusion imaging more feasible and safe to perform.

Currently, the greatest limitations to CT coronary angiography are the presence of severely calcified coronary segments, stents, or other artifacts that limit luminal visualization. Patients with calcified arteries tend to be older and/or have advanced CAD. Their studies are challenging from a diagnostic viewpoint because vulnerable plaques and stenotic lesions may be hidden underneath large amounts of calcium accumulated in the atherosclerotic plaques encompassing one or more segments. While progress in multidetector technology has improved our ability to study such patients, greater coverage and improved temporal resolution are unlikely to eliminate the problem, which is in large part intrinsic to the pathogenesis of atherosclerosis, namely, plaques grow outwardly first and tend to accumulate calcium as part of the healing process, therefore creating a natural shield to X-ray penetration. That is a particular limitation to the study of older persons, patients with advanced CAD, and patients who underwent coronary artery bypass graft surgery or multiple stent implantation, as well as patients with diseases such as chronic renal failure that accelerate plaque calcification.

Furthermore, coronary anatomic information is much more valuable when combined with a functional test, since some decisions regarding treatment are based on the detection of myocardial ischemia [3]. Corresponding perfusion deficit related to an anatomic stenosis also confers worse clinical prognosis [4]. The poor correlation between anatomic modalities such as invasive coronary angiography [5, 6] and MDCT [7] with stress perfusion tests underscores the fact that one cannot substitute for the other.

Myocardial perfusion measurements by MDCT are derived from the upslope differences in contrast enhancement between the ischemic and remote areas (Fig. 12.1). Previous generation 64-detector scanners had limited coverage of the heart, resulting in the base of the heart being scanned earlier in time than the apex, making comparisons in signal intensities between the two areas problematic. In this regard, the introduction of wide coverage MDCT technology allowed the entire heart to be imaged in one gantry rotation (Fig. 12.2) combined with the capability of programming such gated image acquisitions to occur only during specific portions of a given cardiac cycle (Fig. 12.3). This created a brand new horizon of possibilities to reduce radiation exposure enough to enable the performance of combined angiography and myocardial perfusion assessment during stress, which associated with the angiographic and delayed enhanced images, should provide a comprehensive cardiac assessment. Also, with more coverage and faster acquisition,

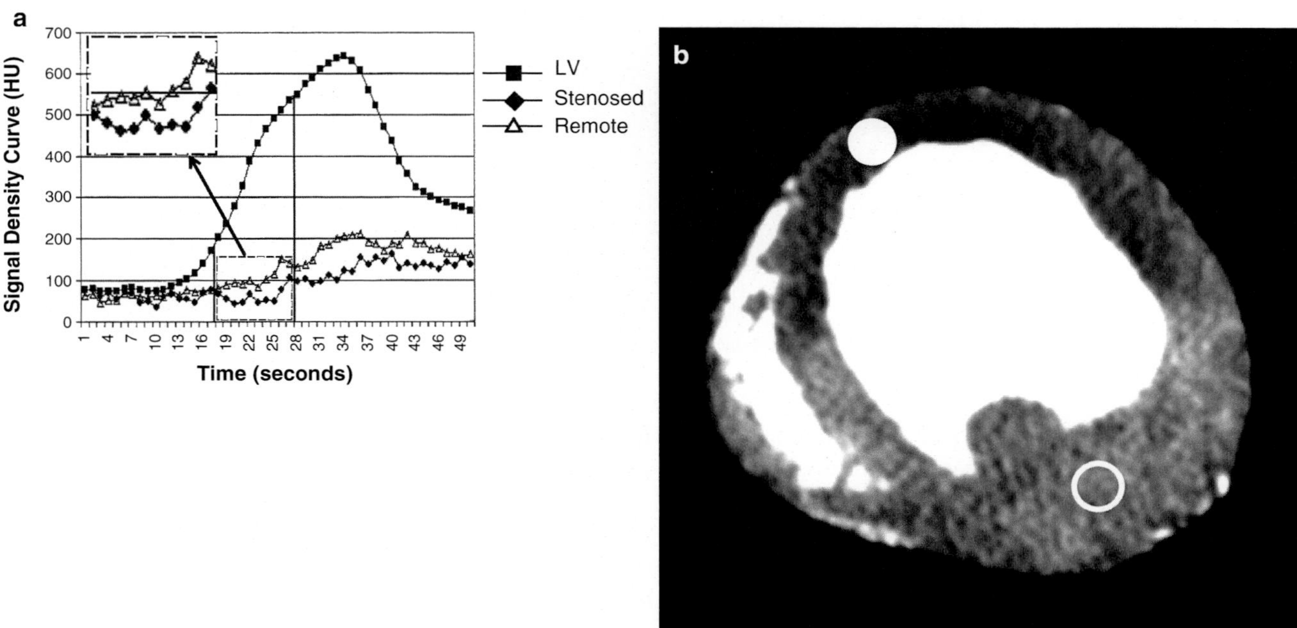

Fig. 12.1 Myocardial enhancement upslope curves for the left ventricular cavity, remote and ischemic region (**a**). The usual timing of a coronary CT angiogram is shown as the region between the vertical bars. following the contrast bolus with an ROI placed at the ischemic (*filled circle*) and remote (*open circle*) areas present a delta in myocardial enhancement intensity (**b**) that can be measured, as shown inside the dashed box (**a**)

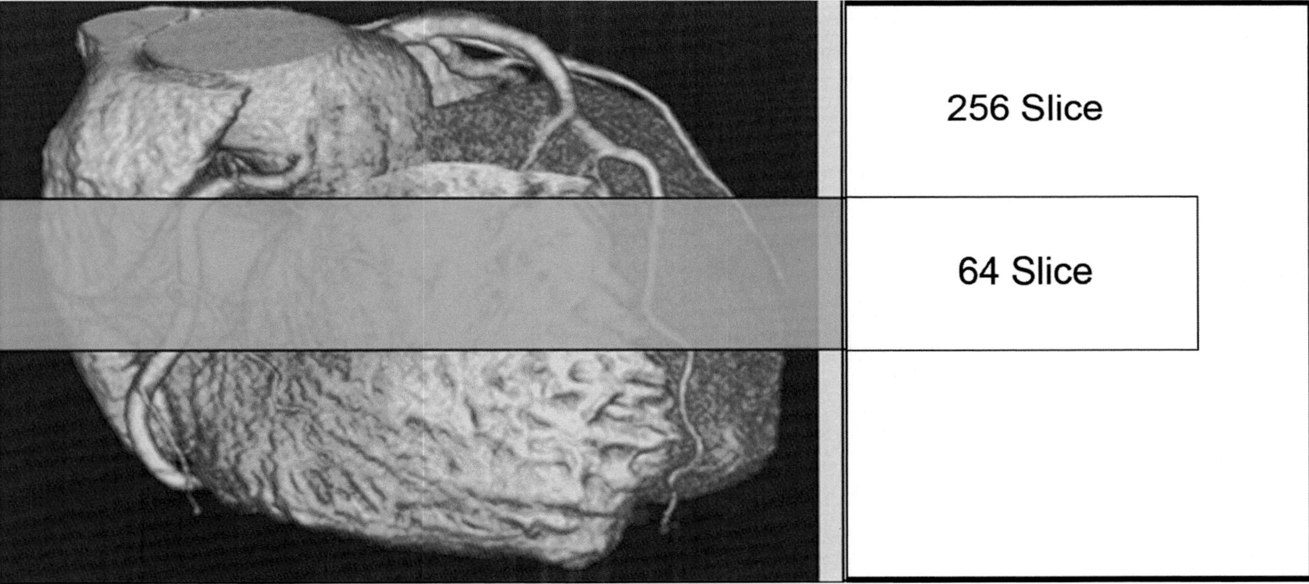

Fig. 12.2 Schematic coverage of a 256-detector as compared to a 64-detector MDCT scanner

scan times have decreased, reducing the amount of contrast material per scan [8]. Such techniques are ideal for the assessment of patients with chest pain who also have calcified coronaries, as well as the follow up of patients with advanced heart disease post coronary artery bypass surgery or multiple stent implantations.

Using iodine molecules as a tracer, current research has demonstrated that by measuring the concentration in time of the tracer in the myocardium, MDCT can determine absolute blood flow in different regions of the myocardium [2]. Recent attention to patients with chest pain but no obstructive epicardial CAD (syndrome X) has demonstrated that in

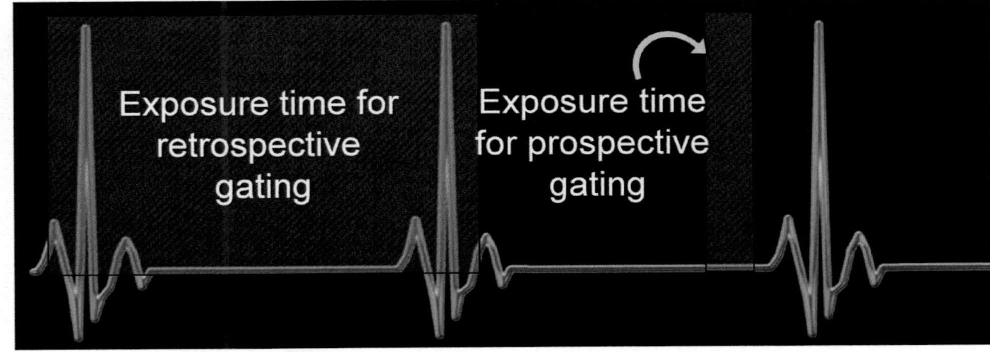

Fig. 12.3 Schematic demonstration of the radiation exposure time differences between retrospective gating (single heart beat) and prospective triggering used in wide coverage MDCT scanners

a substantial proportion of these individuals microvascular processes can be identified by perfusion reserve measurements in association with traditional CAD risk factors such as hypercholesterolemia, hypertension and smoking as well as with diabetes [9]. The possibility of quantifying epicardial coronary plaque while also assessing microvascular disease during maximal vasodilatation enables coronary MDCTA – armored with high spatial resolution – to characterize macrovascular atherosclerosis as well as microvascular dysfunction secondary to atherosclerosis or other disease processes. The capability of quantifying myocardial blood flow by contrast enhanced MDCT represent a "quantum leap" in our ability to assess and characterize the entire process of cardiac atherosclerosis.

Single center studies [10–12] have demonstrated the incremental diagnostic performance of MDCT stress perfusion imaging in addition to coronary CTA in assessing flow-limiting stenosis. Subsequently, the CORE320 study [13], a multicenter, international study also validated improved diagnostic accuracy of coronary CTA plus MDCT perfusion imaging compared to the reference standard of invasive coronary angiography plus a corresponding perfusion deficit on SPECT imaging. On head to head comparison, the ability of stress MDCT perfusion imaging to detect myocardial ischemia was similar to SPECT imaging, with better MDCT sensitivity for left main and multivessel stenoses [14]. This enhanced sensitivity is attributed to better spatial resolution of MDCT and favorable kinetics of iodine dye which serves as a tracer in MDCT perfusion imaging.

Previously limited to single center experience [10, 15–17], current efforts are directed towards expanding this technique to different MDCT scanner systems (including 64-, 128-, 256-, and 320-slice) and across multivendor platform using different stress agents. The ongoing multicenter, multivendor study of Regadenoson in Subjects Undergoing Stress Myocardial Perfusion Imaging Using Multidetector Computed Tomography Compared to Single Photon Emission Computed Tomography [18] (www.clinicaltrials.gov, NCT01334918) is a step in this direction.

MDCT for Detection of Myocardial Fibrosis and Viability

The ability to distinguish dysfunctional but viable myocardium from nonviable tissue after acute or chronic ischemia has important implications for the therapeutic management of patients with coronary artery disease [19, 20]. Image-based characterization of myocardial scar morphology can identify those patients with hibernating myocardium who may achieve functional systolic recovery with revascularization [21]. The assessment of myocardial viability and infarct morphology with delayed contrast-enhanced MRI has been well validated over the past several years and is performed routinely at several clinical cardiac MRI centers.

The recent advent of MDCT technology has expanded its potential for a more comprehensive evaluation of cardiovascular diseases. While hypo attenuation in the non-contrasted scan (due to fatty degeneration of the infarcted area) or during the contrast enhanced coronary angiography scan has been shown to demonstrate areas of previous MI, it is largely underestimated by MDCT [22, 23]. Delayed enhanced MDCT (DE-MDCT) myocardial imaging can accurately identify and characterize morphological features of acute and healed myocardial infarction, including infarct size, transmurality, and the presence of microvascular obstruction and collagenous scar (Fig. 12.4) [24, 25]. Infarcted myocardial tissue by DE-MDCT is characterized by well-delineated hyper-enhanced regions, whereas regions of microvascular obstruction by MDCT are characterized by hypo-enhancement on imaging early after MI [24, 25]. Detection of fibrosis by DE-MDCT has been validated against gold standards such as histology and contrast enhanced MRI [24, 26–28]. In addition, recent studies [29, 30] have also substantiated the utility of contrast enhanced MDCT in assessment of extracellular volume fraction (ECV), a measurement of interstitial myocardial volume expansion which corresponds to diffuse myocardial fibrosis.

Introduction of delayed contrast enhanced MDCT imaging in assessment of hypertrophic cardiomyopathy has been

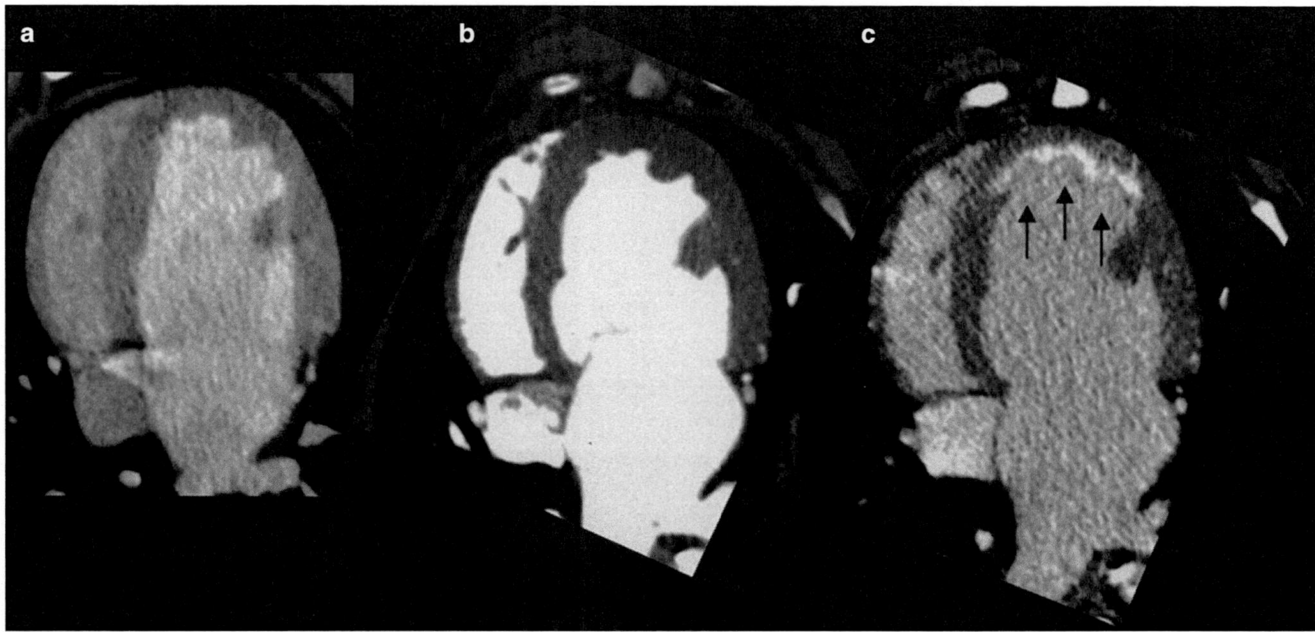

Fig. 12.4 Typical contrast-enhanced myocardial MDCT images showing axial slices (**a**) at baseline (preinfarct) 5 min after contrast, (**b**) postinfarct during first-pass contrast injection, and (**c**) postinfarct 5 min after contrast injection. the infarcted region is represented by the subendocardial anterior hyperintense region (*arrows*)

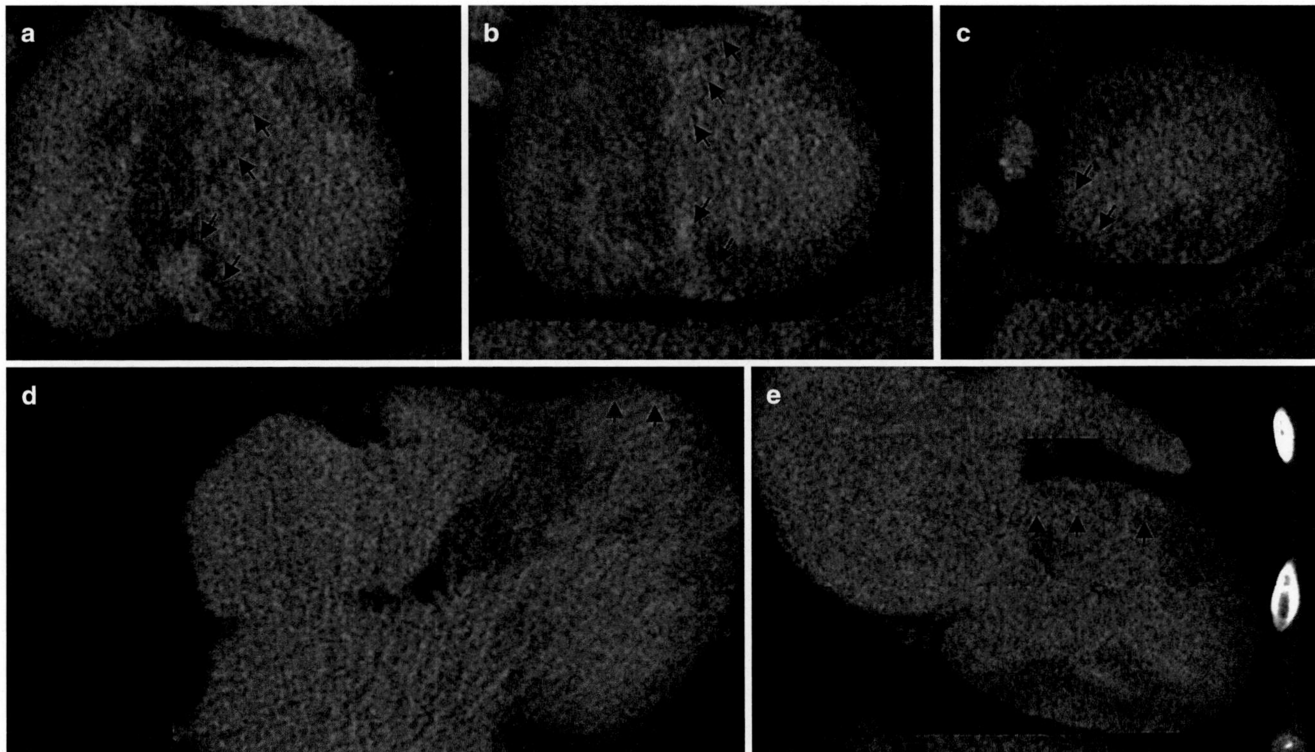

Fig. 12.5 Multiplanar reconstruction of the left ventricular basal (**a**), mid (**b**), and apical short-axis (**c**) views and horizontal (**d**) and vertical long-axis (**e**) views show delayed hyperenhancement in the basal anterior, basal to mid septal, and apical septal walls (*arrows*). A small aneurysm is noted in the apical septum (**c**, **d**) (Reprinted from Gore R et al. [41] with permission from Elsevier)

of particular interest where it has shown comparable accuracy to delayed contrast enhanced MRI in detecting myocardial fibrosis (Fig. 12.5) [31–33]. This has allowed comprehensive evaluation of myocardial tissue characteristics with significant bearing on the management [31], prognosis [34], and follow-up in these patients who may not be ideal candidates for MRI given significant proportion of them have implantable cardiac defibrillator.

The mechanism of myocardial hyperenhancement and hypo-enhancement in acutely injured myocardial territories after iodinated contrast administration is similar to that proposed for delayed gadolinium-enhanced MRI [19]. Under conditions of normal myocyte function, sarcolemmal membranes serve to exclude iodine from the intracellular space. After myocyte necrosis, however, membrane dysfunction ensues, and iodine molecules are able to penetrate the cell. Because 75 % of the total myocardial volume is intracellular, large increases in the volume of distribution are achieved, which results in marked hyperenhancement relative to the non-injured myocytes. The mechanism of hyperenhance-

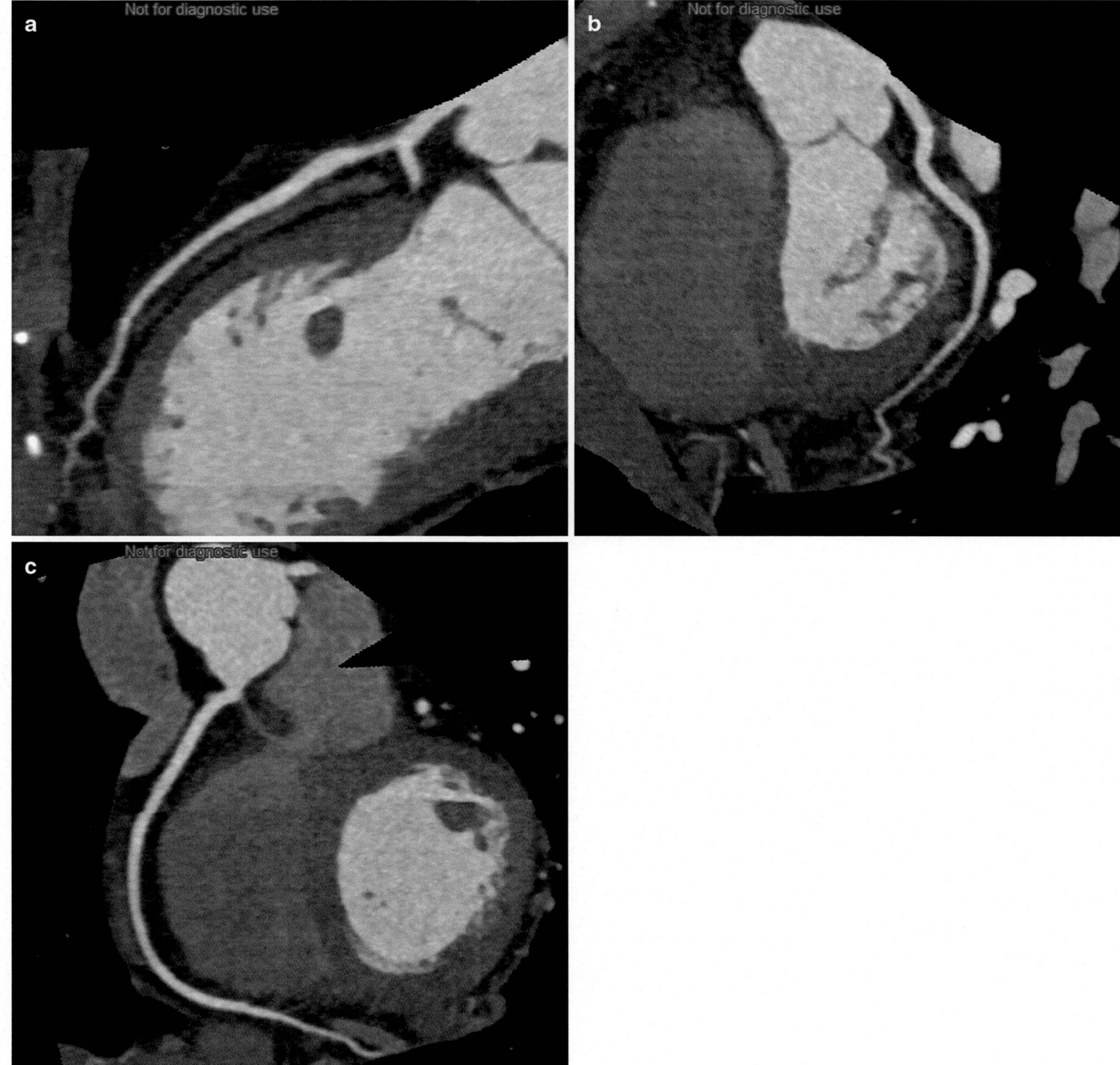

Fig. 12.6 Multiplanar reconstruction images showing normal left anterior descending (**a**), left circumflex (**b**), and right coronary artery (**c**)

ment of healed myocardial infarction or collagenous scar is thought to be related to an accumulation of contrast media in the interstitial space between collagen fibers and thus an increased volume of distribution compared with that of tightly packed myocytes. The low signal intensity of microvascular obstruction regions despite restoration of normal flow through the infarct-related artery is explained by the death and subsequent cellular debris blockage of intramyocardial capillaries at the core of the damaged region. These obstructed capillaries do not allow contrast material to flow into the damaged bed, which results in a region of low signal intensity compared with normal myocardium. In minutes to hours, contrast material is able to penetrate this relatively "no reflow" region, and the necrotic myocytes that reside in that myocardial territory then become hyperenhanced as iodine is internalized by the cell. In weeks the microvascular obstruction area is replaced by collagenous scar tissue and the former dark area now become bright. Since the transmurality of delayed enhancement predicts functional recovery after revascularization [21], the better spatial resolution of MDCT as compared to CMR may influence the accuracy of viability assessment, but no study thus far has tested this hypothesis.

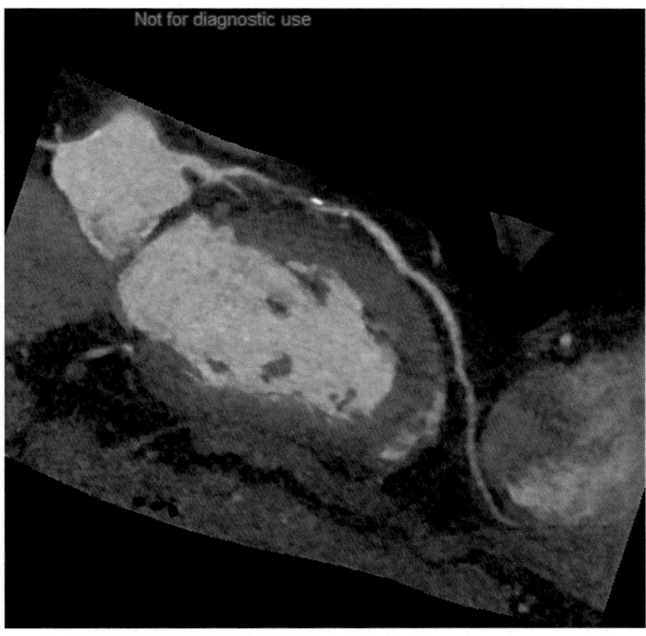

Fig. 12.7 Multiplanar reconstruction image showing obstructive coronary artery stenosis of left anterior descending artery (**a**)

Integrating All Methodologies into One Examination

The number of scans to be performed varies for individual patients, depending on the clinical questions to be answered. For a comprehensive cardiac evaluation, in the future four consecutive scans should be performed, with acceptable radiation dose. The first one would be a low dose prospectively unenhanced calcium score scan (<1 mSv) [35], the second one also prospectively gated and contrasted for the acquisition of coronary angiography and morphology (approximately 1–4 mSv) [36], the third would be the stress perfusion study during maximum vasodilation, which could be performed as a "static" perfusion acquisition, i.e. one acquisition at peak contrast opacification of the myocardium (approximately 1–4 mSv); or alternatively as a "dynamic" perfusion acquisition, i.e. several low dose prospective acquisitions representing the contrast passage through the heart (approximately 3–7 mSv) (Fig. 12.6 and 12.7, Videos 12.1, 12.2, 12.3, and 12.4).[16] Static perfusion has been more validated and can be performed in scanners with 4 cm coverage or more, but dynamic perfusion might improve accuracy, by allowing construction of contrast wash in curves in the myocardium. For that, one would need a scanner with at least 8 cm coverage, multiple "shots" are acquired during contrast administration and at least a large portion of the myocardium needs to be imaged at each "shot". Finally, a low dose prospectively triggered delayed enhancement scan would be performed 5–10 min after the stress study (1–3 mSv) [36]. The final result would be calcium score, coronary anatomy, morphology, stress perfusion and viability in a "one stop shop" scan that lasts around 20 min. (Fig. 12.8) shows a timeline for a comprehensive cardiac evaluation. Employing dose reduction techniques [37] like

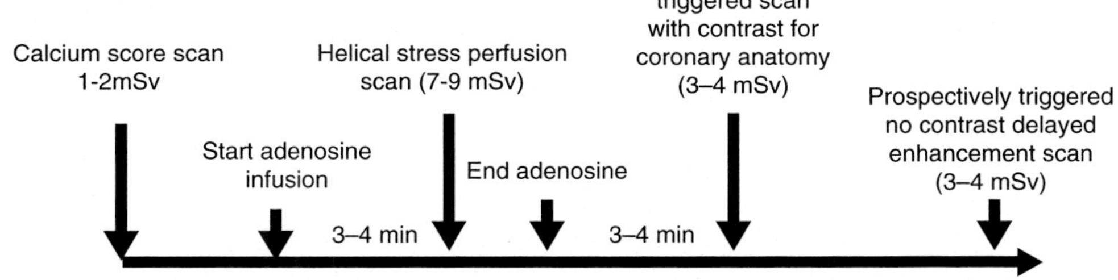

Fig. 12.8 Proposed timeline for a comprehensive MDCT scan

limiting scan length, prospective scan acquisition, post processing methods such as iterative reconstruction and filtered back projection [38], and availability of next generation scanners with faster gantry rotation time and wide volume coverage could result in substantial reduction in the amount of radiation exposure, allowing one to acquire enhanced information at the cost of less than 10 mSv of radiation.

Clinical Pearls DE

1. The optimal contrast dose to be used for DE images is still not defined, but studies in humans [23, 25] showed that the usual amount used for a 16-detector coronary CTA (120–140 ml) provide good enhancement and could be as low as 80–90 ml using advanced scanner system.[31]
2. For optimal contrast between the infarcted and the remote regions, the delayed enhanced scan should be done between 5 and 10 min after contrast injection.[24]
3. Most of the studies done so far reconstructed the images in end-diastole for DE analysis.
4. The delayed enhancement pattern is important to differentiate between ischemic and non-ischemic etiologies, the earlier being found as a wave front from the endocardium to the pericardium. Non-ischemic cardiomyopathies can also result in myocardial scar that appears on DE images, but those tend to be patchy and do not follow the endocardium-to-epicardium pattern seen in ischemic cardiomyopathy.[39]
5. Molecular size of the iodinated contrast material may affect the uptake of the tissue by that agent. Two trials used a smaller molecule with high iodine concentration (iomeprol) [23, 25] while another one used a larger molecule with a lower iodine concentration (iodixanol).[24] It is still unclear which one is the best, if any, or whether other factors (such as ionic polarization) are important.
6. DE imaging by MDCT can be obtained both in patients with an acute MI as well as patients that had infarcts more than 6 months prior to imaging.[23–25]
7. Microvascular obstruction can be imaged in the early phase after MI, and it is gradually replaced by fibrous tissue that appears bright on the DE images 2–4 weeks after the MI.[40]

Clinical Pearls Ischemia

1. MDCT myocardial perfusion is shown to have incremental diagnostic accuracy in identifying or excluding hemodynamically significant stenosis.
2. Adenosine is the drug most often tested for stress perfusion in MDCT, due to its short onset and offset, safety profile and proved efficacy in diverging blood from ischemic to non-ischemic territories. Utility of regadenoson is currently being explored.[18]
3. Since adenosine usually increases heart rate, aggressive beta-blockade should be pursued. Adequate hydration prior to the scan may potentially blunt the reflex increase in heart rate from the adenosine infusion.
4. Nitroglycerin should not be given concomitantly to adenosine, since it can reverse the ischemic effects of the latter, as well as decrease blood pressure and increase heart rate even further.
5. The visual contouring of the underperfused myocardial areas is the method currently being applied in addition to the semi-automated software. However, the best threshold for quantitatively discriminating ischemia from remote myocardium is still not defined.
6. The problem of balanced ischemia will potentially be solved with wide coverage MDCT scanners by allowing absolute quantification of myocardial blood flow.
7. Whether stress perfusion scans will be recommended to everyone or just selected patient populations (such as the ones with high calcium scores) is still under investigation.

References

1. Lerman LO, Siripornpitak S, Maffei NL, Sheedy 2nd PF, Ritman EL. Measurement of in vivo myocardial microcirculatory function with electron beam CT. J Comput Assist Tomogr. 1999;23:390–8.
2. George RT, Jerosch-Herold M, Silva C, Kitagawa K, Bluemke DA, Lima JA, Lardo AC. Quantification of myocardial perfusion using dynamic 64-detector computed tomography. Invest Radiol. 2007;42:815–22.
3. Smith Jr SC, Feldman TE, Hirshfeld Jr JW, Jacobs AK, Kern MJ, King SB, Morrison DA, O'Neil WW, Schaff HV, Whitlow PL, Williams DO, Antman EM, Adams CD, Anderson JL, Faxon DP, Fuster V, Halperin JL, Hiratzka LF, Hunt SA, Nishimura R, Ornato JP, Page RL, Riegel B. ACC/AHA/SCAI 2005 guideline update for percutaneous coronary intervention: a report of the American College of Cardiology/American Heart Association Task Force on Practice Guidelines (ACC/AHA/SCAI Writing Committee to Update 2001 Guidelines for Percutaneous Coronary Intervention. Circulation. 2006;113:166–286.
4. van Werkhoven JM, Schuijf JD, Gaemperli O, Jukema JW, Boersma E, Wijns W, Stolzmann P, Alkadhi H, Valenta I, Stokkel MP, Kroft LJ, de Roos A, Pundziute G, Scholte A, van der Wall EE, Kaufmann PA, Bax JJ. Prognostic value of multislice computed tomography and gated single-photon emission computed tomography in patients with suspected coronary artery disease. J Am Coll Cardiol. 2009;53:623–32.
5. Rodes-Cabau J, Candell-Riera J, Angel J, de Leon G, Pereztol O, Castell-Conesa J, Soto A, Anivarro I, Aguade S, Vazquez M, Domingo E, Tardif JC, Soler-Soler J. Relation of myocardial perfusion defects and nonsignificant coronary lesions by angiography with insights from intravascular ultrasound and coronary pressure measurements. Am J Cardiol. 2005;96:1621–6.
6. Ragosta M, Bishop AH, Lipson LC, Watson DD, Gimple LW, Sarembock IJ, Powers ER. Comparison between angiography and

fractional flow reserve versus single-photon emission computed tomographic myocardial perfusion imaging for determining lesion significance in patients with multivessel coronary disease. Am J Cardiol. 2007;99:896–902.

7. Schuijf JD, Wijns W, Jukema JW, Atsma DE, de Roos A, Lamb HJ, Stokkel MP, Dibbets-Schneider P, Decramer I, De Bondt P, van der Wall EE, Vanhoenacker PK, Bax JJ. Relationship between noninvasive coronary angiography with multi-slice computed tomography and myocardial perfusion imaging. J Am Coll Cardiol. 2006;48:2508–14.
8. Hein PA, May J, Rogalla P, Butler C, Hamm B, Lembcke A. Feasibility of contrast material volume reduction in coronary artery imaging using 320-slice volume CT. Eur Radiol. 2010;20:1337–43.
9. Buchthal SD, den Hollander JA, Merz CN, Rogers WJ, Pepine CJ, Reichek N, Sharaf BL, Reis S, Kelsey SF, Pohost GM. Abnormal myocardial phosphorus-31 nuclear magnetic resonance spectroscopy in women with chest pain but normal coronary angiograms. N Engl J Med. 2000;342:829–35.
10. Cury RC, Magalhaes TA, Borges AC, Shiozaki AA, Lemos PA, Junior JS, Meneghetti JC, Rochitte CE. Dipyridamole stress and rest myocardial perfusion by 64-detector row computed tomography in patients with suspected coronary artery disease. Am J Cardiol. 2010;106:310–5.
11. George RT, Arbab-Zadeh A, Miller JM, Vavere AL, Bengel FM, Lardo AC, Lima JA. Computed tomography myocardial perfusion imaging with 320-row detector computed tomography accurately detects myocardial ischemia in patients with obstructive coronary artery disease. Circ Cardiovasc Imaging. 2012;5:333–40.
12. Rief M, Zimmermann E, Stenzel F, Martus P, Stangl K, Greupner J, Knebel F, Kranz A, Schlattmann P, Laule M, Dewey M. Computed tomography angiography and myocardial computed tomography perfusion in patients with coronary stents: prospective intraindividual comparison with conventional coronary angiography. J Am Coll Cardiol. 2013;62:1476–85.
13. Rochitte CE, George RT, Chen MY, Arbab-Zadeh A, Dewey M, Miller JM, Niinuma H, Yoshioka K, Kitagawa K, Nakamori S, Laham R, Vavere AL, Cerci RJ, Mehra VC, Nomura C, Kofoed KF, Jinzaki M, Kuribayashi S, de Roos A, Laule M, Tan SY, Hoe J, Paul N, Rybicki FJ, Brinker JA, Arai AE, Cox C, Clouse ME, Di Carli MF, Lima JA. Computed tomography angiography and perfusion to assess coronary artery stenosis causing perfusion defects by single photon emission computed tomography: the CORE320 study. Eur Heart J. 2014;35:1120–30.
14. George RT, Mehra VC, Chen MY, Kitagawa K, Arbab-Zadeh A, Miller JM, Matheson MB, Vavere AL, Kofoed KF, Rochitte CE, Dewey M, Yaw TS, Niinuma H, Brenner W, Cox C, Clouse ME, Lima JA, Di Carli M. Myocardial CT perfusion imaging and SPECT for the diagnosis of coronary artery disease: a Head-to-Head comparison from the CORE320 multicenter diagnostic performance study. Radiology. 2014;272:407–16.
15. Rocha-Filho JA, Blankstein R, Shturman LD, Bezerra HG, Okada DR, Rogers IS, Ghoshhajra B, Hoffmann U, Feuchtner G, Mamuya WS, Brady TJ, Cury RC. Incremental value of adenosine-induced stress myocardial perfusion imaging with dual-source CT at cardiac CT angiography. Radiology. 2010;254:410–9.
16. George RT, Arbab-Zadeh A, Miller JM, Kitagawa K, Chang HJ, Bluemke DA, Becker L, Yousuf O, Texter J, Lardo AC, Lima JA. Adenosine stress 64- and 256-row detector computed tomography angiography and perfusion imaging: a pilot study evaluating the transmural extent of perfusion abnormalities to predict atherosclerosis causing myocardial ischemia. Circ Cardiovasc Imaging. 2009;2:174–82.
17. Blankstein R, Shturman LD, Rogers IS, Rocha-Filho JA, Okada DR, Sarwar A, Soni AV, Bezerra H, Ghoshhajra BB, Petranovic M, Loureiro R, Feuchtner G, Gewirtz H, Hoffmann U, Mamuya WS, Brady TJ, Cury RC. Adenosine-induced stress myocardial perfusion imaging using dual-source cardiac computed tomography. J Am Coll Cardiol. 2009;54:1072–84.
18. Cury RC, Kitt TM, Feaheny K, Akin J, George RT. Regadenoson-stress myocardial CT perfusion and single-photon emission CT: rationale, design, and acquisition methods of a prospective, multicenter, multivendor comparison. J Cardiovasc Comput Tomogr. 2014;8:2–12.
19. Wu KC, Lima JA. Noninvasive imaging of myocardial viability: current techniques and future developments. Circ Res. 2003;93:1146–58.
20. Pagley PR, Beller GA, Watson DD, Gimple LW, Ragosta M. Improved outcome after coronary bypass surgery in patients with ischemic cardiomyopathy and residual myocardial viability. Circulation. 1997;96:793–800.
21. Kim RJ, Wu E, Rafael A, Chen EL, Parker MA, Simonetti O, Klocke FJ, Bonow RO, Judd RM. The use of contrast-enhanced magnetic resonance imaging to identify reversible myocardial dysfunction. N Engl J Med. 2000;343:1445–53.
22. Sanz J, Weeks D, Nikolaou K, Sirol M, Rius T, Rajagopalan S, Dellegrottaglie S, Strobeck J, Fuster V, Poon M. Detection of healed myocardial infarction with multidetector-row computed tomography and comparison with cardiac magnetic resonance delayed hyperenhancement. Am J Cardiol. 2006;98:149–55.
23. Mahnken AH, Koos R, Katoh M, Wildberger JE, Spuentrup E, Buecker A, Gunther RW, Kuhl HP. Assessment of myocardial viability in reperfused acute myocardial infarction using 16-slice computed tomography in comparison to magnetic resonance imaging. J Am Coll Cardiol. 2005;45:2042–7.
24. Lardo AC, Cordeiro MA, Silva C, Amado LC, George RT, Saliaris AP, Schuleri KH, Fernandes VR, Zviman M, Nazarian S, Halperin HR, Wu KC, Hare JM, Lima JA. Contrast-enhanced multidetector computed tomography viability imaging after myocardial infarction: characterization of myocyte death, microvascular obstruction, and chronic scar. Circulation. 2006;113:394–404.
25. Gerber BL, Belge B, Legros GJ, Lim P, Poncelet A, Pasquet A, Gisellu G, Coche E, Vanoverschelde JL. Characterization of acute and chronic myocardial infarcts by multidetector computed tomography: comparison with contrast-enhanced magnetic resonance. Circulation. 2006;113:823–33.
26. Bauer RW, Kerl JM, Fischer N, Burkhard T, Larson MC, Ackermann H, Vogl TJ. Dual-energy CT for the assessment of chronic myocardial infarction in patients with chronic coronary artery disease: comparison with 3-T MRI. AJR Am J Roentgenol. 2010;195:639–46.
27. Schuleri KH, Centola M, George RT, Amado LC, Evers KS, Kitagawa K, Vavere AL, Evers R, Hare JM, Cox C, McVeigh ER, Lima JA, Lardo AC. Characterization of peri-infarct zone heterogeneity by contrast-enhanced multidetector computed tomography: a comparison with magnetic resonance imaging. J Am Coll Cardiol. 2009;53:1699–707.
28. Senra T, Shiozaki AA, Salemi VM, Rochitte CE. Delayed enhancement by multidetector computed tomography in endomyocardial fibrosis. Eur Heart J. 2008;29:347.
29. Nacif MS, Kawel N, Lee JJ, Chen X, Yao J, Zavodni A, Sibley CT, Lima JA, Liu S, Bluemke DA. Interstitial myocardial fibrosis assessed as extracellular volume fraction with low-radiation-dose cardiac CT. Radiology. 2012;264:876–83.
30. Nacif MS, Liu Y, Yao J, Liu S, Sibley CT, Summers RM, Bluemke DA. 3D left ventricular extracellular volume fraction by low-radiation dose cardiac CT: assessment of interstitial myocardial fibrosis. J Cardiovasc Comput Tomogr. 2013;7:51–7.
31. Zhao L, Ma X, Delano MC, Jiang T, Zhang C, Liu Y, Zhang Z. Assessment of myocardial fibrosis and coronary arteries in hypertrophic cardiomyopathy using combined arterial and delayed

enhanced CT: comparison with MR and coronary angiography. Eur Radiol. 2013;23:1034–43.

32. Langer C, Lutz M, Eden M, Ludde M, Hohnhorst M, Gierloff C, Both M, Burchert W, Faber L, Horstkotte D, Frey N, Prinz C. Hypertrophic cardiomyopathy in cardiac CT: a validation study on the detection of intramyocardial fibrosis in consecutive patients. Int J Cardiovasc Imaging. 2014;30:659–67.
33. Berliner JI, Kino A, Carr JC, Bonow RO, Choudhury L. Cardiac computed tomographic imaging to evaluate myocardial scarring/fibrosis in patients with hypertrophic cardiomyopathy: a comparison with cardiac magnetic resonance imaging. Int J Cardiovasc Imaging. 2013;29:191–7.
34. Shiozaki AA, Senra T, Arteaga E, Martinelli Filho M, Pita CG, Avila LF, Parga Filho JR, Mady C, Kalil-Filho R, Bluemke DA, Rochitte CE. Myocardial fibrosis detected by cardiac CT predicts ventricular fibrillation/ventricular tachycardia events in patients with hypertrophic cardiomyopathy. J Cardiovasc Comput Tomogr. 2013;7:173–81.
35. Detrano R, Guerci AD, Carr JJ, Bild DE, Burke G, Folsom AR, Liu K, Shea S, Szklo M, Bluemke DA, O'Leary DH, Tracy R, Watson K, Wong ND, Kronmal RA. Coronary calcium as a predictor of coronary events in four racial or ethnic groups. N Engl J Med. 2008;358:1336–45.
36. Chang HJ, George RT, Schuleri KH, Evers K, Kitagawa K, Lima JA, Lardo AC. Prospective electrocardiogram-gated delayed enhanced multidetector computed tomography accurately quantifies infarct size and reduces radiation exposure. JACC Card Imaging. 2009;2:412–20.
37. Halliburton SS, Abbara S, Chen MY, Gentry R, Mahesh M, Raff GL, Shaw LJ, Hausleiter J. SCCT guidelines on radiation dose and dose-optimization strategies in cardiovascular CT. J Cardiovasc Comput Tomogr. 2011;5:198–224.
38. Chen MY, Steigner ML, Leung SW, Kumamaru KK, Schultz K, Mather RT, Arai AE, Rybicki FJ. Simulated 50 % radiation dose reduction in coronary CT angiography using adaptive iterative dose reduction in three-dimensions (AIDR3D). Int J Cardiovasc Imaging. 2013;29:1167–75.
39. Gottlieb I, Macedo R, Bluemke DA, Lima JA. Magnetic resonance imaging in the evaluation of non-ischemic cardiomyopathies: current applications and future perspectives. Heart Fail Rev. 2006;11:313–23.
40. Wu KC, Kim RJ, Bluemke DA, Rochitte CE, Zerhouni EA, Becker LC, Lima JA. Quantification and time course of microvascular obstruction by contrast-enhanced echocardiography and magnetic resonance imaging following acute myocardial infarction and reperfusion. J Am Coll Cardiol. 1998;32:1756–64.
41. Gore R, Abraham T, George RT. CT characterization of myocardial substrate in hypertrophic cardiomyopathy. J Cardiovasc Comput Tomogr. 2014;8(22):166–9.

Cardiovascular CT for Assessment of Pericardial/Myocardial Disease Processes

13

Muhammad Aamir Latif and Khurram Nasir

Abstract

Pericardial and myocardial diseases represent an important cause of morbidity and mortality. Although echocardiography remains the initial standard diagnostic tool for identifying these diseases it has limited detail for the morphological and functional analysis of the pericardium and myocardium. Cardiac CT (CCT) and MR (CMR) are the primary modalities of choice when comprehensive functional assessment of the heart is required. These imaging techniques provide advanced information on anatomy and cardiac function to optimize diagnosis and treatment. However, as CMR is relatively more costly and time consuming, it is often only used when diagnosis is not clear. Due to the volumetric nature of image acquisition, cardiac CT provides an accurate and reproducible method for assessing both myocardial and pericardial morphology and function. The excellent spatial resolution and contrast to noise ratio of CT allows for the detection of mural thrombi in patients with severely reduced left ventricular function. CCT can easily help identify pericardial diseases such as inflammation, effusion, pericardial cyst, benign or malignant masses, as well as pericardial calcification in the case of constrictive pericarditis. CCT is also proficient in diagnosing the functional assessment of the heart. As most of cardiomyopathies have functional compromise, CCT is best suited for cardiomyopathies in terms of functional analysis. With the advancement of CT technology, radiation exposure is minimal, and with continued improvement in post-processing software, it is able to produce a variety of high-quality images in multiple reformats with historically low radiation and contrast dose. The new General Electric (GE) Revolution CT scanner has made it possible to image the heart with abnormal rate and rhythm without compromising image quality. It is especially useful for patients who have contraindications to beta-blockers or who have atrial fibrillation.

Electronic supplementary material The online version of this chapter (doi:10.1007/978-3-319-28219-0_13) contains supplementary material, which is available to authorized users.

M.A. Latif, MD
Department of Medicine, Center for Healthcare Advancement and Outcomes, Baptist Health South Florida, 6262 Sunset Dr. Suite 200, Miami, FL 33143, USA
e-mail: draamirlatif@gmail.com; muhammadl@baptisthealth.net

K. Nasir, MD, MPH (✉)
Department of Medicine, Center for Healthcare Advancement and Outcomes, Baptist Health South Florida, 1691 Michigan Avenue Suite 500, Miami Beach, FL 33139, USA
e-mail: khurramn@baptisthealth.net; knasir1@jhmi.edu

M.J. Budoff, J.S. Shinbane (eds.), *Cardiac CT Imaging: Diagnosis of Cardiovascular Disease*,
DOI 10.1007/978-3-319-28219-0_13

Keywords
Pericardial • Myocardial • Computed Tomography • Cardiomyopathies • Dilated Cardiomyopathy • Restrictive Cardiomyopathy • Takotsubo Cardiomyopathy • Arrhythmogenic Right Ventricular Cardiomyopathy (ARVC)

Introduction

The twenty first century has already seen extensive research to benefit human civilization. Theories and concepts previously considered imaginary and magical are now being implemented in a practical way with the help of technology. Cardiac CT is one such technology. It started as an imaging machine to augment x-ray radiography and give detailed three-dimensional images of the body's internal organs. Cardiac CT use for heart images has received great attention worldwide because previously it was hard to image a continuously moving structure in the body. Cardiac CT is able to freeze the image in each phases of the cardiac cycle and with high temporal and spatial resolution give a detailed anatomical and physiological picture of the heart. Although the current primary clinical use of contrast-enhanced cardiac computed tomography (CCT) remains the exclusion of coronary artery disease in low to intermediate risk symptomatic patients, this modality also offers a unique opportunity to assess both the pericardium and myocardium. Given the associated contrast and radiation exposure, CCT presently serves as an adjunct to echocardiography and cardiac MRI for this purpose. However, CCT provides superb delineation of the pericardium and can precisely localize lesions as well as aid in their characterization. Further, CCT can effectively evaluate morphology and function in various myocardial diseases, including the various cardiomyopathies. The volumetric nature of image acquisition with CCT provides an accurate and reproducible method for quantifying ventricular mass, volumes, and function. This chapter will discuss the application of CCT in the assessment of various myocardial and pericardial disease processes.

Cardiac CT Advancement

Due to the volumetric nature of image acquisition, cardiac CT provides an accurate and reproducible method for assessing both myocardial and pericardial morphology and function. The excellent spatial resolution and contrast to noise ratio of CT allows for the detection of mural thrombi in patients with severely reduced left ventricular function. While echocardiography remains the primary noninvasive imaging modality for evaluation of the myocardium and pericardium, CCT serves as a valuable tool for further evaluation due to its inherently superb spatial resolution and soft tissue contrast. With further improvements in CCT technology, including refinements in temporal resolution and dramatic reductions in radiation exposure, CCT may play a larger role in the evaluation of patients with known or suspected diseases of the myocardium and pericardium. The main concern of cardiac CT is radiation exposure. With recent advancement in technology, radiation exposure has been minimized. Newer CT protocols have been developed to do selective gating images that lower the dose delivered during non-diagnostic portions of the cardiac cycle. Most recently the General Electric Revolution CT scanner has the ability to even further reduce the radiation dose by selective retrospective imaging. Previously for gating purposes, it was required to use either retrospective or prospective gating synchronized with the patient ECG monitor. The newer scanners no longer require a decision for which mode (retrospective or prospective) to be used but rather the focus is primarily on when to image within the cardiac cycle according to the ECG strip as interpreted by the scanner. This has further reduced radiation exposure. Technological advancement has also overcome the dependence on low heart rate, beat-to-beat variability and their relation to image quality. Now excellent image quality can be obtained with heart rates ranging from 70 to 90 bpm by using newer CT protocols. The Revolution CT scanner has robust, high performance cardiac imaging based on three points of excellence: **temporal resolution** (0.28 s gantry rotation, intelligent motion correction), **spatial resolution** and **whole organ coverage** (160 mm detector). With these improvements the cardiac CT exam provides the best possible overall picture of the heart, including the pericardium and myocardium. The cinematic mode is a feature of cardiac CT software to provide functional global assessment of the myocardium. These imaging modalities can also play an important role in prognosis, as well as direct treatment and further management.

CT Imaging of Myocardial Disease

Myocardial diseases or cardiomyopathies can be classified based on their origin, anatomy, physiology, histopathology or genetics. The World Health Organization (WHO) defines the cardiomyopathies as diseases of myocardial tissue associated with cardiac dysfunction and subdivides them mainly into four categories: dilated, restrictive, hypertrophic, and arrhythmogenic right ventricular cardiomyopathy (ARVC) [1]. Non-invasive imaging can determine whether abnormalities are present in the myocardium, valves, pericardium, or vessels. Echocardiography is the most common imaging technique used for the initial diagnosis and management of cardiomyopathy; however, other imaging modalities, including nuclear cardiac imaging, cardiac magnetic resonance imaging, and cardiac computed tomography, may play an important role depending on the underlying etiology of the cardiomyopathy [2].

Dilated Cardiomyopathy

Dilated cardiomyopathy is characterized by ventricular enlargement and decreased systolic function. Besides the reconstructed CT data at specific diastolic (and/or systolic) phases of the cardiac cycle for evaluation of the coronary arteries and cardiac morphology, a multiphase data set, which reconstructs the entire cardiac cycle at 5–10 % intervals, allows for viewing images in cinematic mode. This multiphase reconstruction allows for assessment of left and right ventricular systolic function in any orientation, including all of the standard echocardiographic planes [3]. Thus, CCT can assess myocardial thickness (Video 13.1), ventricular shape and volume, and global and regional ventricular function with excellent correlation to echocardiography and cardiac MRI [4, 5]. Additionally, patients with severely reduced left ventricular function are at risk for the development of mural thrombus. Given its inherently high contrast to noise ratio and excellent spatial resolution, CCT can readily identify such mural thrombi.

Restrictive Cardiomyopathy

Restrictive cardiomyopathy is characterized by increased ventricular stiffness and associated diastolic dysfunction. Ventricular size and systolic function are usually normal, but the atria and systemic veins (superior and inferior vena cavae, hepatic veins, coronary sinus) are often dilated due to increased filling pressures. These features are easily depicted by CCT but are nonspecific. While CCT is not indicated solely for the evaluation of possible restrictive cardiomyopathy, it is useful in differentiating it from constrictive pericarditis by excluding pericardial abnormalities. This distinction leads to important therapeutic consequences.

Hypertrophic Cardiomyopathy

Hypertrophic cardiomyopathy is a genetic disorder of various sarcomeric proteins resulting in cardiac myocyte disarray and left ventricular hypertrophy with or without obstruction. This most commonly involves asymmetric septal hypertrophy, although other variants exist, including apical and mid-ventricular hypertrophy (Fig. 13.1). In patients with dynamic left ventricular outflow obstruction, CCT delineates the systolic anterior motion of the anterior mitral valve leaflet on the multiphase images. While poor acoustic windows may limit echocardiography, CCT can reliably identify all areas of the myocardium and provide accurate, reproducible measurements of wall thickness.

Arrhythmogenic Right Ventricular Cardiomyopathy (ARVC)

ARVC is an unusual cardiomyopathy characterized by abnormal right ventricular function, fibrofatty deposition into the right ventricular myocardium, and abnormal electrocardiographic changes, which predispose these patients to sudden cardiac death. CCT has an advantage over echocardiography in its ability to visualize the right ventricle and thus to evaluate right ventricular morphology and systolic function, similar to MRI. However, MRI has superior tissue characterization capabilities and remains the modality of choice for evaluating suspected ARVC. CCT becomes the modality of choice when metal implants or claustrophobia preclude MRI. When performing CCT in these patients, it is important to ensure adequate opacification of the right ventricle at the time of image acquisition. This can be achieved by either prolonging the contrast administration by several seconds (4–6 s) or by empirically utilizing a shorter delay time. Alternatively, placing a region of interest in the main pulmonary artery and triggering the scan at its peak opacification can consistently achieve preferential right-sided opacification. CCT can reliably characterize right ventricular dimensions as well as focal aneurysms of the myocardium, increased trabeculations, and/or areas of right ventricular dysfunction, all confirmatory findings in RV dysplasia. Importantly, CCT can also detect fatty infiltration as areas of hypoattenuation, confirmed by CT attenuation measurements. However, the finding of fat is sensitive but not specific for ARVC [6]. Hence, CCT findings must be correlated with clinical and electro-cardiographic data to establish the diagnosis of ARVC.

Left Ventricular Noncompaction

Left ventricular noncompaction is a cardiomyopathy characterized by a 2-layered myocardium: a thin compacted layer and a thick noncompacted layer. The ratio of noncompacted to compacted myocardium has been reported to be greater than or equal to 2.3:1 by cardiac MRI in cases of non-compaction [7]. The hypertrabeculations of the noncompacted myocardium, as well as thrombi that may form within the recesses, are easily delineated with CCT due to its favorable contrast-to-noise ratio (Fig. 13.2). Left ventricular noncompaction frequently manifests itself as a dilated cardiomyopathy with

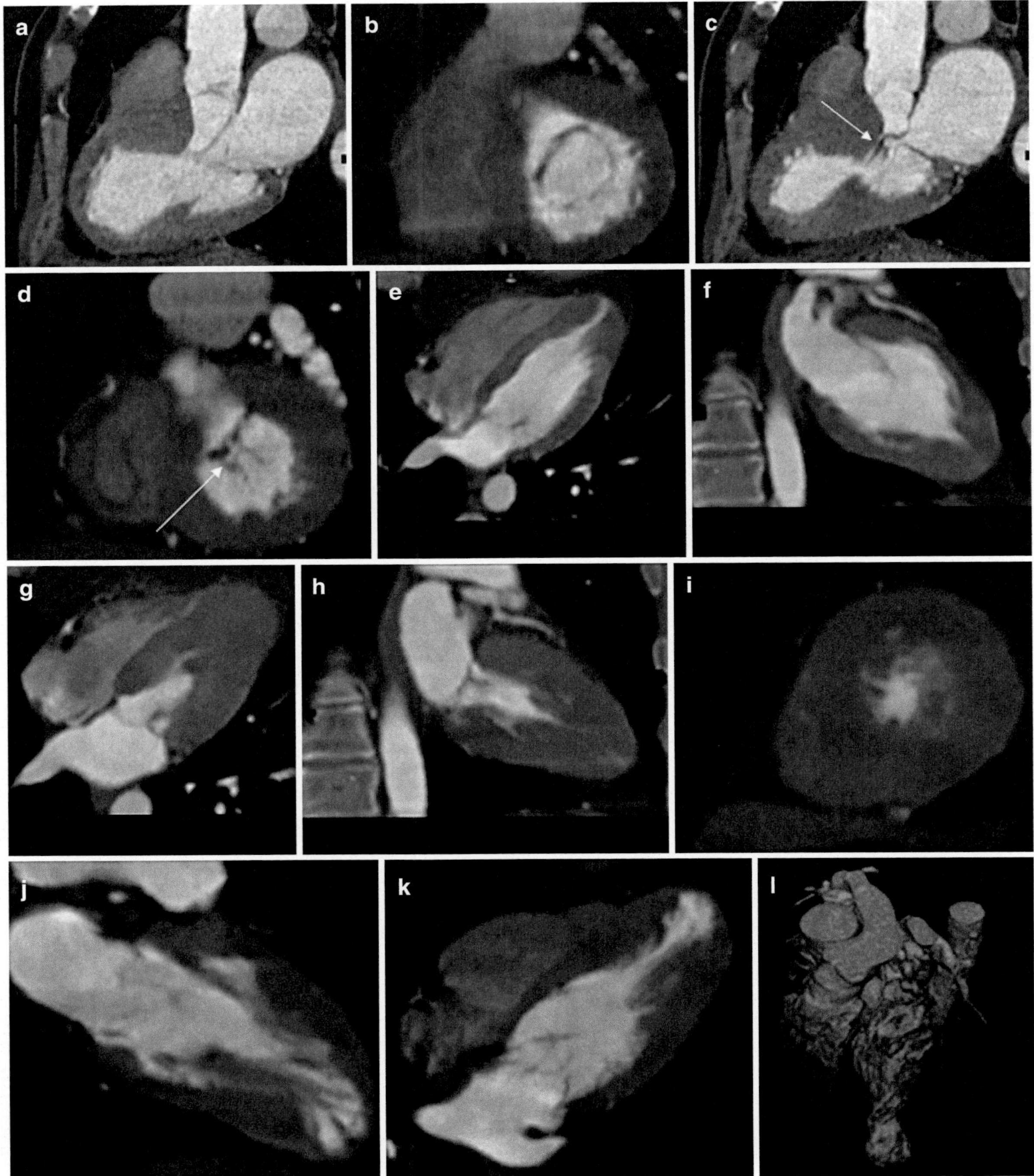

Fig. 13.1 The most common form of hypertrophic cardiomyopathy manifests as asymmetric septal hypertrophy with or without obstruction. This three-chamber view in end-diastole (**a**) demonstrates abnormal thickening of the mid-and basal interventricular septum. The short-axis view in end-diastole (**b**) demonstrates normal mitral valve morphology and opening. In systole, the three-chamber view (**c**) demonstrates systolic anterior motion of the anterior mitral valve leaflet (*arrow*) causing a gradient across the left ventricular outflow tract. This is consistent with hypertrophic obstructive cardiomyopathy. The short-axis view in systole (**d**) also demonstrates systolic anterior motion of the mitral valve as well as incomplete coaptation of the leaflets (*arrow*), causing mitral regurgitation. In the apical form of hypertrophic cardiomyopathy, muscle thickening occurs predominantly at the apex of the left ventricle, as can be seen in end-diastolic images in the four-and two-chamber views (**e**, **f**). The corresponding end-systolic images demonstrate complete obliteration of the left ventricular apex (**g**, **h**). When the left ventricular hypertrophy primarily affects the mid-ventricular level, there can be mid-cavitary obliteration with an associated gradient at the level of obstruction. End-diastolic images in the short-axis (**i**), two-chamber (**j**), and four-chamber (**k**) views, and the 3-D volume-rendered image (**l**) demonstrate prominent thickening at the mid-ventricular level. The corresponding end-systolic images (**m–p**) demonstrate complete obliteration of the mid-cavity and early apical outpouching

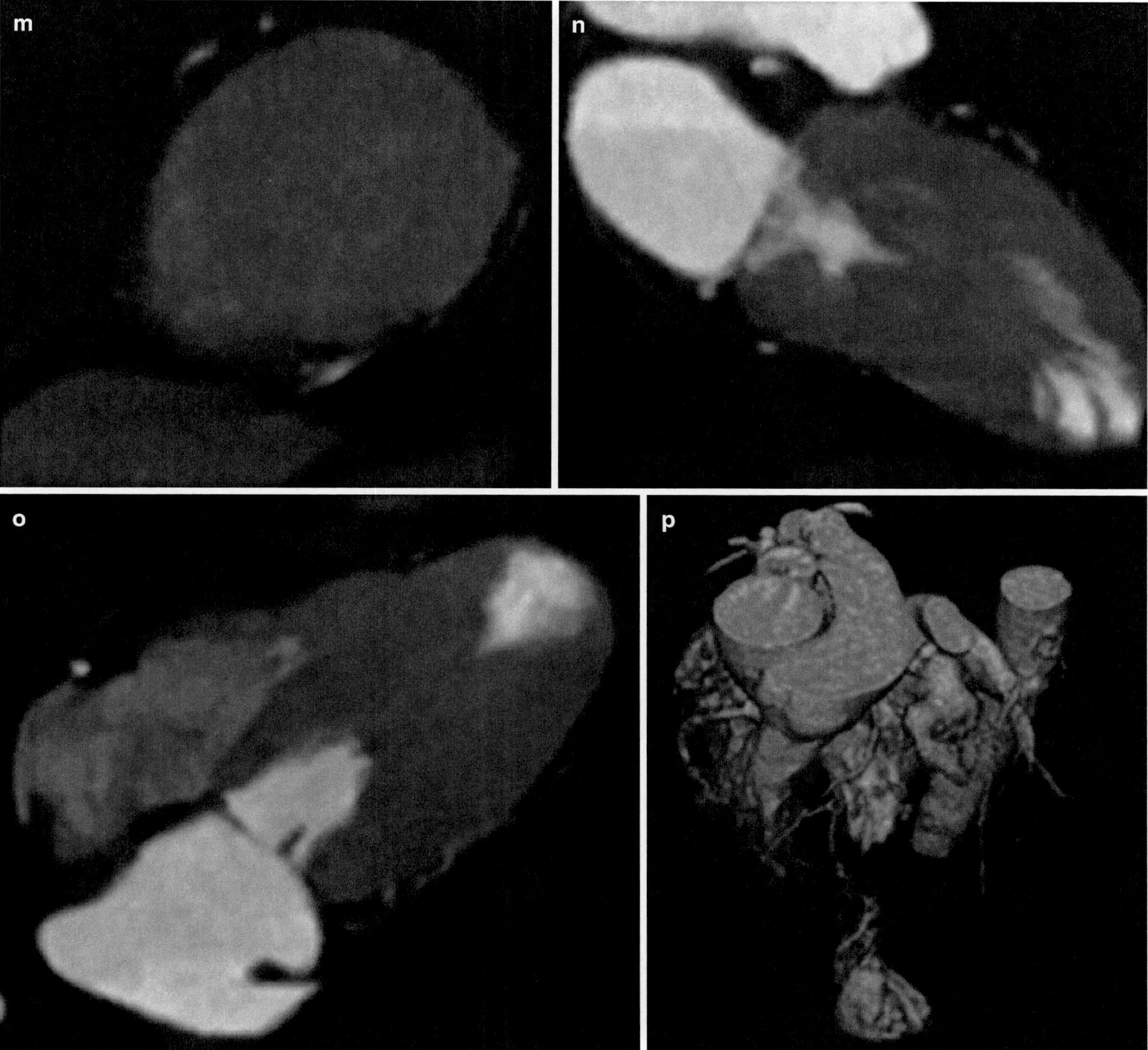

Fig. 13.1 (continued)

reduced left ventricular function, which can also be assessed by CCT. Clinically, noncompaction is associated with both heart failure and sudden death.

Myocardial Inflammation (Myocarditis) on CT Scan

Acute myocarditis is a relatively uncommon disease but may well be under diagnosed. CCT can be helpful in the diagnosis of myocarditis. With the typical history of chest pain and elevated serum troponin-I level in young patients, myocarditis on CCT will show normal epicardial coronary arteries. Due to edema of the myocardium, CCT may also show low attenuation at ventricular wall and interventricular septum [8], which can be confirmed with Cardiac MR as increased signal on T2-weighted imaging. There may also be delayed myocardial enhancement on contrast-enhanced CCT images in acute myocarditis [9]. The morphologic features of the enhancement are similar to the myocardial enhancement of myocarditis with gadolinium contrast on CMR, and different from the enhancement patterns seen in patients with myocardial infarction [9]. On CMR there is a subepicardial delayed contrast enhancement (DCE) pattern typical of acute myocarditis in comparison to an ischemic DCE pattern, which is transmural or subendocardial [10].

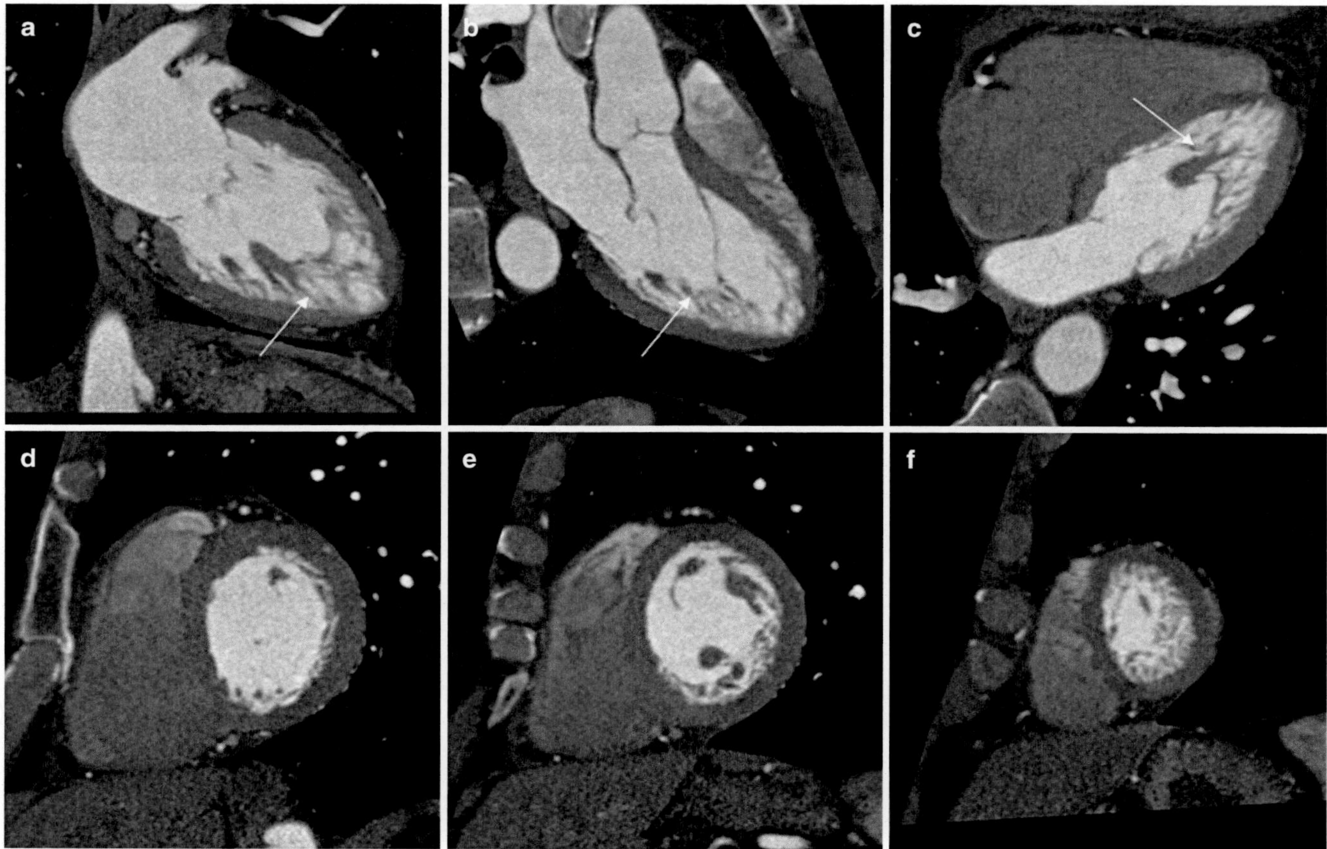

Fig. 13.2 The morphological hallmark of left ventricular noncompaction is the presence of hypertrabeculations. These hypertrabeculations are often most prominent toward the left ventricular apex. End-diastolic images in the two-(**a**), three-(**b**), and four-chamber (**c**) views demonstrate these characteristically prominent trabeculations that form the noncompacted layer (*white arrows*). End-diastolic images in the short-axis view at the base (**d**), mid-ventricular (**e**), and apical levels (**f**) again demonstrate these hypertrabeculations, most prominently at the apex

CT Imaging of Pericardial Disease

Pericardial diseases represent an important cause of morbidity and mortality in patients with cardiovascular disease and constitute a spectrum ranging from benign to malignant causes. Pericardial diseases can present clinically as acute pericarditis, pericardial effusion, cardiac tamponade, and constrictive pericarditis. Patients can subsequently develop chronic or recurrent pericarditis. Structural abnormalities including congenitally absent pericardium and pericardial cysts are usually asymptomatic and are uncommon.

Advances in multimodality noninvasive cardiac imaging have enhanced its role in the management of patients with suspected pericardial disease. Structural and functional information obtained from echocardiography and the anatomic detail provided by cardiac computed tomography and magnetic resonance have led to growing interest in the complementary use of these techniques. Management of the patient with suspected pericardial disease requires expertise with the key imaging modalities and the ability to choose the appropriate imaging tests for each patient.

Anatomy of Pericardium and CT Scan

The pericardium is a double-layered membrane normally measuring <2 mm in thickness that forms a sac which surrounds the heart and the origins of the great vessels (Fig. 13.3) [11]. It is made of two sacs in one. The outer sac is the fibrous pericardium and inner sac is the double-layered serous pericardium. Layers of serous pericardium are divided by the **pericardial space**, which usually only contains 15–50 mL of serous fluid. They have quite different structures—the **fibrous pericardium** is a tough connective tissue continuous with and bound to the central tendon of the diaphragm, the roots of the great vessels, the pretracheal layer of the deep cervical fascia and the sternum via the superior sterno-pericardiac ligaments (to manubrium) and inferior sterno-pericardiac ligaments (to xiphoid process). **The serous pericardium** is composed of a single layer of flattened cells forming a closed sac and in turn also forms two continuous layers. The visceral serous pericardium (or epicardium) covers heart and great vessels. The parietal serous pericardium lines the fibrous pericardium and is inseparable from it.

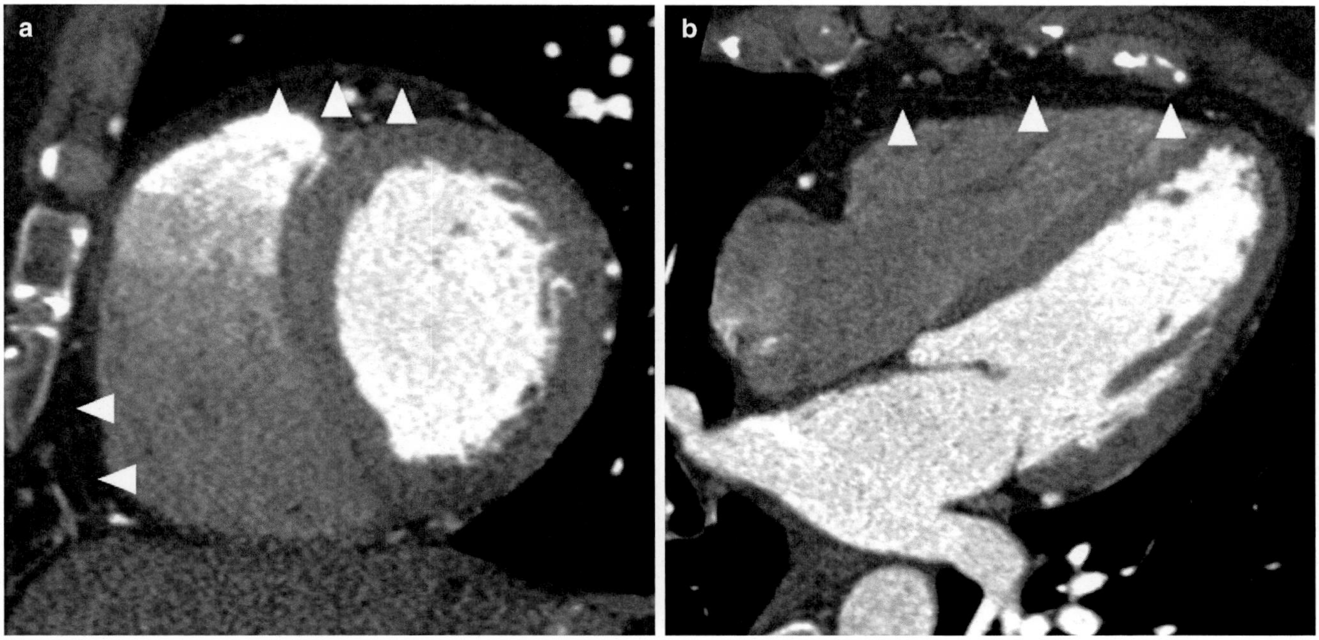

Fig. 13.3 Due to its excellent spatial resolution, cardiac CT can image the pericardium, which is normally <2 mm thick. These short-axis (**a**) and four-chamber (**b**) views demonstrate the normal, thin pericardium (*white arrowheads*). The pericardium is often best visualized over the right side of the heart, as the more abundant epicardial fat located there provides good tissue contrast

The serous pericardium is invaginated by the heart and great vessels to form two sinuses: **the oblique sinus is** formed by the indentations of the superior and inferior vena cavae and the four pulmonary veins (blind-ending) and thus sits posterior to the left atrium where it may be mistaken for an esophageal mass or bronchogenic cyst. The **transverse sinus** lies between the aorta and pulmonary artery anteriorly and the atria posteriorly, surrounding the ascending aorta. It includes several recesses (superior aortic recess, inferior aortic recess, pulmonic recesses and post caval recess) that may be mistaken for dissection or lymphadenopathy [12]. These recesses are important when evaluating for pericardial metastatic disease in oncology patients.

While echocardiography is conventionally used for the evaluation of pericardial diseases, CCT offers a number of distinct advantages. CCT provides a larger imaging field allowing assessment of concomitant pathology. In addition, CCT offers a superior soft tissue contrast, and thus characterization of specific pericardial processes is sometimes possible. CCT is exquisitely sensitive to the detection of calcium and thus can be useful in identifying pericardial calcification, a finding that can be associated with constrictive pericarditis (Fig. 13.4). One of the limitations of CCT in evaluating the pericardium, however, is its occasional difficulty in differentiating pericardial fluid from a thickened pericardium.

With CCT, the normal pericardium (Video 13.2) is best imaged in systole and appears as a line of average thickness of 1.3–2.5 mm (almost always <4 mm). CCT delineates the pericardium as a well-defined, linear structure that is easily detectable in both contrast and noncontrast-enhanced examinations because of its visibility against the low attenuation of the surrounding fat. Visualization of the pericardium varies with location and is sometimes difficult at the lateral, posterior, and inferior left ventricular walls because of a paucity of pericardial fat in these locations.

Inflammation of Pericardium on CT Scan

To evaluate for pericardial inflammation, a noncontrast CT can be performed prior to the contrast-enhanced CT. Enhancement of the pericardium after contrast administration is indicative of pericardial inflammation, and may be seen in cases of pericarditis. The current reference standard for the noninvasive evaluation of pericardial constriction is cardiac MRI. The characteristic anatomic changes associated with constrictive pericardial disease (elongated and narrow RV, enlargement of the right atrium and inferior cava, and pericardial thickening) are clearly identified with both MRI and CCT. However, since patients with true constrictive pericarditis typically present with orthopnea, it is often difficult for them to lie flat in the MRI scanner for up to 1 h. CCT may offer another option for evaluating constrictive pericarditis, with short examination times representing one of its major advantages. The excellent spatial resolution of CCT allows for accurate measurement of

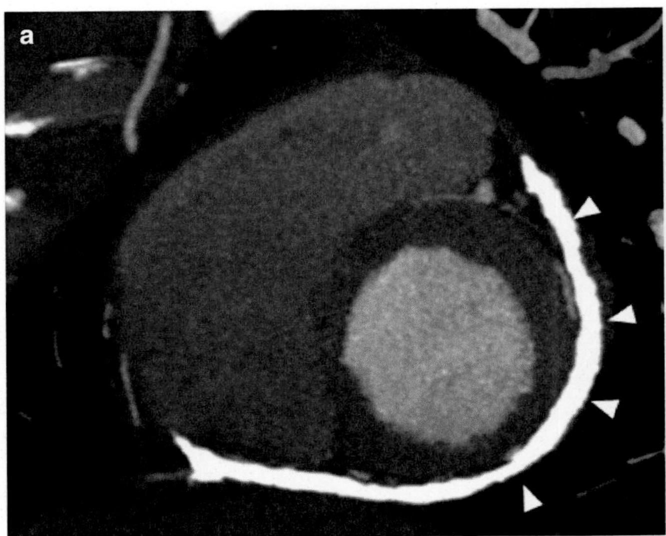

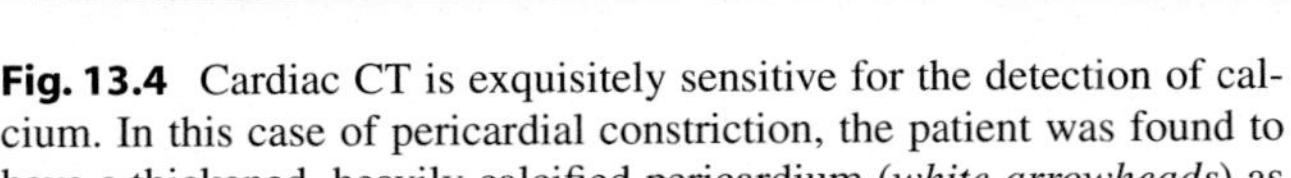

Fig. 13.4 Cardiac CT is exquisitely sensitive for the detection of calcium. In this case of pericardial constriction, the patient was found to have a thickened, heavily calcified pericardium (*white arrowheads*) as noted on the short-axis view (**a**) and 3-D volume-rendered image (**b**). The volume rendered image demonstrates circumferential pericardial calcification at the base

pericardial thickness. A pericardial thickness >4 mm is considered pathological and, in the appropriate clinical context, is suggestive of pericardial constriction [13, 14]. However, it is important to note that neither pericardial calcification nor thickening is diagnostic of constrictive pericarditis. Besides these morphological characteristics, the demonstration of an early diastolic septal bounce on the multiphase cine images is suggestive of constrictive physiology [15].

The normal pericardium is a double-layered membrane that is <2 mm thick. A pericardial thickness >4 mm is considered pathological. Pericardial thickening may be found in the absence of constriction (e.g., acute pericariditis, uremia, collagen vascular diseases). Enhancement of the pericardium, indicative of pericardial inflammation, may be found in cases of pericarditis. Pericardial inflammation can be evaluated by performing CCT with and without contrast. The inflamed pericardium will demonstrate a significant increase in CT attenuation after contrast administration.

Congenital Absence of Pericardium

Rare individuals demonstrate a congenital absence of the pericardium. While this can present as a complete absence of pericardial tissue, most cases demonstrate only partial pericardial defects, typically on the left side (Fig. 13.5a). Clues on CCT that suggest this diagnosis are rotation of the heart to the left, interposition of lung tissue in the aortopulmonary window, and bulging of the left atrial appendage through the pericardial defect. Infrequently, the left atrial appendage can be incarcerated in the defect requiring surgical enlargement or closure.

Pericardial Effusion on CT Scan

Echocardiography remains the modality of choice for the initial evaluation of pericardial effusion (Fig. 13.5b). However, several findings make further evaluation with CCT useful, such as a loculated effusion, hemorrhagic effusion, or equivocal findings on echocardiography. Pericardial effusions may be characterized with CCT by measuring their CT attenuation. A CT attenuation close to water (e.g., 0 Hounsfield Units, HU) suggests a simple pericardial effusion. If the CT attenuation is greater than that of water, the effusion may represent hemorrhage, purulence, or a malignant/cellular process.

Pericardial Masses

Pericardial masses include cysts and neoplasms. Pericardial cysts are congenital and are usually found at the right costophrenic angle [16]. They tend to be asymptomatic smooth-walled simple cysts that do not enhance after contrast administration (Fig. 13.5c). However, sometimes pericardial cyst can present on left side and can compress the left atrium with clinical symptoms of dyspnea [17]. With regard to neoplasms, metastases are far more common than primary pericardial tumors. Neighboring structures, such as the lung and breast, are most commonly the source of metastatic disease to the pericardium. Other findings associated with metastatic disease include pericardial effusion and an irregularly thickened pericardium [18]. Primary neoplasms of the pericardium occur infrequently and may be benign (fibroma, teratoma, lipoma, hemangioma) or malignant (mesothelioma, lymphoma, sarcoma, and liposarcoma) [19].

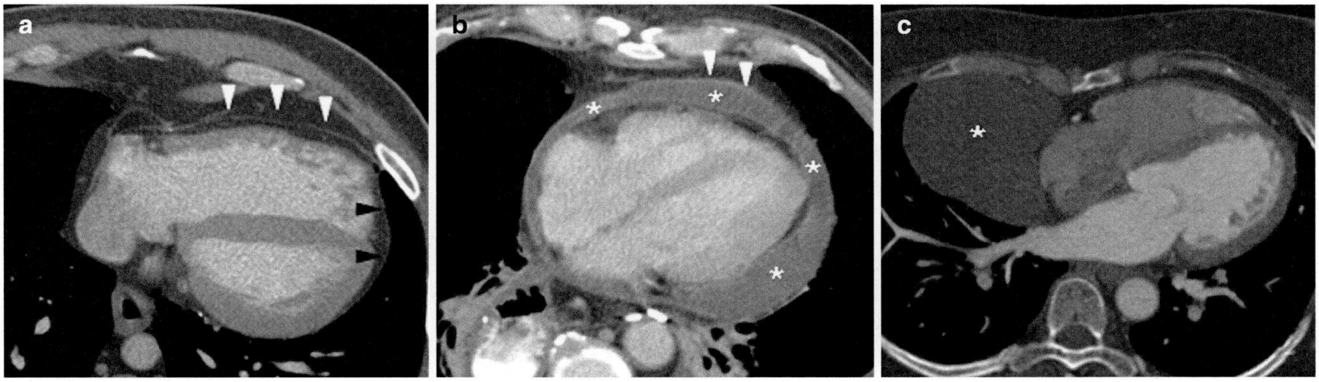

Fig. 13.5 Partial absence of the pericardium (**a**). In this example, normal pericardium is found over the right ventricular free wall (*white arrowheads*), but there is absence of the pericardium over the right ventricular apex and left ventricle (*black arrowheads*). Pericardial effusions (*asterisks*) are often found in the context of pericarditis (**b**). In this case, the pericardium also enhanced after administration of iodinated contrast (*white arrowheads*), suggesting pericardial inflammation. Pericardial cysts (*asterisk*) are benign fluid-filled pericardial masses, typically found at the right cardio-phrenic angle (**c**)

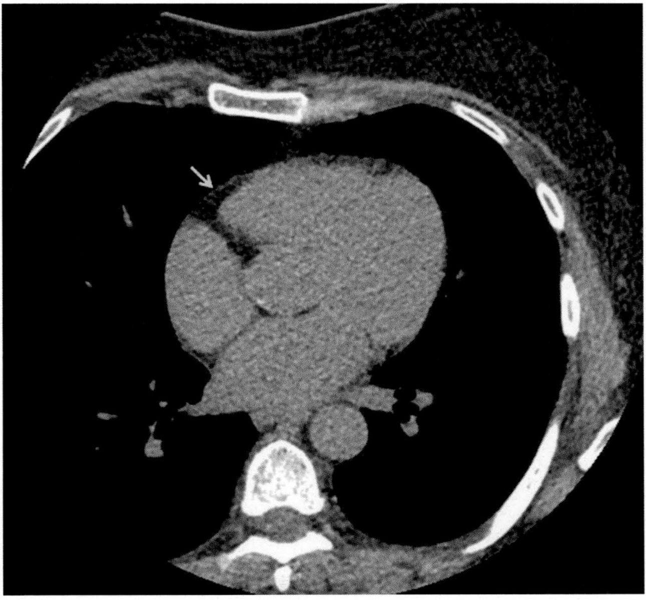

Fig. 13.6 Axial view of heart with normal pericardium on Revolution CT calcium scan (*yellow arrowhead*)

Pericardial Fat Assessment with CT Scan

Recent studies have shown that increased pericardial fat is strongly associated with increased coronary artery calcium, coronary plaque burden and major adverse cardiovascular events (MACE) [20, 21]. These findings suggest that pericardial fat may play a role in causing coronary atherosclerosis [22–26]. Due to distinct attenuation values of fat on CT, fat can be readily measured around the heart with cardiac CT, both with and without contrast [27]. Cardiac CT, with its high spatial resolution, allows accurate measurement of epicardial and thoracic fat distances and volumes (Fig. 13.6).

Volumetric quantification of epicardial fat and thoracic fat require the following steps: demarcation of the heart boundaries on CT images, and tracing of the inner thoracic cavity and pericardium, which can be manual [21, 28] or semi-automated [20]. The superior most slice is typically chosen at the bifurcation of the pulmonary artery. The anatomic landmark for the inferior limit of the heart is typically the most inferior slice of the myocardium [26] or the most inferior slice with the posterior descending artery [29]. With semi-automated measurement, pericardial fat contours are generated by spline interpolation through several control points, which are placed manually on the visceral pericardium [30], and the inner thoracic cavity is segmented automatically [31]. CT uses standard fat attenuation values to define fat attenuation; for non-contrast CT typically an attenuation range of (−30, −190) Hounsfield Units is used. Fat voxels within this attenuation range within the visceral pericardium are classified as epicardial fat, and within the inner thoracic cavity classified as thoracic fat.

Comparison to Other Imaging Modalities

Generally cardiac computed tomography is superior to echocardiography and cardiac MRI because of its superior and ultrasensitive resolution and excellent field of view. Echocardiography is good for a quick assessment of pericardium but it does not give the detail of pericardial disease as clearly as CT/MRI. Cardiac MRI is limited in use because of high cost and time duration of the scan that make it less suitable for emergent pericardial conditions such as cardiac tamponade. Table 13.1 [32, 33] compares pericardial disorder assessment with CCT, echocardiography and CMR. Table 13.2 [34–90] compares myocardial disorder assessment with these imaging modalities.

Table 13.1 Pericardial disorders assessment with cardiac imaging modalities

Pericardial condition	Definition	CT angiographic diagnostic finding	Echocardiographic diagnostic finding	MRI diagnostic finding
Pericarditis	Pericarditis is an inflammation of the pericardium.	Normal pericardial thickness is less than 4 mm and is usually 1–2 mm Pericardial thickening/ enhancement (the most accurate single parameter for pericarditis, with sensitivity of 54–59 % and specificity of 91–96 %) [32].	Only helpful if a pericardial effusion is present with pericarditis. Can determine whether the effusion is limiting the filling of the heart (i.e., causing cardiac tamponade).	Most sensitive method for the diagnosis of acute pericarditis is delayed enhancement of the pericardium on cardiac MR (CMR) [33]. On CMR, the pericardium normally appears black because of its low water content; However, in patients with pericarditis, enhanced gadolinium uptake in the inflamed pericardium is present on delayed images
Cardiac Tamponade	Cardiac Tamponade is a clinical syndrome caused by the accumulation of fluid in the pericardial space, resulting in reduced ventricular filling and subsequent hemodynamic compromise. The condition is a medical emergency, the complications of which include pulmonary edema, shock, and death.	Enlargement of the SVC and IVC Periportal lymphedema Reflux of contrast material within the IVC and azygos vein, and enlargement of hepatic and renal veins. Flattened heart sign. Compression of the coronary sinus. Angulation or bowing of interventricular septum.	RV diameters are reduced. Early diastolic collapse of RV RA free-wall collapse during late diastole. RA isovolumic contraction is prolonged to occupy one third of the cardiac cycle. LA free-wall compression in patients with fluid posterior to the left atrium. LV free-wall may exhibit paradoxical movement SVC & IVC may show congestion (unless patient is relatively volume depleted) IVC is usually greater than 2.2 cm in diameter with less than 50 % inspiratory compression Exaggerated inspiratory effects, especially with pulsus paradoxus, may include RV expansion, interventricular septum shift to the left, and LV compression Mitral changes, with reduced D-E amplitude or E-F slope and delayed mitral opening time Aortic valve with premature closure Echocardiographic stroke volume diminished RV epicardial notching during isovolumic contraction Coarse vibrations of LV posterior wall. Pseudohypertrophy or apparent wall thickening due to compression	CMR has a limited role in the setting of cardiac tamponade owing to the emergent and life-threatening nature of this condition. CMR findings with other imaging modalities include; swinging heart and paradoxical septal bounce seen on short-or long-axis cine MR images. CMR imaging can help differentiate the nature of the pericardial effusion (transudative, exudative, and or hemorrhagic) in addition to the effects on cardiac functioning and diastolic filling.

Constrictive Pericarditis	Constrictive pericarditis is a reduction in the elasticity, or stiffening, of the pericardium, a sack-like covering that surrounds the heart, resulting in impaired filling of the heart with blood.	Diffuse thickening of anterior pericardium upto the vascular root best seen on multiplanar reformats. Size of all 4-heart chambers should be within the normal range. -IVC is dilated to more than double the size of aortic diameter. Poor opacification of liver parenchyma due to congestion and no contrast enhancement in the portal vein. No progression of the contrast-agent bolus through the vascular system, and evidence of significant systolic dysfunction should be absent	Cardiac echograms show normal contraction and systolic function. Special procedures, including an assessment of Doppler velocities across the mitral and tricuspid valves during inspiration and expiration, are needed to demonstrate ventricular interdependence. Newer echocardiographic procedures, such as the evaluation of the early diastolic Doppler myocardial velocity gradients at the posterior wall, echocardiographic TDI, and color M mode flow propagation, have been reported to enhance the differentiation between CP and restrictive cardiomyopathy	Cardiac MRI can detect constrictive physiology. MRI allows precise measurement pericardial thickness; the ideal views for measuring pericardial thickness are short axis views Measure chamber sizes at successive 50-msec delays after the R wave and to determine whether or not a filling plateau is present. Assess volumetric flow and regurgitant flow to the pulmonary veins and the hepatic vein. Fast imaging with deep respiration help to establish whether filling is concordant or discordant. CP restriction creates discordance with reduced left ventricular filling, which corresponds to increased right ventricular filling. MRI shows reversed curvature of the intraventricular septum. MRI does not depict pericardial calcifications.
Pericardial effusion	Pericardial effusion is an abnormal accumulation of fluid in the pericardial cavity. Because of the limited amount of space in the pericardial cavity, fluid accumulation leads to an increased intrapericardial pressure which can negatively affect heart function	Differentiation of the pericardial line from the myocardium is enabled by the presence of a small amount of epicardial and pericardial fat. This fat may be visible on CT scans. CT demonstrates the superior recesses of the pericardium extending over the ascending aorta and lateral to the main pulmonary artery. These recesses may be distended in the presence of a pericardial effusion. Attenuation of the effusion on CT may be helpful in suggesting the etiology.	Echo-free space: (1) posterior to LV (small-to-moderate effusion); (2) posterior and anterior (moderate-to-large effusion); (3) behind left atrium large-to-very large effusion and/or anterior adhesion. Diminished mobility of posterior pericardium-to-lung interface. Enhanced RV wall mobility unmasked in presence of anterior fluid Swinging heart (large effusions, usually tamponade): (1) RV and LV walls move in synchrony; (2) periodicity 1:1 or 2:1 (one or two swings per cardiac cycle); (3) 2:1 swing is characteristic of cardiac Tamponade; (4) pseudoparadoxic motion of LV posterior wall; (5) mitral and/or tricuspid pseudoprolapse; (6) mitral systolic anterior motion; (7) alternating mitral E-F slope and aortic opening excursion; (8) aortic valve exhibiting midsystolic closure; (9) pulmonic valve with midsystolic notch Hemopericardium with blood clots identifiable by echocardiography Inspiratory decrease in LV ejection time (with effusion	On spin-echo images, the pericardial effusion or portions of it may appear as a signal void (dark) sac because of moving fluid in the pericardial cavity. In gradient-echo sequences, effusions are hyperintense. Hemorrhagic effusions have the opposite appearance; they have high signal intensity on T1-weighted spin echo images and low intensity on gradient echo images. Depict pericardial recesses, mediastinal fat, and other similar anatomic structures within the pericardial sac. Dark-blood (double inversion recovery) imaging can measure pericardial thickness accurately. Fat-sensitive imaging (based on chemical shift or on T1 values) can discern pericardial fat from other materials. Dynamic MRI can identify constrictive disease (failure to expand for the last 6/20 frames of diastole). MRI can also assess for adhesions by placing demagnetization stripes to observe for translational motion at the pericardium, and it can assess for restrictive disease by strain mapping.

CT computed tomography, *MRI* magnetic resonance imaging, *CMR* cardiac MR, *SVC* superior vena cava, *IVC* inferior vena cava, *RV* right ventricle, *LV* left ventricle, *RA* right atrium, *LA* left atrium, *CP* Contrictive Pericarditis, *TDI* tissue Doppler imaging

Table 13.2 Myocardial disorder assessment with cardiac imaging modalities

Myocardial condition	Definition	CT Angiographic diagnostic finding	Echocardiographic diagnostic finding	MRI diagnostic finding
Dilated cardiomyopathy	Dilated cardiomyopathy is a condition in which the ventricular chambers show increased systolic and diastolic volume and a low Ejection Fraction (<40 %) [1, 34].	Gated CT scanning is an accurate means of evaluating cardiac function, especially with the use of ultrafast CT scanning and 50-millisecond image acquisition. Only 1 short breath-hold period is required, and definition of the endocardial margins is excellent, allowing a degree of automation for defining the ventricular volumes. Increased in left ventricular end-diastolic and end-systolic volume. Left ventricular wall thinning. Decrease ejection fraction.	Left ventricular spherical dilatation. Normal or reduced wall thickness. Poor systolic wall thickening, and/or reduced inward endocardial systolic motion. All of the systolic indices are reduced, including left ventricular fractional shortening, fractional area change, and ejection fraction. Four chamber cardiac enlargement is often present. On M-mode, additional features related to systolic dysfunction are increased separation of the mitral leaflet E point from the septum, poor mitral valve opening, poor aortic valve opening and early closure from a reduced stroke volume, and poor systolic aortic root motion. Doppler has been used in dilated cardiomyopathy to measure decreased stroke volume	MRI and magnetic resonance angiography (MRA) are the most accurate methods for assessing cardiac anatomy or function. MRI/MRA is used when echocardiography is inadequate, as this study is often not used because of its relatively high cost and limited availability, as well as contraindications if ferromagnetic metallic foreign bodies are present in the patient.

Table 13.2 (continued)

Myocardial condition	Definition	CT Angiographic diagnostic finding	Echocardiographic diagnostic finding	MRI diagnostic finding
Hypertrophic cardiomyopathy	Hypertrophic cardiomyopathy is characterized by left ventricular hypertrophy (wall thickness >12–15 mm) without obvious etiology. Associated right ventricular hypertrophy may be seen in 15 % of cases.	MDCT is an excellent method for observing irregular wall hypertrophy, apical morphology, and wall motion dynamics [35]. Criterion for LV wall hypertrophy is an LV wall thicker than 13-mm. Right ventricular hypertrophy is considered when the right ventricular wall is thicker than 6 mm (Fig. 13.8). Wall thickening during systole can be calculated with MDCT. Most patients (71 %) have decreased wall thickening at the hypertrophic site and normal or increased thickening at the nonhypertrophic site [35]. Late enhancement of the myocardium on EBCT has been reported in approximately 47 % of HCM patients [36]; this finding suggests the presence of abnormal tissue Degree of regional wall thickening also is significantly less in areas of late enhancement, which reflects the abnormal myocardial architecture [37].	LV wall thickness of 13 mm in the anterior septum or posterior wall or 15 mm in the posterior septum or free wall, in the absence of LV dilatation or other cardiac and systemic causes of increased mass [38]. Asymmetric septal hypertrophy (defined as a ratio of septal thickness to posterior wall thickness of at least 1.3–1.5) [39]. Ground-glass appearance is noted either visually or by using quantitative texture analysis in both hypertrophied and nonhypertrophied regions of the ventricle [40], used to distinguish HCM from other causes of secondary hypertrophy [41]. Narrowing or obstruction of the LVOT caused by IVS and the anterior leaflet of the mitral valve, which results in a dynamic pressure gradient. Abnormal systolic anterior motion (SAM) of the anterior leaflet and, occasionally, the posterior leaflet of the mitral valve may be present; severe SAM, with septal-leaflet contact, has been proposed as a major diagnostic criterion. Mitral valve abnormalities in HCM patients include increased leaflet area, elongation of the leaflet, and anomalous insertion of papillary muscle directly into the anterior mitral leaflet. Prasad et al. have reported pitfalls in the echocardiographic diagnosis of HCM [42]. Approximately 70 % of HCM patients have an LV outflow gradient of 30 mmHg (2.7 m/s by Doppler) [43].	Either spin-echo MRI or cine MRA help to views 4 chamber and short axis [44]. Accurately characterize the distribution and degree of myocardial hypertrophy & asymmetric septal hypertrophy. Visualize apical and posterolateral myocardial hypertrophy that is not always evident on 2D echograms [45]. MRI helps to calculate hypertrophic scores [46]. Hypertrophy in HCM is usually asymmetric and is typically most evident in the anteroseptal myocardium [47]. Basal IVS at end diastole is disproportionately thickened, ratio of IVS thickness to posterolateral wall thickness is significantly increased. Decreased systolic myocardial thickening [48]. Long-axis show typical spade-shaped deformity of the LV cavity and the apical distribution of myocardial hypertrophy. Diffuse hypertrophy of RV wall, increased RV wall index [49]. LV mass can be reliably estimated with spin-echo MRI, ECG-gated MRI, or multilevel cine MRA; however, LV mass, indexed to body surface area, is normal in about 20 % of patients with HCM [50]. LVH in HCM often decreases the LV volume and increases the ejection fraction, without significantly changing stroke volume. Cine MRA can be used to calculate these parameters Obstruction of LVOT results in a subaortic pressure gradient (can be detected on cine MRA as signal void). Although areas of physiologic signal void can be seen on scans in healthy individuals, signal voids are larger and persist longer in the cardiac cycle in patients with pathologic conditions that cause obstruction [51]. Mitral regurgitation appears on cine MRAs as a signal void in the left atrium during ventricular systole which may be associated with mitral valve prolapse [52–54]. Gadolinium enhancement can detect myocardial fibrosis [55]. MRI can differentiate between HCM and amyloidosis [56, 57].

(continued)

Table 13.2 (continued)

Myocardial condition	Definition	CT Angiographic diagnostic finding	Echocardiographic diagnostic finding	MRI diagnostic finding
Restrictive cardiomyopathy	Restrictive cardiomyopathy is characterized by a marked decrease in ventricular compliance. It is predominantly a disease of diastolic dysfunction where the systolic (contractile) function of the myocardium is usually unaffected.	CT is not useful in the evaluation of restrictive cardiomyopathy but can help in multi-modality imaging for exclusion of other diagnoses. Presence of pericardial calcification on CT along with appropriate hemodynamics may indicate pericardial constriction [58]. Although calcification of the pericardium is associated with constrictive pericarditis, not with restrictive cardiomyopathy, the absence of calcium is not a diagnostic finding. In 50 % of cases of constrictive pericarditis, there are no findings of a calcified pericardium; however, although a thickened pericardium (>4 mm) is associated with constrictive pericarditis, some patients with restrictive cardiomyopathy also have a mildly thickened pericardium in the absence of calcification (see the image below). Advanced imaging techniques may not be sufficient to make the diagnosis of restrictive cardiomyopathy, necessitating myocardial biopsy.	Echocardiography is often part of the patient's evaluation Normal ventricular size and systolic functions usually are evident in cases of restrictive cardiomyopathy [59–63]. Findings that have been described as helpful in diagnosing restrictive cardiomyopathy include mid-diastolic reversal of flow across the mitral and tricuspid valves. Atrial enlargement with normal left ventricular end-diastolic dimensions may also be seen. Typically, patients with constrictive pericarditis have a thickened pericardium and marked respiratory variation during diastole. One study showed that Doppler myocardial velocity gradients, as measured from the left ventricular posterior wall during the predetermined phases of the cardiac cycle, are lower in patients with restrictive cardiomyopathy than in patients with constrictive pericarditis [60]. Restrictive cardiomyopathy might not be distinguishable from constrictive pericarditis on the basis of echocardiography alone. Inadequate acoustic windows may limit echocardiography, and it may not be sufficient for the evaluation of pericardial thickness. In such cases, use of CT or MRI is the next step.	MRI is a sophisticated, accurate, noninvasive tool that is well suited to the evaluation of the morphology and function of the heart. In restrictive cardiomyopathy, the thickness of the pericardium (<4 mm) is a key finding [64–71]. Diagnosis of constrictive pericarditis (excluding restrictive cardiomyopathy) may be made on the basis of pericardial thickness. The sensitivity is 88 %; the specificity is 100 %; and the accuracy is 93 %. Ventricular hypertrophy is not associated with restrictive cardiomyopathy, but some degree of thickening may be seen on both cross-sectional imaging and echocardiography in cases of infiltrative restrictive cardiac disease (e.g., amyloidosis or hemochromatosis). Patients with a history of cardiac surgery or pericardiotomy may have a thickened pericardium without a constrictive physiologic pattern. Conversely, in the postoperative patient, the visceral pericardium may constrict the heart without being abnormally thick.

Table 13.2 (continued)

Myocardial condition	Definition	CT Angiographic diagnostic finding	Echocardiographic diagnostic finding	MRI diagnostic finding
Arrhythmogenic right ventricular cardiomyopathy (ARVC)	Disorder of the heart muscle of unknown origin. It is characterized by electrical instability of the heart as a result of replacement of the right ventricular myocardium with fatty or fibrous fatty tissue.	Dilatation of the right ventricle is one criterion for diagnosis of ARVC and it is commonly seen in patients with ARVC. Fatty tissue in conspicuous trabeculae of the right ventricle, especially in the anterior wall, apex, and inferior (diaphragmatic) wall; and a scalloped appearance (bulging) of the right ventricular wall are characteristic findings at helical computed tomography (CT) that may be used to diagnose ARVC [72]. Fatty tissue in the left ventricle and ventricular septum is seen relatively frequently in ARVC, and fat in the ventricular septum is another useful finding for diagnosis of ARVC with helical CT. When evaluating dilatation of the right ventricle, it is important to rule out pulmonary hypertension. A dilated right ventricle with an ectatic pulmonary trunk may indicate pulmonary hypertension rather than ARVC [72].	Tricuspid annular measurements are valuable, easy to obtain, and allow quantitative assessment of right ventricular function [73]. ARVC patients showed an abnormal velocity pattern that may be an early but non-specific sign of the disease. Normal right ventricular dimensions do not exclude ARVC, and subjective detection of early changes in wall motion may be difficult [73].	Revised CMR criteria now require presence of both qualitative findings (RV regional akinesia, dyskinesia, dyssynchronous contraction) and quantitative metrics (decreased ejection fraction *or* increased indexed RV end-diastolic volume) [74]. Major criteria (RV ejection fraction ≤40 % *or* indexed RV end-diastolic volume ≥110 mL/m^2 for men and ≥100 mL/m^2 for women) are chosen to achieve approximately 95 % specificity. Cutoffs with high specificity invariably result in lower sensitivity; major CMR criteria have a sensitivity of 68–76 % [75]. Minor criteria (RV ejection fraction 40–45 % *or* indexed RV end-diastolic volume 100–110 mL/m^2 for men and 90–100 mL/m^2 for women) had a higher sensitivity (79–89 %), but a consequently lower specificity (85–97 %) [76].

(continued)

Table 13.2 (continued)

Myocardial condition	Definition	CT Angiographic diagnostic finding	Echocardiographic diagnostic finding	MRI diagnostic finding
Takotsubo cardiomyopathy	Takotsubo cardiomyopathy, also known as transient apical ballooning syndrome is a type of non-ischemic cardiomyopathy in which there is a sudden temporary weakening of the muscular portion of the heart	Normal coronary arteries. Left ventricular apical hypokinesis with systolic ballooning. Useful to rule out acute coronary chest pain causes including the aorta and pulmonary arteries. CT is usually not performed in these patients unless the diagnosis is uncertain.	Echocardiography plays a key role in diagnostic assessment of Takotsubo cardiomyopathy (TTC) [76]. During the acute phase, TTE may detect a large area of dysfunctional myocardium usually extended beyond the territory of distribution of a single coronary artery. Wall motion analysis reveals a typical pattern of LV myocardial contractility characterized by symmetrical regional abnormalities extending equally into the anterior, inferior, and lateral walls. This 'circumferential pattern' can be considered a hallmark of TTC [77]. Echocardiography reveals LV morphology allowing the recognition not only the classic LV apical dysfunction, but also variant forms, such as midventricular dysfunction and apical sparing [76]. It also plays an important role in the early detection of severe potential complications such as right ventricular (RV) involvement (biventricular dysfunction), LVOT obstruction, thrombus formation, MR, and ventricular rupture [77–80]. Helps at follow-up to confirm recovery of LV function. Finally, non-conventional echocardiographic techniques (tissue Doppler, strain imaging, real-time three-dimensional [3D] echocardiography), coronary flow velocity reserve, and myocardial contrast echocardiography may provide new insights in the assessment of LV and RV myocardial function and coronary microcirculation physiopathology [78, 81]. Symmetric pattern of wall motion abnormalities (WMA) characteristic of typical TTC is sometimes difficult to assess by transthoracic echo (use of contrast agent for LV opacification could magnify this pattern). This peculiar pattern of WMA could also be evaluated by myocardial deformation imaging using the speckle tracking method, which demonstrates a transient circular impairment of not only longitudinal LV function but also circumferential and radial LV function as well as LV twist mechanics deficiency [82–84].	Late gadolinium enhancement (LGE) on CMRI is generally absent in stress cardiomyopathy in contrast to myocardial infarction in which intense subendocardial or transmural LGE is seen [85–89]. LGE is also useful in differentiating stress cardiomyopathy from myocarditis, which is characterized by patchy late gadolinium enhancement. However, when a low threshold for LGE is used (e.g., three standard deviations above the mean signal intensity of remote myocardium), LGE is occasionally detected in stress cardiomyopathy [87]. CMR evidence of myocardial edema is commonly seen in stress cardiomyopathy. However, myocardial edema is also seen in acute MI and myocarditis. In one series, 81% of patients had evidence of focal myocardial edema on CMR and these regions corresponded to areas of wall motion abnormality [90]. CMR may also enable identification of thrombus in the left or right ventricle, which may not be detected by echocardiography [90].

CT computed tomography, *MRI* magnetic resonance imaging, *CMR* cardiac MR, *SVC* superior vena cava, *IVC* inferior vena cava, *RV* right ventricle, *LV* left ventricle, *RA* right atrium, *LA* left atrium, *CP* Contrictive Pericarditis, *TDI* tissue Doppler imaging, *MRA* magnetic resonance angiography, *ECG* electrocardiography, *TTE* trans-thoracic echocardiography, *LVOT* left ventricular outflow tract

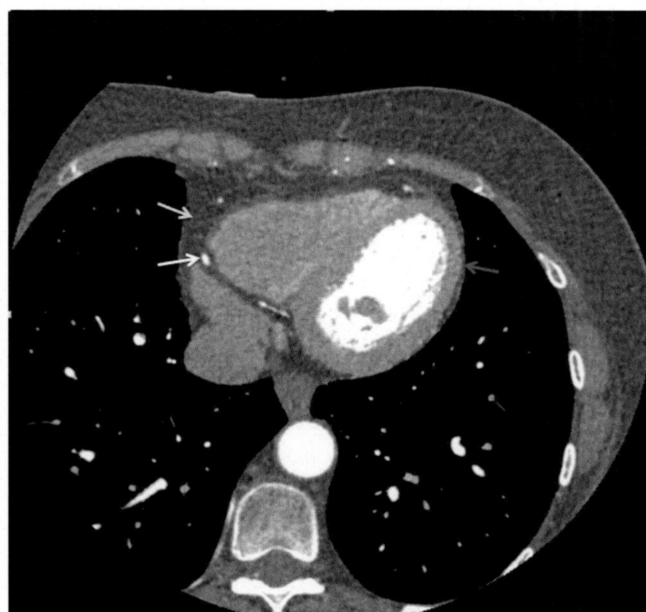

Fig. 13.7 Revolution CT Angiography produces excellent image quality with reduce radiation dose. Thinning of the left ventricular wall (*blue arrowhead*) a sign of dilated cardiomyopathy in this patient. Note the right coronary artery (*white arrowhead*) and pericardium (*yellow arrowhead*)

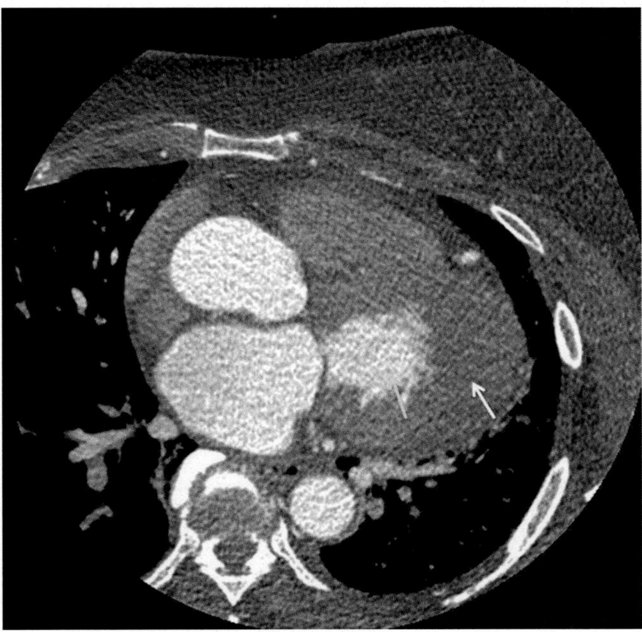

Fig. 13.8 55 year old African American female with zero calcium score (scanning heart rate of 53 beat per minute and body mass index of 43). Apical variant hypertrophic Cardiomyopathy with marked thickening of the apical walls of the left ventricle (*white arrowhead*). Very small left ventricular cavity (*yellow arrowhead*) due to hypertrophy of the left ventricle.

Future Directions

CT scan has revolutionized cardiac diagnostic and prognostic capabilities, not only to diagnose the disease but also to monitor the progression and or regression of the disease. With current advancement of the CT technology, radiation exposure is very limited and continues to diminish with ongoing development of CT protocols. The Revolution CT scanner is one of the newer developments by GE healthcare. It can acquire excellent image quality despite high heart rates and with less radiation and contrast dose than typical CT scanners (Fig. 13.7). The pericardium may be secondarily involved with ischemic or other heart disease. Implementation of CT scanning in ER protocols for chest pain may help identify pericardial disease. Future molecular imaging will be another addition to the current CT protocol for pericardial and myocardial disease evaluation.

References

1. Richardson P, McKenna W, Bristow M, Maisch B, Mautner B, O'Connell J, et al. Report of the 1995 World Health Organization/International Society and Federation of Cardiology Task Force on the definition and classification of cardiomyopathies. Circulation. 1996;93(5):841–2.
2. Tummala LS, Young RK, Singh T, Jani S, Srichai MB. Role of non-invasive imaging in the work-up of cardiomyopathies. Curr Atheroscler Rep. 2015;17(3):486.
3. Cerqueira MD, Weissman NJ, Dilsizian V, Jacobs AK, Kaul S, Laskey WK, et al. Standardized myocardial segmentation and nomenclature for tomographic imaging of the heart. A statement for healthcare professionals from the Cardiac Imaging Committee of the Council on Clinical Cardiology of the American Heart Association. Circulation. 2002;105(4):539–42.
4. Annuar BR, Liew CK, Chin SP, Ong TK, Seyfarth MT, Chan WL, et al. Assessment of global and regional left ventricular function using 64-slice multislice computed tomography and 2D echocardiography: a comparison with cardiac magnetic resonance. Eur J Radiol. 2008;65:112–9. Ireland.
5. Halliburton SS, Petersilka M, Schvartzman PR, Obuchowski N, White RD. Evaluation of left ventricular dysfunction using multiphasic reconstructions of coronary multi-slice computed tomography data in patients with chronic ischemic heart disease: validation against cine magnetic resonance imaging. Int J Cardiovasc Imaging. 2003;19(1):73–83.
6. Tandri H, Bomma C, Calkins H, Bluemke DA. Magnetic resonance and computed tomography imaging of arrhythmogenic right ventricular dysplasia. J Magn Reson Imaging. 2004;19(6):848–58.
7. Petersen SE, Selvanayagam JB, Wiesmann F, Robson MD, Francis JM, Anderson RH, et al. Left ventricular non-compaction: insights from cardiovascular magnetic resonance imaging. J Am Coll Cardiol. 2005;46:101–5. United States.
8. Brett NJ, Strugnell WE, Slaughter RE. Acute myocarditis demonstrated on CT coronary angiography with MRI correlation. Circ Cardiovasc Imaging. 2011;4:e5–6. United States.
9. Brooks MA, Sane DC. CT findings in acute myocarditis: 2 cases. J Thorac Imaging. 2007;22:277–9. United States.
10. Codreanu A, Djaballah W, Angioi M, Ethevenot G, Moulin F, Felblinger J, et al. Detection of myocarditis by contrast-enhanced

MRI in patients presenting with acute coronary syndrome but no coronary stenosis. J Magn Reson Imaging. 2007;25(5):957–64.
11. Roberts WC, Spray TL. Pericardial heart disease: a study of its causes, consequences, and morphologic features. Cardiovasc Clin. 1976;7(3):11–65.
12. Truong MT, Erasmus JJ, Gladish GW, Sabloff BS, Marom EM, Madewell JE, et al. Anatomy of pericardial recesses on multidetector CT: implications for oncologic imaging. AJR Am J Roentgenol. 2003;181(4):1109–13.
13. Soulen RL, Stark DD, Higgins CB. Magnetic resonance imaging of constrictive pericardial disease. Am J Cardiol. 1985;55:480–4. United States.
14. Spodick DH. Pericardial disease. JAMA. 1997;278(9):704.
15. Himelman RB, Lee E, Schiller NB. Septal bounce, vena cava plethora, and pericardial adhesion: informative two-dimensional echocardiographic signs in the diagnosis of pericardial constriction. J Am Soc Echocardiogr. 1988;1(5):333–40.
16. Oyama N, Komuro K, Nambu T, Manning WJ, Miyasaka K. Computed tomography and magnetic resonance imaging of the pericardium: anatomy and pathology. Magn Reson Med Sci. 2004;3:145–52. Japan.
17. Seo GW, Seol SH, Jeong HJ, Seo MG, Song PS, Kim DK, et al. A large pericardial cyst compressing the left atrium presenting as a pericardiopleural efussion. Heart Lung Circ. 2014;23(12):e273–5.
18. O'Leary SM, Williams PL, Williams MP, Edwards AJ, Roobottom CA, Morgan-Hughes GJ, et al. Imaging the pericardium: appearances on ECG-gated 64-detector row cardiac computed tomography. Br J Radiol. 2010;83:194–205. England.
19. Luk A, Ahn E, Vaideeswar P, Butany JW. Pericardial tumors. Semin Diagn Pathol. 2008;25(1):47–53.
20. Dey D, Wong ND, Tamarappoo B, Nakazato R, Gransar H, Cheng VY, et al. Computer-aided non-contrast CT-based quantification of pericardial and thoracic fat and their associations with coronary calcium and Metabolic Syndrome. Atherosclerosis. 2010;209:136–41. Ireland.
21. Ding J, Kritchevsky SB, Harris TB, Burke GL, Detrano RC, Szklo M, et al. The association of pericardial fat with calcified coronary plaque. Obesity (Silver Spring). 2008;16:1914–9. United States.
22. Ding J, Kritchevsky SB, Hsu FC, Harris TB, Burke GL, Detrano RC, et al. Association between non-subcutaneous adiposity and calcified coronary plaque: a substudy of the Multi-Ethnic Study of Atherosclerosis. Am J Clin Nutr. 2008;88:645–50. United States.
23. Mazurek T, Zhang L, Zalewski A, Mannion JD, Diehl JT, Arafat H, et al. Human epicardial adipose tissue is a source of inflammatory mediators. Circulation. 2003;108:2460–6. United States.
24. Greif M, Becker A, von Ziegler F, Lebherz C, Lehrke M, Broedl UC, et al. Pericardial adipose tissue determined by dual source CT is a risk factor for coronary atherosclerosis. Arterioscler Thromb Vasc Biol. 2009;29:781–6. United States.
25. Alexopoulos N, McLean DS, Janik M, Arepalli CD, Stillman AE, Raggi P. Epicardial adipose tissue and coronary artery plaque characteristics. Atherosclerosis. 2009;210:150–4. Ireland: Elsevier Ireland Ltd.
26. Cheng VY, Dey D, Tamarappoo B, Nakazato R, Gransar H, Miranda-Peats R, et al. Pericardial fat burden on ECG-gated noncontrast CT in asymptomatic patients who subsequently experience adverse cardiovascular events. JACC Cardiovasc Imaging. 2010;3:352–60. United States: American College of Cardiology Foundation. Published by Elsevier Inc.
27. Dey D, Nakazato R, Li D, Berman DS. Epicardial and thoracic fat – Noninvasive measurement and clinical implications. Cardiovasc Diagn Ther. 1949–2012;2:85–93. China Republic.
28. Rosito GA, Massaro JM, Hoffmann U, Ruberg FL, Mahabadi AA, Vasan RS, et al. Pericardial fat, visceral abdominal fat, cardiovascular disease risk factors, and vascular calcification in a community-based sample: the Framingham Heart Study. Circulation. 2008;117:605–13. United States.
29. Tamarappoo B, Dey D, Shmilovich H, Nakazato R, Gransar H, Cheng VY, et al. Increased pericardial fat volume measured from noncontrast CT predicts myocardial ischemia by SPECT. JACC Cardiovasc Imaging. 2010;3:1104–12. United States American College of Cardiology Foundation. Published by Elsevier Inc.
30. Saura D, Oliva MJ, Rodriguez D, Pascual-Figal DA, Hurtado JA, Pinar E, et al. Reproducibility of echocardiographic measurements of epicardial fat thickness. Int J Cardiol. 2010;141:311–3. Netherlands.
31. Dey D, Suzuki Y, Suzuki S, Ohba M, Slomka PJ, Polk D, et al. Automated quantitation of pericardiac fat from noncontrast CT. Invest Radiol. 2008;43:145–53. United States.
32. Hammer MM, Raptis CA, Javidan-Nejad C, Bhalla S. Accuracy of computed tomography findings in acute pericarditis. Acta Radiol. 2014;55:1197–202. England: The Foundation Acta Radiologica 2013 Reprints and permissions: sagepub.co.uk/journalsPermissions.nav.
33. Khandaker MH, Espinosa RE, Nishimura RA, Sinak LJ, Hayes SN, Melduni RM, et al. Pericardial disease: diagnosis and management. Mayo Clin Proc. 2010;85:572–93. United States.
34. Boffa GM, Thiene G, Nava A, Dalla VS. Cardiomyopathy: a necessary revision of the WHO classification. Int J Cardiol. 1991;30(1): 1–7.
35. Yoshida M, Takamoto T. Left ventricular hypertrophic patterns and wall motion dynamics in hypertrophic cardiomyopathy: an electron beam computed tomographic study. Intern Med. 1997;36(4): 263–9.
36. Naito H, Saito H, Ohta M, Takamiya M. Significance of ultrafast computed tomography in cardiac imaging: usefulness in assessment of myocardial characteristics and cardiac function. Jpn Circ J. 1990;54(3):322–7.
37. Saito H, Naito H, Takamiya M, Hamada S, Imakita S, Ohta M. Late enhancement of the left ventricular wall in hypertrophic cardiomyopathy by ultrafast computed tomography: a comparison with regional myocardial thickening. Br J Radiol. 1991;64(767): 993–1000.
38. McKenna WJ, Spirito P, Desnos M, Dubourg O, Komajda M. Experience from clinical genetics in hypertrophic cardiomyopathy: proposal for new diagnostic criteria in adult members of affected families. Heart. 1997;77(2):130–2.
39. Maron BJ, Pelliccia A, Spirito P. Cardiac disease in young trained athletes. Insights into methods for distinguishing athlete's heart from structural heart disease, with particular emphasis on hypertrophic cardiomyopathy. Circulation. 1995;91(5):1596–601.
40. Lattanzi F, Spirito P, Picano E, Mazzarisi A, Landini L, Distante A, et al. Quantitative assessment of ultrasonic myocardial reflectivity in hypertrophic cardiomyopathy. J Am Coll Cardiol. 1991;17:1085–90. United States.
41. Naito J, Masuyama T, Tanouchi J, Mano T, Kondo H, Yamamoto K, et al. Analysis of transmural trend of myocardial integrated ultrasound backscatter for differentiation of hypertrophic cardiomyopathy and ventricular hypertrophy due to hypertension. J Am Coll Cardiol. 1994;24:517–24. United States.
42. Prasad K, Atherton J, Smith GC, McKenna WJ, Frenneaux MP, Nihoyannopoulos P. Echocardiographic pitfalls in the diagnosis of hypertrophic cardiomyopathy. Heart. 1999;82 Suppl 3:III8–15.
43. Maron BJ, McKenna WJ, Danielson GK, Kappenberger LJ, Kuhn HJ, Seidman CE, et al. American College of Cardiology/European Society of Cardiology clinical expert consensus document on hypertrophic cardiomyopathy. A report of the American College of Cardiology Foundation Task Force on Clinical Expert Consensus Documents and the European Society of Cardiology Committee for practice guidelines. J Am Coll Cardiol. 2003;42:1687–713. United States.
44. Park JH, Kim YM, Chung JW, Park YB, Han JK, Han MC. MR imaging of hypertrophic cardiomyopathy. Radiology. 1992;185(2): 441–6.

45. Sardanelli F, Molinari G, Petillo A, Ottonello C, Parodi RC, Masperone MA, et al. MRI in hypertrophic cardiomyopathy: a morphofunctional study. J Comput Assist Tomogr. 1993;17(6):862–72.
46. Posma JL, Blanksma PK, van der Wall EE, Hamer HP, Mooyaart EL, Lie KI. Assessment of quantitative hypertrophy scores in hypertrophic cardiomyopathy: magnetic resonance imaging versus echocardiography. Am Heart J. 1996;132:1020–7. United States.
47. Hansen MW, Merchant N. MRI of hypertrophic cardiomyopathy: part I. MRI appearances. AJR Am J Roentgenol. 2007;189:1335–43. United States.
48. Maron BJ, Bonow RO, Cannon 3rd RO, Leon MB, Epstein SE. Hypertrophic cardiomyopathy. Interrelations of clinical manifestations, pathophysiology, and therapy (1). N Engl J Med. 1987;316(13):780–9.
49. Maron MS, Hauser TH, Dubrow E, Horst TA, Kissinger KV, Udelson JE, et al. Right ventricular involvement in hypertrophic cardiomyopathy. Am J Cardiol. 2007;100:1293–8. United States.
50. de Roos A, Doornbos J, Luyten PR, Oosterwaal LJ, van der Wall EE, den Hollander JA. Cardiac metabolism in patients with dilated and hypertrophic cardiomyopathy: assessment with proton-decoupled P-31 MR spectroscopy. J Magn Reson Imaging. 1992;2(6):711–9.
51. Mirowitz SA, Lee JK, Gutierrez FR, Brown JJ, Eilenberg SS. Normal signal-void patterns in cardiac cine MR images. Radiology. 1990;176(1):49–55.
52. Aurigemma G, Reichek N, Schiebler M, Axel L. Evaluation of mitral regurgitation by cine magnetic resonance imaging. Am J Cardiol. 1990;66:621–5. United States.
53. Utz JA, Herfkens RJ, Heinsimer JA, Shimakawa A, Glover G, Pelc N. Valvular regurgitation: dynamic MR imaging. Radiology. 1988;168(1):91–4.
54. Wagner S, Auffermann W, Buser P, Lim TH, Kircher B, Pflugfelder P, et al. Diagnostic accuracy and estimation of the severity of valvular regurgitation from the signal void on cine magnetic resonance images. Am Heart J. 1989;118:760–7. United States.
55. O'Hanlon R, Assomull RG, Prasad SK. Use of cardiovascular magnetic resonance for diagnosis and management in hypertrophic cardiomyopathy. Curr Cardiol Rep. 2007;9(1):51–6.
56. Hansen MW, Merchant N. MRI of hypertrophic cardiomyopathy: part 2, Differential diagnosis, risk stratification, and posttreatment MRI appearances. AJR Am J Roentgenol. 2007;189:1344–52. United States.
57. Fattori R, Rocchi G, Celletti F, Bertaccini P, Rapezzi C, Gavelli G. Contribution of magnetic resonance imaging in the differential diagnosis of cardiac amyloidosis and symmetric hypertrophic cardiomyopathy. Am Heart J. 1998;136:824–30. United States.
58. Mastouri R, Sawada SG, Mahenthiran J. Noninvasive imaging techniques of constrictive pericarditis. Expert Rev Cardiovasc Ther. 2010;8(9):1335–47.
59. Cheitlin MD, Alpert JS, Armstrong WF, Aurigemma GP, Beller GA, Bierman FZ, et al. ACC/AHA guidelines for the clinical application of echocardiography: executive summary. A report of the American College of Cardiology/American Heart Association Task Force on practice guidelines (Committee on Clinical Application of Echocardiography). Developed in collaboration with the American Society of Echocardiography. J Am Coll Cardiol. 1997;29(4):862–79.
60. Palka P, Lange A, Donnelly JE, Nihoyannopoulos P. Differentiation between restrictive cardiomyopathy and constrictive pericarditis by early diastolic doppler myocardial velocity gradient at the posterior wall. Circulation. 2000;102(6):655–62.
61. Rajagopalan N, Garcia MJ, Rodriguez L, Murray RD, Apperson-Hansen C, Stugaard M, et al. Comparison of new Doppler echocardiographic methods to differentiate constrictive pericardial heart disease and restrictive cardiomyopathy. Am J Cardiol. 2001;87:86–94. United States.
62. Sengupta PP, Krishnamoorthy VK, Abhayaratna WP, Korinek J, Belohlavek M, Sundt 3rd TM, et al. Comparison of usefulness of tissue Doppler imaging versus brain natriuretic peptide for differentiation of constrictive pericardial disease from restrictive cardiomyopathy. Am J Cardiol. 2008;102:357–62. United States.
63. McCall R, Stoodley PW, Richards DA, Thomas L. Restrictive cardiomyopathy versus constrictive pericarditis: making the distinction using tissue Doppler imaging. Eur J Echocardiogr. 2008;9:591–4. England.
64. White CS. MR evaluation of the pericardium. Top Magn Reson Imaging. 1995;7(4):258–66.
65. White CS. MR evaluation of the pericardium and cardiac malignancies. Magn Reson Imaging Clin N Am. 1996;4(2):237–51.
66. Celletti F, Fattori R, Napoli G, Leone O, Rocchi G, Reggiani LB, et al. Assessment of restrictive cardiomyopathy of amyloid or idiopathic etiology by magnetic resonance imaging. Am J Cardiol. 1999;83:798–801, A10. United States.
67. Masui T, Finck S, Higgins CB. Constrictive pericarditis and restrictive cardiomyopathy: evaluation with MR imaging. Radiology. 1992;182(2):369–73.
68. Schulz-Menger J, Friedrich MG. Magnetic resonance imaging in patients with cardiomyopathies: when and why. Herz. 2000;25(4):384–91.
69. Shehata ML, Turkbey EB, Vogel-Claussen J, Bluemke DA. Role of cardiac magnetic resonance imaging in assessment of nonischemic cardiomyopathies. Top Magn Reson Imaging. 2008;19:43–57. United States.
70. Westenberg JJ, Braun J, Van de Veire NR, Klautz RJ, Versteegh MI, Roes SD, et al. Magnetic resonance imaging assessment of reverse left ventricular remodeling late after restrictive mitral annuloplasty in early stages of dilated cardiomyopathy. J Thorac Cardiovasc Surg. 2008;135:1247–52; discussion 52–3. United States.
71. Harris SR, Glockner J, Misselt AJ, Syed IS, Araoz PA. Cardiac MR imaging of nonischemic cardiomyopathies. Magn Reson Imaging Clin N Am. 2008;16:165–83, vii. United States.
72. Kimura F, Sakai F, Sakomura Y, Fujimura M, Ueno E, Matsuda N, et al. Helical CT features of arrhythmogenic right ventricular cardiomyopathy. Radiographics. 2002;22(5):1111–24.
73. Lindstrom L, Wilkenshoff UM, Larsson H, Wranne B. Echocardiographic assessment of arrhythmogenic right ventricular cardiomyopathy. Heart. 2001;86(1):31–8.
74. te Riele AS, Tandri H, Bluemke DA. Arrhythmogenic right ventricular cardiomyopathy (ARVC): cardiovascular magnetic resonance update. J Cardiovasc Magn Reson. 2014;16:50. England.
75. Bluemke DA. ARVC: Imaging diagnosis is still in the eye of the beholder. JACC Cardiovasc Imaging. 2011;4:288–91. United States.
76. Citro R, Piscione F, Parodi G, Salerno-Uriarte J, Bossone E. Role of echocardiography in takotsubo cardiomyopathy. Heart Fail Clin. 2013;9(2):157–66, viii.
77. Citro R, Rigo F, Ciampi Q, D'Andrea A, Provenza G, Mirra M, et al. Echocardiographic assessment of regional left ventricular wall motion abnormalities in patients with tako-tsubo cardiomyopathy: comparison with anterior myocardial infarction. Eur J Echocardiogr. 2011;12:542–9. England.
78. Parodi G, Del Pace S, Salvadori C, Carrabba N, Olivotto I, Gensini GF. Left ventricular apical ballooning syndrome as a novel cause of acute mitral regurgitation. J Am Coll Cardiol. 2007;50:647–9. United States.
79. Haghi D, Athanasiadis A, Papavassiliu T, Suselbeck T, Fluechter S, Mahrholdt H, et al. Right ventricular involvement in Takotsubo cardiomyopathy. Eur Heart J. 2006;27:2433–9. England.
80. de Gregorio C, Grimaldi P, Lentini C. Left ventricular thrombus formation and cardioembolic complications in patients with Takotsubo-like syndrome: a systematic review. Int J Cardiol. 2008;131:18–24. Netherlands.
81. Meimoun P, Clerc J, Vincent C, Flahaut F, Germain AL, Elmkies F, et al. Non-invasive detection of tako-tsubo cardiomyopathy vs.

acute anterior myocardial infarction by transthoracic Doppler echocardiography. Eur Heart J Cardiovasc Imaging. 2013;14: 464–70. England.
82. Mansencal N, Abbou N, Pilliere R, El Mahmoud R, Farcot JC, Dubourg O. Usefulness of two-dimensional speckle tracking echocardiography for assessment of Tako-Tsubo cardiomyopathy. Am J Cardiol. 2009;103:1020–4. United States.
83. Meimoun P, Passos P, Benali T, Boulanger J, Elmkies F, Zemir H, et al. Assessment of left ventricular twist mechanics in Tako-tsubo cardiomyopathy by two-dimensional speckle-tracking echocardiography. Eur J Echocardiogr. 2011;12:931–9. England.
84. Heggemann F, Weiss C, Hamm K, Kaden J, Suselbeck T, Papavassiliu T, et al. Global and regional myocardial function quantification by two-dimensional strain in Takotsubo cardiomyopathy. Eur J Echocardiogr. 2009;10:760–4. England.
85. Abe Y, Kondo M, Matsuoka R, Araki M, Dohyama K, Tanio H. Assessment of clinical features in transient left ventricular apical ballooning. J Am Coll Cardiol. 2003;41:737–42. United States.
86. Dec GW. Recognition of the apical ballooning syndrome in the United States. Circulation. 2005;111:388–90. United States.
87. Eitel I, von Knobelsdorff-Brenkenhoff F, Bernhardt P, Carbone I, Muellerleile K, Aldrovandi A, et al. Clinical characteristics and cardiovascular magnetic resonance findings in stress (takotsubo) cardiomyopathy. JAMA. 2011;306:277–86. United States.
88. Handy AD, Prasad A, Olson TM. Investigating genetic variation of adrenergic receptors in familial stress cardiomyopathy (apical ballooning syndrome). J Cardiol. 2009;54:516–7. Japan.
89. Sharkey SW, Maron BJ, Nelson P, Parpart M, Maron MS, Bristow MR. Adrenergic receptor polymorphisms in patients with stress (tako-tsubo) cardiomyopathy. J Cardiol. 2009;53:53–7. Japan.
90. Sharkey SW, Windenburg DC, Lesser JR, Maron MS, Hauser RG, Lesser JN, et al. Natural history and expansive clinical profile of stress (tako-tsubo) cardiomyopathy. J Am Coll Cardiol. 2010;55:333–41. United States: 2010 American College of Cardiology Foundation. Published by Elsevier Inc.

Computed Tomography Evaluation in Valvular Heart Disease

14

Nada Shaban, Javier Sanz, Leticia Fernández Friera, and Mario Jorge García

Abstract

Valvular heart disease commonly affects patients evaluated in the cardiology practice. Although Echocardiography is the primary modality for the evaluation of patients with suspected or known valvular heart disease, cardiac CT has distinct advantage in the evaluation of several anatomical features of the cardiac valves, including the extent of calcification, the geometry of the annulus and the evaluation of biological and mechanical prostheses. It is important for cardiologists, radiologists and other cardiac imaging specialists to recognize the features of normal and abnormal valves in patients who are referred for cardiac CT evaluation.

Keywords

Cardiac valve • Aortic stenosis • Aortic regurgitation • Mitral Stenosis • Mitral Regurgitation • Bioprosthetic valves • Mechanical prosthetic valves • Trans-aortic valve replacement (TAVR)

Introduction

Valvular heart disease (VHD) affects 2.5 % of U.S. adults and predominantly involves the left cardiac chambers. Regurgitant lesions are more common than stenotic, and mitral regurgitation (MR) is the most prevalent abnormality [1]. Doppler echocardiography is the initial imaging modality of choice, allowing for comprehensive diagnosis in the majority of patients [2, 3]. In cases of poor acoustic window and/or disparate results regarding disease severity, additional tests may be required. Cardiac catheterization is a time-honored modality, but is limited by its invasive nature. Magnetic resonance imaging (MRI) has become an excellent noninvasive alternative for both valvular insufficiency and stenosis [4]. Due to the need for radiation and contrast, computed tomography (CT) has a limited role for the evaluation of VHD as the primary indication. It may occasionally be employed as such when echocardiographic results are inconclusive and the patient is not a good candidate for MRI. Table 14.1 outlines the strengths and weaknesses of the different imaging modalities used to assess VHD [5]. CT is increasingly being used for preoperative evaluations for noninvasive coronary angiography and for workup for transcatheter heart valve replacement. Useful information on valve anatomy and function can simultaneously be obtained from a coronary CT examination.

Electronic supplementary material The online version of this chapter (doi:10.1007/978-3-319-28219-0_14) contains supplementary material, which is available to authorized users.

N. Shaban, MD
Department of Medicine, Division of Cardiology, North Shore University Hospital, Manhasset, NY, USA

J. Sanz, MD
Department of Medicine, Division of Cardiology, Mount-Sinai Medical Center, New York, NY, USA

L.F. Friera, MD
Department of Medicine, Division of Cardiology, Mount-Sinai Medical Center, New York, NY, USA

Centro Nacional de Investigaciones Cardiovasculares, Madrid, Spain

M.J. García, MD, FACC, FACP (✉)
Division of Cardiology, Montefiore Medical Center, 111 East 210th St, Bronx, NY 10467, USA
e-mail: mariogar@montefiore.org

M.J. Budoff, J.S. Shinbane (eds.), *Cardiac CT Imaging: Diagnosis of Cardiovascular Disease*, DOI 10.1007/978-3-319-28219-0_14

Table 14.1 Strengths and weaknesses of the different imaging modalities used to assess VHD

Parameter	Transthoracic echocardiography	Transesophageal echocardiography	Cardiac CT	Cardiac MRI
Spatial resolution	Very good. Pixel size 1–2 mm.	Excellent. Pixel sizes 0.5–1.0 mm.	Excellent. Pixel sizes 0.6–0.75 mm	Good. In plane resolution is good, but through-plane resolution is fair, 6–8 mm.
Temporal resolution	Excellent. 30–60 frames/s in real time.	Excellent. 30–60 frames/s in real time.	Dependent on scanner technology. 10–20 frames per beat if ECG gating applied.	Depends on pulse sequence and heart rate. 20–30 frames per beat if ECG gating applied.
Flow velocity and volume measurements	Excellent with Doppler ultrasound.	Excellent with Doppler ultrasound.	Poor. No current validated clinical method for measuring flow velocity or flow volume at CT.	Good with cine phase-contrast imaging. Not as widely used or standardized as Doppler measurements.
Patient specific limitations	Poor acoustic windows in some patients.	Invasive and requires sedation.	Images are easily acquired in many patients, but uses radiation and contrast material, which limits use.	Requires compliant patient. Claustrophobia limits uses. Cannot be used with pacemakers or defibrillators.
Ancillary information	Good. Cardiac dimensions can be measured, although with less precision than with CT or MRI.	Good. Cardiac dimensions can be measured, although with less precision than with CT or MRI.	Excellent. Quantitatively measures left ventricular dimensions and volumes.	Superior.

General Considerations

A diagram summarizing the potential applications of CT for the evaluation of patients with VHD is shown in Fig. 14.1. The Society for Computed Cardiac Tomography recently released consensus guidelines for the appropriate use of cardiac CT to evaluate non-coronary structures including cardiac valves. It is appropriate to use cardiac CT to evaluate native and prosthetic valves with suspected clinically significant valvular dysfunction if the images from other noninvasive methods are inadequate. It is not recommended as the initial imaging modality to assess valvular anatomy and function [6].

Valvular assessment includes the detection of calcification on non-contrast scans and of other aspects of valvular anatomy and cardiac function using contrast enhancement. Quantification of valve calcification follows the same principles as coronary calcium scoring, and the "Agatston", volumetric and mass scores have been proposed. Regarding contrast-enhanced CT, detailed evaluation of valvular function and anatomy is possible for both regurgitant and, particularly, stenotic lesions through planimetry of the valve area.

CT also allows for accurate quantification of ventricular volumes, ejection fraction and mass [7], all of which carry important prognostic and therapeutic implications in patients with VHD. In isolated regurgitant lesions, the regurgitant volume and regurgitant fraction can be derived from the difference between the left and right stroke volumes [8]. Stenosis or regurgitation of the atrioventricular valves usually results in atrial enlargement. Significant regurgitation of any valve eventually causes ipsilateral ventricular dilatation, often accompanied by eccentric hypertrophy. Stenotic lesions of the semilunar (aortic and pulmonary) valves lead to concentric hypertrophy and later may also lead to ventricular dilatation. Post-stenotic dilatation of the pulmonary trunk or the ascending aorta may be present as well.

CT can provide important information regarding hemodynamic repercussions of valvular lesions. Enlargement of the right heart chambers can be caused by tricuspid/pulmonary abnormalities or secondary pulmonary hypertension, and typically leads to posterior rotation of the cardiac axis (Fig. 14.2). Pulmonary vein dilatation and interstitial and alveolar lung edema are all signs of increased left atrial pressures and left-sided heart failure. Similarly, dilatation of the pulmonary arteries, right heart chambers, superior and inferior vena cava, pleuro-pericardial effusions and ascites, are suggestive of pulmonary hypertension and/or right ventricular heart failure [9].

Cardiac CT has had a major emergence in the realm of preoperative assessment of transcatheter aortic valve replacement (TAVR). It is crucial in the assessment of annular area (Fig. 14.3), diameter, valve leaflet morphology/calcification (Fig. 14.4), optimum deployment angles, and peripheral vascular assessment (Figs. 14.5 and 14.6). The severity of the aortic valve Agatston calcium score, calculated by cardiac CT, has been shown to correlate with degree of paravalvular leak following transcatheter heart valve implantation.

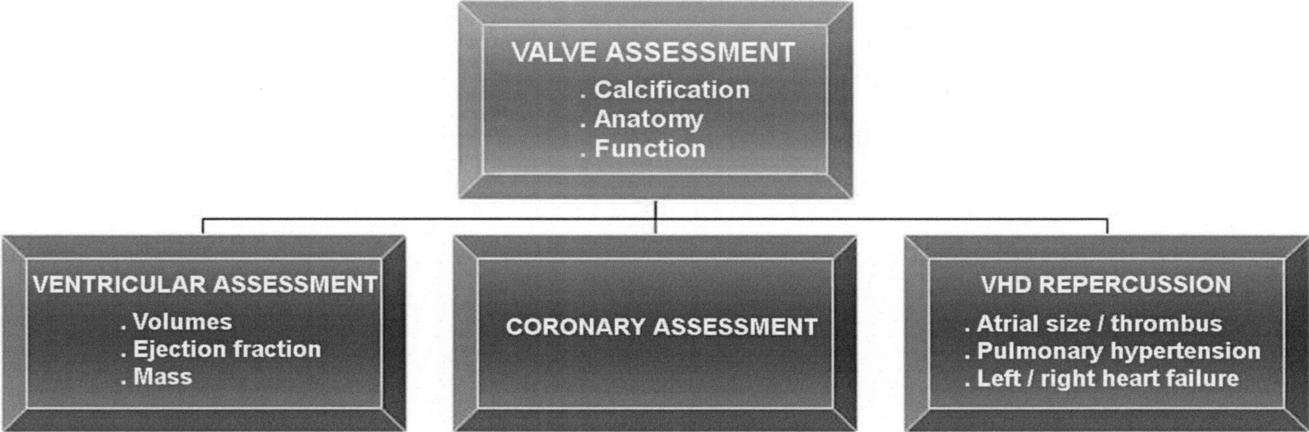

Fig. 14.1 Comprehensive evaluation of valvular heart disease (*VHD*) with CT

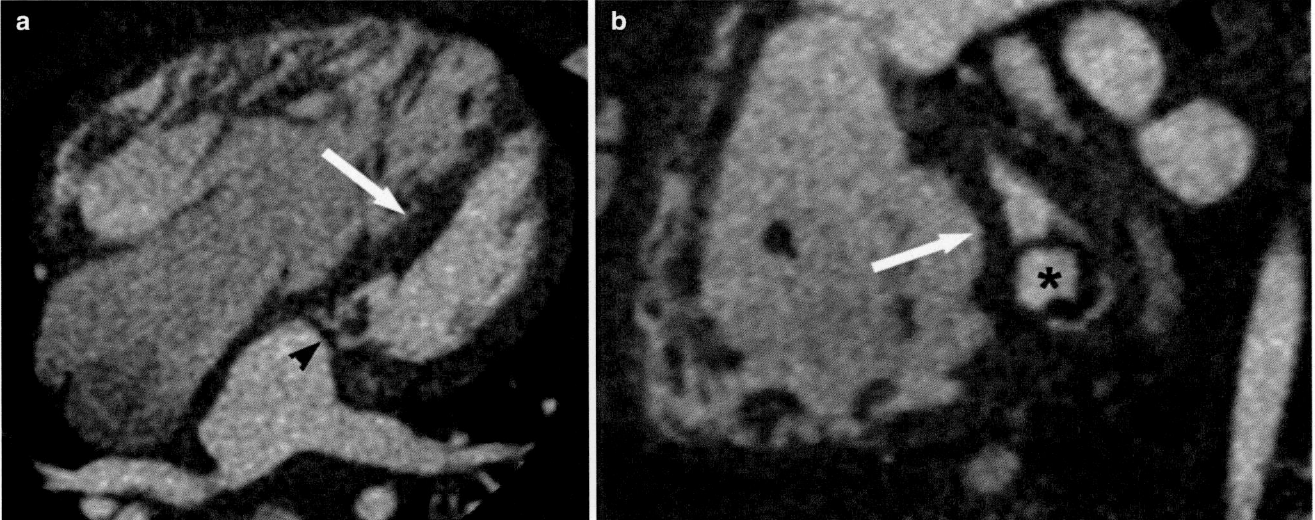

Fig. 14.2 Four chamber (panel **a**) and short-axis (panel **b**) views of a contrast-enhanced CT scan in an young patient with congenital mitral stenosis ("parachute mitral valve"; *arrowhead* and *asterisk*) and secondary pulmonary hypertension. There is severe right ventricular hypertrophy and enlargement, together with abnormal interventricular septal bowing indicative of right ventricular pressure/volume overload (*arrows*)

CT coronary angiography for preoperative evaluation in VHD is also increasingly being used. A high accuracy for the detection of significant coronary stenoses has been reported, with slightly lower diagnostic yield in cases of aortic stenosis (AS) due to frequent aortic and coronary calcifications [10–13]. These studies have demonstrated high negative and moderate positive predictive value; thus, patients referred for valvular surgery without significant coronary stenoses by CT may safely avoid the need for invasive angiography [14]. On the other hand, patients with greater than a mild degree of luminal stenosis or extensive calcifications need to have a confirmatory catheterization. For this reason, it seems prudent to consider CT for this application only in selected patients with low or intermediate pre-test probability.

A typical imaging protocol is summarized in Table 14.2. Contrast infusion is routinely followed by saline, resulting in a more compact bolus and easier evaluation of the right coronary artery; however, it may also impair the visualization of right chambers and valves. This can be overcome by employing dual- or triple-phase injection protocols [15, 16]. Retrospective ECG gating is advantageous in patients with VHD at the expense of higher radiation dose. ECG-based tube current modulation can be used, but it may limit the assessment of both ventricles and valves, particularly in obese patients and in the cardiac phases with lower output. If such evaluation is intended, it may be necessary to avoid its use.

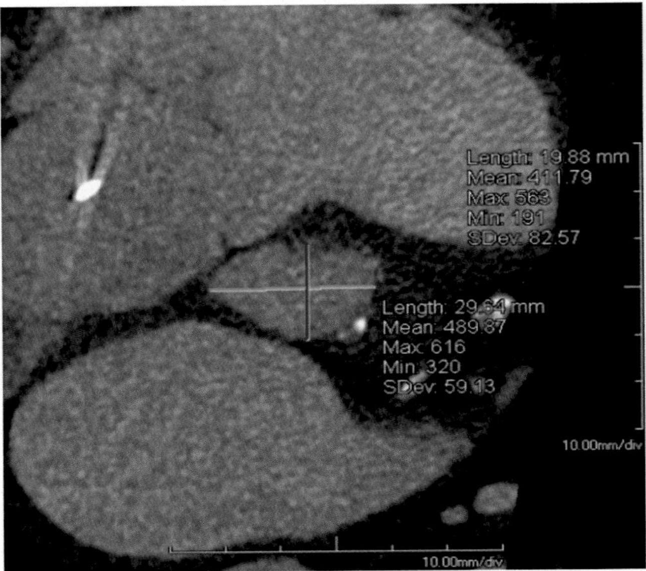

Fig. 14.3 Axial-oblique image of the aortic annulus in a patient evaluated for trans-aortic valve replacement (TAVR) demonstrating an elliptical geometry. *Green* is antero-posterior and *blue* is transverse diameter of the LV outflow tract

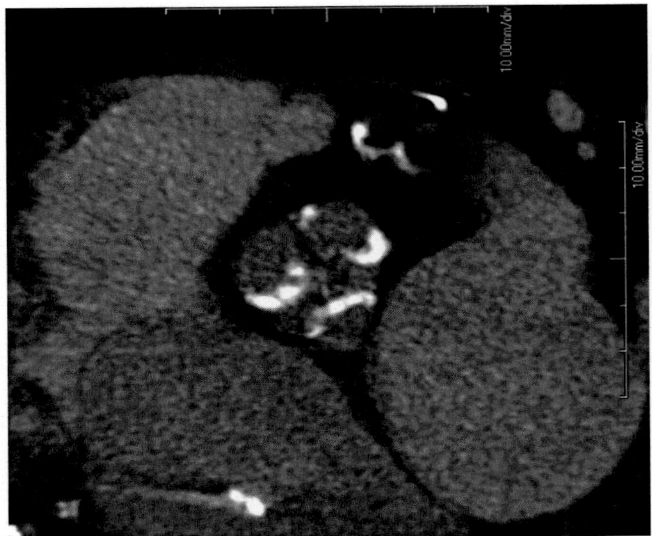

Fig. 14.4 Axial-oblique image of the aortic valve in a patient evaluated for trans-aortic valve replacement (TAVR) demonstrating moderate leaflet calcification

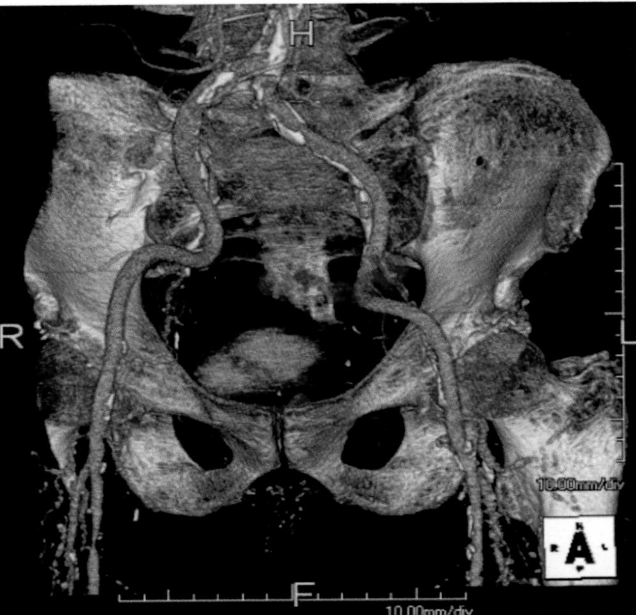

Fig. 14.5 3-D Volume-rendered image of the iliac and femoral arteries in a patient evaluated for trans-aortic valve replacement (TAVR) demonstrating moderate calcification and tortuosity

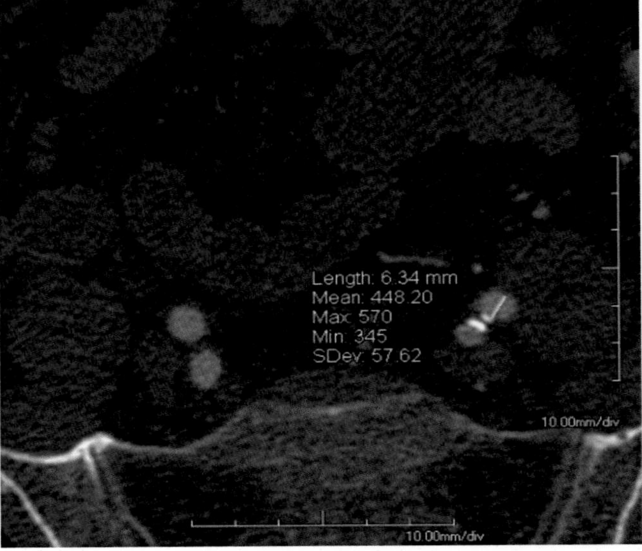

Fig. 14.6 Axial image of the proximal femoral arteries in a patient evaluated for trans-aortic valve replacement (TAVR)

Specific Valvular Abnormalities

Aortic Stenosis

Aortic stenosis (AS) is often accompanied by cusp calcification and tends to occur in patients with trileaflet valves above 65 years of age or in younger patients with congenital abnormalities (i.e. bicuspid valves). Severe calcification associated with faster rates of stenosis progression and increased cardiac event rates [17]. Aortic valve calcification can be accurately quantified using CT (Fig. 14.7), and interscan reproducibility is >90 % [18–20]. The amount of calcification is directly correlated with the severity of AS [19–22], although the relationship is curvilinear with stenosis severity increasing more rapidly at lower than higher calcium loads.

Table 14.2 Imaging protocol

Scanning protocol (for a 256-slice scanner)	
Tube voltage (kV)	100–120
Tube output (mA)	500–800
Detector number	128
Detector collimation (mm) ECG gating	0.6 Retrospective/Prospective
Helical pitch[a]	0.16–0.18
Rotation time (ms)	270–330
Tube current modulation[a]	
(HR ≤ 65) (HR > 65)	On Off
Contrast protocol (370 mgI/cc)	
Contrast amount (cc)	80–100
Contrast infusion rate (cc/s)	4–5
Saline amount (cc)	50
Saline infusion rate (cc/s)	4–5
Image reconstruction	
Reconstruction filter	Intermediate
Slice width (mm)	0.6
Increment (mm)	0.3 mm
Matrix	512 × 512
Reconstruction interval	Every 5–10 %
Image analysis: Axial images, MPR, MIP (cine loops and still frames)	

Typical scanning protocol for MDCT coronary angiography employed in our institution
ECG electrocardiogram, *HR* heart rate, *MPR*: multiplanar reformation, *MIP* maximum intensity projection
[a]If retrospective gating

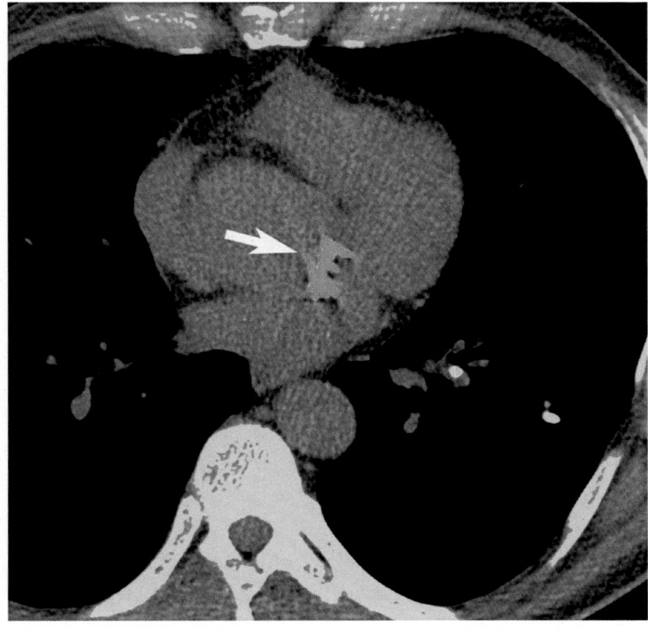

Fig. 14.7 Axial, non-contrast CT image in a patient with moderate aortic stenosis, demonstrating the quantification of aortic valve calcium (*arrow*) using the same approach as for coronary calcium scoring. The valvular calcium score ("Agatston") was 2227

The incremental value of the information derived from the aortic valve calcium score may be particularly useful in patients with low cardiac output and reduced transvalvular gradients.

Contrast-enhanced CT can precisely evaluate valve morphology, accurately differentiating trileaflet from bicuspid valves (Fig. 14.8a, b). Planimetric determinations of the aortic valve area (Fig. 14.8c) have shown excellent correlation with echocardiographic and invasive measurements [23–29].

CT has emerged as the integral imaging modality for transcatheter heart valve replacement. As opposed to conventional aortic valve replacement, direct visualization of the valve and annulus is lacking during the TAVR procedure. As a result, imaging is necessary to allow for appropriate valve sizing. CT is used to assess valve morphology, location and degree of calcification, annular sizing, optimum deployment angles, and for presence of peripheral vascular disease. These assessments play a role in predicting success of valve implantation and risk of paravalvular leak in these patients.

Expert consensus documents have been released on the use of CT before TAVR stating that CT should be used in the

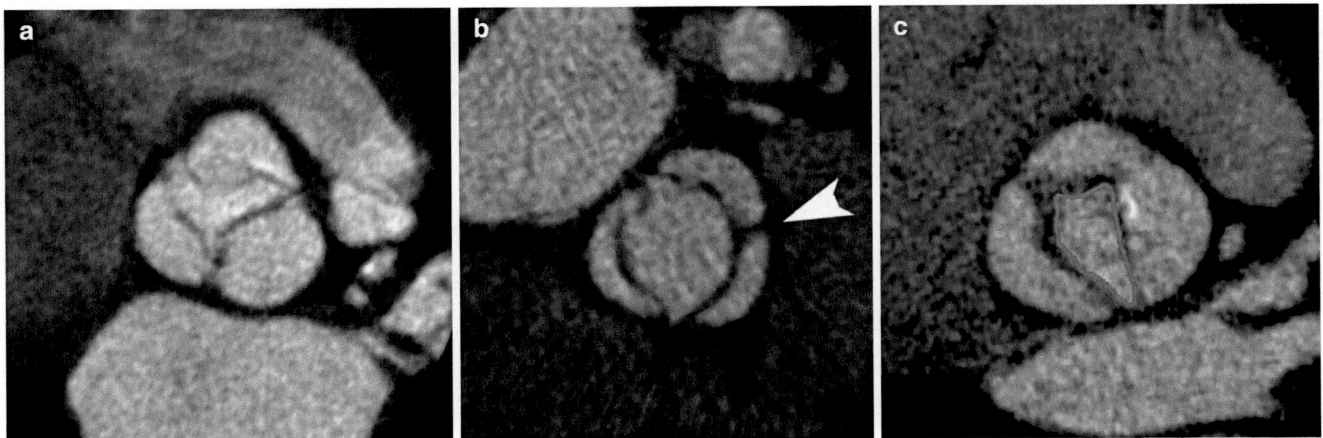

Fig. 14.8 Double oblique systolic reconstructions of contrast-enhanced CT scans showing a tri-leaflet (panel **a**) and a bicuspid aortic valve (the *arrowhead* indicates the fusion of the right and left coronary sinuses; panel **b**). Planimetry of the valve can be performed subsequently (red contour, panel **c**): the figure shows a bicuspid aortic valve with moderate stenosis (valve area = 1.2 cm^2)

assessment of all patients being considered for TAVR unless contraindicated and that datasets should be interpreted jointly within a multidisciplinary team [30].

Aortic Regurgitation

CT may be useful in evaluating the mechanism leading to aortic regurgitation (AR). AR caused by degenerative valve disease is characterized by thickened and/or calcified leaflets, and the area of lack of coaptation may be visualized in diastolic phase reconstructions centrally or at the commissures. In cases of AR secondary to enlargement of the aortic root, the regurgitant orifice is typically located centrally (Fig. 14.9). Other etiologies that can be depicted include interposition of an intimal flap in cases of dissection, valve distortion or perforation in cases of endocarditis, or leaflet prolapse observed in dissection and in Marfan syndrome. Regurgitant orifice areas measured by planimetry using MDCT correlate well with echocardiographic parameters of AR severity, such as the vena contracta width and the ratio of regurgitant jet to left ventricular outflow tract height, and allow for the detection of moderate and severe AR with high accuracy [31–33].

Mitral Stenosis

As in the case of aortic valve calcification, the presence of calcium in the mitral annulus is associated with systemic atherosclerosis and carries negative prognostic implications. The amount of mitral annular calcium can also be quantified with CT (Fig. 14.10), although reproducibility appears to be somewhat lower [18]. In rheumatic mitral stenosis (MS), calcification can extend to the leaflets, commissures, sub-valvular apparatus or even the left atrial wall. MS is often accompanied by marked atrial enlargement involving the appendage. The presence or absence of thrombus in the left atrial appendage can be determined after contrast administration with very high sensitivity although lower specificity since slow flow may impair opacification, which may be increased by adding delayed imaging [34, 35]. Planimetry of mitral valve opening by CT provides accurate assessment of MS severity (Fig. 14.11) [36].

Mitral Regurgitation

Both echocardiography and cardiac CT have high sensitivities (92.3 % and 84.6 %, respectively) and specificities (100 % each) for assessing mitral valve abnormalities compared with intraoperative findings, and echocardiography is more sensitive than CT for depicting each prolapsed leaflet of the mitral valve [37]. Echocardiography has been considered the reference imaging modality for mitral valve evaluation given the radiation dose exposure and inferior temporal resolution of CT. In mitral valve prolapse, for example, the use of echocardiography alone to identify the exact site of prolapse is clinician dependent and sometimes difficult, even for those with expertise, because of the limited acoustic window and the complex structure of the mitral apparatus.

In patients with mitral valve prolapse, CT can demonstrate the presence of leaflet thickening or the degree and location of prolapse (Fig. 14.12 and Video 14.1). In cases of MR secondary to annular enlargement, often accompanying dilated cardiomyopathy, dimensions of the annulus can be accurately quantified, and a central area of insufficient leaflet coaptation may be observed. Although quantifying MR degree may be difficult, preliminary data suggests that

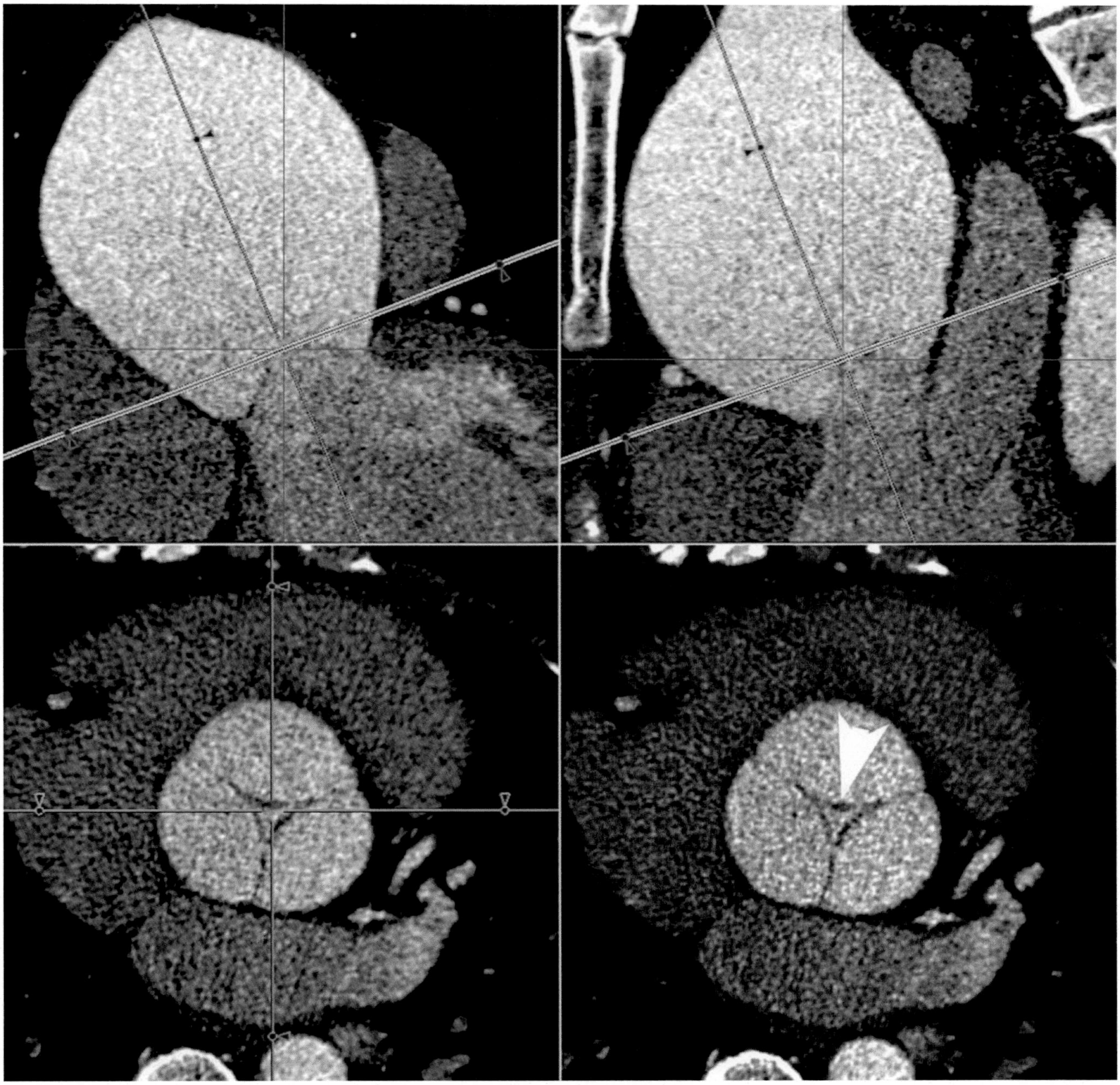

Fig. 14.9 Contrast-enhanced MDCT in a patient with an aneurysmal aorta and aortic insufficiency. The valvular plane (*yellow line*; *left lower panel*) is oriented perpendicular to two orthogonal planes aligned with the ascending aorta (*red and green lines*). A large, central area of insufficient leaflet coaptation during diastole (*right lower panel*; *arrowhead*) can be visualized

planimetry of the regurgitant orifice by CT correlates well with echocardiographic grading of severity [38].

Pulmonic Valve Disease

Pathology of the pulmonic valve, whether from idiopathic causes, infective endocarditis, thrombus, regurgitation/stenosis, or secondary to congenital heart disease is difficult to evaluate by echocardiography in the adult patient. Therefore, CT and MRI, due to their good spatiotemporal resolution, large field of view, and multiplanar reconstruction techniques, are playing increasingly important roles in the evaluation of this valve.

For visualizing the pulmonary valve, the CT intravenous contrast medium injection protocol should be optimized to ensure that there is adequate contrast opacification in the right cardiac chambers. For morphological evaluation of the valve, prospective electrocardiography (ECG) triggered acquisition should be used to minimize radiation dose. However, if functional analysis of the valve or the RV is desired, retrospective ECG-gated multi-phasic acquisition with tube current modulation is the ideal scanning mode [39].

Infective Endocarditis

Studies have shown that cardiac-gated CTA has excellent sensitivity, specificity, and positive predictive and negative predictive values in the preoperative evaluation for suspected infective endocarditis, in addition to excellent correlations with preoperative TEE and intraoperative findings [40].

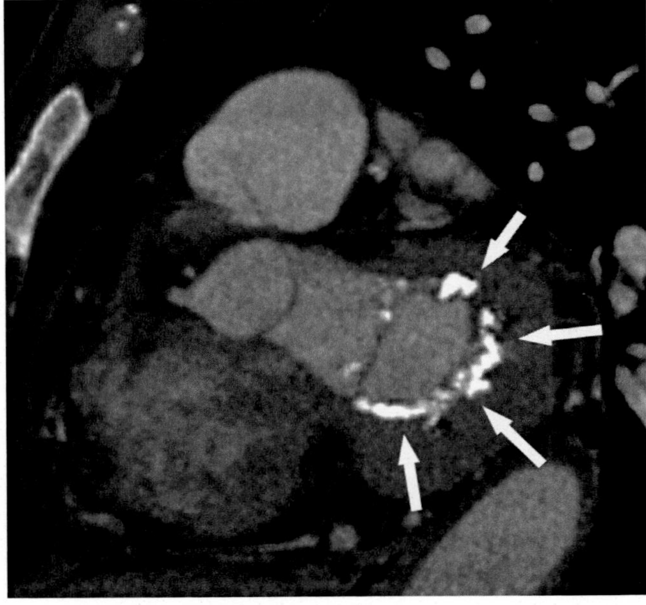

Fig. 14.10 Short-axis view at the level of the mitral valve, showing extensive annular calcification (*arrows*)

Vegetations are often mobile and tend to be on the atrial aspect of atrioventricular valves, and on the ventricular aspect of semilunar valves (Fig. 14.13). CT can be particularly useful in the demonstration of perivalvular abscesses as fluid-filled collections (Fig. 14.14) that may retain contrast in delayed imaging [41]. In a recent study, MDCT correctly identified 26 out of 27 (96 %) patients with valvular vegetations and 9 out of 9 (100 %) patients with abscesses, which were better characterized by MDCT than with transesophageal echocardiography [42]. Intravascular contrast administration should be optimized, and intravascular attenuation can be further accentuated by the use of 100-kV scan protocols whenever possible. Although the maximal temporal resolution of a scanner cannot be altered, the reconstruction frame of the dataset can and should be optimized when assessing valvular function. Reconstruction of 20- or 25-phase datasets (at 5 % or 4 % increments of the R-R interval) provides improved temporal depiction of valve motion that facilitates cine evaluation of valvular pathology, such as hypermobile vegetations. In addition, advanced image processing techniques, such as blood pool inversion (BPI) volume-rendering, can be used to allow 3-Dimensional/4-Dimensional (3-D/4-D) assessment of valvular structure and function [43]. In patients with aortic valve endocarditis with highly mobile vegetations, CT may be especially attractive as an alternative to invasive coronary angiography for preoperative evaluation.

Prosthetic Valves

Many of the aforementioned features of native VHD apply also to the evaluation of cardiac bioprostheses. Transthoracic echocardiography is useful for prosthetic valve evaluation, but can be limited by acoustic shadowing and poor acoustic windowing. Recently, cardiac CT has been recognized as a viable alternative to evaluation of prosthetic valve complications

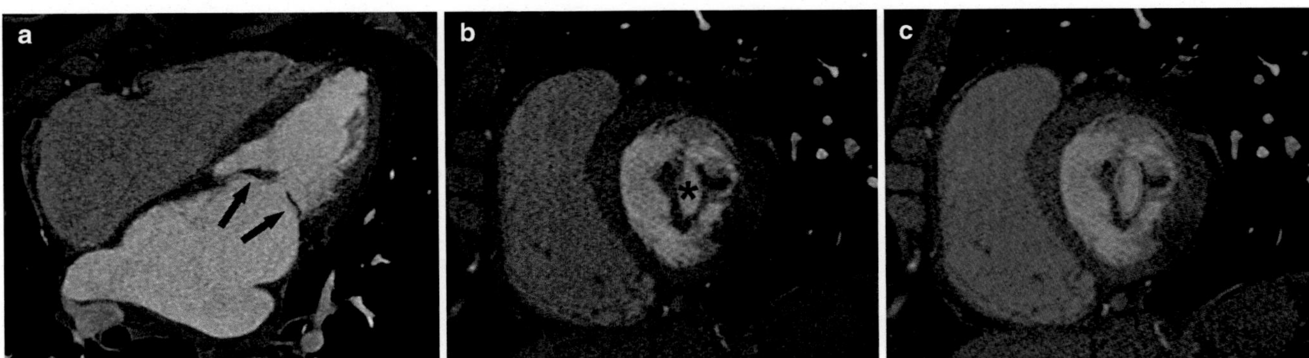

Fig. 14.11 Contrast-enhanced CT scan in the four-chamber and short-axis views (panels **a** and **b**, respectively) from a patient with rheumatic mitral stenosis. The typical thickening and restricted dome-shaped opening of the leaflets can be observed (*arrows* and *asterisk*). Planimetry of the valve (panel **c**) demonstrated moderate stenosis (*red contour*; area = 1.3 cm^2)

including valve thrombosis, dehiscence, pannus development, endocarditis, and paravalvular leak. However, careful attention to CT technique, achieving prescan target heart rates, extensive windowing adjustments, and awareness of normal postoperative paravalvular structures is imperative. Some valves, such as ball in cage valves, are not readily evaluable by CT because of extreme beam hardening artifact from the thicker metal struts found in these models. Whereas evaluation of most other valves using a very soft window with considerable windowing adjustments is to minimize beam hardening is certainly possible [44].

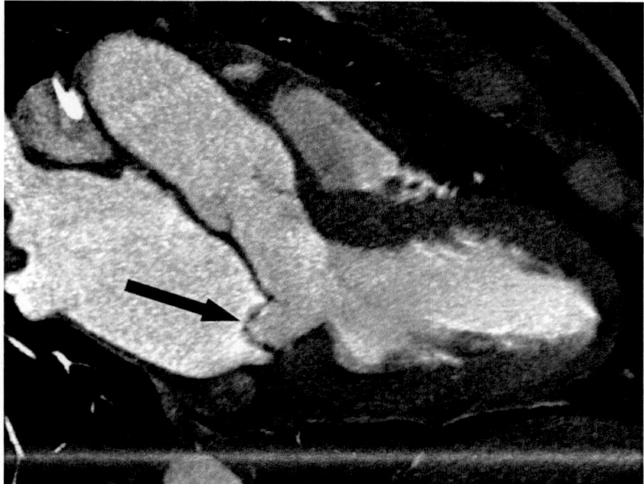

Fig. 14.12 End-systolic three-chamber view of the left ventricle demonstrating prolapse of the posterior mitral leaflet (*arrow*)

Recent work suggests iterative reconstructions may reduce beam-hardening artifact from prosthetic valves compared with filtered back projection reconstruction techniques [45]. Motion artifact can be adequately reduced by administration of beta-blockade to achieve heart rates between 50 and 60 bpm. Motion artifact is worst for aortic valve prosthesis during ventricular systole and for mitral valve prosthesis during end-diastole. Thus, it has been found that imaging in mid-diastole is the most ideal for prosthetic valve evaluation [46]. CT is particularly useful for the evaluation of some types of mechanical valves. In Prostheses with two discs should open symmetrically (Fig. 14.15 and Video 14.2). In those with a single disc, the angle of opening can also be measured [47]. Finally, heterografts and homografts can be evaluated completely, including the distal anastomosis and the patency of the coronary arteries if these were reimplanted.

Imaging Pearls

- Plan ahead; as this will allow for imaging protocol optimization if valvular evaluation will be attempted.
- If simultaneous assessment of the right heart structures is intended, the contrast protocol should be optimized. An initial bolus of 80–100 cc followed by a mixture of

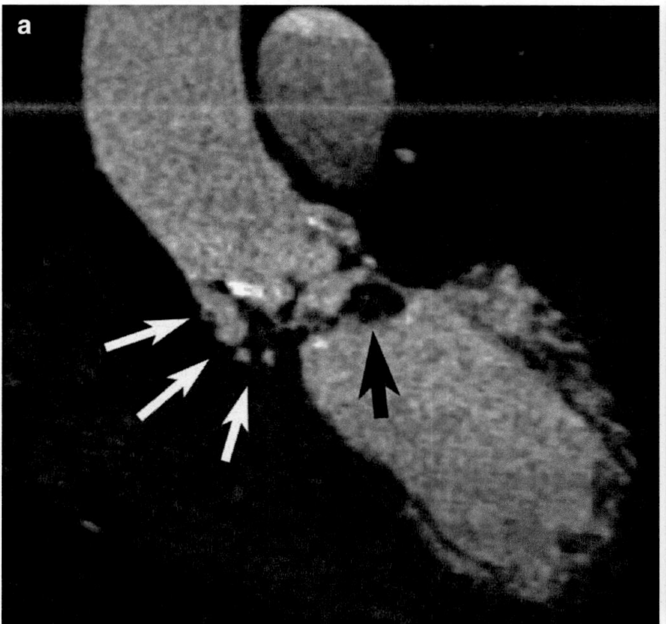

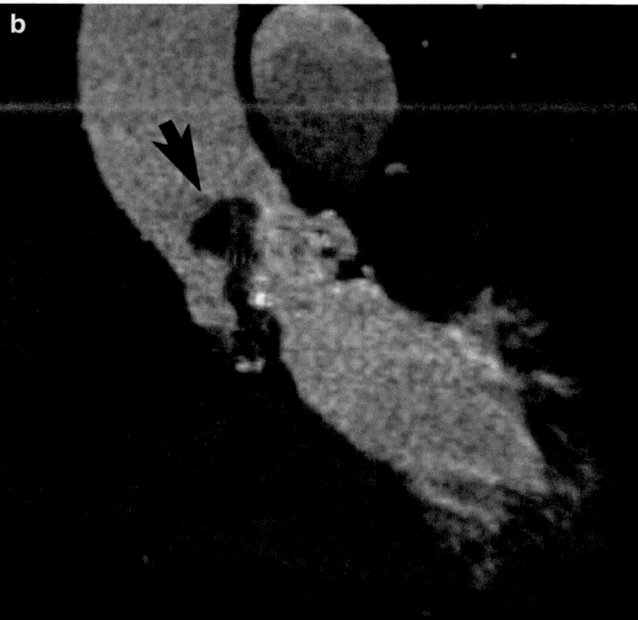

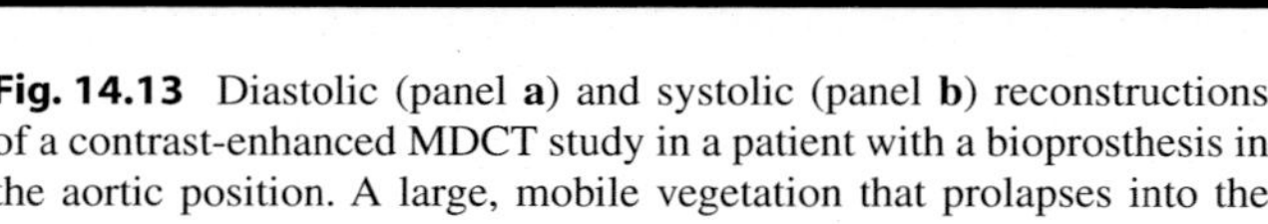

Fig. 14.13 Diastolic (panel **a**) and systolic (panel **b**) reconstructions of a contrast-enhanced MDCT study in a patient with a bioprosthesis in the aortic position. A large, mobile vegetation that prolapses into the ascending aorta in systole can be noted (*black arrows*). In addition, perivalvular thickening and fluid-filled collections can be noted (*white arrows*) indicating the presence of a perivalular abscess

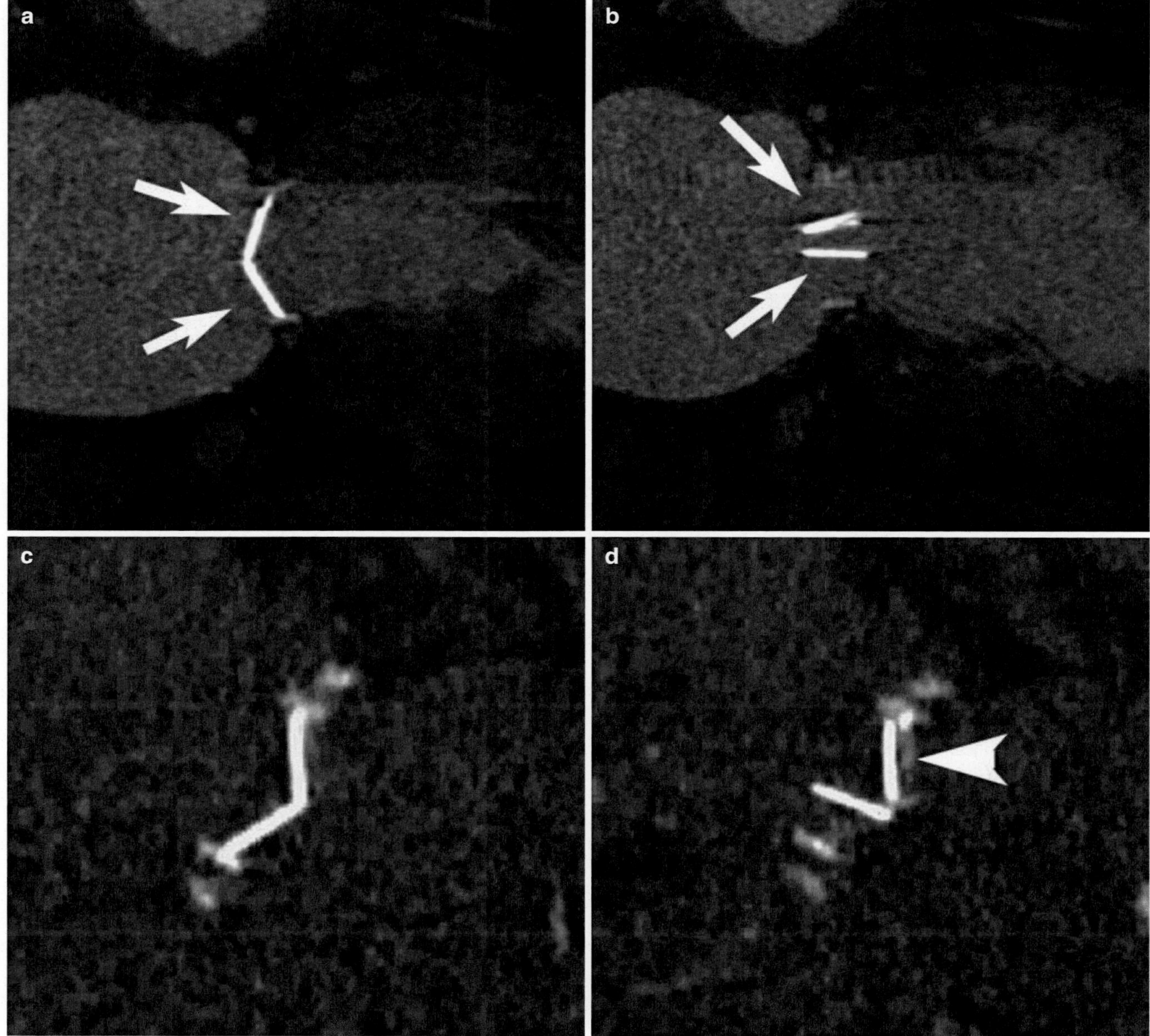

Fig. 14.14 Evaluation of mechanical prostheses by CT. The top row shows contrast-enhanced images (systole, panel **a**; diastole, panel **b**) of a normal-functioning mechanical prosthesis in the mitral position. The two discs close and open completely and symmetrically (*white arrows*) during the cardiac cycle. Comparable systolic (panel **c**) and diastolic (panel **d**) reconstructions of a non-contrast CT evaluation of a dysfunctional mitral prosthesis. One of the discs does not open in diastole (*white arrowhead*). Subsequent surgical intervention demonstrated prosthetic thrombosis

contrast and saline (1:1) at 4–5 cc/s will result in adequate coronary evaluation and sufficient right-heart opacification without excessive enhancement. Alternatively, a second infusion of contrast administered at a slower rate (2–3 cc/s) can be employed [15, 16].

- Quantification of ventricular end-systolic volumes and the degree of MR and AS requires adequate image quality during systole. It may be necessary to avoid tube current modulation in these cases. Alternatively, the maximal tube output can be timed to end-systole, which will provide adequate depiction of mitral closure and aortic opening, as well as potentially motionless coronary images, particularly at higher heart rates.
- If the entire thoracic aorta needs to be imaged (i.e. in cases of aneurysm with associated AR) and coronary evaluation is not required, using thicker detector collimation will enable reductions in radiation dose and breath-hold duration.

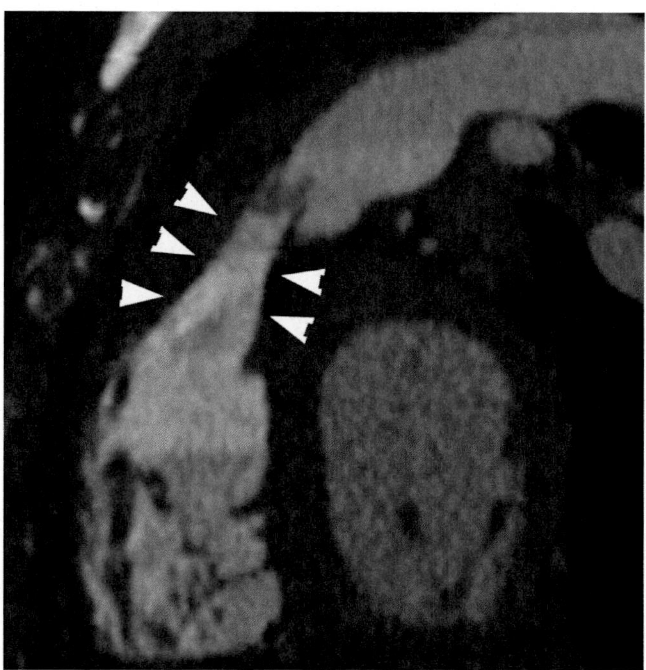

Fig. 14.15 Contrast-enhanced CT in a patient with pulmonary infundibular stenosis (*arrowheads*). The contrast protocol was optimized to provide adequate opacification of right heart chambers

- Most patients with VHD can tolerate beta-blockers for optimal coronary evaluation. However, caution and smaller doses are recommended in cases with severe degrees of left ventricular dysfunction/dilatation, AS, AR or pulmonary hypertension.
- Atrial fibrillation is common in patients with VHD. It may lead to a decrease in image quality and accuracy of valvular and ventricular assessment, although this is typically more significant for evaluation of the coronary arteries.
- For the evaluation of ventricular or valvular function with MDCT, reconstructions at every 10 % of the RR interval are usually sufficient. In specific cases, a more detailed evaluation of the valve can be obtained by reconstructing images at smaller intervals (i.e. every 5 %) in the cardiac phase of interest (for example, during systole for AS) [48].
- The combination of cine loops and still frames facilitates the detection of valvular abnormalities.
- CT imaging in the evaluation for TAVR should include imaging of the aortic root, aorta, and iliac, as well as common femoral arteries. To achieve the desired accuracy and to allow for adequate motion-free images, imaging of the aortic root must be synchronized to the electrocardiogram (ECG) either by retrospective ECG gating or by prospective ECG triggering, depending on patient characteristics. It is not necessary to image the entire aorta and iliofemoral arteries with ECG synchronization. For these sections, non-gated acquisitions will allow lower radiation exposure and faster volume coverage requiring lower contrast volumes. Since detailed dimensions of the aortic root and of the iliofemoral arteries must be obtained, spatial resolution must be high enough to provide adequate imaging. The optimal acquisition protocol is that which obtains a reconstructed slice width of <1.0 mm throughout the entire imaging volume.
- Variability of the quantification of aortic valve calcium is lowest in mid-diastole [49].
- A valvular "Agatston" score ≥1100 resulted in respective sensitivity and specificity of 93 and 82 % for the diagnosis of severe AS [20]. A score >3700 has a positive predictive value of near 100 % [25].
- The optimal plane to perform planimetry of the valvular area is parallel to the annulus as determined from two orthogonal double-oblique views perpendicular to the valve plane. The optimal level of that plane is the one showing the smallest area during the phase of maximum valve opening (Fig. 14.9).
- Quantification of the regurgitant volume/fraction from the difference in right and left stroke volumes is only accurate for isolated regurgitant lesions.
- A score evaluating leaflet mobility and thickening, subvalvular thickening and calcification, as well as the presence of left atrial thrombus, may determine whether MS can be treated percutaneously or surgically. CT can provide useful information for all of these features.
- The mitral valve is divided into the anterolateral commissure, posteromedial commissure, anterior leaflet and posterior leaflet. The leaflets are subdivided into three segments each (A1, A2 and A3; and P1, P2, and P3, from lateral to medial). Determination of which segments are affected and to what degree determines in part the likelihood of successful surgical repair in mitral valve prolapse.
- Sharper reconstruction filters and increasing window level of the image display facilitates evaluation of mechanical prosthetic valves.
- Optimum valve evaluation for both aortic and mitral prosthetic valves is best achieved during mid-diastole.

References

1. Nkomo VT, Gardin JM, Skelton TN, Gottdiener JS, Scott CG, Enriquez-Sarano M. Burden of valvular heart diseases: a population-based study. Lancet. 2006;368(9540):1005–11.
2. Nishimura RA, Otto CM, Bonow RO, Carabello BA, Erwin JP 3rd, Guyton RA, O'Gara PT, Ruiz CE, Skubas NJ, Sorajja P, Sundt TM 3rd, Thomas JD. 2014 AHA/ACC guideline for the management of

patients with valvular heart disease: executive summary: a report of the American College of Cardiology/American Heart Association Task Force on Practice Guidelines. J Am Coll Cardiol 2014;63(22): 2438–88.

3. Bonow RO, Carabello BA, Chatterjee K, de Leon Jr AC, Faxon DP, Freed MD, et al. 2008 Focused update incorporated into the ACC/AHA 2006 guidelines for the management of patients with valvular heart disease: a report of the American College of Cardiology/American Heart Association Task Force on Practice Guidelines (Writing Committee to Revise the 1998 Guidelines for the Management of Patients With Valvular Heart Disease): endorsed by the Society of Cardiovascular Anesthesiologists, Society for Cardiovascular Angiography and Interventions, and Society of Thoracic Surgeons. Circulation. 2008;118(15):e523–661.
4. Cawley PJ, Maki JH, Otto CM. Cardiovascular magnetic resonance imaging for valvular heart disease: technique and validation. Circulation. 2009;119(3):468–78.
5. Bennett CJ, Maleszewski JJ, Araoz PA. CT and MR imaging of the aortic valve: radiologic-pathologic correlation. Radiographics Rev Publ Radiol Soc North Am Inc. 2012;32(5):1399–420.
6. Taylor AJ, Cerqueira M, Hodgson JM, Mark D, Min J, O'Gara P, et al. ACCF/SCCT/ACR/AHA/ASE/ASNC/NASCI/SCAI/SCMR 2010 appropriate use criteria for cardiac computed tomography. A report of the American College of Cardiology Foundation Appropriate Use Criteria Task Force, the Society of Cardiovascular Computed Tomography, the American College of Radiology, the American Heart Association, the American Society of Echocardiography, the American Society of Nuclear Cardiology, the North American Society for Cardiovascular Imaging, the Society for Cardiovascular Angiography and Interventions, and the Society for Cardiovascular Magnetic Resonance. J Am Coll Cardiol. 2010;56(22):1864–94.
7. Orakzai SH, Orakzai RH, Nasir K, Budoff MJ. Assessment of cardiac function using multidetector row computed tomography. J Comput Assist Tomogr. 2006;30(4):555–63.
8. Reiter SJ, Rumberger JA, Stanford W, Marcus ML. Quantitative determination of aortic regurgitant volumes in dogs by ultrafast computed tomography. Circulation. 1987;76(3):728–35.
9. Boxt LM. CT of valvular heart disease. Int J Cardiovasc Imaging. 2005;21(1):105–13.
10. Gilard M, Cornily JC, Pennec PY, Joret C, Le Gal G, Mansourati J, et al. Accuracy of multislice computed tomography in the preoperative assessment of coronary disease in patients with aortic valve stenosis. J Am Coll Cardiol. 2006;47(10):2020–4.
11. Meijboom WB, Mollet NR, Van Mieghem CA, Kluin J, Weustink AC, Pugliese F, et al. Pre-operative computed tomography coronary angiography to detect significant coronary artery disease in patients referred for cardiac valve surgery. J Am Coll Cardiol. 2006;48(8):1658–65.
12. Reant P, Brunot S, Lafitte S, Serri K, Leroux L, Corneloup O, et al. Predictive value of noninvasive coronary angiography with multidetector computed tomography to detect significant coronary stenosis before valve surgery. Am J Cardiol. 2006;97(10):1506–10.
13. Scheffel H, Leschka S, Plass A, Vachenauer R, Gaemperli O, Garzoli E, et al. Accuracy of 64-slice computed tomography for the preoperative detection of coronary artery disease in patients with chronic aortic regurgitation. Am J Cardiol. 2007;100(4):701–6.
14. Russo V, Gostoli V, Lovato L, Montalti M, Marzocchi A, Gavelli G, et al. Clinical value of multidetector CT coronary angiography as a preoperative screening test before non-coronary cardiac surgery. Heart (Br Cardiac Soc). 2007;93(12):1591–8.
15. Litmanovich D, Zamboni GA, Hauser TH, Lin PJ, Clouse ME, Raptopoulos V. ECG-gated chest CT angiography with 64-MDCT and tri-phasic IV contrast administration regimen in patients with acute non-specific chest pain. Eur Radiol. 2008;18(2):308–17.
16. Takakuwa KM, Halpern EJ. Evaluation of a "triple rule-out" coronary CT angiography protocol: use of 64-Section CT in low-to-moderate risk emergency department patients suspected of having acute coronary syndrome. Radiology. 2008;248(2):438–46.
17. Rosenhek R, Binder T, Porenta G, Lang I, Christ G, Schemper M, et al. Predictors of outcome in severe, asymptomatic aortic stenosis. N Engl J Med. 2000;343(9):611–7.
18. Budoff MJ, Takasu J, Katz R, Mao S, Shavelle DM, O'Brien KD, et al. Reproducibility of CT measurements of aortic valve calcification, mitral annulus calcification, and aortic wall calcification in the multi-ethnic study of atherosclerosis. Acad Radiol. 2006;13(2):166–72.
19. Koos R, Kuhl HP, Muhlenbruch G, Wildberger JE, Gunther RW, Mahnken AH. Prevalence and clinical importance of aortic valve calcification detected incidentally on CT scans: comparison with echocardiography. Radiology. 2006;241(1):76–82.
20. Messika-Zeitoun D, Aubry MC, Detaint D, Bielak LF, Peyser PA, Sheedy PF, et al. Evaluation and clinical implications of aortic valve calcification measured by electron-beam computed tomography. Circulation. 2004;110(3):356–62.
21. Koos R, Mahnken AH, Sinha AM, Wildberger JE, Hoffmann R, Kuhl HP. Aortic valve calcification as a marker for aortic stenosis severity: assessment on 16-MDCT. AJR Am J Roentgenol. 2004;183(6):1813–8.
22. Shavelle DM, Budoff MJ, Buljubasic N, Wu AH, Takasu J, Rosales J, et al. Usefulness of aortic valve calcium scores by electron beam computed tomography as a marker for aortic stenosis. Am J Cardiol. 2003;92(3):349–53.
23. Alkadhi H, Wildermuth S, Plass A, Bettex D, Baumert B, Leschka S, et al. Aortic stenosis: comparative evaluation of 16-detector row CT and echocardiography. Radiology. 2006;240(1):47–55.
24. Bouvier E, Logeart D, Sablayrolles JL, Feignoux J, Scheuble C, Touche T, et al. Diagnosis of aortic valvular stenosis by multislice cardiac computed tomography. Eur Heart J. 2006;27(24):3033–8.
25. Cowell SJ, Newby DE, Burton J, White A, Northridge DB, Boon NA, et al. Aortic valve calcification on computed tomography predicts the severity of aortic stenosis. Clin Radiol. 2003;58(9):712–6.
26. Feuchtner GM, Dichtl W, Friedrich GJ, Frick M, Alber H, Schachner T, et al. Multislice computed tomography for detection of patients with aortic valve stenosis and quantification of severity. J Am Coll Cardiol. 2006;47(7):1410–7.
27. Feuchtner GM, Muller S, Bonatti J, Schachner T, Velik-Salchner C, Pachinger O, et al. Sixty-four slice CT evaluation of aortic stenosis using planimetry of the aortic valve area. AJR Am J Roentgenol. 2007;189(1):197–203.
28. LaBounty TM, Sundaram B, Agarwal P, Armstrong WA, Kazerooni EA, Yamada E. Aortic valve area on 64-MDCT correlates with transesophageal echocardiography in aortic stenosis. AJR Am J Roentgenol. 2008;191(6):1652–8.
29. Lembcke A, Thiele H, Lachnitt A, Enzweiler CN, Wagner M, Hein PA, et al. Precision of forty slice spiral computed tomography for quantifying aortic valve stenosis: comparison with echocardiography and validation against cardiac catheterization. Invest Radiol. 2008;43(10):719–28.
30. Achenbach S, Delgado V, Hausleiter J, Schoenhagen P, Min JK, Leipsic JA. SCCT expert consensus document on computed tomography imaging before transcatheter aortic valve implantation (TAVI)/transcatheter aortic valve replacement (TAVR). J Cardiovasc Comput Tomogr. 2012;6(6):366–80.
31. Alkadhi H, Desbiolles L, Husmann L, Plass A, Leschka S, Scheffel H, et al. Aortic regurgitation: assessment with 64-section CT. Radiology. 2007;245(1):111–21.
32. Feuchtner GM, Dichtl W, Muller S, Jodocy D, Schachner T, Klauser A, et al. 64-MDCT for diagnosis of aortic regurgitation in patients

referred to CT coronary angiography. AJR Am J Roentgenol. 2008;191(1):W1–7.

33. Jassal DS, Shapiro MD, Neilan TG, Chaithiraphan V, Ferencik M, Teague SD, et al. 64-slice multidetector computed tomography (MDCT) for detection of aortic regurgitation and quantification of severity. Invest Radiol. 2007;42(7):507–12.
34. Kim YY, Klein AL, Halliburton SS, Popovic ZB, Kuzmiak SA, Sola S, et al. Left atrial appendage filling defects identified by multidetector computed tomography in patients undergoing radiofrequency pulmonary vein antral isolation: a comparison with transesophageal echocardiography. Am Heart J. 2007;154(6):1199–205.
35. Hur J, Kim YJ, Lee HJ, Ha JW, Heo JH, Choi EY, et al. Left atrial appendage thrombi in stroke patients: detection with two-phase cardiac CT angiography versus transesophageal echocardiography. Radiology. 2009;251(3):683–90.
36. Messika-Zeitoun D, Serfaty JM, Laissy JP, Berhili M, Brochet E, Iung B, et al. Assessment of the mitral valve area in patients with mitral stenosis by multislice computed tomography. J Am Coll Cardiol. 2006;48(2):411–3.
37. Ghosh N, Al-Shehri H, Chan K, Mesana T, Chan V, Chen L, et al. Characterization of mitral valve prolapse with cardiac computed tomography: comparison to echocardiographic and intraoperative findings. Int J Cardiovasc Imaging. 2012;28(4):855–63.
38. Alkadhi H, Wildermuth S, Bettex DA, Plass A, Baumert B, Leschka S, et al. Mitral regurgitation: quantification with 16-detector row CT--initial experience. Radiology. 2006;238(2):454–63.
39. Rajiah P, Nazarian J, Vogelius E, Gilkeson RC. CT and MRI of pulmonary valvular abnormalities. Clin Radiol. 2014;69(6):630–8.
40. Gahide G, Bommart S, Demaria R, Sportouch C, Dambia H, Albat B, et al. Preoperative evaluation in aortic endocarditis: findings on cardiac CT. AJR Am J Roentgenol. 2010;194(3):574–8.
41. Gilkeson RC, Markowitz AH, Balgude A, Sachs PB. MDCT evaluation of aortic valvular disease. AJR Am J Roentgenol. 2006; 186(2):350–60.
42. Feuchtner GM, Stolzmann P, Dichtl W, Schertler T, Bonatti J, Scheffel H, et al. Multislice computed tomography in infective endocarditis: comparison with transesophageal echocardiography and intraoperative findings. J Am Coll Cardiol. 2009;53(5): 436–44.
43. Entrikin DW, Gupta P, Kon ND, Carr JJ. Imaging of infective endocarditis with cardiac CT angiography. J Cardiovasc Comput Tomogr. 2012;6(6):399–405.
44. O'Neill AC, Martos R, Murtagh G, Ryan ER, McCreery C, Keane D, et al. Practical tips and tricks for assessing prosthetic valves and detecting paravalvular regurgitation using cardiac CT. J Cardiovasc Comput Tomogr. 2014;8(4):323–7.
45. Sucha D, Willemink MJ, de Jong PA, Schilham AM, Leiner T, Symersky P, et al. The impact of a new model-based iterative reconstruction algorithm on prosthetic heart valve related artifacts at reduced radiation dose MDCT. Int J Cardiovasc Imaging. 2014;30(4):785–93.
46. Symersky P, Budde RP, Westers P, de Mol BA, Prokop M. Multidetector CT imaging of mechanical prosthetic heart valves: quantification of artifacts with a pulsatile in-vitro model. Eur Radiol. 2011;21(10):2103–10.
47. Konen E, Goitein O, Feinberg MS, Eshet Y, Raanani E, Rimon U, et al. The role of ECG-gated MDCT in the evaluation of aortic and mitral mechanical valves: initial experience. AJR Am J Roentgenol. 2008;191(1):26–31.
48. Abbara S, Pena AJ, Maurovich-Horvat P, Butler J, Sosnovik DE, Lembcke A, et al. Feasibility and optimization of aortic valve planimetry with MDCT. AJR Am J Roentgenol. 2007;188(2):356–60.
49. Ruhl KM, Das M, Koos R, Muhlenbruch G, Flohr TG, Wildberger JE, et al. Variability of aortic valve calcification measurement with multislice spiral computed tomography. Invest Radiol. 2006;41(4):370–3.

15 Transcatheter Aortic Valve Implantation (TAVI)

Chesnal Dey Arepalli, Christopher Naoum, Philipp Blanke, and Jonathon A. Leipsic

Abstract

Computerized tomography (CT) plays a pivotal role in selection of patients', appropriate device size and pre-procedural guidance in successful outcome of transcatheter aortic valve implantation (TAVI). CT based vascular and non-vascular evaluation and integration of relevant measurements into TAVI work up has been shown to reduce morbidity and mortality. Post-procedural device assessment and complications could also be reliably evaluated with CT. Utilization of CT is not just confined to TAVI but it is also increasingly being used for any transcatheter valvular assessment.

Keywords

AS – Aortic Stenosis • AVC – Aortic Valvular Calcifications • AA – Aortic Annulus • SOV – Sinus of Valsalva • Coronary Artery Ostium • PAR – Paravalvular Regurgitation • CT – Computerized tomography • TTE – Transthoracic Echocardiography • TEE – Transesophageal Echocardiography • TAVI – Transcatheter Aortic Valve Implantation

Introduction

Transcatheter aortic valve implantation (TAVI) is an alternative treatment option for symptomatic severe aortic stenosis (AS) patients who are deemed inoperable or at high risk for surgical aortic valve replacement (AVR). TAVI as the name suggests is a procedure where in a bio-prosthetic device is implanted without removing the diseased valve via a transcatheter approach.

C.D. Arepalli, MBBS, DNB • C. Naoum, MBBS, FRACP
Department of Radiology, St Paul's Hospital UBC, Vancouver, BC, Canada

P. Blanke, MD
Department of Medicine, St Paul's Hospital UBC, Vancouver, BC, Canada

J.A. Leipsic, MD, FRCPC, FSCCT (✉)
Department of Radiology, St. Paul's Hospital, Room P2214 – 2nd Floor Providence Building 1081 Burrard Street, Vancouver, BC V6Z 1Y6, Canada
e-mail: jleipsic@providencehealth.bc.ca

The most common cause for AS is age related progressive calcification of a normal aortic valve (Fig. 15.1a–c) [1, 2]. Additionally, congenital causes like bicuspid aortic valve or inflammatory conditions like rheumatic heart disease are also common causes of AS [1]. The prevalence of senile AS is increasing as the mean age of Western societies is increasing [3, 4]. Current data has documented the prevalence of AS in the elderly population (age $\geq$ 75 years) as 12.4 % and severe AS is 3.4 % [3]. Although senile or degenerative aortic stenosis occurs primarily in the elderly population, with mean age of 65–70 years, congenital bicuspid aortic valve (BAV) with significant aortic stenosis tends to occur slightly earlier between 15 and 65 years of age (Fig. 15.1d) [5, 6]. In one study it was observed that BAV was the commonest cause of AS between the ages of 60 and 75 years (59 % of cases) and those aged less than 60 years, BAV was a causative factor in 40 % [7]. BAV AS were found to require AVR 5 years before than those with a tricuspid valve [8].

Importantly, the natural clinical progression of symptomatic AS is rapid and associated with a poor clinical

M.J. Budoff, J.S. Shinbane (eds.), *Cardiac CT Imaging: Diagnosis of Cardiovascular Disease*,
DOI 10.1007/978-3-319-28219-0_15

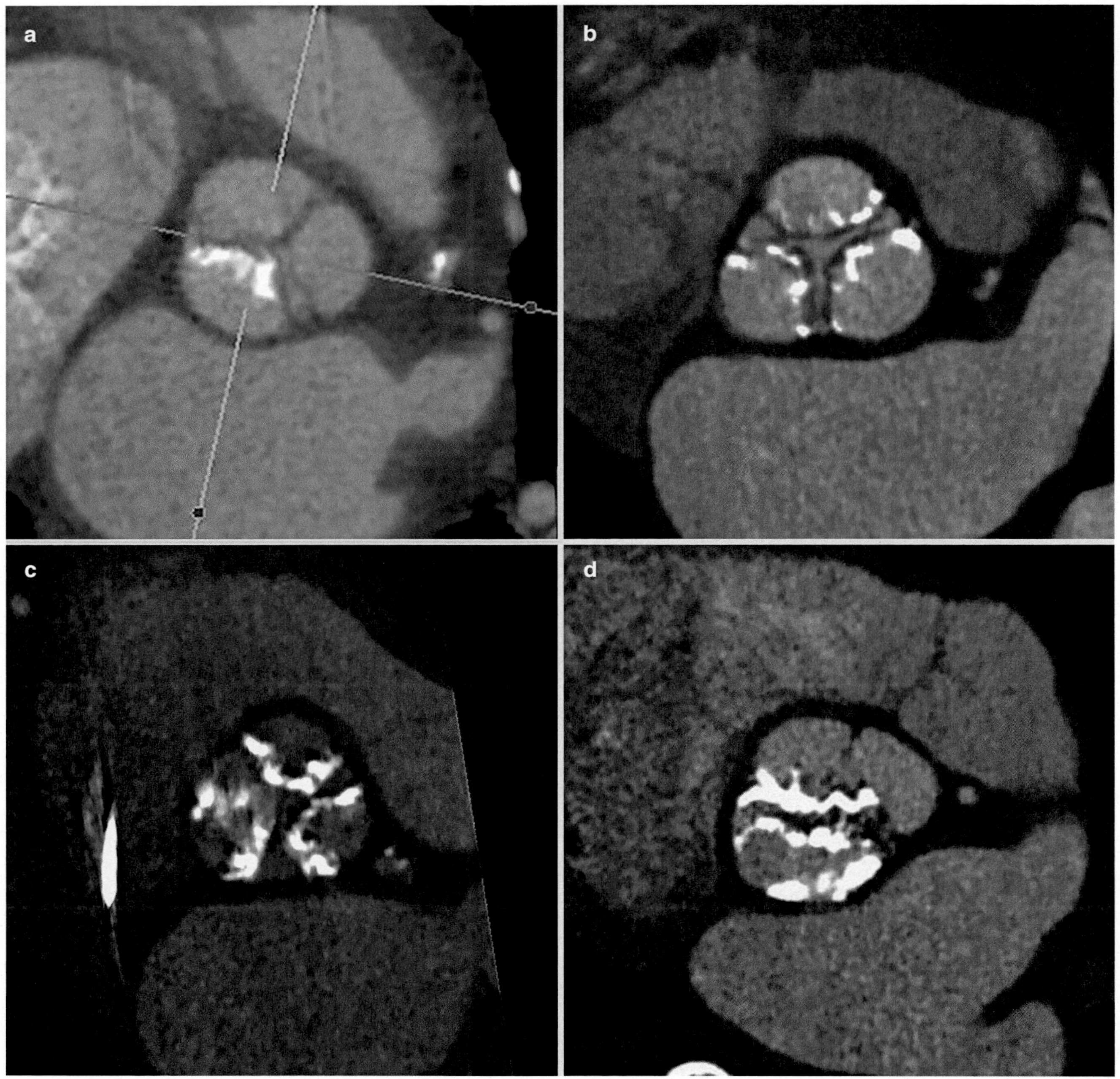

Fig. 15.1 Aortic valvular calcification (AVC). AVC of varying degrees – (**a**) mild, (**b**) moderate, (**c**) severe, (**d**) Bicuspid aortic valve (BAV) with calcification. Note the asymmetry of the cusps with a larger non-coronary cusp and raphae between the right and the left coronary cusps in keeping with a Type 1 A Bicuspid Valve

outcome with an average time of death shown to be within 5 years after onset of angina, 3 years after onset of syncope and within 1–2 years after onset of heart failure symptoms [9].

Until the advent of TAVI, the sole effective treatment option for symptomatic AS was surgical AVR. Medical treatment alone had very poor prognosis with a mortality rate of 50 % at 2 years. Unfortunately, many patients with severe symptomatic AS are denied this surgery owing to associated co-morbidities in the elderly population that make surgical risk prohibitive [3, 10].

TAVI is a new alternate therapy that has been shown through many registries, meta-analyses, and a number of randomized trials to be an effective therapy for severe symptomatic AS who were deemed inoperable and high risk surgical patients [11, 12]. TAVI was first pioneered by Cribier et al. in 2002 through transvenous transeptal approach [13]. However, over the past decade, alternative procedures have been developed and at present retrograde transarterial transfemoral path, first described by Webb and colleagues in 2005, is the most favored approach.

As opposed to surgical AVR where it is possible to directly visualize and measure the size of the aortic root; TAVI relies indirectly on imaging measurements before implantation. Based on these measurements; device selection and the procedural approach are planned. Pre-procedural imaging plays a critical role in ensuring the success of the procedure and also to minimize the peri and post-procedural complications.

Imaging Modalities

Historically, TAVI imaging was reliant on measurements derived form 2-dimensional echocardiography and invasive angiography. However, multidetector computed tomography (MDCT) has grown to become an essential tool for the assessment of aortic root/annulus, evaluation of thoracic and abdominal aorta and ilio-femoral vessels. Moreover, MDCT is being used to predict optimal co-planar projection angles for device deployment.

Current state of the art CT scanners acquire data volumetrically with isotropic spatial and high temporal resolution. Post processing of data provide multiplanar and curved planar reformations (MPR and CPR), volume rendered technique images (VRT), minimum and maximum intensity projections (MIP_{min} and MIP_{max} respectively) which are essential to accurately size the aortic annulus, aortic root and other vascular access sites. Integration of CT data into sizing algorithms and work flow has consistently demonstrated significant reduction in the incidence of paravalvular and vascular complications [14–16]. Thus CT has become an accepted integral part in the overall work flow of TAVI patients. Of late, CT has also been shown to play an important additional role in valve in valve procedures.

The role of MDCT for valvular intervention can be broadly discussed under three headings:

(a) Pre-procedural,
(b) Peri-procedural and
(c) Post procedural.

Although the focus of this chapter is on pre-procedural role of CT; it is equally pertinent to understand the peri and post procedural complications as they play an important role in understanding the dynamics of TAVI and thus indirectly influence the pre-procedural work up.

Before one can proceed with CT based 'Sizing of the aortic annulus' and procedural planning in the work up of TAVI patients, it is important to understand the complex aortic valve and root anatomy. Knowledge of the 3 dimensional (3 D) complex aortic root geometry and consideration of various anatomical measurements are critical in the determination of patient eligibility, bioprosthesis size, procedural planning and to anticipate procedural complications.

Anatomy

Aortic Root

The Aortic root is a further extension of the left ventricular outflow tract (LVOT). As a result, the LVOT should be considered an anatomical segment between the left ventricle and ascending aorta.

As the aortic root is a complex dynamic structure; understanding the morphology and kinesis of the aortic root subcomponents helps in better appreciation of interplay of different sub-components with each other and also with adjacent structures. This not only helps in procedural success but also has the potential in refinement of the bio-prosthesis devices.

Aortic root sub-components include aortic annulus (AA), aortic sinus and the valvular leaflets, the coronary ostia and the sinotubular junction.

Aortic Annulus

Broadly, two terms define the aortic annulus – (a) anatomic annulus and (b) virtual basal ring. The Anatomical Aortic annulus is more of a histological demarcation that is defined as a fibrous structure that attaches the aortic root to the left ventricle. It consists of three coronets like structures that support the valvular leaflets. The Virtual basal annulus is defined by nadir (lowest depth) plane of each of the coronets and it corresponds to the aortic-ventricular junction.

Although the term annulus suggests a circular shape, with the use of 3-D MDCT imaging , it has been found to be fairly consistently to be of a non-circular geometry with often elliptical and sometimes oval shaped configuration [17, 18].

It has been also observed that there are considerable variations in shape, size and direction of the annulus during the cardiac cycle (Fig. 15.2). These are influenced by deformation, stretch, compliance of the aortic root as well as left ventricular geometry, mitral valve anatomy and pathology [19, 20]. Further, Nakai et al. [21] showed that there is cranial displacement of aortic annulus during early systole and in diastole whereas in rest of the systole and in isovolumetric relaxation there is caudal displacement. It has been observed in multiple studies, that the aortic annulus measurements in cohorts without and with aortic stenosis show largest size (area) and diameter in systole and smallest measurements during diastole due to cyclical changes [22–26].

Imaging Modalities and Aortic Annulus Assessment

Strengths and Limitations of Echocardiography and MDCT

Accurate and reproducible pre-operative measurements of annulus are of paramount importance that helps in patient selection, device selection and size for TAVI procedure and also forecasting the outcome of the geometrical configuration of aortic annulus-prosthesis after implantation. In addition, better understanding of the aortic root complex and precise measurements would help in predicting and mitigating peri and post procedural complications.

Owing to the complex 3D aortic root geometry, measurements in a single plane have been shown to lead to both under or overestimation (depending upon the plane used) and have therefore been shown to be limited value for TAVI sizing. Two dimensional (2D) measurements as provided by transthoracic echocardiography (TTE) and transesophageal echocardiography (TEE) are routinely used. In fact, the current TAVI device sizes provided by vendors are based on 2D echocardiography measurements. However, it was noted in several studies that echocardiography measurements underestimated the true aortic annular size and were smaller in size when compared to MDCT.

In a meta-analysis, MDCT aortic annulus diameter measurements on coronal view were 25.3 ± 0.52 mm which were larger than sagittal view measurements by MDCT (22.7 ± 0.37 mm), TTE (22.6 ± 0.28 mm), and TEE (23.1 ± 0.32 mm) [27]. In a study by Mizia-Stec at el, the mean aortic annulus diameter on TTE was 24 ± 3.6 mm, 26 ± 4.2 mm using TEE, and 26.9 ± 3.2 mm on MDCT ($P = 0.04$ vs. TTE) [28]. Messika-Zeitoun and colleagues [29] observed larger differences between CT and TTE (1.22 ± 1.3 mm) or TEE (1.52 ± 1.1 mm) than the difference between TTE and TEE (0.6 ± 0.8 mm; and $p < 0.0001$, respectively $p = 0.03$).

Early experiences with the integration of CT not only documented differences in annular measurements between

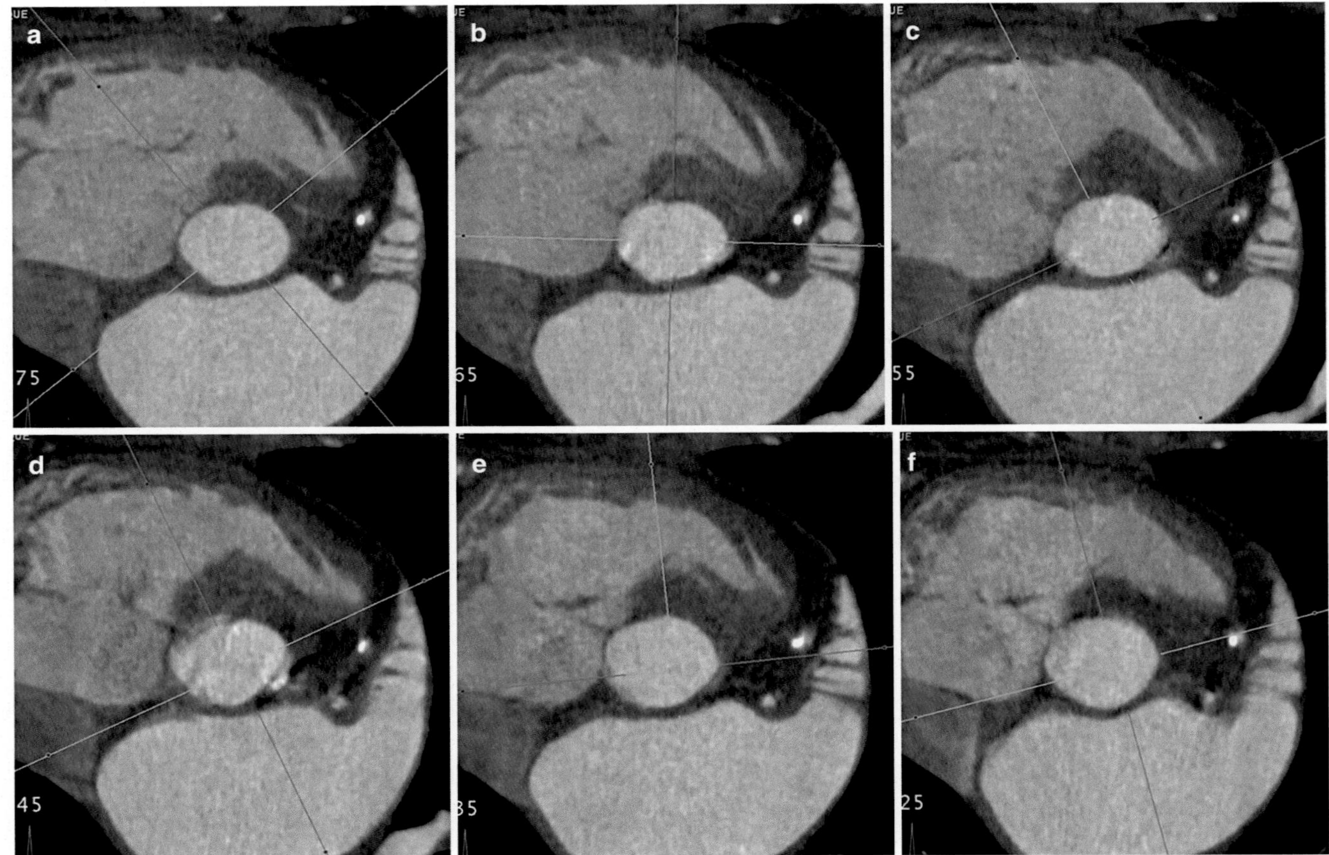

Fig. 15.2 Dynamic nature of Aortic Annulus over the course of cardiac cycle (75–25 %) (**a–f**) and corresponding measurements (**g–l**). Note the variation in the shape and size of the aortic annulus from diastole (65–75 %) through systole (25–35 %). Measurement of aortic annulus is usually performed in systole. The Geometrical shape of the aortic annulus changes from elliptical in diastole (75 %) to near circular in systole (25 %). The perimeter size increased from 74 to 79 mm (~5 mm difference – ~6 %) variation, whereas area size increased from 4.24 to 4.84 cm^2 (~0.6 cm^2 difference – ~variation of 13 %)

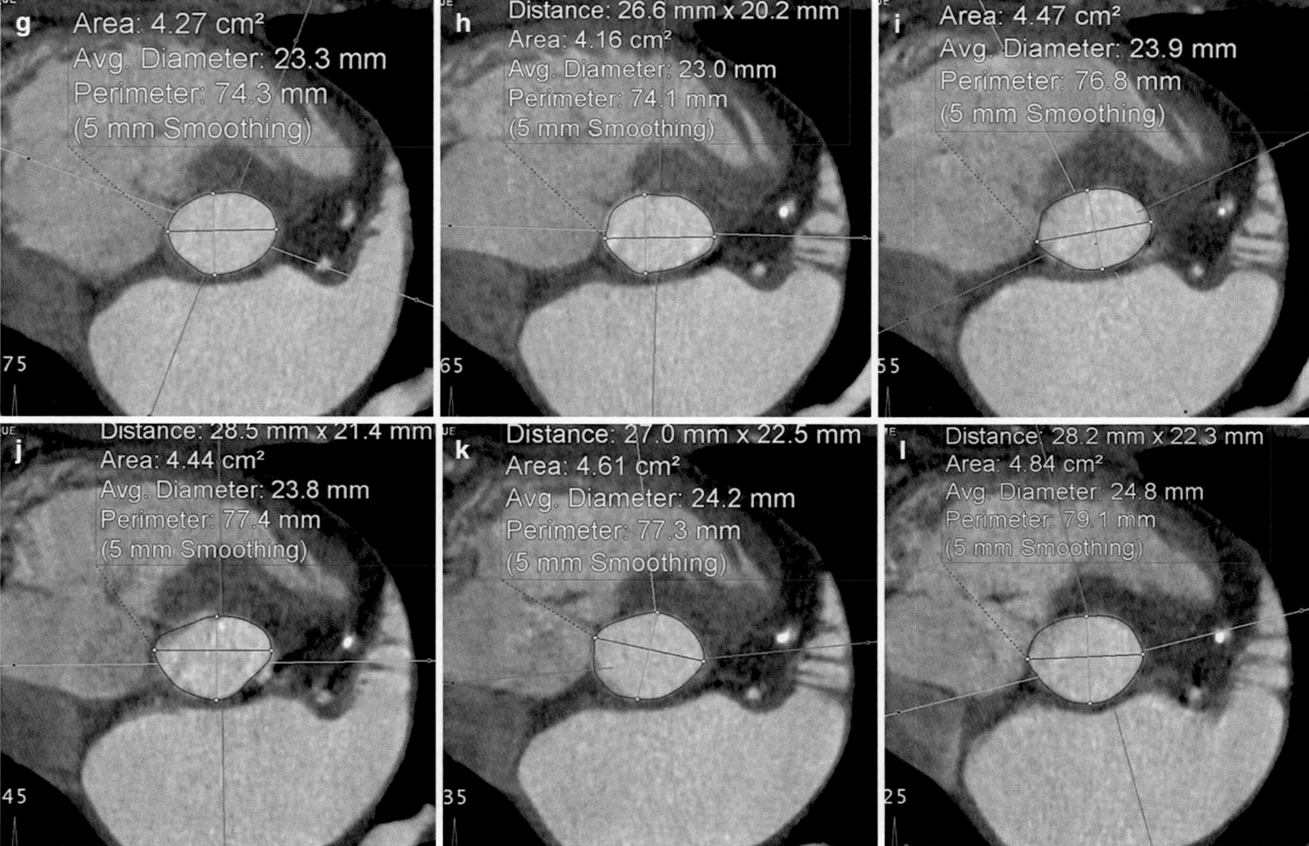

Fig. 15.2 (continued)

MDCT and echocardiography but also differences in potential sizing recommendations. Koos et al. evaluated the impact of 3D imaging methods (Cardiac magnetic resonance – CMR and dual source CT – DSCT) versus 2D TEE methods on TAVI selection [30]. In their cohort of 58 patients, different measurements would have changed TAVI strategy in 22–24 % patients. DSCT coronal measurements when compared to 2D TEE would have changed strategy in 16 patients. Further in 14/16 of those patients, the prosthesis size would have been larger and in the rest of the two, it was too large to implant. In a related similar study of 45 patients comparing 2D TTE and TEE and MSCT measurements, Messika-Zeitoun et al. observed that a decision based on MSCT would have modified TAVI strategy in 40–42 % [29].

The limitations of 2-D imaging largely reflect the complex almost uniformly non-circular configuration of the annulus. It is not that 2-D diameters derived from echocardiography or MSCT are inaccurate but it is simply a geometrical reality that the complex morphology of a non-circular structure cannot be accurately characterized with a single 2-D measurement. The growing appreciation of the limitations of 2-D imaging has driven and increased focus on the utilization of 3D modalities in measurement of aortic root including aortic annulus and left ventricular outflow tract.

Ng et al. evaluated 2D circular, 3D circular and 3D planimetered annular and LVOT areas by TEE and compared with MSCT planimetered areas [23]. In their cohort, the mean annular area by MSCT planimetry was 4.65 ± 0.82 cm^2 whereas by 2D TEE circular (3.89 ± 0.74 cm^2, $P < 0.001$), 3D TEE circular (4.06 ± 0.79 cm^2, $P < 0.001$), and 3D TEE planimetered annular areas (4.22 ± 0.77 cm^2, $P < 0.001$). They observed 3D TEE derived planimetered annular areas had the narrowest limits of agreement and least bias when compared to MDCT. Although the circular geometric assumptions made by 2D and 3D circular measurements were overcome by 3D TEE; Ng et al. observed 3D TEE when compared to MDCT still underestimated annular areas by up to 10 %.

MSCT has also been shown to be highly discriminatory of those patients that historically experienced paravalvular regurgitations owing to undersizing secondary to device sizing on the basis of 2-dimensional echocardiography. Willson and colleagues noted that the annular area in particular on MDCT was highly discriminatory of PAR [31]. This was important knowledge as it has been well established the paravalvular regurgitation is associated with increased morbidity and mortality [28–30, 32, 33].

Building upon this retrospective knowledge multiple groups have shown that the integration of MDCT in device selection allows for the reduction in the burden of PAR. Jilaihawi et al, prospective integration of CT guided algorithm reduced worse than mild paravalvular regurgitation (PAR) from 21.9 to 7.5 % when compared to 2D TEE [24]. Building upon this single center data Binder et al. in a prospective, multicenter controlled trial, evaluated the effects of the integration of an area based sizing algorithm on the clinical outcomes post TAVI [34]. With a non-randomized trial design half of the subjects (n = 133) underwent TAVI with the integration of MDCT measurements and sizing recommendations and the other half underwent TAVI without the integration of MDCT. They observed more than mild PAR (primary endpoint) was present in 5.3 % (7 of 133) of the MDCT group and in 12.8 % (17 of 133) in the control group ($p = 0.032$). The combined secondary endpoint (composite of in-hospital death, aortic annulus rupture, and severe PAR) occurred in 3.8 % (5 of 133) of the MDCT group and in 11.3 % (15 of 133) of the control group ($p = 0.02$). Finally the recently published large multicenter high risk CoreValve (Medtronic, Minneapolis, MN) trial showed excellent clinical outcomes as compared to surgical aortic valve replacement with the THV selection supported almost exclusively by MDCT perimeter measurements [35].

Dynamism of the Aortic Annulus

It is to be noted that aortic annulus is a dynamic structure with variation during systole and diastole phases of the cardiac cycle. The aortic annulus is often elliptical and assumes more circular shape during systole (Fig. 15.2). Further, it has been observed that there is increased asymmetrical deformation during diastole which especially affects the right coronary cusp portion of the annulus [36]. The ellipticity index (EI) defined as ratio of maximum to minimum diameters substantially decreased from diastole to systole due to significant increase in antero-posterior minor diameter [25]. Significant changes in area and radius were observed in both non-diseased annulus and stenotic annulus [37]. This has been attributed to annular reshaping than stretch with corresponding increase in systolic area [25].

Although cross-sectional area (CSA) derived measurements varied during cardiac cycle, it was found perimeter based diameter measurements show negligible increase in patients with calcified valves (0.56 ± 0.85 %; $p < 0.001$) and very small changes in normal subjects (2.2 ± 2.2 %, $p = 0.01$) [25]. In another study by Aspern et al., no significant difference was observed with perimeter-derived effective diameters (ED) (mean difference: 0.2 ± 0.4; $p = 0.07$), however, area derived ED showed a significant mean difference (0.4 ± 0.6 mm; $p = 0.009$), thus reconfirming influence of the cardiac cycle on aortic annulus area measurements [38]. It is likely that the diseased valves/tissues leave little scope for stretch and therefore perimeter derived aortic annulus measurements are least subjected to variation in cardiac cycle (Fig. 15.2). However, it is being noted smoothing algorithms used for perimeter derived measurements are inconsistent across work station platforms and might cause measurement errors. Although area based ED measurements are smaller than perimeter derived ED, both approaches showed good agreement [38].

Whether perimeter or area is chosen for transcatheter heart valve (THV) selection it is essential to understand the impact that the geometrical variable (area or perimeter derived measurements) may have on the prosthesis size that would be selected. Blanke et al. showed assuming a perfect circle with ellipticity index of 1, with increase in nominal diameter, area increases exponentially whereas perimeter increases proportionally [39]. Thus, for e.g. 10 % diameter oversizing would translate to 10 % increase in perimeter whereas it would increase area by 21 %. These geometrical truths are essential to understand and of clinical importance when certain degree of annular oversizing is contemplated during TAVI.

In summation, 3D MDCT measurements play a critical role in annular sizing and THV selection. MDCT measurements are accurate, reproducible and choice of area or perimeter derived measurements need to be tailored depending upon the choice of prosthesis devices, allowing for dynamism of the aortic annulus and based on the available tools (software) available at the sites.

MDCT Measurement of the Aortic Annulus

Approach to Aortic Annulus Measurement

We recommend using the phase of the cardiac cycle with best image quality and in systolic phases (25–45 %) to allow for consistent assessment of the annulus when it is the largest. Aortic annulus measurements are performed orthogonally in relation to the plane of 3 hinge points on a dedicated work station. Manual multiplanar reformats of the annulus is preferred as it helps in better understanding of the annulus and the annular plane rather than relying on automated tools which should ideally only be used by highly experienced operators. Briefly, the steps to achieve 'optimal' sizing of the aortic annulus are mentioned below (Fig. 15.3), however, reader should look into expert consensus documents/recommendations for further in-depth information [15, 40].

The first step is to lock the orthogonal planes at 90° to each other. The cross hairs in the coronal and sagittal images

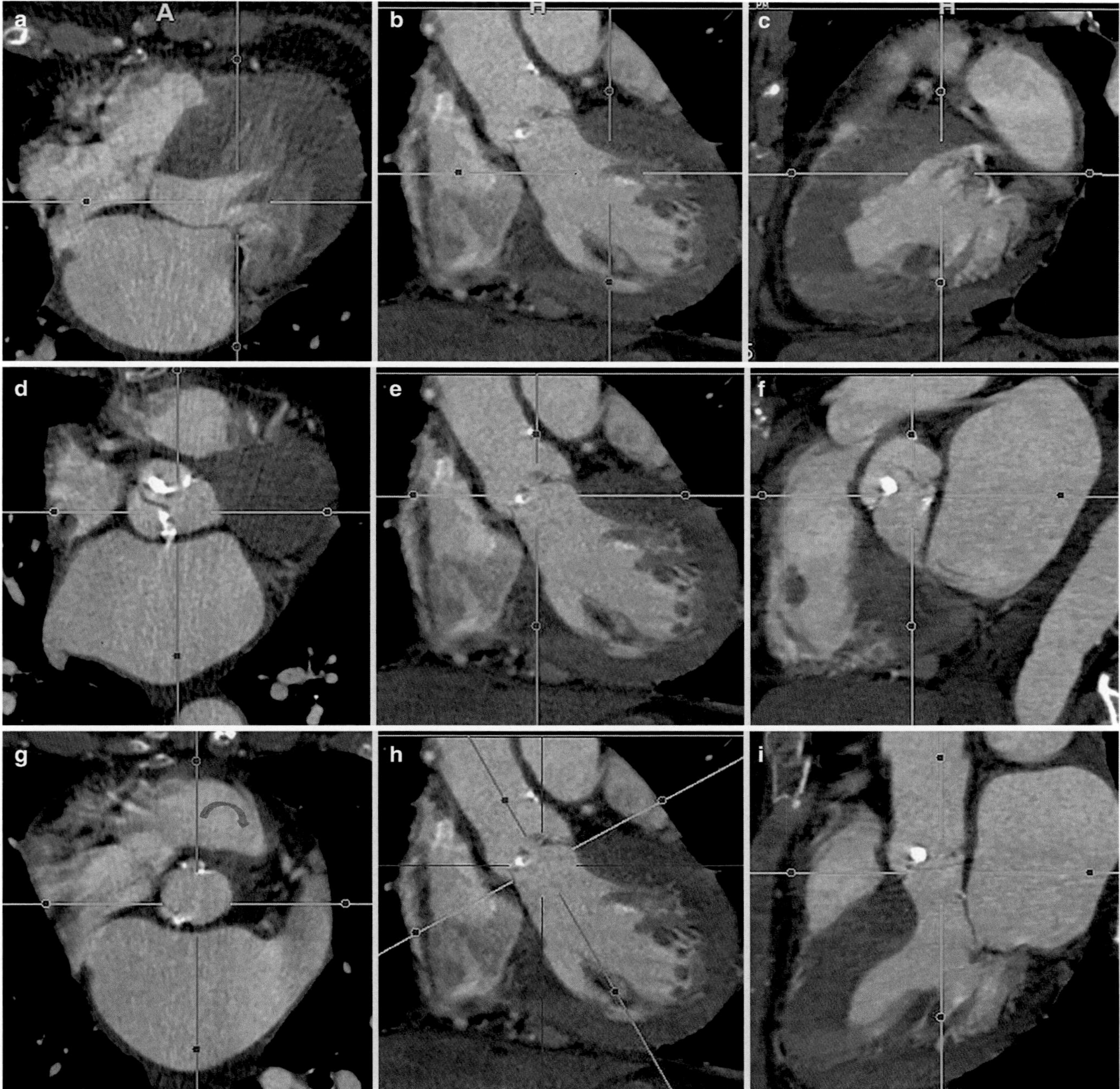

Fig. 15.3 Steps to achieve optimal sizing of aortic annulus. Step 1: Volumetric data is loaded onto the workstation and in a standard 3D format (*panel 1*), the views are transverse (**a**), Coronal (**b**) and sagittal (**c**). The first step is to lock the orthogonal planes at 90° to each other (**a–c**). Step 2: The cross hairs in the coronal and sagittal images are moved to the level of aortic valves and adjusted so that the cross hairs on the transverse plane are positioned at the level of aortic valve (*panel 2* – **d–f**). Step 3: Then the cross hairs on the coronal and sagittal views are rotated and adjusted so as to correspond to the aortic annulus plane (*panel 3*). Now the corresponding views are oblique set of images, for e.g. transverse/coronal/sagittal oblique (**g–i**). Step 4: The cross hairs on the transverse oblique are rotated either clockwise or anticlockwise (*panel 3* **g**) so as to check whether the cross hairs correspond to aortic annular plane i.e. nadir point of the coronary cusps (*panel 4* – **j–l**). In this panel views, the cross hairs cuts across the cusp rather than located at the hinge/nadir point (*panel 4* – **k**). Step 5: The cross hairs are further adjusted by placing the cross hairs at the aortic annular plane (*panel 5* – **m–o**). Once again the cross hair on the transverse oblique view is rotated and again investigated to see the cross hairs on the rest of the two oblique planes correspond to aortic annulus plane (*panel 6* – **p–r**). Any adjustments, if necessary, are made by following the above steps. Step 6: Once a satisfactory plane is achieved (*panel 7* – **s–u**), it is further confirmed by toggling the transverse oblique set of images cranially and caudally across the aortic root (*panel 7* – **s** and *panel 8* – **v**, *red arrows*). If a true aortic annular plane has been achieved, then one would observe that the valve hinge points would disappear or appear symmetrically all at once (*panels 7* – **s–u** and *8* – **v–x**). Utmost focus is given so that cross hairs are just touching the nadir points (*panel 7* – **s–u**). If this plane is not achieved, then the coronal (*panel 7* – **t**) and sagittal oblique (*panel 7* – **u**) planes needs to be further fine-tuned so as to achieve desired plane and again cross checked by rotating the cross hairs on the transverse oblique view (*panel 7* – **s**). Step 7: Once an optimal view is achieved then the cross hairs are at the true aortic annular plane (*panel 9* – **y, z, A**). Then a ROI trace is made along the circumference of the aortic annulus to calculate the major and minor diameters, mean diameters, area and circumference of the aortic annulus (*panel 9* – **y**). Corresponding coronal and sagittal oblique planes are shown (*panel 9* – **z, a**)

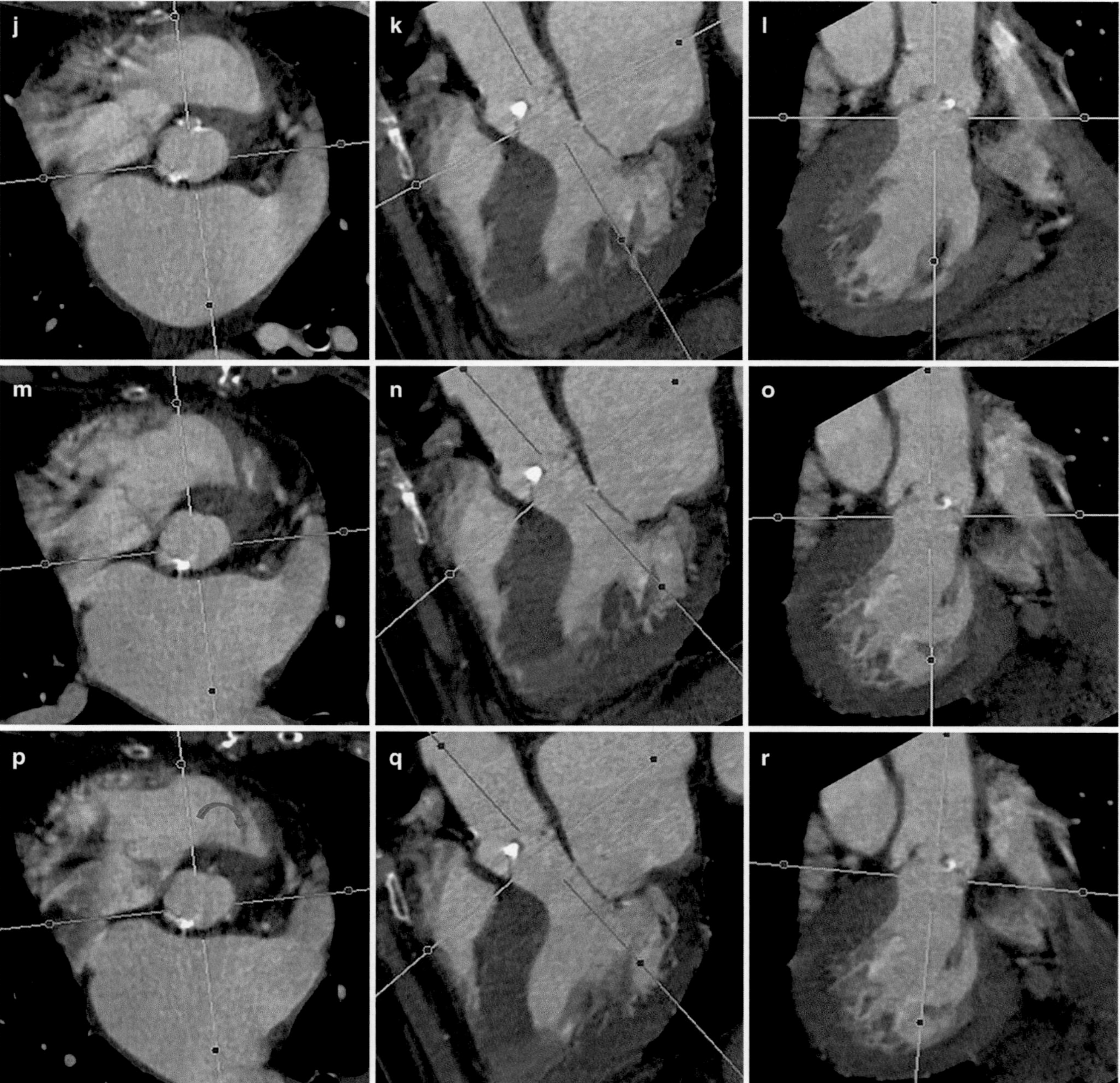

Fig. 15.3 (continued)

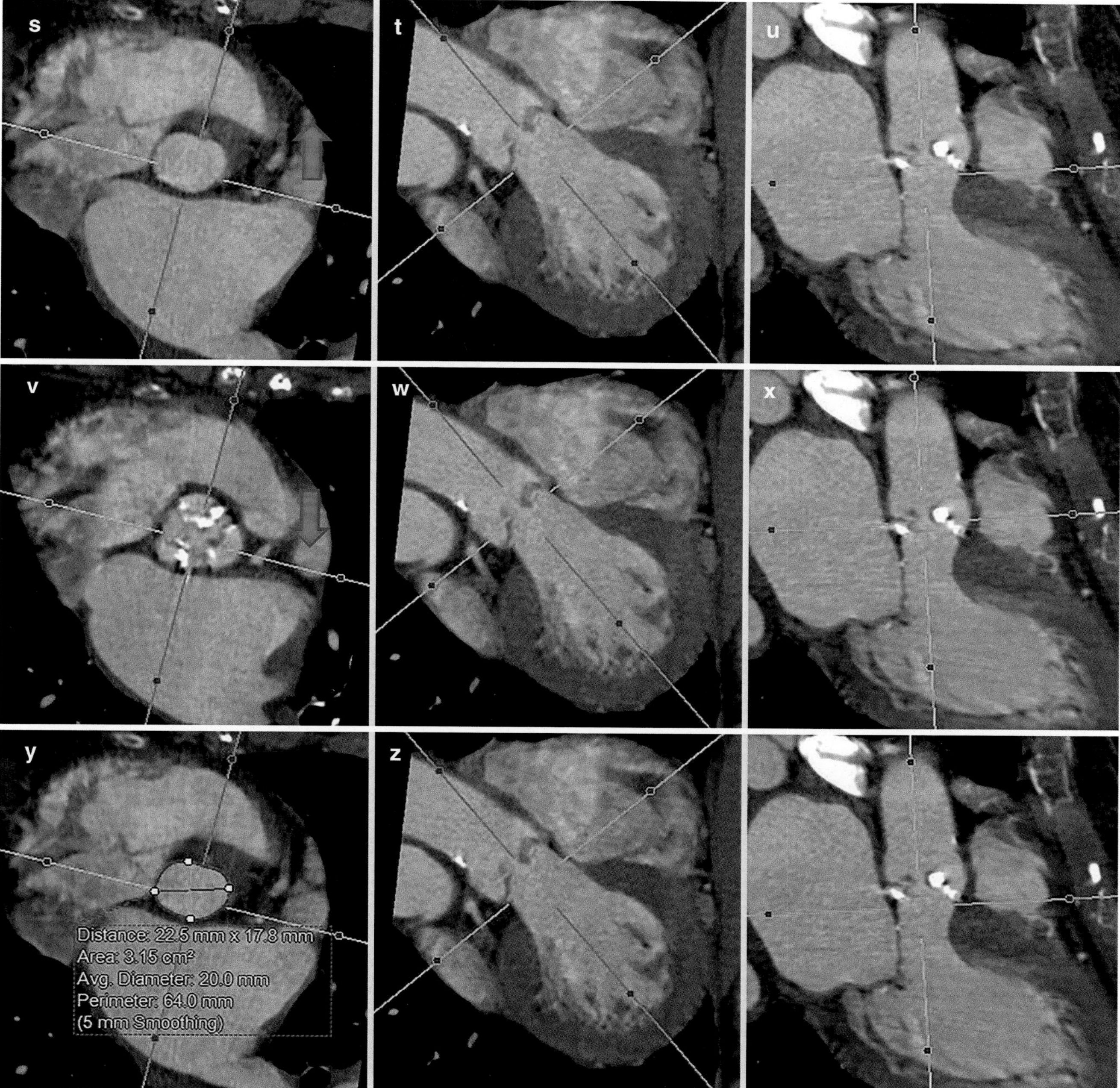

Fig. 15.3 (continued)

should be moved to the level of aortic valves and adjusted so that the transverse plane is positioned at the level of aortic valve. This would correspond to coronal and sagittal oblique planes respectively. Next the transverse oblique plane is moved up and down across the aortic root so as to visualize the valve hinge points. The valve hinge points should disappear or appear symmetrically all at once, if not, coronal and sagittal oblique planes need to be further fine-tuned so as to achieve desired plane. Again, the cross hairs are rotated across the transverse oblique so that to visualize the nadir point of the valves in coronal oblique and sagittal oblique planes. Utmost focus is given so that cross hairs are just touching the nadir points and they disappear equally in all planes. Once this is confirmed, the specific position of aortic annulus in the transverse oblique plane is identified and a ROI trace is made along the circumference of the aortic annulus. Majority of the present day work stations have automatic tools that would calculate diameters (D) – Dmin,

Dmax, Dmean, area and perimeter once the tracing is made. If these features are not available, diameter (D) can be calculated from circumference (D=circumference / π). (π=Pi). Area is calculated from $\pi.D^2/4$.

Implantation View – CO Planar Angle Prediction

The Aortic annulus is not orthogonal to the body axis/planes. For a successful implantation, the prosthetic device needs to be deployed coaxially to the centerline of the aorta. Inappropriate deployment might lead to complications [41]. This plane can be achieved on both CT workstation and fluoroscopy units. However to achieve the same plane in fluoroscopy unit, multiple aortograms are to be performed in a stepwise approach.

This situation offers an opportunity for pre-procedural CT to help predict the co-planar angles of deployment prior to the procedure. At here are innumerable co-planar angles of deployment typically ranging from RAO Caudal to LAO Cranial. Pre-procedural co-planar angle guidance has been shown to help reduce procedure fluoroscopy time and the volume of contrast needed for the procedure [42, 43]. Binder et al. have demonstrated significant correlation ($r=0.682$, $p<0.001$) between the predicted optimal deployment projections using 3D angiographic projections and MDCT of aortic root [44]. It is important to recognize that correlation with the fluoroscopic angles in the hybrid operating room relies on comparable positioning at the time of CT and during the procedure.

Evaluation of Aortic Annulus and Aortic Valve Leaflets

Apart from annulus sizing, assessment of the aortic annulus, left ventricular outflow tract and aortic valve leaflets is equally important for a successful TAVI procedure. Valve calcifications may be distributed focally or diffusely over the surface of the valve cusps or they may present along the leaflet edges. Presence of severe calcium is likely to cause important peri and post procedural complications. Post dilatation techniques might need to be employed in patients with severe calcification.

In TAVI cohorts, it is not uncommon to see sub annular or LVOT calcification (Figs. 15.4 and 15.5) or aorto-mitral calcification as a continuum (Fig. 15.4a, b). Distribution of calcium in each of these locations has been shown to have important prognostic implications. In a study by Barbanti et al., 31 consecutive TAVI patients who had LVOT/annular/aortic contained/noncontained rupture were caliper-matched to control group of 31 patients without annular injury [45]. They observed at least 2 features were significantly associated with

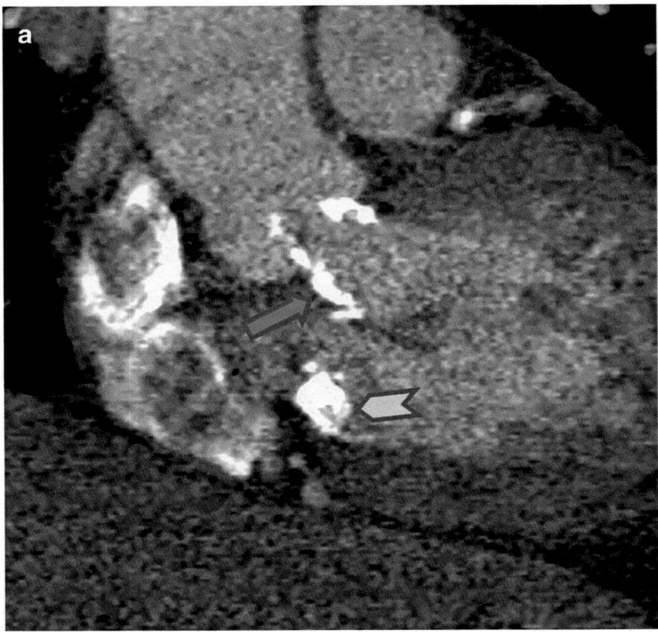

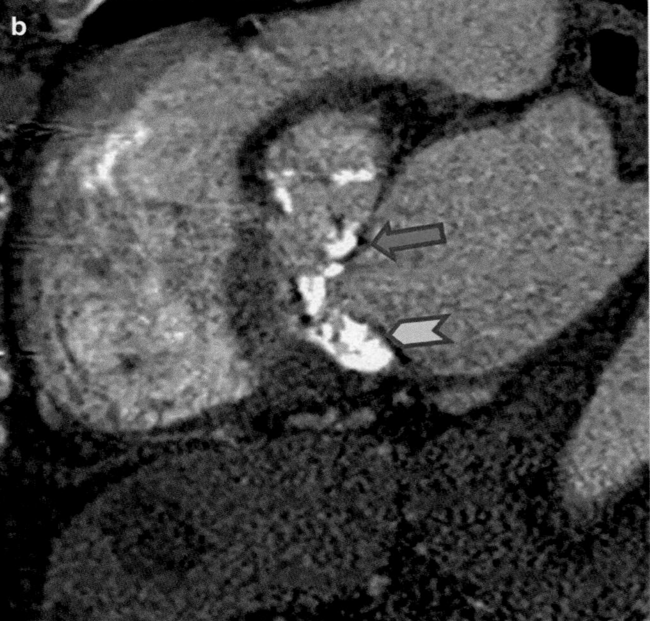

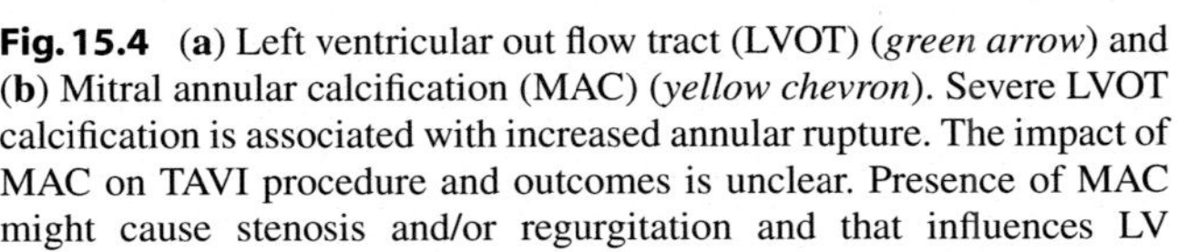

Fig. 15.4 (**a**) Left ventricular out flow tract (LVOT) (*green arrow*) and (**b**) Mitral annular calcification (MAC) (*yellow chevron*). Severe LVOT calcification is associated with increased annular rupture. The impact of MAC on TAVI procedure and outcomes is unclear. Presence of MAC might cause stenosis and/or regurgitation and that influences LV function and geometry. It should be noted that deployment of a balloon expandable prosthesis is contraindicated in concomitant significant mitral stenosis with significant mitral annular calcification. *LVEF* left ventricle ejection fraction

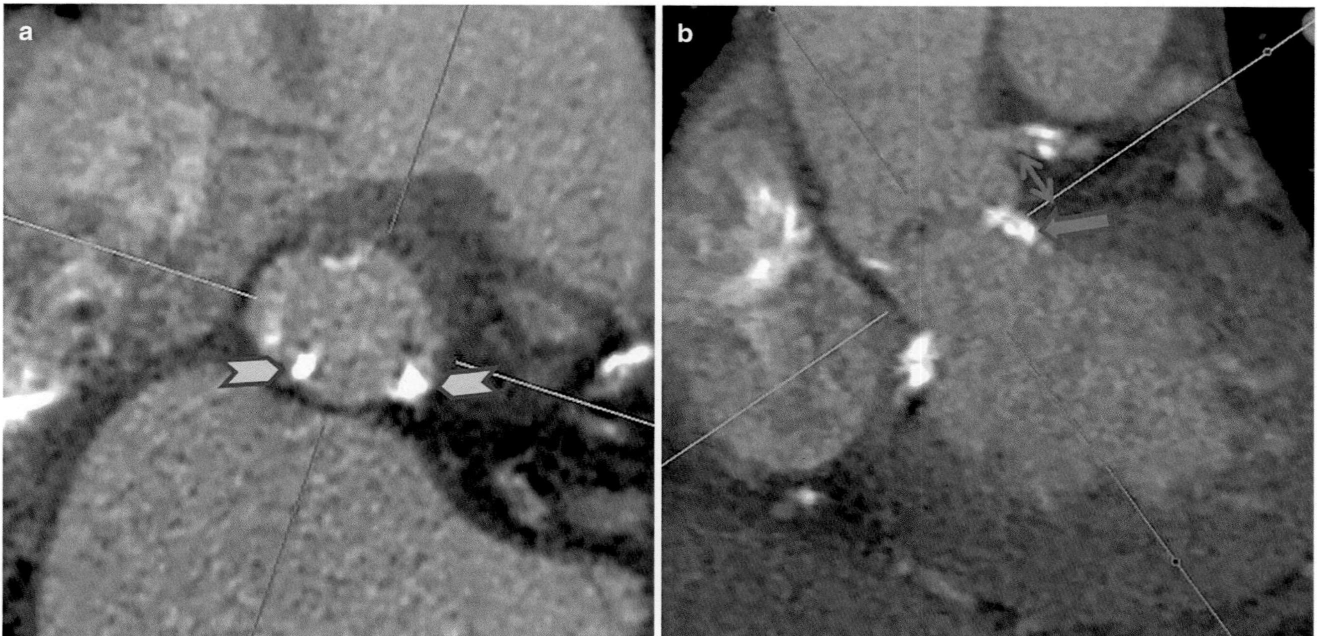

Fig. 15.5 Factors influencing annular rupture. (**a**) Subannular (*yellow chevrons*) and (**b**) LVOT calcification (*green arrow*). Note the relatively low left coronary ostial-aortic annulus height (measured 9.6 mm) (*red double arrow*)

annular rupture: 1. Moderate/severe LVOT/subannular calcification ((odds ratio, 10.92; 95 % CI, 3.23–36.91; P<0.001) and 2. ≥20 % area oversizing (odds ratio, 8.38; 95 % CI, 2.67–26.33; P=<0.001). Area oversizing ≥20 % was found to be the strongest predictor of aortic rupture and presence of significant LVOT/subannular calculation seems to compound to increased risk. Additionally, presence and characteristics of annular calcification such as protruding, round and asymmetrical distribution at the coronary cusps seems to predict PAR (Fig. 15.5a). In a study by Feuchtner et al., protruding annular calcification >4 mm, adherent annular calcification >6 mm predicted significant PAR (p=0.03 and 0.009 respectively). Further, it was observed total left and non-coronary and left coronary calcium size score predicted relevant leaks (p=0.004 and p=0.001, resp.) but not right or non-coronary cusps calcium [46].

During the procedure, severe calcification may offer resistance to the expansion caused by balloon or self-expandable devices and may prevent appropriate alignment and/or complete apposition of the sealing skirt to the native commissures. Further, incomplete apposition of the device with commissures may potential lead to development of paravalvular regurgitation (PAR). It has been shown that even mild paravalvular leaks are associated with increased mortality [47, 48]

Aortic valve calcifications (AVC) distribution is better visualized on the cross-sectional view of the sinus of Valsalva. AVC can be assessed qualitatively as mild, moderate or severe (Fig. 15.1a–c) or could also be quantified analogous to the concept of the Agatston score that is being used in assessment of coronary artery calcifications.

Haensig et al. assessed for association between native AVC and paravalvular leak in 120 consecutive patients who proceeded with Edwards SAPIEN prosthesis. No paravalvular leaks (n=66) were noted with mean AVC score of 2704±1510, mild paravalvular leaks (n=31) with 3804±2739 (P=0.05); and moderate paravalvular leaks (n=4) with AVC score of 7387±1044 (P=0.002) [48]. A significant association between the AVC score and paravalvular leaks [odds ratio [(OR; per AVC score of 1000), 11.38; 95 % confidence interval (CI) 2.33–55.53; P=0.001)] was noted. It is not only the amount of calcification but location/distribution at each separate cusp or commissure has been found to be associated with PAR [48]. Their study identified significant association for the right and left coronary cusp, for right-left and left non coronary commissure, and there was no significant association for non-coronary right commissure and for non-coronary cusp. Interestingly a number of other studies evaluating patients who underwent TAVI using a self-expanding system,, did not find an association between PAR and the degree of calcification [49, 50]. It is likely the distribution of radial force at different locations due to the nature of the device with balloon expandable at the annulus whereas the self-expandable at the ascending aorta cause varied propensity towards development of PAR.

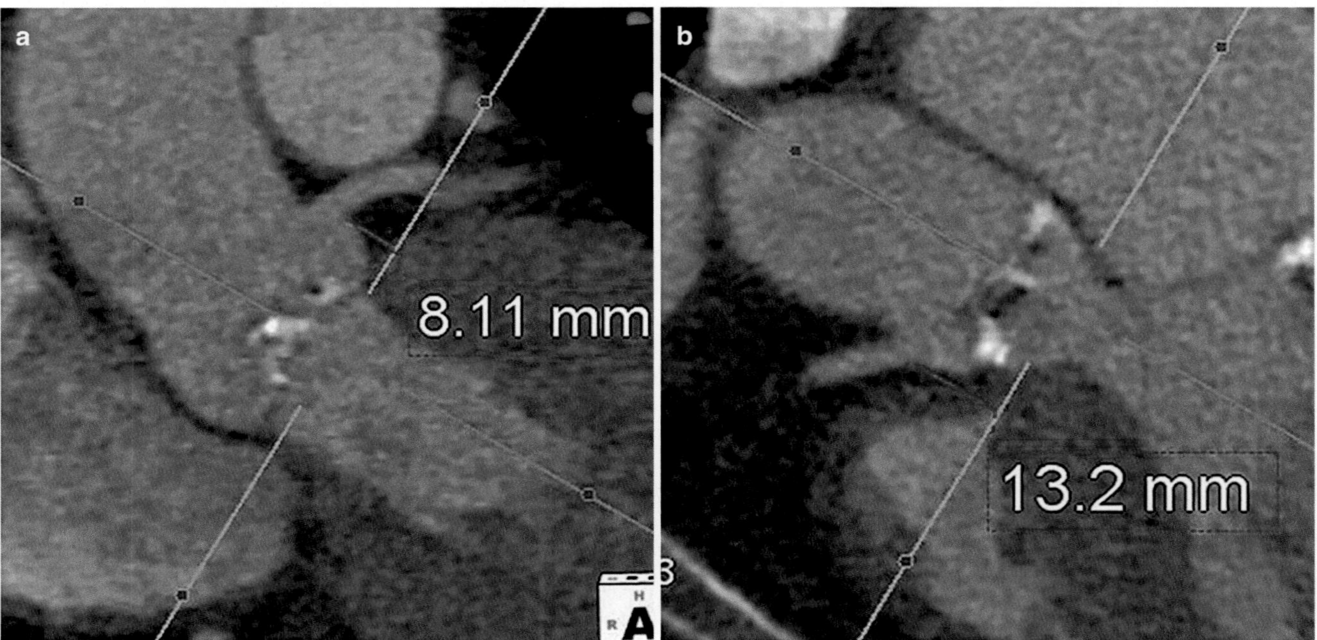

Fig. 15.6 Coronary ostial-aortic annulus heights. (**a**) Low left coronary ostial height (~8 mm) and (**b**) adequate right coronary ostial height (~13 mm)

Coronary Arteries and Ostial Heights

In general, the right and left coronary arteries arise from their respective right and left coronary cusps. They usually arise below the sinotubular junction with the right coronary artery typically at a higher level than left. Given the nature of TAVI, where in the native aortic leaflets are displaced and the bioprosthesis is implanted in the aortic root; the coronary ostial height clearance measurement is important to understand and discriminate those at risk of coronary arterial occlusion. Coronary ostial height measurements are performed in a perpendicular fashion from the annular plane to the coronary ostia (Fig. 15.6a, b).

A coronary ostial cut off of 10 mm was suggested by the American College of Cardiology Foundation/American Association for Thoracic Surgery/Society for Cardiovascular Angiography and Interventions/Society of Thoracic Surgeons expert consensus [15, 51]. However, in a study of reported cases of coronary obstruction, the mean height was 10.3 mm (range 7–12 mm) and 60 % of cases with obstruction had a height >10 mm [52]. In a multicenter registry study, it was observed majority of the patients who had coronary obstruction (~80 % overall and 96 % of women) had a left ostial height <12 mm [53]. Further, adding to the complexity and importance of ostial measurements, in the same registry study, even though the coronary ostial heights were more than >12 mm, 21.4 % had a coronary obstruction implying that there are factors beyond 'safety cutoff' of coronary ostial height that might predispose to coronary obstruction. This registry allowed the field to understand mechanisms of coronary occlusion beyond coronary height that the majority of patients (~ 65 %) who had coronary obstruction had aortic root effacement and also SOV diameter of <30 mm when compared to the control group. Coronary artery obstruction was more frequently observed in female patients (>80 %) likely related to the female anatomy with smaller aortic root/shallow aortic sinus and also relatively due to low lying coronary ostia (Figs. 15.5b and 15.6a). In addition, a significant difference in SOV/AA ratios was also observed between those who had coronary obstruction when compared to control groups (1.25+_0.04 vs. 1.34+_0.03; p=0.003) [53].

It is also interesting to note that coronary obstruction was more often observed in patients with balloon expandable devices than those who had self-expandable devices [53, 54]. It is unknown whether makeup of the device or mechanism of deployment has any role in the observed obstructions. Other causes which predispose to coronary obstruction include bulky calcification of the native aortic leaflets, long mobile leaflets and specifically presence of leaflet length more than the coronary ostial heights.

Although, at present there are no standard guidelines for a 'safe' coronary ostial height; various factors that predispose to coronary obstruction need to be taken into account. These include patient's sex, the size of the aortic root, sinus of Valsalva diameter, coronary ostial heights, and the ratio of SOV/AA (Fig. 15.7).

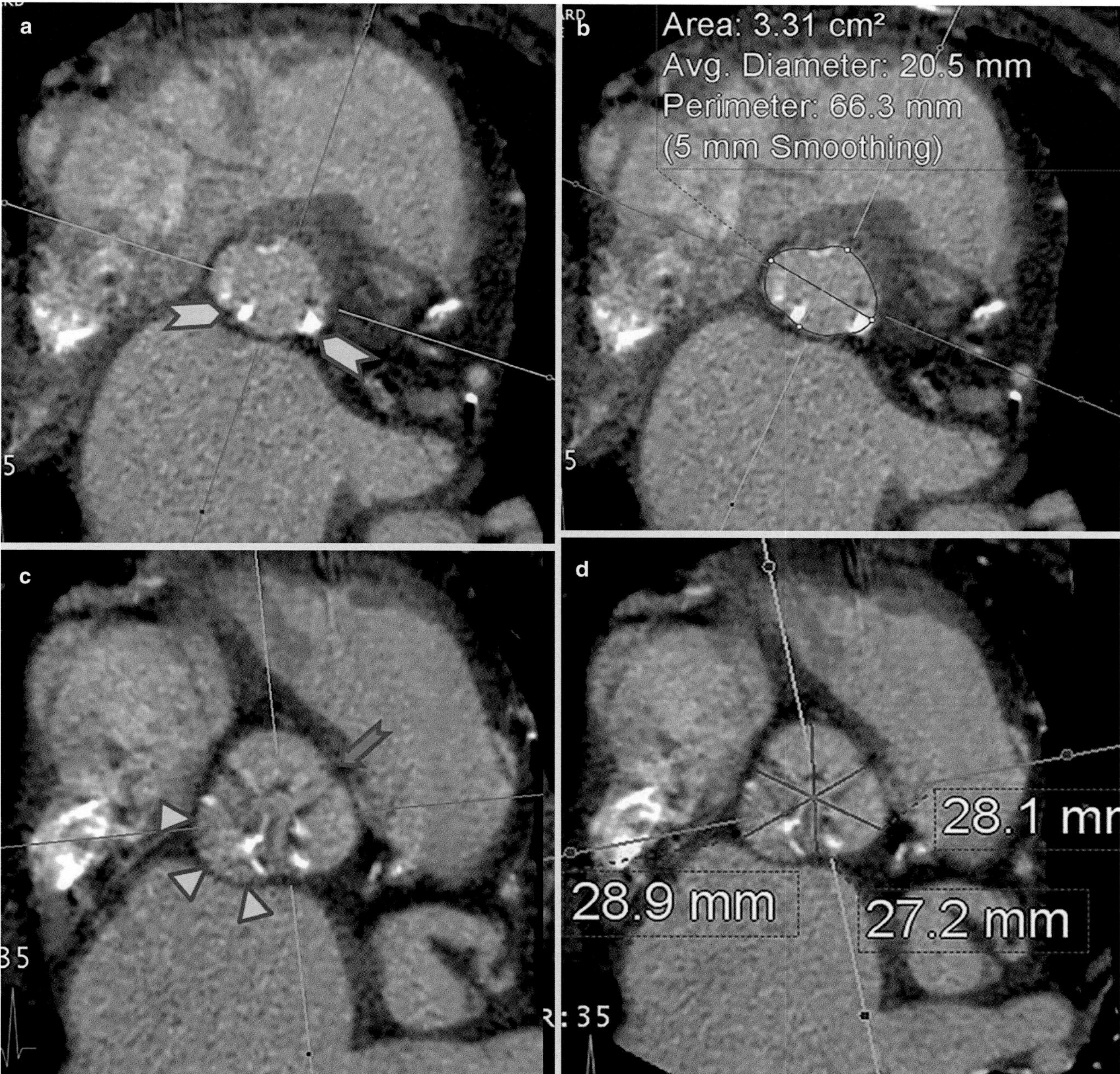

Fig. 15.7 Unfavorable anatomy of aortic root (same patient as in Fig. 15.5). (**a**, **b**) Aortic annulus is smaller in size and it shows subannular and LVOT calcification (*yellow chevron's*). (Even though aortic valvular calcification is of mild degree (**c**), the aortic sinus is shallow as it measures <30 in all cusp-commissure diameters (**d**) (Cusp – yellow triangles, Commissure – notched *green arrow*). This TAVI patient is female and there is relatively low left coronary ostial height (9.6 mm) (Fig. 15.5b). Multiple confounding factors increase risk of peri-procedural complications

Evaluation of Aortic Arch, Thoraco-Abdominal Aortic Assessment and Ilio-Femoral Arterial Assessment

Vascular related complications are one of the most frequent adverse events associated with TAVI procedure [11, 12, 55–59]. TAVR related complications are defined by Valve Academic Research Consortium (VARC) [60, 61]. In a meta-analysis study of 16 outcomes based on VARC 2011, the pooled estimated rate for major and minor vascular complications were 11.9 % (range 5–23.3 %) and 9.7 % (range 5.6–28.3 %) with an overall vascular complication rate of 18.8 % (range 9.5–51.6 %) [56]. Occurrence of major vascular complication was associated significantly with higher rates of 30 day and 1 year all-cause and cardiac mortality Owing to the increased risk associated with vascular injury the assessment of the vascular pathway and risk factors for vascular injury are important steps in pre-TAVI work up.

Peripheral Vascular Accesses

Access routes can be broadly classified into retrograde (transfemoral [TF], transaortic, transsubclavian etc.), antegrade (tranapical) approach or a combination of both (transcaval-transaortic). Each of the access sites for delivery of TAVI has advantages and limitations.

The risk factors for vascular injury include small caliber vessels (Fig. 15.8), presence of significant occlusive disease, burden and pattern of calcification, excessive iliac tortuosity. Dual plane angiography can be used in the assessment of vessel caliber and also for presence of significant stenosis; however, it is limited in the evaluation of plaque burden and vessel tortuosity. Similarly, although ultrasound could be used in the assessment of plaque burden and assessment of luminal diameter, it is limited in evaluation of tortuosity and if the calcific plaque burden is high. MDCT with its superior spatial and temporal resolution, volumetric acquisition and relatively simple post-processing techniques helps in evaluation of the risk factors for vascular injury and thus is considered gold standard modality for vascular screening.

Arterial Lumen Diameter Assessment

Ideally the delivery system needs to be smaller than vascular luminal diameter. Due to relatively larger delivery systems that are used (>18 F), accurate assessment of the vascular access and pathway is critical. As most TAVI cohorts are elderly, it is not uncommon to see vessels which are tortuous and have considerable atherosclerotic burden. In a study of 100 TAVI patients for peripheral artery disease, one-third (35 %) had at least one criterion of unsuitable iliofemoral anatomy and out of those more than 75 % had a luminal diameter of less than 8 mm [62]. The other unfavorable factors included severe circumferential calcification at the iliac bifurcation (>60 %), and severe angulation of the iliac arteries (<90°).

Although the arterial lumen can be assessed on the source axial or transverse set of images, assessment in this view tends to inaccurately measure the true minimal luminal diameter. Areas of significant stenosis can be under appreciated due tortuous course of the vessels. Further, the presence of dense calcium causes blooming artifacts which tend to overestimate stenosis.

Accurate measurements of lumen diameter are obtained through multiplanar reformations. Due to MDCT volumetric acquisition, orthogonal planes to the center line of arterial lumen can be obtained to determine the true short and long axis diameter measurements. Modern post processing work stations have curved planar reformations tool which would help in extracting the entire course of the vessel and thus a visual and quantitative measurements could be obtained. A potential limitation in assessment of arterial lumen arises

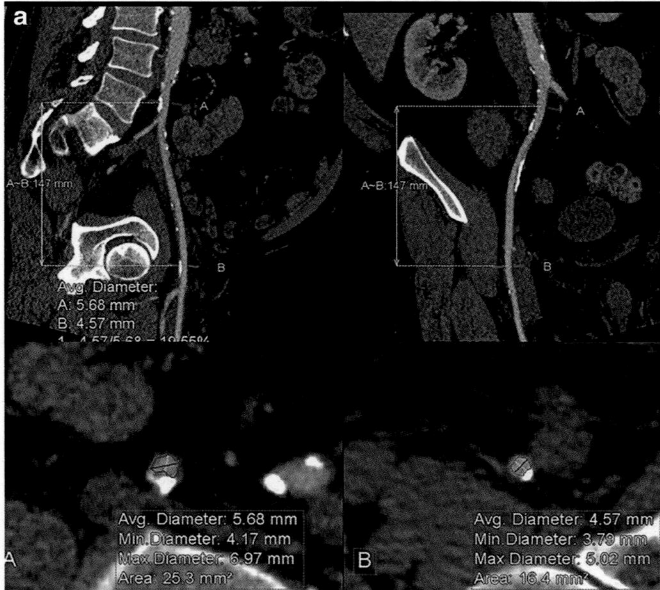

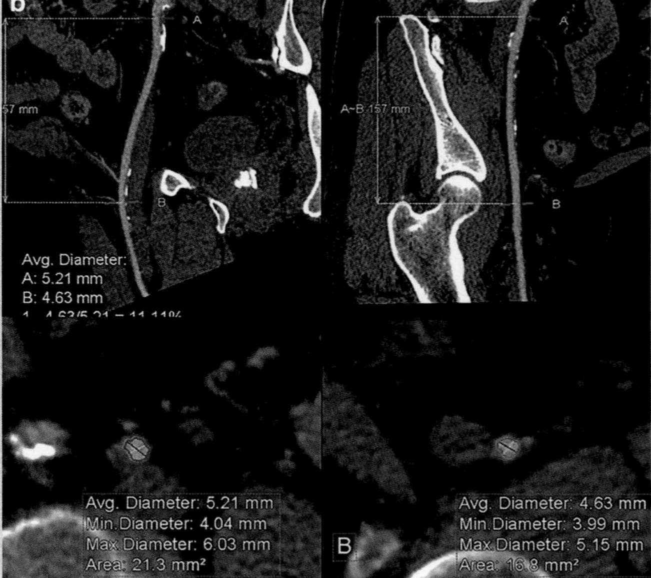

Fig. 15.8 Narrow Ilio-femoral luminal diameters. Although calcification in the ilio-femoral arteries is minimal; bilateral ilio-femoral arteries show narrow minimal lumen diameter. Common iliac arteries measure <6 mm and the common femoral arteries access sites measures <5 mm. Alternative access sites need to be considered in this patient

in the presence of dense calcium which tends to overestimate stenosis and thus undermines the luminal diameter. This is overcome by choosing proper window level and width settings or by using bone algorithm settings during measurements. Some of the modern work stations have a full width half maximum built in tool which could be used for accurate diameter measurements. Hayashida et al. were the first to introduce the concept of sheath to femoral artery ratio (SFAR) and defined it as the ratio of the sheath outer diameter (in millimeters-mm) to the minimal femoral artery diameter (in mm) [58]. In their study, a SFAR threshold of 1.05 (area under the curve = 0.727) predicted a higher rate of VARC major complications (30.9 % vs. 6.9 %, p = 0.001) and 30-day mortality (18.2 % vs. 4.2 %, p = 0.016). A SFAR ≥1.05 was also associated with an increased incidence of 30-day mortality (18.2 % vs. 2.8 %, p = 0.004). Using this SFAR threshold, the minimal femoral artery diameter necessary for the 19- and 18-F introducer sheaths was calculated as 7.1 and 6.9 mm, respectively.

Another series looked into both SFAR and sheath: femoral artery area ratio (SFAAR – sheath area to the femoral minimal lumen area [MLA]) in 255 patients and found SFAAR of 1.35 was predictive of vascular complications (sensitivity 78.6 %, specificity 62.9 %) [63]. In comparison, although a diameter ratio cutoff of 1.45 was predictive but it had lower sensitivity and specificity (64.2 % and 67.4 %, respectively). These findings highlight the importance of lumen diameter and area measurements and their relation to sheath diameter/areas in predicting vascular complications.

Vessel Wall Calcifications

Arterial luminal or area measurements need to be determined in concurrence with the presence of atherosclerotic plaques, more specifically calcifications. Calcifications are broadly defined as follows: 0-no calcification; 1-mild calcification; 2-moderate calcification; and 3-severe calcification (Fig. 15.9) [64]. Presence of circumferential calcification (>75 % vessel circumference) and/or horseshoe (>180°) calcifications with decreased luminal diameter are at a higher risk of complications. In a study of 132 patients, the presence

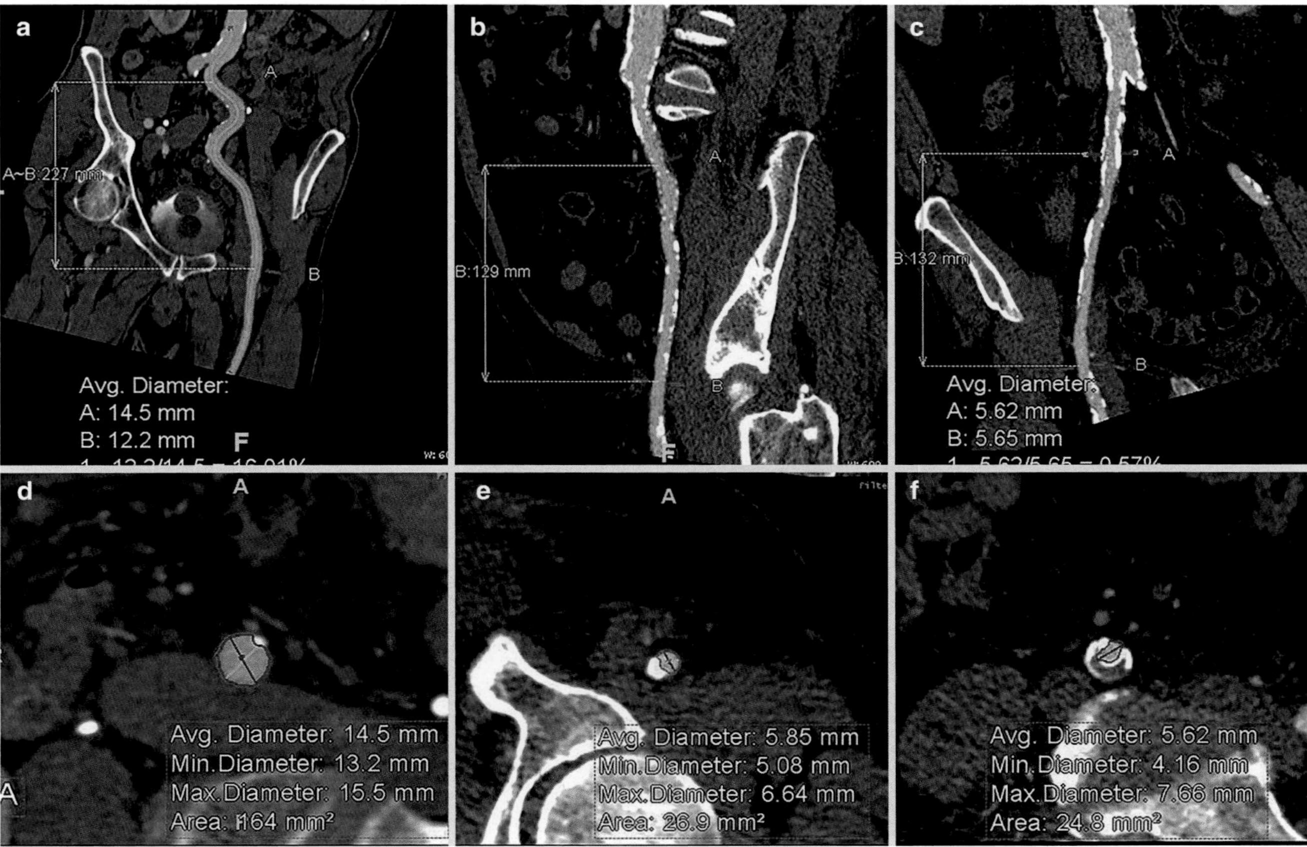

Fig. 15.9 Iliofemoral calcifications. They are broadly classified as: 0-no calcification; (**a**) 1-mild calcification; (**b**) 2-moderate calcification; and (**c**) 3-severe calcification [66]. Presence of horseshoe or circumferential calcification increases risk of vascular complications. Further, the diameter and area measurements derived from MDCT (**d**–**f**) could be used to calculate SFAR and SFAAR depending upon the sheath device used. SFAR > 1.05 and SFAAR > 1.35 were associated with increased vascular complications. *SFAR* Sheath to Femoral Artery Ratio (Diameter), *SFAAR* Sheath Area to Femoral Minimal Lumen Area Ratio

of circumferential ilio-femoral calcifications was an important risk factor for vascular complications and also an independent predictor of increased mortality after TF-TAVI [65]. Further, incorporation of this MSCT derived parameter in the workup algorithm of patients with a sheath-to-iliofemoral artery ratio – SIFAR ≥1 on angiographic screening improved the specificity for prediction of major vascular complications to 62 % without altering the sensitivity (100 %).

In another series, arterial calcification (Grade > 2) at puncture site was found to be independent predictor of major vascular complication, p < 0.001 [66] . The authors also noted despite the use of a pigtail catheter for an ideal puncture, arterial wall calcification could not be evaluated by fluoroscopy and recommended assessment through MDCT. Kurra et al. proposed presence of more than 60 % circumferential calcification at the external–internal iliac bifurcation as an unsuitable iliofemoral anatomy [62].

Iliofemoral Arterial Tortuosity

Iliofemoral Arterial Tortuosity have implications for transfemoral TAVI approach as excess tortuosity might increase the access site complication rates and thus would affect procedural success. The degree of tortuosity could be graded as – 0-no tortuosity; 1-mild tortuosity (30–60°); 2-moderate tortuosity (60–90°); and 3-severe tortuosity (≥90°) (Fig. 15.10) [62, 64].

Although it was observed that iliofemoral tortuosity alone does not predict vascular complications [58, 67]; Vavuranakis et al. in their study incorporated total arterial tortuosity/access vessel diameter (TT/AD) index and observed that a value 27.89 predicts vascular complications with 50.8 % sensitivity and 70.6 % specificity (AUC: 0.22, P = 0.008) [66]. TT/AD ratio defined as sum of angles (TT) divided by the minimum femoral arterial diameter (AD) at the access site. Even though, the indexed values were primarily based on 2D invasive angiography, nevertheless, a small subset of their cohort were evaluated with 3D MDCT and found to have good correlation (r = 0.66, p = 0.013).

Chiam et al. assessed iliofemoral dimensions and characteristics by ultrasonography in 549 Asian patients [68]. They observed female gender, lower body surface area, and presence of diabetes mellitus; dyslipidemia and smoking history were independent factors for smaller iliofemoral dimensions. Thus for the same degree of tortuosity, a smaller intraluminal diameter might predispose to increased vascular risk, if TT/AD index is incorporated.

Alternative Access

Alternative access routes should be considered in patients where reconstructed CT images reveal unfavorable ilio-femoral anatomy. Description of various access sites is beyond the scope of this chapter; however, the underlying principles would remain the same as mentioned above. Access routes need to be assessed holistically depending upon patient's condition and also the device that is likely to be deployed with minimal complications (Fig. 15.11).

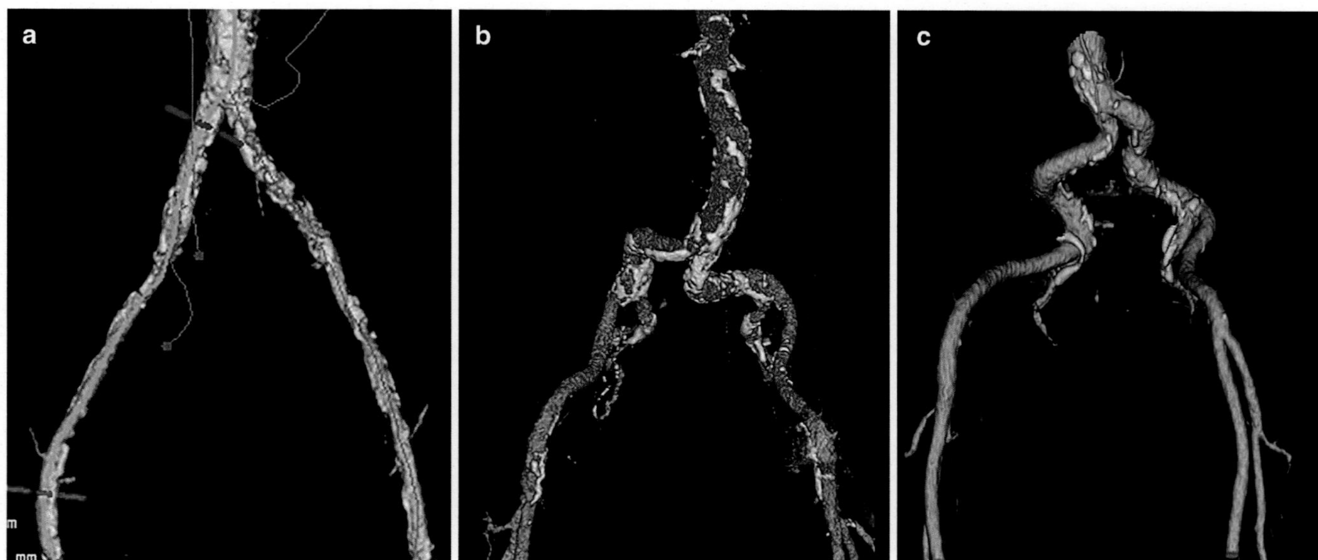

Fig. 15.10 Ilio-femoral tortuosity. Multiple panels show mild, moderate and severe tortuosity of peripheral vascular access (**a–c**). Degree of tortuosity is graded as: 0-no tortuosity; (**a**) 1-mild tortuosity (30–60°); (**b**) 2-moderate tortuosity (60–90°); and (**c**) 3-severe tortuosity (≥90°) [64, 66]. Although, the degree of tortuosity per se might not significantly influence increased risk for vascular complications; a combination of increased tortuosity and small luminal diameter predisposes to vascular risk

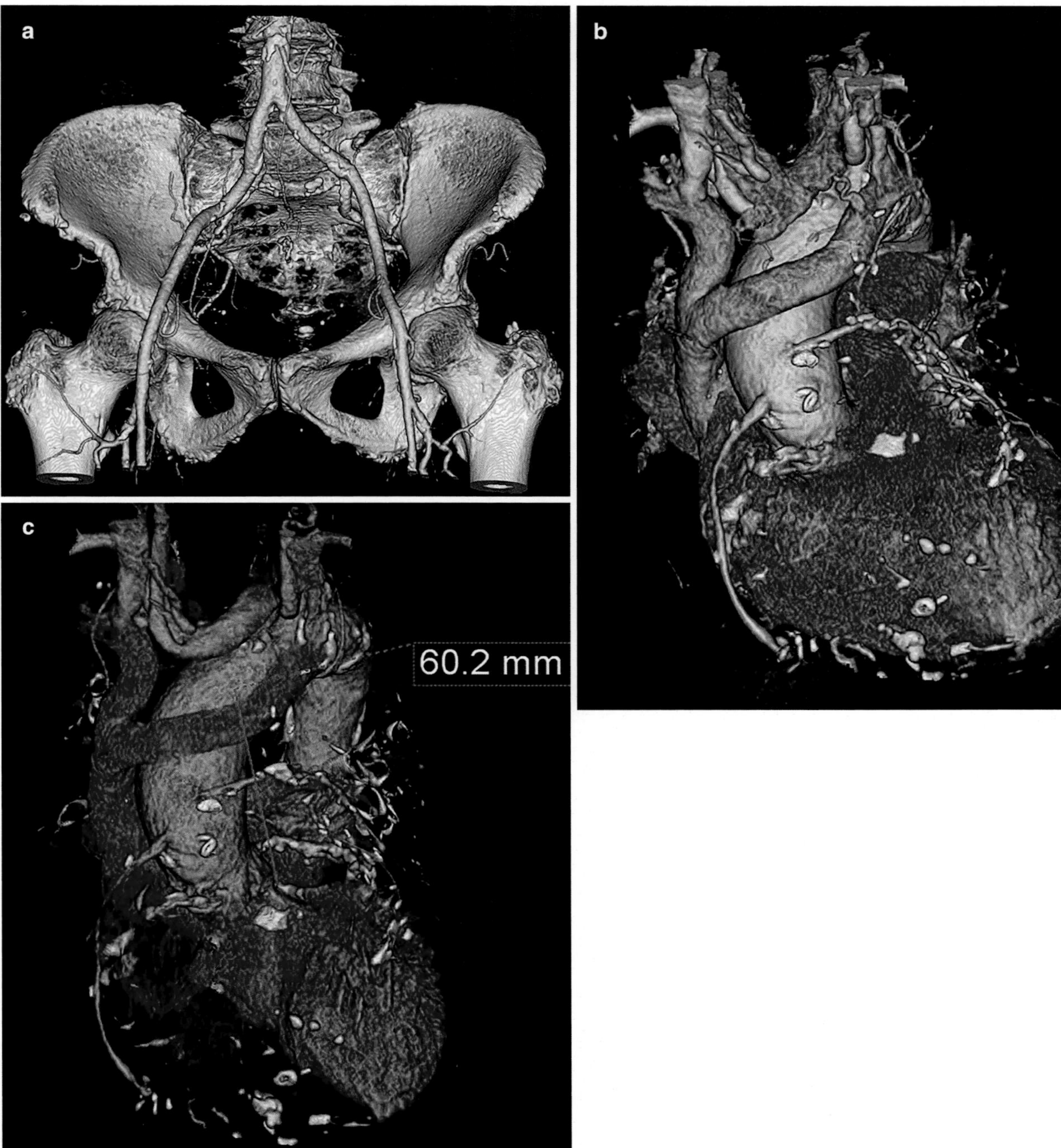

Fig. 15.11 Structural overlay of peripheral access sites. MDCT volumetric acquisition provides VRT images which help in better anatomical understanding of the overlying structures. For e.g. (**a**). Overlay of Iliofemoral arteries against the backdrop of pelvic bones helps in easy assessment of tortuosity. In another TAVI patient, an unfavorable iliofemoral access was noted and hence alternate vascular access sites were assessed (**b**, **c**). VRT images provide visual depiction of prior bypass graft procedure and presence of left brachiocephalic vein overlying the ascending aorta (**b**, **c**). If a transaortic access is contemplated relevant knowledge of anatomy and their relations to each other help in proper planning. *VRT* volume rendered technique

Conclusion

The integration of computed tomography into transcatheter aortic valve replacement planning and guidance has seen rapid progression over the last 5 years. CT has gone from simply being a tool for the assessment of iliofemoral access to now being the non-invasive test of choice for pre-procedural annular sizing and transcatheter heart valve selection. With ongoing evolution of the transcatheter devices and the procedure, as well as the introduction of other transcatheter valvular solutions CT will almost certainly grow in its utilization and help us further understand how to appropriately size transcatheter devices and hopefully reduce procedural related complications.

References

1. Go AS, Mozaffarian D, Roger VL, Benjamin EJ, Berry JD, Borden WB, et al. Heart disease and stroke statistics – 2013 update: a report from the American Heart Association. Circulation. 2013;127(1):e6–245. Epub 2012/12/15.
2. Thaden JJ, Nkomo VT, Enriquez-Sarano M. The global burden of aortic stenosis. Prog Cardiovasc Dis. 2014;56(6):565–71. Epub 2014/05/20.
3. Osnabrugge RL, Mylotte D, Head SJ, Van Mieghem NM, Nkomo VT, LeReun CM, et al. Aortic stenosis in the elderly: disease prevalence and number of candidates for transcatheter aortic valve replacement: a meta-analysis and modeling study. J Am Coll Cardiol. 2013;62(11):1002–12. Epub 2013/06/04.
4. Nkomo VT, Gardin JM, Skelton TN, Gottdiener JS, Scott CG, Enriquez-Sarano M. Burden of valvular heart diseases: a population-based study. Lancet. 2006;368(9540):1005–11. Epub 2006/09/19.
5. Fedak PW, Verma S, David TE, Leask RL, Weisel RD, Butany J. Clinical and pathophysiological implications of a bicuspid aortic valve. Circulation. 2002;106(8):900–4. Epub 2002/08/21.
6. Beppu S, Suzuki S, Matsuda H, Ohmori F, Nagata S, Miyatake K. Rapidity of progression of aortic stenosis in patients with congenital bicuspid aortic valves. Am J Cardiol. 1993;71(4):322–7. Epub 1993/02/01.
7. Pomerance A. Pathogenesis of aortic stenosis and its relation to age. Br Heart J. 1972;34(6):569–74. Epub 1972/06/01.
8. Mautner GC, Mautner SL, Cannon 3rd RO, Hunsberger SA, Roberts WC. Clinical factors useful in predicting aortic valve structure in patients >40 years of age with isolated valvular aortic stenosis. Am J Cardiol. 1993;72(2):194–8. Epub 1993/07/15.
9. Ross Jr J, Braunwald E. Aortic stenosis. Circulation. 1968;38(1 Suppl):61–7. Epub 1968/07/01.
10. Salinas P, Moreno R, Lopez-Sendon JL. Transcatheter aortic valve implantation: current status and future perspectives. World J Cardiol. 2011;3(6):177–85. Epub 2011/07/21.
11. Panchal HB, Ladia V, Desai S, Shah T, Ramu V. A meta-analysis of mortality and major adverse cardiovascular and cerebrovascular events following transcatheter aortic valve implantation versus surgical aortic valve replacement for severe aortic stenosis. Am J Cardiol. 2013;112(6):850–60. Epub 2013/06/13.
12. Cao C, Ang SC, Indraratna P, Manganas C, Bannon P, Black D, et al. Systematic review and meta-analysis of transcatheter aortic valve implantation versus surgical aortic valve replacement for severe aortic stenosis. Ann Cardiothorac Surg. 2013;2(1):10–23. Epub 2013/08/27.
13. Cribier A, Eltchaninoff H, Bash A, Borenstein N, Tron C, Bauer F, et al. Percutaneous transcatheter implantation of an aortic valve prosthesis for calcific aortic stenosis: first human case description. Circulation. 2002;106(24):3006–8. Epub 2002/12/11.
14. Leipsic J, Yang TH, Min JK. Computed tomographic imaging of transcatheter aortic valve replacement for prediction and prevention of procedural complications. Circ Cardiovasc Imaging. 2013;6(4):597–605. Epub 2013/07/19.
15. Achenbach S, Delgado V, Hausleiter J, Schoenhagen P, Min JK, Leipsic JA. SCCT expert consensus document on computed tomography imaging before transcatheter aortic valve implantation (TAVI)/transcatheter aortic valve replacement (TAVR). J Cardiovasc Comput Tomogr. 2012;6(6):366–80. Epub 2012/12/12.
16. Neragi-Miandoab S, Michler RE. A review of most relevant complications of transcatheter aortic valve implantation. ISRN Cardiol. 2013;2013:956252. Epub 2013/07/12.
17. Tops LF, Wood DA, Delgado V, Schuijf JD, Mayo JR, Pasupati S, et al. Noninvasive evaluation of the aortic root with multislice computed tomography implications for transcatheter aortic valve replacement. JACC Cardiovasc Imaging. 2008;1(3):321–30. Epub 2009/04/10.
18. Schultz CJ, Moelker A, Piazza N, Tzikas A, Otten A, Nuis RJ, et al. Three dimensional evaluation of the aortic annulus using multislice computer tomography: are manufacturer's guidelines for sizing for percutaneous aortic valve replacement helpful? Eur Heart J. 2010;31(7):849–56. Epub 2009/12/10.
19. Blanke P, Russe M, Leipsic J, Reinohl J, Ebersberger U, Suranyi P, et al. Conformational pulsatile changes of the aortic annulus: impact on prosthesis sizing by computed tomography for transcatheter aortic valve replacement. JACC Cardiovasc Interv. 2012;5(9):984–94. Epub 2012/09/22.
20. Ng AC, Yiu KH, Ewe SH, van der Kley F, Bertini M, de Weger A, et al. Influence of left ventricular geometry and function on aortic annular dimensions as assessed with multi-detector row computed tomography: implications for transcatheter aortic valve implantation. Eur Heart J. 2011;32(22):2806–13. Epub 2011/07/26.
21. Nakai H, Takeuchi M, Yoshitani H, Kaku K, Haruki N, Otsuji Y. Pitfalls of anatomical aortic valve area measurements using two-dimensional transoesophageal echocardiography and the potential of three-dimensional transoesophageal echocardiography. Eur J Echocardiogr. 2010;11(4):369–76. Epub 2009/12/22.
22. Bertaso AG, Wong DT, Liew GY, Cunnington MS, Richardson JD, Thomson VS, et al. Aortic annulus dimension assessment by computed tomography for transcatheter aortic valve implantation: differences between systole and diastole. Int J Cardiovasc Imaging. 2012;28(8):2091–8. Epub 2012/02/10.
23. Ng AC, Delgado V, van der Kley F, Shanks M, van de Veire NR, Bertini M, et al. Comparison of aortic root dimensions and geometries before and after transcatheter aortic valve implantation by 2- and 3-dimensional transesophageal echocardiography and multislice computed tomography. Circ Cardiovasc Imaging. 2010;3(1):94–102. Epub 2009/11/19.
24. Jilaihawi H, Kashif M, Fontana G, Furugen A, Shiota T, Friede G, et al. Cross-sectional computed tomographic assessment improves accuracy of aortic annular sizing for transcatheter aortic valve replacement and reduces the incidence of paravalvular aortic regurgitation. J Am Coll Cardiol. 2012;59(14):1275–86. Epub 2012/03/01.
25. Hamdan A, Guetta V, Konen E, Goitein O, Segev A, Raanani E, et al. Deformation dynamics and mechanical properties of the aortic annulus by 4-dimensional computed tomography: insights into the functional anatomy of the aortic valve complex and implications for transcatheter aortic valve therapy. J Am Coll Cardiol. 2012;59(2):119–27. Epub 2012/01/10.
26. Buellesfeld L, Stortecky S, Kalesan B, Gloekler S, Khattab AA, Nietlispach F, et al. Aortic root dimensions among patients with severe aortic stenosis undergoing transcatheter aortic valve replacement. JACC Cardiovasc Interv. 2013;6(1):72–83. Epub 2013/01/26.
27. Zhang R, Song Y, Zhou Y, Sun L. Comparison of aortic annulus diameter measurement between multi-detector computed tomography and echocardiography: a meta-analysis. PLoS One. 2013;8(3):e58729. Epub 2013/03/22.

28. Mizia-Stec K, Pysz P, Jasinski M, Adamczyk T, Drzewiecka-Gerber A, Chmiel A, et al. Preoperative quantification of aortic valve stenosis: comparison of 64-slice computed tomography with transesophageal and transthoracic echocardiography and size of implanted prosthesis. Int J Cardiovasc Imaging. 2012;28(2):343–52. Epub 2011/02/01.
29. Messika-Zeitoun D, Serfaty JM, Brochet E, Ducrocq G, Lepage L, Detaint D, et al. Multimodal assessment of the aortic annulus diameter: implications for transcatheter aortic valve implantation. J Am Coll Cardiol. 2010;55(3):186–94. Epub 2010/02/02.
30. Koos R, Altiok E, Mahnken AH, Neizel M, Dohmen G, Marx N, et al. Evaluation of aortic root for definition of prosthesis size by magnetic resonance imaging and cardiac computed tomography: implications for transcatheter aortic valve implantation. Int J Cardiol. 2012;158(3):353–8. Epub 2011/02/15.
31. Willson AB, Webb JG, Labounty TM, Achenbach S, Moss R, Wheeler M, et al. 3-dimensional aortic annular assessment by multidetector computed tomography predicts moderate or severe paravalvular regurgitation after transcatheter aortic valve replacement: a multicenter retrospective analysis. J Am Coll Cardiol. 2012;59(14):1287–94. Epub 2012/03/01.
32. Altiok E, Koos R, Schroder J, Brehmer K, Hamada S, Becker M, et al. Comparison of two-dimensional and three-dimensional imaging techniques for measurement of aortic annulus diameters before transcatheter aortic valve implantation. Heart (Br Cardiac Soc). 2011;97(19):1578–84. Epub 2011/06/28.
33. Husser O, Rauch S, Endemann DH, Resch M, Nunez J, Bodi V, et al. Impact of three-dimensional transesophageal echocardiography on prosthesis sizing for transcatheter aortic valve implantation. Catheter Cardiovasc Interv. 2012;80(6):956–63. Epub 2012/03/16.
34. Binder RK, Webb JG, Willson AB, Urena M, Hansson NC, Norgaard BL, et al. The impact of integration of a multidetector computed tomography annulus area sizing algorithm on outcomes of transcatheter aortic valve replacement: a prospective, multicenter, controlled trial. J Am Coll Cardiol. 2013;62(5):431–8. Epub 2013/05/21.
35. Adams DH, Popma JJ, Reardon MJ, Yakubov SJ, Coselli JS, Deeb GM, et al. Transcatheter aortic-valve replacement with a self-expanding prosthesis. N Engl J Med. 2014;370(19):1790–8. Epub 2014/04/01.
36. Lehmkuhl L, Foldyna B, Von Aspern K, Lucke C, Grothoff M, Nitzsche S, et al. Inter-individual variance and cardiac cycle dependency of aortic root dimensions and shape as assessed by ECG-gated multi-slice computed tomography in patients with severe aortic stenosis prior to transcatheter aortic valve implantation: is it crucial for correct sizing? Int J Cardiovasc Imaging. 2013;29(3):693–703. Epub 2012/09/19.
37. de Heer LM, Budde RP, van Prehn J, Mali WP, Bartels LW, Stella PR, et al. Pulsatile distention of the nondiseased and stenotic aortic valve annulus: analysis with electrocardiogram-gated computed tomography. Ann Thorac Surg. 2012;93(2):516–22. Epub 2011/12/06.
38. von Aspern K, Foldyna B, Etz CD, Hoyer A, Girrbach F, Holzhey D, et al. Effective diameter of the aortic annulus prior to transcatheter aortic valve implantation: influence of area-based versus perimeter-based calculation. Int J Cardiovasc Imaging. 2015;31: 163–9. Epub 2014/08/29.
39. Blanke P, Willson AB, Webb JG, Achenbach S, Piazza N, Min JK, et al. Oversizing in transcatheter aortic valve replacement, a commonly used term but a poorly understood one: dependency on definition and geometrical measurements. J Cardiovasc Comput Tomogr. 2014;8(1):67–76. Epub 2014/03/04.
40. Kasel AM, Cassese S, Bleiziffer S, Amaki M, Hahn RT, Kastrati A, et al. Standardized imaging for aortic annular sizing: implications for transcatheter valve selection. JACC Cardiovasc Imaging. 2013;6(2):249–62. Epub 2013/03/16.
41. Kurra V, Kapadia SR, Tuzcu EM, Halliburton SS, Svensson L, Roselli EE, et al. Pre-procedural imaging of aortic root orientation and dimensions: comparison between X-ray angiographic planar imaging and 3-dimensional multidetector row computed tomography. JACC Cardiovasc Interv. 2010;3(1):105–13. Epub 2010/02/05.
42. Gurvitch R, Wood DA, Leipsic J, Tay E, Johnson M, Ye J, et al. Multislice computed tomography for prediction of optimal angiographic deployment projections during transcatheter aortic valve implantation. JACC Cardiovasc Interv. 2010;3(11):1157–65. Epub 2010/11/23.
43. Leipsic J, Gurvitch R, Labounty TM, Min JK, Wood D, Johnson M, et al. Multidetector computed tomography in transcatheter aortic valve implantation. JACC Cardiovasc Imaging. 2011;4(4):416–29. Epub 2011/04/16.
44. Binder RK, Leipsic J, Wood D, Moore T, Toggweiler S, Willson A, et al. Prediction of optimal deployment projection for transcatheter aortic valve replacement: angiographic 3-dimensional reconstruction of the aortic root versus multidetector computed tomography. Circ Cardiovasc Interv. 2012;5(2):247–52. Epub 2012/03/23.
45. Barbanti M, Yang TH, Rodes Cabau J, Tamburino C, Wood DA, Jilaihawi H, et al. Anatomical and procedural features associated with aortic root rupture during balloon-expandable transcatheter aortic valve replacement. Circulation. 2013;128(3):244–53. Epub 2013/06/12.
46. Feuchtner G, Plank F, Bartel T, Bonaros N, Müller S, Leipsic J, et al. TCT-836 prediction of paravalvular leaks after transcatheter aortic valve implantation by valvular or annular calcification? J Am Coll Cardiol. 2012;60(17_S).
47. Kodali SK, Williams MR, Smith CR, Svensson LG, Webb JG, Makkar RR, et al. Two-year outcomes after transcatheter or surgical aortic-valve replacement. N Engl J Med. 2012;366(18):1686–95. Epub 2012/03/27.
48. Haensig M, Lehmkuhl L, Rastan AJ, Kempfert J, Mukherjee C, Gutberlet M, et al. Aortic valve calcium scoring is a predictor of significant paravalvular aortic insufficiency in transapical-aortic valve implantation. Eur J Cardiothorac Surg. 2012;41(6):1234–40. discussion 40-1. Epub 2012/01/14.
49. John D, Buellesfeld L, Yuecel S, Mueller R, Latsios G, Beucher H, et al. Correlation of Device landing zone calcification and acute procedural success in patients undergoing transcatheter aortic valve implantations with the self-expanding CoreValve prosthesis. JACC Cardiovasc Interv. 2010;3(2):233–43. Epub 2010/02/23.
50. Koos R, Mahnken AH, Dohmen G, Brehmer K, Gunther RW, Autschbach R, et al. Association of aortic valve calcification severity with the degree of aortic regurgitation after transcatheter aortic valve implantation. Int J Cardiol. 2011;150(2):142–5. Epub 2010/03/31.
51. Holmes Jr DR, Mack MJ, Kaul S, Agnihotri A, Alexander KP, Bailey SR, et al. 2012 ACCF/AATS/SCAI/STS expert consensus document on transcatheter aortic valve replacement: developed in collaboration with the American Heart Association, American Society of Echocardiography, European Association for Cardio-Thoracic Surgery, Heart Failure Society of America, Mended Hearts, Society of Cardiovascular Anesthesiologists, Society of Cardiovascular Computed Tomography, and Society for Cardiovascular Magnetic Resonance. J Thorac Cardiovasc Surg. 2012;144(3):e29–84. Epub 2012/08/18.
52. Ribeiro HB, Nombela-Franco L, Urena M, Mok M, Pasian S, Doyle D, et al. Coronary obstruction following transcatheter aortic valve implantation: a systematic review. JACC Cardiovasc Interv. 2013; 6(5):452–61. Epub 2013/04/23.
53. Ribeiro HB, Webb JG, Makkar RR, Cohen MG, Kapadia SR, Kodali S, et al. Predictive factors, management, and clinical outcomes of coronary obstruction following transcatheter aortic valve

implantation: insights from a large multicenter registry. J Am Coll Cardiol. 2013;62(17):1552–62. Epub 2013/08/21.

54. Khatri PJ, Webb JG, Rodes-Cabau J, Fremes SE, Ruel M, Lau K, et al. Adverse effects associated with transcatheter aortic valve implantation: a meta-analysis of contemporary studies. Ann Intern Med. 2013;158(1):35–46. Epub 2013/01/02.
55. Genereux P, Webb JG, Svensson LG, Kodali SK, Satler LF, Fearon WF, et al. Vascular complications after transcatheter aortic valve replacement: insights from the PARTNER (Placement of AoRTic TraNscathetER Valve) trial. J Am Coll Cardiol. 2012;60(12):1043–52. Epub 2012/08/14.
56. Genereux P, Head SJ, Van Mieghem NM, Kodali S, Kirtane AJ, Xu K, et al. Clinical outcomes after transcatheter aortic valve replacement using valve academic research consortium definitions: a weighted meta-analysis of 3,519 patients from 16 studies. J Am Coll Cardiol. 2012;59(25):2317–26. Epub 2012/04/17.
57. Mwipatayi BP, Picardo A, Masilonyane-Jones TV, Larbalestier R, Thomas S, Turner J, et al. Incidence and prognosis of vascular complications after transcatheter aortic valve implantation. J Vasc Surg. 2013;58(4):1028–36.e1. Epub 2013/09/03.
58. Hayashida K, Lefevre T, Chevalier B, Hovasse T, Romano M, Garot P, et al. Transfemoral aortic valve implantation new criteria to predict vascular complications. JACC Cardiovasc Interv. 2011; 4(8):851–8. Epub 2011/08/20.
59. Lange R, Bleiziffer S, Piazza N, Mazzitelli D, Hutter A, Tassani-Prell P, et al. Incidence and treatment of procedural cardiovascular complications associated with trans-arterial and trans-apical interventional aortic valve implantation in 412 consecutive patients. Eur J Cardiothorac Surg. 2011;40(5):1105–13. Epub 2011/04/26.
60. Leon MB, Piazza N, Nikolsky E, Blackstone EH, Cutlip DE, Kappetein AP, et al. Standardized endpoint definitions for Transcatheter Aortic Valve Implantation clinical trials: a consensus report from the Valve Academic Research Consortium. J Am Coll Cardiol. 2011;57(3):253–69. Epub 2011/01/11.
61. Kappetein AP, Head SJ, Genereux P, Piazza N, van Mieghem NM, Blackstone EH, et al. Updated standardized endpoint definitions for transcatheter aortic valve implantation: the Valve Academic Research Consortium-2 consensus document. J Am Coll Cardiol. 2012;60(15):1438–54. Epub 2012/10/06.
62. Kurra V, Schoenhagen P, Roselli EE, Kapadia SR, Tuzcu EM, Greenberg R, et al. Prevalence of significant peripheral artery disease in patients evaluated for percutaneous aortic valve insertion: preprocedural assessment with multidetector computed tomography. J Thorac Cardiovasc Surg. 2009;137(5):1258–64. Epub 2009/04/22.
63. Krishnaswamy A, Parashar A, Agarwal S, Modi DK, Poddar KL, Svensson LG, et al. Predicting vascular complications during transfemoral transcatheter aortic valve replacement using computed tomography: a novel area-based index. Catheter Cardiovasc Interv. 2014;84(5):844–51. Epub 2014/03/25.
64. Eltchaninoff H, Kerkeni M, Zajarias A, Tron C, Godin M, Sanchez Giron C, et al. Aorto-iliac angiography as a screening tool in selecting patients for transfemoral aortic valve implantation with the Edwards SAPIEN bioprosthesis. EuroIntervention. 2009;5(4):438–42. Epub 2009/09/17.
65. Reinthaler M, Aggarwal SK, De Palma R, Landmesser U, Froehlich G, Yap J, et al. Predictors of clinical outcome in transfemoral TAVI: Circumferential iliofemoral calcifications and manufacturer-derived recommendations. Anadolu kardiyoloji dergisi: AKD Anatol J Cardiol. 2015;15:297–305. Epub 2014/11/22.
66. Vavuranakis M, Kariori M, Voudris V, Kalogeras K, Vrachatis D, Aznaouridis C, et al. Predictive factors of vascular complications after transcatheter aortic valve implantation in patients treated with a default percutaneous strategy. Cardiovasc Ther. 2013;31(5):e46–54. Epub 2013/06/15.
67. Toggweiler S, Gurvitch R, Leipsic J, Wood DA, Willson AB, Binder RK, et al. Percutaneous aortic valve replacement: vascular outcomes with a fully percutaneous procedure. J Am Coll Cardiol. 2012;59(2):113–8. Epub 2012/01/10.
68. Chiam PT, Koh AS, Ewe SH, Sin YK, Chao VT, Ng CK, et al. Iliofemoral anatomy among Asians: implications for transcatheter aortic valve implantation. Int J Cardiol. 2013;167(4):1373–9. Epub 2012/04/24.

Assessment of Cardiac and Thoracic Masses

16

Jabi E. Shriki, Patrick M. Colletti, and Suresh Maximin

Abstract

Cardiac masses are uncommonly encountered, but can pose a perplexing diagnostic dilemma when present. Familiarity with cross-sectional imaging of the heart can provide a number of tools to enable diagnosis. In this chapter, we discuss the varied appearances of cardiac masses. Thrombi tend to occur in characteristic locations include the left atrial appendage and left ventricular apex. Benign neoplastic masses, tend to be pedunculated and have narrow attachments to the myocardial walls. For example, atrial myxomas tend to have narrow attachments at the left atrial side of the interatrial septum. Malignant neoplastic masses tend to grow in an infiltrative pattern with broad attachments to the myocardium.

Keywords

Myocardial masses • Cardiac mass • Thrombus • Myxoma • Angiosarcoma • Cardiac metastases

Overview

Excellent spatial and contrast resolution make cardiovascular computed tomographic angiography (CCTA) an ideal method for the detection and evaluation of cardiac masses and masses adjacent to the heart. Suspended respiration and cardiac gating techniques employed with CCTA enhance delineation of planes between masses and normal structures. While many cardiac masses are well demonstrated with non-gated CT, the ability to freeze cardiac motion enables clearer evaluation of tissue attenuation and enhancement characteristics of normal myocardium and of masses. Two approaches to cardiac gating may be applied: prospective ECG triggering and retrospective ECG gating [1].

Pre-contrast CT imaging may help to identify some features, such as calcifications, which appear as foci of punctuate or coarse hyperattenuation, typically in the range of 130 Hounsfield units (HU), and hemorrhage, which may have a more modest and ill-defined hyperattenuation relative to normal myocardium. CT without contrast is the imaging modality of choice for demonstrating calcification. Demonstration of low attenuation prior to contrast administration may be helpful

The amount of iodinated contrast agent required for satisfactory CT evaluation of cardiac masses depends on patient mass, with 0.5–1.0 g of iodine per kilogram body mass as the usual dose [2]. Most clinically used contrast agents have low osmolality, with concentrations of 300–400 mg iodine/ml. Typically, 100 ml of contrast agent is administered at 4–5 ml/s via a programmable injector system. This is followed by a bolus flush of 50 ml of normal saline [3].

Timing CT image acquisition to the arrival of the contrast bolus in the left atrium or left ventricle is typically

J.E. Shriki, MD (✉)
Department of Radiology, Puget VA Health System, University of Washington, 1660 S. Columbian Way, Seattle, WA 98101, USA
e-mail: shriki@uw.edu

P.M. Colletti, MD
Department of Radiology, University of Southern California, Los Angeles, CA, USA

S. Maximin, MD
Department of Radiology, University of Washington, Seattle, WA, USA

M.J. Budoff, J.S. Shinbane (eds.), *Cardiac CT Imaging: Diagnosis of Cardiovascular Disease*,
DOI 10.1007/978-3-319-28219-0_16

identical to the timing used for coronary artery CT examinations [4]. Optimal left atrial appendage enhancement may, however, be somewhat difficult, since the left atrial appendage may opacify somewhat more slowly or heterogeneously. In addition, there may be considerable variability in circulation time from patient to patient, particularly in patients with cardiac tumors or thrombi. The time between intravenous contrast injection and appearance of contrast in the aorta can be determined using a small volume test contrast agent bolus of 20 ml and rapid, repeated imaging of a single trans-aortic plane [5]. Alternatively, with bolus tracking, a Hounsfield unit (HU) threshold may be set such that the volume acquisition is triggered to begin once a certain HU value is detected in the ascending aorta. A uniform, programmed injection requires 10–25 s for delivery of intravenous contrast agent and up to 50 additional seconds for the saline flush. One potential pitfall in employing automatic bolus detection in cardiac masses is that it is possible to inadvertently place the bolus detection region of interest (ROI) within a chamber or a vessel which contains internal thrombus or tumor. Such an error may result in failure to detect the bolus as shown in Fig. 16.1.

Opacification of the right heart with contrast may be more challenging. Without appropriate acquisition timing for right heart visualization, there may be insufficient contrast for delineation of right atrial and right ventricular endocardial borders. Excessive contrast within the right heart may result in streaking and obscuration of subtle masses. Even when the right heart is well opacified, there is frequently swirling of contrast with non-opacified blood arriving from the inferior vena cava. The mixture of opacified and non-opacified blood can make delineation of masses in the right heart difficult. Optimal timing and technique for right heart examination usually differs from that used for routine CCTA. In most patients, optimal right ventricular opacification is achieved by placing the ROI for bolus tracking in the main pulmonary artery.

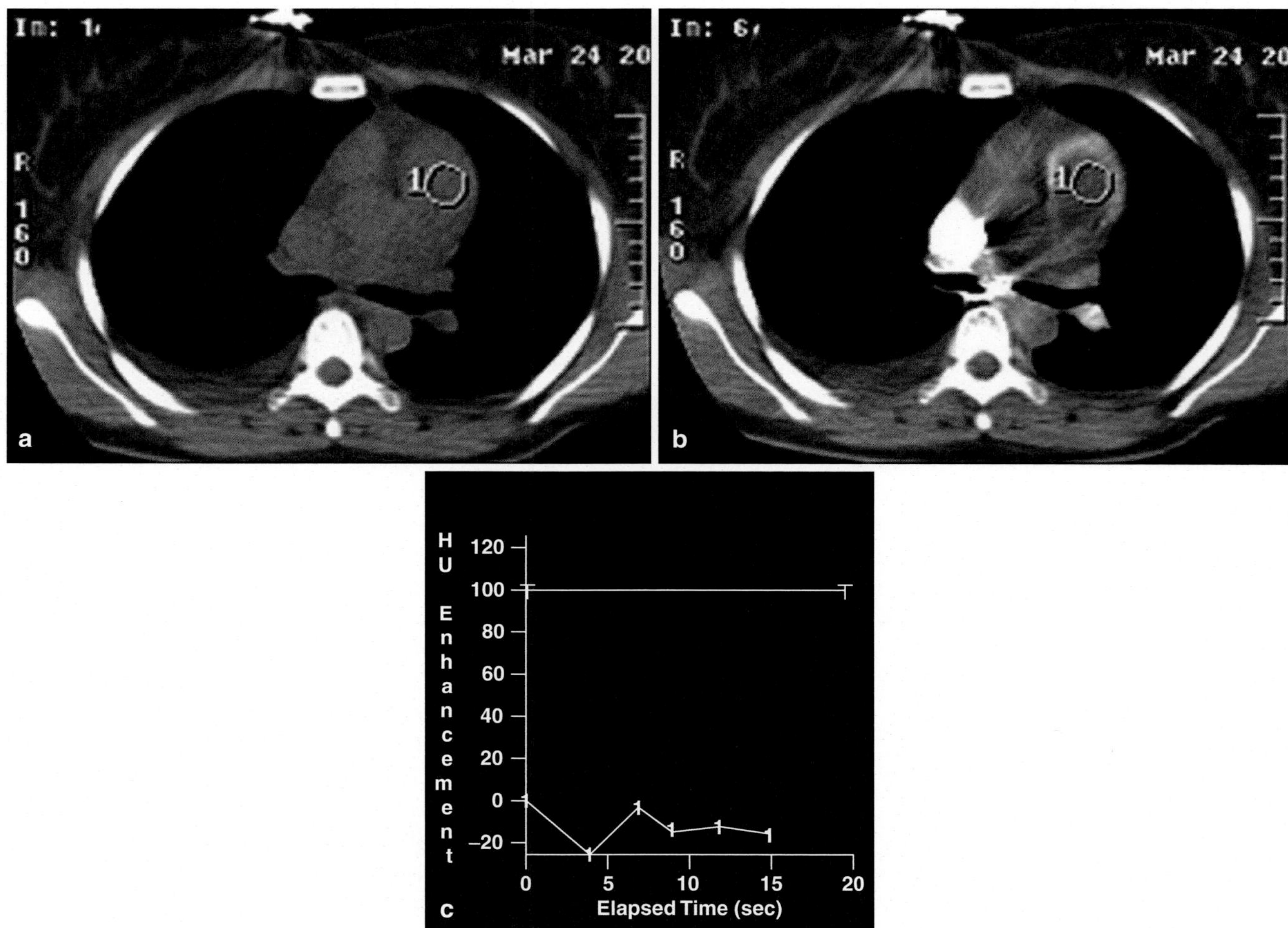

Fig. 16.1 (**a**, **b**) Pitfall of automated bolus detection. Automatic bolus detection fails due to tumor replacing the blood pool in the selected region-of-interest in the main pulmonary artery

Right ventricular delineation in congenital heart disease with transposition or other abnormal great vessel relationships requires some a priori knowledge of the anatomy and relevant surgical history to select the correct region for timing prescription. When opacification of multiple chambers is needed, more complex injection protocols can be utilized with multiphasic contrast administration, including injection of mixtures of saline and contrast [6].

One advantage cardiac magnetic resonance imaging (CMR) holds over cardiac CT for cardiac masses is the ability to obtain excellent contrast for both the right ventricle and left ventricle in the same examination due to the ability to image the heart in multiple phases of contrast administration, with no radiation dose. Venous or equilibrium phase imaging on CMR can help to homogeneously opacify the right heart chambers.

Clinical [7–19] and imaging [20–28] features of cardiac masses are summarized in Tables 16.1, 16.2, 16.3, and 16.4.

Interpreting Cardiac Masses: Key Descriptors

Location

Lesion location relative to the specific, involved chambers should be noted and may provide a hint as to the nature of a particular mass. Masses related to the heart itself which are cardiac in origin have a unique differential diagnosis. Masses immediately adjacent to the heart and intimately involving the pericardium should be described as pericardial (Fig. 16.2). Masses which are external to the heart should be described as paracardial (within the mediastinum, adjacent to the heart). For lesions within the mediastinum, a separate set of diagnostic possibilities should be included in the differential. A full discussion of mediastinal masses, however, is beyond the scope of this text. Although some tumors may violate planes and make identification of the organ of origin difficult, in most cases, cardiac masses, pericardial masses, and mediastinal masses can be separated.

Table 16.1 Benign cardiac neoplasms

	Location	Features
Myxoma (40 % of all benign tumors) (Fig. 16.16)	LA septum 75 %; RA 18 %; ventricles 7 %; multiple 5 %	10 % calcified; frequent systemic emboli; may protrude through mitral valve during diastole
Fibroelastoma Lipoma	Arise from valves; project into aorta or MPA Varies	Derived from endocardium; may be multiple; often an incidental finding at surgery
		Encapsulated adipose tissue (fat attenuation); asymptomatic; negative CT density; 25 % are multiple; consider tuberous sclerosis; should not be confused with fat in paracardiac folds
Lipomatous hypertrophy	Atrial septum; protrudes into RA	Fat attenuation
Fibroma	Myocardium	Well delineated, calcified; enhance minimally
Hemangioma	Myocardium	Calcifications; delayed enhancement
Lymphangioma	Myocardium	Diffuse proliferation; minimally enhancing
Paraganglioma, dysembryoma, pheochromocytoma	Paracardiac; AV groove	Sympathetic plexus; hyper-enhancing; correlate with urinary catecholamines; alpha-and beta-blockade for surgery
Teratoma	Pericardial; attach to the aorta or PA roots	Multi-cystic; frequently calcify; moderate enhancement

Table 16.2 Cystic cardiac masses

	Location	Features
Pleuro-pericardial cyst	75 % in right paracardiac angle	Asymptomatic (avascular/calcified); unilocular, sharply marginated, 20–40 HU; may communicate with pericardium; change shape with body position
Echinococcal cysts	Myocardial or pericardial	(Avascular/calcific rim); nearly always also in liver, lung, eyes, brain
Tuberculoma	Myocardial or pericardial	Calcified; constrictive pericarditis
Hematoma	Posterior recesses at the aortic root or left atrium	Acutely hyper-dense; may calcify; traumatic or post-surgical
Thrombosed coronary aneurysm	Course of coronary arteries	Calcified rim; thrombus

Table 16.3 Malignant cardiac tumors

	Location	Features
Metastasis (20×as common as primary tumor) (Fig. 16.2)	Pericardial; intravascular; intra-myocardial	Seen in 10 % of end-stage cancers; lung (36 %), breast (7 %), esophagus (6 %); lymphoma, melanoma, Kaposi's sarcoma, leukemia (20 %); modes of dissemination: direct or lymphatic; hematogenous; direct venous extension (pulmonary veins or inferior vena cava)
Lung, breast, melanoma, sarcoma, leukemia, thyroid, kidney	Pericardial; direct or lymphatic; hematogenous; direct venous extension	Lung cancer may extend to the left atrium along the pulmonary veins
Renal, urothelial, hepatocellular, adrenal, retroperitoneal sarcoma	Extend up the inferior vena cava to the right atrium	Enhancing intravascular mass; primary tumor identified
Lymphoma	Pericardium; myocardium; commonly basal in location	May infiltrate epicardial fat; 50 % associated with HIV
Angiosarcoma (Fig. 16.1)	Pericardium; RV, RA, myocardium	Angiosarcoma of the pericardium or right ventricle is most common; poor prognosis; distribution is similar to lymphoma
Osteosarcoma	RA, RV	Ossification
Rhabdomyosarcoma, fibrosarcoma	Myocardium	Most common primary cardiac malignancy in infants and children
		Always involves the myocardium; pericardial involvement is typically in the form of nodular masses rather than sheet-like spread
Mesothelioma	Pericardium	Intra-pericardial mass; effusions; constrictive physiology

Table 16.4 Other cardiac masses

	Location	Features
Endo-myocardial fibrosis	Pericardium; myocardium	Thickened pericardium; thickened myocardium with patchy enhancement restrictive and constrictive physiology
Erdheim-Chester disease	Pericardium; myocardium	Thickened pericardium; thickened (non-langherans fibrosis) myocardium with patchy enhancement restrictive and constrictive physiology
RA thrombus (Fig. 16.12)	Right atrium	Associated with indwelling catheters and devices
RV thrombus	Right ventricle	Associated with severe coagulopathy; dilated cardiomyopathy
LA thrombus (Fig. 16.11)	Left atrium	Seen in atrial fibrillation and mitral stenosis; attached to posterior or superior atrial wall; may be calcified
LV thrombus (Fig. 16.8)	Left ventricle	Common complication of myocardial infarction (20–40 % of anterior MIs); contiguous to akinetic myocardium; most common at the apex
Vegetations	Valves; catheters	EKG-triggered cine views of valves helpful

Chamber Involvement

The chamber of origin and location within the chamber should be noted. For example, a mass in the left atrium attached along the interatrial septum has a higher chance of being an atrial myxoma. A mass in the left atrial appendage has a higher probability of being a thrombus. Some authors have suggested that, on imaging, metastases are more common in the right heart.

However, this could be due to the earlier detection of right heart masses, since the wall of the right ventricle is thinner than the wall of the left ventricle. A mass in the left ventricle may be neoplastic, if it is felt to be arising from the wall. A mass at the apex of the left ventricle, which appears separate from the wall, has a higher probability of being a thrombus. Attention should be given to associated wall motion abnormalities or aneurysms. Severe metastatic involvement of the myocardial wall may result in a wall motion abnormality. However, a thrombus may present as a mass closely associated with a wall motion abnormality such as dyskinetic aneurysmal segment. Transiently, thromboemboli with a peripheral origin, such as deep vein thrombi, may be seen in the right atrium and right ventricle (Fig. 16.3), and are called "in transit thrombi". A mass which arises from the crista terminalis of the right atrium may be a prominent network of Chiari. Elastofibromas are

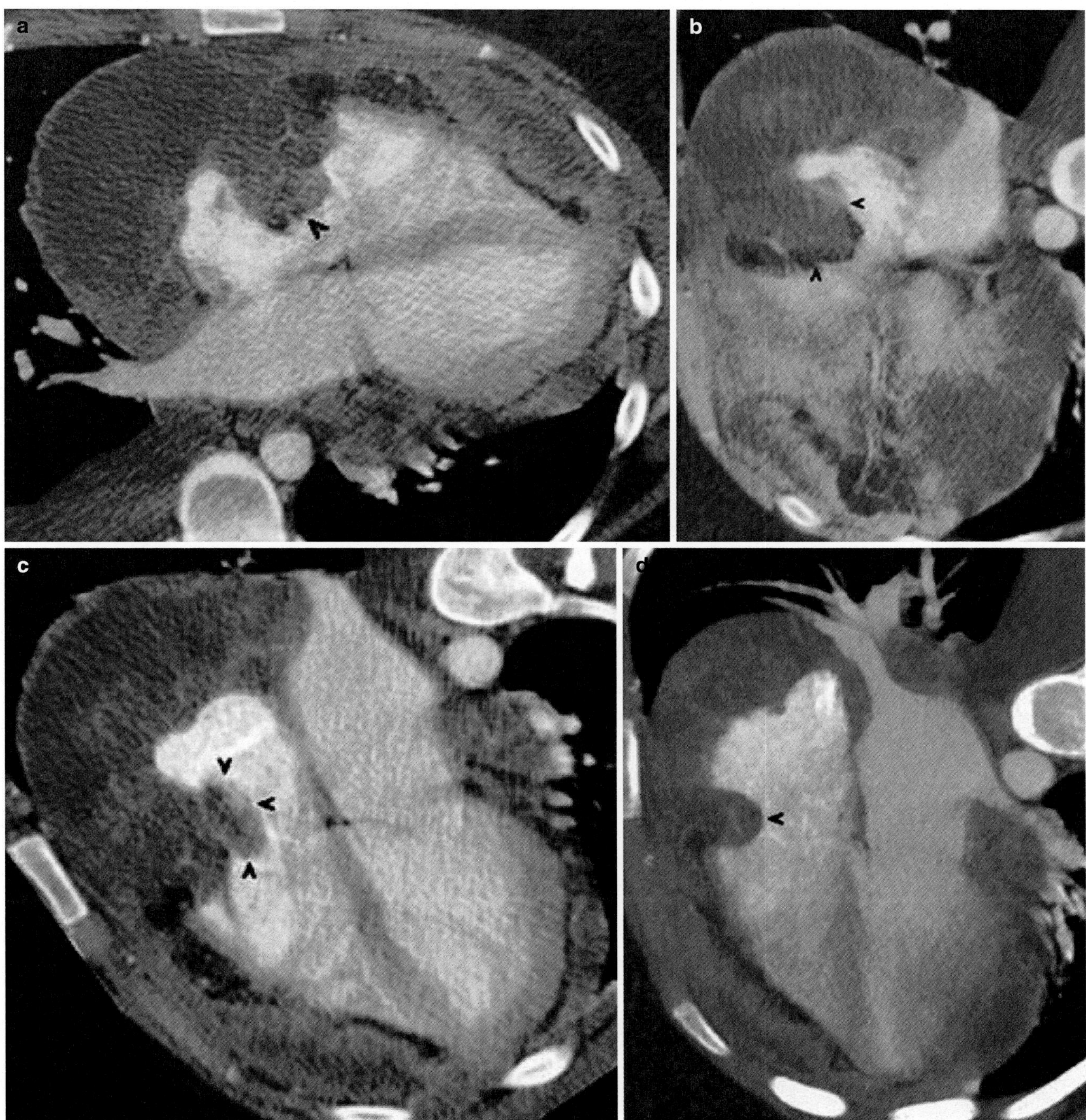

Fig. 16.2 A 22-year-old female with a primary pericardial primitive neuroectodermal tumor. Images obtained are obtained as part of a post-contrast non-gated CT scan of the chest. Transverse and oblique 4-chamber views are shown (**a–d**). In this case, the tumor was causing restriction of cardiac motion, and as a result artifacts due to cardiac motion are mild. There is heavy neoplastic infiltration of the atrioventricular groove with invasion of the right atrium and ventricle (*black arrowheads*)

common lesions which occur along the valve surfaces, but are usually small and not well-seen on CCTA. Valvular vegetations may rarely grow to a size where they may mimic a cardiac mass, although this diagnosis should be considered in some cases where a mass is closely related to a valve. An example of valvular pathology mimicking a cardiac mass is caseous mitral annular calcification, where an ovoid mass of caseous calcifications develops in close proximity to the mitral annulus as a result of liquefactive necrosis of mitral valvular calcifications (Fig. 16.4).

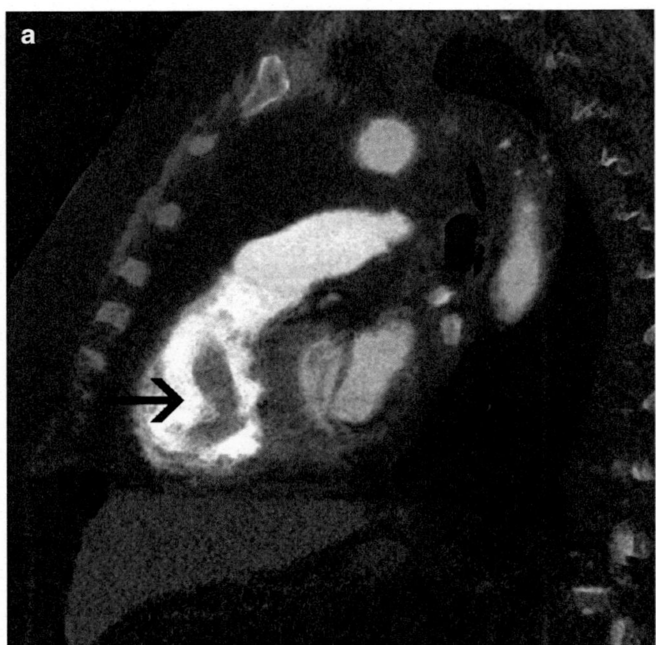

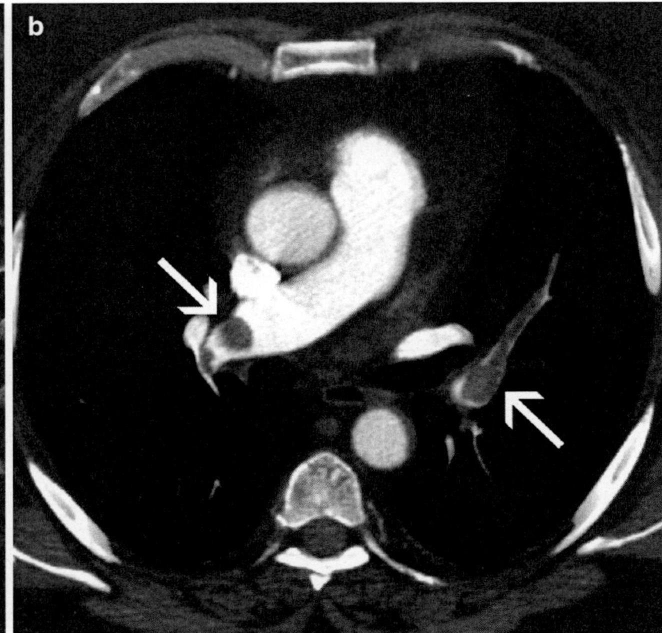

Fig. 16.3 A 44 year-old female with shortness of breath. The sagittal, minimum intensity projection (MinIP) view shows a vermiform, low-attenuation filling defect (*black arrow*, **a**), representing a thrombus in the right ventricle, which had likely migrated from the lower extremities or from the pelvic venous system. MinIP views are useful in demonstrating low attenuation structures, when surrounded by relatively high attenuation. A transverse view on the same study shows multiple, separate pulmonary emboli (*white arrows*, **b**)

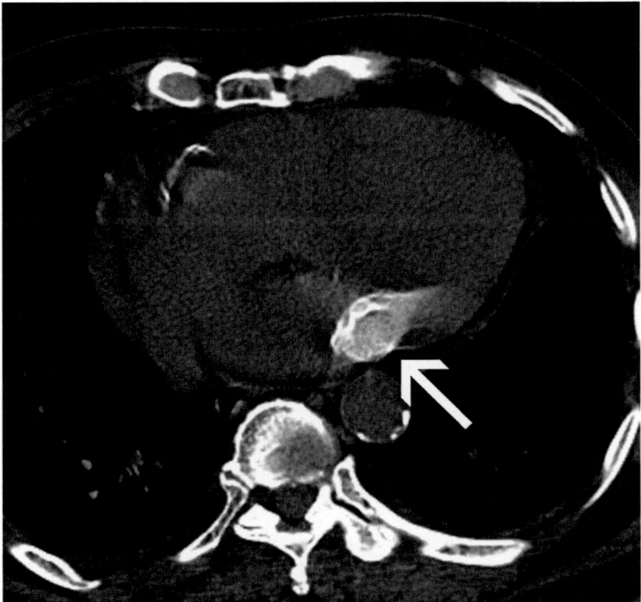

Fig. 16.4 An 81 year-old male with caseous mitral annular calcifications. A mass was seen near the region of the mitral annulus on echocardiography. CT was performed for further evaluation. A non-contrast, transverse image shows the classic morphology of caseous mitral annular calcifications, with central homogeneous hyperattenuation representing liquified calcifications and denser, peripheral shell-like calcifications (*white arrow*)

Lesion Morphology

Masses should also be described as intramural (within the myocardial wall) or intracameral (within the cardiac chamber). Metastatic and malignant primary tumors usually have a significant intramural component or a very broad-based attachment to the wall of the myocardium, whereas benign masses are more commonly pedunculated and intracameral, often having a narrow attachment. Masses arising from the myocardium tend to have more obtuse angles with the endocardial surface, whereas masses within chambers or with pedunculated attachments tend to have more acute angles with the endocardium. This rubric is commonly helpful in identifying pedunculated masses as benign. Thrombi which are adherent to the internal wall of the ventricle are, however, an important exception to this rule. Lesion shape is less helpful as both benign and malignant masses may be lobulated or appear round.

Attenuation

Attenuation can be characterized by Hounsfield unit (HU) measurement. Care should be taken to ensure that cardiac gating is adequate, as the presence of motion may alter or artifactually elevate measured attenuation. Attenuation values from −100 to −10 HU are generally associated with fatty masses such as intracardiac lipomas or lipomatous hyperplasia of the interatrial septum. Frequently, measurement of attenuation is not needed. For example, fatty intracardiac masses can be compared to the attenuation of subcutaneous or mediastinal fat. Cystic masses will tend to have attenuation values between −10 and 10 HU. Calcifications have an attenuation value of 130 HU or greater. Coarse calcifications may be seen in myxomas, although many other lesions may calcify, including some thrombi and many treated metastases. Attenuation relative to muscle or specifically myocardium is frequently used to describe lesions as hypoattenuating or hyperattenuating. Frequently, attenuation relative to the blood pool is also described, although it should be noted that patients with anemia may have depressed pre-contrast attenuation values within vascular structures.

Enhancement

Enhancement should be reported with respect to the degree of enhancement and to the phase at which enhancement is seen. Lesions which show no or minimal enhancement are more likely to be benign. This is true of thrombi, which usually show no enhancement. Myxomas usually show minimal or mild post-contrast enhancement, particularly in the arterial phase of contrast administration, when CCTA imaging is performed. Angiosarcomas, the most common malignant primary neoplasm of the heart, may have very avid enhancement, to the extent that the borders of these masses may be indistinguishable from contrast within the chamber of the heart. Other neoplastic lesions, including metastases, may show more modest enhancement.

Involvement of Other Vascular Structures

Numerous masses may invade the heart from the great vessels. Tumors of the upper abdomen may grow into the right atrium via the inferior vena cava (Fig. 16.5). Hepatocellular carcinoma, adrenocortical carcinoma, and renal cell carcinoma are among the most common tumors of the upper abdomen to invade into the right atrium. Bronchogenic carcinomas may invade into the heart through the pulmonary veins and present as a left atrial mass. Mediastinal tumors and bronchogenic carcinomas that involve the mediastinum may extend into the heart via the superior vena cava. Tumors of the mediastinum may grow directly into the heart with external myocardial invasion. Thrombi along catheters may track along venous structures, most commonly the superior vena cava.

Lesion Number

Multiple lesions are more likely to be due to metastatic disease or to multiple thrombi. Metastatic disease typically appears as multiple lesions in the myocardial wall in different locations. Multiple thrombi may be encountered as well, especially when masses are located in characteristic locations, such as the left atrial appendage or the left ventricular apex.

Commonly Encountered Masses

Although a complete discussion of all cardiac masses is beyond the scope of this chapter, familiarity with the most common causes of cardiac masses assists in arriving at the correct diagnosis.

Thrombi

Thrombi are the most common cause of intracardiac masses. On pre-contrast CT, thrombi may either present as hypoattenuating or hyperattenuating masses relative to blood pool (Figs. 16.6 and 16.7). Attenuation relative to blood pool is influenced by the patient's hematocrit, since more anemic patients will have relatively lower attenuation of blood pool. The degree of attenuation within a thrombus may also be dependent on thrombus age. Most thrombi will show no enhancement after administration of contrast. However, some chronic thrombi, described as being more organized, have been reported to have some peripheral enhancement after contrast administration [29]. This is most commonly seen in the setting of chronic thrombi adherent to the wall, and has been reported mostly on MRI. On CCTA, essentially no contrast enhancement will be shown within thrombi. In the case of small thrombi, Hounsfield units may be elevated after administration of contrast when comparison between pre- and post-contrast CCTA is made, although this is more likely related to pseudoenhancement, whereupon beam hardening effects cause false elevation of attenuation values due to adjacent hyperattenuating structures or contrast. Pseudoenhancement tends to occur in lesions less than 1 cm in size. On MRI, thrombi are most commonly dark on all sequences. Thrombi can also be recognized by the characteristic locations in which they occur, including at the left ventricular apex and in the left atrial appendage.

Ventricular thrombi can be recognized by their characteristic location, most commonly at the apex of the left ventricle (Fig. 16.8). Morphologically, they may either present as one or many ovoid structures within the chamber or may appear pedunculated (Fig. 16.9). Many thrombi may also

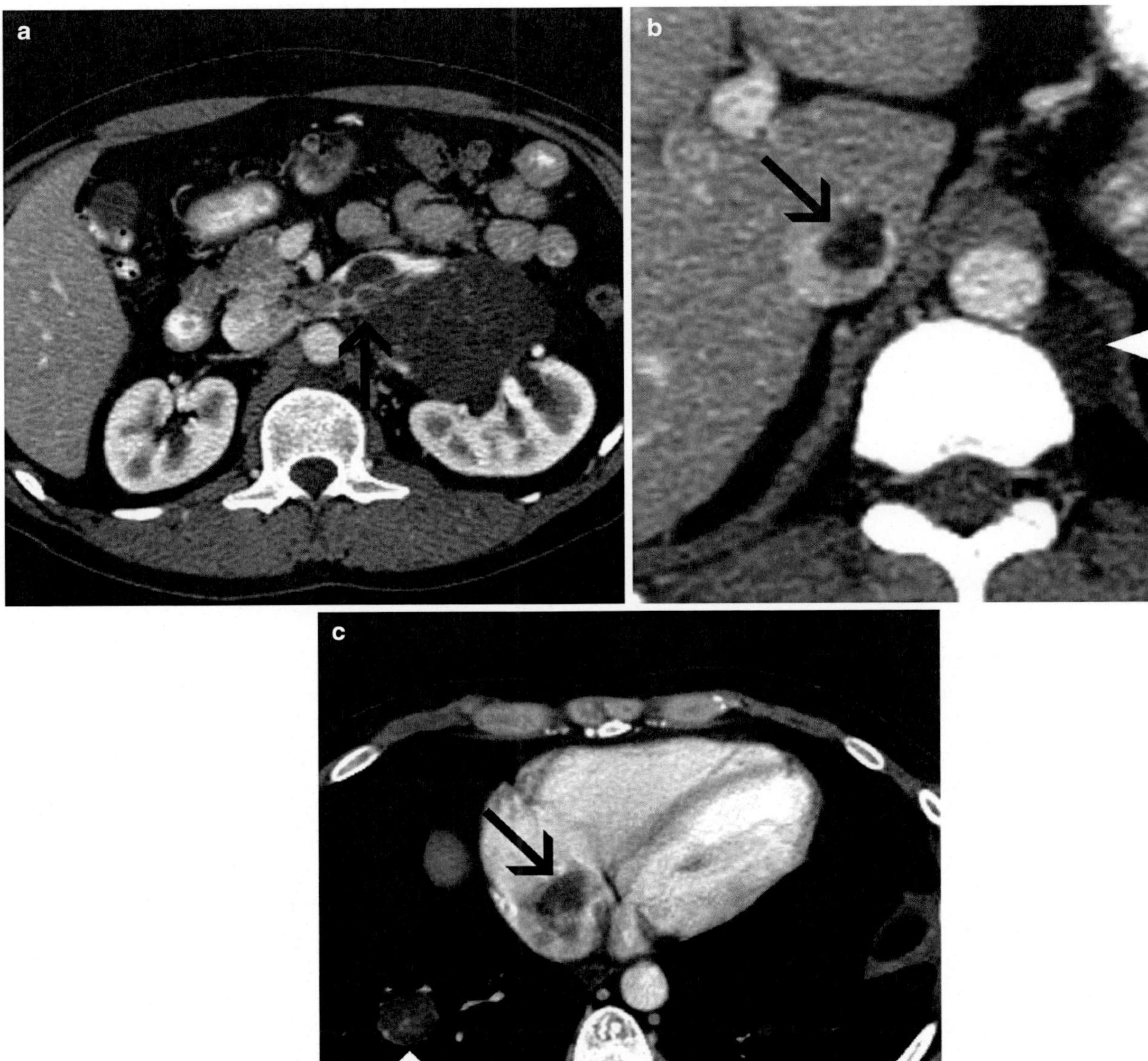

Fig. 16.5 A 24 year-old male with retroperitoneal malignant germ cell tumor. Post-contrast CT images are obtained of the abdomen in the portal venous phase and are shown from caudal (**a**) to cranial (**c**). There is extensive left periaortic lymphadenopathy, with invasion of tumor into the left renal vein (*black arrow* on **a**). There is also extension of tumor into the inferior vena cava and right atrium (*black arrows* on **b** and **c**, respectively). Note other sites of metastatic disease including a right lower lobe metastasis (*white arrow*, **c**) and a left retrocrural lymph node (*white arrowhead*, **b**). This tumor exhibits a common appearance of metastatic disease from germ cell tumor with low internal attenuation

be flat and layered against the endocardial surface of the left ventricular wall. Association with an underlying wall motion abnormality, such as an area of aneurysm formation or an area of infarction, is also an important hint to the correct diagnosis. Ventricular thrombi have been reported in up to one third of transmural infarctions [30], and are associated much more commonly with apical and anterior infarctions, in comparison to inferior infarctions [30, 31]. Visualization of multiple thrombi is not uncommon in the post-infarction setting.

Atrial thrombi can be very problematic to confidently diagnose, particularly when present in the left atrial appendage, where contrast opacification is often nonuniform. Patients at risk for atrial thrombi commonly have

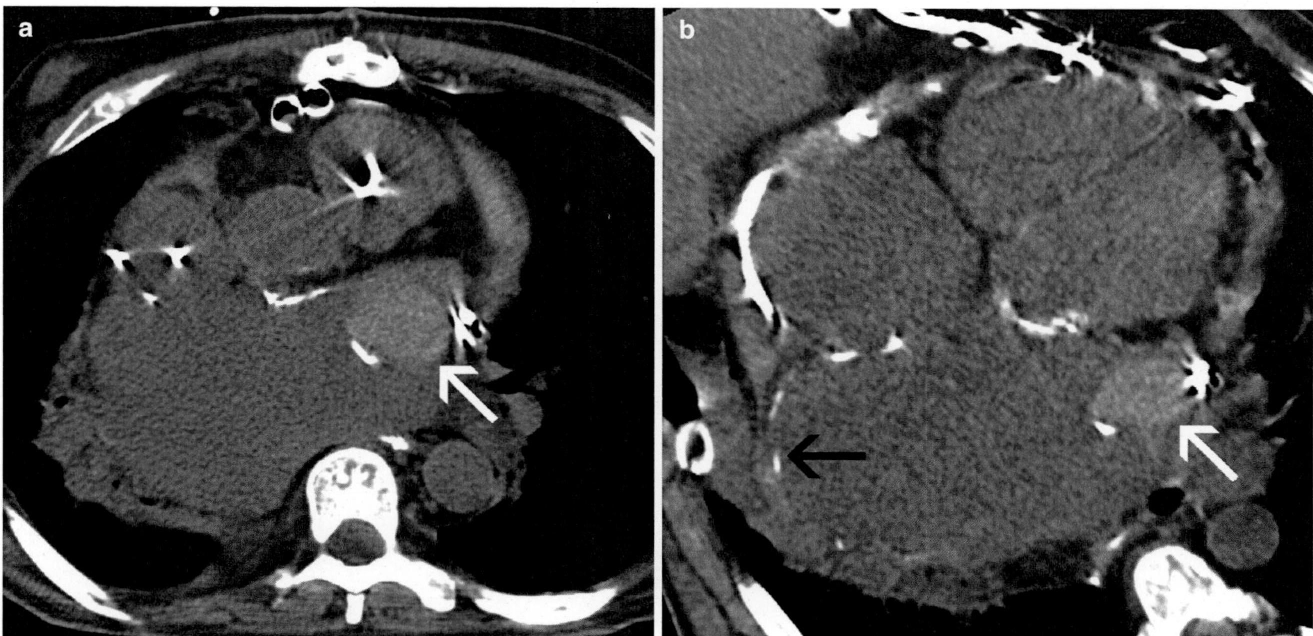

Fig. 16.6 A 56 year-old male with rheumatic heart disease and a hyperattenuating left atrial appendage thrombus. Oblique MPR views are shown from a non-contrast scan (**a**, **b**). A focal mass with hyperattenuation is present in the left atrial appendage, which was also seen on echocardiogram (not shown) and was consistent with an atrial thrombus (*white arrows*). Note the presence of atrial wall calcifications, which are encountered commonly in the setting of rheumatic heart disease. The left atrium is massively enlarged and forms the right heart border (**a**)

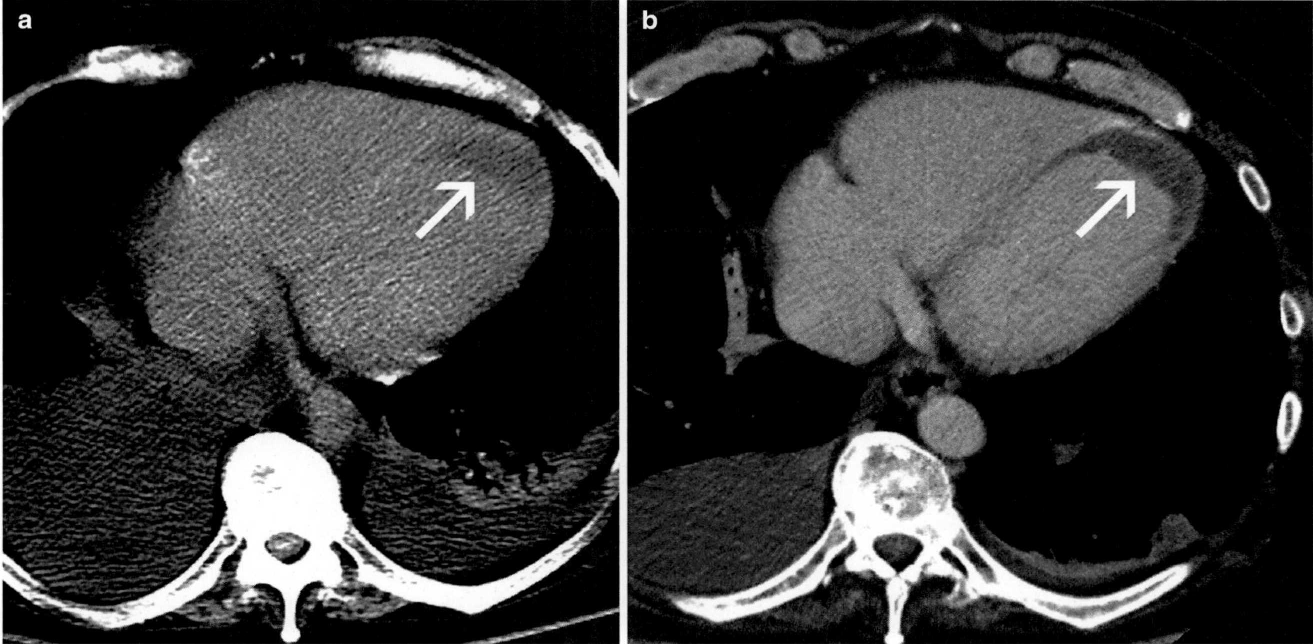

Fig. 16.7 A 62 year-old male admitted with a recent myocardial infarction with a hypoattenuating left ventricular thrombus. A transverse, non-contrast view (**a**) obtained to evaluate the extent of pleural effusion demonstrates an area of low attenuation at the left ventricular apex (*white arrow*). A thrombus was suspected. A repeat scan 1 week later obtained with a small amount of intravenous contrast (**b**) demonstrates clear delineation of the large thrombus at the left ventricular apex (*white arrow*)

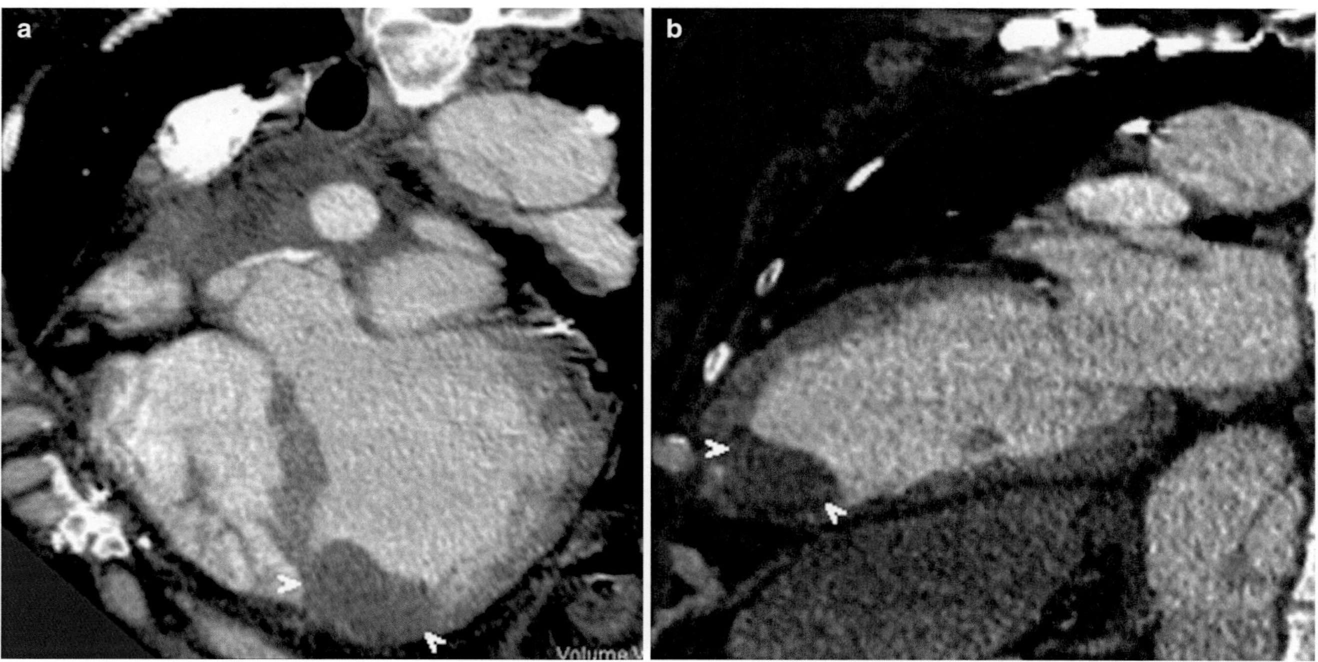

Fig. 16.8 A 45-year-old woman with a recent myocardial infarction. Four-chamber (**a**) and two-chamber (**b**) views from a cardiac CT show a left ventricular apical aneurysm with thrombus

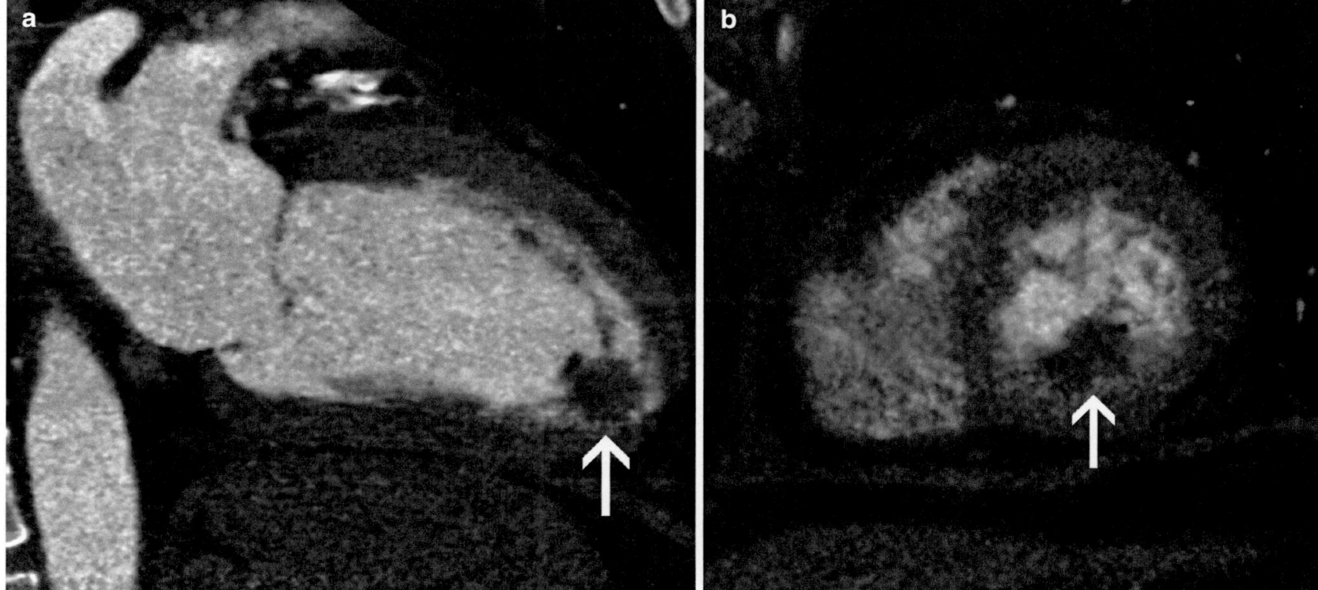

Fig. 16.9 A 55 year-old male with a mass at the ventricular apex on transthoracic echocardiogram. Images from a cardiac CT scan obtained in the two-chamber (**a**) and short axis (**b**) planes are shown. A mobile, intracameral, low attenuating, non-enhancing, apical mass is seen, consistent with a thrombus. A small area of apical septal late gadolinium enhancement was demonstrated on the patient's CMR (not shown)

enlarged atria with heterogeneous enhancement as a result of circulatory stasis within the left atrium. This smoke-like enhancement can be especially prominent in the left atrial appendage, and, in patients with severe atrial enlargement, this poor opacification of the chamber and appendage may make exclusion of thrombus very difficult (Fig. 16.10). As a result, transesophageal echocardiography is still considered the gold standard for the evaluation of a thrombus in the left atrium or left atrial appendage. Imaging protocols with a delayed phase or with the patient

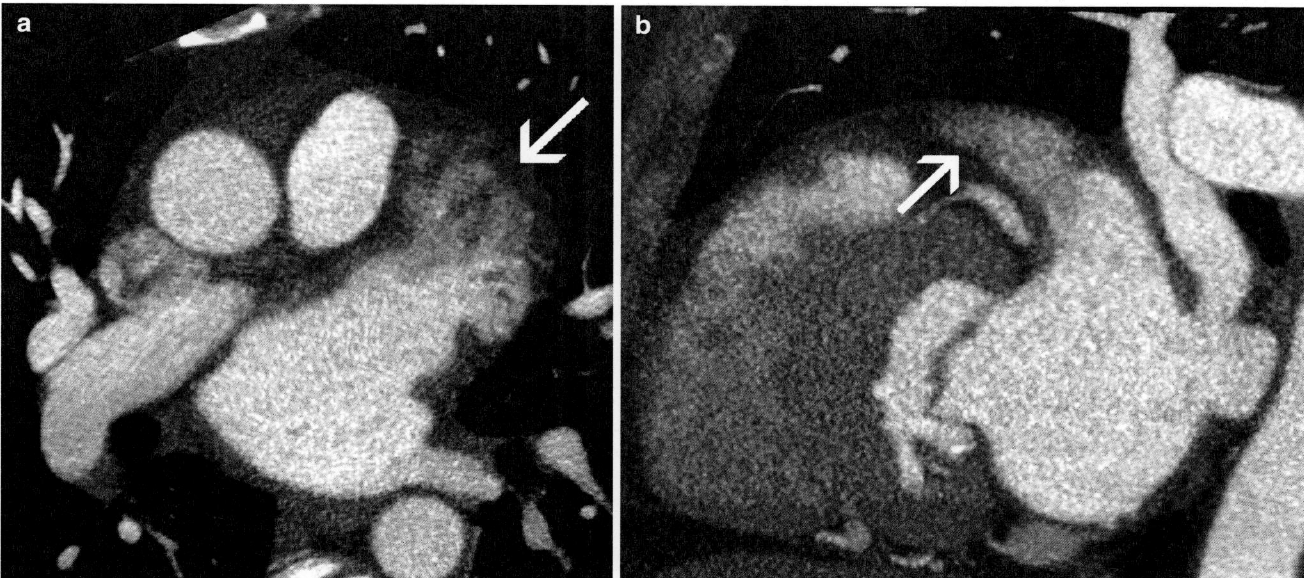

Fig. 16.10 A 47 year-old female with atypical chest pain. Orthogonal MPR views of the left atrium from a CCTA (**a**, **b**) demonstrate left atrial enlargement with heterogeneous enhancement of the left atrial appendage. No thrombus was identified on echocardiography. Heterogeneous opacification of the left atrial appendage is a significant pitfall in the identification or exclusion of atrial thrombi on CCTA

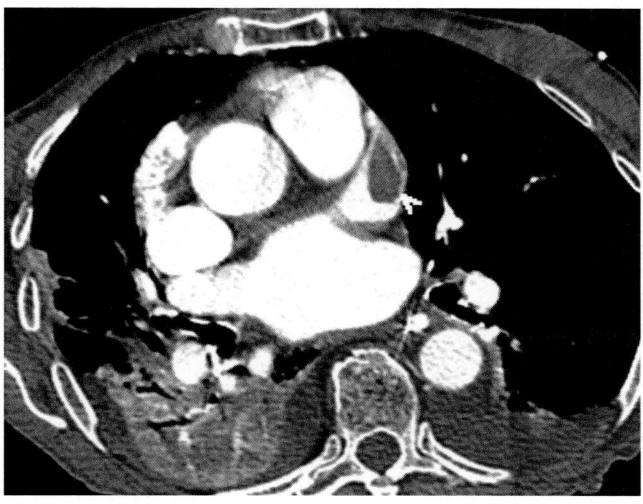

Fig. 16.11 A 48 year-old female with left atrial enlargement and atrial fibrillation. On a contrast-enhanced CT scan, a filling defect is clearly identified in the left atrial appendage (*white arrowhead*). When such a defect is clearly delineated by contrast as in this case, thrombus can be more definitively identified

in the prone position have been reported as techniques for improved opacification of the atrial appendage, although these techniques are not yet widely employed [32, 33]. When a non-enhancing filling defect is clearly delineated by contrast, however, a left atrial appendage thrombus can be more easily diagnosed (Fig. 16.11). Differentiation of atrial thrombus from other cardiac masses is usually made on the clinical basis in patients with known atrial enlargement and dysfunction. Right atrial thrombi may form in the atrial appendage, and can be difficult to delineate due to the inherently heterogeneous opacification of the normal right heart (Fig. 16.12). There are however lower risks of thrombus development in the right atrial appendage, since this structure tends to be flatter and more broad-based, compared to the left atrial appendage, which is a more lobulated or tubular structure and has a neck. These morphologic differences make the left atrial appendage more prone to the development of thrombi compared to the right atrial appendage.

Metastatic Disease

Metastatic disease is the most common cause of a malignant neoplastic mass in the heart. Metastatic disease has been reported as more common in the right heart, but, as previously mentioned, this may be due to the earlier recognition of metastatic lesions in the right ventricle, since the wall is thinner than that of the left ventricular wall. Most metastatic lesions are isoattenuating to the myocardium on pre-contrast CT imaging. Contrast enhancement of metastatic lesions is somewhat variable depending on the degree of vascularity of the neoplasm. Most metastases enhance less than the myocardium initially after administration of contrast, but will slowly accumulate and retain contrast. Metastases may also show retention of contrast on late-phase imaging. This pattern of enhancement may be less well-characterized on CT, since multiphasic imaging with

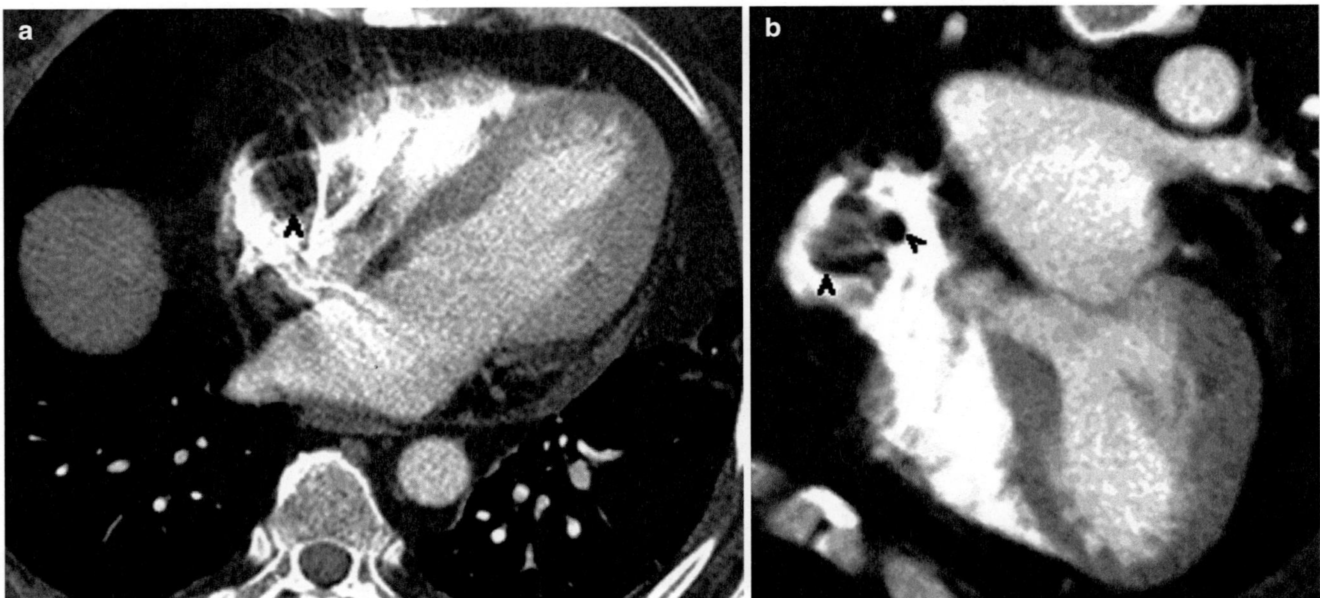

Fig. 16.12 A 38 year-old female with recent resection of gastric carcinoma. Transverse (**a**) and four-chamber (**b**) views are shown from a CT scan of the chest. There is some heterogeneous opacification of the right atrium with some streaking, although the thrombus can be seen through these artifacts (*black arrowheads*, (**a**) and (**b**)). The patient also had a large parenchymal hepatic hematoma, related to her recent surgery, which may have contributed to the development of a right atrial thrombus. CMR (not shown) demonstrated features consistent with a thrombus, and this structure resolved on subsequent studies

CT is uncommonly performed (Fig. 16.13). It should also be noted that the optimal phase for CCTA during coronary arterial enhancement is earlier than the optimal phase for demonstrating myocardial wall enhancement. As a result, the differential enhancement between a metastatic lesion and normal myocardium may not be as clearly seen on CCTA (Fig. 16.14).

The most common morphology of cardiac metastatic disease is an intramural mass or a mass with a broad-based attachment, in contradistinction to benign masses, which tend to be intracameral and have a narrow attachment. Many metastases which invade the heart from the adjacent mediastinal or pericardial spaces may, however, involve the epicardium first, and subsequently invade into the myocardium. Metastatic disease to the heart is found in up to 10 % of patients with a primary malignancy at the time of autopsy [34]. Although numerous neoplasms have been reported to be metastatic to the heart, the lung is the most common site of a primary tumor, occurring in up to 36.7 % of patients [35]. Melanoma is however, an important source of hematogenous spread of disease to the heart from a distant primary site [36]. An example of metastases involving the right ventricle is shown in Fig. 16.15.

Myxomas

Myxomas are the most common benign neoplasm of the heart and comprise 50 % of all primary cardiac masses. Myxomas characteristically occur in the atria, and are more commonly left atrial rather than right atrial, with a reported predominance of 80 % in the left atrium compared to 20 % in the right atrium. Masses which arise in the atria may also prolapse into the ventricular chambers [14]. Myxomas have also, however, been reported to occur in both ventricles. The most common imaging appearance is that of a lobulated mass with pre-contrast hypoattenuation relative to blood pool and relative to myocardium. Masses are commonly lobulated in appearance and predominantly intracameral. The most common site of attachment for either right or left atrial myxomas is at the fossa ovalis, a feature which can be helpful in arriving at the correct diagnosis [9]. Correct identification of the site of attachment is also helpful in presurgical planning. Atrial myxomas commonly demonstrate punctate or coarse calcifications, which is also useful in establishing the diagnosis. Pre-contrast hypoattenuation is commonly seen relative to blood pool and normal myocardium (Fig. 16.16). Rarely, atrial myxomas may be diffusely and densely calcified [17].

The classic triad of clinical symptoms reported with myxomas includes constitutional symptoms, manifestations of obstructive valvular disease, and embolic phenomenon. Constitutional symptoms include fever, malaise, weight loss, and anemia, among others. These symptoms are likely related to an autoimmune response initiated by the tumor [37]. Cardiac-related symptoms of atrial myxomas vary depending on the chamber of involvement. Atrial myxomas have been commonly reported to mimic mitral valve disease

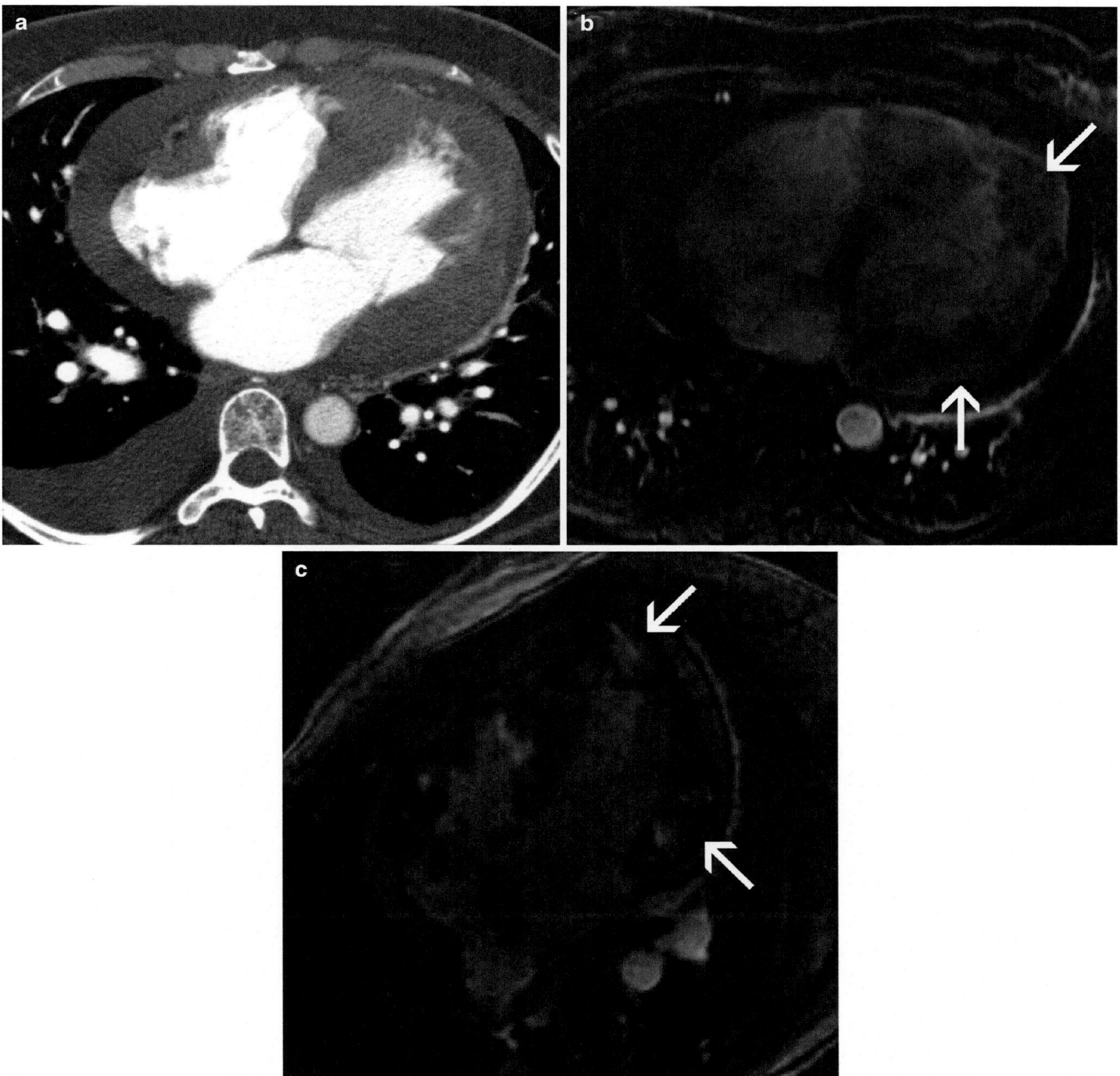

Fig. 16.13 A 45 year-old female with metastatic melanoma. A transverse view from a contrast-enhanced CT scan (**a**) shows irregular thickening of the ventricular walls and a moderate-sized pericardial effusion. The ventricular metastases are not well-delineated due to the early phase of contrast administration, which was in part, due to the patient's poor cardiac function. A post-contrast CMR sequence obtained at 70 s after intravenous injection of gadolinium (**b**) demonstrates areas of relatively decreased enhancement related to the perfused myocardium (*white arrows*). A delayed, 4-chamber view obtained 10 min after contrast administration (**c**) demonstrates late enhancement within the cardiac metastases (*white arrows*)

and rheumatic heart disease by clinical presentation [38]. Involvement of other valves may, however, produce manifestations of aortic, pulmonic, or tricuspid valvular disease. Embolization is another common feature of myxomas, and may occur to either the pulmonic or systemic circulation, depending on the chamber of involvement. Up to 35 % of left atrial myxomas and up to 10 % of right atrial myxomas may embolize, although this difference in embolization rate could be related to the more apparent manifestations of systemic emboli [39].

A genetic predisposition to myxomas has been postulated and suggested by case reports of families with multiple members with myxomas and in patients with several myxomas [40]. Notably, Carney's Syndrome may be associated

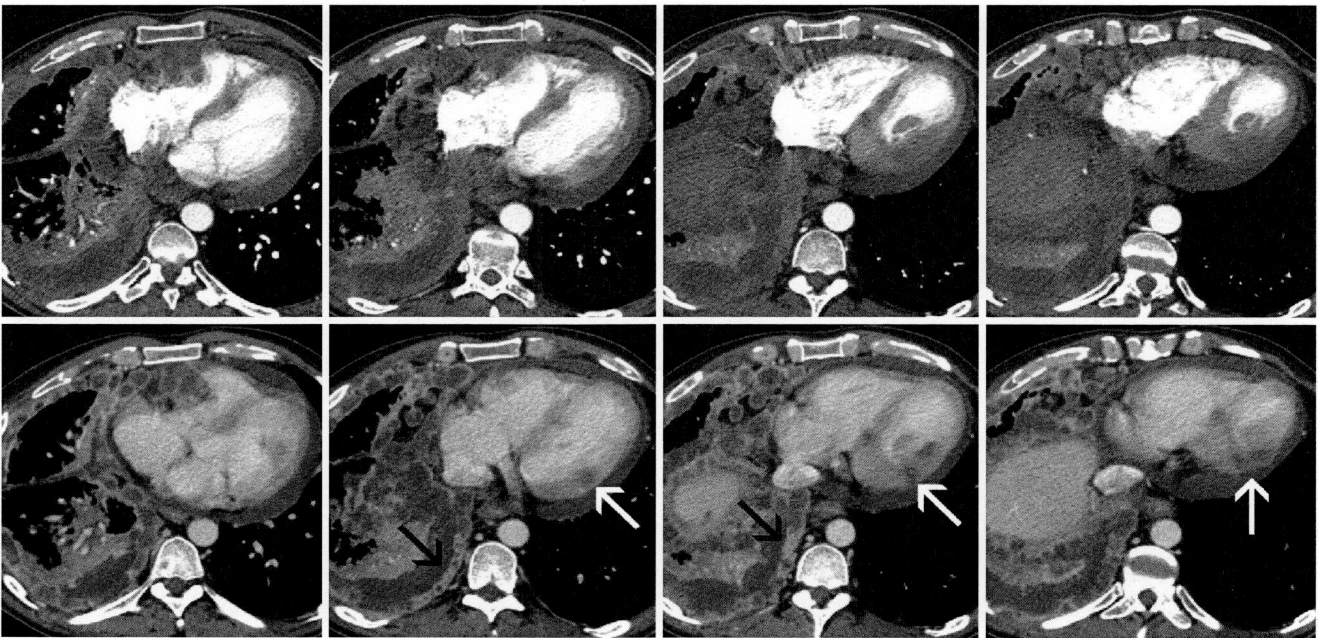

Fig. 16.14 A 56 year-old male with high-grade urothelial malignancy and cardiac metastases. Transverse views from an arterial phase of a post-contrast CT scan (*top row*) faintly show metastases to the left ventricular myocardium (*white arrows*). These areas of hypoenhancement are better seen in the portal venous phase images (*bottom row*), where the myocardium is more well-enhanced. Note that other metastases are also better seen on the later phase study, including pleural metastases (*black arrows*)

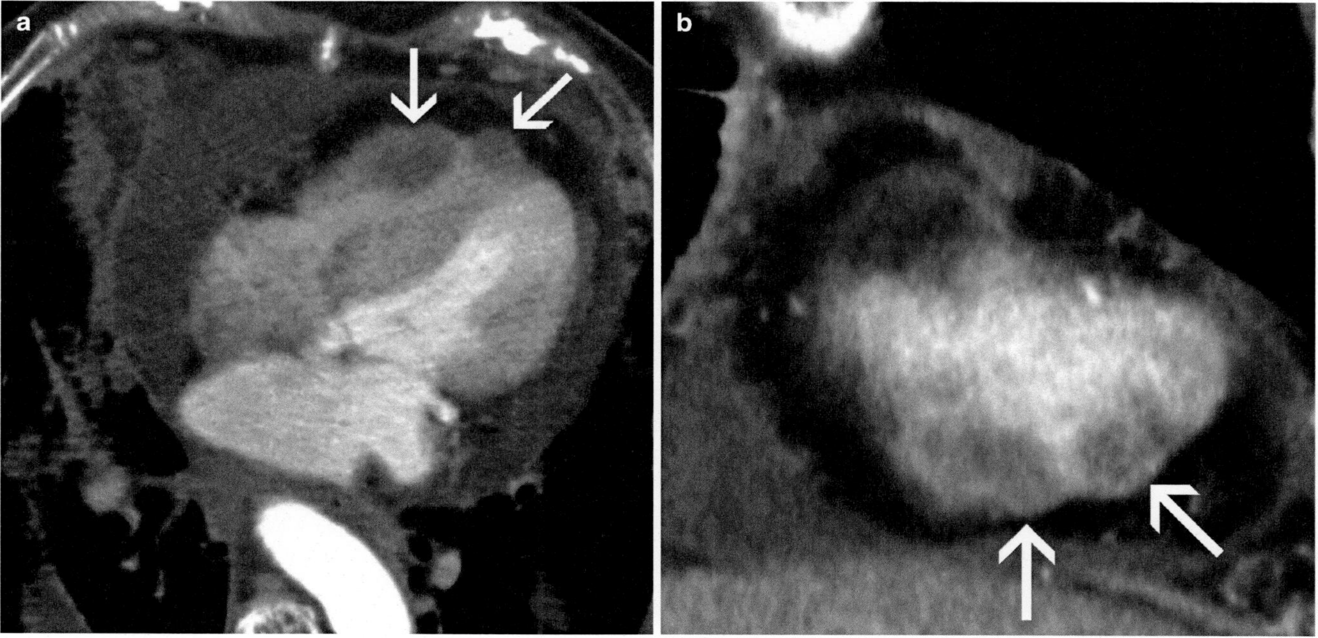

Fig. 16.15 A 48 year-old female with right ventricular metastases due to thymic carcinoma. Transverse (**a**) and coronal (**b**) views from a post-contrast CT scan show large masses arising from the wall of the right ventricle, with broad-based attachments to the ventricular wall, consistent with metastatic disease

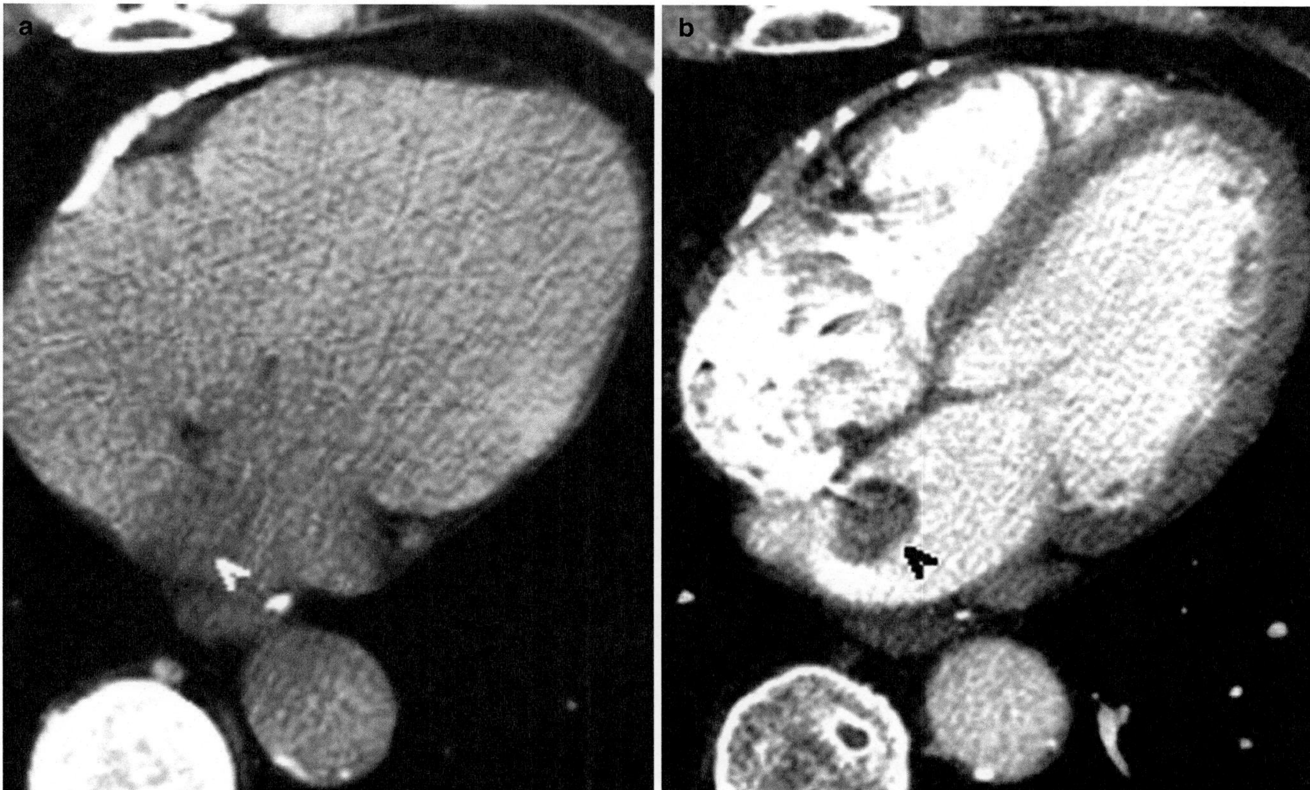

Fig. 16.16 A 52 year-old male with treated colorectal carcinoma and a left atrial mass. A pre-contrast CT scan (**a**) demonstrates the low attenuation left atrial mass. The post-contrast study (**b**) shows no enhancement, and delineates the pedunculated nature of the mass, which arises from the region of the fossa ovalis

with atrial myxomas, occurring in two thirds of patients, in addition to other manifestations including mammary myxoid fibroadenomas, pigmented cutaneous lesions, endocrine disorders, testicular tumors, and schwannomas [41].

Cardiac Sarcomas

Cardiac sarcomas comprise the most common primary malignant tumors of the heart, but are a rare entity overall, with a prevalence at autopsy as low as 0.0001 % [42]. Metastases to the heart outnumber malignant primary lesions by a ratio of 20–40 to 1. Among subtypes of sarcoma, angiosarcomas are most common, comprising approximately 37 %. This tumor subtype in particular tends to occur commonly in the right atrium. Other subtypes tend to arise most commonly from the left atrium, although all types of sarcomas may occur in any chamber [13]. For most cardiac sarcomas, survival is reported as very poor, with metastases commonly detected shortly after clinical presentation [10].

On CCTA and CMR, angiosarcomas may show areas of hemorrhage and necrosis and may appear heterogeneous. Avid enhancement is commonly seen (Fig. 16.17), and tumors may be difficult to delineate from the ventricular chamber on later phases due to bright enhancement. Venous lakes and linear vascular structures within masses may be seen, resulting in what has been likened to a "sunray pattern" [43]. Two morphological appearances of angiosarcomas have been reported, including a focal mass arising from the myocardium itself or a diffuse infiltrating process involving the myocardium and pericardium [44, 45]. Undifferentiated sarcomas are tumors with no specific histological staining patterns. The nature and definition of tumors in this category has changed over time as histological techniques have improved. Similar to angiosarcomas, these tumors may either present as a focal mass or as a diffusely infiltrative myocardial and pericardial process. The common site of origin is the left atrium, with a predisposition reported at 80 % [13]. A propensity for valvular involvement has also been reported [46–48]. Rhabdomyosarcomas are very uncommon in adults, but are the most common form of cardiac sarcomas and the most common primary cardiac malignancy in pediatric populations [13]. Embryonal rhabdomyosarcomas occur in pediatric patients, whereas tumors in adults tend to be more pleomorphic [49]. Osteosarcomas of the heart are rare neoplasms, and are distinguished by their propensity to form

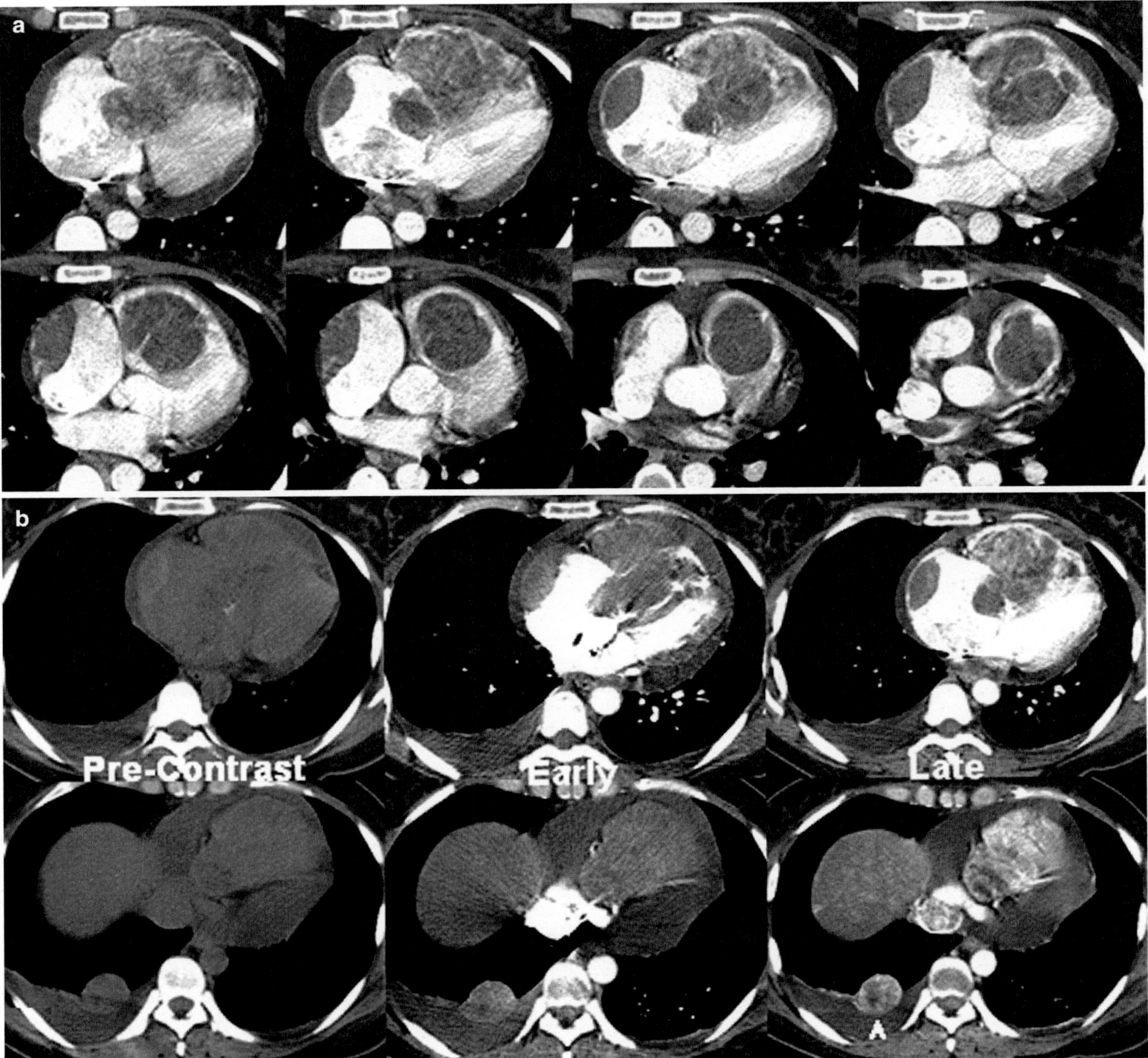

Fig. 16.17 (**a**, **b**) A 33 year-old female with angiosarcoma. Sequential pre-contrast, early, and late contrasted images demonstrate vascular enhancement within the angiosarcoma. Note the enhancing right lower lobe pulmonary nodule (*arrowhead*), consistent with a metastasis

dense calcifications [50], although some tumors of this type may demonstrate only minimal calcification [13]. Other tumor subtypes include leiomyosarcoma, fibrosarcoma, and liposarcoma, although these are even rarer than the aforementioned neoplasms.

Cardiac Lymphoma

Cardiac lymphoma is a very rare entity, and in a series of 533 cardiac tumors and cysts, it accounted for only 1.3 % of tumors [11]. These tumors are rare since there are no true intracardiac lymph nodes. Tumors likely arise from primitive, totipotential mesenchymal cells, and usually consist of high grade B-cell lymphomas. Strictly defined, cardiac lymphoma includes lymphoma involving the heart and pericardium without other areas of lymphomatous involvement. Anecdotal reports suggest that there is increased risk for cardiac lymphoma in AIDS and in other immune deficiency states [51]. Given the rarity of this entity, the radiologic findings are not well-established, although reports indicate that tumors are usually relatively isoattenuating on CT and isointense on CMR, with heterogeneous enhancement after contrast administration [52].

Lipoma

Cardiac lipomas are the second most common cause of a benign cardiac neoplasm, after myxomas. Lipomas are easily recognized as benign by the homogeneously low, pre-contrast attenuation consistent with fat, which demonstrate essentially no enhancement after contrast administration. Tumors are soft and may be large at the time of initial diagnosis. Symptoms are usually due to mass effect, although commonly cardiac lipomas are detected incidentally and prior to onset of clinical manifestations. Some tumors may encase coronary arteries, resulting in mass effect and displacement, making resection difficult [53]. Although there is seldomly diagnostic uncertainty, some entities may mimic lipomas, including lipomatous hypertrophy of the interatrial septum (Fig. 16.18). Rarely, lipomatous metaplasia within chronic myocardial infarctions may be misdiagnosed as a lipoma [54].

Papillary Fibroelastoma

Papillary fibroelastomas, also known as Lambl's excrescences, are avascular masses comprised of fronds of dense connective tissue. These masses may be either reactive in nature or may be related to a hamartoma [55]. The true prevalence of this entity is not known, and these tumors have been postulated to be under-recognized and under-diagnosed due to their small size. Most sources refer to these lesions as the third most common benign neoplasms behind myxomas and lipomas. Ninety percent of papillary fibroelastomas occur on valves, with the aortic valve being the most common location. When associated with the atrioventricular valves, these tumors tend to occur along the atrial side, which may help to differentiate these lesions from thrombi [56]. Associated valvular dysfunction is common, although many of these lesions are detected incidentally [57]. An additional, common presentation is the occurrence of embolic phenomenon to the systemic or pulmonary circulation [58]. These tumors are, however, uncommonly reported on CCTA, and as a result no characteristic CCTA features of this entity have emerged.

Pediatric Cardiac Masses

In pediatric patients who present with cardiac masses, a separate set of diagnostic possibilities should be considered. Pediatric patients will less commonly present for CCTA evaluation, due to radiation concerns. Additionally, since there is sparse literature on CCTA in pediatric patients, the typical appearances of many masses are difficult to delineate. However, some familiarity with masses which may present in pediatric patients is useful to physicians involved in cardiac imaging.

In infants and children, the most common masses encountered are rhabdomyomas. These masses tend to occur in the walls of the ventricles, and the vast majority of these masses

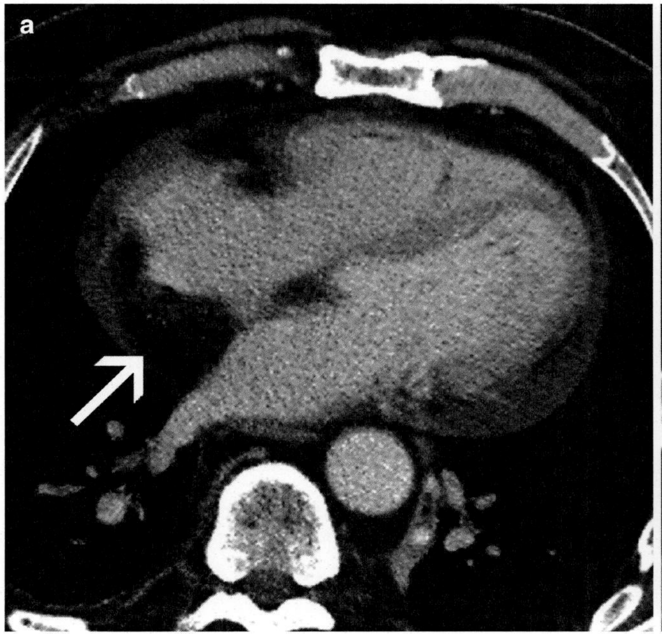

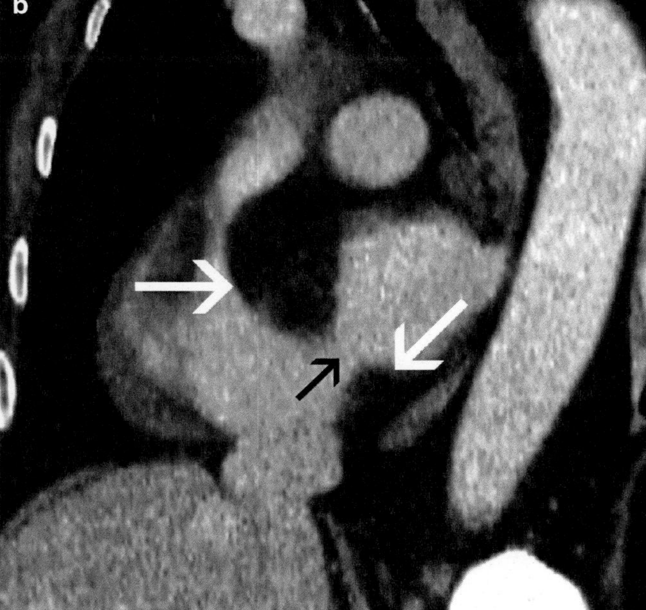

Fig. 16.18 A 78 year-old male with lipomatous hypertrophy of the interatrial septum. Images from a CT scan of the chest obtained in the transverse plane (**a**) and in the short axis plane of the heart (**b**) show lipomatous hypertrophy in the wall of the interatrial septum (*white arrows*). Note the characteristic sparing of the region of the fossa ovalis (*black arrow*)

are multiple. A strong association with tuberous sclerosis is present, although many patients do not manifest other signs of tuberous sclerosis until many years later. Spontaneous regression of tumors is common, although the initial clinical presentation may be severe. When these lesions regress, they may leave behind foci of myocardial fat attenuation [59]. Cardiac fibromas constitutes the second most common cause of pediatric cardiac masses, and usually are seen as large, solitary lesions. Some of these may grow to an enormous size. Symptoms may include heart failure, chest pain, arrhythmias, and sudden cardiac death [60]. Myxomas are very rare in the pediatric population, but have been reported in large series in older pediatric patients and adolescents [17]. As described earlier, the most common malignant neoplasm in pediatric patients is a cardiac rhabdomyosarcoma, which often has embryonal features at histology. Additional rare tumors are encountered in pediatric populations including cardiac angiomas, cardiac teratomas, and Purkinje cell tumors.

Mimics of Cardiac Masses

Several normal structures in the heart may mimic a mass even to an experienced reader. Misidentification of normal structures as masses can lead to unnecessary biopsies, surgeries, and subsequent morbidity. Notably, in the right atrium, a prominent crista terminalis may mimic a cardiac mass. When a small and reticulated mass is present along this structure in the right atrium, a network of Chiari may be present. Uncommonly, prominence of the Eustachian valve or juxtacaval lipomatous tissue may mimic a lower right atrial mass. Usually, the contrast timing for the right ventricle is such that some saline is being injected at the time of scanning of the heart. However, in some cases, unopacified blood flow entering the right atrium from the inferior vena cava may simulate a mass when the right atrium is otherwise filled with contrast. In the left atrium, the "coumadin ridge," located between the atrial appendage ostium and the superior pulmonary vein, may appear mass-like.

References

1. Desjardins B, Kazerooni EA. ECG-gated cardiac CT. Am J Roentgenol. 2004;182:993–1010.
2. Newhouse JH, Murphy RX. Tissue distribution of soluble contrast: effect of dose variation and changes with time. Am J Roentgenol. 1981;136:463–7.
3. Cademartiri F, Mollet N, van der Lugt A, et al. Non-invasive 16-row multislice CT coronary angiography: usefulness of saline chaser. Eur Radiol. 2004;14:178–83.
4. Awai K, Hiraishi K, Hori S. Effect of contrast material injection duration and rate on aortic peak time and peak enhancement at dynamic CT involving injection protocol with dose tailored to patient weight. Radiology. 2004;230(1):142–50.
5. Cademartiri F, Nieman K, van der Lugt A, et al. Intravenous contrast material administration at 16-detector row helical CT coronary angiography: test bolus versus bolus-tracking technique. Radiology. 2004;233:817–23.
6. Bae KT, Tran HQ, Heiken JP. Uniform vascular contrast enhancement and reduced contrast medium volume achieved by using exponentially decelerated contrast material injection method. Radiology. 2004;231:732–6.
7. Boyd DB. Computerized transmission tomography of the heart using scanning electron beams. In: Higgins CH, editor. Computed tomography of the heart and great vessels. Mount Kisco/New York: Futura Publishing Company; 1983. p. 45–55.
8. Newhouse JH. Fluid compartment distribution of intravenous iothalamate in the dog. Invest Radiol. 1977;12:364–7.
9. Prichard RW. Tumors of the heart. Arch Pathol. 1951;51:98–128.
10. Glancy DL, Morales JB, Roberts WC. Angiosarcoma of the heart. Am J Cardiol. 1968;21:413–9.
11. McAllister HA, Fenoglio Jr JJ. Tumors of the cardiovascular system: atlas of tumor pathology, vol. 2. Washington, DC: Armed Forces Institute of Pathology; 1978.
12. Lund JT, Ehman RL, Julsrud PR, et al. Cardiac masses: assessment by MR imaging. AJR Am J Roentgenol. 1989;152(3):469–73.
13. Burke AP, Cowan D, Virmani R. Primary sarcomas of the heart. Cancer. 1992;69:387–95.
14. Tazelaar HD, Locke TJ, McGregor CG. Pathology of surgically excised primary cardiac tumors. Mayo Clin Proc. 1992;67(10):957–65.
15. Lam KY, Dickens P, Chan AC. Tumors of the heart. A 20-year experience with a review of 12,485 consecutive autopsies. Arch Pathol Lab Med. 1993;117(10):1027–31.
16. Marx GR. Cardiac tumors. In: Emmanouilides GC, Gutgesell HP, Riemenschneider TA, Allen HD, editors. Moss and Adams heart disease in infants, children, and adolescents: including the fetus and young adult, vol. 2. 5th ed. Baltimore: Williams & Wilkins; 1995. p. 1773–86.
17. Burke A, Virmani R. Tumors of the heart and great vessels: atlas of tumor pathology. Fasc 16, ser 3. Washington, DC: Armed Forces Institute of Pathology; 1996.
18. Takach TJ, Reul GJ, Ott DA, Cooley DA. Primary cardiac tumors in infants and children: immediate and long-term operative results. Ann Thorac Surg. 1996;62(2):559–64.
19. Ludomirsky A. Cardiac tumors. In: Bricker JT, Fisher DJ, editors. The science and practice of pediatric cardiology, vol. 2. 9th ed. Baltimore: Williams & Wilkins; 1998. p. 1885–93.
20. Araoz PA, Eklund HE, Welch TJ, Breen JF. CT and MR imaging of primary cardiac malignancies. Radiographics. 1999;19(6):1421–34.
21. Chiles C, Woodard PK, Gutierrez FR, Link KM. Metastatic involvement of the heart and pericardium: CT and MR imaging. Radiographics. 2000;20:1073–103.
22. Grebenc ML, Rosado de Christenson ML, Burke AP, Green CE, Galvin JR. Primary cardiac and pericardial neoplasms: radiologic–pathologic correlation. Radiographics. 2000;20:1073–103; quiz 1110–1071, 1112.
23. Grebenc ML, Rosado-de-Christenson ML, Green CE, Burke AP, Galvin JR. Cardiac myxoma: imaging features in 83 patients. Radiographics. 2002;2(3):673–89.
24. Piazza N, Chughtai T, Toledano K, et al. Primary cardiac tumours: eighteen years of surgical experience on 21 patients. Can J Cardiol. 2004;20(14):1443–8.
25. Tatli S, Lipton MJ. CT for intracardiac thrombi and tumors. Int J Cardiovasc Imaging. 2005;21(1):115–31.
26. Butany J, Nair V, Naseemuddin A, et al. Cardiac tumours: diagnosis and management. Lancet Oncol. 2005;6(4):219–28.

27. Leipsic JA, Heyneman LE, Kim RJ. Cardiac masses and myocardial diseases. In: McAdams HP, Reddy GP, editors. Cardiopulmonary imaging syllabus—2005. Leesburg: American Roentgen Ray Society; 2005. p. 1–13.
28. Sparrow PJ, Kurian JB, Jones TR, Sivananthan MU. MR imaging of cardiac tumors. Radiographics. 2005;25:1255–76.
29. Barkhausen J, Hunold P, Eggebrecht HH, et al. Detection and characterization of intracardiac thrombi on MR imaging. AJR Am J Roentgenol. 2002;179:1539–42.
30. Weinreich DJ, Burke JF, Ferrel JP. Left ventricular mural thrombi complicating acute myocardial infarction long-term follow-up with serial echocardiography. Ann Intern Med. 1984;100(6):789–94.
31. Asinger RW, Mikell FL, Elsperger J, Hodges M. Incidence of left ventricular thrombosis after acute transmural myocardial infarction: serial evaluation by two-dimensional echocardiography. N Engl J Med. 1981;305(6):297–302.
32. Hur J, Kim YJ, Nam JE, Choi EY, Shim CY, Choi BW, et al. Thrombus in the left atrial appendage in stroke patients: detection with cardiac CT angiography--a preliminary report. Radiology. 2008;249(1):81–7.
33. Hur J, Kim YJ, Lee HJ, et al. Left atrial appendage thrombi in stroke patients: detection with two-phase cardiac CT angiography versus transesophageal echocardiography. Radiology. 2009;251(3):683–90.
34. Abraham KP, Reddy V, Gattuso P. Neoplasms metastatic to the heart: review of 3314 consecutive autopsies. Am J Cardiovasc Pathol. 1990;3:195–8.
35. Klatt EC, Heitz DR. Cardiac metastases. Cancer. 1990;65:1456–9.
36. MacGee W. Metastatic and invasive tumours involving the heart in a geriatric population: a necropsy study. Virchows Arch A Pathol Anat Histopathol. 1991;419:183–9.
37. Bjessmo S, Ivert T. Cardiac myxoma: 40 years' experience in 63 patients. Ann Thorac Surg. 1997;63:697–700.
38. Markel ML, Waller BF, Armstrong WF. Cardiac myxoma: a review. Medicine. 1987;66:114–25.
39. Castells E, Ferran V, Octavio-de-Toledo MC. Cardiac myxomas: surgical treatment, long-term results and recurrence. J Cardiovasc Surg. 1993;34:49–53.
40. Carney JA. Differences between nonfamilial and familial cardiac myxoma. Am J Surg Pathol. 1985;9:53–5.
41. Carney JA, Gordon H, Carpenter PC, Shenoy BV, Go VW. The complex of myxomas, spotty pigmentation and endocrine overactivity. Medicine. 1985;64:270–83.
42. McCallister Jr HA. Primary tumors of the heart and pericardium. Curr Probl Cardiol. 1979;4:1–51.
43. Yahata S, Endo T, Honma H, et al. Sunray appearance on enhanced magnetic resonance image of cardiac angiosarcoma with pericardial obliteration. Am Heart J. 1994;127:468–71.
44. Bruna J, Lockwood M. Primary heart angiosarcoma detected by computed tomography and magnetic resonance imaging. Eur Radiol. 1998;8:66–8.
45. Jannigan DT, Husain A, Robinson NA. Cardiac angiosarcomas: a review and a case report. Cancer. 1986;57:852–9.
46. Herhusky MJ, Gregg SB, Virmani R, Chun PKC, Bender H, Gray Jr GF. Cardiac sarcoma presenting as metastatic disease. Arch Pathol Lab Med. 1985;109:943–5.
47. Ludomirsky A, Vargo TA, Murphy DJ, Gresik MV, Ott DA, Mullins CE. Intracardiac undifferentiated sarcoma in infancy. J Am Coll Cardiol. 1985;6:1362–4. Abstract 37.
48. Itoh K, Matsumura T, Egawa Y, et al. Primary mitral valve sarcoma in infancy. Pediatr Cardiol. 1998;19:174–7.
49. Hwa J, Ward C, Nunn G, et al. Primary interventricular cardiac tumors in children: contemporary diagnostic and management options. Pediatr Cardiol. 1994;15:233–7.
50. Chaloupka JC, Fishman EK, Siegelman SS. Use of CT in the evaluation of primary cardiac tumors. Cardiovasc Intervent Radiol. 1986;9:132–5.
51. Holladay AO, Siegel RJ, Schwartz DA. Cardiac malignant lymphoma in acquired immune deficiency syndrome. Cancer. 1997;70(8):2203–7.
52. Dorsay TA, Ho VB, Roviera MJ, Armstrong MA, Brissette MD. Primary cardiac lymphoma: CT and MR findings. J Comput Assist Tomogr. 1993;17:978–81.
53. Hananouchi GI, Goff WB. Cardiac lipoma: six-year follow-up with MRI characteristics, and a review of the literature. Magn Reson Imaging. 1990;8(6):825–8.
54. Banks KP, Lisanti CJ. Incidental finding of a lipomatous lesion involving the myocardium of the left ventricular wall. AJR Am J Roentgenol. 2004;182:261–2.
55. Rubin MA, Snell JA, Tazelaar HD, Lack EE, et al. Cardiac papillary fibroelastoma: an immunohistochemical investigation and unusual clinical manifestations. Mod Pathol. 1995;8:402–7.
56. Klarich KW, Enriquez-Sarano M, Gura GM, et al. Papillary fibroelastoma: echocardiographic characteristics for diagnosis and pathologic correction. J Am Coll Cardiol. 1997;30:784–90.
57. Edward FH, Hale D, Cohen A, et al. Primary cardiac valve tumors. Ann Thorac Surg. 1991;52:1127–31.
58. McFadden PM, Lacy JR. Intracardiac papillary fibroelastoma: an occult cause of embolic neurologic deficit. Ann Thorac Surg. 1987;43:667–9.
59. Bosi G, Lintermans JP, Pellegrino PA, et al. The natura history of cardiac rhabdomyoma with and without tuberous sclerosis. Acta Paediatr. 1996;85:928–31.
60. Turi GK, Albala A, Fenoglio Jr JJ. Cardiac fibromatosis: an ultrastructural study. Hum Pathol. 1980;11:577–9.

Part IV

CT Vascular Angiography

CT Angiography of the Peripheral Arteries

17

Jabi E. Shriki, Leonardo C. Clavijo, and Gale L. Tang

Abstract

The application of CT angiography to the systemic vascular tree poses a number of unique challenges, but offers the ability to noninvasively depict a wide array of arterial pathology. CT of the peripheral arterial tree also has a number of specific advantages relative to other modalities, including conventional angiography, MRI, and ultrasound. Peripheral CT angiography has particularly important applications in imaging extremities in the setting of acute ischemia or trauma. While some of the skills in performing CT angiography in other body parts are applicable to peripheral CT angiography, several technical considerations should be recognized in incorporating peripheral imaging into a CT angiography practice.

Keywords

Peripheral computed tomography • Peripheral vascular ct angiography • Peripheral angiogram • Peripheral vascular disease • Systemic arterial disease • Vascular cta • Peripheral ct angiogram

Introduction

CT angiography is a useful modality in imaging the peripheral arterial tree and has become an integral component in many cardiovascular imaging practices. Large portions of the arterial system can be easily imaged with excellent spatial resolution, low radiation dose, and minimal risk to the patient. Peripheral CT angiography has particular advantages as a non-invasive means of depicting the systemic arterial tree and is able to demonstrate a number of disease entities. Additionally, the skills of 3-D data manipulation useful in evaluation of coronary arteries and vascular structures elsewhere in the body can be translated into skills in interpreting peripheral CT angiographic studies. Advancements in CT angiography, including the dissemination of multislice, dual source, and dual energy scanners, have made submillimeter isotropic voxel resolution possible, and have enabled more detailed visualization of arterial structures. Simultaneous increases in computational speed and widespread availability of dedicated 3-D software make visualization and evaluation of peripheral arterial anatomy much more facile.

Acquisition and Scanning Techniques

Special Considerations Regarding Peripheral CT Angiography

Several technical considerations should be recognized in making the transition from cardiac to peripheral vascular CT

J.E. Shriki, MD (✉)
Department of Radiology, Puget VA Health System, University of Washington, 1660 S. Columbian Way, Seattle, WA 98101, USA
e-mail: shriki@uw.edu

L.C. Clavijo, MD, PhD, FACC, FSCAI, FSVM
Department of Medicine, Division of Cardiovascular Medicine, Department of Clinical Medicine, University of Southern California, Los Angeles, CA, USA

G.L. Tang, MD
Department of Surgery, University of Washington, Seattle, WA, USA

M.J. Budoff, J.S. Shinbane (eds.), *Cardiac CT Imaging: Diagnosis of Cardiovascular Disease*, DOI 10.1007/978-3-319-28219-0_17

angiography. First, while the coronary arteries are usually opacified along with the aorta even in the presence of stenoses, the peripheral vasculature may have a variable relationship with aortic opacification. In patients with severe atherosclerotic disease, the presence of stenoses, occlusions, and aneurysms may delay optimal opacification of the peripheral arteries. In thoracic, abdominal, and neuroimaging applications, higher detector row CT scanners provide a number of advantages. However, for peripheral CT angiography, the high speed of scanning with multi-detector row CT scanners may result in outpacing of the bolus of contrast, with images obtained prior to arrival of the contrast bolus into the area of interest. As a result, the timing of peripheral CT angiography has separate considerations that differ from scanning other, more proximal, body parts (Fig. 17.1).

Also, the reconstructed field of view for peripheral applications is frequently larger in transverse axial dimension than that employed for cardiac CT. This is because of the wider distribution of peripheral arterial structures in the transverse plane. As a result, images may have lower in-plane spatial resolution. This loss of in-plane resolution may be offset by the use of separate, reconstructed fields of view for each lower extremity or for different parts of the anatomy scanned. When imaging the lower extremities, the feet should be kept straight and positioned as closely together as possible, so that the reconstructed field of view closely matches the anatomy being imaged. This can be achieved by securing the feet into a table extension or harness, which is usually attachable or built into the table (Fig. 17.2).

In comparison to cardiac CT, there is a longer craniocaudal extent of anatomy imaged with peripheral CT angiography. As a result, data sets may be much larger for comparable slice thickness. For example, whereas a single phase of a cardiac CT reconstruction at 0.5 mm may comprise 1–200 or more images, a data set from a peripheral CT angiogram of the lower extremities might include several thousand images, due to the craniocaudal extent of imaging from the diaphragm to the toes. As a result, some readers prefer thicker slices or coronal plane images for initial evaluation, and reserve the use of thin slices for a more limited, adjunctive role in problem solving. Alternatively, most 3-D workstations have options for subvolume selection, which enables evaluation of the arterial tree in an incremental fashion, allowing larger data sets to be evaluated, with enhanced multiplanar reformatting capabilities.

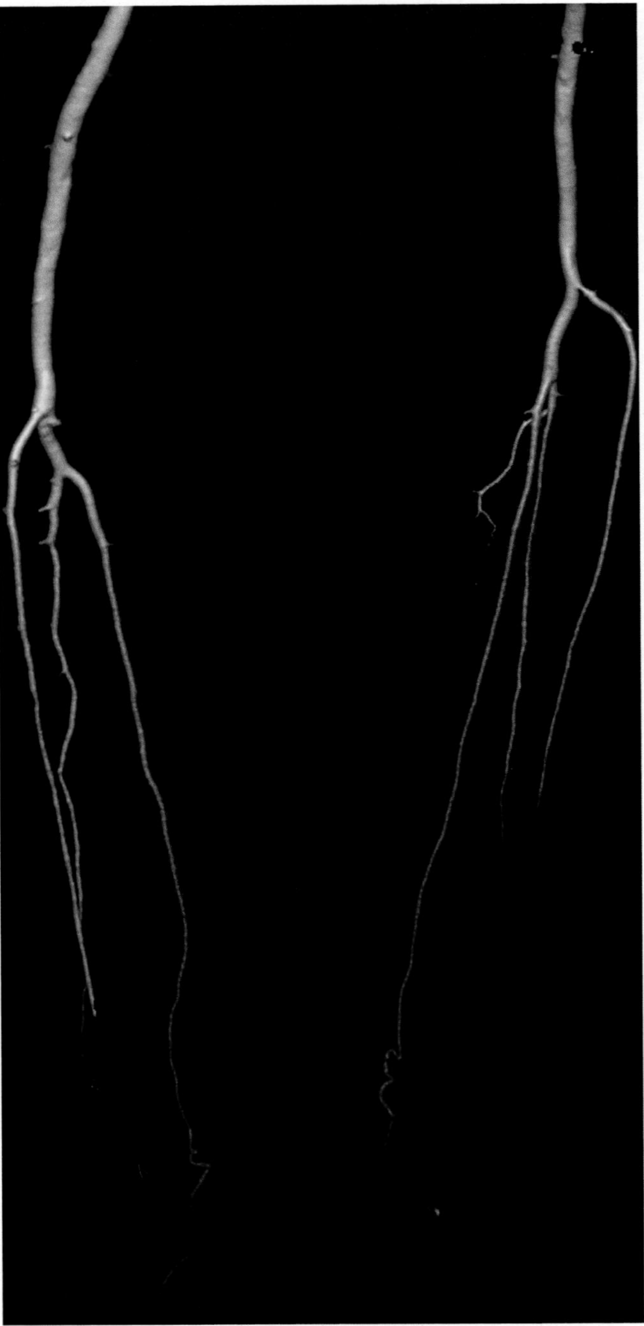

Fig. 17.1 A 3-D reconstruction demonstrating that the run-off vessels are less well opacified than the popliteal arteries, likely related to slight outpacing of the contrast bolus by the speed of the scanner

Dual Energy and Dual Source CT

The advent of dual source and dual energy scanning has enabled a new set of advantages of CT imaging for the peripheral vascular tree. It should be noted that the descriptors of "dual energy" and "dual source" CT are sometimes used interchangeably, although there are differences between the terms. Dual source CT is a technique of scanning with orthogonally positioned CT acquisition systems (including x-ray source and x-ray detector) mounted to the same gantry. This enables fast and essentially simultaneous acquisition of scan data with two separate energies. The main advantage of dual source CT is that scanning at two different energies can

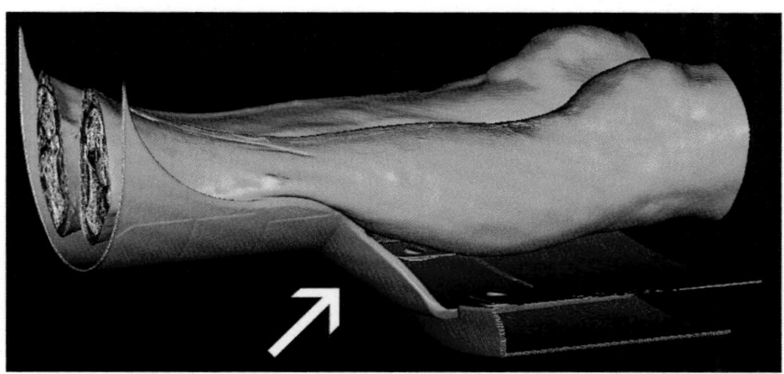

Fig. 17.2 Reconstructed volume projections can demonstrate the soft tissue anatomy. The lower extremities should be closely apposed to one another in order to minimize the dimensions of the reconstructed field of view. In this case, this is achieved by use of a table extension (*white arrow*)

be obtained rapidly, resulting in excellent temporal resolution with minimal mismatch between acquisitions. However, dual source CT scanning is one means of obtaining scan data at two different energies, and is therefore, best considered a subtype of dual energy CT. Other means of scanning at two energies are available, including rapid switching of kilovolt potentials (kVp) of the x-ray generating tube, or selective detector arrays which are sensitive to different types of radiation.

Dual energy scanning using sequential scanning with two different energies has been a research tool since soon after the advent of CT [1]. The development of more advanced CT acquisition techniques has enabled dual energy CT using dual source CT scanners and other techniques to be commercially available since 2006 [2]. A further, more extensive discussion of the physics of dual energy and dual source CT is beyond the scope of this chapter, but typically, the two energies during which scanning is performed are 80 and 140 kV.

There are several potential advantages of dual energy CT, including plaque characterization and improvement of contrast visualization. In peripheral CT angiography, the main advantage of scanning at two energies is that higher energy scan data can be obtained, resulting in selective subtraction of higher attenuation materials, such as calcium or stent material [3]. As a result, the contrast column within the vessel can be depicted more easily, without obscuration or blooming from high attenuation calcium or stent wall (Fig. 17.3).

Contrast Administration

As with imaging other vasculature, rapid rates of contrast administration are critical in obtaining optimal peripheral vascular opacification. Consequently, a more central, large bore, venous access line (usually consisting of an 18-gauge catheter in the antecubital fossa) is highly preferable to a smaller or more peripheral venous access site. Most studies for peripheral CT angiography report contrast rates of 3.5–4.0 ccs per second as optimal [4–6]. Since the area scanned in imaging the peripheral arterial tree is significantly larger in craniocaudal extent compared to the coronary tree, a more prolonged bolus of contrast, with a slightly slower rate of delivery is preferable to ensure homogeneous, persistent, bright opacification of the peripheral arteries. This injection rate is slightly slower than the rate employed for imaging the heart, which may be as high as 5–6 ccs per second [7], since the aim of peripheral CT angiography is a sustained peak of bright opacification, whereas in coronary CT, prolongation of peak contrast opacification is a less important factor. Patients are usually given a formulation of intravenous contrast with 300–400 mg of iodine per mL, with 120–180 ccs of contrast given depending on each patient's body surface area [8]. The total amount of contrast, however, may be reduced when scanners with higher numbers of detectors are used [9, 10]. Higher iodine concentrations have been demonstrated to have higher attenuation levels when the aortic enhancement is compared [11]. Larger amounts of contrast are needed in patients who are taller or are more obese [8].

Administration of a saline chaser is useful in ensuring a higher degree of opacification, and also in prolonging the plateau of attenuation once the peak is reached. A saline chaser is also useful in diminishing the total amount of contrast needed for optimal opacification [12, 13]. Saline injection can also clear residual contrast from the central venous system. Central venous? stasis of contrast can impede imaging of the central upper extremity arteries due to streaking as a result of dense contrast in the superior vena cava, brachiocephalic veins, or other venous structures. When imaging the upper extremities, contrast injection should be made via the extremity contralateral to the area of interest to avoid this pitfall. Optimal timing for acquisition varies significantly in each patient. In patients with normal cardiac function, a rapid acquisition of images may outpace the bolus of contrast. In patients with depressed cardiac function or arterial pathology, the scanning time should be prolonged to ensure scanning is not performed before arrival of the contrast bolus [14]. At our institution, in patients with suspected atherosclerotic disease, the lower extremities are scanned twice, with a second acquisition beginning just above the knees and timed immediately after the first acquisition. This second acquisition enhances visualization of arterial structures, although there may be significant venous contamination at the time of a second scan, which may make 3-D reconstructions somewhat difficult to evaluate.

Several techniques for ensuring optimal arterial timing may be employed. A timing bolus utilizes injection of a small amount of contrast with serial images through a region of interest (ROI) in order to predict the timing of bolus arrival. This is somewhat problematic in evaluating the

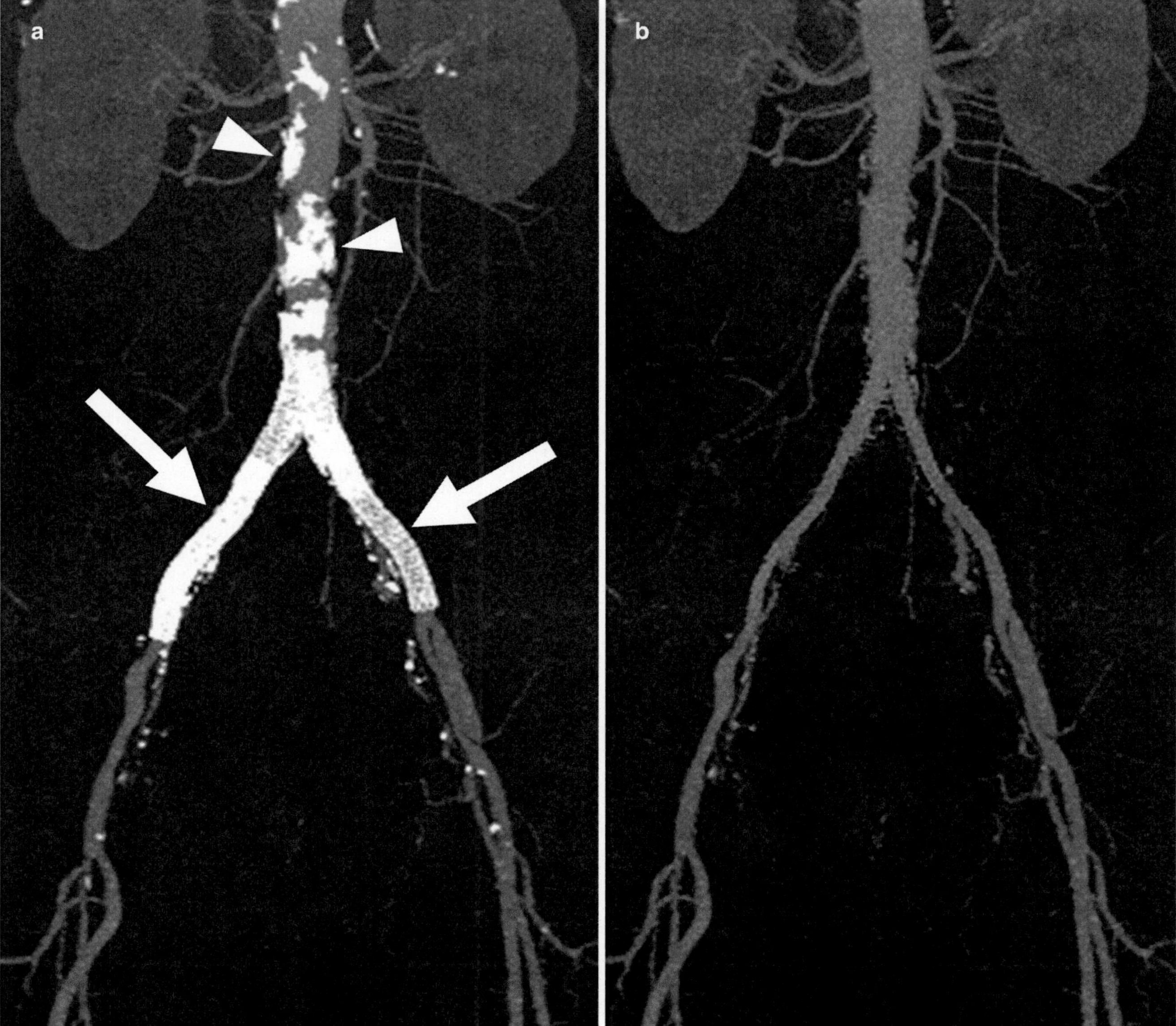

Fig. 17.3 Frontal, thick volume, maximum intensity projection CT images are shown with bone removal. The scan is obtained with dual energy CT, enabling subtraction imaging. Images are shown before (**a**) and after (**b**) subtraction of high attenuation materials, including the bilateral common iliac artery stents (*white arrows*) and calcified plaque in the aorta (*white arrowheads*). Subtraction of high attenuation structures, including stents and vascular calcifications is one of the advantages of dual energy, dual source CT

peripheral arterial tree, since different portions may be opacified at different times, depending on the degree of upstream disease. This technique also necessitates two separate injections with an initial, small bolus. Because only a small, initial dose of contrast is used though, the total amount of contrast is generally not significantly impacted. This technique may also help in preparing the patient for the clinical, physiologic manifestations such as sensory warmth and a metallic taste which commonly ensue after contrast administration.

Alternatively, bolus tracking can be performed with the main contrast injection. With this technique, an ROI within the aorta is serially scanned during the injection of contrast. When the attenuation value reaches a particular, preset threshold, scanning of the remainder of the field of view is initiated. At our institution, for peripheral CT angiography of the lower extremities, an attenuation value of 180 Hounsfield units (HU) is employed, and the ROI is placed in the infrarenal aorta. Alternatively, the ROI can also be placed in the lower extremity arteries, such as the femoral arteries. This technique has the pitfall of being affected by patient motion, and may require some technologist expertise in identifying the vessel. When bolus triggering is used, the ROI is generally positioned to include approximately half of the diameter of the vessel. Different vendor-specific protocols are available for automated contrast monitoring. For slower scanners, a lower threshold (100 HU) may be used to ensure that the speed of scanning matches arrival of the contrast bolus [15]. A significant limitation of the bolus tracking technique is that the ROI may be placed within an area of thrombus or in the false lumen of a dissection. If this occurs, opacification within the ROI may not be achieved, and scanning might be incorrectly delayed.

Preset timing of scanning uses a fixed time interval between initiation of contrast administration and scanning. This is less commonly employed at most institutions, especially for imaging peripheral arteries. This technique may be especially problematic in patients with atherosclerotic disease and in patients with low cardiac output, where the bolus will be circulated through the arteries more slowly. For the upper extremities, scanning may be initiated 20 s after the start of contrast injection. For the lower extremities, scanning may be initiated 50 s after the beginning of injection [16].

Techniques for Interpreting Studies

Several studies have demonstrated an excellent accuracy of CT in comparison to conventional digital subtraction angiography (DSA), based solely on evaluation of transverse images [17, 18]. In many early studies, only the transverse axial data set was evaluated. The transverse plane of the body is in a relatively perpendicular axis to the long arteries of the extremities, resulting in views which approximate the short axis plane of much of the vascular tree with minimal technical manipulation of data sets. For a more accurate interpretation, final review of studies at a dedicated 3-D workstation is commonly employed. Key images for demonstrating stenoses or other vascular pathology are subsequently also sent to archiving and communication systems (PACS) to illustrate important findings.

In addition to the evaluation of transverse axial data sets, review of long and short axis planes utilizing multiplanar reformatted views (MPR), thick maximum intensity projection views (MIP) (Fig. 17.4), and curvilinear plane reformatted views (CPR) (Fig. 17.5) result in a more thorough assessment of the peripheral vascular tree and in improved sensitivity and specificity for depicting disease [19]. Review of the transverse axial views is the usual starting point for most readers. Reformatting data along the plane of the vessel utilizing MPR views introduces few artifacts, as long as scans are obtained using isotropic voxels. MIP views generally demonstrate the higher attenuation values within a thick slab of the data set, and are useful for demonstrating the

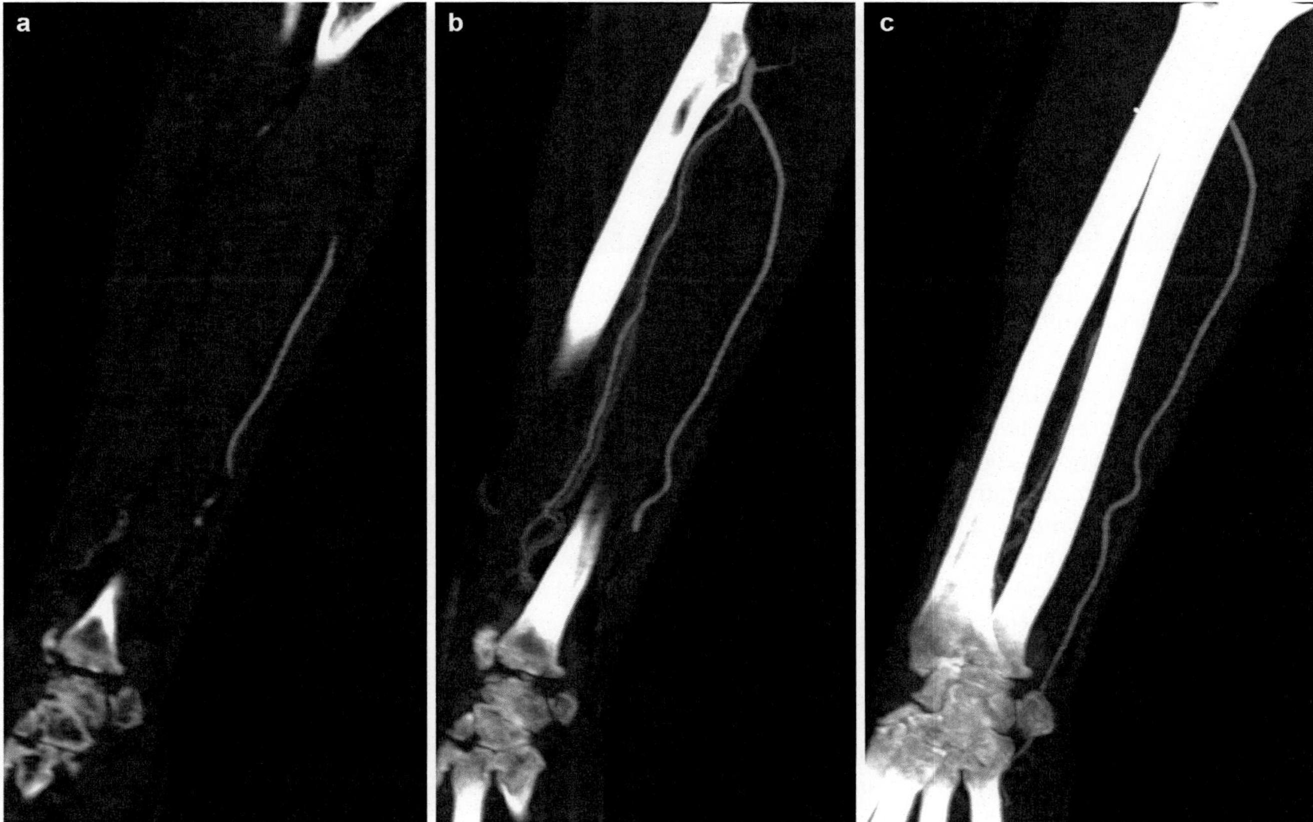

Fig. 17.4 A reformatted view through the radial artery is shown (**a**). On the progressively thicker maximum intensity projection (MIP) views obtained with a thickness of 2 cm (**b**) and 4 cm (**c**), a greater length of the arterial anatomy is demonstrated. MIP views are also useful for demonstrating high attenuation structures such as bones and stents

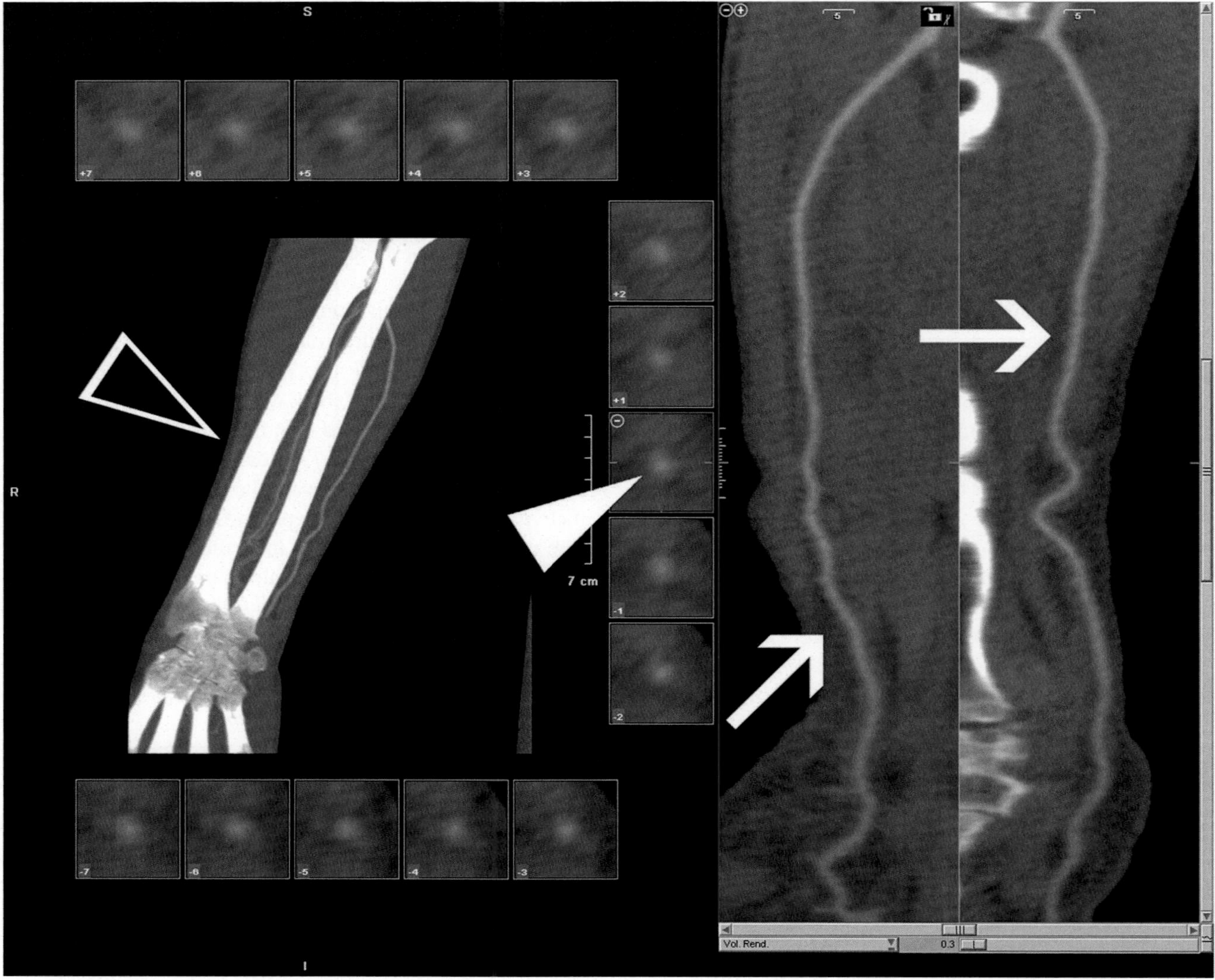

Fig. 17.5 Curved planar reformatted views show the long axis, orthogonal (*white arrows*) and short axis (*closed arrowhead*) of arterial structures. This is contrasted with the MIP MPR view (*open arrowhead*)

course of a tortuous vessel. MIP views are also useful for demonstrating other high attenuation structures such as stents (Fig. 17.6a), surgical clips, calcifications, and osseous structures. CPR images introduce some potential artifacts, as computer algorithms select the center line to be followed. Frequently, computer-generated center lines may drift into an area of calcification in the wall, and may make a stenosis appear more severe. User-directed CPR images may be created, but are commonly time consuming and require some expertise to generate. Unlike evaluation of the coronary arteries, CPR images are less susceptible to artifacts in the large vessels of the extremities, where arteries course in relatively straight planes. Three-dimensional views are usually demonstrated with a lit projection and are helpful in demonstrating anatomic relationships, though they are problematic for demonstrating or grading stenoses (Fig. 17.6b).

Newer tools enable color-coding of vessels to bring attention to areas of plaque. Techniques are also available for characterization of atherosclerotic lesions with respect to attenuation values in order to classify lesions as fatty, fibrous, or calcified. These tools may be used adjunctively to the techniques described earlier, but have yet to be rigorously evaluated or validated.

Validation of Peripheral CT Angiography

Advancement in CT technology has been rapid, with the recent advent of isotropic voxel imaging and multi-detector CT. The pace of technological advancement has surpassed the rate at which newer technologies are validated. For this reason, large multicenter studies and meta-analyses likely underestimate the accuracy of CT angiography as a tool.

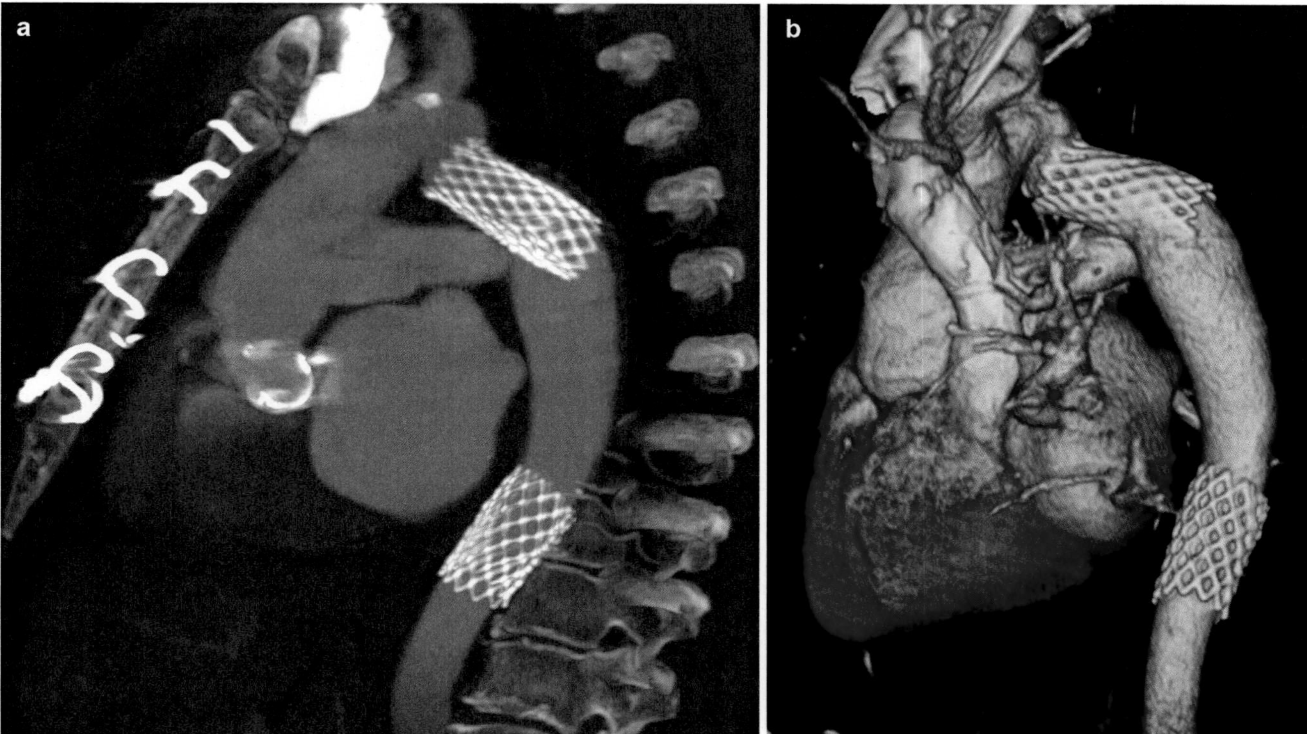

Fig. 17.6 The thick MIP view (**a**) demonstrates the aortic stents. They are also well-seen on the volume rendered view (**b**) in this patient who is status post aortic stenting after repair for aortic coarctation and a bicuspid aortic valve

Large studies have, however, demonstrated several significant advantages of CT angiography in comparison to DSA, including a fourfold lower radiation dose and a much lower risk of complications. Moreover, studies have shown an excellent accuracy for the diagnosis of atherosclerotic disease as well as excellent correlation with DSA [20]. Diagnostic CT angiography performs comparably to DSA and favorably compares to duplex ultrasound and MR angiography for the evaluation in patients with chronic peripheral arterial disease or traumatic vascular injuries [21].

Compared to other non-invasive imaging modalities such as ultrasonography and MRA, CTA possesses several advantages. CTA reproducibility does not significantly depend on variability of technical skills as is oftentimes the limitation of ultrasonography. In patients with multilevel peripheral arterial disease, ultrasonography assessment has poor specificity to localize lesions, and is hindered by an impractical amount of time consumed in such extensive clinical evaluation. MRI angiography may have limitations in patients with stents, surgical clips, or other devices, and is problematic in patients with non-MR conditional cardiac devices.

A study evaluating CT angiography with 64-row detector scanners for the detection of peripheral vascular disease evaluated 840 segments of the systemic arteries in 28 patients with lower extremity claudication. This study found an overall diagnostic accuracy of 98 % in the detection of lesions with a degree of stenosis of 50 % or higher. The sensitivity and specificity for detecting stenoses by CT angiography were 99 % and 98 %, respectively [21]. Moreover, the use of advanced imaging tools, including 3-D reconstructions and multiplanar reformatted views, provide detailed visualization of stenotic lesions, normal vasculature, or previously revascularized lower extremity arteries along with nearby extravascular structures. Augmenting axial images with reformatted views has been shown to improve accuracy of interpretation [22].

Due to the speed and accessibility of imaging, CTA is also extremely useful in diagnosing acute limb ischemia and critical limb ischemia, helping clinicians to promptly and effectively formulate treatment plans. CTA also possesses advantages in depicting peripheral vascular aneurysms, providing clear, comprehensive images and precise dimensions along with delineating involvement of adjacent vessels and structures. Thus, CTA is a useful diagnostic and surveillance tool for aneurysm detection and follow-up.

Role of Peripheral CT Angiography for the Vascular Physician

The most important application of CT angiography for the vascular interventional specialist is pre-procedure planning, including: selection of patients best treated with endovascular intervention versus open surgical procedures, identification of vascular access sites, pre-procedure selection of

Table 17.1 Advantages of CT angiography in patients with peripheral arterial disease prior to endovascular interventions

1. Selection of patients for endovascular versus open surgical revascularization.
2. Vascular access selection.
3. Lesion characterization (thrombus, degree of calcification, lesion length, vessel size).
4. Arterial vascular inflow and outflow.
5. Selection of interventional angiographic views and angulations.
6. Equipment selection based on lesion characteristics and vessel size (thrombolysis, sheaths, wires, balloons, stents, atherectomy, distal embolic protection).
7. Decreased contrast use.
8. Decreased radiation exposure.
9. Evaluation of extravascular arterial disease (popliteal entrapment, cystic adventitial disease, bony exostosis, thoracic outlet syndrome).

appropriate angiographic views, and pre-procedural lesion characterization (thrombus burden, dissection, calcification, tortuosity, etc.). CT angiography also provides valuable information for tailoring the most appropriate endovascular therapy, including: thrombolysis, laser, directional or orbital atherectomy, reentry device, distal embolic protection device, balloon angioplasty, self-expanding or balloon expandable stents, and covered stents (Table 17.1).

Patients who undergo intervention for peripheral arterial disease have a higher incidence of vascular access site complications compared to patients who undergo percutaneous coronary intervention [23]. Patients with peripheral atherosclerotic disease commonly have a high burden of diffuse, often densely calcified, atherosclerotic plaques. As a result, vascular access selection is important to ensure safe and successful peripheral interventions. The atherosclerotic burden in some patients may prevent adequate hemostasis, which predisposes these patients to hemorrhagic complications at access sites. CT angiography offers an overall view of the arterial system and, therefore, may allow for identification of the most appropriate access site for peripheral interventions. In patients with severe, diffuse disease, alternative access sites or techniques (brachial, popliteal, antegrade, bypass grafts) may be utilized.

CT angiography also helps in the decision to use distal embolic protection devices, especially in cases where there is heavy atherosclerotic burden, soft or unstable plaque, or thrombus. The choice of an appropriate device for the protection against distal embolization may be guided by vessel anatomy, tortuosity, and landing zone anatomy.

Normal Peripheral Arterial Anatomy and Variants

Symptomatic manifestations of arterial diseases may appear in the distal extremities, but may also arise from disease which is proximal and remote to the site of symptoms. For example, non-healing ulcers in the toes as a result of ischemia may arise from stenosis as far proximal as the aorta. Since disease anywhere in the arterial tree may produce symptoms, knowledge of normal anatomy of the entire arterial tree is necessary in order to accurately interpret peripheral CT angiography.

Upper Extremities

The normal upper extremity arterial supply begins with the subclavian arteries. The left subclavian artery typically arises directly from the aortic arch. The right subclavian artery most commonly arises from the brachiocephalic (innominate) artery, which typically gives off a right common carotid artery as well a right subclavian artery. In 15 % of patients, the innominate artery also gives off the left common carotid artery, a variant described as a bovine arch. In these patients, the left common carotid artery commonly arises as the first vessel off of the bovine innominate, although it may arise more cranially as a trifurcation vessel of the innominate artery [24].

Other commonly encountered variants of aberrant origination of the subclavian artery exist. An aberrant right subclavian artery may either arise from a left sided aortic arch, as the last major vessel from the arch (left arch with aberrant right subclavian artery) (Fig. 17.7). In the case of a right aortic arch, the left subclavian artery may arise as the last major vessel from the arch (right arch with aberrant left subclavian artery). In either case, the aberrant subclavian artery usually takes a course posterior to the esophagus and may produce dysphagia, which is commonly referred to as dysphagia lusoria. A double aortic arch may also cause dysphagia lusoria [25]. In addition, an aberrant subclavian artery may arise from a dilated trunk, termed a diverticulum of Kommerel. This is a true aneurysm that likely results from an embryological remnant of a separate, incompletely formed aortic arch. Both the double aortic arch and the right arch with an aberrant left subclavian artery represent vascular rings. In the latter case, the ring is completed by the ligamentum arteriosum. Clinically significant atherosclerotic occlusive complication rates resulting from aberrant subclavian arteries are likely similar to rates of atherosclerotic complications observed in normal arteries, although aberrant subclavian arteries are more prone to aneurysmal degeneration.

Anatomically, the subclavian artery is divided into proximal, middle, and distal portions. The proximal portion of the subclavian artery is defined as the portion medial to the anterior scalene muscle. The mid portion of the subclavian artery is located posterior to the anterior scalene muscle and usually contains the most cranial portion of the subclavian arch. The distal portion of the subclavian artery lies lateral to the lateral border of the anterior scalene muscle and ends at the lateral border of the first rib. At this point the subclavian artery changes name to become the axillary artery.

The vertebral artery is usually the first vessel that arises from the subclavian artery and most commonly arises from the

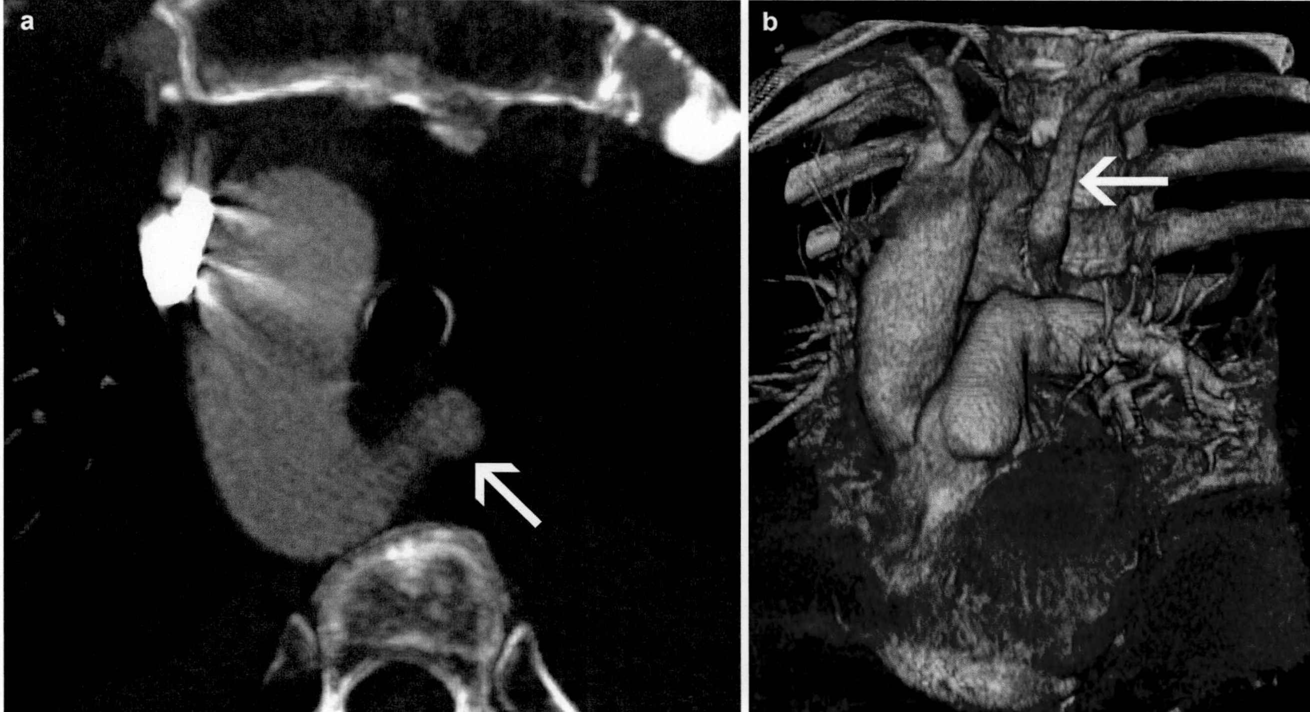

Fig. 17.7 On this CT scan of the chest performed to evaluate for an etiology of shortness of breath, a right-sided aortic arch with an aberrant left subclavian artery (*white arrow*) is incidentally noted. This is shown on the transverse view (**a**) and volume rendered (**b**) view

first portion of the subclavian artery, usually within 1.2–2.5 cm of the vessel origin. The other vessels include the internal mammary artery (Fig. 17.8), thyrocervical trunk, and costocervical trunk. These vessels also most commonly arise from the first portion of the subclavian artery and are usually clustered near the medial border of the anterior scalene muscle.

At the lateral border of the first rib, the subclavian artery transitions to become the axillary artery, which proceeds to predominantly supply arterial blood flow to the upper chest wall and the proximal portion of the upper extremity. In the case of axillary artery occlusion proximal to the origin of the subscapular artery, collateral flow may be provided through chest wall and scapular collaterals. By definition, the axillary artery ends at the lateral border of the teres major, where it changes name to become the brachial artery. The axillary artery is surrounded by the brachial plexus.

The brachial artery is the main vessel to the upper extremity. Most commonly, the brachial artery gives off a profunda branch in the upper portion of the upper extremity. Below the elbow, the brachial artery usually trifurcates into a radial artery laterally and a common trunk that gives off an interosseous artery and an ulnar artery medially. In 15 % of patients, the brachial artery gives off the radial artery proximal to the elbow as it courses in the upper arm. The radial or ulnar artery may rarely arise aberrantly from the axillary artery. There is a close relationship with the median nerve which normally runs just medial to the brachial artery throughout the upper arm. The median nerve may overlie the brachial artery rendering it vulnerable to injury during brachial artery access.

Lower Extremity

The aortic bifurcation most commonly occurs at the level of the L4 vertebral body, although some patients may have an unusually high aortic bifurcation as a normal variant. The common iliac arteries are usually 4–5 cm in length, although the right common iliac artery is usually slightly longer than the left. The common iliac arteries course medial to the psoas muscles and beneath the ureters to the inferior pelvic brim before bifurcating into external and internal branches. The common iliac artery may give rise to an iliolumbar trunk, which can be a source of endoleak in patients who have undergone aortic aneurysm repair. Accessory renal arteries may rarely arise from the common iliac arteries, especially when a pelvic or ptotic kidney is present.

The internal iliac artery runs posteriorly from the common iliac artery, and subsequently gives off anterior and posterior divisions. The main branch of the posterior division is the superior gluteal artery, which exits the sciatic foramen. The posterior division may also give rise to an iliolumbar artery. The anterior division gives off several important branches including the internal pudendal artery, and the uterine artery in women. The external iliac artery courses more anteriorly in comparison to the internal iliac artery. Below the inguinal ligament, it changes name to become the common femoral artery. Vascular landmarks for the inguinal ligament are the origins of the deep circumflex iliac artery and the inferior extent of the inferior epigastric artery, which also mark the delineation between external iliac artery and

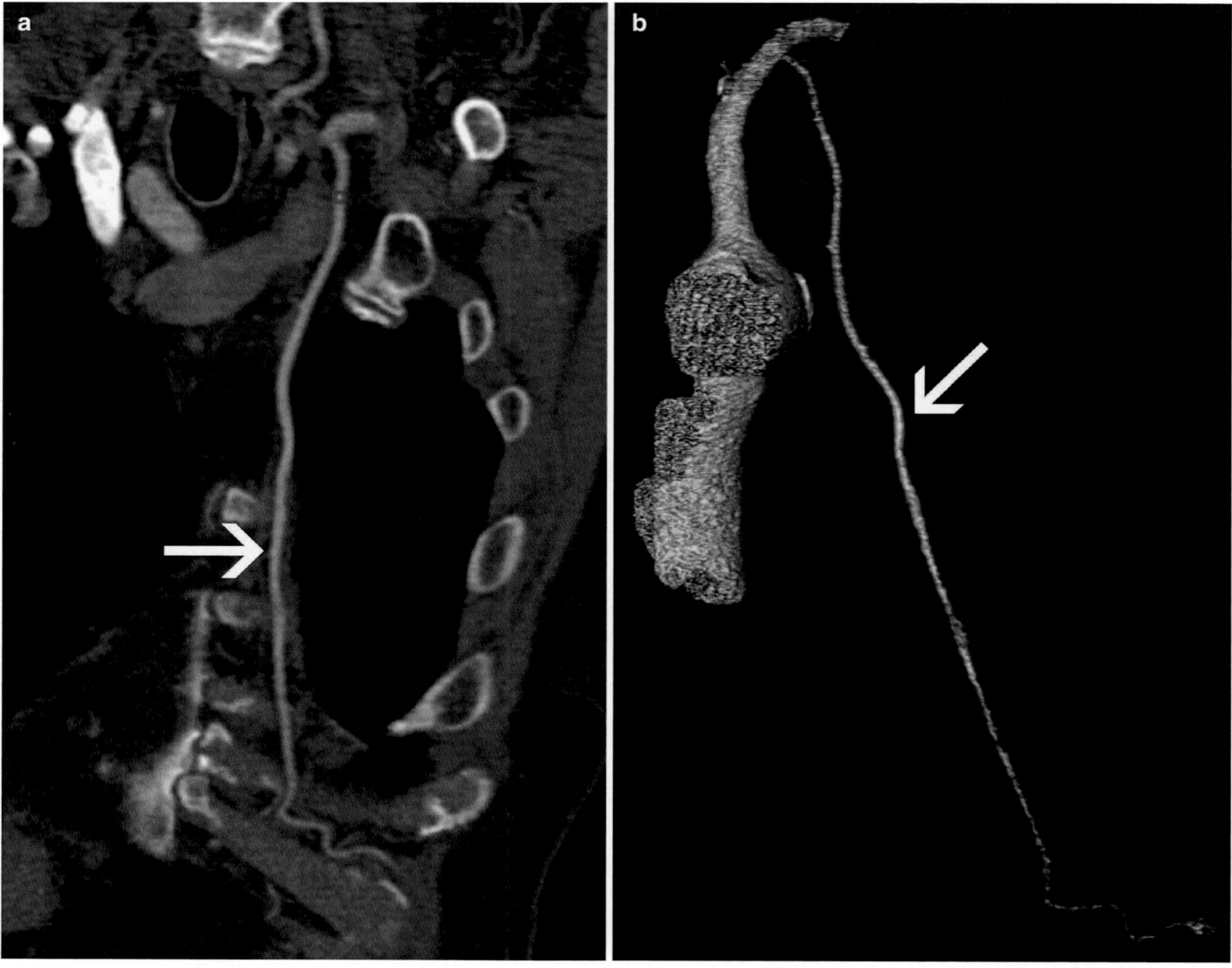

Fig. 17.8 CT angiography is useful in demonstrating the internal mammary arteries in patients in whom aortocoronary bypass is planned. The course of the left internal mammary artery (*white arrows*) is demonstrated on the curved plane reformatted view (**a**) and also on the volume rendered view (**b**). In evaluating the subclavian artery and its branches, injection of contrast should be made via the contralateral extremity in order to ensure that streaking from dense venous contrast does not occur

common femoral artery. The external iliac artery gives off other small branches, such as small muscular branches and the cremasteric artery, which runs in the spermatic cord.

The common femoral artery, which begins below the inguinal ligament, is a short vessel which usually has a length of 4 cm and gives off the superficial femoral artery and deep femoral artery at approximately the level of the lesser trochanter of the femur. Most commonly, there is also a slightly more lateral branch given off at the same level, which is the circumflex femoral artery. The term "superficial femoral artery" is still used commonly by physicians, whereas anatomists favor the name "femoral artery". In regard to femoral venous anatomy, there has been some shift in nomenclature among physicians in order to avoid confusion when thrombi of the vein are reported. Drop of the descriptor "superficial" from the femoral vein can avoid confusion as the vein is part of the deep venous system.

The femoral artery courses anteromedially in the thigh. In the middle third of the thigh, the femoral artery enters the adductor canal or eponymously, Hunter's canal. This is a frequent site of atherosclerotic disease. At the junction of the middle and lower third of the thigh, the femoral artery exits the adductor canal and changes name to the popliteal artery. The popliteal artery is a common site of several unique diseases including cystic adventitial disease and popliteal artery entrapment syndrome. Knee dislocation injuries may damage the popliteal artery. At approximately the level of the knee, the popliteal artery gives off medial and lateral geniculate branches. These branches may serve as important collaterals for reconstitution of the popliteal artery from the profunda using geniculate collateral pathways in the setting of femoral artery occlusion.

The popliteal artery continues behind the knee and gives off the anterior tibial artery. In most patients, the anterior tibial artery gives off the dorsalis pedis artery, which courses along the dorsal aspect of the foot. The other main branch of the popliteal artery is the tibioperoneal trunk. This divides into the posterior tibial artery and peroneal artery. Variations in this conventional anatomy occur approximately 10 % of the time, with the most common variant being a high takeoff of the anterior tibial at or above the level of the knee joint. A true trifurcation followed by a hypoplastic or absent posterior tibial artery are the next most common variants, while high origin of the posterior tibial artery is rare. The peroneal artery runs in the deep compartment of the lower portion of the lower extremity and usually terminates above the ankle in collateral branches to the posterior tibial and dorsalis pedis arteries. The posterior tibial artery runs posterior to the medial maleolus of the ankle and frequently can be palpated at this point. The plantar arch is an arcade of vessels which may be primarily served by either the dorsalis pedis artery or the posterior tibial artery. The main vessel supplying the plantar arch should be noted and included in CT angiography reports.

CT has an advantage in comparison to conventional angiography in demonstrating 3-D vascular anatomy and variants in the context of muscular and osseous anatomy. Variants which contribute to clinically significant arterial disease are rare and some variants may not cause significant vascular pathology. Rarely, for example, the external iliac artery may be absent, and the common femoral artery arises from the internal iliac artery (Fig. 17.9). This common variant would not be expected to cause clinically significant manifestations of arterial disease [26].

Rarely, the main lower extremity artery may arise from the internal iliac artery, and courses posteriorly to the ischial tuberosity. This variant is known as a persistent sciatic artery. The anomalous course of the artery along the ischial tuberosity can result in premature atherosclerotic disease (Fig. 17.10) and also in formation of aneurysms (Fig. 17.11). Typically, occlusion or aneurysm formation occurs where the artery courses behind the ischial tuberosity. Vascular pathology is thought to occur due to repetitive underlying trauma due to impact of the ischial tuberosity onto the artery [27].

For variants where abnormal muscular anatomy may contribute to pathology, the arterial tree may be better imaged with MRI. In general imaging of the muscular structures of the extremities, MRI has advantages relative to CT angiography,

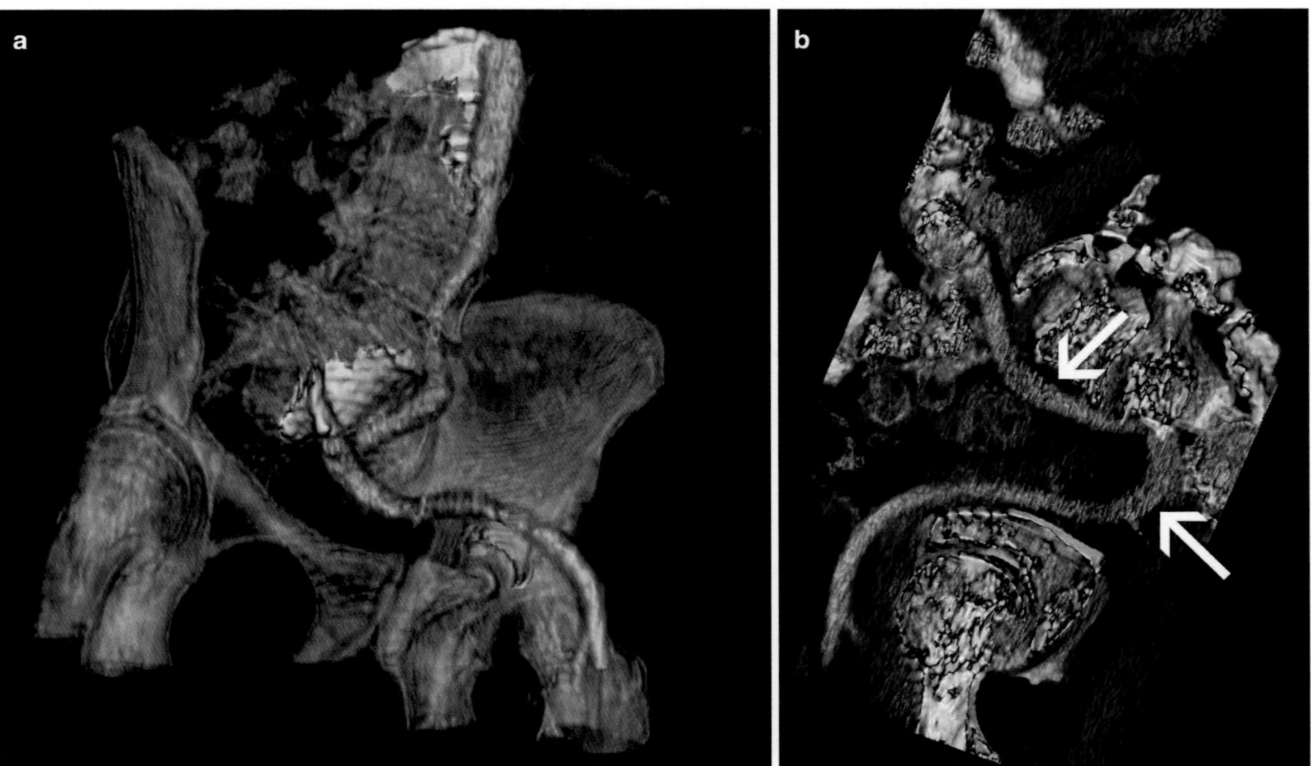

Fig. 17.9 (**a**, **b**) An unusual variant is shown in which there is congenital absence of the external iliac artery. The internal iliac artery (*white arrow*) in this case takes a course posteriorly to give off the anterior and posterior divisions, before continuing anteriorly to give off the common femoral artery

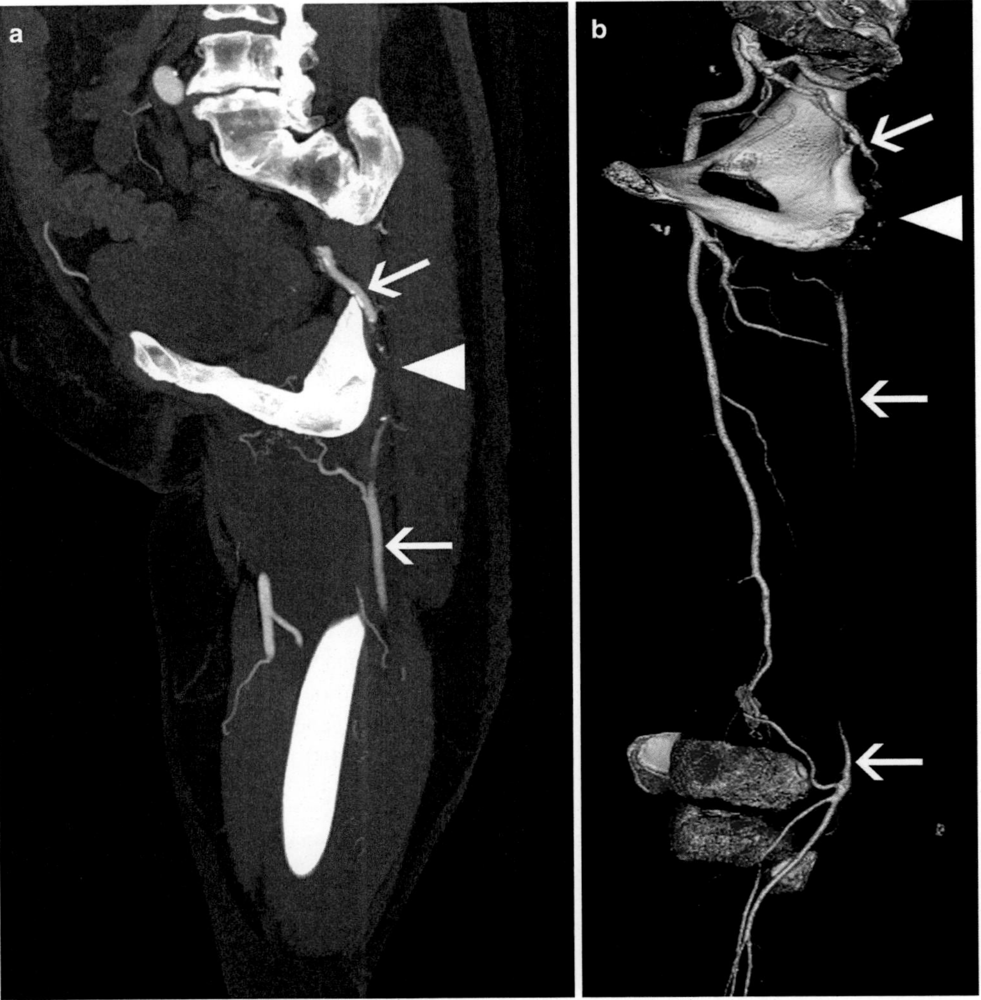

Fig. 17.10 (**a**, **b**) Images of the right lower extremity are shown in a patient with bilateral persistent sciatic arteries. Note that the persistent sciatic artery (*white arrows*) is occluded at the level of the ischial tuberosity (*white arrowhead*). There is also a second long segment of probable occlusion of the persistent sciatic artery in the thigh. There is, however, reconstitution of the vessel via large profunda collaterals after both occlusions

including better resolution of soft tissue structures such as musculature and joints. Non-contrast MR angiography techniques also permit imaging with the extremity in different positions, without the use of ionizing radiation.

Abnormalities and Diseases of the Peripheral Arteries

Atherosclerotic Disease

Atherosclerosis is by far the most common disease of the peripheral arterial tree [28]. At times, patients may present with concomitant cerebrovascular disease and coronary atherosclerotic disease, although some patients with atherosclerotic disease may present with peripheral ischemia as their initial manifestation. The presence of peripheral arterial disease significantly contributes to worsened morbidity and mortality, likely because it is a marker of systemic atherosclerotic disease burden. Patients with peripheral arterial disease have a four to fivefold increase in risk of myocardial infarction or stroke [29, 30].

Peripheral arterial disease is a common condition, occurring in 10–25 % of patients over the age of 55. The incidence increases with age at a rate of 0.3 % per year in men aged 40–55 and at a rate of 1 % per year in men over the age of 75. Up to 70–80 % of affected individuals are symptomatic, although only a minority of patients will eventually require revascularization. Twenty five percent of patients with peripheral arterial disease will require some medical or surgical treatment. Because of their increased morbidity and mortality, all patients with peripheral arterial disease should

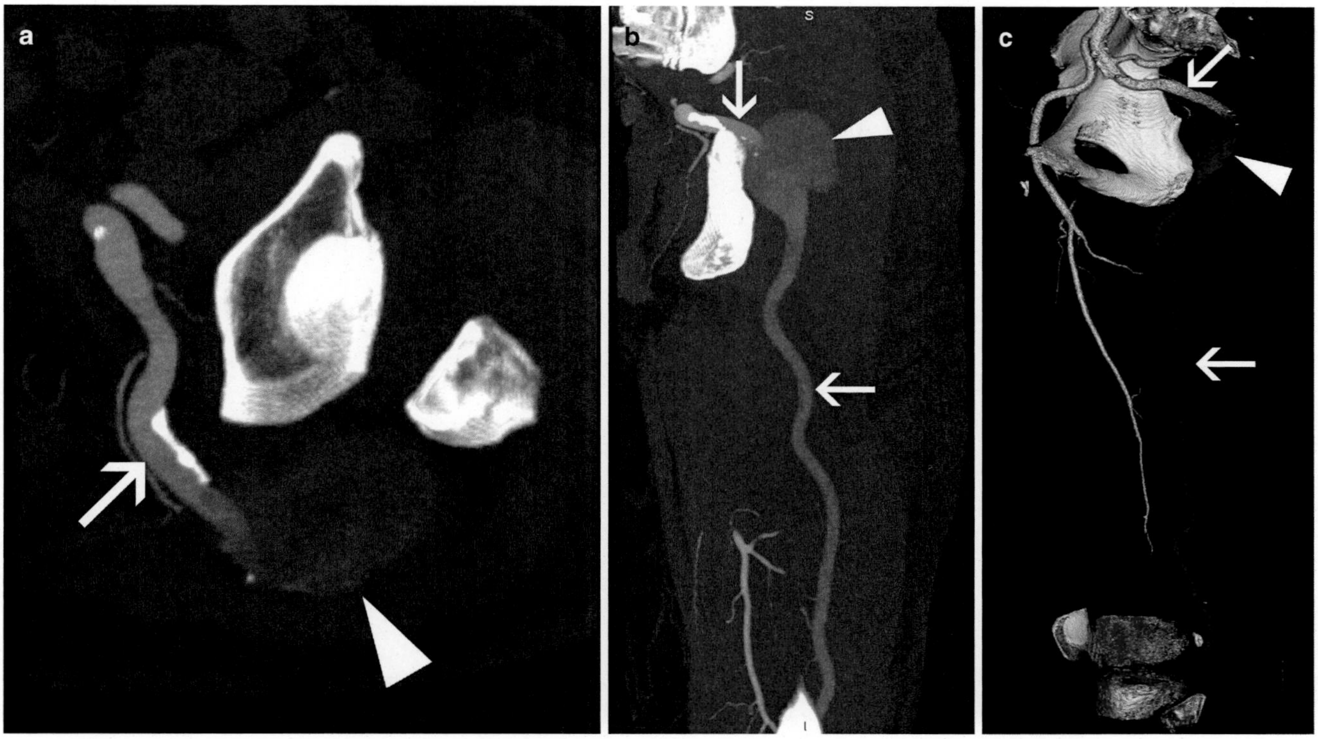

Fig. 17.11 (Same patient as in Fig. 16.9). (**a–c**) Images of the left lower extremity are shown in a patient with bilateral persistent sciatic arteries (*white arrows*). Note the presence of a large aneurysm extending just above the ischial tuberosity (*white arrowhead*). Note also that the vessel is less well opacified distal to the aneurysm due to stagnant flow

have aggressive control of their atherosclerotic risk factors; however, only about 25 % of patients are actually treated [31, 32].

Peripheral CT angiography can demonstrate atherosclerosis at a very early stage in the disease process. Low attenuation plaques, likely related to an early phase of plaque evolution, may be seen [33]. Plaques may be calcified or non-calcified, and may not cause stenosis until very late in the disease course (Fig. 17.12). Densely calcified atherosclerotic plaques in the peripheral arterial tree may somewhat degrade CT angiography image quality, although this is less of a concern when imaging the extremities compared to the coronary arteries due to the larger caliber of vessels and the lower potential for motion and other artifacts.

Atherosclerotic plaques may be present throughout the vascular tree. Typically aortic atherosclerotic disease begins in the infrarenal aorta and becomes more severe closer to the aortic bifurcation. A rarer variant in some patients with atherosclerotic disease is the development of arborified, endoaortic calcified plaques, which predominantly protrude into the lumen, and are usually most pronounced in the juxtamesenteric and juxtarenal aorta. This variant has been termed a "coral reef" aorta (Fig. 17.13) [34]. Recognition of this variant of atherosclerotic disease is important since patients with endoaortic calcific proliferation are at higher risk for post-catheterization embolic phenomenon. It has been suggested that patients with a 'coral reef aorta' should not undergo endovascular interventions which necessitate crossing of the juxtamesenteric aorta should be avoided in patients with a "coral reef aorta" [35, 36].

In the peripheral tree, atherosclerotic disease may be multifocal and usually consists of mixed attenuation plaques. CT angiography is useful in demonstrating stenoses of 50 % or greater, which may contribute to patient symptoms. Specific features of each plaque that should be described include the location of the lesion, degree of stenosis, and length of the plaque. When CT angiography is used for plaque characterization, descriptors for plaque attenuation may be added, with reporting of plaques as calcified, non-calcified, or mixed plaque. Further evaluation of lesions with stenoses is commonly pursued with catheterization for measurement of pressure gradients. Specific criteria for intervention have also been delineated, based on the degree of patient symptoms [37].

Atherosclerotic disease may cause a number of symptoms depending on the site of involvement. Several syndromes have been characterized based on the distribution of atherosclerotic disease. For example, subclavian steal syndrome results from proximal stenosis in the subclavian artery (Fig. 17.14). As a result of stenosis, the distal subclavian artery may receive collateral flow from the vertebral arteries. Reversal of flow through the ipsilateral vertebral artery commonly ensues. Because of the relatively rich brain collateral

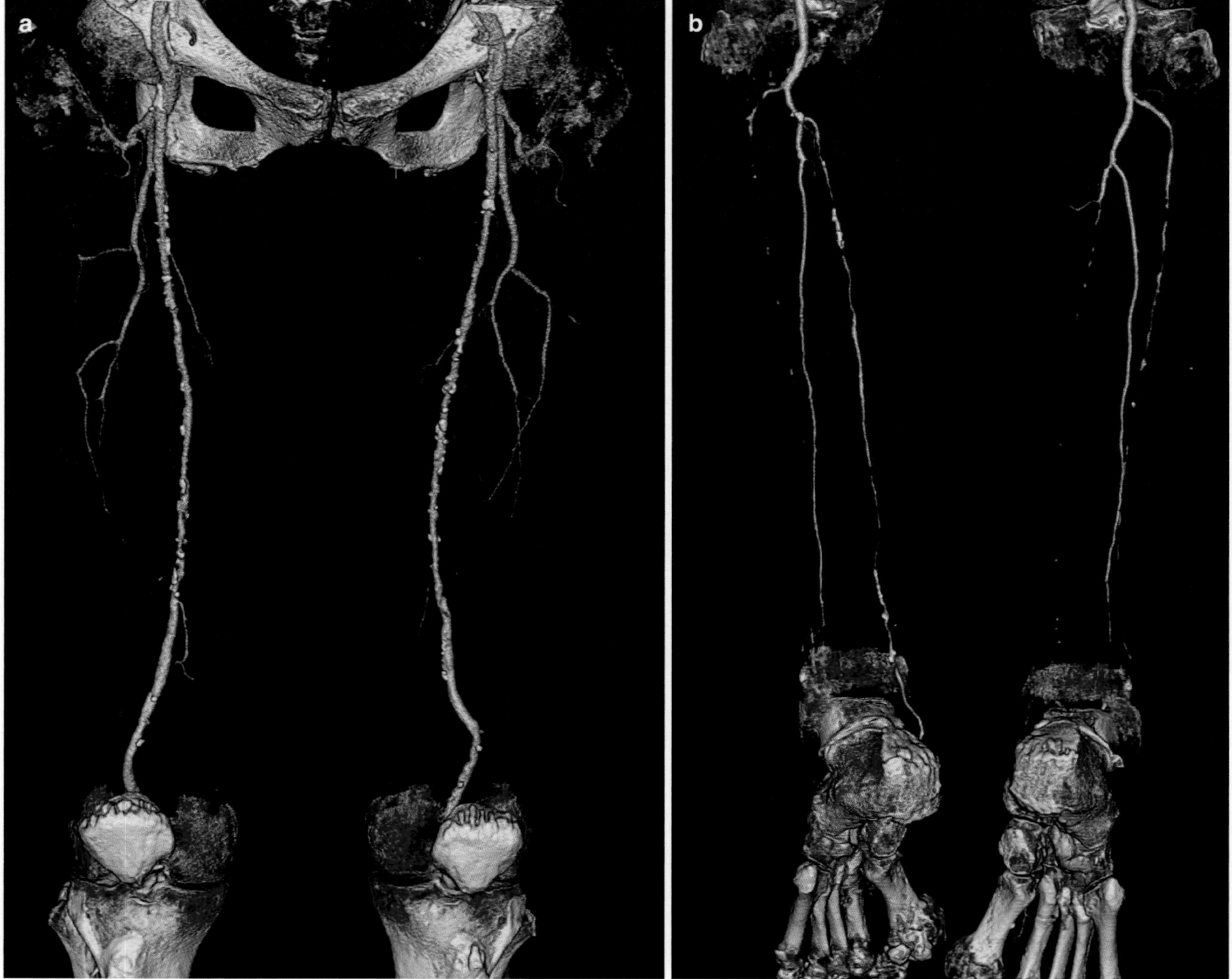

Fig. 17.12 (**a**, **b**) Multifocal atherosclerosis is demonstrated on these volume rendered views of the lower extremities. The femur, tibia, and fibula have been subtracted from the field of view in order to better demonstrate the arterial anatomy

system, only a small percentage of patients with this reversal of flow will present with symptoms related to vertebrobasilar insufficiency. These symptoms are commonly worsened during exercise of the upper extremity, which results in increased flow to the extremity and worsened steal from the cerebrovascular circulation. Leriche syndrome is a constellation of symptoms which results from aortic and bilateral iliac artery disease, including gluteal and lower extremity claudication, penile impotence, and lower extremity atrophy.

Similar to assessment of aortic aneurysms, duplex ultrasound is the most cost effective strategy for surveillance of popliteal or femoral aneurysms. CT angiography, however, is also favored over other imaging modalities for accurate sizing of the proximal and distal arterial landing zones prior to endovascular peripheral aneurysm repair. Evaluation of thrombus and patency of runoff vessels is also easily accomplished by preoperative CT angiography.

Grafts and Stents in the Arterial Tree

In addition to being a non-invasive modality with excellent spatial resolution, CT angiography has several other advantages in the evaluation of the treated vascular system. In comparison to MRI and MR angiography, CT angiography is advantageous for visualization of stents. On MRI, stents may be visualized only as artifacts and the internal lumen may be non-visualized due to susceptibility effects. Even when the internal lumen is visualized, the stented segment generally is incompletely evaluated by MR angiography. Other metallic structures including surgical clips may also induce artifacts on MRI, including signal void and failure of fat saturation, whereas artifacts from surgical devices are generally less significant on CT. Dual source or dual energy CT further potentiates visualization of high attenuation, metallic structures with

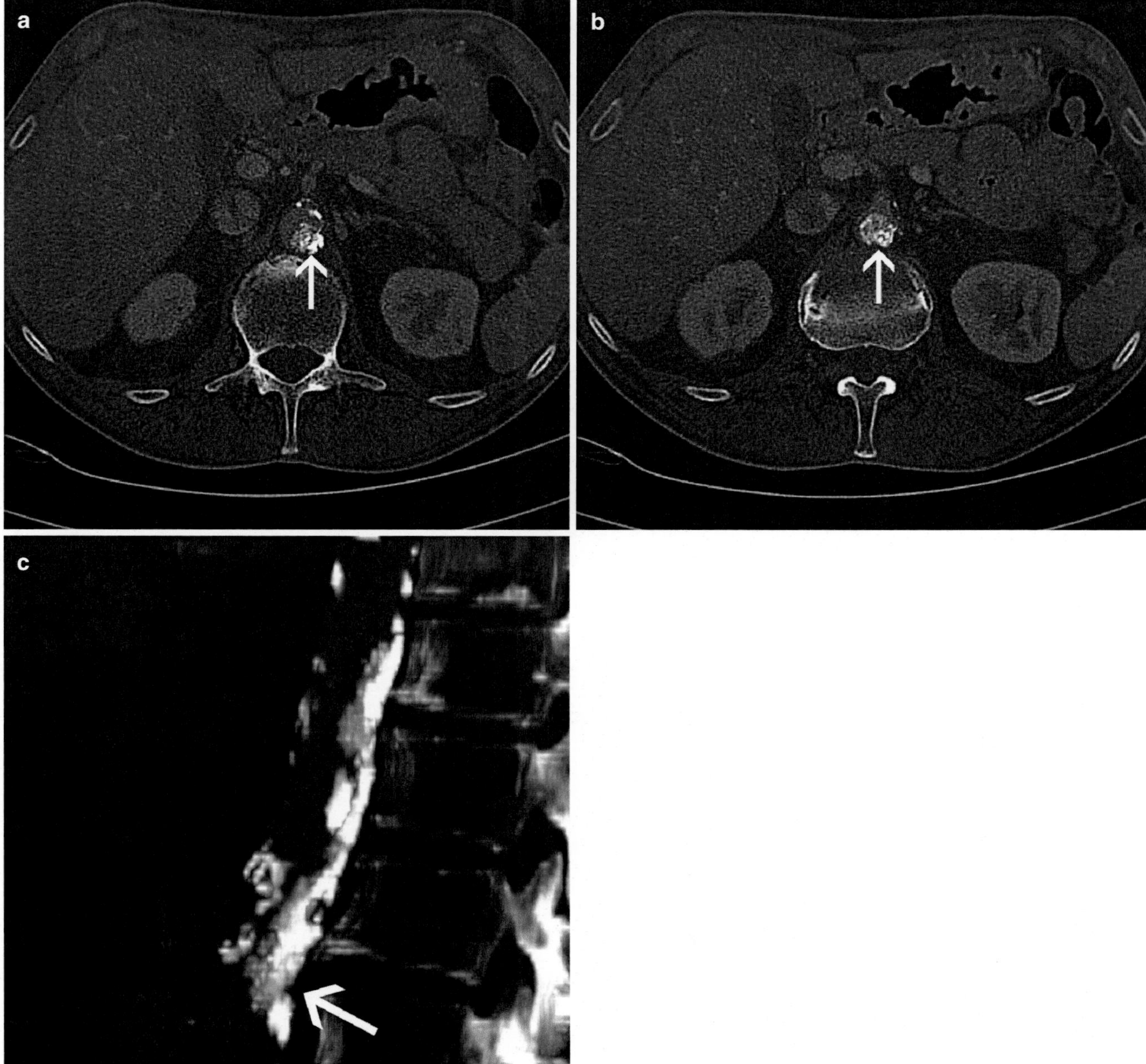

Fig. 17.13 Views from a CT angiogram of the abdomen are shown with transverse (**a**, **b**) and sagittal (**c**) images shown. A "coral reef" aorta is present with dense endoaortic calcific proliferation. Densely calcified, endoluminal, arborified plaques are present (*white arrows*) in the juxtamesenteric aorta

less significant obscuration of adjacent anatomy due to minimizing of streaking.

Stents in peripheral arterial structures are typically well-seen using thick MIP images (Fig. 17.15). This allows visualization of stent struts and exclusion of strut fractures. Stents are easily depicted as high attenuation structures. Stents are frequently well-evaluated on post-contrast and non-contrast images. In the short axis view, stent struts are frequently seen as regularly spaced, hyper-attenuating foci at the rim of the artery, commonly in a hexagonal array (Fig. 17.16). Because of the relatively high attenuation of metallic stents, and because of the phenomenon of "blooming" on CT, a very bright stent may appear to be outside the confines of the wall of a vessel. The limitations of stent depiction on coronary CT are less significant in evaluation of the peripheral arterial tree due to the larger internal diameter of stents commonly employed in the peripheral vessels and also due to the absence of motion and other artifacts that can limit the evaluation of stented coronary arteries. In-stent restenosis in the peripheral vasculature is usually easily evaluated using CT angiography.

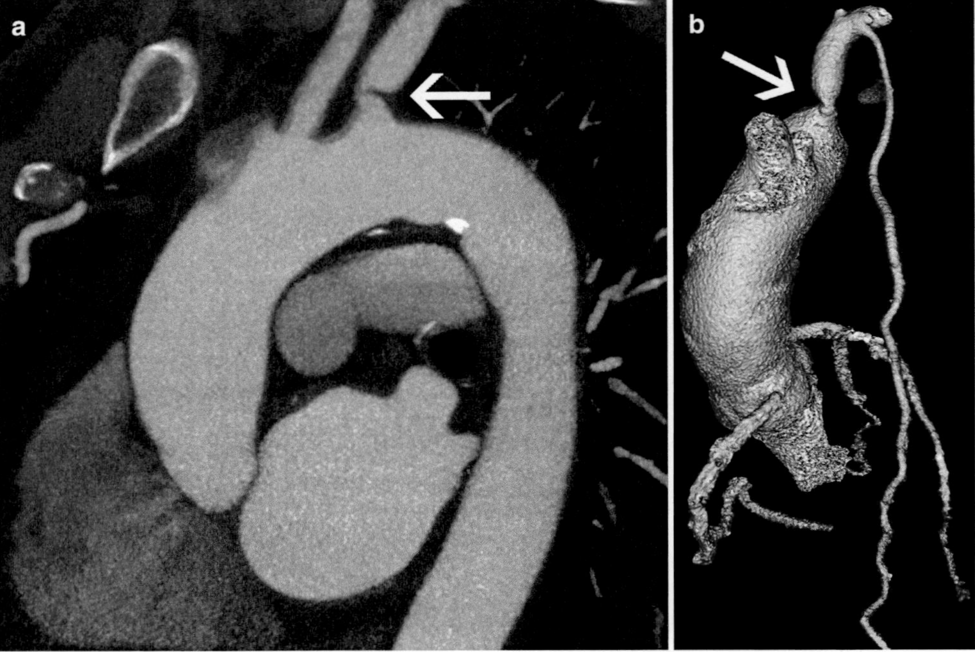

Fig. 17.14 Images from a CT angiogram are shown in a patient with known coronary artery disease and concomitant symptoms of subclavian steal. The oblique sagittal (**a**) and volume rendered (b) views show a focal, shelf-like area of narrowing near the origin of the left subclavian artery (*arrow*, (**a**) and (**b**)). In this case, identification of this stenosis was useful as an explanation of the patient's symptoms. Preoperative identification of subclavian stenosis is also important in patients in whom aortocoronary bypass is planned, as this condition may impede optimal flow through the internal mammary artery

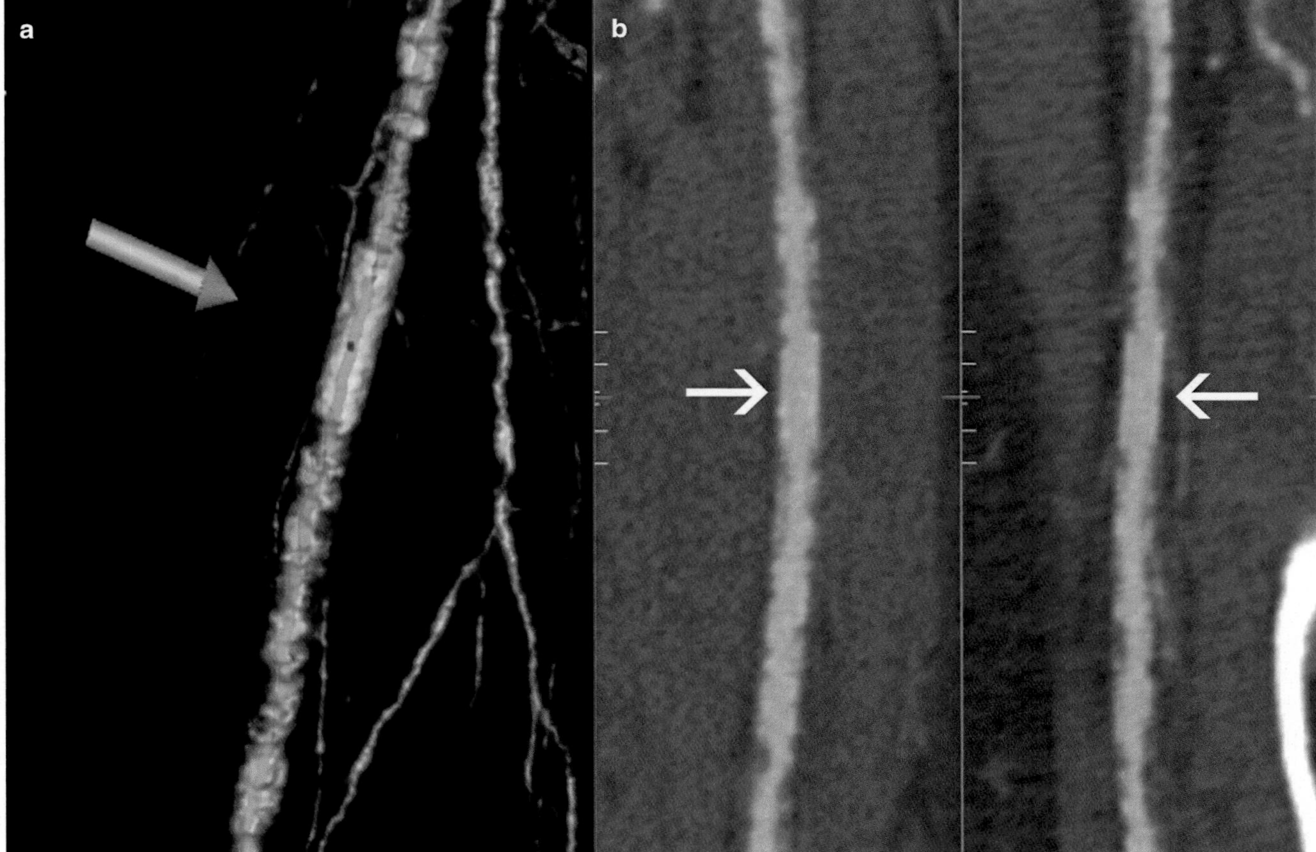

Fig. 17.15 Stents are well-depicted on CT angiography. In this case, the stent is seen on the volume rendered view (*yellow arrow*, **a**) and also on the orthogonal, curved plane reformatted views (*white arrows*, **b**)

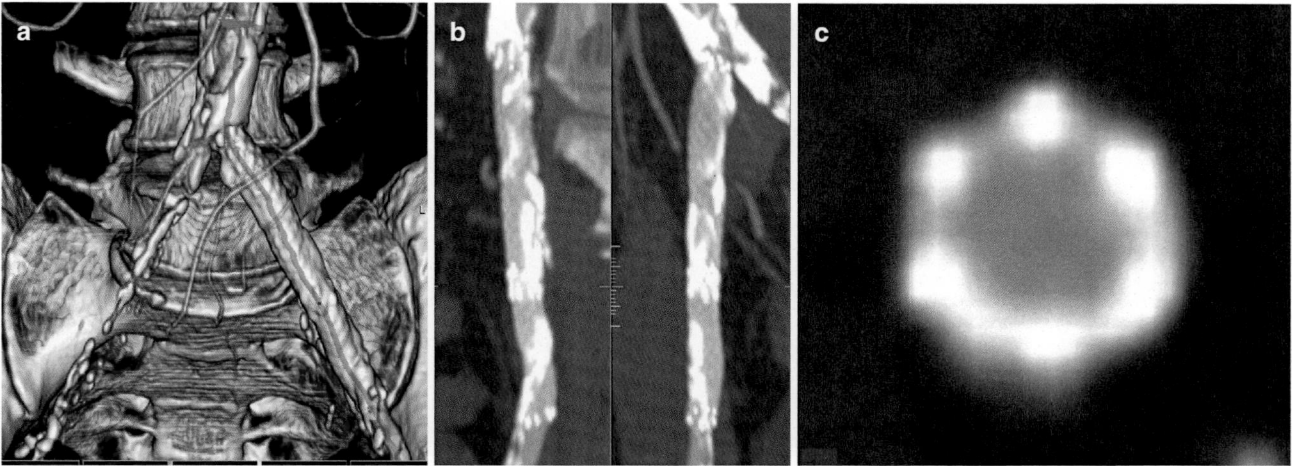

Fig. 17.16 A stent is the left common iliac artery is shown. The stent is present on the volume rendered view (**a**) and also on the curved plane reformatted views (**b**). Note that, in the short axis of the vessel (**c**), the stent is seen as a hexagonal array of hyperattenuating struts

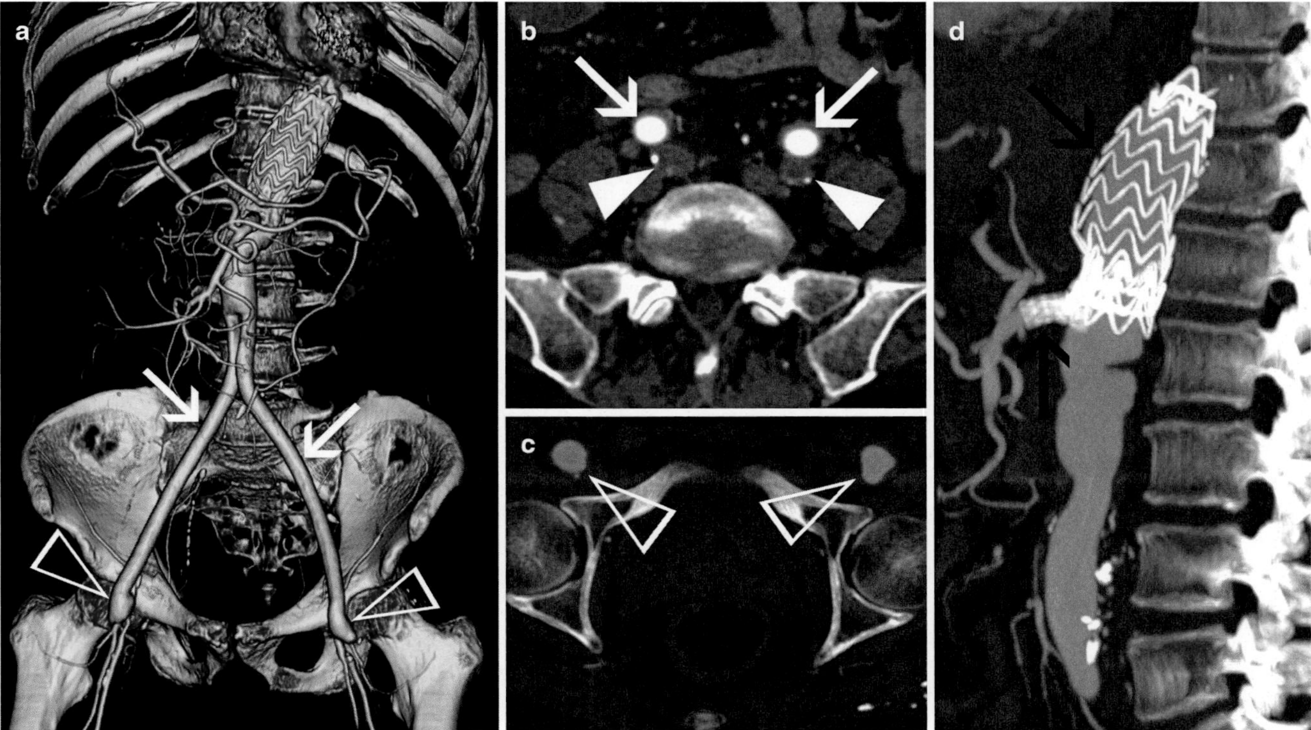

Fig. 17.17 Bilateral, aortofemoral bypass grafts are present (*white arrows*) and are seen as unusually smooth appearing structures connecting portions of the vascular tree. The occluded, native vessels are visualized on the transverse view (**b**, *white arrowheads*), but are not visualized on the volume rendered view (**a**) since the native arteries are not opacified. Enlargement and irregularity may be present at anastomotic sites as shown in this transverse CT image taken at the level of the patient's anastomoses (*white*, *open arrowheads*, **c**). Note that the patient also has aortic and celiac stents (*black arrows*, **d**)

Graft material is also well evaluated on CT. Bypass grafts are commonly recognized as long, smooth, branchless tubes connected to the native vasculature on 3-D colored, lit projections (Fig. 17.17). On axial views, the excluded, unopacified, native vessels are frequently visible. The connections between graft material and native vessel lumen may be enlarged and irregular, as a result of the patch angioplasty frequently performed at anastomosis sites. Grafts commonly are comprised of either interposed veins, Dacron, or expanded polytetrafluoroethylene (PTFE). In some cases, where increased torsional effects are anticipated and may compromise grafts, reinforced graft material is commonly

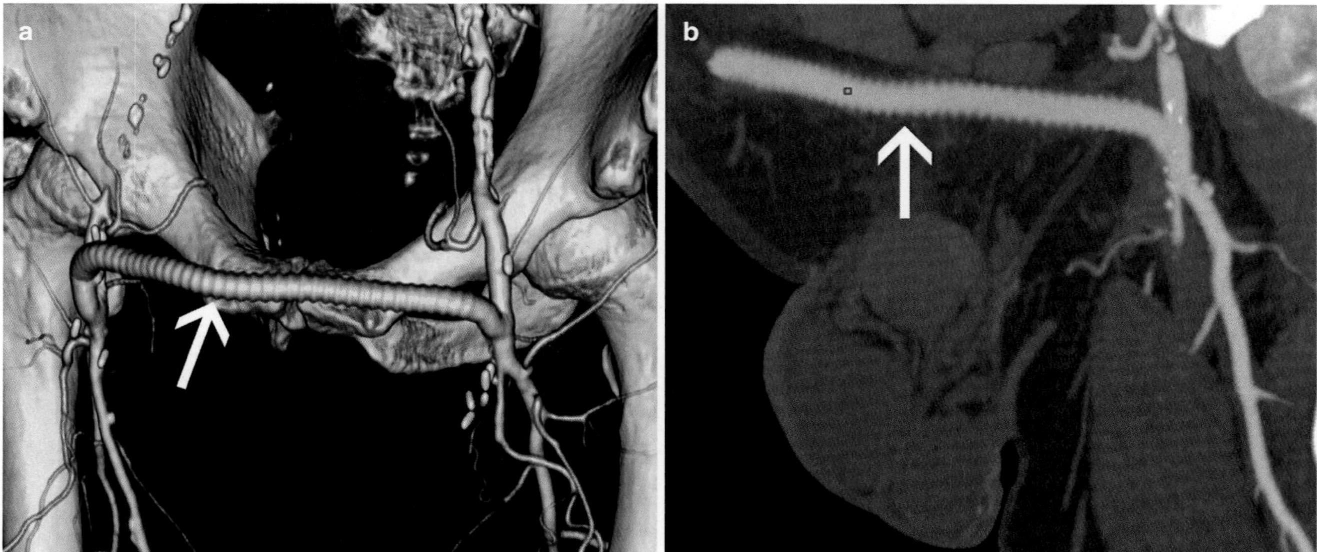

Fig. 17.18 A bifemoral bypass graft (*white arrows*) is evident with a typical, corrugated appearance, which is well seen on the volume rendered view (**a**) and the curved planar reformatted view (**b**)

employed. The rings of such grafts are typically visible as corrugated on CT angiography (Fig. 17.18).

Trauma

CT angiography as a modality has multiple features that make it ideal for imaging of the arterial tree in the setting of trauma. First, intimal flaps and abnormalities of the wall of the artery are better depicted by CT angiography compared to MR angiography, and may be better seen on CT than on ultrasound, especially within the bony pelvis where bowel gas and patient body habitus may limit duplex evaluation. CT angiography is also useful in demonstrating the entire arterial tree in a less time-intensive fashion than ultrasound or MR angiography. Concomitant post-traumatic deformities to the muscles and bones may also be simultaneously demonstrated on CT (Fig. 17.19).

CT signs of arterial injury include contrast extravasation, vessel non-opacification, abrupt vessel occlusion, focal vessel narrowing/spasm, pseudoaneurysm, intimal flap, or arteriovenous fistula. Traumatic injury to vessels may ensue after blunt or penetrating trauma and may be seen in association with fractures which displace vessels [16].

Fibromuscular Dysplasia

Although fibromuscular dysplasia is a common cause of stenosis in the renal or carotid arteries, it is less commonly encountered elsewhere in the peripheral arterial tree. When involving the peripheral arteries, fibromuscular dysplasia most commonly occurs in the external iliac artery, which is the third most common site of fibromuscular dysplasia in the body. As in other parts of the body, the classification system for fibromuscular dysplasia is based on the layer of the artery involved, with medial fibroplasia being the most common form. The most typical appearance of fibromuscular dysplasia is apparent beading of the vessel and is due to several, closely approximated weblike areas of narrowing with intervening outpouchings of the vessel from post-stenotic dilatation (Fig. 17.20) [38]. Other forms of fibromuscular dysplasia may have a variety of appearances [39]. Conventional angiography may have an advantage in demonstrating this entity compared with CT, due to the inherently higher spatial resolution of conventional angiographic images.

Other Diseases of the Systemic Arteries

Cystic adventitial disease is a rare entity, which may affect any artery adjacent to a joint and presents as a smooth narrowing without atherosclerotic disease. The narrowing is accompanied by cystic structures along the course of the artery. The most common artery affected is the popliteal. MRI is the preferred modality for depicting the cysts which occur along the vessel, although low attenuation cysts are commonly observed on CT [40, 41].

Popliteal artery entrapment syndrome can occur due to a number of abnormalities in the relationship between the popliteal artery and the muscles of the popliteal space. The most common abnormal muscle in this case is the medial

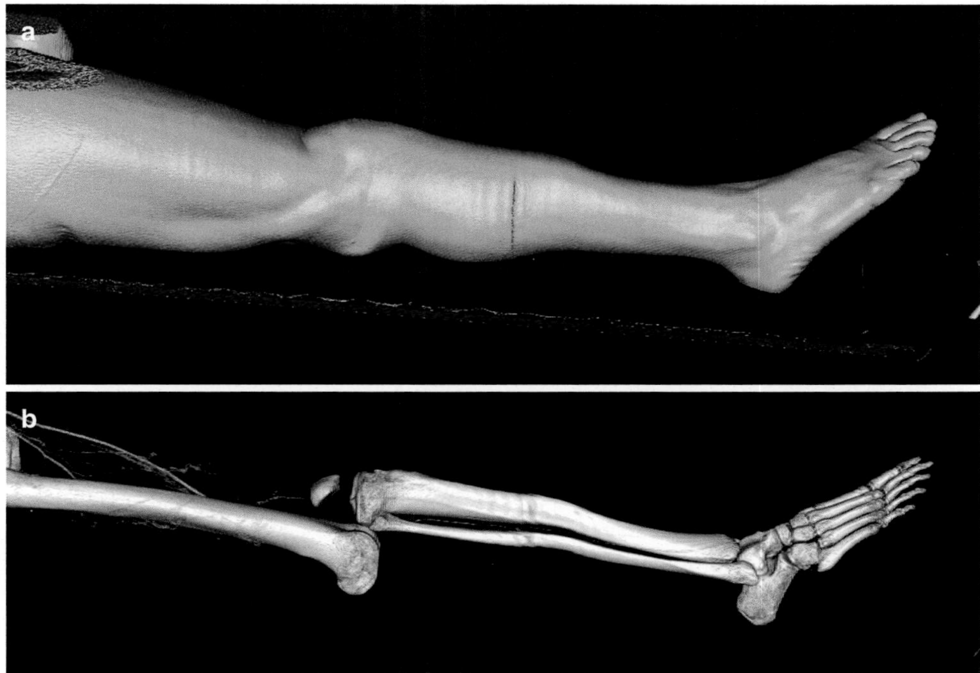

Fig. 17.19 CT angiography is useful in the setting of trauma. A surface-rendered view (**a**) shows the deformity in the outer contour of the extremity. CT angiography simultaneously demonstrates osseous structures, demonstrating a dislocation at the knee (**b**, **c**). The osseous structures may be subtracted, however, in order to better demonstrate the underlying arterial anatomy (**d**). In this case, resultant occlusion of the popliteal artery is also present (*white arrow*, **d**)

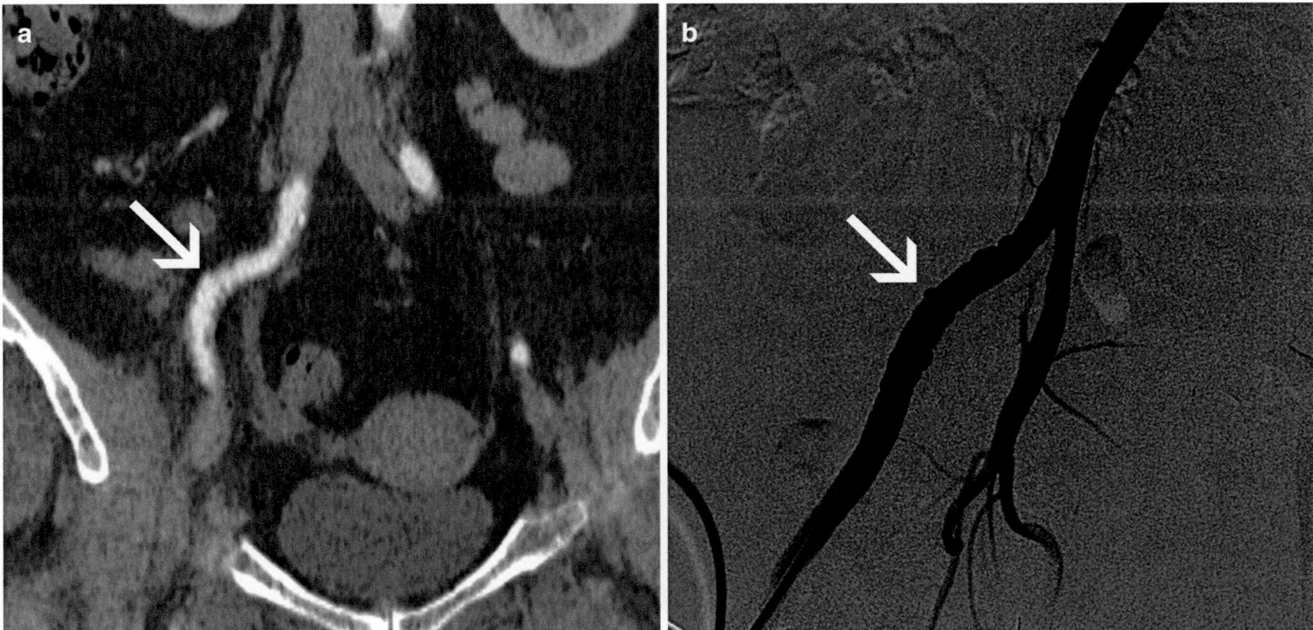

Fig. 17.20 Fibromuscular dysplasia is shown in the external iliac artery, which is the third most common site for this entity, following the internal carotid and renal arteries. The classic, beaded appearance of the external iliac artery (*arrow*) is demonstrated on a reformatted view from the patient's abdominal CT (**a**), but is more clearly demonstrated on the conventional angiography (**b**), due to the higher spatial resolution

head of the gastrocnemius, although a number of abnormal relationships have been described. This syndrome usually causes some degree of fixed narrowing of the popliteal artery, although there is commonly a dynamic component of narrowing, usually during plantar flexion or dorsiflexion. Repetitive trauma to the artery as a result of the abnormal relationship to the muscle may cause aneurysmal dilatation, thrombosis, or thromboembolism. MRI is useful in demonstrating popliteal artery entrapment syndrome, where an abnormal muscular slip courses medial to the popliteal artery. In this case, the lower extremity may need to be imaged in several positions including dorsiflexion and plantarflexion [40]. This is also more easily performed with MR angiography, since MR angiography is less sensitive to optimal vascular opacification and images can be obtained at different time-points. Also, as non-contrast means of performing MRA become more robust, some vascular pathology may be imaged without the administration of contrast.

Since the common femoral artery is a common site of vascular access, it is subject to iatrogenic complications including chiefly pseudoaneurysm and arteriovenous fistula formation. Because of the focal nature of these complications, and because the portion of the artery involved is frequently very superficial, ultrasound with Doppler is usually an adequate modality for the diagnosis and follow-up of iatrogenic femoral artery complications. On the other hand, when a deep or retroperitoneal hematoma is suspected, CT may be a more robust technique than ultrasound.

Other Modalities for Imaging the Peripheral Arteries

Advancements in imaging of the peripheral arteries have occurred in virtually every modality. As a result, the decision between modalities is more complex. Physical exam and ankle-brachial index measurement is an adequate means of making an initial diagnosis of peripheral arterial disease [37]. Further evaluation with ultrasound is also useful in demonstrating and localizing atherosclerotic disease. Complete evaluation of the entire extremity with ultrasound is, however, very time-intensive and detection of disease is technologist dependent. Detection and measurement of stenoses with ultrasound is also dependent on technical factors, such as the angle of insonation employed. Evaluation of the pelvic vasculature by ultrasound is much more difficult, and portions of the vasculature may not be easily demonstrated with ultrasound due to overlying bowel gas and osseous structures. In very obese patients, ultrasound may be significantly limited. Heavy or circumferential calcification, such as that found within patients with diabetes or renal insufficiency also significantly limits ultrasound. Determination of severity of disease by ultrasound also has difficulty in determining the severity of disease in arterial segments distal to a high-grade stenosis.

MRI and MR angiography have several advantages in patients, including the ability to perform imaging without contrast. Non-contrast MR angiography techniques have advanced dramatically, although there is still considerable variability between institutions and MR technology. Clinically useful imaging of tibial and pedal vessels using non-contrast MR is generally not possible except in highly specialized centers. Because calcium does not interfere with contrast-enhanced MR angiography, evaluation of tibial vessels with MRA, when a separate tibial imaging bolus is used instead of a bolus-chase technique, is frequently superior to CTA in patients with critical limb ischemia. In particular, the adequacy of MR sequences for imaging the arterial tree are dependent on the scanner, sequences, and vendor-specific techniques used. MR angiography has significant limitations in evaluating the post-surgical arterial tree, due to artifacts such as failure of fat saturation and susceptibility artifacts due to surgical clips, stents, or other foreign material. MR angiography is also contra-indicated in patients with non-MR conditional pacemakers or ICDs. Likewise, certain stents and stent-grafts are MR conditional, such that patients with these implants cannot undergo MR in 3 T machines. Patients with claustrophobia or significant back pain may not tolerate lying still for the hour-long exam. Because of these limitations MR is contraindicated in approximately 30 % of patients.

In the past, MR has been preferable in patients with renal disease due to relatively lower nephrotoxicity of gadolinium, compared to iodinated contrast media. However, the recent recognition of nephrogenic systemic fibrosis as a complication of gadolinium administration has decreased the utility of MR angiography in patients with chronic, severe renal disease [42]. Gadolinium should generally not be given to patients with a creatinine clearance of 30 ccs per minute or less. In patients who are already dialysis-dependent, iodinated contrast may be a better choice. CT has an advantage to MR angiography in superior spatial resolution and depiction of smaller vessels. Evaluation of the patency of circumferentially calcified tibial vessels remains challenging for CTA, however, and is one of the few circumstances where DSA may be required.

Radiation Dose in Peripheral CT Angiography

The radiation dose in CT angiography remains high and is increasingly a consideration in most CT applications. Concerns of radiation are somewhat mitigated by the fact that the extremities contain less radiosensitive tissues. When imaging the extremities, breast and abdominal shielding can easily be employed with no compromise to image quality. Shielding significantly decreases scatter and is under-utilized in patients undergoing CT in general, including peripheral CT angiography.

The radiation dose for conventional angiography is, however, much higher than for CT angiography [43]. This is in contradistinction to radiation doses in the heart, where catheterization results in lower radiation doses compared to CT. One study found that for a 16-slice CT scanner, the average radiation dose for a peripheral CT angiogram was 3.0 mSv in men, whereas the radiation dose for a conventional angiogram had an average of 11.0 mSv. Other studies have shown similar results, with CT angiography generally found to have a fourfold lower radiation dose in comparison with peripheral angiography [44]. Although peripheral CT angiography has a relatively low radiation dose and relatively less radiosensitive tissues are exposed, the risks of radiation should not be taken lightly.

References

1. Chiro GD, Brooks RA, Kessler RM, et al. Tissue signatures with dual-energy computed tomography. Radiology. 1979;131:521–3.
2. Flohr TG, McCollough CH, Bruder H, et al. First performance evaluation of a dual-source CT (DSCT system). Eur Radiol. 2005;16(2):256–68.
3. Kau T, Eicher W, Reiterer C, et al. Dual-energy CT angiography in peripheral arterial occlusive disease-accuracy of maximum intensity projections in clinical routine and subgroup analysis. Eur Radiol. 2011;21(8):1677–86.
4. Rubin GD, Schmidt AJ, Logan LJ, Sofilos MC. Multi-detector row CT angiography of lower extremity arterial inflow and runoff: initial experience. Radiology. 2001;221:146–58.
5. Ofer A, Nitecki SS, Linn S, et al. Multidetector CT angiography of peripheral vascular disease: a prospective comparison with intraarterial digital subtraction angiography. Am J Roentgenol. 2003;180:719–24.
6. Jakobs TF, Wintersperger BJ, Becker CR. MDCT-imaging of peripheral arterial disease. Semin Ultrasound CT MR. 2004; 25:145–55.
7. Johnson PT, Pannu HK, Fishman EK. IV contrast infusion for coronary artery CT angiography: literature review and results of a nationwide survey. Am J Roentgenol. 2009;192:W214–21.
8. Bae KT, Seeck BA, Hildebolt CF, et al. Contrast enhancement in cardiovascular MDCT: effect of body weight, height, body surface area, body mass index, and obesity. Am J Roentgenol. 2008; 190:777–84.
9. Fleischmann D. Aorto-popliteal bolus transit time in peripheral CT angiography: can fast acquisition outrun the bolus? Eur Radiol. 2003;13:S268.
10. Heuschmid M, Krieger A, Beierlein W, et al. Assessment of peripheral arterial occlusive disease: comparison of multislice-CT angiography (MS-CTA) and intraarterial digital subtraction angiography (IA-DSA). Eur J Med Res. 2003;8:389–96.
11. Cademartiri F, Mollet NR, Van der Lugt A, et al. Intravenous contrast material administration at helical 16–detector row CT coronary angiography: effect of iodine concentration on vascular attenuation. Radiology. 2005;236:661–5.
12. Orlandini FA, Boini S, Iochum-Duchamps S, et al. Assessment of the use of a saline chaser to reduce the volume of contrast medium in abdominal CT. Am J Roentgenol. 2006;187:511–5.
13. Cademartiri F, Mollet NR, Van der Lugt A, et al. Non-invasive 16-row multislice CT coronary angiography: usefulness of saline chaser. Eur Radiol Vol. 2004;14(2):178–83.
14. Becker CR, Wintersperger B, Jakobs TF. Multi-detector-row CT angiography of peripheral arteries. Semin Ultrasound CT MR. 2003;24:268–79.
15. Fleischmann D. Use of high concentration contrast media: principles and rationale—vascular district. Eur J Radiol. 2003;45:S88–93.
16. Miller-Thomas MM, West OC, Cohen AM. Diagnosing traumatic arterial injury in the extremities with CT angiography: pearls and pitfalls. Radiographics. 2005;25:S133–42.
17. LawrenceJ A, Kim D, Kent KC, et al. Lower extremity spiral CT angiography versus catheter angiography. Radiology. 1995; 194:903–8.
18. Rieker O, Duber C, Schmiedt W, et al. Prospective comparison of CT angiography of the legs with intraarterial digital subtraction angiography. AJR Am J Roentgenol. 1996;166:269–76.
19. Otah KE, Takase K, Igarashi K, et al. MDCT compared with digital subtraction angiography for assessment of lower extremity arterial occlusive disease: importance of reviewing cross-sectional images. AJR Am J Roentgenol. 2004;182:201–9.
20. Willman JK, Baumert T, Chandler P. Aortoiliac and lower extremity assessed with 16 detector row CT angiography respective comparison with distal subtraction angiography. Radiology. 2005;236: 1083–93.
21. Shareghi S, Gopal A, Gul K, et al. Diagnostic accuracy of 64 multidetector computed tomographic angiography in peripheral vascular disease. Catheter Cardiovasc Interv. 2010;75:23–31.
22. Fishman EK, Ney DR, Heath DG, et al. Volume rendering versus maximum intensity projection in CT angiography: what works best, when, and why. Radiographics. 2006;26:905–22.
23. Shammas MW, Lemke JH, Dipple EG. In-hospital complications of peripheral vascular interventions using fractionated heparin as the primary anticoagulant. J Invasive Cardiol. 2003;15:242–6.
24. Lippert H, Pabst R. Aortic arch. In: Arterial variations in man: classification and frequency. Munich: JF Bergmann-Verlag; 1985. p. 3–10.
25. Janssen M, Baggen MGA, Veen HF, et al. Dysphagia lusoria: clinical aspects, manometric findings, diagnosis, and therapy. Am J Gastroenterol. 2000;95:1411–6.
26. Koyama T, Tadanori T, Kitanaka Y, Katagiri K, et al. Congenital anomaly of the external iliac artery: a case report. J Vasc Surg. 2003;37(3):683–5.
27. Brantley SK, Rigdon EE, Raju S. Persistent sciatic artery: embryology, pathology, and treatment. J Vasc Surg. 1993;18(2):242–8.
28. Mesurolle B, Qanadli SD, El Hajjam M, Goeau-Brissonniere OA, Mignon F, Lacombe P. Occlusive arterial disease of abdominal aorta and lower extremities: comparison of helical CT angiography with transcatheter angiography. Clin Imaging. 2004;28:252–60.
29. Ness J, Aronow WS. Prevalence of coexistence of coronary artery disease, ischemic stroke, and peripheral arterial disease in older persons, mean age 80 years, in an academic hospital-based geriatrics practice. Brief reports. J Am Geriatr Soc. 1999;47(10):1255–6.
30. Newman AB, Shemanski L, Manolio TA, et al. Ankle-arm index as a predictor of cardiovascular disease and mortality in the cardiovascular health study. Arterioscler Thromb Vasc Biol. 1999; 19:538–45.
31. "Peripheral arterial disease prevention and prevalence". Peripheral arterial disease. 2007. http://www.3-rx.com/ab/more/peripheral-arterial-disease-prevention-and-prevalence/. Retrieved on 03 Sept 2009.
32. Sharrett AR. "Peripheral arterial disease prevalence". Peripheral arterial disease. 2007. http://www.health.am/vein/more/peripheral-arterial-disease-prevalence/. Retrieved on 03 Sept 2009.
33. Cordeiro M, Lima J. Atherosclerotic plaque characterization by multidetector row computed tomography angiography. J Am Coll Cardiol. 2006;47(8):C40–7.
34. Rosenberg GD, Killewich LA. Case report: blue toe syndrome from a "coral reef" aorta. Ann Vasc Surg. 1995;9(6):561–4.

35. Levien LJ, Veller MG. Popliteal artery entrapment syndrome: more common than previously recognized. J Vasc Surg. 1999; 30(4):587–98.
36. Qvarfordt PG, Reilly LM, Sedwitz MM, Ehrenfeld WK, Stoney RJ. "Coral reef" atherosclerosis of the suprarenal aorta: a unique clinical entity. J Vasc Surg. 1984;1(6):903–9.
37. Hirsch AT, et al. ACC/AHA guidelines for the management of patients with peripheral arterial disease (lower extremity, renal, mesenteric, and abdominal aortic). J Vasc Interv Radiol. 2006;17(9):1383–98.
38. Walter JF, Stanley JC, Mehigan JT, et al. External iliac artery fibrodysplasia. Am J Roentgenol. 1978;31(1):125–8.
39. Sauer L, Reilly LM, Goldstone J, et al. Clinical spectrum of symptomatic external iliac fibromuscular dysplasia. J Vasc Surg. 1990;12(4):488–95. Discussion 495–6.
40. Elias DA, White LM, Rubenstein JD, et al. Pictorial essay, clinical evaluation and MR imaging features of popliteal artery entrapment and cystic adventitial disease. Am J Roentgenol. 2003;180: 627–32.
41. Tsolakis CS, Walvatne CS. Cystic adventitial disease of the popliteal artery: diagnosis and treatment I.A. Eur J Vasc Endovasc Surg. 1998;15(3):188–94.
42. Sadowski EA, Bennett LK, Chan MR, et al. Nephrogenic systemic fibrosis: risk factors and incidence estimation. Radiology. 2007;243:148–57.
43. Kocinaja D, Cioppaa AA, Ambrosinia GT, et al. Radiation dose exposure during cardiac and peripheral arteries catheterization. Int J Cardiol. 2006;113(2):283–4.
44. Martin ML, Tay KH, Borys F, et al. Multidetector CT angiography of the aortoiliac system and lower extremities: a prospective comparison with digital subtraction angiography. Am J Roentgenol. 2003;180:1085–91.

18 Aortic, Renal, Mesenteric and Carotid CT Angiography

Anas Alani and Matthew J. Budoff

Abstract

Computed tomography angiography has an increasing role in vascular imaging of the aorta, renal, mesenteric, and carotid arteries. There has been tremendous improvement in computed tomography technology that has made such images the preferred choice for diagnosing various acute and chronic vascular diseases and replacing non-invasive and invasive tests.

Keywords

Computed Tomography Angiography • Aorta CT Angiography • Renal CT Angiography • Mesenteric CT Angiography • Carotid CT Angiography • Vascular CT Angiography • Aortic Dissection • CT Angiography Acquisition and Protocol

Introduction

Computed tomographic angiography (CTA) of vascular beds is significantly easier to perform and interpret than coronary studies. There is no cardiac motion to contend with, so gating is most often not necessary. The exception is the ascending aorta, where pseudodissections (an appearance of a dissection caused by motion of the aortic root – Fig. 18.1) have plagued earlier studies with single-slice computed tomography (CT) due to motion artifacts [1]. Most of the large vessels of interest (the carotid, renal, and mesenteric arteries) have significantly larger diameters than coronary arteries, as well as less tortuous courses. The renal and carotid arteries are usually straight structures, so reconstructions are significantly less complicated than coronary imaging. Also, due to the increased speed of newer systems (electron beam tomography (EBT) and 16+ row multidetector computed tomography (MDCT)), venous enhancement is less common, so it is easier to see the arteries without superimposed contrast-filled structures (venous contamination). This is another reason why CT is most often superior to magnetic resonance imaging (MRI) in these vascular beds.

In regard to the aorta, CTA can diagnose aneurysm, dissection, and wall abnormalities such as ulceration, calcification, or thrombus throughout the full length of the aorta, as well as the involvement of branch vessels. Disease of the aorta or great vessels can present with a broad clinical spectrum of symptoms and signs. The accepted diagnostic gold standard, selective digital subtraction angiography, is now being challenged by state-of-the-art CTA and magnetic resonance (MR) angiography. Currently, in many centers, cross-sectional imaging modalities are being used as the first line of diagnosis to evaluate the vascular system, and conventional angiography is reserved for therapeutic intervention.

A. Alani, MD
Department of Medicine, University of Florida – Gainesville, Gainsville, FL, USA

Los Angeles Biomedical Research Institute at Harbor-UCLA, 1124 W Carson Street, Torrance, CA 90502, USA
e-mail: aaj.alani@gmail.com

M.J. Budoff, MD (✉)
David Geffen School of Medicine at UCLA, Los Angeles Biomedical Research Institute, Torrance, CA USA
e-mail: mbudoff@labiomed.org

M.J. Budoff, J.S. Shinbane (eds.), *Cardiac CT Imaging: Diagnosis of Cardiovascular Disease*, DOI 10.1007/978-3-319-28219-0_18

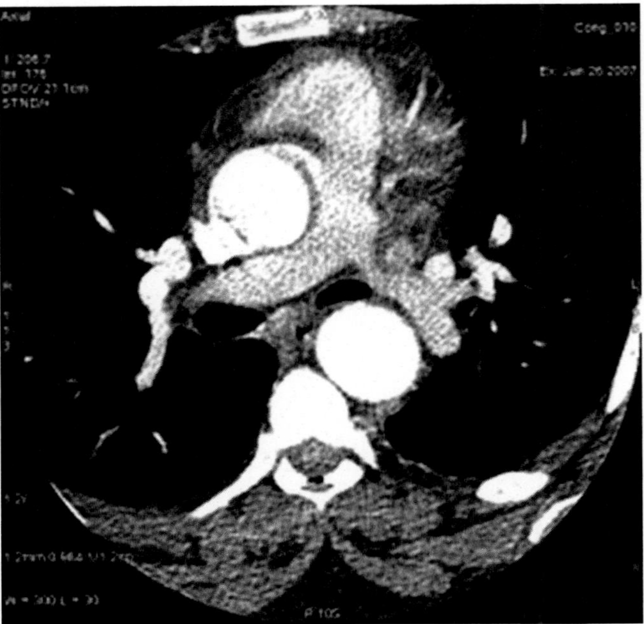

Fig. 18.1 Axial view of pseudo-dissection of aorta caused by motion artifact in an ungated computed tomography (CT) scan of the chest

Principles of Imaging

In aortic imaging, the volume coverage capabilities of MDCT have come to full use without having to compromise on resolution or detail [2, 3]. With the current configuration of 64-row (or greater) CT scanners, the entire abdominal aorta and the iliac arteries can be covered within seconds and with isotropic resolution (Chap. 1). Investigation of the dataset can now be done on the anteroposterior (coronal) and lateral (sagittal) planes, which has been the convention with invasive angiography. A few important technical advances have further improved aorta imaging using CTA. First is the increased number of detector rows for the acquisition of images over greater z-axis lengths with one gantry rotation. With up to 320 detectors, volume coverage per rotation is as much as 160 mm. The typical distance needed for the abdominal aorta is on the order of 400 mm, so two to three rotations would cover the entire abdomen. Using a rotation speed of <500 ms, this could be accomplished in 1–2 s. Second, the use of dual-source technology allows for further reduction of acquisition times, since the entire aorta can be scanned in one breath hold. This technology has considerably improved temporal resolution compared to single-source acquisition (for which resolution approaches 0.4 mm) [4].

CT Technique

Understanding the principles of CTA techniques is essential to acquire diagnostic images consistently. This section reviews current CTA methods used in the evaluation of great vessels. The following broad approach is a guide to CT scan acquisition for various scanners. For peripheral imaging, where electrocardiogram (ECG) gating is not required, 16–320-slice scanners are more than adequate to image the entire volume. In addition, there is no need for the speed that is required for cardiac work (temporal resolution or rotation speed).

1. Intravenous injection of 35–70 mL of a nonionic contrast agent (300–370 mg I/mL), decreasing with scanners with higher numbers of detectors.
2. Monophasic or biphasic injection rate: most commonly a monophasic injection at 4 mL/s (followed by a saline bolus). Three phase injections (pure contrast, followed by mixed contrast saline and pure saline) are more important and common with cardiac applications.
3. Scan delay is determined by test injection (10 mL at 4 mL/s) or by automated triggering (to achieve imaging to coincide with contrast arrival in the aortic root close to the area of interest). The scan delay should be determined near the start of the section being imaged (transverse aorta for carotids, abdominal aorta for renals or runoffs).
4. Pitch:
   - For 16-detector MDCT: 16×0.625 mm detector configuration with 1.25-mm reconstruction thickness and pitch = 1.7 (table speed 17.5 mm/rotation divided by 10-mm detector coverage (16×0.625 = 10 mm)), reconstructed retrospectively with 0.37-mm intervals for 3D and multi-planar reconstruction (MPR).
   - For 64-detector MDCT: 64×0.625 mm detector configuration with 0.625–1.25-mm reconstruction thickness and pitch = 1 (moving the table 40 mm and covering 40 mm with each rotation) up to a pitch of 1.375 (table speed 55 mm/rotation divided by 40-mm detector width), reconstructed retrospectively with 0.3-mm intervals for 3D and MPR (the 40-mm detector width coverage per rotation used is currently available in the GE and Phillips 64 systems. The Siemens single- or dual-source has a collimation of 19.2–38.4 mm, increasing with the Philips 256 (128 detectors of 0.625 mm allowing 80 mm of coverage per rotation; the Toshiba 320 allows 160 mm of coverage per rotation)).

Aortic CTA

The speed and ease of modern CTA make it the technique of choice for diagnosing chronic and acute aortic pathologic findings, such as intramural hematoma, aneurysm, traumatic injuries, atherosclerosis, and dissection (Fig. 18.2). With the current configuration of 64-row CT scanners, the entire abdominal aorta and the iliac arteries can be covered with isotropic resolution. Moreover, the high scan speed allows substantial reduction of the amount of contrast material used in earlier studies, hence reducing the adverse effects.

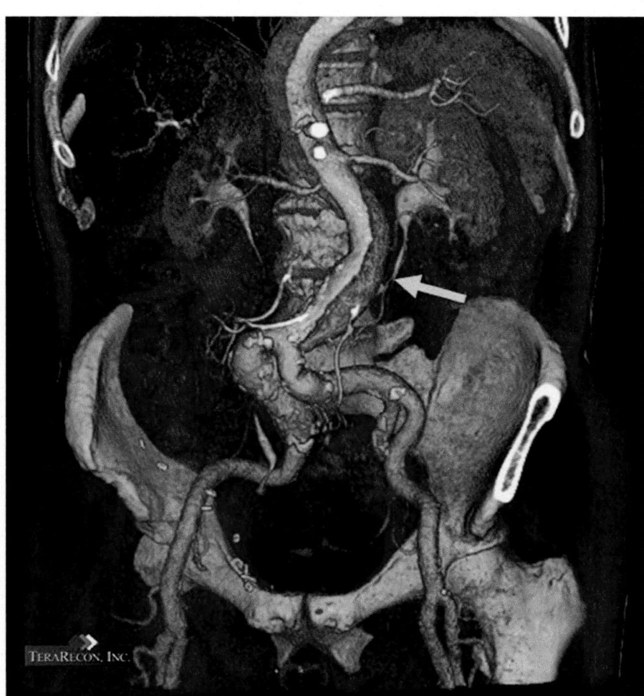

Fig. 18.2 A volume-rendered image depicting an aortic dissection involving the abdominal aorta (*arrow*), starting below the renal arteries and ending prior to the iliac arteries

Gated vs. Non-ECG Gated CTA

Non-gated CTA allows for very fast acquisition, and interpretation is significantly less complicated. Without ECG gating or breath-holding, artifacts such as misregistration do not occur, which improves image quality compared to cardiac studies. Non-ECG-gated CT is performed in parts of the aorta without much aortic dynamics, such as the abdominal aorta. ECG gating means that the scan is synchronized to the cardiac beat. This will lead to decreased motion artifacts from cardiac movement and aortic dynamics [5] (Fig. 18.1). Such motion artifacts may mimic the appearance of a dissection in the ascending aorta and lead to misdiagnosis [6]. This ECG triggering should be considered in the ascending aorta, the aortic arch, and the descending thoracic aorta [7]. ECG-gated CTA requires longer acquisition to obtain the specific phase of the ECG cycle, which will result in more contrast media [8]. The possibility of applying ECG-controlled X-ray-tube dose modulation is another step forward for reducing radiation exposure rates.

Challenges

CTA application can be limited due to radiation doses and nephrotoxicity. Of course, the requirements of radiation (which are more significant for carotid imaging due to radiation-sensitive organs such as the thyroid and orbits) and contrast (which is more significant for renal artery imaging due to the frequent coexistence of renal insufficiency and renal artery stenosis) make MR more attractive for selective cases. New scanners with more detectors reduce contrast, since the imaging territory is covered in a shorter period. If there is no ECG gating, contrast requirements are minimal (30–40 cc per study). Another technique to minimize contrast is using saline to flush the contrast through the system (Chap. 2). The saline chaser offers two significant benefits with CTA imaging. One is that the contrast is forced from the tubing and extremity veins into the central circulation, allowing for a reduction in the total contrast dose. A second benefit is that the contrast sitting in the vein during imaging can cause partial volume (beam hardening) artifacts. Moving the contrast out of the venous system is important for cardiac imaging (where the scatter from the superior vena cava can cause artifacts in the right atrium and right coronary artery), carotid imaging (obscuring the proximal brachiocephalic artery or carotid base), and pulmonary imaging.

With fast imaging, the venous circulation is not filled; reducing venous contamination (large veins obscuring smaller arteries). This could be problematic in renal beds and runoff studies, as is often seen with MRI. Thus, using new scanners, large areas can be scanned with minimal contrast use. The most common protocols employed increase the image acquisition time from 100 ms per image to 200–300 ms per image to improve tissue penetration and reduce image noise. Still, 50–60 mL of contrast at most is all that is necessary to complete a thoracic and abdominal aortic study.

The radiation dose of CTA has improved dramatically over the last few years [9]. Using a low and reasonably achievable dose to obtain a diagnostic image can be done by decreasing tube current, tube voltage, scan coverage, and other dose-saving strategies. Newer-generation scanners with a large detector array can cover a larger area of the aorta with each gantry rotation and provide prospective triggering over a larger span of the aorta, resulting in less radiation.

Aortic Dissection

The superior temporal resolution of current MDCT systems significantly improves imaging of the aorta, because motion artifacts are eliminated in the ascending aorta. CT is often considered a superior method over other imaging methods for the identification of aortic dissection, as the intimal flap is usually well delineated, even in branches of the aorta. The 3D nature and the ability to see the outer wall, false lumens, and the presence of a clot make this technique superior to even invasive angiography for the evaluation of dissection (Fig. 18.3). The extent of the dissection, including the proximal entry and distal re-entry sites, the involvement of

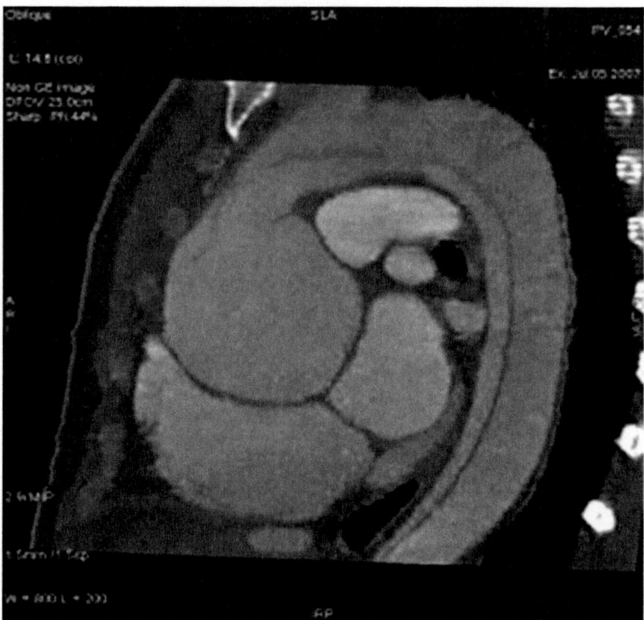

Fig. 18.3 Spiral aortic dissection seen on a sagittal view of a gated 64-multidetector computed tomography (MDCT) cardiac scan

adjacent branch vessels, and the potential comprise of the true lumens are thoroughly evaluated.

The ability to visualize the great vessels in the transverse aorta, neck, and arms makes CT significantly more robust than transthoracic and transesophageal echocardiographic imaging and tolerance by patients is significantly better. Transthoracic echocardiography visualizes the aortic root well but is poor at imaging the mid-ascending and descending thoracic aorta. Transesophageal echocardiography is minimally invasive but does not image the distal ascending thoracic aorta or arch well. Because imaging protocols for MDCT can be performed in less than 10 min (significantly shorter than MR or transesophageal echocardiography), even unstable patients can be evaluated and triaged quickly. With the use of flow modes (usually used for timing of contrast), assessing luminal flow in the true and false lumens is possible.

Thoracic Imaging

Diseases of the thoracic aorta present a diagnostic challenge. Many aortic conditions such as aneurysms typically cause no symptoms and often go clinically unrecognized until a life-threatening complication occurs. CT is the primary means of imaging the lung, thoracic trauma (blunt and penetrating), aneurysms, and aortic dissections [10]. CT is playing an increasingly important role in the diagnosis and management of thoracic aortic pathology [11, 12]. Once aortic disease is detected, a comprehensive evaluation of the entire thoracic aorta is indicated to demonstrate the maximal aortic diameter and to detect associated disease in other segments of the aorta. In the situation of an acute life-threatening event, CT can provide extensive information concerning the heart, aorta, and great vessels with a single scan protocol (Fig. 18.4). In addition, during the same examination, the brain and spinal canal can be evaluated if necessary. The entire global CT examination (head, cervical spine, chest, abdomen, and pelvis) can be completed on modern MDCT systems with scan times of 20 s and exam times of <15 min [13].

Comparison to Other Methods

Although MRI and transesophageal echocardiography can provide excellent and unique information, the robust nature of CT often makes it preferable. Advantages are the ability to image the entire aorta and beyond, the demonstration of surrounding structures and organs, quantitative measures of aneurysm size and location, and a rapid examination time. Limitations are the negative effects of iodinated contrast on renal function, the rare adverse reactions to iodinated contrast, and the inability to directly measure blood flow (which is useful for determining true and false lumens). A current MDCT protocol for CTA provides high-resolution arterial phase images from the thoracic inlet to the femoral arteries. This coverage incorporates the entire aorta, as well as the organs of the chest, abdomen, and pelvis. Beyond classifying dissections as involving the ascending (Stanford type A) or descending (type B), CT can demonstrate associated findings that are critical to patient care, such as mediastinal hematoma, pericardial effusions, pseudoaneurysm formation, and active extravasation of contrast from the aorta. Quantitative measurement of aneurysm size, location, and relation to branch vessels can be used for planning operative or intravascular repair and for monitoring post-procedure anatomy.

The need for precise and quantitative measurements with CT has become more critical with continued advancements in endovascular repair with stent grafts [14, 15]. CTA is less operator-dependent than transesophageal echocardiography, it allows for complete organ visualization, and it is faster and more convenient for patients than MRI and digital subtraction angiography. The latter issues are especially important with severely ill patients. In the setting of blunt and penetrating trauma, CT of the chest can be extremely useful in diagnosis and as an aid to surgical management [16]. Another major advantage over MR is that these examinations are performed in critically ill patients who may require mechanical ventilation, invasive monitoring, intravenous infusion pumps, and cardiac pacing.

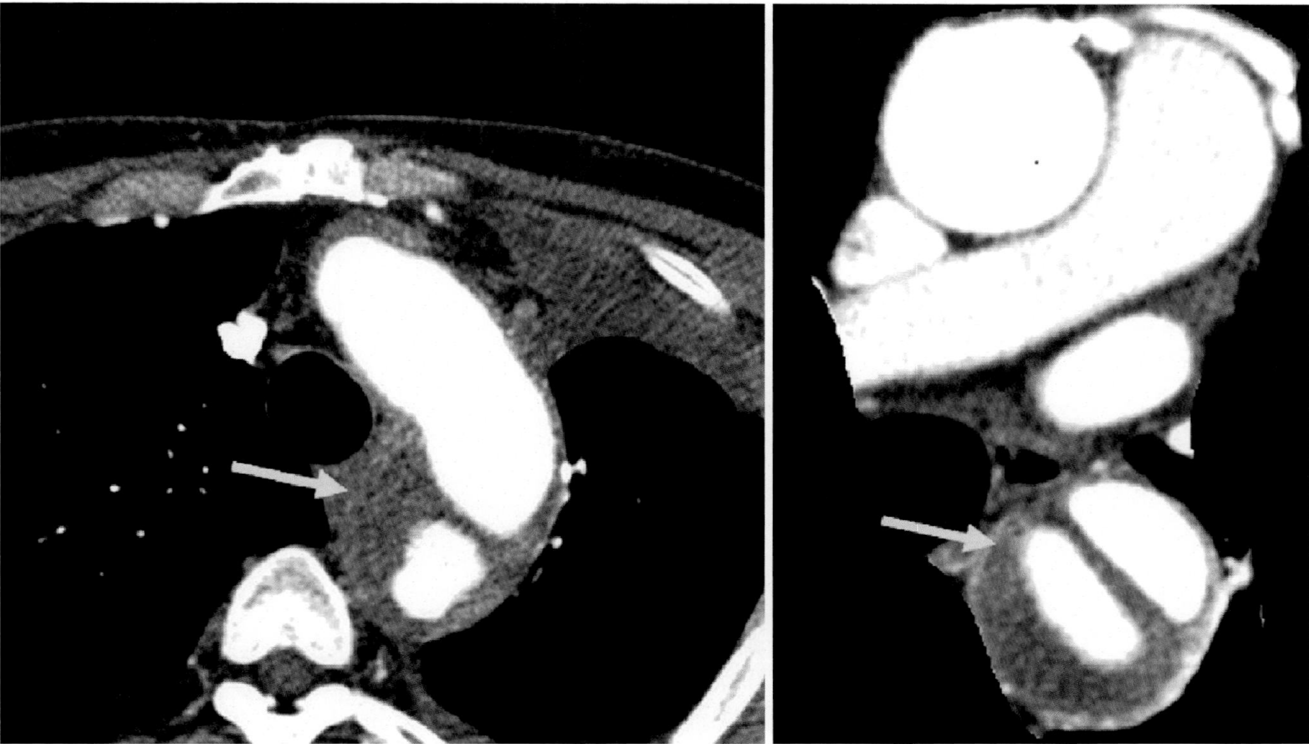

Fig. 18.4 Thoracic aortic dissection extending into the transverse aorta (*left*) and descending thoracic aorta (*right*). The intramural thrombus is easily identified by the *arrow*

Abdominal Aorta

Aortic aneurysm is associated with risk of sudden death due to aortic dissection or ruptures. It can occur in association with connective tissue disorders or acquired cardiovascular disease [17]. The ability to measure the diameter, wall thrombus, and calcification makes CT an ideal modality for sequentially following patients and making accurate assessments for surgical planning or medical therapy (Fig. 18.5). Aortic endovascular stenting is gaining acceptance as an alternative to traditional open surgical repair for abdominal aortic aneurysms. CT imaging is the predominant method used for preoperative planning to assess the feasibility of endovascular aortic stenting and to select the appropriate aortic stent graft. The abdominal aorta is usually scanned before and following intravenous contrast enhancement, which enables detection of calcification of the arterial wall that will be partly obscured following contrast enhancement. It also provides a baseline for evaluating any vascular injury with hemorrhage or thrombus that will be seen in the post-contrast acquisition. 3D sagittal and coronal reconstructions are routinely performed (Figs. 18.6 and 18.7). Maximum intensity projection (MIP) provides images similar to conventional angiography and is useful to visualize calcification and the relationship of the aneurysm to adjacent vessels.

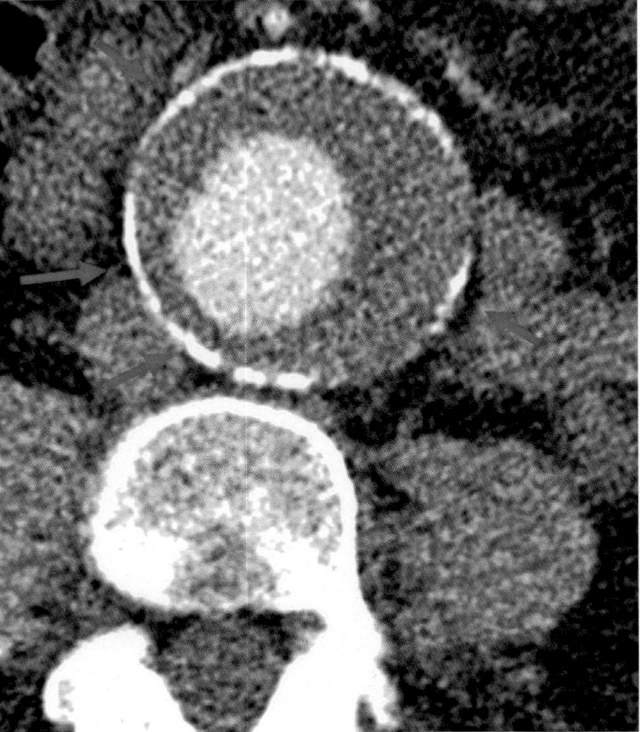

Fig. 18.5 Aortic wall calcification (*arrow*) and aneurysm on an axial image at the level of abdominal aorta

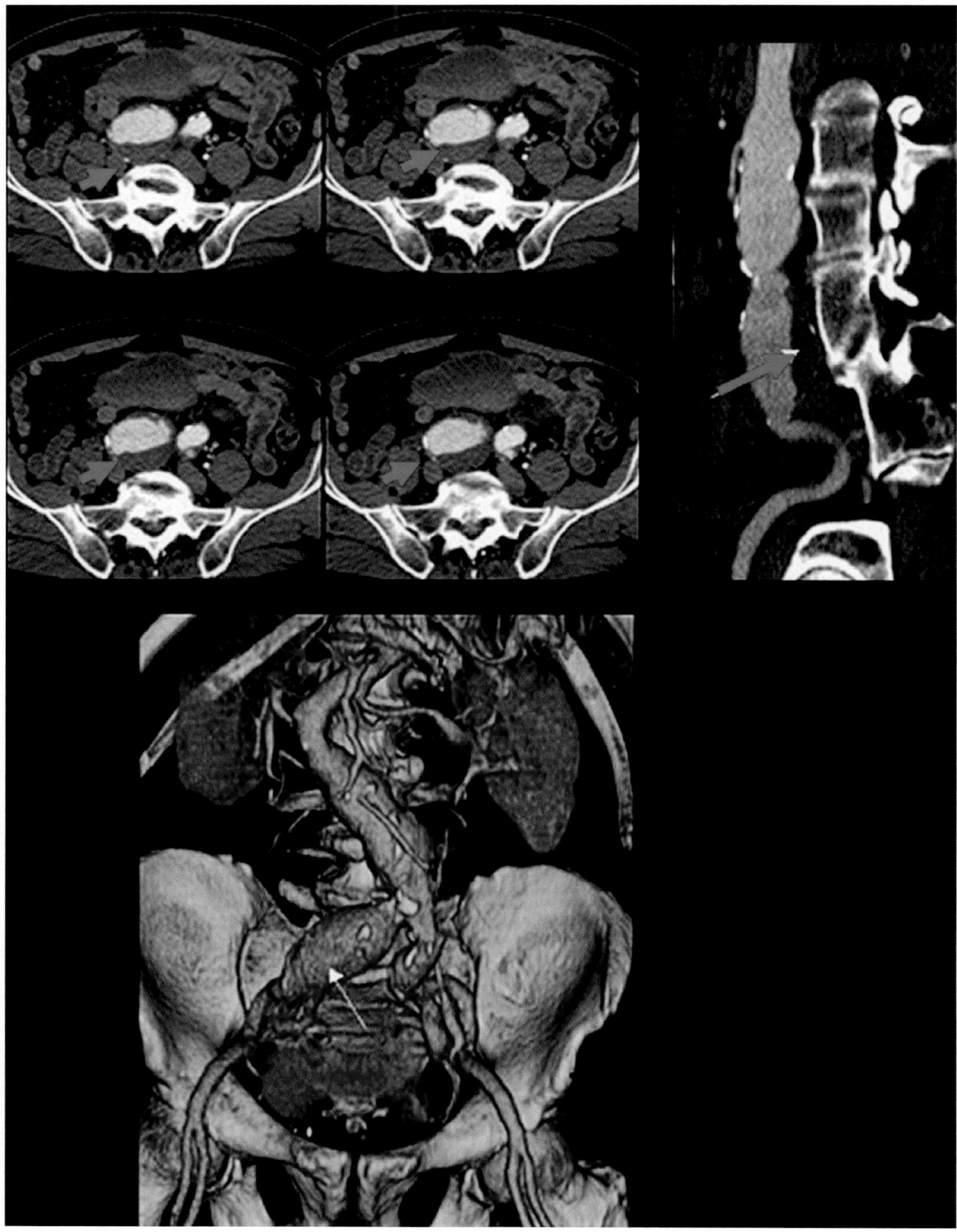

Fig. 18.6 A representation of the 2D axial images (*top left*), curved multiplanar reformat (*top right*), and volume-rendered images (*bottom*) of a patient with an abdominal aortic aneurysm. The iliacs and femoral bifurcations can be seen best in their true anatomic 3D orientation with the volume-rendered image. The thrombus, however, is only visible on the 2D images and curved MIP image (*green arrows*). The *white arrow* demonstrates the iliac aneurysm

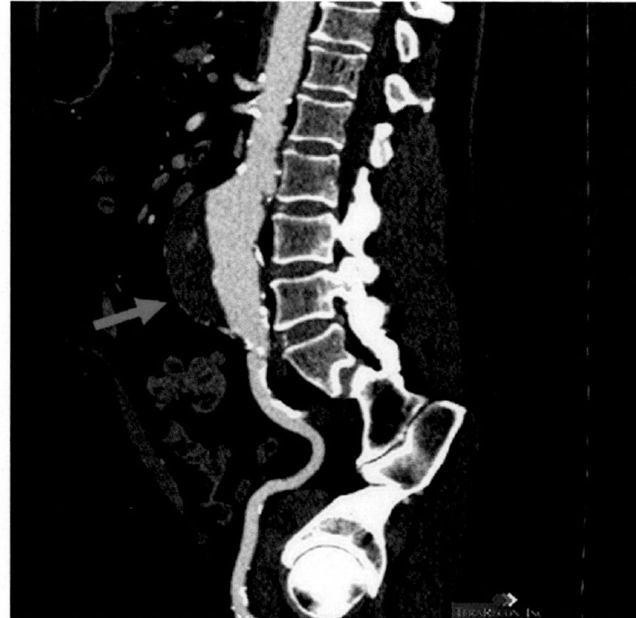

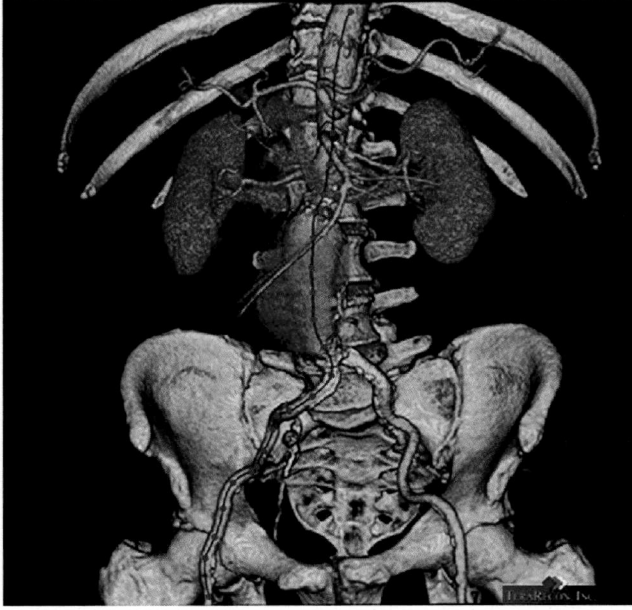

Fig. 18.7 Abdominal aortic aneurysm with large intramural thrombus, seen on maximal intensity projection image (*top, green arrow*) and volume-rendered (*bottom, blue structure*)

Common Indications for CTA of Abdominal Aorta

1. Detection and depiction of atherosclerotic occlusive disease or aneurysmal dilatation of the abdominal aorta and iliac arteries.
2. Preoperative assessment of aortoiliac aneurysms to determine whether open repair or stent grafting is indicated.
3. Preoperative measurement of the aneurysm for selecting the appropriate stent graft.
4. Follow-up for the size and progression or regression of abdominal aortic aneurysms.
5. Diagnosis of the presence and severity of complications following aortic stent-graft placement, including endoleaks, aneurysm expansion, rupture, and pseudoaneurysm, thrombus, and graft migration [18].
6. Detection and depiction of aortic dissection.
7. Detection of the presence of aortic aneurysm rupture.

Accurate measurements of the aortic root diameter can be made easily, and the extent of the aneurysm can be defined. Luminal thrombus is easily identified by differences in tissue density during contrast enhancement. The tomographic format of CT provides excellent definition of the relationship of aortic aneurysms to adjacent structures. Blood leakage from the aneurysm or stent may be recognizable with contrast enhancement of surrounding tissues.

The 2D images (axial data), MIP, and multiplanar imaging allow accurate measurement of the length, location, and diameter of aneurysms. The involvement of branch vessels (renals, mesenterics, iliacs, etc.) is also easily assessed with minimal contrast requirements. CTA has become the first-line modality for evaluation to plan stent-graft deployment (Fig. 18.7) and post-procedural assessment (Fig. 18.8). Cephalocaudal coverage from the celiac trunk to the proximal thighs provides a suitable study volume to detect aortic disease. Although the preoperative assessment requires a true early arterial phase to investigate all preoperative necessities (e.g., aortic neck diameters, angle and distance from the renal arteries), postoperative study requires a biphasic scan protocol for more detailed inspection of the perigraft space to rule out possible endoleaks. High-resolution thin-slice protocols are preferable, especially for the post-processing task.

Comparison to Other Modalities

Like CT, magnetic resonance angiography (MRA) of the abdomen is always acquired as part of a routine lower-extremity runoff procedure most commonly performed for symptoms of claudication. With CT, the renals can be routinely evaluated during an abdominal aorta study. For MR, the evaluation of the renal arteries for characterizing potential renal artery stenosis in patients with hypertension must be done as a separate procedure with different imaging protocols. This is also true for the evaluation of a potential renal donor. In these patients, dedicated abdominal MRA acquisition is required with greater contrast enhancement, which is not feasible when the legs and feet must also be imaged at the same time. This is because there is a limit on the total volume of gadolinium, which is usually 30–45 mL for an adult. An abdominal MRA performed for the indications listed is often scanned as part of the same procedure as a thoracic MRA, as it is for CT.

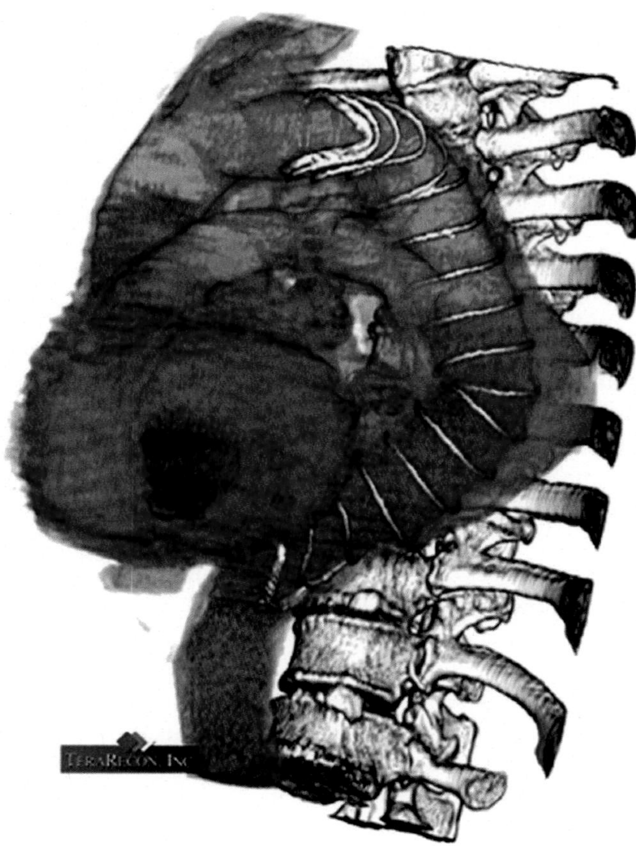

Fig. 18.8 A patient status post repair of a thoracic aortic aneurysm. The stent can be seen without scatter artifact or partial volume effect

Triple Rule-Out CTA

CTA can be used as the first choice in the emergency room to rule out aortic dissection, acute coronary syndrome, pulmonary embolism, and adjacent intrathoracic structure pathology in patients with chest pain in an appropriate clinical setting. Triple rule-out requires an ECG-gated study. This can eliminate further testing in 75 % of the patients and provide a cost-effective evaluation [19].

CTA Accuracy in Diagnosis of Aortic Disease

Several studies have demonstrated the accuracy of CT for the diagnosis of aortic diseases. Hayter et al. [20] investigated 373 patients who underwent CTA in the emergency room for suspected aortic disorders. The diagnosis of acute aortic disorder was confirmed using surgical/pathologic diagnoses or any imaging as the reference standard (aortography, MRA, or echocardiography). In total, there were 23 acute aortic dissections, 14 acute aortic intramural hematomas, 20 acute penetrating aortic ulcers, 44 new or enlarging aortic aneurysms, and 11 acute aortic ruptures, and 305 cases were interpreted as negative for acute aortic disorder. The resulting sensitivity was 99 % (67 of 68), specificity was 100 % (304 of 304), the positive predictive value was 100 % (67 of 67), the negative predictive value was 99.7 % (304 of 305), and the accuracy was 99.5 % (371 of 373). Stueckle et al. [21] compared conventional angiography to CTA in the diagnosis of morphologic changes in the abdominal aorta and its branches in 52 patients who underwent both MDCT and invasive angiography before surgical treatment. All CT examinations were performed after the administration of 100 mL of contrast medium with a collimation of 4 × 1 mm and a pitch of 7. All aneurysms, occlusions, stenoses, and calcifications were diagnosed correctly by CTA in axial and multiplanar projections (sensitivity 100 %; specificity 100 %). The degree of stenosis was overestimated in three cases when using axial projections. 3D volume-rendered (VR) CTA showed a sensitivity of 91 % for aneurysms, 82 % for stenoses, 75 % for occlusions, and 77 % for calcifications. The specificity was 100 % in all cases.

With more detector systems, imaging improves. Multislice CTA is similar to invasive angiography for abdominal vessels if multiplanar projections are used. Yoshida et al. [22] evaluated 57 individuals who underwent emergency CTA and surgery for type A aortic dissection or intramural hematoma. The diagnosis by CTA was correct as type A aortic dissection (45 patients) or intramural hematoma (12 patients) according to surgical pathology. The accuracy of CTA was 100 % (57 of 57), the sensitivity was 100 % (49 of 49), and the specificity was 100 % (eight of eight). In addition, all values were 100 % for diagnosis of aortic arch anomalies.

These findings demonstrated that CTA is a highly accurate imaging method in all kinds of thoracic and abdominal aorta diseases. CTA produces excellent 3D images that are competitive in quality with interventional angiography. In some instances, CTA images can give more information about the aortic diseases due to visualization of lumen, thrombus, and wall disease simultaneously as compared to interventional angiography.

Conclusion

The simultaneous acquisition of multiple thin collimated slices in combination with enhanced gantry rotation speed offers thin-slice coverage of extended volumes without any loss in spatial resolution. Early limitations of four-slice scanners required restricting the scan volume and focusing on dedicated abdominal vessel territories in order to provide high spatial resolution (1–2 mm). 16+ detector-row technology now enables full abdominal coverage from the diaphragm to the groin without compromising spatial resolution. This technique enables the evaluation of the whole arterial visceral vasculature (e.g., hepatic vessels, mesenteric vessels, renal arteries) and the aortic-iliac axis in a single data acquisition. More detectors allow faster volume coverage (and reduce the contrast requirements).

Renal CT Angiography

Important indications for directed renal artery imaging comprise the assessment of patients with suspected renal vascular hypertension to exclude hemodynamically significant renal artery stenosis, as well as a complete preoperative assessment for renal transplant candidates. Current CT systems with 64+ channels permit rapid acquisition of large volumes of submillimeter data with isotropic resolution (equal resolution in the X, Y, and Z dimensions). This allows 3D data to be reconstructed in any plane. Wide ranges of functional techniques are now available with CTA, which may help us to identify patients who would or would not benefit from renal artery revascularization [23]. CTA of the renal arteries is performed with a high-resolution protocol (with thickness as low as 0.5–0.625 mm). Achieving adequate coverage to encompass the entire kidneys and the origins of accessory renal arteries is easily accomplished in a scan with a duration of <3 s, or as part of the aortic evaluation (described previously). With adequate selection of the acquisition parameters (thin collimation), high-spatial-resolution volumetric datasets for subsequent 2D and 3D reformation can be acquired (Fig. 18.9). Whereas fast acquisitions allow for a reduction of total contrast volume in the setting of CTA, this is not the case when CTA is combined with a second-phase abdominal MDCT acquisition for parenchymal (e.g., hepatic) imaging.

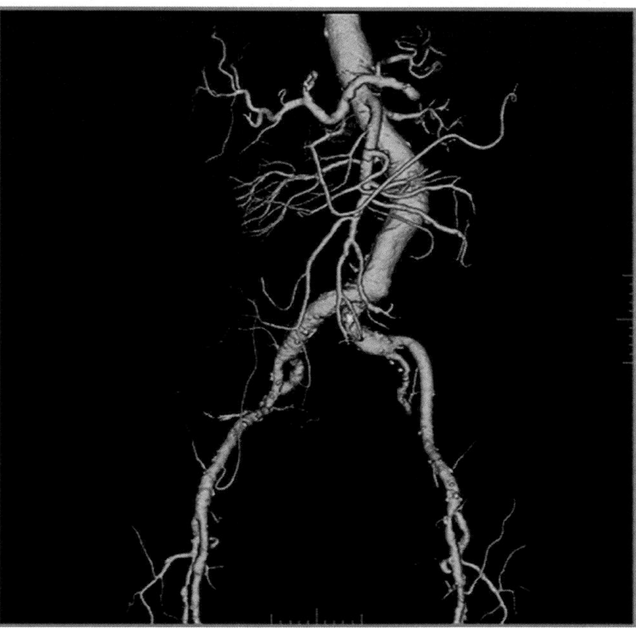

Fig. 18.9 A volume-rendered image of the abdominal aorta and vessels (including exquisite detail of the mesenteric and iliac arteries) using 64-detector MDCTA

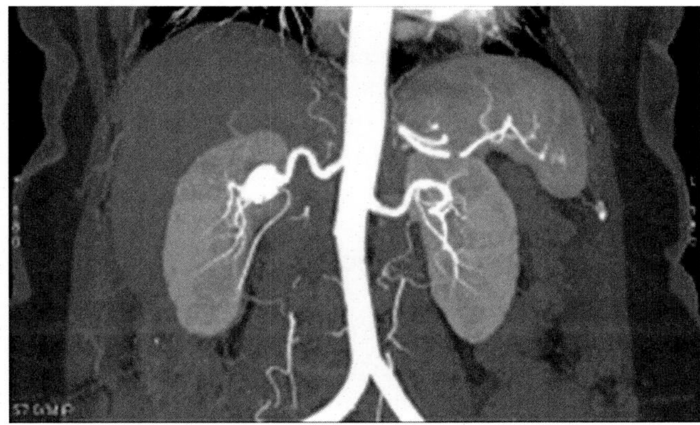

Fig. 18.10 Renal artery aneurysm

Comparison to Other Modalities

Although renal artery duplex ultrasound (US) is often the first examination performed, there are a number of well-recognized limitations, the most important of which is the challenge of optimally visualizing these vessels in obese patients. Catheter angiography has been the traditional gold standard for renal artery evaluation [24], but limitations include invasiveness of the procedure, contrast allergy, nephropathy, and plaque embolization. The improvements in spatial resolution and image quality of cross-sectional techniques have allowed MR and CTA to replace this invasive examination in most circumstances. MRA has also benefited from a number of recent developments, including improvements in gradient hardware and the recent introduction of parallel imaging, both of which permit reduced acquisition times and improved spatial resolution. However, thicker slices with MRA require acquisition in the plane of interest, making scanning protocols much more complicated. Renal CTA is an accurate and reliable test for visualizing vascular anatomy (Fig. 18.10) and renal artery stenosis, and it is therefore a viable alternative to MRA in the assessment of patients with renovascular hypertension and in potential living related renal donors.

CTA Accuracy in Diagnosis of Renal Artery Stenosis

Several studies investigated the diagnostic accuracy of CTA in the diagnosis of renal artery stenosis. CTA has been reported as having 94–100 % sensitivity and 79–97 % specificity [25]. Rountas et al. [26] compared the diagnostic accuracy of renal artery duplex US, CTA, and MRA to the gold standard, digital subtraction angiography, for the detection of renal artery stenosis in 58 patients with clinically suspected renovascular hypertension. There were 132 renal arteries. The sensitivity and specificity were 75 % and 89.6 % for renal artery duplex US, 94 % and 93 % for CTA, and 90 % and 94.1 % for MRA, respectively. Willmann et al. [27] obtained excellent-quality CT angiograms (92 % sensitivity and 99 % specificity) for the detection of hemodynamically significant arterial stenosis of aortoiliac and renal arteries. In this study, they used a half-second MDCT scanner and a nominal section thickness of 1 mm. Compared to MRA, there is no statistically significant difference between 3D MRA and CTA in the detection of hemodynamically significant arterial stenosis of the aortoiliac and renal arteries. This study also demonstrated that patient acceptance of the CT study is higher than that of either invasive angiography or MRA.

Methods of Renal CTA

As a rule of thumb, the injection duration should match the acquisition time in routine clinical practice. Biphasic injection protocols with an initially high injection rate followed by a slower continuing injection phase ensure optimal opacification of the renal arteries (Chap. 2). Note that high-concentration contrast material requires only moderate injection flow rates (with a maximum of 4.5 mL/s) to achieve high iodine administration rates [28].

Image Post-processing Techniques

While most vascular beds have demonstrated an advantage of MIP imaging over VR for accurate stenosis detection (especially coronary artery imaging), renal vasculature seems more amenable to quantitation with VR. One study specifically compared overall image quality and vascular delineation in MIP and VR images. The authors found that all main and accessory renal arteries depicted in invasive angiography were also demonstrated in MIP and VR images [29]. VR performed slightly better than MIP for quantification of stenoses >50 % (VR: $r^2=0.84$, $p<0.001$; MIP: $r^2=0.38$, $p=0.001$) and significantly better for severe stenoses (VR: $r^2=0.83$, $p<0.001$; MIP: $r^2=0.21$, $p=0.1$). For detection of stenosis, VR yielded a substantial improvement in positive predictive value (for stenoses >50 and 70 %, VR: 95 and 90 %; MIP: 86 and 68 %, respectively). The image quality obtained with VR was not significantly better than that with MIP, but vascular delineation in VR images was significantly better (Fig. 18.11). The VR technique of renal MRA enabled more accurate detection and quantification of renal artery stenosis than MIP, with significantly improved vascular delineation.

Tepe et al. [30] used 3D EBT angiography to evaluate renal artery lesions as well as vascular variants that are crucial to detect before surgery. Forty patients underwent EBT (GE-Imatron, C 150 ultrafast CT scanner, San Francisco, CA) of the renal arteries. The study demonstrated that both MIP and VR images were excellent in demonstrating stenosis of the renal arteries. Accessory and main renal arteries were easily depicted, and stenosis was shown with high accuracy. Among 40 renal angiography patients, 21 had stenosis of the renal arteries with different percentages. A total of 12 accessory renal arteries (five left, seven right) were detected. With its noninvasive VR and MIP techniques, CT is easy to apply and is functional and accurate for neoplasms, renal vascular anatomy, and renal artery stenosis.

Another study evaluated findings in 50 main and 11 accessory renal arteries [31]. All arteries depicted in conventional angiograms were visualized in MIP and VR images. Receiver operating characteristic (ROC) analysis for MIP and VR images demonstrated excellent discrimination for the diagnosis of stenosis of at least 50 % (area under the ROC curve, 0.96–0.99). Sensitivity was not significantly different for VR and MIP (89 % vs. 94 %, $p>0.1$), and specificity was greater with VR (99 % vs. 87 %, $p=0.008$–0.08). Stenosis of at least 50 % was overestimated with CTA in four accessory renal arteries, but three accessory renal arteries that were not depicted in conventional angiography were depicted in CTA. In the evaluation of renal artery stenosis, CTA with VR is faster and more accurate than CTA with MIP. Accessory arteries that were not depicted with conventional angiography were depicted with both CT angiographic algorithms.

Conclusion

CTA is a highly reliable technique for the detection of renal artery stenosis and for morphologic assessment. CTA can surpass conventional angiography in terms of diagnostic accuracy and reduced exposure to iodinated contrast (Fig. 18.11). In patients with renal insufficiency, color-coded duplex US or gadolinium-enhanced MRA should remain as the initial examination performed, depending on local expertise and availability. However, new warnings regarding systemic fibrosis with gadolinium make this agent contraindicated in patients with glomerular filtration rates of <30 mg/mL/mm^2.

Mesenteric CT Angiography

CTA has become a valuable minimally invasive tool for the visualization of normal vascular anatomy and its variants, as well as for pathologic conditions affecting the mesenteric vessels (Figs. 18.12 and 18.13) [32, 33]. CTA is considered the first-line imaging test in the diagnosis of mesenteric ischemia [34]. Indications for CTA include not only acute and chronic ischemia, aneurysm, and dissection, but also preoperative vascular assessment for patients undergoing liver lesion embolization and in the setting of liver transplantation [35, 36]. In addition, mesenteric CTA can assist in the evaluation of abdominal pain by ruling out other intra-abdominal pathology.

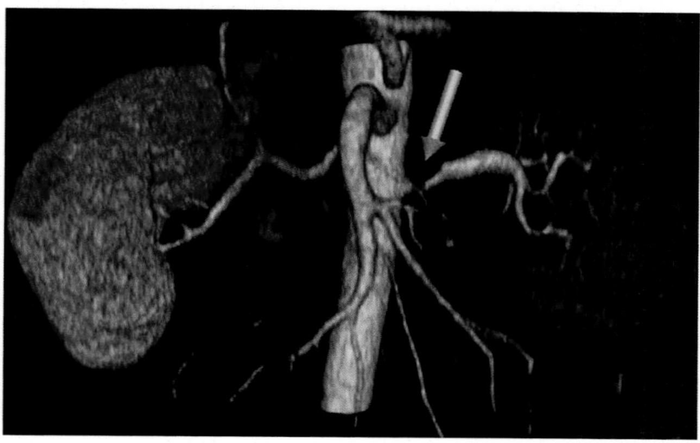

Fig. 18.11 A volume-rendered electron beam tomography (EBT) study of the renal arteries, depicting a high-grade stenosis of the left renal artery (*arrow*). The left kidney also opacifies less (*darker color*) than the right kidney, suggesting decreased blood flow and significance of the visualized stenosis

CTA Accuracy in Diagnosis of Mesenteric Ischemia

According to a recent review and meta-analysis that included eight studies, CTA has a high diagnostic accuracy in the diagnosis of mesenteric ischemia. Sensitivity ranged from 83 to 100 % with a pooled sensitivity of 94 %, and specificity ranged from 67 to 100 % with a pooled specificity of 95 % [37].

Methods and Image Post-processing Techniques

Protocols for typical aortic imaging (described previously) are used to image the mesenteric vasculature. Mesenteric CTA has been facilitated by rapid image acquisition with 64-slice scanners, which reduce artifacts from respiratory variation. This allows for the visualization of lesions at the mesenteric orifice and evaluation of distal reconstitution. Multiple axial images and rotational views may be necessary to evaluate mesenteric lesions at the aortic orifice. The reconstructed images allow for easy evaluation of all abdominal vasculature. VR is most often used, predominantly due to complex anatomy that makes MIP imaging more difficult (Fig. 18.13). Since the arteries are highly tortuous, leaving the 2D plane often (and traveling both caudally and

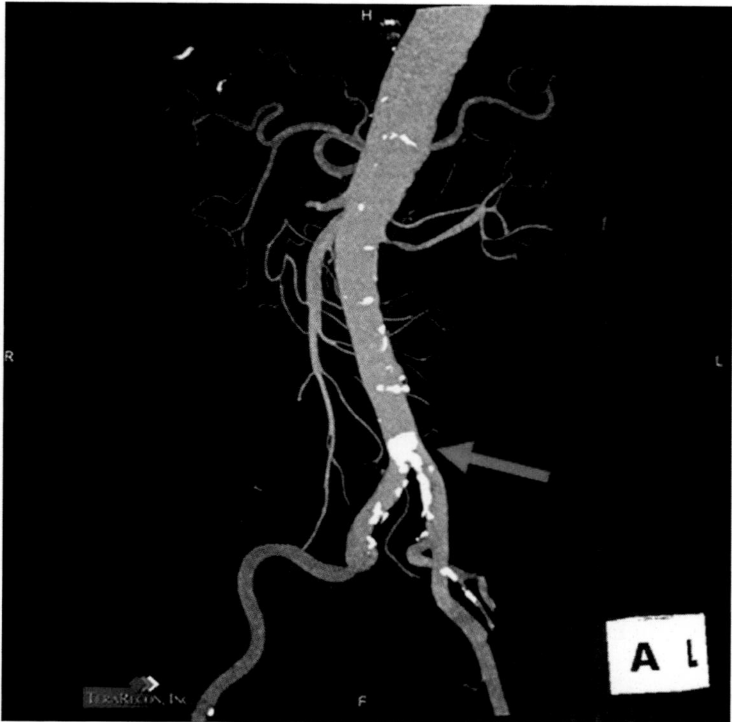

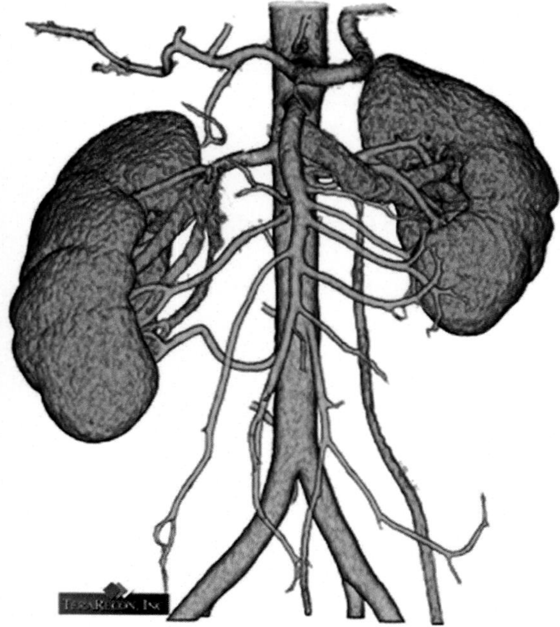

Fig. 18.12 Maximal intensity projection of the abdominal aorta, demonstrating severe calcifications at the iliac bifurcation (*arrow, left image*). The right image demonstrates a normal arterial bed in another patient, displayed using volume rendering (VR)

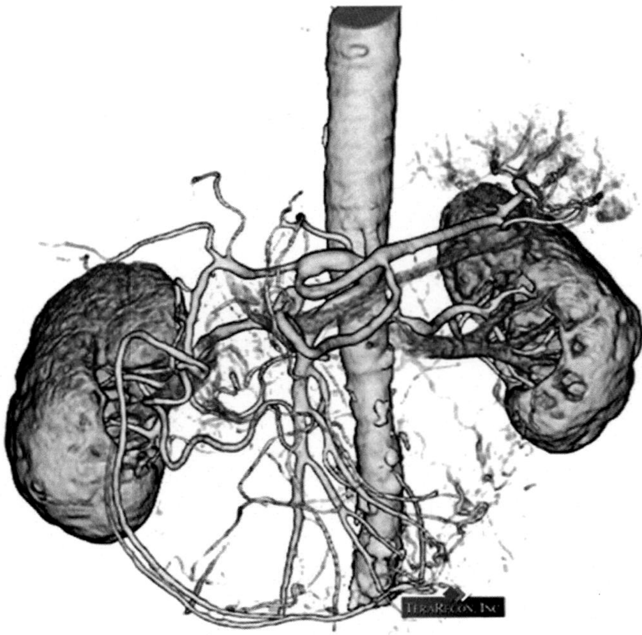

Fig. 18.13 3D image demonstrating the ability of CT to visualize the abdominal arteries, including the gastric arteries in this case

cranially at different times), these vessels pose the most challenge with axial interpretations. With coronary imaging, the arteries run cranial to caudal, without significant exception. Thus, interpreting with MIP or axial imaging is fairly straightforward, as the operator needs to systematically start from the most cranial images to the most caudal to follow the respective arteries. With mesenteric imaging, the arteries commonly turn both cranially and caudally, and VR enables visualization of the entire dataset with one reconstruction. No studies of the diagnostic potential of the different reconstruction methods have been reported.

Comparison to Other Modalities

Invasive angiography allows for diagnosis and treatment in a single test and is thus considered the reference standard test to evaluate acute and chronic mesenteric ischemia [38]. CTA and contrast-enhanced MRA are excellent noninvasive screening techniques for patients suspected of having mesenteric ischemia from all causes. CTA has higher spatial resolution and faster acquisition times, allowing assessment of the peripheral visceral branches and the inferior mesenteric artery with greater accuracy than contrast-enhanced MRA. In addition, it allows for the identification of calcified plaques. Contrast-enhanced MRA has a longer examination time that may result in delay therapeutic intervention. In addition, it has limited use in the diagnosis of distal stenosis and nonocclusive mesenteric ischemia [39]. MRA is therefore the clear second choice in this clinical setting, but the lack of radiation and iodinated contrast agents make it the best technique for children and patients with azotemia [40].

Carotid Artery CT Angiography

Ischemic cerebrovascular events are often due to atherosclerotic narrowing of the carotid bifurcation (Fig. 18.14) [41]. Carotid disease contributes to stroke, transient ischemic attacks, amaurosis figax through sudden occlusion, and cerebral or ocular embolization. Invasive angiography is the current reference standard for the evaluation of obstructive carotid artery disease. CTA is a robust technique in assessing carotid artery stenosis, allowing for excellent visualization of the lumen of the carotid artery using intravenous contrast (Fig. 18.15). Subsequent refinement of US, CT, and MRI techniques has led to changes in clinical practice, such that many centers have now abandoned conventional angiography in favor of safer imaging modalities [42].

CTA offers details of the entire relevant neurovascular axis by excluding significant carotid disease and intracranial disease [43]. Coupling non-contrast-enhanced cranial CT imaging with CT perfusion imaging and CTA of the entire cerebrovascular axis is both safe and feasible [44]. The eventual ability to preemptively identify asymptomatic plaques with high likelihood to produce symptoms is the most practical goal of the CTA imaging technique, which would allow for appropriate intervention prior to a disabling or fatal neurologic event. CTA and gadolinium-enhanced MRA have both proved to be reliable and fast techniques to evaluate the degree of internal carotid artery (ICA) stenosis [45]. Apart from a hemodynamically significant luminal stenosis, complexities in extracranial carotid artery plaque morphology have also been shown to increase the risk of thromboembolic events, including surface irregularities/ulcerations due to plaque rupture, calcification, fibrous cap thinning, intraplaque hemorrhage, and the presence of necrotic core. Out of all the modalities, luminal surface irregularities and ulcerations are most frequently seen in CTA.

The North American Symptomatic Carotid Endarterectomy Trial and European Carotid Surgery Trial demonstrated a large reduction in strokes by performing carotid endarterectomy [46, 47] in symptomatic patients with a stenosis of more than 70 %. Thus, an accurate assessment of carotid disease is important. Furthermore, endarterectomy in patients with a symptomatic moderate carotid stenosis of 50–69 % produced a moderate reduction in the risk of stroke [33]. Current practice is to use CTA to facilitate patient triage and provide specific information to rule out large vessel stenosis in patients with transient ischemic attacks, suspected stroke, or carotid bruits (Fig. 18.16) [42]. Common indications include evaluation of patients with carotid bruits, symptoms of vertebral insufficiency, borderline carotid US examinations, or insufficient

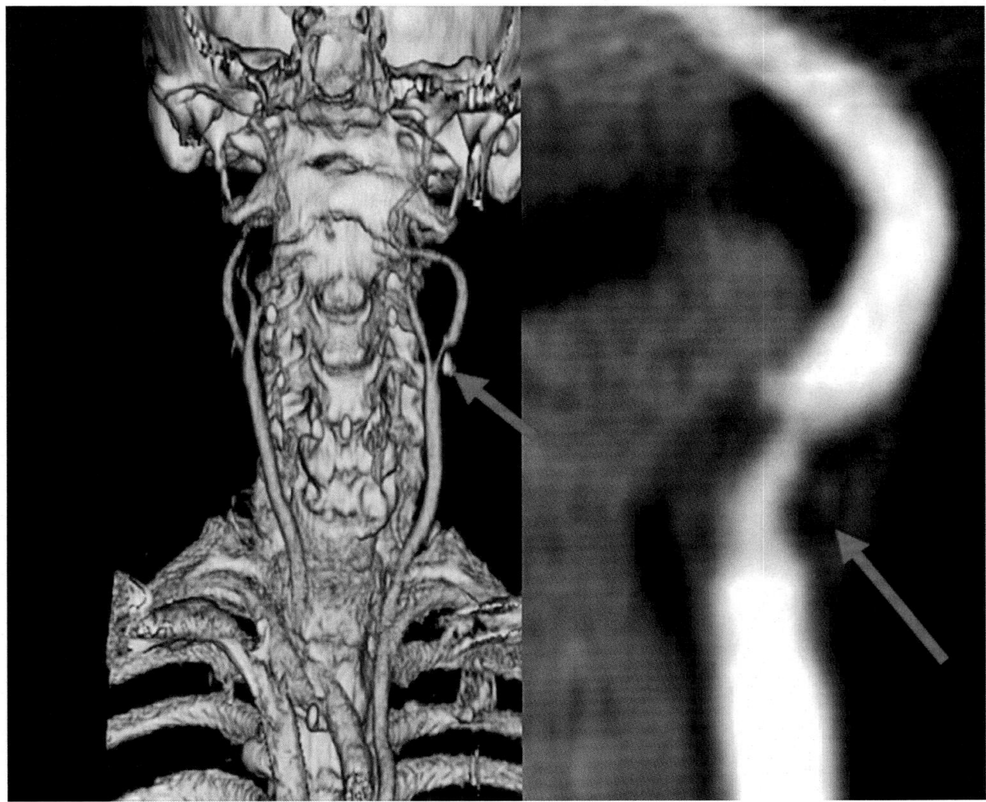

Fig. 18.14 Two patients with carotid stenosis at the bifurcation. The *left image* is a volume- rendered image, with a high-grade stenosis at the proximal portion of the internal carotid, with a dense calcification also seen (*arrow*). The *right image* demonstrates a maximal intensity projection image of the same region, with a tight stenosis and thrombus present (*arrow*)

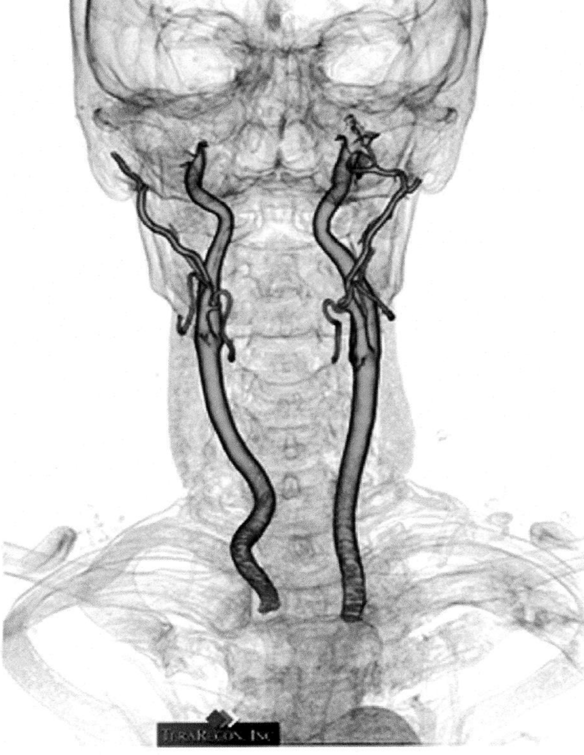

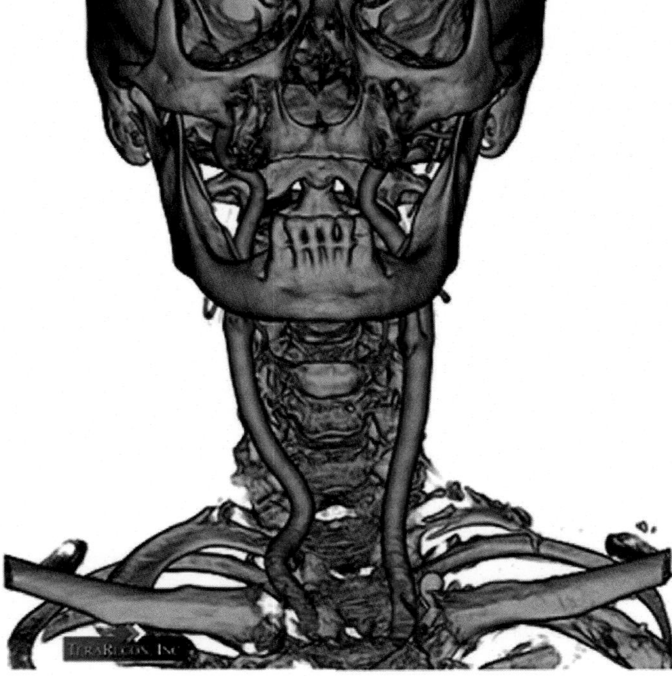

Fig. 18.15 3D images of normal carotid arteries bilaterally

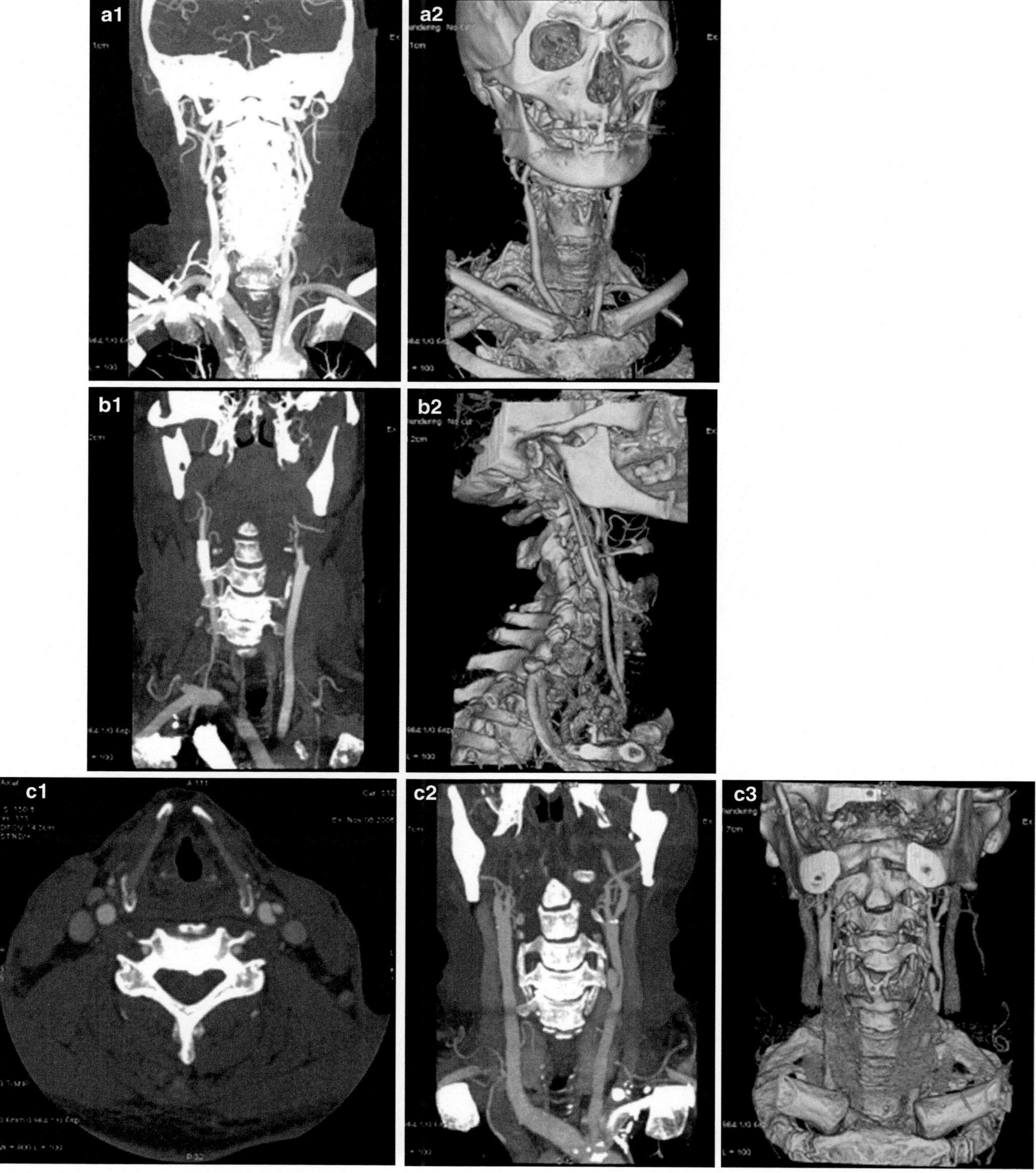

Fig. 18.16 (**a1**) Right external carotid artery stenosis. (**a2**) Volume rendered image of right external carotid artery stenosis. (**b1**) Coronal view of right internal carotid artery (ICA) stent. (**b2**) Volume rendered image of right ICA stent. (**c1**) Axial view of left carotid artery dissection. (**c2**) Coronal view of left carotid artery dissection. (**c3**) Volume rendered image of left carotid artery dissection

MRA examinations of the carotid system. Many vascular surgeons will not operate based upon carotid US, requiring confirmation with either CTA or invasive angiography.

Given that a large proportion of patients with carotid artery disease will be evaluated for potential carotid artery stenting, CT imaging should focus on assessment of the following: (1) stenosis severity, (2) disease within the aortic arch and at the origin of the common carotid arteries, (3) the size of the common carotid artery at the lesion location, (4) the size of the distal ICA, and (5) the presence of contralateral disease.

CTA Accuracy in Diagnosis of Carotid Artery Stenosis

According to previous research and reviews that included old CT scanners, contrast-enhanced MRA is more accurate than MDCT in diagnosing carotid artery stenosis [48, 49]. However, MDCT is quickly developing, and more high-quality images are being produced. A recent prospective study by Anzidei et al. evaluated 170 patients with suspected carotid artery disease. They compared the diagnostic accuracy of US Doppler, steady-state contrast-enhanced MRA, and CTA with invasive angiography as the reference standard. CTA has slightly better accuracy, sensitivity, and specificity than MRA (97 %, 95 %, and 98 % vs. 95 %, 93 %, and 97 %, respectively). CTA has a greater accuracy than US (97 % vs. 76 %). Moreover, CTA and MRA have an identical ability in plaque morphology and composition analysis with no statistical difference between the two tests [50].

Methods for Carotid CTA

Carotid CT angiographic images are obtained with patients placed in the supine position with the head tilted back as far as possible to avoid inclusion of dental hardware. Spiral data can be acquired with a slice thickness of 0.5–0.625 mm starting at the seventh cervical vertebra and proceeding as far cephalad as required. Transverse source images are reconstructed in 1-mm increments using a small field of view (15 cm). These parameters allowed for a spatial resolution of $0.3 \times 0.3 \times 0.6$ mm. Total coverage was approximately 18 cm. In general, good image quality is essential. A CT angiographic image of good quality is easily obtained if the patient does not move during the study. Given the faster scan times with increased detector systems, this is even easier. A breath-hold acquisition is not necessary. Compared with invasive angiography and CTA, a major limitation of gadolinium-enhanced MRA is spatial resolution.

With a power injector, 30–40 mL of nonionic contrast medium is injected at a rate of 2.5 mL/s into an antecubital vein. Administration of each bolus was followed immediately by a 20-mL saline flush. The acquisition is initiated after the start of the administration of contrast medium, the time of which was determined by a test of circulation time. By using automatic triggering with detection of the contrast material bolus, it is straightforward to selectively obtain an arterial phase image. Previous studies [51] have shown that a combination of optimal tracking volume placement and adjustment of tracking volume size ensures optimal sensitivity to the contrast material bolus. By choosing a 20-mm tracker volume placed in the aortic arch, bolus arrival was always detected. Careful timing is very important, with arterial enhancement being critical. It is vital to make sure that there is no venous filling when images are obtained. Obtaining images too early will lead to non-enhanced images, and obtaining images late allows for venous enhancement. Large jugular veins filled with contrast in close proximity to the carotid arteries can make the interpretation of carotid arteries more difficult.

Image Post-processing Techniques

Precision in the length and degree of stenosis has been reported to depend more on measurement technique than on acquisition parameters [52]. The accuracy of stenosis measurement depends on the scanning plane, which ideally should be perpendicular to the carotid artery used to obtain magnified transverse oblique images. Most authors consider MIP or curved multiplanar reconstructions as the most accurate techniques for measurements. VR is considered the least accurate technique for measurement. CTA allows data to be reconstructed into 2D and 3D images with cross-sectional views that can accurately depict plaque morphology. The images are analyzed with axial images and MIP or curved multiplanar reconstruction. Total post-processing is now done in real time (<1 min). MIP techniques allow data to be reconstructed into images that closely resemble conventional catheter-based angiograms that can be rotated 360° to be viewed from any angle. This helps to delineate the unstable plaques that are less stenotic but at high risk of producing symptomatic embolization or carotid occlusion.

Plaque Composition

Plaques that are more prone to disruption fracture or fissuring may be associated with a higher risk of embolization, occlusion, and consequent ischemic neurologic events [53]. The degree of arterial stenosis is the main determinant of stroke risk in carotid artery disease, and it has been used to select patients who will benefit from surgical intervention [54]. However, with recent advances in MRI and CTA imaging, there has been interest in atherosclerotic plaque features (vulnerable plaque) beyond the degree of stenosis in risk stratification for stroke. Wintermark el al. [55] found a good correlation between the plaque composition evaluated by CTA and histopathological findings.

A recent study by Gupta et al. [56] evaluated patients with high-grade ICA disease. There was a strong relation between increasing soft plaque thickness measurements and ipsilateral ischemic stroke (each 1-mm increase in plaque thickness corresponded to 2.7 times more likelihood of ipsilateral ischemic events). A cutoff thickness of 3.5 mm of the soft plaque can differentiate between asymptomatic and symptomatic individuals. In contrast, calcified plaque was associated with a lower risk of disease, with maximum thickness substantially higher in asymptomatic patients. Acute carotid ischemic events were associated certain plaque morphology found by CT imaging. Increased wall volume, a thinner fibrous cap, a greater number of lipid clusters, and lipid clusters closer to the lumen were associated with increased risk of stroke [57].

Comparison to Other Modalities

Invasive angiography has long been considered the standard for evaluation of carotid stenosis, but it has well-known risks and limitations. Invasive angiography allows only a limited number of views, which can lead to an underestimation of the degree of stenosis by as much as 40 % [58] compared with histological correlation. Invasive angiography is also a relatively expensive technique that uses numerous resources. Most importantly, there is a small but definite risk of major complications secondary to the procedure itself. The Asymptomatic Carotid Atherosclerosis Study Committee reported a 1.2 % risk of persisting neurologic deficit or death following invasive angiography, while the surgical risk was 1.5 %. The risks associated with CTA are markedly lower with similar or lower radiation exposures and no catheter-induced risks.

Carotid artery CTA has substantial benefits, including its accuracy, lack of invasiveness [59], and improved spatial and temporal resolution compared with MRA. Gadolinium-enhanced MRA is an appropriate technique for evaluating ICA stenosis [60–62]. Clinically relevant stenosis and occlusions of the ICA were correctly detected with good sensitivity, specificity, and interobserver agreement. Most studies with gadolinium-enhanced MRA demonstrate overestimation of the degree of stenosis [53, 61, 62]. Artifacts due to the excessive section thickness necessary with current MR systems cause a partial volume effect [58, 63]. The signal loss can also be explained by the presence of hemodynamic modifications. The decreased flow caused by stenosis leads to a reduced concentration of contrast agent in the distal arterial lumen, which may also explain why overestimation of stenosis with gadolinium-enhanced MRA can occur [64], especially for evaluating the degree of stenosis in small-vessel lumens. MRA can replace invasive angiography in most patients. However, it has been proved that CTA is highly accurate and can replace invasive angiography [44, 64].

In contrast to the other two modalities, CTA allows direct visualization of the arterial wall and atheromatous plaque, making the measurement of stenosis much easier. Almost all authors consider that calcified plaque is a limitation of CTA. This can be minimized by using multiplanar volume reconstruction to visualize the entire bifurcation initially with a large-volume reconstruction. By reducing volume reconstruction, we can clearly visualize the residual lumen at the maximal part of stenosis, even when circumferential calcified plaques are present. Moreover, CTA is able to differentiate mural calcifications and contrast material, because the attenuations of intraluminal contrast and calcifications are not similar. Therefore, calcifications should not be considered limitations of CTA [64]. In addition, carotid arteries tend to calcify less than either coronary or peripheral arteries (perhaps because carotid arteries are more elastic and less muscular), so dense circumferential calcifications occur less frequently in this vascular bed.

Detection of ulcerated plaques may prove to be important, since it has been suggested that the presence of plaque ulceration is a risk factor for embolism [65]. Most studies suggest that CTA is the best modality for analyzing plaque morphology. Plaque irregularities are more frequent in CTA than in invasive angiography or contrast-enhanced MRA. However, the inability of invasive angiography to depict plaque ulceration is well documented [65, 66], partly because of the limited number of views typically obtained. The case of CTA depicting an ulceration that is not depicted in gadolinium-enhanced MRA could be due to a lack of spatial resolution in gadolinium-enhanced MRA.

Conclusion

Carotid CTA has matured and can be used to quantify stenoses more precisely than US, to detect tandem stenoses, and for the workup of acute stroke patients. The newer scanners and multiple dose-saving strategies have the additional advantage of a very low radiation profile, allowing for minimal risk to the patient and maximum visualization of the arteries in question.

Vertebral Artery CT Angiography

Although conventional intra-arterial angiography remains the gold standard method for imaging the vertebral artery, noninvasive modalities such as MDCT, MRA, and US are constantly improving and are playing an increasingly important role in diagnosing vertebral artery pathology in clinical practice. Normal anatomy, normal variants, and a number of pathologic entities such as vertebral atherosclerosis, arterial dissection, arteriovenous fistula, subclavian steal syndrome, and vertebrobasilar dolichoectasia can be seen.

Chapter Summary

During the past decade, we have been witness to a tremendous development in the field of CT imaging. CTA has gained remarkably by improvements in scan time and image quality, replacing diagnostic angiography in many cases of aorta, renal, mesenteric, and carotid angiography. In addition, there has been an exciting advance in techniques for reducing radiation dose that have achieved dramatic results and decreased radiation concerns. These vascular beds suffer from fewer motion artifacts (except for the ascending aorta), so imaging with CTA is ideal. CTA is less expensive and less invasive, and it allows for simultaneous visualization of large anatomic areas from multiple angles using 3D display.

References

1. Stanford W, Rooholamini SA, Galvin JR. Ultrafast computed tomography in the diagnosis of aortic aneurysms and dissections. J Thorac Imaging. 1990;5(4):32–9.
2. Katz DS, Hon M. CT angiography of the lower extremities and aortoiliac system with a multi-detector row helical CT scanner: promise of new opportunities fulfilled. Radiology. 2001;221(1):7–10.
3. Kim JK, et al. Living donor kidneys: usefulness of multi-detector row CT for comprehensive evaluation. Radiology. 2003;229(3):869–76.
4. Kalender WA, Quick HH. Recent advances in medical physics. Eur Radiol. 2011;21(3):501–4.
5. Roos JE, et al. Thoracic aorta: motion artifact reduction with retrospective and prospective electrocardiography-assisted multidetector row CT. Radiology. 2002;222(1):271–7.
6. Qanadli SD, et al. Motion artifacts of the aorta simulating aortic dissection on spiral CT. J Comput Assist Tomogr. 1999;23(1):1–6.
7. Gotway MB, Dawn SK. Thoracic aorta imaging with multisclice CT. Radiol Clin North Am. 2003;41(3):521–43.
8. Blanke P, et al. Thoracic aorta: prospective electrocardiographically triggered CT angiography with dual-source CT--feasibility, image quality, and dose reduction. Radiology. 2010;255(1):207–17.
9. Raff GL. Radiation dose from coronary CT angiography: five years of progress. J Cardiovasc Comput Tomogr. 2010;4(6):365–74.
10. Fishman JE. Imaging of blunt aortic and great vessel trauma. J Thorac Imaging. 2000;15(2):97–103.
11. Kouchoukos NT, Dougenis D. Surgery of the thoracic aorta. N Engl J Med. 1997;336(26):1876–88.
12. Rubin GD. Helical CT angiography of the thoracic aorta. J Thorac Imaging. 1997;12(2):128–49.
13. Rubin GD, et al. Aorta and iliac arteries: single versus multiple detector-row helical CT angiography. Radiology. 2000;215(3):670–6.
14. Galla JD, et al. Identification of risk factors in patients undergoing thoracoabdominal aneurysm repair. J Card Surg. 1997;12(2 Suppl):292–9.
15. Semba CP, et al. Acute rupture of the descending thoracic aorta: repair with use of endovascular stent-grafts. J Vasc Interv Radiol. 1997;8(3):337–42.
16. Zinck SE, Primack SL. Radiographic and CT findings in blunt chest trauma. J Thorac Imaging. 2000;15(2):87–96.
17. Lu B, et al. Electron beam tomography with three-dimensional reconstruction in the diagnosis of aortic diseases. J Cardiovasc Surg (Torino). 2000;41(5):659–68.
18. Hobo R, Buth J, EUROSTAR Collaborators. Secondary interventions following endovascular abdominal aortic aneurysm repair using current endografts. A EUROSTAR report. J Vasc Surg. 2006;43(5):896–902.
19. Halpern EJ. Triple-rule-out CT angiography for evaluation of acute chest pain and possible acute coronary syndrome. Radiology. 2009;252(2):332–45.
20. Hayter RG, et al. Suspected aortic dissection and other aortic disorders: multi-detector row CT in 373 cases in the emergency setting. Radiology. 2006;238(3):841–52.
21. Stueckle CA, et al. Multislice computed tomography angiography of the abdominal arteries: comparison between computed tomography angiography and digital subtraction angiography findings in 52 cases. Australas Radiol. 2004;48(2):142–7.
22. Yoshida S, et al. Thoracic involvement of type A aortic dissection and intramural hematoma: diagnostic accuracy – comparison of emergency helical CT and surgical findings. Radiology. 2003;228(2):430–5.
23. Glockner JF, Vrtiska TJ. Renal MR and CT angiography: current concepts. Abdom Imaging. 2007;32(3):407–20.
24. Kim D, et al. Renal artery imaging: a prospective comparison of intra-arterial digital subtraction angiography with conventional angiography. Angiology. 1991;42(5):345–57.
25. Sarkodieh JE, Walden SH, Low D. Imaging and management of atherosclerotic renal artery stenosis. Clin Radiol. 2013;68(6): 627–35.
26. Rountas C, et al. Imaging modalities for renal artery stenosis in suspected renovascular hypertension: prospective intraindividual comparison of color Doppler US, CT angiography, GD-enhanced MR angiography, and digital substraction angiography. Ren Fail. 2007;29(3):295–302.
27. Willmann JK, et al. Aortoiliac and renal arteries: prospective intraindividual comparison of contrast-enhanced three-dimensional MR angiography and multi-detector row CT angiography. Radiology. 2003;226(3):798–811.
28. Fleischmann D. Multiple detector-row CT angiography of the renal and mesenteric vessels. Eur J Radiol. 2003;45 Suppl 1:S79–87.
29. Mallouhi A, et al. 3D MR angiography of renal arteries: comparison of volume rendering and maximum intensity projection algorithms. Radiology. 2002;223(2):509–16.
30. Tepe SM, Memisoglu E, Kural AR. Three-dimensional noninvasive contrast-enhanced electron beam tomography angiography of the kidneys: adjunctive use in medical and surgical management. Clin Imaging. 2004;28(1):52–8.
31. Johnson PT, et al. Renal artery stenosis: CT angiography – comparison of real-time volume-rendering and maximum intensity projection algorithms. Radiology. 1999;211(2):337–43.
32. Laghi A, et al. Multislice spiral computed tomography angiography of mesenteric arteries. Lancet. 2001;358(9282):638–9.
33. Lawler LP, Fishman EK. Celiomesenteric anomaly demonstration by multidetector CT and volume rendering. J Comput Assist Tomogr. 2001;25(5):802–4.
34. Oliva IB, et al. ACR Appropriateness Criteria (R) imaging of mesenteric ischemia. Abdom Imaging. 2013;38(4):714–9.
35. Erbay N, et al. Living donor liver transplantation in adults: vascular variants important in surgical planning for donors and recipients. AJR Am J Roentgenol. 2003;181(1):109–14.
36. Byun JH, et al. Evaluation of the hepatic artery in potential donors for living donor liver transplantation by computed tomography angiography using multidetector-row computed tomography: comparison of volume rendering and maximum intensity projection techniques. J Comput Assist Tomogr. 2003;27(2):125–31.
37. Cudnik MT, et al. The diagnosis of acute mesenteric ischemia: a systematic review and meta-analysis. Acad Emerg Med. 2013;20(11):1087–100.

38. Brandt LJ, Boley SJ. AGA technical review on intestinal ischemia. American Gastrointestinal Association. Gastroenterology. 2000;118(5):954–68.
39. Laissy JP, Trillaud H, Douek P. MR angiography: noninvasive vascular imaging of the abdomen. Abdom Imaging. 2002;27(5):488–506.
40. Shih MC, Hagspiel KD. CTA and MRA in mesenteric ischemia: part 1, role in diagnosis and differential diagnosis. AJR Am J Roentgenol. 2007;188(2):452–61.
41. Kannel WB. Current status of the epidemiology of brain infarction associated with occlusive arterial disease. Stroke. 1971;2(4):295–318.
42. North American Symptomatic Carotid Endarterectomy Trial Collaborators. Beneficial effect of carotid endarterectomy in symptomatic patients with high-grade carotid stenosis. N Engl J Med. 1991;325(7):445–53.
43. Smith WS, et al. Safety and feasibility of a CT protocol for acute stroke: combined CT, CT angiography, and CT perfusion imaging in 53 consecutive patients. AJNR Am J Neuroradiol. 2003;24(4):688–90.
44. Na DG, et al. Multiphasic perfusion computed tomography in hyperacute ischemic stroke: comparison with diffusion and perfusion magnetic resonance imaging. J Comput Assist Tomogr. 2003;27(2):194–206.
45. Runge VM, Kirsch JE, Lee C. Contrast-enhanced MR angiography. J Magn Reson Imaging. 1993;3(1):233–9.
46. MRC European carotid surgery trial: interim results for symptomatic patients with severe (70-99%) or with mild (0-29%) carotid stenosis. European Carotid Surgery Trialists' Collaborative Group. Lancet. 1991;337(8752):1235–43.
47. Barnett HJ, et al. Benefit of carotid endarterectomy in patients with symptomatic moderate or severe stenosis. North American Symptomatic Carotid Endarterectomy Trial Collaborators. N Engl J Med. 1998;339(20):1415–25.
48. U-King-Im JM, Young V, Gillard JH. Carotid-artery imaging in the diagnosis and management of patients at risk of stroke. Lancet Neurol. 2009;8(6):569–80.
49. Chappell FM, et al. Carotid artery stenosis: accuracy of noninvasive tests – individual patient data meta-analysis. Radiology. 2009;251(2):493–502.
50. Anzidei M, et al. Diagnostic accuracy of colour Doppler ultrasonography, CT angiography and blood-pool-enhanced MR angiography in assessing carotid stenosis: a comparative study with DSA in 170 patients. Radiol Med. 2012;117(1):54–71.
51. Castillo M, Wilson JD. CT angiography of the common carotid artery bifurcation: comparison between two techniques and conventional angiography. Neuroradiology. 1994;36(8):602–4.
52. Cinat M, et al. Helical CT angiography in the preoperative evaluation of carotid artery stenosis. J Vasc Surg. 1998;28(2):290–300.
53. Cronqvist M, et al. Evaluation of time-of-flight and phase-contrast MRA sequences at 1.0 T for diagnosis of carotid artery disease. I. A phantom and volunteer study. Acta Radiol. 1996;37(3 Pt 1):267–77.
54. Halliday A, et al. 10-year stroke prevention after successful carotid endarterectomy for asymptomatic stenosis (ACST-1): a multicentre randomised trial. Lancet. 2010;376(9746):1074–84.
55. Wintermark M, et al. High-resolution CT imaging of carotid artery atherosclerotic plaques. AJNR Am J Neuroradiol. 2008;29(5):875–82.
56. Gupta A, et al. Evaluation of computed tomography angiography plaque thickness measurements in high-grade carotid artery stenosis. Stroke. 2014;45(3):740–5.
57. Wintermark M, et al. Carotid plaque computed tomography imaging in stroke and nonstroke patients. Ann Neurol. 2008;64(2):149–57.
58. Levy RA, Prince MR. Arterial-phase three-dimensional contrast-enhanced MR angiography of the carotid arteries. AJR Am J Roentgenol. 1996;167(1):211–5.
59. Marro B, et al. Computerized tomographic angiography scan following carotid endarterectomy. Ann Vasc Surg. 1998;12(5):451–6.
60. Leclerc X, et al. Contrast-enhanced three-dimensional fast imaging with steady-state precession (FISP) MR angiography of supraaortic vessels: preliminary results. AJNR Am J Neuroradiol. 1998;19(8):1405–13.
61. Slosman F, et al. Extracranial atherosclerotic carotid artery disease: evaluation of non-breath-hold three-dimensional gadolinium-enhanced MR angiography. AJR Am J Roentgenol. 1998;170(2):489–95.
62. Scarabino T, et al. MR angiography in carotid stenosis: a comparison of three techniques. Eur J Radiol. 1998;28(2):117–25.
63. Remonda L, Heid O, Schroth G. Carotid artery stenosis, occlusion, and pseudo-occlusion: first-pass, gadolinium-enhanced, three-dimensional MR angiography – preliminary study. Radiology. 1998;209(1):95–102.
64. Randoux B, Marro B, Marsault C. Carotid artery stenosis: competition between CT angiography and MR angiography. AJNR Am J Neuroradiol. 2004;25(4):663–4; author reply 664.
65. Hatsukami TS, et al. Carotid plaque morphology and clinical events. Stroke. 1997;28(1):95–100.
66. Comerota AJ, et al. The preoperative diagnosis of the ulcerated carotid atheroma. J Vasc Surg. 1990;11(4):505–10.

Assessment of Pulmonary Vascular Disease

19

Bradley S. Messenger and Ronald J. Oudiz

Abstract

Pulmonary hypertension (PH) is defined as an abnormal elevation of pulmonary arterial pressure (PAP), with a mean PAP ≥25 mmHg. A classification system organizes this heterogeneous patient population into five groups based on the underlying etiology, pathogenesis, and pathophysiology associated with the PH. A thorough diagnostic workup is necessary to determine the precise etiology, treatment strategy, and prognosis for patients with PH. Cardiac Computed Tomography is a useful tool in PH for detection of disease, workup, and characterization of the underlying etiologies as it describes the cardiac structures and functional abnormalities seen with PH.

Keywords

Pulmonary Arterial Hypertension • Pulmonary Artery • Right Ventricle • Pulmonary Embolism • Right Heart Catheterization • Cardiac Structure

Pulmonary hypertension (PH) is defined as an abnormal elevation of the pulmonary arterial pressure with diverse etiologies and pathogenesis. It is hemodynamically defined as a mean pulmonary artery pressure ≥25 mm Hg and pulmonary vascular resistance >3 Wood units. The presence of PH typically leads to the right ventricular failure syndrome [1] of dyspnea, fluid overload, and untimely death, and is responsible for millions of US hospital admissions annually.

Diseases of the pulmonary circulation span a variety of disease entities including pulmonary arterial hypertension (PAH), pulmonary venous hypertension, chronic thromboembolic pulmomary hypertension (CTEPH), pulmonary arteriovenous malformation, pulmonary arterial stenosis, pulmonary arterial aneurysm, pulmonary venoocclusive disease, and pulmonary capillary hemangiomatosis. (See section "Classification of PH", below) In this chapter, we provide an overview of PH characteristics seen on cardiac CT.

B.S. Messenger, MD (✉)
Division of Cardiology, Department of Medicine,
Harbor-UCLA Medical Center,
k1000 West Carson Street, Torrance, CA 90502, USA
e-mail: Bradley.messenger@gmail.com

R.J. Oudiz, MD
Department of Medicine, Los Angeles Biomedical Research Institute, The David Geffen School of Medicine at UCLA, Harbor-UCLA Medical Center, Torrance, CA, USA

Classification of PH

The simplicity of defining pulmonary hypertension with hemodynamic data belies the challenges of diagnosing and managing this disorder. The patient population is heterogeneous with multiple potential etiologies, prognoses, and treatment options. The modified classification from the 5th World Symposium on PH held in Nice, France in 2013 (revised from the previous revision in 2008) divides PH into five groups, shown in Table 19.1. The largest groups in the Western world are Groups 2 and 3, respectively the left sided heart disease and hypoxic lung disease [2].

Group 1 PH: PAH

Group 1 pulmonary hypertension is referred to as pulmonary arterial hypertension (PAH), a disease of the precapillary

M.J. Budoff, J.S. Shinbane (eds.), *Cardiac CT Imaging: Diagnosis of Cardiovascular Disease*,
DOI 10.1007/978-3-319-28219-0_19

Table 19.1 Summary of CT findings in pulmonary hypertension

Pulmonary arteries
Enlarged proximal vessels
Pruning of the distal vessels
Calcification of the proximal pulmonary arteries
Thrombosis
Aneurysms
Heart
RA, RV, and IVC dilation
RV hypertrophy
Decreased RV systolic function
Flattened interventricular septum ("D-shaped" and undersized left ventricle)
Pericardial thickening and/or effusion
Others
Hypertrophy of bronchial arteries
Segmental bronchial artery to bronchus ratio > 1:1 in 3 or 4 lobes
Retrograde opacification of the inferior vena cava or hepatic vein

pulmonary circulation due to a complex process intrinsic to the pulmonary vasculature. As many entities clinically mimic PAH, it is a diagnosis of exclusion, requiring a thorough workup and proper consideration of more common etiologies such as left-sided heart disease and hypoxic lung disease. PAH, like PH, is similarly defined hemodynamically as a mean pulmonary artery pressure ≥25 mmHg at rest and PVR >3 Wood units, but the pulmonary capillary wedge pressure measures ≤15 mmHg [3].

The natural history of PAH is variable based upon etiology but it typically follows a progressive course with a poor prognosis if left untreated [4]. Most patients with PAH present with exertional dyspnea that worsens over months to years. Exertional angina, syncope, and peripheral edema appear later in the course when increasing pulmonary vascular resistance strains and ultimately impairs right ventricular function. The diagnosis of PAH is often delayed due to the nonspecific symptoms and subtle findings on physical examination {5].

Idiopathic and Heritable PAH

Idiopathic PAH (IPAH) is a diagnosis of exclusion in which no etiology nor family history can account for the disease. The incidence of IPAH is rare, with an estimated incidence of 1–2 cases per million per year worldwide [6]. The disorder is approximately 4 times more common in women [7, 8], presenting in the third decade for women and in the fourth decade for men without racial or ethnic predisposition [6].

PAH has a familial component is some patients. Germline mutations in the bone morphogenetic protein receptor type 2 (*BMPR2*) gene can be detected in approximately 70 % of cases [8, 9]. Mutations in activin receptor-like kinase type 1 (ALK-1 or endoglin have been found in familial PH with a strong association for concomitant hereditary hemorrhagic telangiectasia. *BMPR2* mutations, however, have also been detected in 11 % to 40 % of apparently idiopathic cases without a family history [10, 11], so the distinction between idiopathic and familial *BMPR2* mutations may be artificial. Interestingly, in up to 30 % of families with PAH, no *BMPR2* mutation has been identified. Thus, heritable forms of PAH include IPAH with germline mutations and familial cases with or without identified germline mutations [12, 13]. Genetic testing is not mandatory in heritable PAH, genetic testing should only be performed after genetic counseling, with a discussion of the risks, benefits, and limitations of such testing [14].

PAH Associated with Connective Tissue Diseases

The prevalence of PAH has been well established for patients with systemic sclerosis (SSc). Two recent prospective studies using echocardiography as a screening method and right heart catheterization for confirmation found a prevalence of PAH in SS of between 7 % and 12 % [15, 16]. The prevalence of PAH in systemic lupus erythematosis and mixed connective tissue disease remains unknown; although its incidence is greater than IPAH, it occurs less frequently than in SSc [17–20]. In the absence of fibrotic lung disease, PAH has also been reported infrequently in Sjögren syndrome [21], polymyositis [22], and rheumatoid arthritis [23]. Approximately one half of patients with PH and connective tissue diseases will die within 1 year if left untreated [24]. PH is also a frequent complication of idiopathic pulmonary fibrosis (IPF). IPF patients with concomitant PH have a two to threefold increase in mortality compared to IPF patients with normal pulmonary arterial pressures [25]. However, the presence or severity of PH does not correlate with the level of IPF disease seen on high resolution CT [26]. It is increasingly being recognized that PH in patients with IPF is the sequelae of a "primary" occlusive pulmonary vasculopathy, rather than being purely secondary to fibrotic destruction of the vascular bed [27].

PAH Associated with Congenital Heart Disease (CHD)

PAH related to CHD results from the effects of a longstanding abnormal increase in pulmonary blood flow which leads to pathologic changes in the pulmonary vasculature, particularly in the smaller vessels. This results in increased pulmonary vascular resistance, which in turn has deleterious effects upon the heart and larger pulmonary vascular structures. Direct shunts can increase pulmonary blood flow and pressure (patent ductus arteriosis) (Fig. 19.1).

Eisenmenger syndrome is defined as CHD with an initially large systemic-to-pulmonary shunt that induces progressive pulmonary vascular disease and PAH, resulting in reversal of the shunt and central cyanosis [28, 29]. Eisenmenger syndrome represents the most advanced form

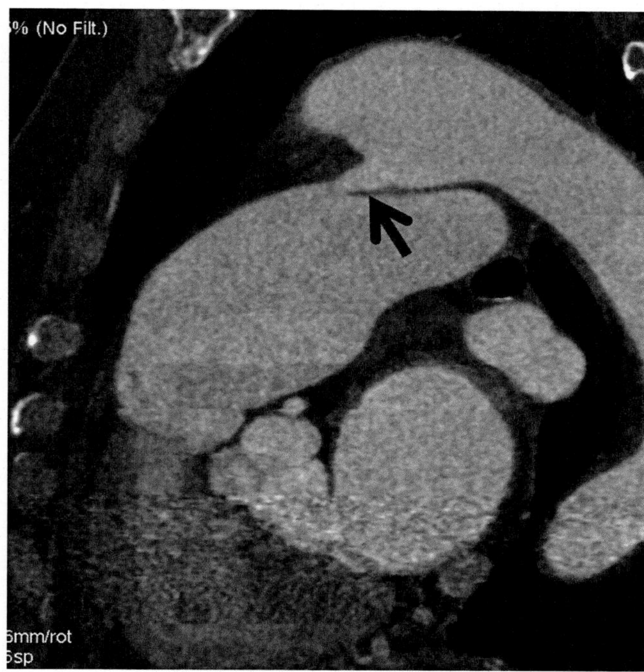

Fig. 19.1 64 slice multi-detector CT in a 20 year-old woman with patent ductus arteriosis (*black arrow*), seen well in this sagittal view with resultant dilation of the main pulmonary artery

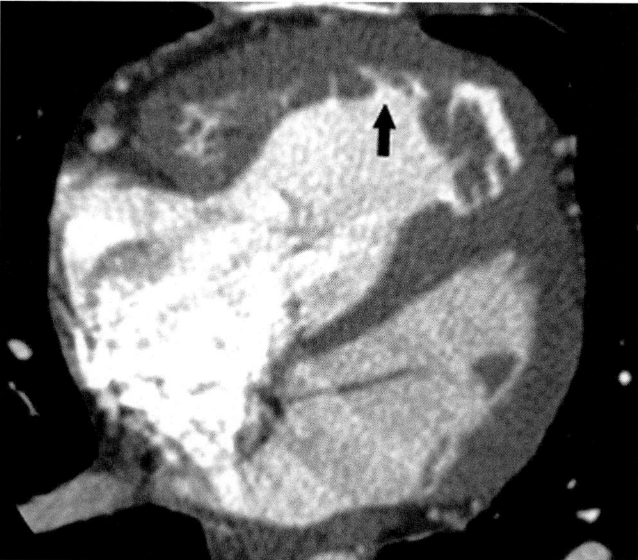

Fig. 19.2 CT scan in a 22 year-old woman with Eisenmenger syndrome due to atrial septal defect and pulmonary hypertension. Right cardiac chambers are enlarged with marked right ventricular hypertrophy (*black arrow*)

of PAH associated with CHD (Fig. 19.2). A large proportion of patients with CHD develop some degree of PAH [30–32]. The prevalence of PAH associated with congenital systemic-to-pulmonary shunts in Europe and North America ranges between 1.6 and 12.5 cases per million adults, with 25–50 % of this population affected by Eisenmenger syndrome [33].

PAH Associated with Schistosomiasis

Though not prominent in industrialized nations, schistosomiasis may be the most common cause of PAH in the world given the expected 200 million people infected with the parasite [34]. The mechanism of PH is probably multifactorial, and includes mechanical obstruction, local vascular inflammation related to eggs, and portal hypertension [35, 36]. These cases can have a similar clinical presentation to IPAH [37], with similar histopathologic findings [38], and thus similar radiographic appearance. PAH occurs almost exclusively in the 10 % of infected patients who develop hepatosplenic schistosomiasis [39].

Pulmonary Veno-Occlusive Disease and Pulmonary Capillary Hemangiomatosis

Pulmonary veno-occlusive disease (PVOD) accounts for a small number of pulmonary hypertension cases, most commonly in children and young adults [40]. The estimated annual incidence rate is 0.1–0.2 cases of PVOD per million persons in the general population [41, 42].

Patients with PH due to PVOD frequently present with congestive heart failure symptoms of dyspnea on exertion, peripheral edema, and radiographic signs of pulmonary edema with Kerley B lines that is expected with post-capillary PH. However, the hemodynamics at right heart catheterization similar to pre-capillary PH and may lead clinicians to diagnose idiopathic PH [40]. Vasodilator therapy, as used to treat a subset of idiopathic PH patients, can cause acute pulmonary edema, so distinguishing PVOD from IPAH has important clinical significance.

CT imaging may help raise a clinician's suspicion for PVOD. The CT findings of the disease includes smooth septal thickening, diffuse or mosaic ground-glass opacities, multiple small nodules, and pleural effusion [43–47]. PVOD and pulmonary capillary hemangiomatosis (PCH) also show the presence of crackles and clubbing on physical examination, hemosiderin-laden macrophages on bronchoalveolar lavage [48], as well as lower carbon monoxide diffusing capacity and PaO_2 [47]. In a comparison study, PVOD patients had peripheral ground glass opacities (GGO) in 93 % of cases compared with 13 % incidence of GGO in patients with PAH [49]. Thickened interlobular septa and mediastinal adenopathy were also strongly correlated with PVOD compared with PAH patients [41].

The only effective treatment for PVOD is lung transplant with most diagnoses being made at time of transplant or autopsy.

Group 2 PH: Pulmonary Hypertension due to Left Heart Disease

One of the most commonly seen forms of PH is pulmonary hypertension due to left heart disease. Since the etiology of their PH is distal to the pulmonary arterial system, Group 2 patients have "post-capillary" PH. Like other forms of PH, it manifests clinical signs and symptoms of the right heart failure syndrome. Group II PH includes patients with preserved or reduced ejection fraction, valvular heart disease and certain forms of congenital heart disease affecting left ventricular flow and/or performance.

Group 3 PH: Pulmonary Hypertension due to Lung Diseases and/or Hypoxia

A subcategory of lung disease characterized by a mixed obstructive and restrictive pattern includes chronic bronchiectasis, cystic fibrosis [50], and a newly identified syndrome characterized by the combination of pulmonary fibrosis, mainly of the lower zones of the lung, and emphysema, mainly of the upper zones of the lung [51]. The prevalence of PH in all of these conditions remains largely unknown. However, in a recent retrospective study of 998 patients with chronic obstructive pulmonary disease who underwent right heart catheterization, only 1 % had severe pulmonary hypertension (mean PA pressure >40 mm Hg) [52]. In the syndrome of combined pulmonary fibrosis and emphysema, the prevalence of PH is almost 50 % [51].

Group 4 PH: Chronic Thromboembolic Pulmonary Hypertension (CTEPH)

Pulmonary embolism (PE) is an obstruction of a pulmonary artery caused by a blood clot, air, fat, or tumor tissue. The most common cause of the obstruction is a blood clot (thrombus) usually from a peripheral vein. The average annual incidence of venous thromboembolism (VTE) in the United States is 1 per 1000, with about 250,000 incident cases occurring annually [53–55]. The challenge in understanding the real disease is that an additional equal number of patients are diagnosed with PE at autopsy [53, 56]. It is estimated that between 650,000 and900,000 fatal and nonfatal VTE events occur in the US annually [57]. The classic triad of signs and symptoms of PE (hemoptysis, dyspnea, chest pain) are neither sensitive nor specific, and many patients with PE are initially asymptomatic; most patients who have symptoms often have atypical and/or nonspecific symptoms.

Diagnostic Workup of PE

Many diagnostic tests have been suggested for the evaluation of patients with suspected VTE. These include the history and physical examination to the electrocardiogram, chest radiography, echocardiography, ventilation-perfusion scintigraphy, pulmonary angiography, CT and MR angiography, lower-extremity venography, and sonography. Although the diagnostic accuracy of laboratory tests such as D-dimer has increased (a negative result in combination with a low-probability clinical assessment provides reasonable certainty for excluding PE), radiographic imaging plays an important role in the diagnosis of PE, especially with the development of multi-detector CT (MDCT) and increased use of CT pulmonary angiography.

Although normal chest x-ray findings are observed in 24 % of patients with PE, an elevated hemidiaphragm can be observed in 20 % of patients with acute PE [58]. An elevated hemidiaphragm, consolidation, pleural effusion, or atelectasis occurs in about 2/3 of patients with acute PE. Especially in a massive PE (Fig. 19.3), local hyperlucency is seen when a lobar or segmental artery is occluded (Westermark sign), and engorgement of a major hilar artery (Fleischner sign) can be detected [59, 60]. Abrupt tapering or termination of a pulmonary vessel (knuckle sign), a pleural-based density or costophrenic density (Hampton's hump), and alveolar or interstitial pulmonary edema may occur. Most of the above chest x-ray findings are nonspecific. Nuclear scintigraphy (ventilation-perfusion or V/Q scanning) is useful if multidetector CT angiography (MDCTA) is not available. The V/Q scan in a patient with an acute PE will demonstrate an area

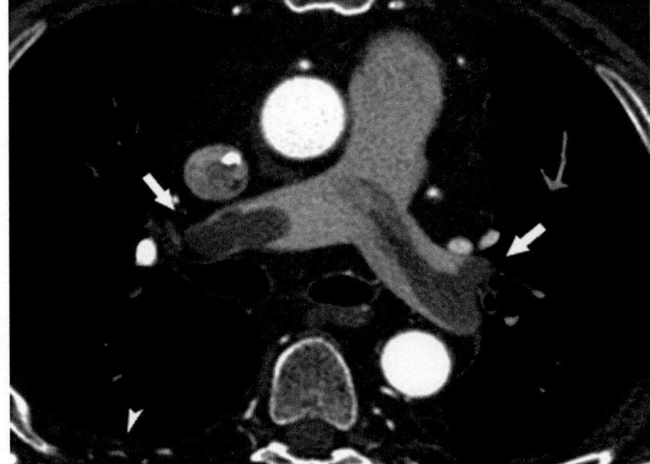

Fig. 19.3 64 slice multi-detector CT in a patient with pulmonary embolism. An axial section at the level of the main pulmonary artery shows the filling defect (*white arrows*) of bilaterally enlarged pulmonary arteries with massive thromo-emboli. A small amount of right pleural effusion (*white arrowhead*) is observed

distal to thrombus that is not properly per fused, increasing the V/Q mismatch.

Perfusion defects appear the same on a VQ scan whether the pulmonary embolus is acute or chronic. In contrast, CT findings of acute versus chronic emboli differ. In CTEPH, there may be intraluminal thrombi and dilated bronchial arteries. Furthermore, a mosaic pattern of hyperattenuation and hypoattenuation is frequently seen, representing the variation in perfusion between pulmonary segments [40]. Other evidence of CTEPH on CT includes abrubt narrowing of vessels, intimal irregularities, or total occlusions. Yet, there is greater concern that CT findings may be difficult to detect. A study from Tunariu, et al. found a sensitivity of 51 % for CTPA compared with 96 % sensitivity for VQ scans [61]. The specificity of CTPA can also be limited by the subtly distinct mosaic pattern of hyperattenuation and hypoattenuation found in Group 1 PAH. With improved ECG-gated CT imaging, recent studies have shown much improved sensitivity. He, et al found the sensitivity of VQ scan to be 100 % if high and intermediate risk results were interpreted as positive for a PE with sensitivity declining to 96 % but specificity rising to 95 % if only high risk results were counted as abnormal [62]. CT had a sensitivity of 92 % with specificity of 95 % in the same patient cohort [62]. While V/Q scan remains slightly more sensitive, CT imaging now serves as a viable alternative given improvements in sensitivity and specificity with newer scanners.

Pulmonary angiography, the gold standard for diagnosing PE, is being replaced in many institutions with MDCTA, which is less invasive, easier to perform, and has high sensitivity (83 %-100 %) and specificity (89 %-97 %) [63–65]. The PIOPED studies (large multicenter trials for CCTA in suspected PE) report negative predictive values as high as 99 %.

The newest noninvasive method for the evaluation and diagnosis of PE is MRI. Although not as extensively studied as other imaging techniques, it can be utilized for the patients with renal dysfunction or an iodine contrast allergy. CT angiographic findings are shown (Figs. 19.3 and 19.4).

Chronic thromboembolic pulmonary hypertension (CTEPH) represents a frequent cause of PH (Fig. 19.4). The incidence of CTEPH is uncertain; however, it is known to occur in up to 4 % of patients after an acute pulmonary embolism [66, 67]. It is strongly recommended that patients with suspected or confirmed CTEPH be referred to a center with expertise in the management of this disease to consider the feasibility of performing pulmonary thromboendarterectomy, currently the only curative treatment. The decision depends on the location of the obstruction (central vs. more distal pulmonary arteries), the correlation between hemodynamic findings, and the degree of mechanical obstruction.

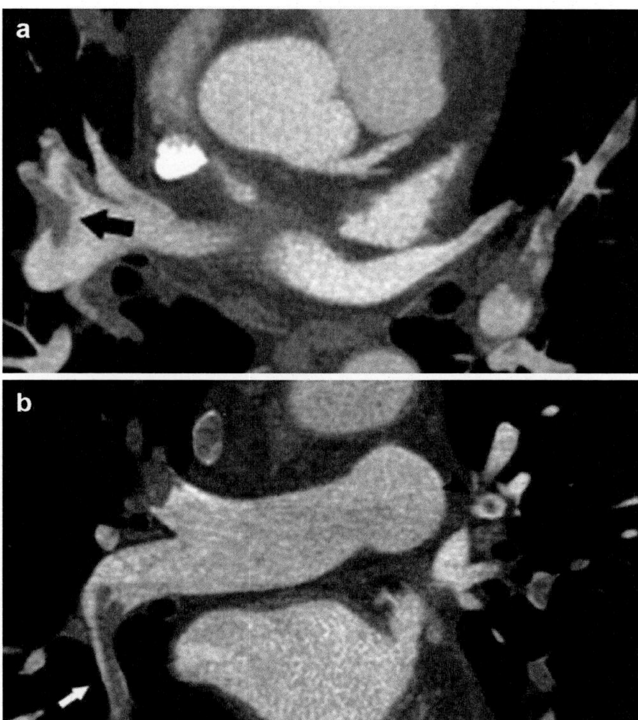

Fig. 19.4 64 slice multi-detector CT in a 58 year-old man with multiple bilateral pulmonary embolism. (**a**) "Saddle embolus" (*black arrow*) at the bifurcation of right pulmonary Artery (PA). (**b**) "Tram line" (*white arrow*) and "ring shape" (*black arrowhead*) features of emboli at both peripheral PAs

Methods of Detecting and Characterizing PH

The appropriate classification of patients with suspicion of PAH requires a rigorous diagnostic approach. PH symptoms are nonspecific and progress slowly over months to years. Exertional dyspnea is the most common symptom with fatigue occurring in a minority of cases. Manifestations of syncope, peripheral edema, and angina may be more concerning and frequently appear in patients with evidence of impaired right ventricular function. Clinicians should have a higher index of suspicion for PAH in patients using amphetamines or diet pills, a history of autoimmune disease, or a known family history of PH.

Guidelines put forth from the AHA/ACCF recommend a rigorous workup for pulmonary hypertension which includes the diagnostic algorithm as shown in Table 19.2 [3]. Transthoracic echocardiography (TTE) is often used as a first-line screening test to exclude or identify patients with severe PH by estimating systolic PA pressure and looking for evidence of the cardiac hemodynamic perturbations seen with PAH, such as right-sided cardiac and great vessel

Table 19.2 Clinical classification of pulmonary hypertension

1. Pulmonary arterial hypertension (PAH)
1. Idiopathic PAH
2. *Heritable*
BMPR2 mutation (familial or isolated)
ALK1, endoglin (with or without hereditary hemorrhagic telangiectasia)
Unknown
3. Drug- and toxin-induced
4. Associated with
Connective tissue diseases
HIV infection
Portal hypertension
Congenital heart diseases
Schistosomiasis
Chronic hemolytic anemia
5. Persistent pulmonary hypertension of the newborn
6. *Pulmonary veno-occlusive disease (PVOD) and/or pulmonary capillary hemangiomatosis (PCH)*
2. Pulmonary hypertension due to left heart disease
1. *Systolic dysfunction*
2. *Diastolic dysfunction*
3. Valvular disease
3. Pulmonary hypertension due to lung diseases and/or hypoxia
1. Chronic obstructive pulmonary disease
2. Interstitial lung disease
3. *Other pulmonary diseases with mixed restrictive and obstructive pattern*
4. Sleep-disordered breathing
5. Alveolar hypoventilation disorders
6. Chronic exposure to high altitude
7. Developmental abnormalities
4. Chronic thromboembolic pulmonary hypertension (CTEPH)
5. Pulmonary hypertension with unclear multifactorial mechanisms
1. Hematologic disorders: myeloproliferative disorders, splenectomy
2. Systemic disorders: sarcoidosis, pulmonary Langerhans cell histiocytosis, lymphangioleiomyomatosis, neurofibromatosis, vasculitis
3. Metabolic disorders: glycogen storage disease, Gaucher disease, thyroid disorders
4. Others: tumoral obstruction, fibrosing mediastinitis, chronic renal failure on dialysis

ALK1 activin receptor-like kinase type1, *BMPR2* bone morphogenetic protein receptor type2

chamber enlargement and dysfunction, flattening of the interventricular septum, and pericardial effusion. Echocardiography is also useful for evaluating congenital heart disease and left-sided heart disease.

Suggested radiographic imaging includes a chest x-ray and, depending on the need, CT radiography. The chest radiographic findings of PH are hilar fullness characteristic of dilated central pulmonary arteries, pruning of the peripheral arteries, and right-sided cardiac chamber enlargement [3, 5]. The chest radiograph may suggest an underlying cause for PH and is thus recommended in the workup of suspected PH.

Right-sided heart catheterization (RHC) is the most accurate test for determining cardiopulmonary hemodynamics and remains the gold standard by which the diagnosis of PH is made and hemodynamic severity is calculated. A RHC is required not only to confirm the presence and the severity of PH, but also to exclude left-sided heart disease, potentially correctable intracardiac left-to-right shunting, and to perform acute vasodilator testing.

Because the signs and symptoms of PH are non-specific and there is no reliable non-invasive test for its detection, patients often undergo computed tomography (CT) as part of their diagnostic work-up. CT is able to evaluate the lung parenchyma (for interstitial or emphysematous changes), the pulmonary artery (calcification, dilation, embolism, patent ductus), the pulmonary veins, the cardiac chambers (hypertrophy, dysplasia, enlargement, thrombus, septal defects), the coronary vessels, and the IVC simultaneously.

It is important to be aware of the CT findings that may suggest the diagnosis of PH, such as an enlarged main pulmonary artery (Figs. 19.5). Radiographically, PH is said to be more likely when the main pulmonary artery diameter (MPAD) is ≥29 mm (sensitivity 69 %, specificity 100 %) [6, 7] and/or the ratio of the main pulmonary artery to ascending aorta diameter is >1 (sensitivity 70.8 % and specificity 76.5 %) [8, 68]. Others have reported that the most specific CT findings for the presence of PH were both a MPAD ≥29 mm and segmental artery-to-bronchus ratio of >1:1 in three or four lobes (specificity 100 %) [9]. In addition, the MPAD correlates with the severity of pulmonary hypertension; two studies have defined the upper limit of normal for main pulmonary artery diameter as 32 mm [6, 10]. An additional feature of PH is rapid tapering or "pruning" of the distal pulmonary vessels (Fig. 19.5).

With improvements in ECG-gated CT technology, newer methods have been developed with similar accuracy in predicting the presence of PH. Revel et al. demonstrated that a reduction in distensibility of the right pulmonary artery has a high specificity for PH[69]. Distensibility is determined by evaluating the change in cross-sectional area of the right PA during systole compared with diastole. The difference in maximum area from the minimum area is divided by the maximum area and multiplied by 100 to get a percentage of distensibility. A value of less than 16.5 % had 86 % sensitivity and 96 % specificity for PH [69]. RV thickness is a known finding in PH with RV free wall thickness >6 mm (81 % sensitivity and 91 % specificity), RV/LV lumen ratio >1.28 (sensitivity of 85 % and specificity of 86 %), and RV wall/LV wall ratio >0.32 as accurate predictors of PH [70]. With a high degree of specificity, CT imaging provides important

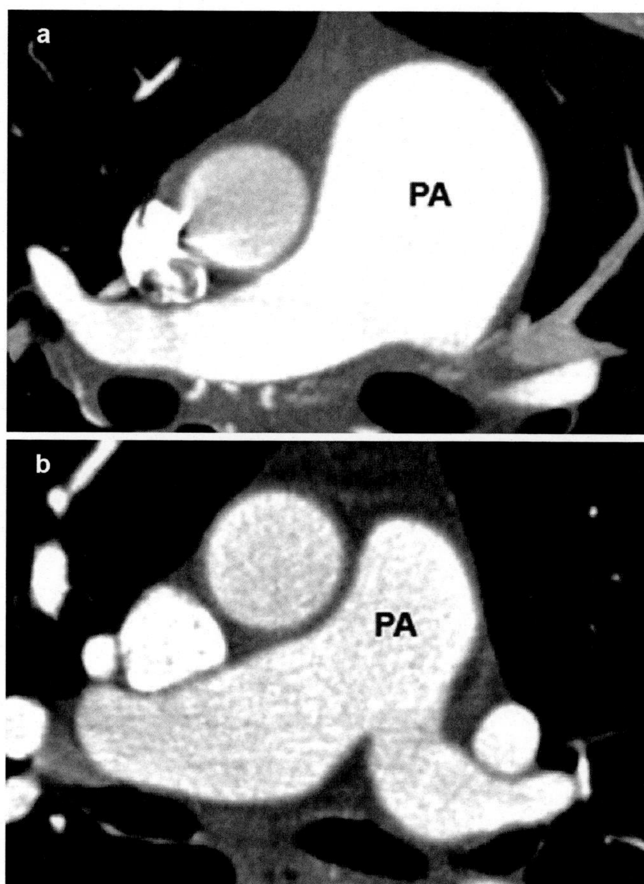

Fig. 19.5 Electron Beam CT scan in a 22 year-old woman (**a**) and 64 slice multi-detector CT in a 40 year-old man (**b**), both with pulmonary hypertension. Pulmonary arteries (*PA*) are enlarged and tapering distally, with an increased main PA to aorta ratio

evidence for pulmonary hypertension that should prompt clinicians to pursue a workup for pulmonary hypertension.

The presence of calcification in the pulmonary arteries suggests more severe disease [9], as does pericardial thickening and/or effusion [12]. Some studies have reported that hypertrophy of the bronchial artery occurs frequently in patients with idiopathic PAH (IPAH) and Eisenmenger's syndrome [13, 14]. These studies also reported that pulmonary artery thromboses and aneurysms were common in patients with congenital heart disease (CHD) as compared to patients with IPAH, while dilation and mural calcification was seen in similar frequency in both groups [13].

It is generally accepted that in patients with chronic, unrepaired systemic-to-pulmonary shunts the CT findings can appear very similar to those found in precapillary pulmonary hypertension such as IPAH and PAH associated with connective tissue disease, portal hypertension, and HIV infection. Commonly, right (or pulmonic) ventricular hypertrophy is seen, with right ventricular enlargement and associated right atrial enlargement (Fig. 19.6).

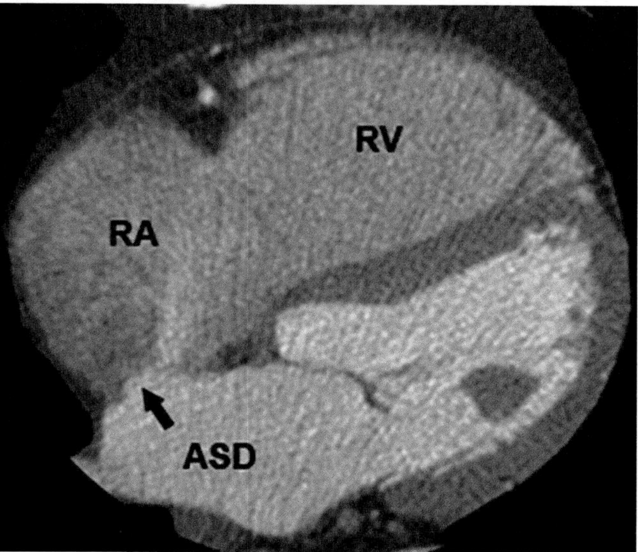

Fig. 19.6 64 slice multi-detector CT in a 44 year-old man with secondum atrial septal defect (*ASD*) and pulmonary hypertension demonstrating right atrial (*RA*) and right ventricular (*RV*) enlargement

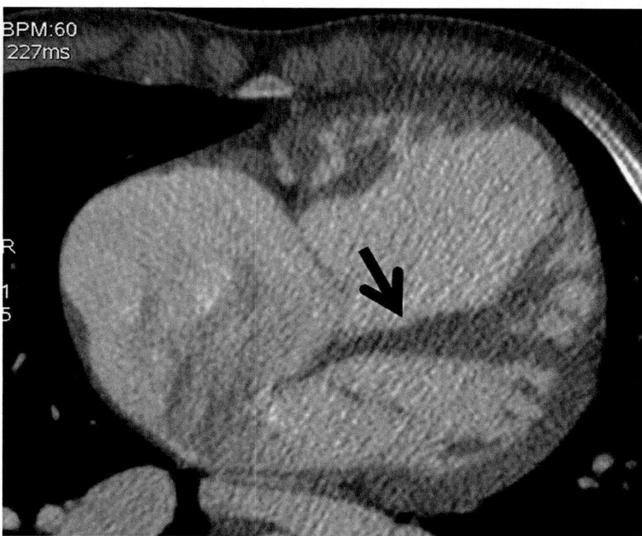

Fig. 19.7 64 slice multi-detector CT in a 31 year-old man with sinus venosum atrial septal defect (ASD) and pulmonary hypertension demonstrating right atrial (RA) dilation and right ventricular (RV) hypertrophy, and flattening of the inter-ventricular septum (*black arrow*), indicating high right sided pressures

As the right ventricle enlarges, the interventricular septum becomes flattened (Fig. 19.7) and eventually convex to the left side [15–17], and thus septal flattening is a commonly noted cardiac abnormality found in patients with PH [18]. If cine-CT is performed, reduced right ventricular systolic function may also be present. The presence of retrograde opacification of the inferior vena cava or hepatic vein during contrast-enhanced CT may be a nonspecific sign of

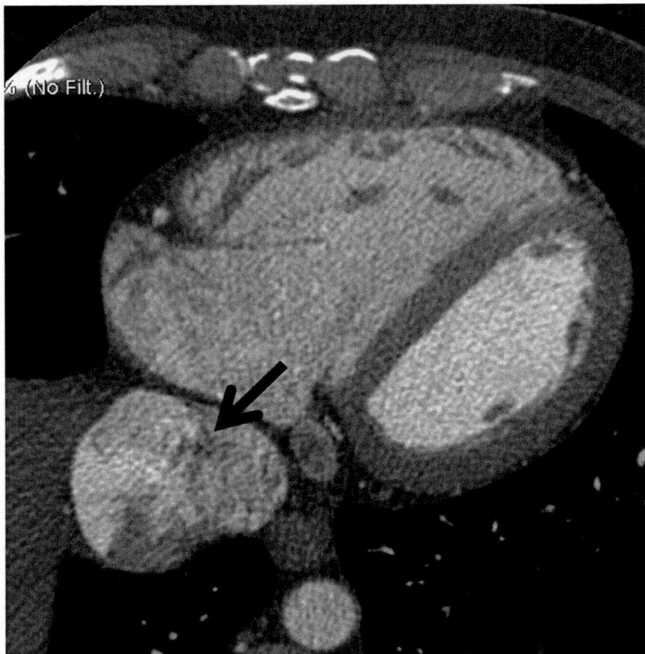

Fig. 19.8 64 slice multi-detector CT in a 26 year-old man with anolamous pulmonary venous return and pulmonary hypertension demonstrating right atrial dilation and right ventricular hypertrophy, and dilated inferior vena cava with swirling of white contrast (*black arrow*), indicating severe tricuspid regurgitation

significant pulmonary hypertension and/or right ventricular dysfunction [19] (Fig. 19.8).

Although hemodynamics cannot be directly measured with CT, the sequelae of chronic pulmonary hypertension can be seen with structural cardiac changes. The increased pulmonary vascular resistance that occurs with PH places greater strain on the right ventricle. Right ventricular hypertrophy (>6 mm thickness) is a common finding, and as the RV begins failing in the setting of persistently elevated afterload, an increased in RV end diastolic volume will occur [71]. RV enlargement leads to increasing RV pressure and volume, which are reflected in the bowing of the interventricular septum. CT findings of RV/LV >1 and LV septal flattening are sensitive and specific markers for PH. In small studies by Contractor et al and Lim et al, found these signs had a sensitivity of 78 %–92 % and a specificity of 100 % for echocardiographic findings of RV dysfunction. [71–73] Systolic eccentricity index (sEi) correlates well with pulmonary hypertension severity [74]. In normal conditions, the LV cavity is shaped like a circle. With increasing RV pressure and volume overload, the septal wall flattening leads to a deformed, D-shaped left ventricle. The length of the septum (D1) becomes longer than the width of the LV cavity (D2), with a ratio of D1/D2 >1 (normal score is 1) that is the eccentricity score [74]. Most studies have evaluated sEi with echocardiographic data, but cine-CT provides the necessary axial images of the LV in systole and diastole to calculate the index.

Although CT imaging of the great vessels is a simple and straightforward noninvasive methodology, it has not gained widespread acceptance as a screening test for PH [1]. Table 19.1 summarizes the CT findings of PH. While CT cannot diagnose pulmonary hypertension, clinicians should be aware that a wealth of information regarding the end result of the chronic hemodynamic effect of PH upon cardiovascular anatomy. A diagnosis and its underlying etiology may be highly suggested by closely evaluating the pulmonary vasculature and cardiac anatomy on CT imaging.

References

1. Vonk-Noordegraaf A, Haddad F, Chin KM, Forfia PR, Kawut SM, Lumens J, Naeije R, Newman J, Oudiz RJ, Provencher S, Torbicki A, Voelkel NF, Hassoun PM. Right heart adaptation to pulmonary arterial hypertension: physiology and pathobiology. J Am Coll Cardiol. 2013;62(25 Suppl):D22–33.
2. Simonneau G, Gatzoulis MA, Adatia I. Updated clinical classification of pulmonary hypertension. J Am Coll Cardiol. 2013;62(25_S):D34–41.
3. McLaughlin VV, Archer SL, Badesch DB, et al. ACCF/AHA 2009 expert consensus document on pulmonary hypertension a report of the American College of Cardiology Foundation Task Force on Expert Consensus Documents and the American Heart Association developed in collaboration with the American College of Chest Physicians; American Thoracic Society, Inc.; and the Pulmonary Hypertension Association. J Am Coll Cardiol. 2009;53:1573–619.
4. McLaughlin VV, Presberg KW, Doyle RL. Prognosis of pulmonary arterial hypertension: ACCP evidence-based Clinical Practice Guidelines. Chest. 2004;126(1_suppl):78S–92.
5. Brown LM, Chen H, Halpern S, Taichman D, McGoon MD, Farber HW, Frost AE, Liou TG, Turner M, Feldkircher K, Miller DP, Elliott CG. Delay in recognition of pulmonary arterial hypertension: factors identified from the REVEAL Registry. Chest. 2011;140:19–26.
6. Rich S, Dantzker DR, Ayres SM, et al. Primary pulmonary hypertension: a national prospective study. Ann Intern Med. 1987; 107:216–23.
7. Loyd JE, Butler MG, Foroud TM, Conneally PM, Phillips JA, Newman JH. Genetic anticipation and abnormal gender ratio at birth in familial primary pulmonary hypertension. Am J Respir Crit Care Med. 1995;152:93–7.
8. Cogan JD, Pauciulo MW, Batchman AP, et al. High frequency of BMPR2 exonic deletions/duplications in familial pulmonary arterial hypertension. Am J Respir Crit Care Med. 2006;174:590–8.
9. Aldred MA, Vijayakrishnan J, James V, et al. BMPR2 gene rearrangements account for a significant proportion of mutations in familial and idiopathic pulmonary arterial hypertension. Hum Mutat. 2006;27:212–3.
10. Machado RD, Aldred MA, James V, et al. Mutations of the TGF- β type II receptor BMPR2 in pulmonary arterial hypertension. Hum Mutat. 2006;27:121–32.
11. Thomson JR, Machado RD, Pauciulo MW, et al. Sporadic primary pulmonary hypertension is associated with germline mutations of the gene encoding BMPR-II, a receptor member of the TGF-β family. J Med Genet. 2000;37:741–5.

12. Chaouat A, Coulet F, Favre C, et al. Endoglin germline mutation in a patient with hereditary haemorrhagic telangiectasia and dexfenfluramine associated pulmonary arterial hypertension. Thorax. 2004;59:446–8.
13. Trembath RC, Thomson JR, Machado RD, et al. Clinical and molecular genetic features of pulmonary hypertension in patients with hereditary hemorrhagic telangiectasia. N Engl J Med. 2001;345:325–34.
14. McGoon M, Gutterman D, Steen V, et al. Screening, early detection, and diagnosis of pulmonary arterial hypertension: ACCP evidencebased clinical practice guidelines. Chest. 2004;126:14S–34.
15. Hachulla E, Gressin V, Guillevin L, et al. Early detection of pulmonary arterial hypertension in systemic sclerosis: a french nationwide prospective multicenter study. Arthritis Rheum. 2005;52:3792–800.
16. Mukerjee D, St George D, Coleiro B, et al. Prevalence and outcome in systemic sclerosis associated pulmonary arterial hypertension: application of a registry approach. Ann Rheum Dis. 2003; 62:1088–93.
17. Tanaka E, Harigai M, Tanaka M, Kawaguchi Y, Hara M, Kamatani N. Pulmonary hypertension in systemic lupus erythematosus: evaluation of clinical characteristics and response to immunosuppressive treatment. J Rheumatol. 2002;29:282–7.
18. Asherson RA, Higenbottam TW, Dinh Xuan AT, Khamashta MA, Hughes GR. Pulmonary hypertension in a lupus clinic: experience with twenty-four patients. J Rheumatol. 1990;17:1292–8.
19. Burdt MA, Hoffman RW, Deutscher SL, Wang GS, Johnson JC, Sharp GC. Long-term outcome in mixed connective tissue disease: longitudinal clinical and serologic findings. Arthritis Rheum. 1999;42:899–909.
20. Jaïs X, Launay D, Yaici A, et al. Immunosuppressive therapy in lupus- and mixed connective tissue disease-associated pulmonary arterial hypertension: a retrospective analysis of twenty-three cases. Arthritis Rheum. 2008;58:521–31.
21. Launay D, Hachulla E, Hatron PY, Jaïs X, Simonneau G, Humbert M. Pulmonary arterial hypertension: a rare complication of primary Sjögren syndrome: report of 9 new cases and review of the literature. Medicine (Baltimore). 2007;86:299–315.
22. Bunch TW, Tancredi RG, Lie JT. Pulmonary hypertension in polymyositis. Chest. 1981;79:105–7.
23. Dawson JK, Goodson NG, Graham DR, Lynch MP. Raised pulmonary artery pressures measured with doppler echocardiography in rheumatoid arthritis patients. Rheumatology (Oxford). 2000;39:1320–5.
24. Coghlan JG, Handler C. Connective tissue associated pulmonary arterial hypertension. Lupus. 2006;15:138–42.
25. Lettieri CJ, Nathan SD, Barnett SD, et al. Prevalence and outcomes of pulmonary arterial hypertension in advanced idiopathic pulmonary fibrosis. Chest. 2006;129:746–52.
26. Corte TJ, et al. Pulmonary hypertension in idiopathic pulmonary fibrosis: a review. Sarcoidosis Vasc Diffuse Lung Dis. 2009; 26:7–19.
27. Zisman DA, Karlamangla AS, Ross DJ, et al. High-resolution chest CT findings do not predict the presence of pulmonary hypertension in advanced idiopathic pulmonary fibrosis. Chest. 2007; 132:773–9.
28. Eisenmenger V. Die angeborene defecte der kammersheidewand das herzen. Z Klin Med. 1897;132:131.
29. Wood P. The Eisenmenger syndrome or pulmonary hypertension with reversed central shunt. Br Med J. 1958;2:701–9.
30. Daliento L, Somerville J, Presbitero P, et al. Eisenmenger syndrome: factors relating to deterioration and death. Eur Heart J. 1998;19:1845–55.
31. Besterman E. Atrial septal defect with pulmonary hypertension. Br Heart J. 1961;23:587–98.
32. Hoffman JI, Rudolph AM. The natural history of ventricular septal defects in infancy. Am J Cardiol. 1965;16:634–53.
33. Galiè N, Manes A, Palazzini M, et al. Management of pulmonary arterial hypertension associated with congenital systemic-to pulmonary shunts and Eisenmenger's syndrome. Drugs. 2008;68:1049–66.
34. Fernandes C, Jardim C, Honanian A, Hoette S, Morinaga LK, Souza R. Schistosomiasis and Pulmonary Hypertension. *Pulmonary Vascular Disorders*. Prog Respir Res. Basel. Karger. 2012;41:143–8.
35. Shaw AP, Ghareed A. The pathogenesis of pulmonary schistosomiasis in Egypt with special reference to Ayerza's disease. J Pathol Bacteriol. 1938;46:401–24.
36. de Cleva R, Herman P, Pugliese V, et al. Prevalence of pulmonary hypertension in patients with hepatosplenic mansonic schistosomiasis- prospective study. Hepatogastroenterology. 2003;50: 2028–30.
37. Lapa MS, Ferreira EV, Jardim C, Martins Bdo C, Arakaki JS, Souza R. Clinical characteristics of pulmonary hypertension patients in two reference centers in the city of Sao Paulo. Rev Assoc Med Bras. 2006;52:139–43.
38. Chaves E. The pathology of the arterial pulmonary vasculature in Manson's schistosomiasis. Chest. 1966;50:72–7.
39. Papamatheakis DG, Mocumbi AOH, Kim NH, Mandel J. Schistosomiasis-associated pulmonary hypertension. Pulmonary Circulation. 2014;4:596–611.
40. Grosse C, Grosse A. CT findings in diseases associated with pulmonary hypertension: a current review. Radiographics. 2010;30(7): 1753–77.
41. Mandel J, Mark EJ, Hales CA. Pulmonary veno-occlusive disease. Am J Respir Crit Care Med. 2000;162:1964–73.
42. Frazier AA, Franks TJ, Mohammed TL, Ozbudak IH, Galvin JR. From the archives of the AFIP: pulmonary veno-occlusive disease and pulmonary capillary hemangiomatosis. Radiographics. 2007;27:867–82.
43. Holcomb Jr BW, Loyd JE, Ely EW, Johnson J, Robbins IM. Pulmonary veno-occlusive disease: a case series and new observations. Chest. 2000;118:1671–9.
44. Resten A, Maitre S, Humbert M, et al. Pulmonary hypertension: CT of the chest in pulmonary veno-occlusive disease. Am J Roentgenol. 2004;183:65–70.
45. Lantuéjoul S, Sheppard MN, Corrin B, Burke MM, Nicholson AG. Pulmonary veno-occlusive disease and pulmonary capillary hemangiomatosis: a clinicopathologic study of 35 cases. Am J Surg Pathol. 2006;30:850–7.
46. Ozsoyoglu AA, Swartz J, Farver CF, Mohammed TL. High resolution computed tomographic imaging and pathologic features of pulmonary veno-occlusive disease: a review of three patients. Curr Probl Diagn Radiol. 2006;35:219–23.
47. Montani D, Achouh L, Dorfmuller P. Pulmonary venoocclusive disease: clinical, functional, radiologic, and hemodynamic characteristics and outcome of 24 cases confirmed by histology. Medicine(Baltimore). 2008;87:220–33.
48. Rabiller A, Jaïs X, Hamid A, et al. Occult alveolar haemorrhage in pulmonary veno-occlusive disease. Eur Respir J. 2006;27:108–13.
49. Resten A, Maitre S, Humbert M, Rabiller A, Sitbon O, Capron F, Simonneau G, Musset D. Pulmonary hypertension: CT of the chest in pulmonary venoocclusive disease. AJR Am J Roentgenol. 2004;183:65–70.
50. Fraser KL, Tullis DE, Sasson Z, Hyland RH, Thornley KS, Hanly PJ. Pulmonary hypertension and cardiac function in adult cystic fibrosis: role of hypoxemia. Chest. 1999;115:1321–8.
51. Cottin V, Nunes H, Brillet PY, et al. Combined pulmonary fibrosis and emphysema: a distinct underrecognised entity. Eur Respir J. 2005;26:586–93.

52. Chaouat A, Bugnet AS, Kadaoui N, et al. Severe pulmonary hypertension and chronic obstructive pulmonary disease. Am J Respir Crit Care Med. 2005;172:189–94.
53. Silverstein MD, Heit JA, Mohr DN, Petterson TM, O'Fallon WM, Melton 3rd LJ. Trends in the incidence of deep vein thrombosis and pulmonary embolism: a 25-year population-based study. Arch Intern Med. 1998;158:585–93.
54. Tapson VF. Acute pulmonary embolism. N Engl J Med. 2008;358:1037–52.
55. Heit JA. The epidemiology of venous thromboembolism in the community. Arterioscler Thromb Vasc Biol. 2008;28:370–2.
56. Sandler DA, Martin JF. Autopsy proven pulmonary embolism in hospital patients: are we detecting enough deep vein thrombosis? J R Soc Med. 1989;82:203–5.
57. Kumar A, Ouriel K. Handbook of endovascular interventions. New York: Springer Science & Business Media; 2012. p. 404.
58. Elliott CG. Chest radiographs in acute pulmonary embolism: results from the international cooperative pulmonary embolism registry. Chest. 2000;118:33–8.
59. Stein PD, Terrin ML, Hales CA, Palevsky HI, Saltzman HA, Thompson BT, Weg JG. Clinical, laboratory, roentgenographic and electrocardiographic findings in patients with acute pulmonary embolism and no pre-existing cardiac or pulmonary disease. Chest. 1991;100:598–603.
60. Stein PD, Willis III PW, DeMets DL, Greenspan RH. Plain chest roentgenogram in patients with acute pulmonary embolism and no pre-existing cardiac or pulmonary disease. Am J Noninvas Cardiol. 1987;1:171–6.
61. Tunariu N, Gibbs SJ, Win Z, Gin-Sing W, Graham A, Gishen P, Al-Nahhas A. Ventilation-perfusion scintigraphy is more sensitive than multidetector CTPA in detecting chronic thromboembolic pulmonary disease as a treatable cause of pulmonary hypertension. J Nucl Med. 2007;48:680–4.
62. He J, Fang W, Lv B, et al. Diagnosis of chronic thromboembolic pulmonary hypertension: comparison of ventilator/perfusion scanning and multidetector computed tomography pulmonary angiography with pulmonary angiography. Nucl Med Commun. 2012;33:459–63.
63. Stein PD, Fowler SE, Goodman LR, et al. Multidetector computed tomography for acute pulmonary embolism. N Engl J Med. 2006;354:2317–27.
64. Qanadli SD, Hajjam ME, Mesurolle B. Pulmonary embolism detection. Prospective evaluation of dual-section helical CT versus selective pulmonary arteriography in 157 patients. Radiology. 2000;217:447–55.
65. Winer-Muram HT, Rydberg J, Johnson MS, et al. Suspected acute pulmonary embolism: evaluation with multi-detector row CT versus digital subtraction pulmonary arteriography. Radiology. 2004;233:806–15.
66. Tapson VF, Humbert M. Incidence and prevalence of chronic thromboembolic pulmonary hypertension: from acute to chronic pulmonary embolism. Proc Am Thorac Soc. 2006;3:564–7.
67. Pengo V, Lensing AW, Prins MH, et al. Incidence of chronic thromboembolic pulmonary hypertension after pulmonary embolism. N Engl J Med. 2004;350:2257–64.
68. Wells JM, Dransfield MT. Pathophysiology and clinical implications of pulmonary arterial enlargement in COPD. Int J Chron Obstruct Pulmon Dis. 2013;8:509–21.
69. Revel MP, Faivre JB, Remy-Jardin M, Delannoy-Deken V, Duhamel A, Remy J. Pulmonary hypertension: ECG-gated 64-section CT angiographic evaluation of new functional parameters as diagnostic criteria. Radiology. 2009;250:558–66.
70. Chan AL, Juarez MM, Shelton DK, MacDonald T, Li CS, Lin C, Albertson TE. Novel computed tomographic chest metrics to detect pulmonary hypertension. BMC Med Imaging. 2011;11:7.
71. Ghaye B, Ghuysen A, Bruyere PJ, D'Orio V, Dondelinger RF. Can CT pulmonary angiography allow assessment of severity and prognosis in patients presenting with pulmonary embolism? What the radiologist needs to know. Radiographics. 2006;26:23–39.
72. Contractor S, Maldjian PD, Sharma VK, Gor DM. Role of helical CT in detecting right ventricular dysfunction secondary to acute pulmonary embolism. J Comput Assist Tomogr. 2002;26:587–91.
73. Lim KE, Chan CY, Chu PH, Hsu YY, Hsu WC. Right ventricular dysfunction secondary to acute massive pulmonary embolism detected by helical computed tomography pulmonary angiography. Clin Imaging. 2005;29:16–21.
74. López-Candales A, Bazaz R, Edelman K, Gulyasy B. Apical systolic eccentricity index: a better marker of right ventricular compromise in pulmonary hypertension. Echocardiography. 2010; 27:534–8.

Part V

Multidisciplinary Topics

Value Based Imaging for Coronary Artery Disease: Implications for Nuclear Cardiology and Cardiac CT

20

Daniel S. Berman, Alan Rozanski, Piotr Slomka, Rine Nakanishi, Damini Dey, John D. Friedman, Sean W. Hayes, Louise E.J. Thomson, Reza Arsanjani, Rory Hachamovitch, James K. Min, Leslee J. Shaw, and Guido Germano

Abstract

Technology in cardiac computed tomography (CT) and nuclear cardiology is constantly improving. In single photon emission CT (SPECT), new cameras, reconstruction methods, and protocols have dramatically reduced radiation doses to patients. In positron emission tomography (PET), application of quantitative measurements of myocardial perfusion reserve is improving assessment of prognosis. PET/CT is routinely performed in conjunction with coronary artery calcium (CAC) scanning in many centers, extending the ability of myocardial perfusion imaging (MPI) studies to impact patient management. In cardiac CT, marked improvements in equipment and reconstruction software have also dramatically reduced the patient radiation associated with cardiac testing, and have reduced the frequency of non-diagnostic studies. New methods for combining anatomic and functional assessment with CT—CT perfusion and FFR_{CT} measurements—are beginning to be used clinically. With the expanding capabilities of each technology, their opportunities to provide value increases. Given the changing reimbursement paradigm from a volume-based to a value-based system, the applications of each technology that will survive are those that improve relationship between outcomes and costs. With respect to coronary artery disease (CAD), a growing body of evidence exists regarding the value of specific tests in the various clinical settings in which CAD is considered. For prevention, data is strong in that CAC scanning can provide value by improving outcomes. In the patient with acute chest pain, CCTA appears to be able to shorten time in the hospital and reduce costs. In patients with

D.S. Berman, MD (✉) • P. Slomka, PhD • D. Dey, PhD
J.D. Friedman, MD • S.W. Hayes, MD • L.E.J. Thomson, MBChB
R. Arsanjani, MD • G. Germano, PhD
Departments of Imaging and Medicine,
Cedars-Sinai Medical Center and the Cedars-Sinai Heart Institute,
Los Angeles, CA, USA
e-mail: bermand@cshs.org

A. Rozanski, MD
Division of Cardiology, Mt. Sinai Saint Luke's
and Roosevelt Hospitals, New York, NY, USA

R. Nakanishi, MD, PhD
Department of Medicine, Los Angeles Biomedical Research
Institute at Harbor-UCLA, Torrance, CA, USA

R. Hachamovitch, MD
Department of Nuclear Medicine, Cleveland Clinic,
Heart and Vascular Institute, Cleveland, OH, USA

J.K. Min, MD, FACC
Department of Radiology, Dalio Institute of Cardiovascular Imaging,
Weill Cornell Medical College and the NewYork Presbyterian
Hospital, New York, NY, USA

L.J. Shaw, PhD
Department of Medicine, Emory Clinical Cardiovascular
Research Institute, Emory University School of Medicine,
Atlanta, GA, USA

M.J. Budoff, J.S. Shinbane (eds.), *Cardiac CT Imaging: Diagnosis of Cardiovascular Disease*,
DOI 10.1007/978-3-319-28219-0_20

suspected stable ischemic heart disease and an intermediate pre-test likelihood of CAD, the use of CCTA appears to be valuable. In patients who have known CAD or in whom a nondiagnostic CCTA is likely, improvement in outcomes based on CCTA is less likely and testing for ischemia may be preferred. In patients with a very high likelihood of CAD or known CAD, registry data suggests that ischemia testing, such as that provided by SPECT- or PET-MPI studies, may improve outcomes by improving selection of patients for revascularization. The ISCHEMIA trial will test whether a strategy basing decisions for revascularization on noninvasive assessment of ischemia improves outcomes. Test selection is highly dependent on accurate pretest risk assessment. An updated method for assessment of pre-test risk has developed which may lead to improved utilization of cardiac imaging procedures. In all of the applications of noninvasive imaging, value can only be achieved if the appropriate patients are selected for testing and if the test result changes management, such that outcomes can be improved or costs reduced.

Keywords
SPECT-MPI • PET-MPI • Myocardial perfusion imaging • Single photon emission computed tomography • Positron emission tomography • Cardiac CT • Coronary CT angiography • Coronary artery calcium scanning

Introduction

The rapid evolution of new medical technologies and therapies and the increasing numbers of patients being studied or treated based on these developments are leading to an unsustainable increase in health care costs. In the United States, through legislation such as the Affordable Care Act, a transition from a volume-based health care reimbursement to a value-based reimbursement. Over the past few decades, there has been a rise in the use of imaging that parallels that of the overall rise in healthcare costs. While efforts such as implementation of Appropriate Use Criteria have slowed the rise in these expenses, a continued increase in overall imaging costs is still occurring. It is virtually inevitable that value-based medical care reimbursement will be increasingly the norm and will apply to most of the use of medical imaging.

What is value in imaging? Inherently, as with any commodity, value is a function of quality and cost (Fig. 20.1). In cardiology, quality ultimately implies improvement in patient outcomes. In the patient with coronary artery disease (CAD), these outcomes might reduce cardiac events such as death or myocardial infarction or improvement in quality of life. Other measures of quality include accuracy of diagnosis, efficiency of service for the patient, and reduction of any harm that might be associated with the care such as radiation, or complications from unnecessary invasive diagnostic or therapeutic procedures. Value is inversely related to costs, which are not only the costs of the imaging studies themselves, but all of the costs related to the study, including cost increases due to downstream testing and therapies and cost decreases due to more efficient care from reduced unnecessary downstream testing and therapies. In the future, whether the payer is the government, insurance companies, or the patients themselves, it is likely that only those approaches that provide value will be purchased. In imaging, this implies an increasing penetrance of value-based imaging, with growth in testing in areas of proven value and reduction of testing in areas in which value has not been shown.

In this chapter, we review the technologic developments in the nuclear cardiology and cardiac CT in light of advances that are likely to improve value and then to explore the potential "value proposition" of these modalities in the various clinical settings of suspected or known CAD in which they are applied.

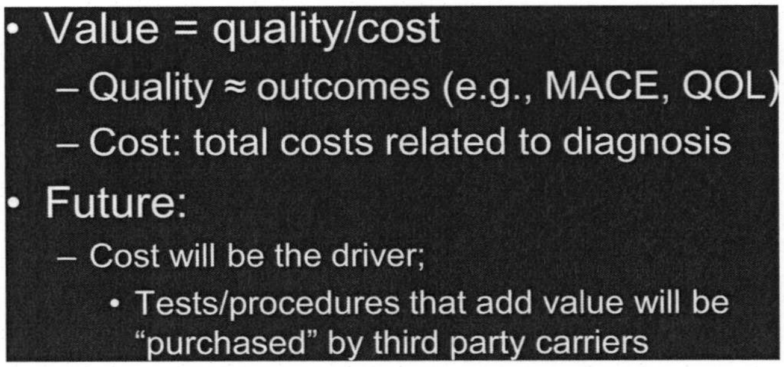

- Value = quality/cost
  - Quality ≈ outcomes (e.g., MACE, QOL)
  - Cost: total costs related to diagnosis
- Future:
  - Cost will be the driver;
    - Tests/procedures that add value will be "purchased" by third party carriers

Fig. 20.1 Value-based imaging: concepts

Technologic Developments

Nuclear Cardiology

In the last several years, there have been several advances in the technology of nuclear cardiology including single photon emission computed tomography (SPECT) and positron emission tomography (PET) for myocardial perfusion imaging (MPI). One of the primary areas of advantage of nuclear cardiology methods is the degree to which automated, objective quantitative analysis is available and implemented in practice. These methods are becoming increasingly automatic. They reduce the dependence on local expertise in interpretation, leading to increased reliability of the measurements across laboratories. Importantly, automated assessment has a dramatic effect on reproducibility of measurements, which is highly important in serial assessment. While the reproducibility of subjective visual assessment is poor, very high reproducibility of quantitative measurements has been shown by documented in multiple patient populations [1–3]. Recently, advanced automated quantitation has been shown to improve accuracy of diagnosis of CAD compared to expert visual interpretations [4]. Further, the introduction of machine learning, in which the computer is provided all of the variables available to the clinician, SPECT MPI has been shown to provide greater accuracy for CAD detection than either expert visual or quantitative perfusion defect assessment [4] (Fig. 20.2; Courtesy Ref. [4]). It is likely that quantitative analysis with machine learning will become routine in nuclear cardiology laboratories.

Specifically pertinent to SPECT, recent camera and computer developments have been introduced that improve image quality [5]. The introduction of CZT detector cameras has resulted in increased counting efficiency (sensitivity), which can be employed to reduce time of procedures or administered radiation doses, while at the same time improving resolution [6]. With these cameras, the ability to perform SPECT MPI with as little as 3 mCi of Tc-99m has been reported, with an associated radiation dose of approximately 1 mSv to the patient [7, 8]. One of these cameras has been shown to be accurate for detection of CAD even in the morbidly obese patient (Fig. 20.3; Courtesy Ref. [9]), allowing cardiac imaging of patients up to 500 lb—perhaps unachievable with any other modality at this time [9]. New approaches to reconstruction of raw data have also become available for use with standard sodium-iodide detector Anger cameras, which allow for shorter imaging time or reduced radiation dose [10, 11]. Protocols have also changed, with stress first sequences, as were used in the initial SPECT imaging applications with Tl-201, becoming more common. With these, stress only studies become possible. To accomplish this, either attenuation correction imaging or two view (prone supine or upright/supine) is important to reduce the effects of soft tissue attenuation, particularly important when a rest and stress examination cannot be compared [12, 13]. Numerous publications have documented that a normal stress only study is associated with excellent patent prognosis, which is equal to that associated with rest/stress studies (Fig. 20.4; Courtesy Ref. [14]) [14, 15]. In 2015 at Cedars-Sinai, stress only studies, with a radiation dose to the patients of <2 mSv, was performed in nearly 40 % of cases.

Added value of machine learning combining supine and prone SPECT-MPI and clinical data

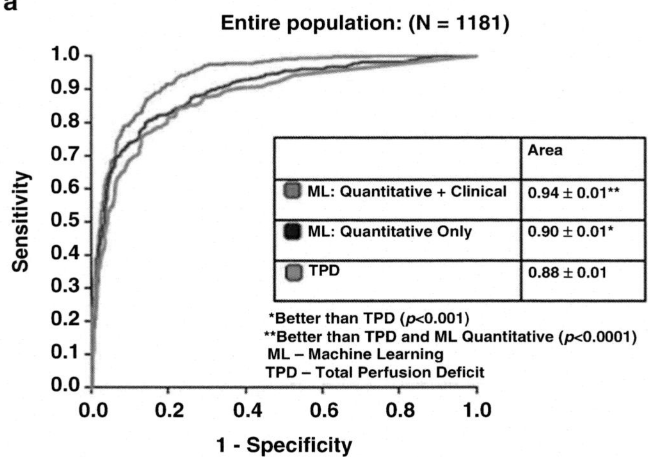

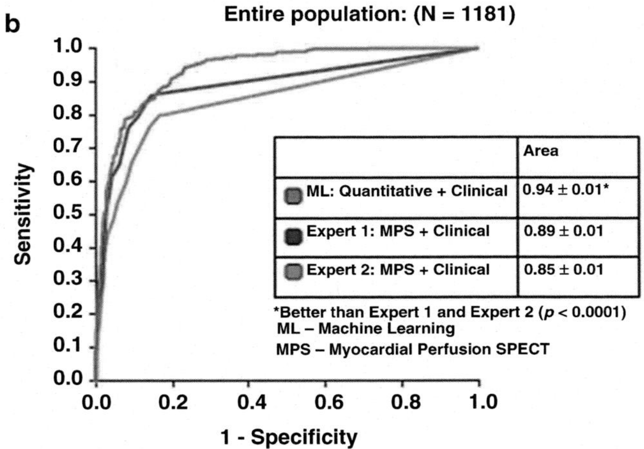

Fig. 20.2 ROC curves comparing the machine learning (*ML*) algorithm of quantitative+clinical data (*red*): (**a**): vs ML of quantitative SPECT-MPI data alone (*blue*) and total perfusion deficit alone (*green*). (**b**): vs expert visual analysis of supine and prone SPECT-MPI (MPS) including clinical data by expert 1 (*blue*) and expert 2 (*green*) for the detection of obstructive coronary artery disease (Reprinted from Arsanjani et al. [4] with permission from Springer)

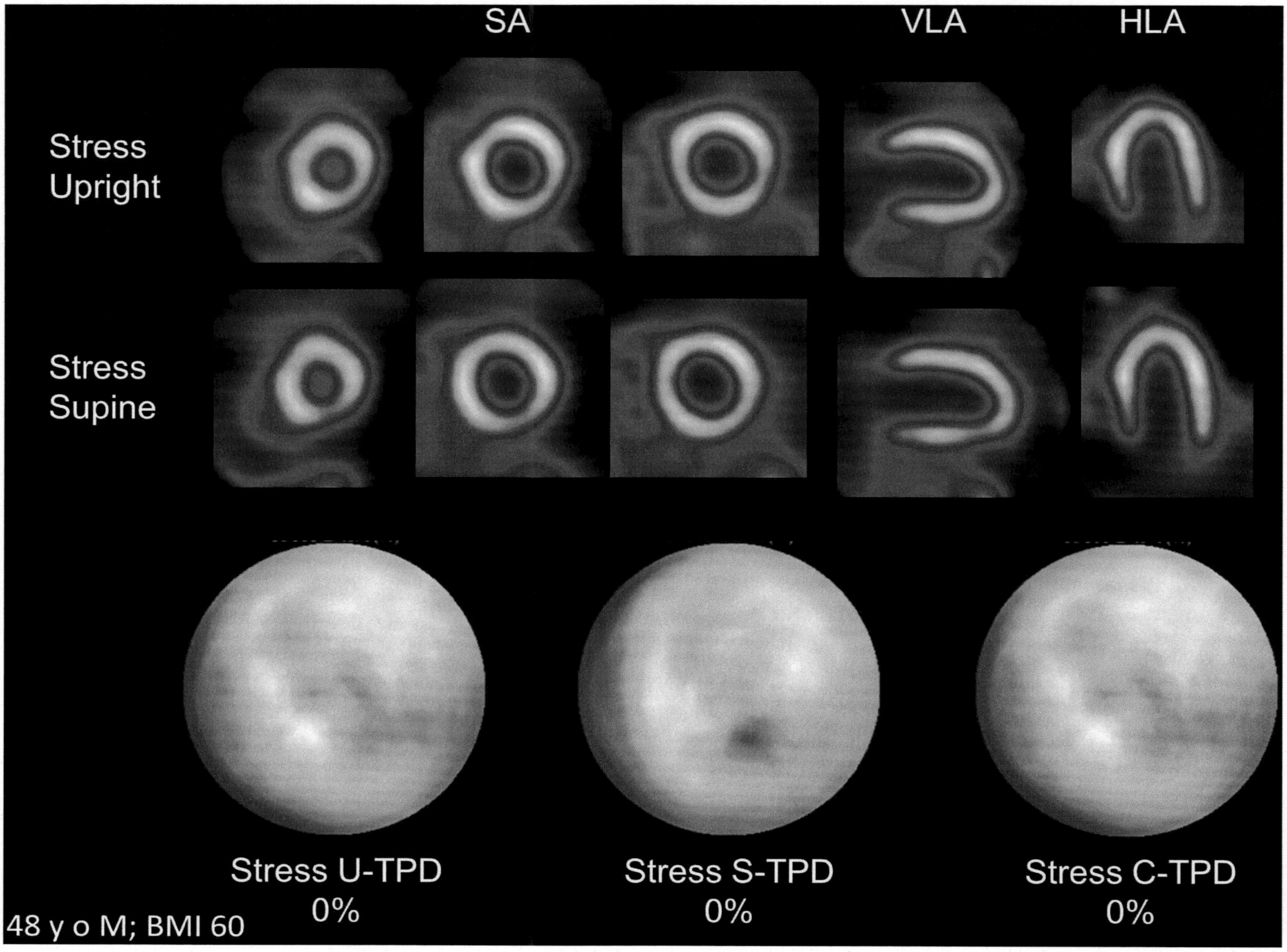

Fig. 20.3 Case example of high SPECT-MPI image quality obtained with a CZT camera using moving detectors in a 48 year old male with body mass index (BMI) 60. *U* upright; *S* supine; *TPD* total perfusion deficit (Reprinted from Nakazato et al. [9] with permission from Springer)

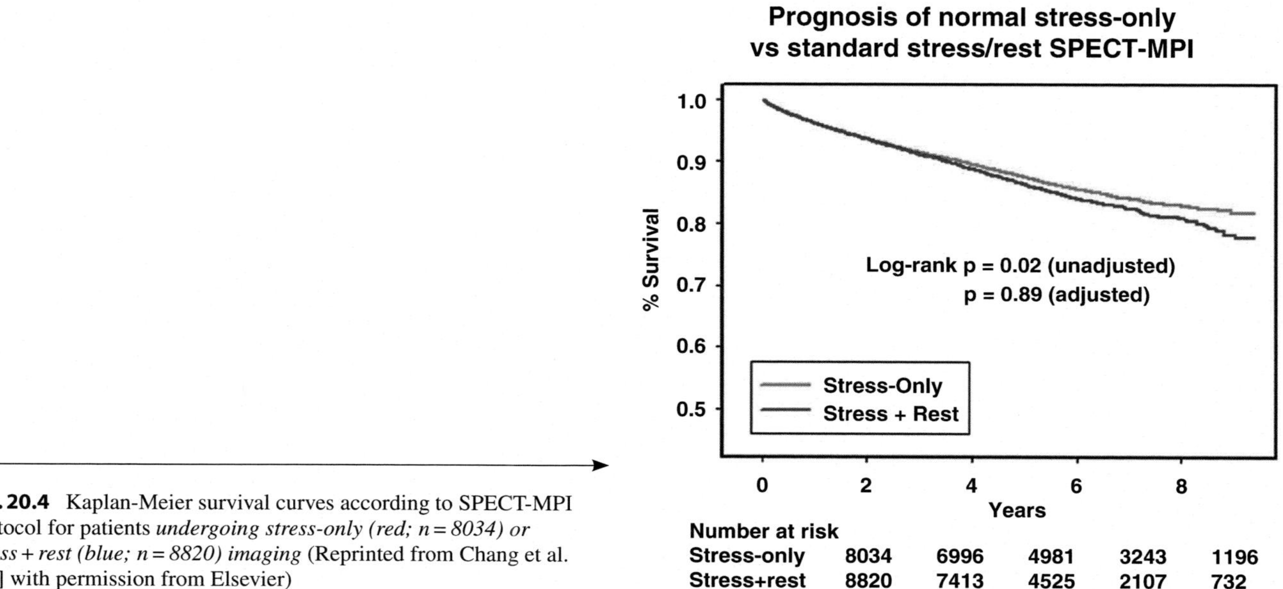

Fig. 20.4 Kaplan-Meier survival curves according to SPECT-MPI protocol for patients *undergoing stress-only (red; n = 8034) or stress + rest (blue; n = 8820) imaging* (Reprinted from Chang et al. [14] with permission from Elsevier)

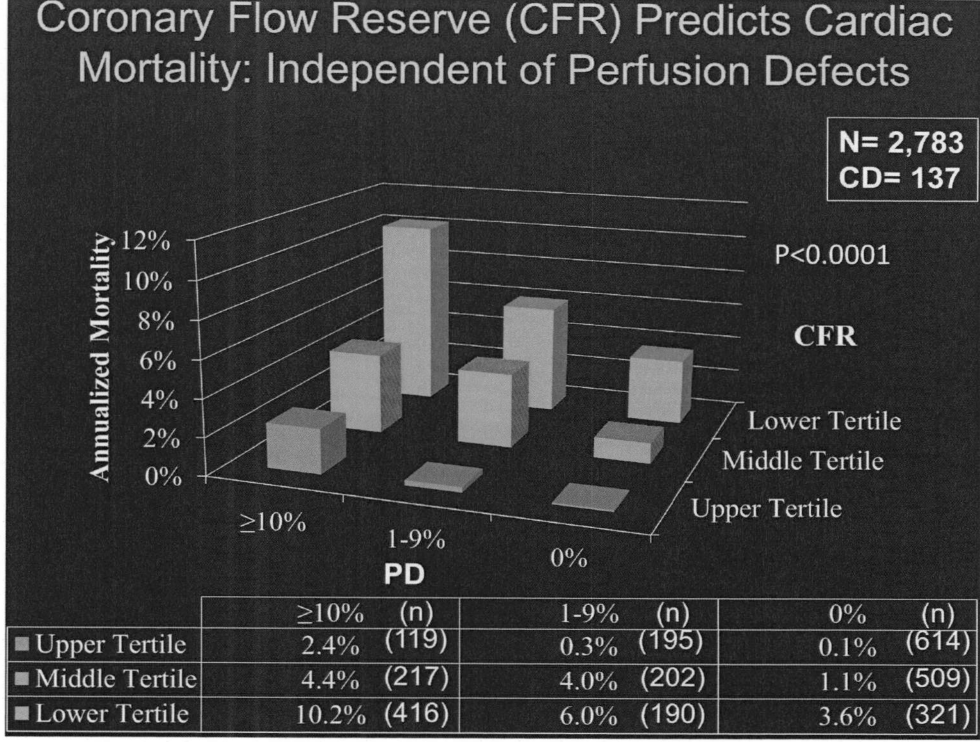

	≥10% (n)	1-9% (n)	0% (n)
Upper Tertile	2.4% (119)	0.3% (195)	0.1% (614)
Middle Tertile	4.4% (217)	4.0% (202)	1.1% (509)
Lower Tertile	10.2% (416)	6.0% (190)	3.6% (321)

Fig. 20.5 Unadjusted annualized cardiac mortality by tertiles of CFR and categories of stress PET-MPI perfusion defect (*PD*). *CD* cardiac mortality. 9 (Reprinted from Murthy et al. [18] with permission from Wolters Kluwer Health, Inc)

Important advances have also been made in PET. For PET-MPI, perhaps the most important of these has been the incorporation of absolute quantitative myocardial perfusion measurement. Referred to as myocardial perfusion reserve (MFR) or coronary flow reserve (CFR)—or absolute peak stress perfusion measurements—these assessments have now become available through the major software vendors and excellent correlation between the methods has been shown [16, 17]. These methods, using the widely available tracer Rb-82, have also validated by comparison with N-13 ammonia PET [17]. The prognostic value of these absolute flow measurements has been documented in a large number of clinical studies. Importantly, the added prognostic value of these measurements when combined with standard relative perfusion PET-MPI assessments has been shown [18, 19]. For any degree of relative perfusion defect abnormality, mortality has been shown to increase according to the degree of abnormality of MFR (Fig. 20.5; Courtesy Ref. [18]). These absolute flow measurements provide added value in many respects, including the ability to recognize when there has been inadequate vasodilation stimulus due to caffeine intake by the patient—seen as no increase in flow between rest and stress. These measurements provide an overall assessment of myocardial perfusion, which is related not only to the presence of significant epicardial stenosis or stenoses, but also the status of the microvasculature. This capability provides information that is complementary to the assessment of fractional flow reserve (FFR), allowing the identification of diffuse epicardial disease and microvascular dysfunction, which have their own prognostic and therapeutic implications beyond those associated with assessment of an individual coronary lesion [20, 21].

The existing PET or SPECT myocardial perfusion tracers are not ideal. One problem of the existing myocardial perfusion tracers is that their uptake in the myocardium is not linear with respect to flow at high flow rates. A new radiopharmaceutical currently in clinical trials overcomes this and other limitations of the currently used tracers. Flurpiridaz F-18 is linearly extracted across the range of flow, providing greater contrast within a perfusion defect compared to a normal zone than is achieved with Tc-99m sestamibi [22–24] (Fig. 20.6; Courtesy Ref. [24]). This is also likely to be true with respect to Rb-82, which has shown a similar plateauing of uptake with respect to flow as the SPECT agents. F-18 provides superior resolution compared to Rb-82, and due to its 110 min half-life can be used with exercise. It also lends itself to stress only application and does not require an on-site cyclotron [23] or expensive generator. It has the potential, depending on pricing, to become the PET-MPI agent of choice.

Increasingly, PET-MPI and SPECT-MPI are combining functional and anatomic assessment of patients with suspected CAD. PET-MPI is currently almost exclusively performed with PET/CT scanners [10]. SPECT/CT scanners are also growing in their use. The use of these hybrid scanners provides the capability to routinely measure and report the

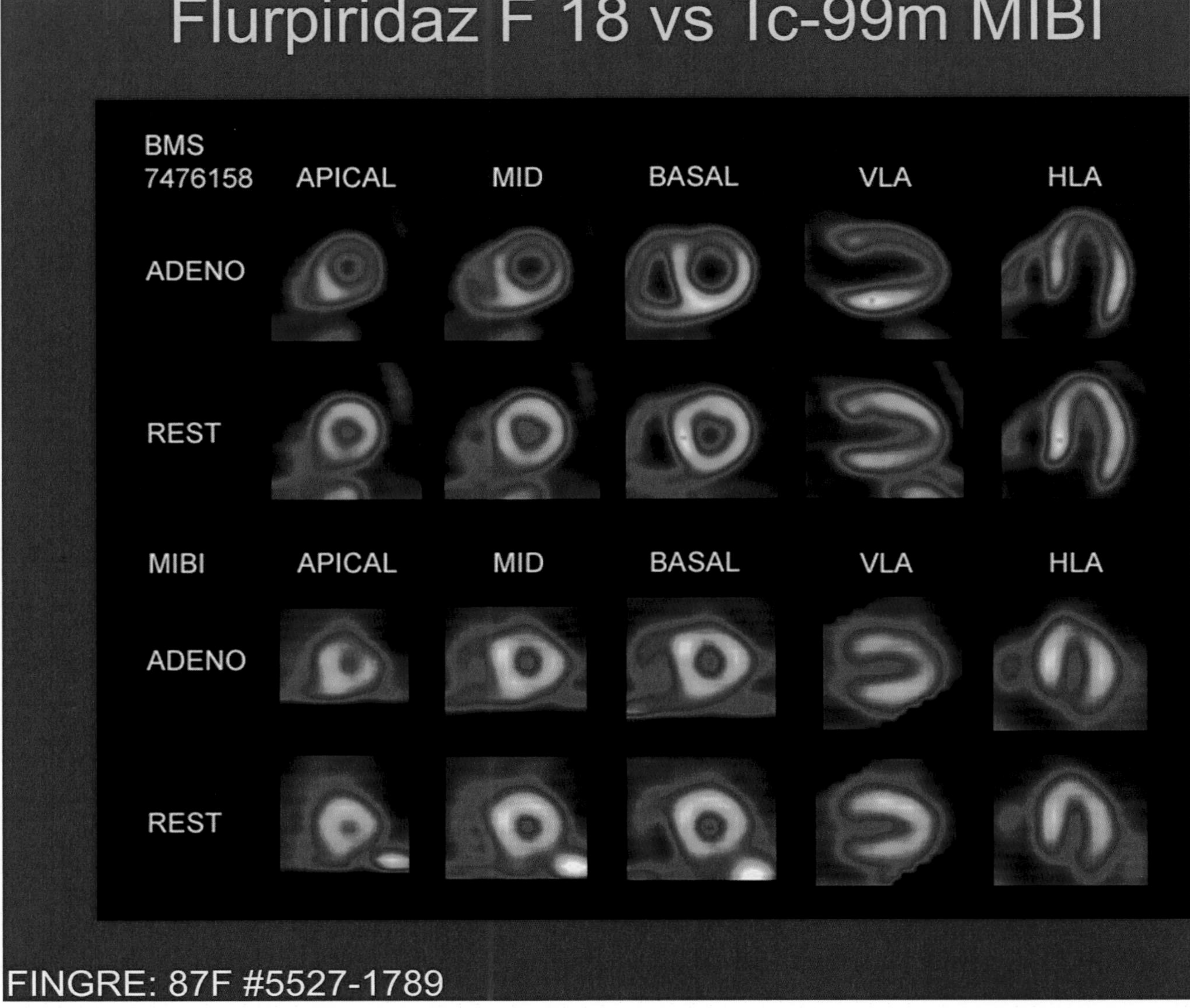

Fig. 20.6 Case example of Flurpiridaz F 18 PET (*top two rows*) vs Tc-99m rest SPECT (*bottom two rows*). The patients was an 87 year old woman with shortness of breath 3 months after stenting the left anterior descending coronary artery. An anterior wall stress perfusion defect is seen on both types of scans but is shows greater contrast on the Flurpiridaz F 18 images. Coronary angiography subsequently demonstrated subtotal in-stent stenosis. *ADENO* adenosine; *VLA* vertical long axis; *HLA* horizontal long axis; *MIBI* sestamibi (Reprinted with permission from Berman et al. [24] with permission from Elsevier)

coronary artery calcium (CAC) score on patients undergoing MPI. This addition of the CAC score has several major advantages. From the standpoint of interpretation, the presence of CAC and its extent provide additional powerful information which can improve the accuracy of interpretation of MPI when borderline perfusion defects are noted: when the CAC score is 0, the interpreter is able to be confident in considering an "equivocal" perfusion scan as "probably normal", while when the CAC is high, the equivocal scan can be considered to be "probably abnormal" (Fig. 20.7). Perhaps most importantly, combining CAC with PET- or SPECT-MPI assessments overcomes one of the major limitations of MPI in detection of epicardial CAD: its reliance on the presence of a hemodynamically significant lesion. Over a decade ago, it was recognized that high CAC scores are common in patients with normal SPECT-MPI [25]. By adding CAC assessment, the combined MPI/CAC study allows both the assessment of the coronary atherosclerotic burden as well as the flow limiting disease [26–28].

Finally, molecular imaging is an area of particular strength for nuclear cardiology, taking advantage of the ability of minute amounts of tracer to be employed, such that the administered tracer has no effect on the physiologic effect of the molecule. Virtually any biologically active molecule can

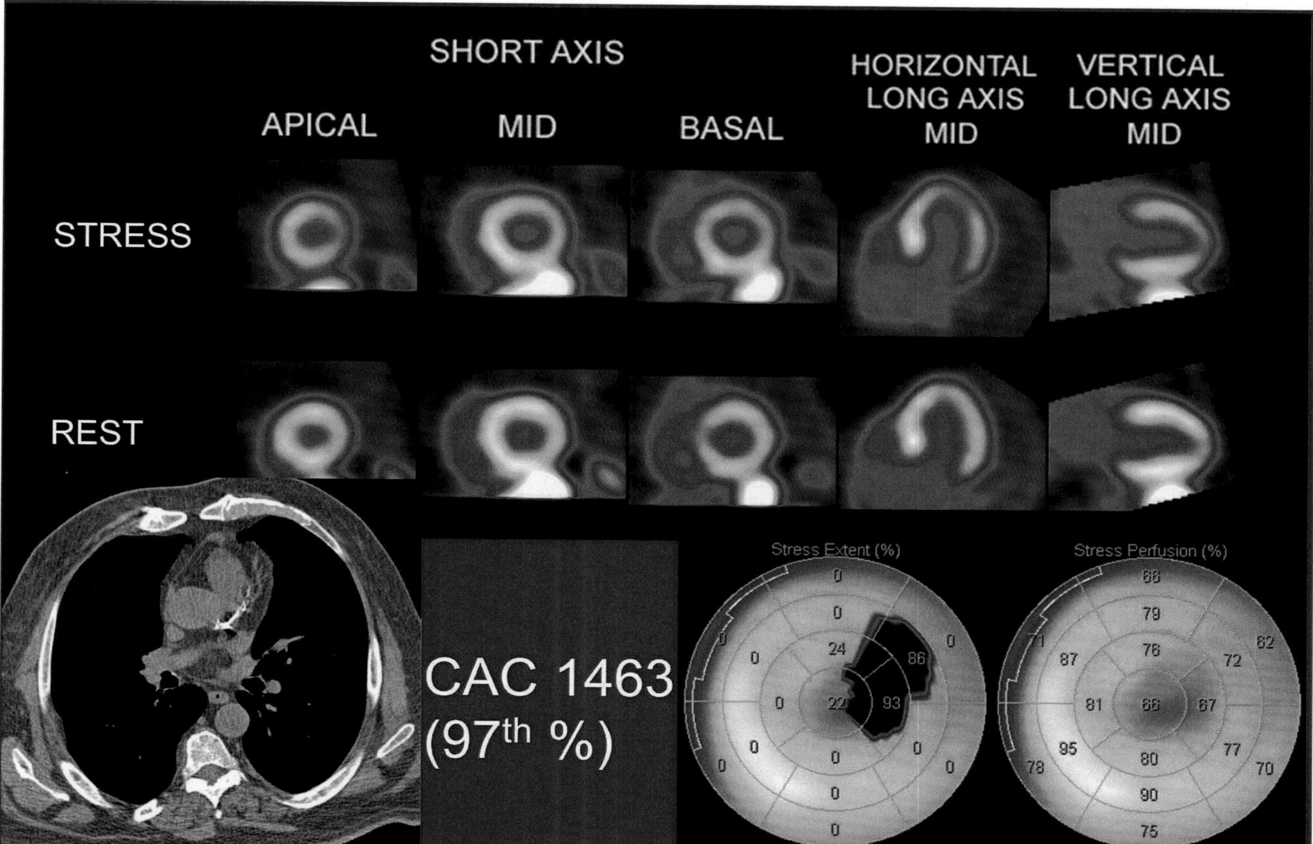

Fig. 20.7 Case example of combined SPECT-MPI and coronary artery calcium scanning (*CAC*). The patient was a 57 year old male. The SPECT-MPI study was considered probably abnormal based on the perfusion study alone. The finding that the CAC score was 1463 (97th percentile) resulted in increased observer certainty in interpreting the study as abnormal

be labelled with a PET radioisotope, providing the opportunity for PET molecular imaging (and for some molecules SPECT imaging) to provide unique insights into pathophysiologic processes. From a practical perspective of broad application in medicine, it must be realized that each tracer developed would need to go through a long and costly development to reach standard clinical use. However, there are two tracers that are approved by the FDA and widely available that can be applied to the assessment of the patient with atherosclerosis. F-18 FDG is widely used for assessment of cancer. It has also been used for over 30 years for the assessment of myocardial viability. Multiple studies have shown that F-18 FDG can also be used for imaging of arterial inflammation, with well-developed application in carotid imaging [29]. While not yet a routine clinical tool, FDG carotid assessment is already playing an important role in assessing novel therapies [30, 31]. F-18 FDG can also be effective in imaging of infection, including infected cardiac devices and intravenous lines.

One of the problems of CAD that is not routinely addressed by any of the standard imaging methods is that they do not assess the activity of disease. It is widely recognized that coronary inflammation plays a pivotal role in the development of plaque rupture—the process that triggers most myocardial infarctions [32]. Severe coronary stenoses can be completely stable, with only fibrous or calcified plaque, and have minimal likelihood of causing a coronary thrombosis. On the other hand large inflamed plaques may not cause a coronary stenosis, but could be at high risk of rupture [33] (Fig. 20.8). Imaging of coronary plaque inflammation with PET has the potential to assess the activity of CAD. Recently, exciting development has been reported with the use of the simple salt-F-18 sodium fluoride—for identification of high risk coronary artery plaque [34, 35]. This agent was used over 40 years ago as a bone scanning tracer. It tracks the active deposition of calcium. In a series of reports, Dweck, Joshi, and Newby have reported that F-18 fluoride can localize in coronary plaque. In an important study of F-18 fluoride imaging in 80 patients, these investigators studied 40 patients with acute ischemic syndromes (ACS) and 40 with stable angina [35]. The found that 93 % of the patients with ACS had F-18 fluoride uptake in the area

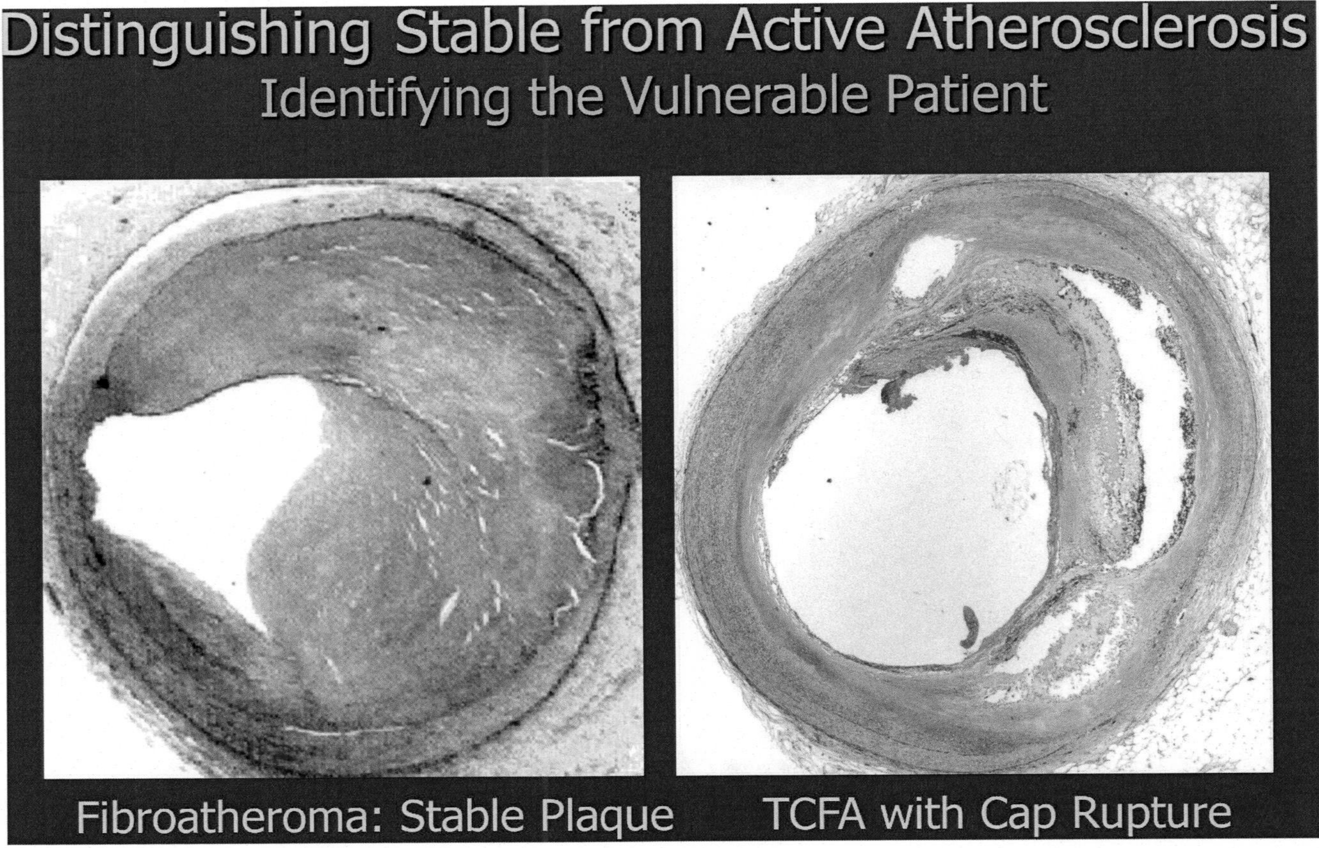

Fig. 20.8 *Left*: Cross-section of a stable atheroma associated with high grade coronary stenosis. *Right*: Cross-section of an fatal inflamed, lipid rich plaque which had ruptured, associated with a mild coronary stenosis (Reprinted from Moreno et al. [33] with permission from Elsevier)

found to be the culprit plaque on invasive coronary angiography (ICA) (Fig. 20.9; Courtesy Ref. [27]). In the patients with stable angina, 45 % had F-18 fluoride uptake, in each corresponding to a lesion with adverse plaque characteristics on IVUS. The current paradigm for guiding revascularization of patients with stable ischemic heart disease (SIHD) is to revascularize based on the presence of hemodynamically significant stenosis. It is possible that if CAD can be characterized by the degree of inflammation associated with it, that patients with stenoses but inactive disease might be safely guided toward conservative management rather than toward revascularization.

Cardiac CT

Cardiac CT has been employed for 20 years for CAC measurements—performed with minimal radiation, in a single breath, and no contrast. As discussed below, this is a powerful tool for prevention in CAD. Coronary CT angiography (CCTA) is a younger method—with its use being accepted only in 64 detector row scanners or more, scanners that were introduced in 2005. This method provides exquisite images of the coronary arteries. Beyond allowing assessment of coronary stenosis, not possible with non-contrast CT, CCTA allows assessment of noncalcified plaque. Motoyama et al. demonstrated that certain adverse characteristics of coronary plaques were associated with increased ACS events [36] (Fig. 20.10). Subsequently, considering positive remodeling and low attenuation plaque (associated with lipid content and the size of the necrotic core), these authors demonstrated in a series of over 1000 patients without obstructive CAD that patients with the number of adverse plaque features as associated with the frequency of ACS events [37]. Shmilovich et al. demonstrated that adverse plaque characteristics added to % stenosis in prediction of myocardial ischemia [38] (Fig. 20.11 Shmilovich). Subsequently, Nakazato et al. demonstrated that the aggregate plaque volume on CCTA added to diameter stenosis in prediction of reduced FFR in intermediate coronary lesions [39]. More recently, Park et al. demonstrated that positive remodeling on CCTA was associated with ischemia-causing lesions across the degrees of coronary artery stenosis [40]. These adverse plaques characteristics can be appreciated visually, but their manual measurement is time consuming and tedious, and not likely to become commonly performed. Importantly, automated software approaches to assessment of coronary plaque have been developed allowing assessing of a wide variety of plaque

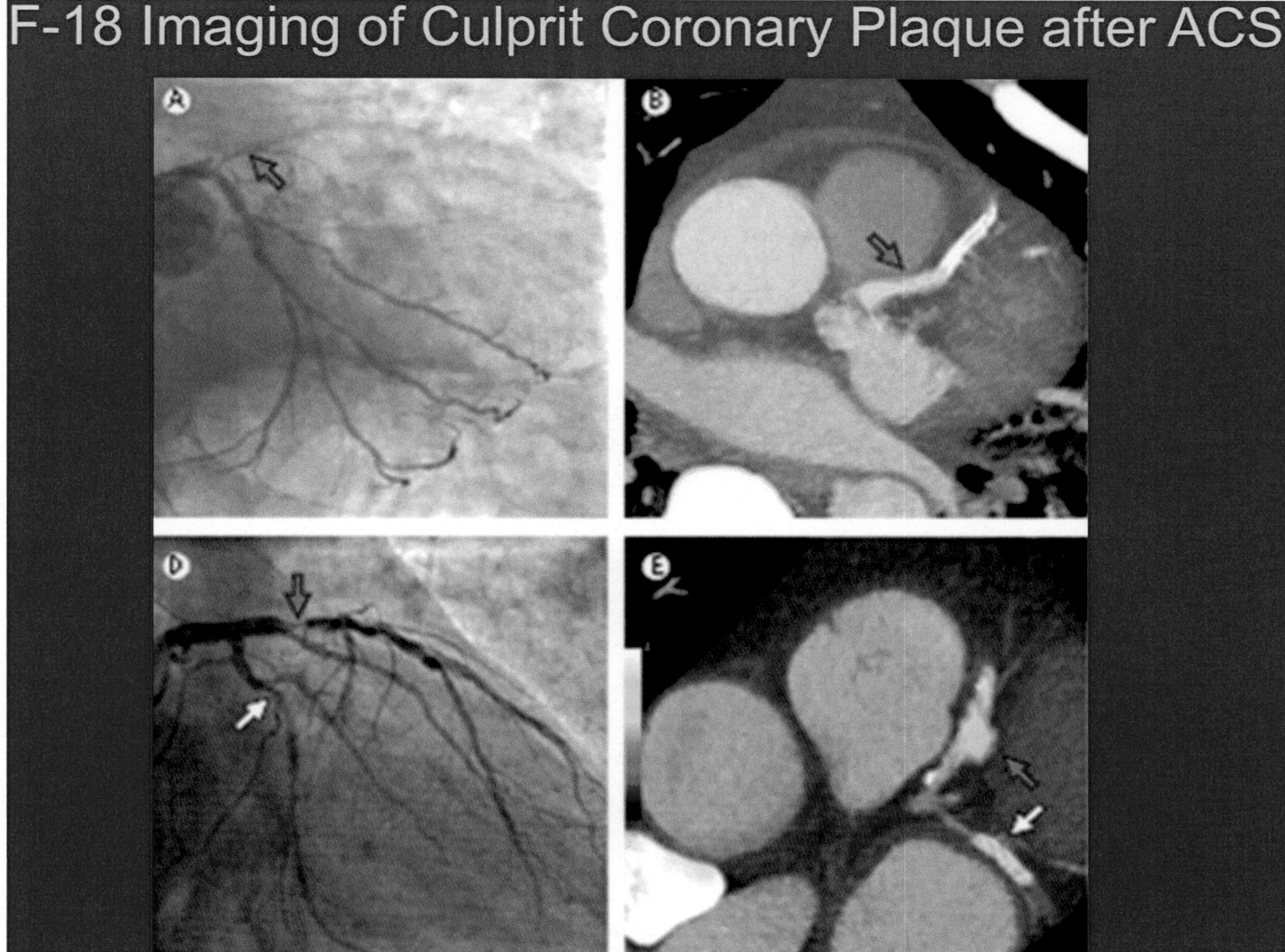

F-18 Imaging of Culprit Coronary Plaque after ACS

Fig. 20.9 Illustration of F-18 NaF uptake superimposed on CCTA (*right*) and corresponding culprit lesions on invasive coronary angiograms (*left*) in a patient with recent anterior ST elevation MI (*top*) and non-ST elevation MI (*bottom*). Intense uptake of F-18 NaF (*orange/red*) is seen at the site of the culprit plaques (*red arrows*). A bystander lesion in the left circumflex coronary artery that was stented but was not the culprit vessel had no increase in uptake of F-18 NaF (*white arrows, lower panel*) (Reprinted from Joshi et al. [35] with permission under a Creative Commons Attribution license)

characteristics (Fig. 20.12 Dey). Automated assessment of plaque characteristics (Autoplaq®; Cedars-Sinai Medical Center, Los Angeles, California) has been shown by Dey et al. to correlate highly with measurements by intravascular ultrasound [41]. More recently, Diaz-Zamudio, Dey and associates have shown these automated plaque measurements to be predictive of abnormal FFR and more predictive than stenosis grading in intermediate coronary lesions, with total, noncalcified, and low-attenuation being significant predictors of ischemia [42]. The automated assessments have the potential of becoming practical clinical tools that could augment the assessment of coronary stenosis by CCTA.

Beyond the anatomic assessments of plaque and stenosis, CCTA acquisitions can be used to assess physiologic processes. Two major developments have been recently reported in this regard. The first is the assessment of myocardial perfusion with CT (CT perfusion or CTP). CTP has its origins in digital subtraction angiography initially evaluated in the 1970s. With cardiac CT, it has now been applied to assess perfusion defects at rest and during vasodilator stress, providing assessments of regional hypoperfusion. The approach has recently been assessed in two large multicenter trials. The CORE64 study evaluated rest/adenosine CTP using the combination of stenosis ≥50 % on ICA and SPECT myocardial perfusion defect as the comparator of hypoperfusion. A high receiver operating characteristic (ROC) curve area was reported [43]. Comparable accuracy for detection of ICA stenosis was subsequently reported in the trial between adenosine CTP and pharmacologic SPECT assessments. In another multicenter trial, Cury et al. reported a high ROC curve area for the assessment of perfusion defect comparing regadenoson CTP to regadenoson SPECT [44]. These reports suggest that CCTA might effectively be used clinically for assessment of vasodilator stress myocardial perfusion and

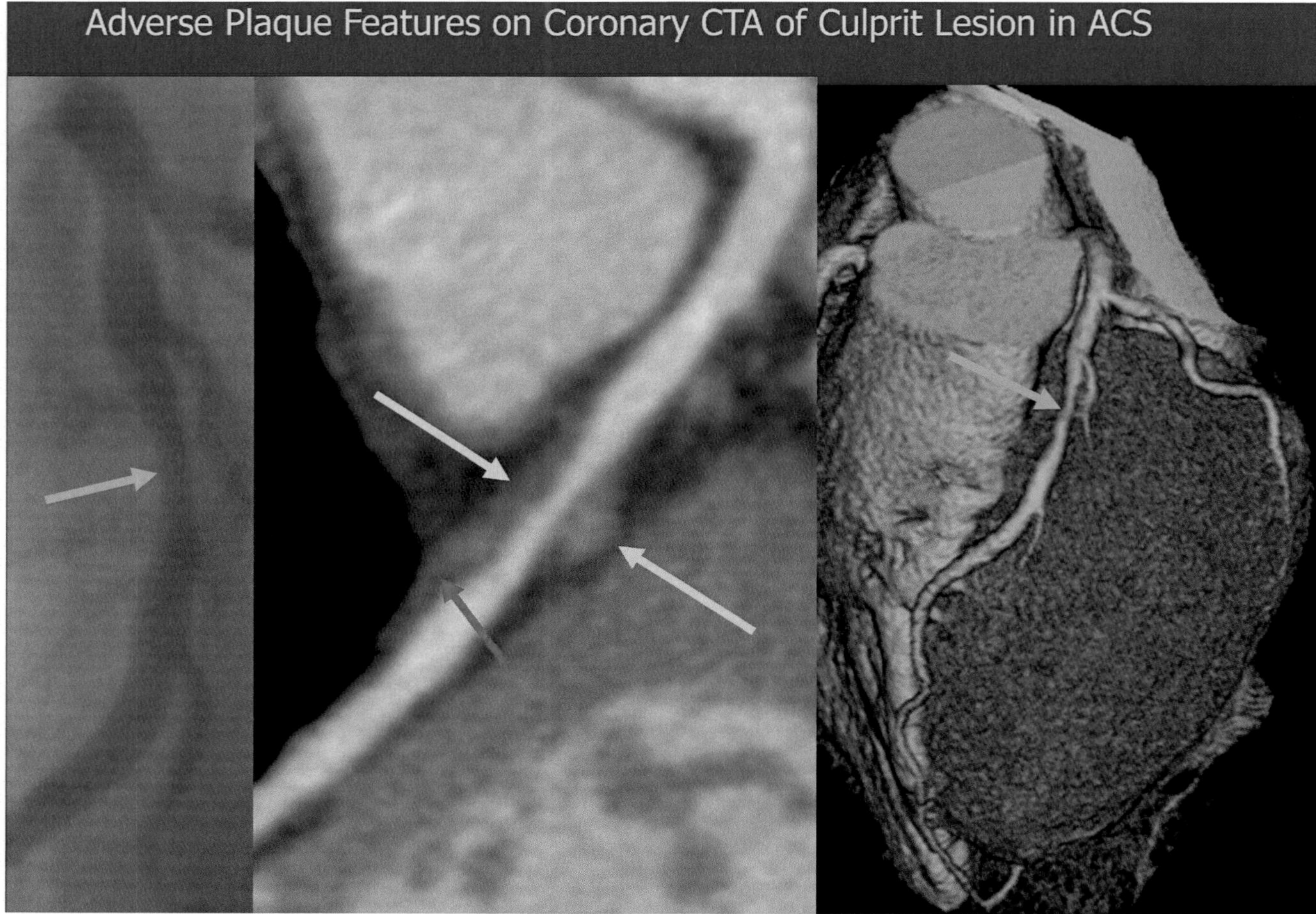

Fig. 20.10 CCTA (volume rendering, right; curved multiplanar reconstruction (*middle*) and ICA showing adverse plaque characteristics associated with moderate stenosis in a culprit left anterior descending coronary artery lesion in a 40-year-old male patient presenting with acute coronary syndrome. The *blue arrow* on ICA shows the site of maximal luminal obstruction. On CCTA the plaque is seen to be large, with positive remodeling (*yellow arrows*; remodeling index 1.43) and to have a low attenuation component (*red arrow*), consistent with lipid in necrotic core (Reprinted from Motoyama et al. [36] with permission from Elsevier)

coronary plaque and stenosis. Potentially, this combination could allow adjudication of borderline stenoses with respect to their hemodynamic significance without need for a second stress test on a separate occasion.

An exciting even more recent development has been that of estimating FFR from a resting CCTA study FFR_{CT}. This approach uses computational fluid dynamics, assessing the CCTA studies through the use of an off-site supercomputer. The method does not require a second acquisition with its attendant radiation and work-flow complexity, and has no additional contrast or radiation, since it uses the standardly acquired CCTA study (Fig. 20.13). Three large multicenter trials have demonstrated the high accuracy of this method in predicting FFR by ICA [45–47]. In the NXT study, the accuracy of FFR_{CT} exceeded that of coronary stenosis measured by ICA in prediction of FFR [47] (Fig. 20.14; Courtesy NXT). This promising technique could be of high value to interventionalists in determining the need for revascularization and potentially allowing them to reduce the need for FFR measurements in the catheterization laboratory as well as to reduce the proportion of times that ICA is performed and revascularization is not needed. How well the approach will perform in standard clinical practice is currently undergoing evaluation.

Value-Based Imaging

All of these assessments now available due to the technologic assessments must now be addressed in terms of how they will fit in with the migration to value-based imaging. In this section, we address consideration of the "value proposition" in four different settings in which CAD is considered or being evaluated: prevention, detection/assessment of ACS, assessment of patients with suspected or known SIHD, and patients with heart failure related to CAD.

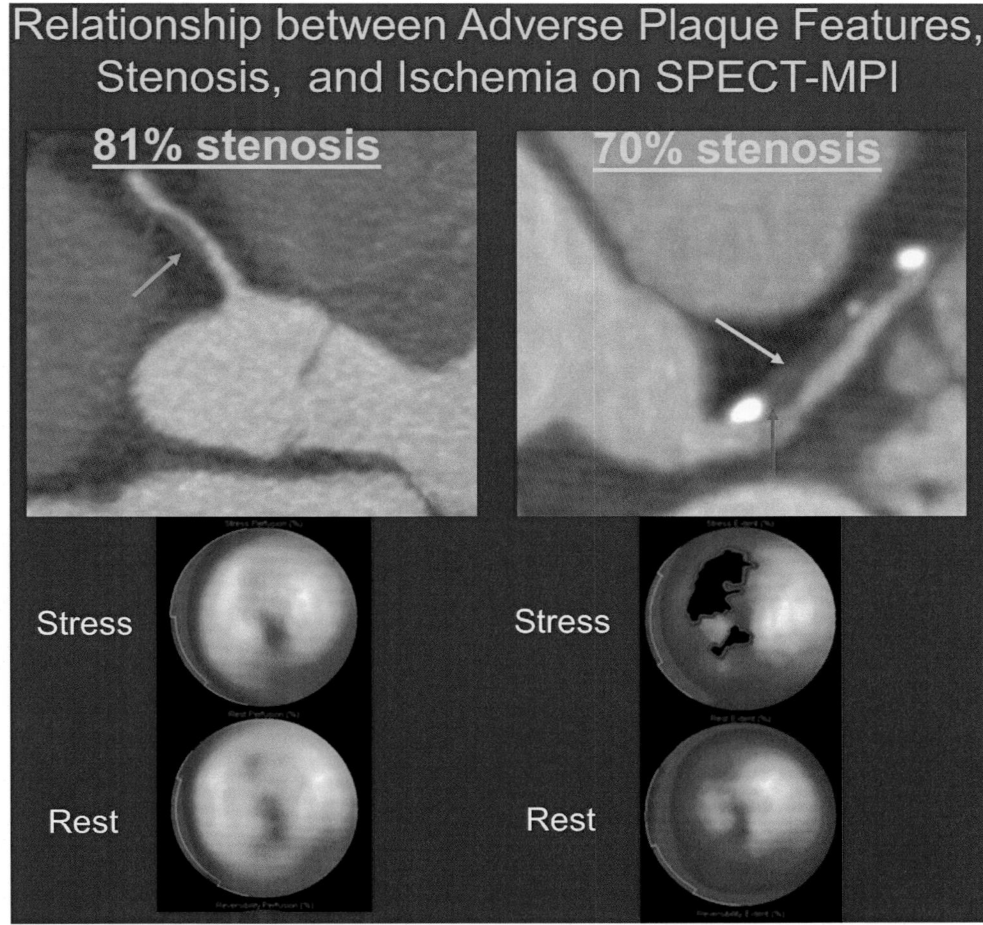

Fig. 20.11 Case examples illustrating the relationship of coronary stenosis on CCTA (*top*) to ischemia on SPECT-MPI polar maps (*bottom*) in patients with high grade coronary stenosis by quantitative coronary analysis (*QCA*). The patient on the left had an 81 % stenosis, associated with a plaque without adverse features (*green arrow*) and had no evidence of ischemia. The patient on the right had a 70 % stenosis by QCA, associated with a plaque with adverse characteristics of large volume, positive remodeling (*yellow arrow*) and low attenuation plaque (*red arrow*) and demonstrated clear evidence of ischemia (Reprinted from Shmilovich et al. [38] with permission from Elsevier)

Automated quantitative plaque characterization

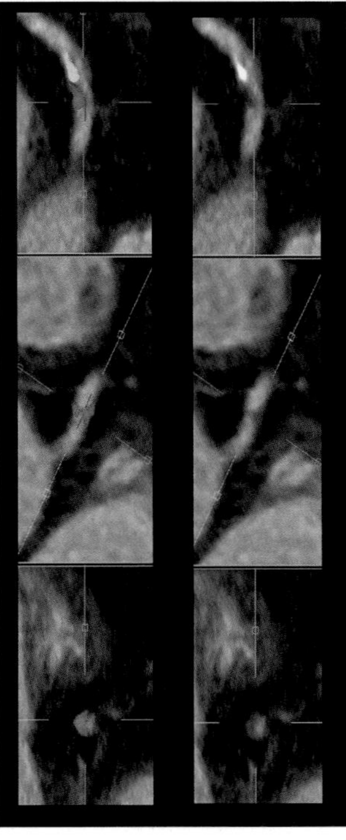

- % Diameter Stenosis
- % Area Stenosis
- NCP volume
- CP volume
- % NCP/Total volume
- % CP/Total Volume
- % Aggregate plaque volume
- Remodeling index
- “Spotty” calcification

Fig. 20.12 Features which can be assessed by automated quantitative plaque characterization (AutoPlaq®; Cedars-Sinai Medical Center; Los Angeles, California). *NCP* non-calcified plaque, *CP* calcified plaque (Reprinted from Dey et al. [41] copyright RNSA® with permission from the Radiological Society of North America)

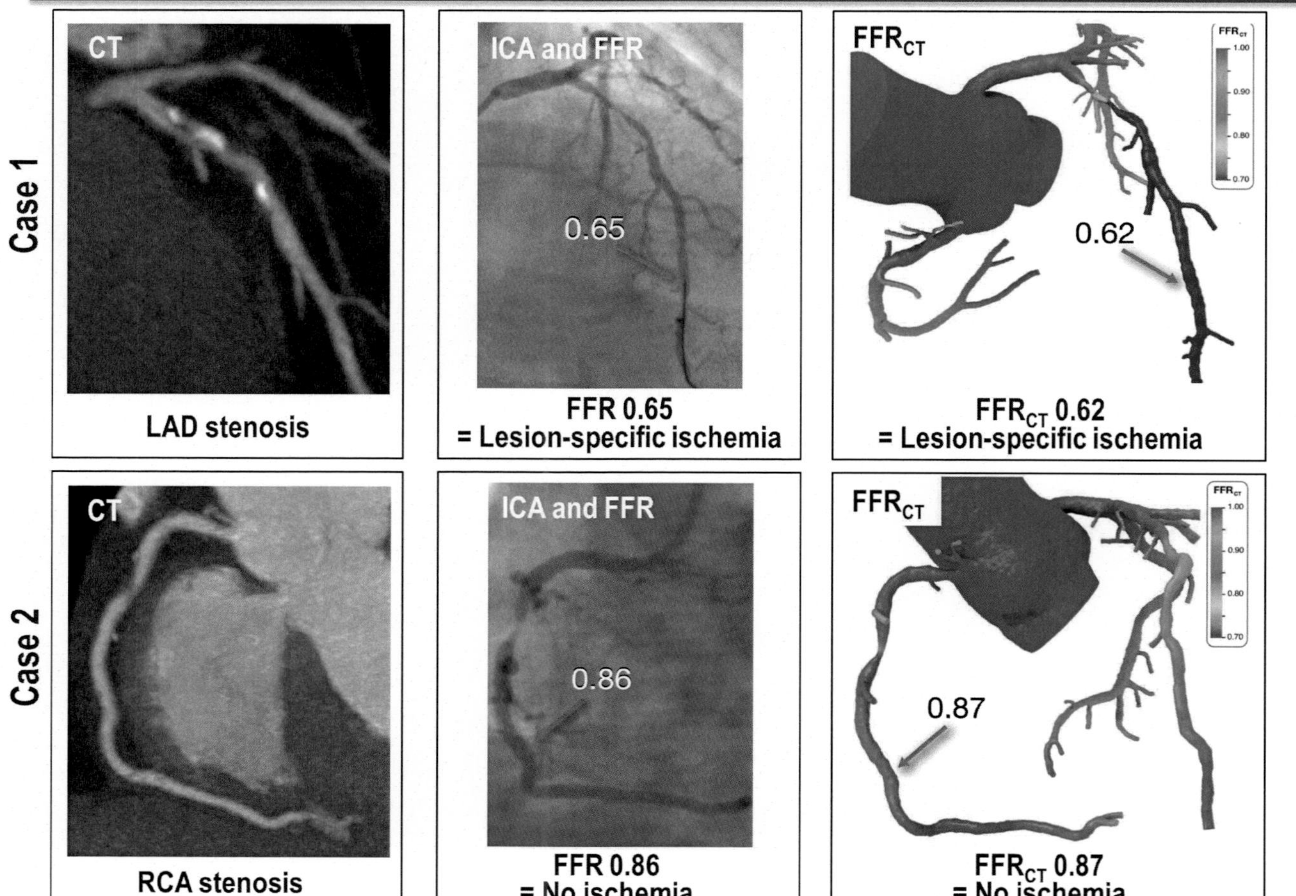

Fig. 20.13 Illustration of CCTA (*left*) ICA (*middle*) and FFR_{CT} (*right*) in: a patient with a moderate coronary stenosis (*top*) associated with a reduced FFR and FFR_{CT} (*top*) and a patient with a higher grade coronary stenosis associated with a normal FFR and FFR_{CT} (*bottom*). Note the correspondence between the FFR and the FFR_{CT} measurements and the discordance with the visually appreciated degree of stenosis (*red arrows*) (Reprinted from Min et al. [45] with permission from the American Medical Association)

Prevention

More lives could be saved by appropriate implementation of preventive therapies such as the use of statin and aspirin than through the use of revascularization. Yet the manner in which prevention strategies are chosen is imprecise. Increasingly, modern concepts are that medicine is migrating toward "precision medicine," in which the therapy for a patient is chosen based on the characteristics of that individual. The standard guidelines for implementation of aggressive prevention strategies employ the use of global risk scores, such as the Framingham Risk Score (FRS) to place patients into treatment groups. These scores are based on risk factors that are known in populations to be independently associated with atherosclerotic cardiovascular disease (ASCVD) [48]. The current ACC/AHA guidelines from 2014 essentially result in nearly 100 % of men over age 55 having a recommendation for being on statin and aspirin therapy [48, 49]. There are multiple limitations in the use of global risk scores in the individual patient. They do not take into account individual variations of the biologic effects of the risk factor, the chronicity of the factor, and cannot account for all risk factors. On the other hand, the CT CAC score is a marker of CAD in an individual patient, representing the integrated effect of all risk factors on the individual's coronary vasculature. It thus overcomes the imprecision of the global risk scores. Recent analysis of patients from the Multi-Ethnic Subclinical Atherosclerosis (MESA) study has shown that the new AHA-ACC-ASCVD score overestimated risk by 25–115 %, with substantial implications for individual patients and the health care system [50].

Hundreds of studies have evaluated the prognostic value of the CAC in asymptomatic subjects. They have consistently documented that CAC score provides incremental

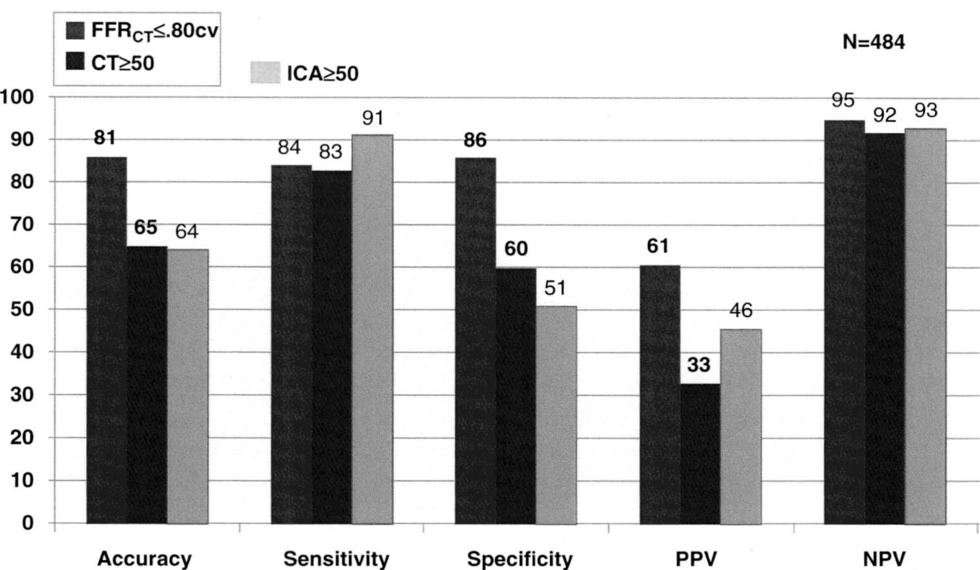

Fig. 20.14 Accuracy, sensitivity, and specificity of FFR_{CT} (*red*) and percent diameter stenosis [*black*: CCTA; *pink*: ICA] in prediction of invasive FFR (Reprinted with permission from Nørgaard et al. [47] with permission from Elsevier)

information over a global risk scores, mainly the FRS. Among most important of these studies to date are the MESA study [51] and the Heinz-Nixdorf Recall study [52]. These were large, population based studies in which CAC and multiple other tests were compared to global risk scores for assessing patient prognosis. The results of the trials were very similar. They showed strong incremental value of CAC over the FRS, and a high net reclassification index (NRI). Each trial has had numerous substudies reported. In a recent report from the MESA trial, the CAC score was the only assessment of many including CRP to add to the FRS in assessment of prognosis [53]. Further interesting work from the MESA trial has been to show that the CAC score could be used to more effectively target statin and aspirin therapy than the FRS. With respect to aspirin, Miedema et al. [54] demonstrated from MESA that in patients with a low FRS (<10 %), the use of aspirin would result in net patient harm, whereas the use of aspirin in patients with CAC >100 would be associated with patient benefit. Similarly, regarding statin therapy, it was projected that it is both cost-saving and more effective to scan intermediate-risk patient for CAC and to treat those with CAC ≥1 with a statin than basing treatment on standard risk-assessment guidelines [55].

The CAC scan can affect the degree to which the patient adopts heart healthy behaviors including improvement in risk factor profile [56], intensification of Rx [57], better adherence to Rx [58], dietary modifications [58], and increased exercise [59]. Interesting work from MESA demonstrated that improvement in healthy lifestyle behavior including regular exercise, healthy diet, smoking avoidance, and weight maintenance was associated with lower coronary calcium incidence, slower calcium progression, and lower all-cause mortality over 7.6 years [60].

The largest randomized trial to date assessing the value of CAC scanning is the Early Identification of Subclinical Atherosclerosis by Noninvasive Imaging Research (EISNER) trial [56]. It was designed to test the primary hypothesis that performing CAC scanning would lead to a beneficial sustained 4-year effect on individuals' CAD risk factors—using the FRS as a composite of these—as a surrogate for improved outcomes. Secondarily, we assessed the impact of CAC scanning on downstream medical resource utilization and healthcare costs. The trial involved assigning 2137 volunteers to groups that did versus did not undergo CAC scanning before risk factor counseling (2:1 scan/control randomization). Compared to the no-scan group, the scan group showed a net favorable change in systolic blood pressure ($p=0.02$), LDL-cholesterol ($p=0.04$), waist circumference for those with increased abdominal girth ($p=0.01$), and tendency to weight loss among overweight subjects ($p=0.07$). While mean FRS rose in the no-scan group, it remained static in the scan group (0.7 ± 5.1 versus 0.002 ± 4.9, $p=0.003$). Within the scan group, increasing baseline CAC score was associated with a dose–response improvement in systolic and diastolic blood pressure ($p<0.001$), total cholesterol ($p<0.001$), LDL-cholesterol ($p<0.001$), triglycerides ($p<0.001$), weight ($p<0.001$) and FRS ($p=0.003$). Downstream medical testing and costs in the scan group were comparable versus the no-scan group, balanced by lower and higher resource utilization for those with normal CAC scans and CAC scores ≥400, respectively. Improvement in the global risk score, associated with no increase in overall costs, provided evidence that there is value in testing this population at intermediate risk. Of note, this study had several components that were acting to underestimate the potential of the CAC scan to improve outcomes. The only difference between the control and treatment groups was a one-time counselling session in which the patients in the scan group were shown their scans and a nurse practitioner discussed the scan implications (those that were known at that early time) along with the patients risk factor profile with the patient, while the control group patients received the risk factor counseling alone. There were no treatments recommended by the nurse practitioner; specifically, the only treatment guidelines that were discussed were those of the NCEP III—with no specific recommendation for change in treatment based on scanning. Subsequently, patients were sent by mail an anonymized report of their study; however, their physicians were not sent reports.

Application in Diabetes

Assessment of the asymptomatic patient with diabetes is an important subgroup with generally a higher risk of cardiac events than patients in most other asymptomatic groups. Comparing the potential value of the various noninvasive tests in these patients casts further light on their effectiveness in the asymptomatic patient population. CAC scanning may be of value in this application.

Extensive data has shown that a CAC score of 0 is found in a high proportion of adult asymptomatic diabetics—38 % in the MESA study [61]. The possibility that this finding might improve patient outcomes, particularly in the psychologic well being of the diabetic patient, if of interest in this regard. There is a greater increase of risk of events in every category of increased CAC score when compared to the non-diabetic population. CAC scanning has the potential of defining a high risk group that might benefit from ischemia testing.

Randomized clinical trials (RCTs) have suggested that routine SPECT-MPI in the asymptomatic diabetic patient may not be of value. In the Detection of Ischemia in Asymptomatic Diabetics (DIAD) study [62], 1143 asymptomatic diabetics were randomized to either a screening approach using SPECT-MPI (n=522), or a non-imaging regimen. The patients were not selected to be high risk. Over a 4.8 year follow-up, the cardiac event rates were low and there was no outcome benefit in the group undergoing SPECT-MPI. While the prevalence of any perfusion or LV function abnormality was 22 %, a moderate-to-large perfusion defect was present in ischemia only 6 %. In the small group that did have moderate-to-large perfusion defects, the event rate was elevated. The Basel Asymptomatic High-risk Diabetes Outcome (BARDOT) trial [63] studied 400 patients with type 2 diabetes who had no history or symptoms of CAD, but who were defined as high risk. Baseline SPECT-MPI was abnormal in 22 %, concordant with the results of the DIAD study. Major adverse cardiac events (MACE, defined as cardiac death, myocardial infarction, or symptom-driven coronary revascularization) occurred in 2.9 % of patients with normal baseline SPECT-MPI compared to 9.8 % of patients with an abnormal MPI (p=0.011). Patients with abnormal SPECT-MPI were randomized to an approach of catheterization with intended revascularization vs noninvasive management; there was no difference in outcomes in those randomized to medical therapy only vs combined medical therapy and revascularization. Overall, the findings suggest a lack of outcome benefit of stress testing of asymptomatic diabetic patients. Whether such testing might have been beneficial if the definition of high-risk had been based on elevated CAC levels would be of interest.

A recent multicenter RCT has evaluated the application of CCTA in the high risk asymptomatic diabetic patient. In this regard, the FACTOR-64 trial evaluated whether routine coronary CTA screening of high risk asymptomatic diabetics affects changes in treatment that leads to a reduction in cardiac events [64]. Nine hundreds patients were randomized to CT screening (n=452) with protocol specific recommendations for management after testing or standard care (n=448). CCTA showed no CAD in 31 %, mild plaque <50 % stenosis in 46 %, moderate stenosis in 12 %, and severe stenosis in 11 % of the patients. CCTA prompted a stress test in 14 % of the cases, and angiography in 8 %, of whom 53 % underwent subsequent PCI and 19 % underwent coronary artery bypass graft (CABG). There was a trend for a lower rate of events in the CT group: for the primary composite endpoint of death, MI, or hospitalization for unstable angina, the rate was 6.2 % in the CT arm vs. 7.6 % in the standard care group (HR 0.80, 95 % CI 0.49–1.32, p=0.38). At the end of the trial, the CT group showed improvements in statin use and intensity, lipid fractions, and blood pressure levels. The composite primary end point was less than half of expected and there was a non-significant trend toward lower composite events. While not yet proven statistically in this trial, the results suggest that a strategy based on screening high risk asymptomatic diabetics using CCTA might be of value.

Value of Noninvasive Imaging for Prevention

Given the plethora of CAC studies demonstrating the adverse prognosis of a high CAC score, it is questionable whether a sufficiently powered randomized clinical trial demonstrating that CAC improves outcomes be performed. Nonetheless, a vast amount of consistent observational data suggest that CAC scanning in the appropriate asymptomatic patient at low to intermediate risk would result in improved outcomes that would outweigh any increase in costs associated with the test and downstream testing and treatments, thus providing value (Fig. 20.15). The possibility that coronary CTA or stress myocardial perfusion imaging might prove of value in very high risk asymptomatic patients has not been fully explored.

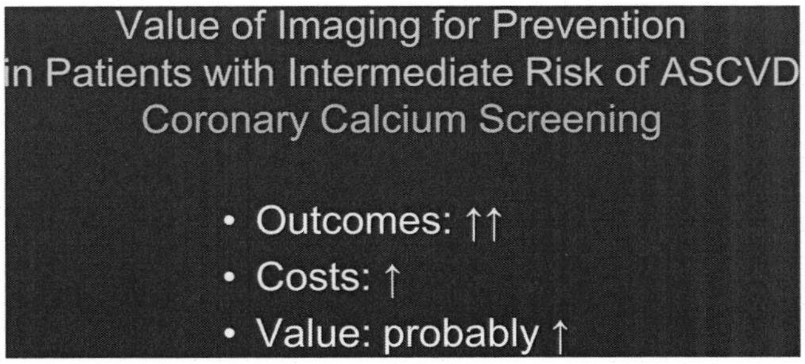

Value of Imaging for Prevention
in Patients with Intermediate Risk of ASCVD
Coronary Calcium Screening

- Outcomes: ↑↑
- Costs: ↑
- Value: probably ↑

Fig. 20.15 Hypothesized value of using CAC scanning for prevention in patients with an intermediate risk of ASCVD

Evaluation of the Symptomatic Patient

In the symptomatic patient without known CAD, the first question that arises addresses what is the cause of the symptoms (i.e., establishing the diagnosis) and, after it is answered, what is the appropriate treatment, which involves assessment of short term as well as long term risk. While use of 50 % stenosis on ICA for establishing diagnosis of CAD as the cause of symptoms is questioned, it has been the usual standard for establishing the presence of "significant" CAD—a standard that might be common to assessment of the patients with either acute or stable chest pain syndromes. In this regard, the sensitivity and specificity for detection of "angiographically significant" CAD has long been a standard for test assessment. Extensive evidence has shown that direct visualization of the coronary stenosis with CCTA is superior to all other forms of noninvasive testing, on a per patient, per vessel, and per segment basis [65–68]. Beyond detection of stenosis, CCTA has been studied extensively in risk prediction and effect on patient outcomes.

Evaluation of Patient with Acute Chest Pain

Almost eight million individuals are evaluated each year for acute chest pain in the emergency department (ED) [69]. Despite standardized protocols and high vigilance, between 2 and 6 % of patients are erroneously discharged with missed myocardial infarction [70] with higher mortality rates than patients who are hospitalized. For patients with normal or nondiagnostic initial ECGs and troponin levels on presentation to the ED, an important clinical problem is to distinguish those with acute coronary syndromes requiring hospital admission from those who may be safely discharged. It is now standard in many EDs and chest pain centers to evaluate such patients with a "rule-out myocardial infarction" strategy followed by stress testing and/or cardiac imaging; however, it has been estimated that the diagnosis of acute ED chest pain costs $10–$12 billion annually in the United States [69].

Use of SPECT-MPI in the Evaluation of Acute Chest Pain

Noninvasive imaging has become part of the standard of care in assessing patients with low to intermediate risk of an ACS in the ED. A common approach is to use rest or rest/stress Tc-99m sestamibi or tetrofosmin SPECT-MPI for this purpose. A 99 % negative predictive value of rest SPECT-MPI, when the radiopharmaceutical is injected during or shortly after chest pain, has been reported [69]. A prospective, randomized, controlled multicenter trial examined whether incorporating acute rest SPECT-MPI into an ER evaluation strategy of patients presenting with suspected acute ischemia improved initial ER triage [71]. A significant reduction in hospitalization was noted in patients with normal SPECT-MPI studies. When the radiopharmaceutical is injected after pain has subsided and the SPECT-MPI study is normal, stress SPECT-MPI studies or stress only SPECT-MPI protocols are common and have been shown to be effective [72]. The comparative use of SPECT-MPI to CCTA is discussed below. Below, evidence that CCTA may be superior in this application will be presented; however, there are settings in which CCTA would be expected to be nondiagnostic in which SPECT-MPI might be preferred. These include patients with known dense coronary calcification, elderly patients in whom dense coronary calcifications are likely, patients with prior bypass surgery, possibly with prior percutaneous coronary intervention (PCI), and known ischemic cardiomyopathy, and with contraindications to CCTA.

Use of CCTA in the Evaluation of Acute Chest Pain

Three large randomized clinical trials have evaluated the application of CCTA to patients in with suspected ACS in the emergency department in comparison to a standard of care approach (SOC). In all of these studies, the patients evaluated were defined as being in a low to intermediate group regarding the likelihood of having an ACS at the time of their ED visit. The first of these was the CT-STAT trial comparing CCTA to rest/stress SPECT-MPI [73]. In 16 centers, 699 patients were randomly assigned to CCTA (n=361) or MPI (n=338) as the index noninvasive test. CCTA resulted in a 54 % reduction in time to diagnosis (2.9 h vs. 6.3 h) compared with MPI ($p < 0.0001$). Costs of care were 38 % lower ($p < 0.0001$). The diagnostic strategies had no difference in major adverse cardiac events after normal index testing (0.8 % in the CCTA arm vs. 0.4 % in the MPI arm, p=0.29). The ACRIN-PA trial [74] evaluated 1392 low-to-intermediate risk patients (TIMI score 0–2) presenting to the ED to CCTA or the physician elected traditional approach to standard care in a 2:1 ratio. Patients evaluated with coronary

CTA had a shorter mean hospital stay and were also discharged more rapidly (total length of stay 18 vs 25 h; p <0.0001) and more frequently (50 vs 23 %) than patients undergoing the standard care evaluation. Of 640 patients with a negative CCTA examination, none died or had a myocardial infarction within 30 days [74]. The ROMICAT II trial [75] randomly assigned patients 40–74 years of age with symptoms suggestive of acute coronary syndromes but without ischemic electrocardiographic changes or an initial positive troponin test to early CCTA or to standard evaluation in the emergency department. The rate of acute coronary syndromes among 1000 patients with a mean (±SD) age of 54±8 years (47 % women) was 8 %. Compared with standard evaluation, in the CCTA group, the mean length of hospital stay was reduced by 7.6 h (p <0.001). Fifty percent of the patients in the CCTA arm were discharged by 8.6 vs 26.7 h in the standard ED evaluation arm (p <0.001). A higher proportion of patients were discharged directly from the emergency department (47 vs. 12 %, p <0.001). Sixty-two percent of patients were in the ED for 12 h or less in the CCTA arm vs 21 % in the control arm. There were no significant differences in major adverse cardiovascular events at 28 days. The cumulative mean cost of care was similar in the CCTA group and the standard-evaluation group ($4289 and $4060, respectively; p=0.65).

The CT-COMPARE trial [76] was a single center large randomized trial comparing CCTA to exercise ECG testing (ExECG) in 562 patients with low-intermediate risk chest pain subjects. ACS occurred in 24 (4 %) patients. Despite higher odds of downstream testing in the CCTA arm (OR 2.0), 30 day per-patient cost was significantly lower in the CCTA group ($2193 vs $2704, p<0.001). The length of stay of patients in the CCTA arm was significantly shorter (p <0.0005). No patient had post-discharge cardiovascular events at 30 days.

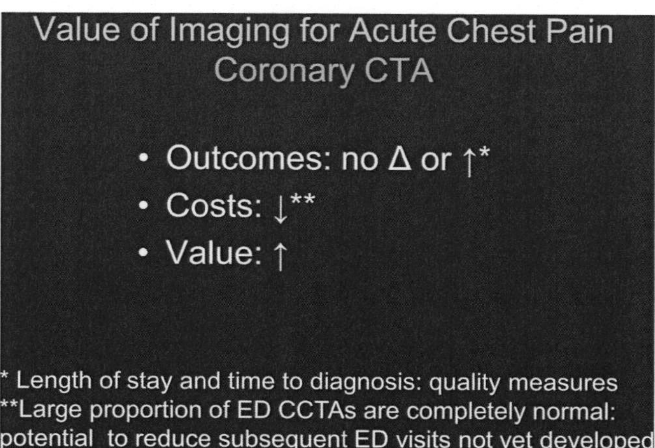

Fig. 20.16 Hypothesized value of using CCTA in patients with acute chest pain. *ED* emergency department

Value of CCTA in the Patient with Suspected ACS

How might the results of these four trials be interpreted with respect to "value"? In aggregate, the results are consistent with respect to the major findings. Overall, both CCTA and standard of care approaches are successful in assuring a low risk of missed events or of early events after discharge. Regarding outcomes, while "hard outcomes" of death or myocardial infarction were not different, improved outcomes would include the patient benefit of rapid discharge and the effect of their rapid discharge on improved care of other patients in a busy ED environment. An effect that has not yet been adequately assessed is the potential of the CCTA approach to reduce both short term and long term costs. Since extensive data has now shown that patients with completely normal CCTA studies have an extremely low rate of subsequent ACS over a prolonged period of time, there may be fewer repeat visits to the ED by patients with normal studies, who might be less concerned about their recurrent chest symptoms. In this regard, the downstream long term effects of knowledge about the presence of non-obstructive CAD—if effectively explained to the patient—may have the effect of increasing preventive treatment and improving outcomes. Thus, the "value proposition" for the use of CCTA in the ED is likely to be positive for application in the correctly selected patient (Fig. 20.16). It is of great interest, however, that as of 2015, the largest insurance carrier in the United States—Wellpoint—has a national medical policy (with effective date 10/08/2013) that the use of CCTA "is considered investigational and not medically necessary for…diagnosis of CAD, in individuals with acute or non-acute symptoms" [77] (reference "Anthem; Medical Policy #: RAD 00035 Last Review Date: 02/05/2015").

Evaluation of the Symptomatic Patient with Suspected Stable Ischemic Heart Disease (SIHD)

Chest discomfort or other symptoms raising the possibility of angina are among the most common problems confronting primary care physicians and cardiologists. While stress testing, usually with imaging, is the most common manner in which patients with suspected SIHD are evaluated, the use of CCTA is rapidly growing in this setting. In these patients, the reason for testing is twofold: (1) establishing the diagnosis explaining the symptoms so as to institute the appropriate medical therapy and (2) assessing potential benefit from revascularization. Despite the youth of the method—with CCTA being introduced with 64 slice scanners only in 2005—an impressive body of evidence has been accumulated documenting the effectiveness of CCTA not only for establishing the diagnosis but in assessing the risk of events.

As noted above, CCTA has higher sensitivity and specificity for angiographically significant disease noted above when compared to other forms of testing. Regarding risk of cardiac events, strong prognostic power of CCTA has been consistently demonstrated. A large number of manuscripts have been published from the CONFIRM registry, which as of 2015 was comprised of more than 32,000 patients evaluated in six countries, in whom comprehensive clinical, scan, and outcome data were recorded [78]. Data elements included risk factors, symptom type, CCTA results interpreted in 16 coronary segments for plaque, plaque type, and stenosis severity (0 = normal; 1 = 1 to <50 % stenosis; 2 = 50 to <70 % stenosis, and 3 = ≥70 % stenosis). The number of vessels with ≥50 % stenosis, a modified Duke score which added the location of the stenosis, a segment involvement score (SIS)—the number from 0 to 16 of segments with plaque, and a summed severity score (SSS), accounting for the severity of stenosis and the number of segments involved, ranging from 0 to 48. In the seminal article from CONFIRM, Min et al. reported analysis of 23,854 patients without known CAD who underwent a 2.3 year follow-up [78]. This early study demonstrated that the mortality rate in patients with entirely normal CCTA studies was extremely low, and that with every degree of increasing abnormality, mortality rate increased. Importantly, there was significant increase in mortality in the patients with non-obstructive CAD progressively increasing according to anatomic extent and severity of non-obstructive CAD (Fig. 20.17). This increase was noted for the number of vessels with greater than 50 % stenosis, the modified Duke score, the SIS, and the SSS. These increases in mortality with each increasing degree of anatomic abnormality were observed in men and women. Since this publication, consistent findings have been reported from CONFIRM across multiple patient subgroups, ranging from patients with no risk factors [79] to patients with abnormal left ventricular function [80]. In a group of 15,187 patients from CONFIRM in whom MACE events were recorded (death, myocardial infarction, and late revascularization), this graded relationship between events and observed degree of CAD by CCTA was also seen [81]. A long "warranty period" for patients with a normal has been described: the annual event rate of patients with a normal CCTA study has been reported in multiple studies to be less than 0.25 %.

Two large randomized clinical trials comparing CCTA to a SOC approach have recently been reported. The Scot-Heart Trial [82] examined 4138 patients aged 18–75 presenting to 12 rapid access chest pain centers in Scotland who were randomized to CCTA vs a SOC approach. The median follow up time was 1.7 years. Of note, 85 % of the patients had already had stress ECG testing at the time of randomization. The primary endpoint was certainty of the diagnosis of angina secondary to coronary heart disease at 6 weeks. From 2010 to 2014, the study randomized 4146 (42 %) of 9849 patients who had been referred for assessment of suspected angina due to CHD. At baseline, 47 % of participants had a clinic diagnosis of CHD and 36 % were considered to have angina

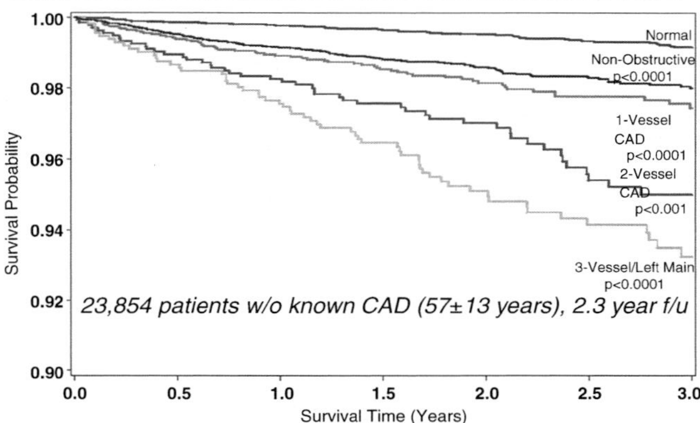

Fig. 20.17 Unadjusted All-Cause Kaplan-Meier Survival by the presence, extent, and severity of CAD by CCTA. Note the dose-response relationship of mortality to increasing numbers of vessels with obstructive coronary artery disease (*CAD*). *f/u* follow-up (Reprinted from Min et al. [78] with permission from Elsevier)

due to CHD. At 6 weeks, CTCA reclassified the diagnosis of CHD in 558 (27 %) patients and the diagnosis of angina due to CHD in 481 (23 %) patients (p <0.0001). Regarding the presence of CHD, physician certainty increased (p < 0.0001) and the frequency of CHD increased (p = 0·0172). Regarding diagnosis of angina due to CHD, the certainty increased (p < 0.0001). The findings changed planned investigations (in 15 vs 1 %; p <0.0001) and treatments (23 vs 5 %; p <0.0001) (Fig. 20.18), but did not affect 6-week symptom severity or subsequent admittances to hospital for chest pain. After 1.7 years, CTCA was associated with a 38 % reduction in fatal and non-fatal myocardial infarction (26 vs 42, HR 0.62, 95 % CI 0.38–1.01; p = 0.053), close to, but missing, statistical significance (Fig. 20.18). The overall conclusion of the trial was the CCTA changed and clarified diagnosis in one of four patients, altered subsequent investigations in one of six, changed treatment in one of four and showed a trend toward reduction of fatal and non-fatal MI.

The PROMISE trial [83] evaluated 10,003 symptomatic patients (60.8 ± 8.3 years, 52.7 % were women, 87.7 % symptomatic) with no prior CAD who were referred for noninvasive testing, randomizing them to CCTA (n = 4686) or functional testing (n = 4692) with stress nuclear (67.3 %), stress echo (22.5 %), or stress ECG alone (10.2 %). The composite primary end point was death, myocardial infarction, hospitalization for unstable angina, or major procedural complication. Secondary end points included invasive cardiac catheterization that did not show obstructive CAD and radiation exposure. The mean pretest likelihood of obstructive CAD by the Diamond-Forrester classification was 53.3 ± 21.4 %. However, the observed prevalence of ≥50 % stenosis on CCTA in the CCTA arm was only 11.3 %. Over a median follow-up period of 25 months, a primary

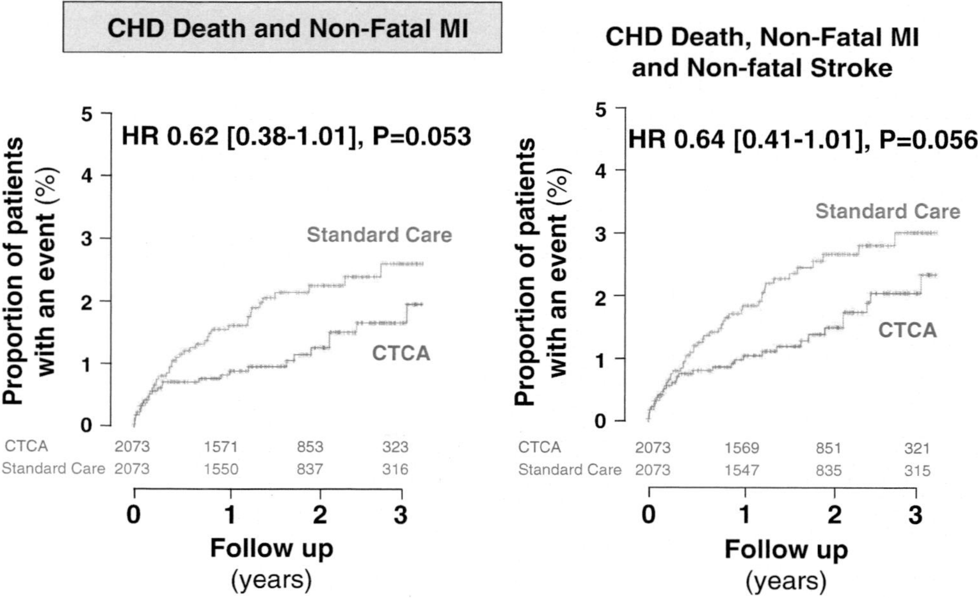

Fig. 20.18 Results of the Scot Heart Trial. Kaplan-Meier curves for CHD death and myocardial infarction (*left*) and CHD death, myocardial infarction, and stroke (*right*) in patients assigned to CTCA (*blue*) and standard care (*red*) (Adapted with permission from the Newby et al. *Lancet*, 2015 under a Creative Commons Attribution license)

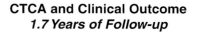

end-point event occurred in 3.3 % of the CCTA group and 3.0 % in the functional-testing group (p = ns). No significant difference was also shown in subsequent death or non-fatal MI. While invasive coronary angiography was more common within 90 days after testing in the CCTA group (12.2 vs. 8.1 %), CCTA was associated with fewer catheterizations showing no obstructive CAD than was functional testing (3.4 vs. 4.3 %, P = 0.02). Although the trial was not powered for non-inferiority, this large trial suggests that a strategy of initial CCTA is not inferior to the more commonly employed functional strategy with respect to short term cardiac events in a relatively low risk, symptomatic population.

The influence of CCTA on subsequent management is illustrated in case examples on Fig. 20.19. When the findings of CCTA are completely normal, treatment and subsequent testing is clear. The very high negative predictive value—the definitive ability to rule out CAD and the associated long "warranty period"—is a principal driving force in the application of CCTA. As with CAC scanning, the finding of non-obstructive CAD may prompt the use of aggressive preventive measures, which is likely to ultimately improve long term outcomes. When a proximal high grade stenosis is found, direct referral for invasive coronary angiography would likely follow. Stress imaging after CCTA may be useful in guiding the decisions in patients with borderline coronary stenosis (50–69 %), non-diagnostic CCTA results, and possibly patients with significant but not critical stenosis to evaluate the presence and extent and severity of ischemia as a guide to potential benefit from revascularization. As discussed above, FFR_{CT} is an alternative approach to assessment of lesions associated with diagnostic uncertainty. An approach to the symptomatic patient with an intermediate pretest likelihood of CAD, based on using CCTA as the initial test is shown schematically in Fig. 20.20.

Value of CCTA and Stress Imaging in the Patient with Suspected Stable Ischemic Heart Disease

How might the results of these the current evidence be interpreted with respect to "value" of CCTA and stress imaging in suspected SIHD? A conceptual approach to the symptomatic patient with an intermediate pretest likelihood of CAD, based on using CCTA as the initial test, is shown in Fig. 20.21. The value will likely depend on the correct selection of patients for testing. Consistent large registry data provide evidence of excellent risk stratification by CCTA. The Scot-Heart trial suggested a possible benefit with respect to outcomes, and important changes in confidence of diagnosis and changes in therapy. The PROMISE trial provided evidence that CCTA has similar outcomes compared to a functional approach in a patient group with a low prevalence of CAD. It is reasonable to hypothesize that in the low-intermediate likelihood of obstructive CAD group, there may be an outcome benefit as suggested by Scot-Heart, or outcomes might be unchanged as suggested by PROMISE. CCTA strategy will likely be less costly than a functional strategy, despite an increase in the rate of revascularization (Fig. 20.21). The greatest cost savings might be in patients with entirely normal studies—as the benign prognosis associated with the completely normal study, commonly seen in the patients being sent for testing, becomes more widely appreciated. In these patients, it is likely that the frequency repeat functional tests will be lower than with the functional

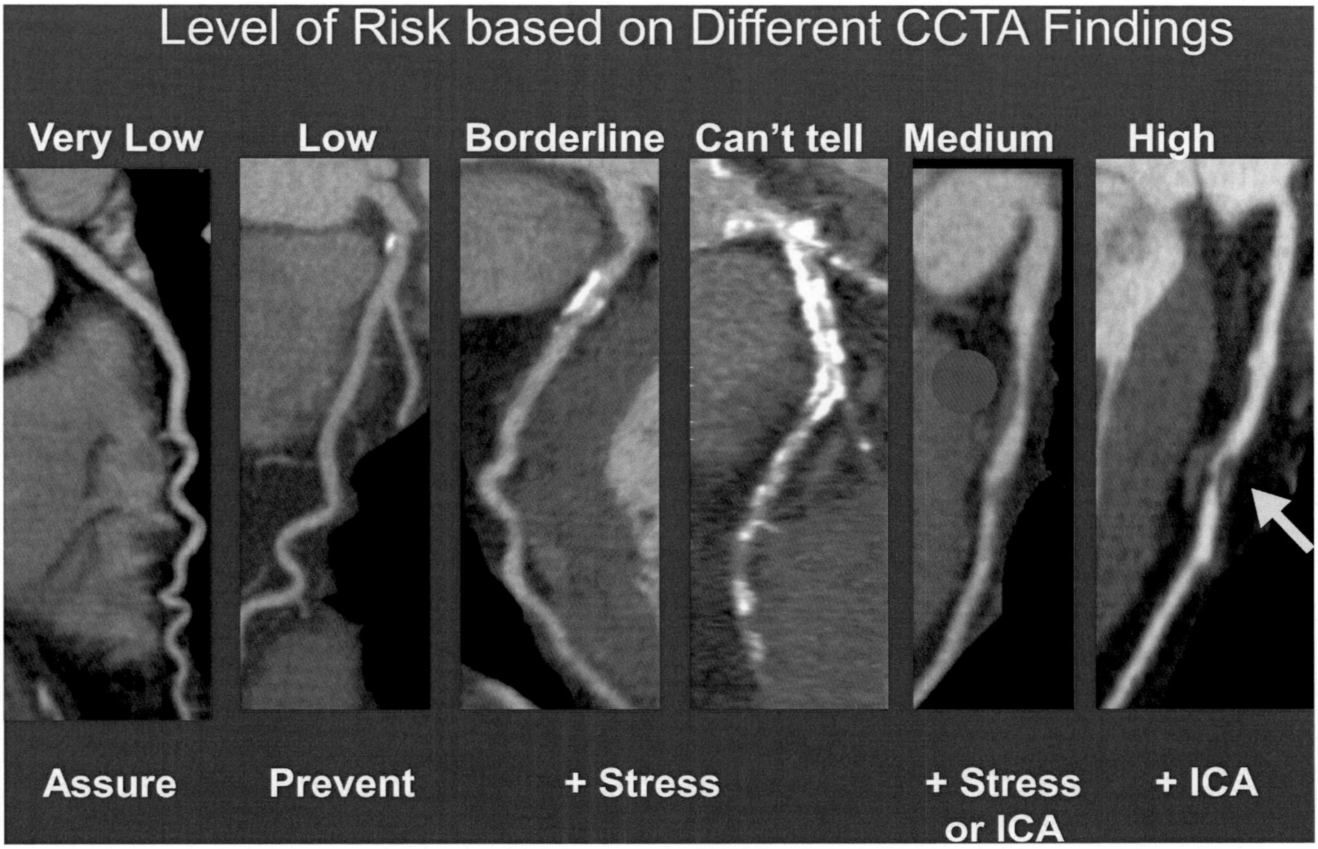

Fig. 20.19 Curved multiplanar reconstructions of CCTA from patients representing different levels of risk based on CCTA findings (*top*) and possible subsequent management. The *arrow* points to an intermediate-to-high finding on CCTA. *ICA* invasive coronary angiography

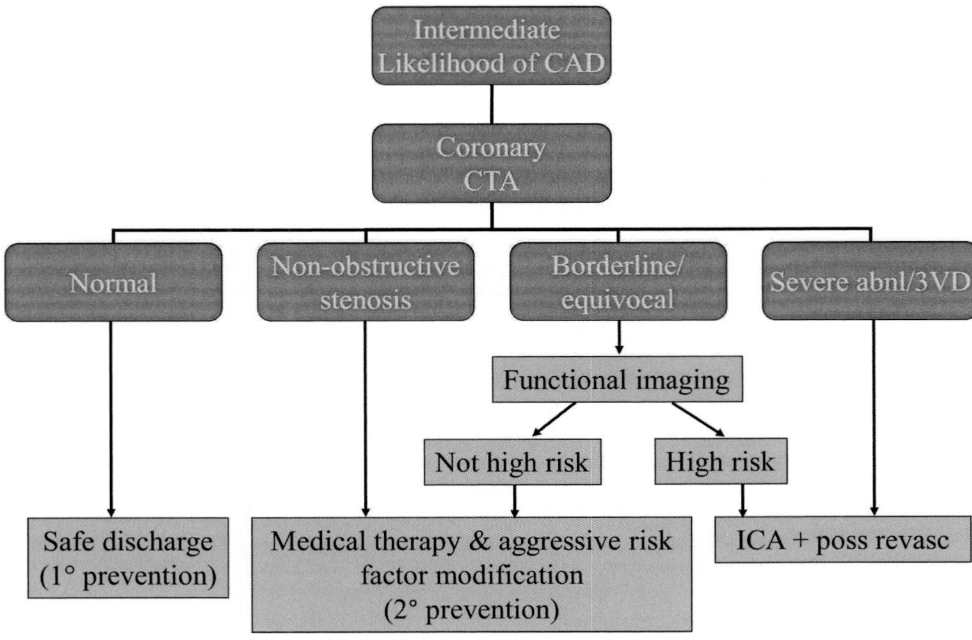

Fig. 20.20 Conceptual approach based on initial CCTA to diagnosis and management of coronary artery disease in symptomatic patients with an intermediate pre-test likelihood of CAD. *Abnl* abnormal, *revasc* revascularization (Adapted from Schuijf et al. [84] with permission from Springer)

testing approach—unless functional testing is combined with anatomic assessment such as performing an adjunctive CAC scan—potentially often stopping a cycle of multiple repeat tests. The cost-effectiveness CCTA in this patient population has recently been reviewed [85]. At the other end of the spectrum of likelihood of hemodynamically significant disease, a reasonable hypothesis would be that if anatomic approach to assessment of CCTA alone is used—not taking advantage of functional information that might be derived from CCTA—CCTA might not prove to be of value (Fig. 20.21). For example, if a very high CAC score is present in a substantial proportion of patients—leading to a high proportion of nondiagnostic studies—CCTA might be associated with an increase in downstream testing, either functional testing or invasive coronary angiography, potentially not changing outcomes compared to a functional approach but increasing costs. Adding "functional" information to CCTA—such as stress CT perfusion or FFR_{CT} might extend the population in whom the initial CCTA approach will likely be of value.

Suspected SIHD
Hypothesis: Value of Coronary CTA
Depends on Pre-test Risk

Low-to-Intermediate	High
• Outcomes: no Δ or ↑	• Outcomes: no Δ
• Costs: ↓	• Costs: ↑
• Value: ↑	• Value: ↓

Fig. 20.21 Hypothesized value of using CCTA in symptomatic patients with suspected stable ischemic heart disease (*SIHD*)

Stress imaging with SPECT-MPI remains by far the most common approach to testing of the patient with an intermediate likelihood of hemodynamically significant CAD. Given the wide availability of stress imaging methods compared to the current less widely available CCTA imaging, the predominance of the stress imaging approach is likely to remain for a considerable amount of time (Fig. 20.22). With the initial stress imaging approach, CCTA could be used as a second test when the results of stress testing are equivocal or discordant (e.g., severe ST depression with a normal MPI study) [86].

A drawback of stress imaging without anatomic assessment in patients with an intermediate likelihood of CAD is that the methods detect only patients with hemodynamically significant lesions and fail to identify patients with subclinical atherosclerosis in whom aggressive medical and lifestyle modification might prevent subsequent cardiac events. While SPECT-MPI assessment of ischemia is an excellent test of short-term prognosis, CAC scanning may be a better test of long-term prognosis. Over a decade ago, it was recognized that high CAC scores are common in patients with normal SPECT-MPI [25] (Fig. 20.23). Thus, patients with non-obstructive CAD, previously unknown, could be afforded effective preventive therapies, such as statins and aspirin. In this regard, the coupling of CAC scanning with SPECT- or PET-MPI discussed above could provide an effective alternative to the CCTA as a first choice approach to management of the patient with suspected SIHD. It has further been suggested [87] that a powerful, inexpensive alternative that may prove to be of value

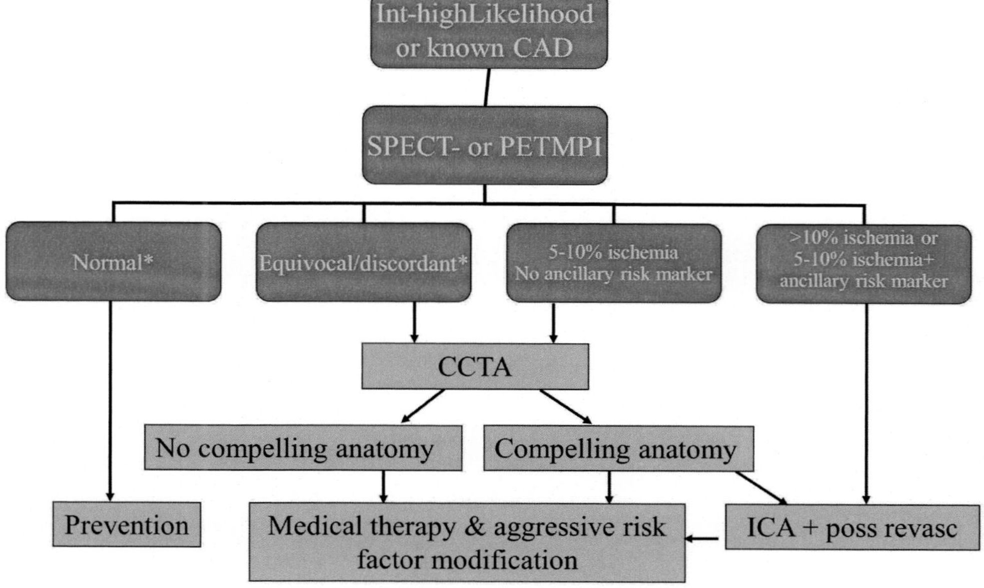

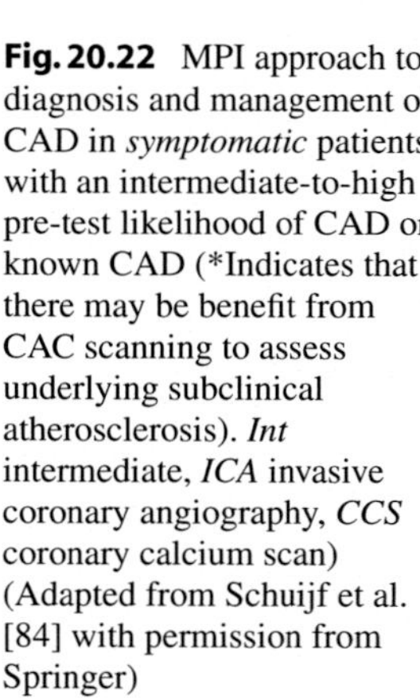

Fig. 20.22 MPI approach to diagnosis and management of CAD in *symptomatic* patients with an intermediate-to-high pre-test likelihood of CAD or known CAD (*Indicates that there may be benefit from CAC scanning to assess underlying subclinical atherosclerosis). *Int* intermediate, *ICA* invasive coronary angiography, *CCS* coronary calcium scan) (Adapted from Schuijf et al. [84] with permission from Springer)

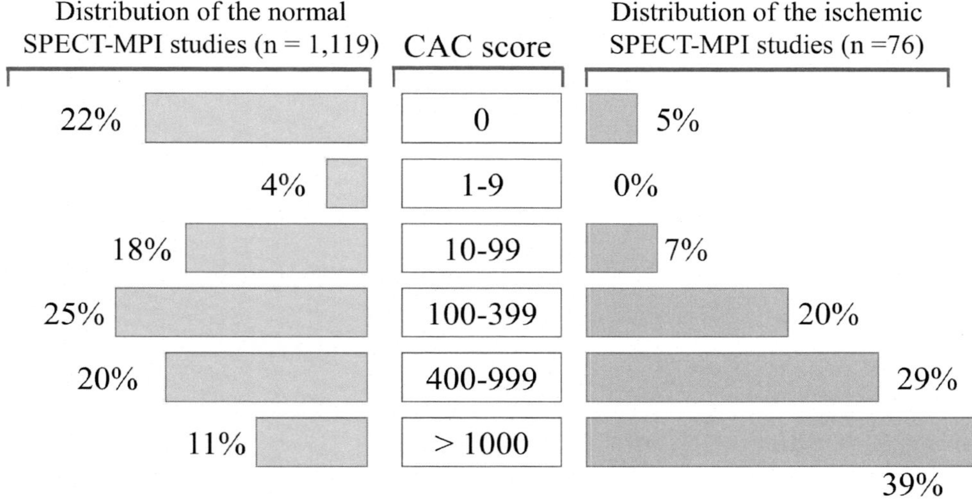

Fig. 20.23 Distribution of coronary artery calcium (*CAC*) scores for 1119 patients manifesting a normal myocardial perfusion single-photon emission computed tomography (*MPS*) (*left*) and the 76 patients with an ischemic MPS (*right*) (Adapted from Berman et al. [25] with permission from Elsevier)

is the combination of an ECG stress test without imaging with a CAC scan—the "coronary calcium treadmill test."

Patients with a High Likelihood of CAD or Known CAD

In contrast to patients with an intermediate likelihood of CAD, patients with a high likelihood of CAD are generally considered by their clinicians to have CAD and are treated accordingly. If limiting symptoms are present, the patient is usually directly sent for invasive angiography. In patients without limiting symptoms, stress imaging is performed to assess the extent and severity of ischemia in order to guide the decision for revascularization. An extensive body of information has demonstrated the prognostic power of ischemia testing with SPECT- or PET-MPI as well as with stress echocardiography and stress cardiac magnetic resonance imaging [88–91]. For SPECT and PET, risk has been shown to increase as a function of stress perfusion abnormality in virtually all subsets of patients with known or suspected CAD [89, 92]. Importantly, as noted above, these include the categories of patients in whom CCTA is contraindicated or likely to be non-diagnostic.

Large randomized clinical trials have suggested that anatomic assessment of disease alone does not provide evidence of revascularization benefit in most patients [93]. Most frequently quoted in this regard are the results of the COURAGE trial [94] and the BARI 2D trial [95] which did not demonstrate benefit over optimal medical therapy as an initial strategy.

There is evidence, however, that an ischemia guided approach to revascularization can be of benefit. Noteworthy in this regard are the results of the FAME studies. The FAME trial provided evidence that a revascularization strategy based on the use of ischemia testing as assessed by invasive FFR—with a cut-off of ≤0.80 considered as the criterion to perform PCI—resulted in improved outcomes in patients with multivessel CAD compared to a strategy based on anatomic assessment alone [96, 97]. Patients with FFR guided revascularization had a lower event rate (death, non-fatal MI, repeat revascularization) than the group in the angiographically guided strategy. Subsequently, the FAME II trial randomized stable patients with FFR ≤0.80 to PCI vs medical management [98]. The trial was stopped before reaching its target sample size due to excessive events—death, non-fatal MI, and unstable angina—in the medical therapy arm. While there were no differences between the FFR guided and the medical management approaches with respect to hard events alone, the results demonstrated an outcome benefit of ischemia driven decisions for revascularization using the composite endpoint ($p < 0.001$). The ability of an FFR-guided approach to reduce cardiac events was also demonstrated in a large registry of 7358 patients with stable disease studied at the Mayo Clinic [99].

Registry data with SPECT-MPI has provided evidence that supports the approach of ischemia driven revascularization. The potential that the amount of ischemia on SPECT-MPI to predict benefit with revascularization was first described in a single center registry by Hachamovitch et al. in 1998 [100]. Subsequently, this benefit was documented in a larger population of 10,627 patients without prior CAD who underwent SPECT MPI. A "proof-of-principle" question was asked: can imaging identify appropriate and beneficial treatment strategies and at what threshold of abnormality does therapeutic efficacy shift [101]. After adjusting for differences between medically treated and revascularized patients—including a propensity score adjustment to correct for differences in referral patterns to treatment options—patients with extensive myocardial ischemia by SPECT MPI exhibited a survival benefit with myocardial revascularization for the intermediate-term occurrences of cardiac death (Fig. 20.24). By contrast, among those with no myocardial ischemia, the cardiac death rate was higher with myocardial

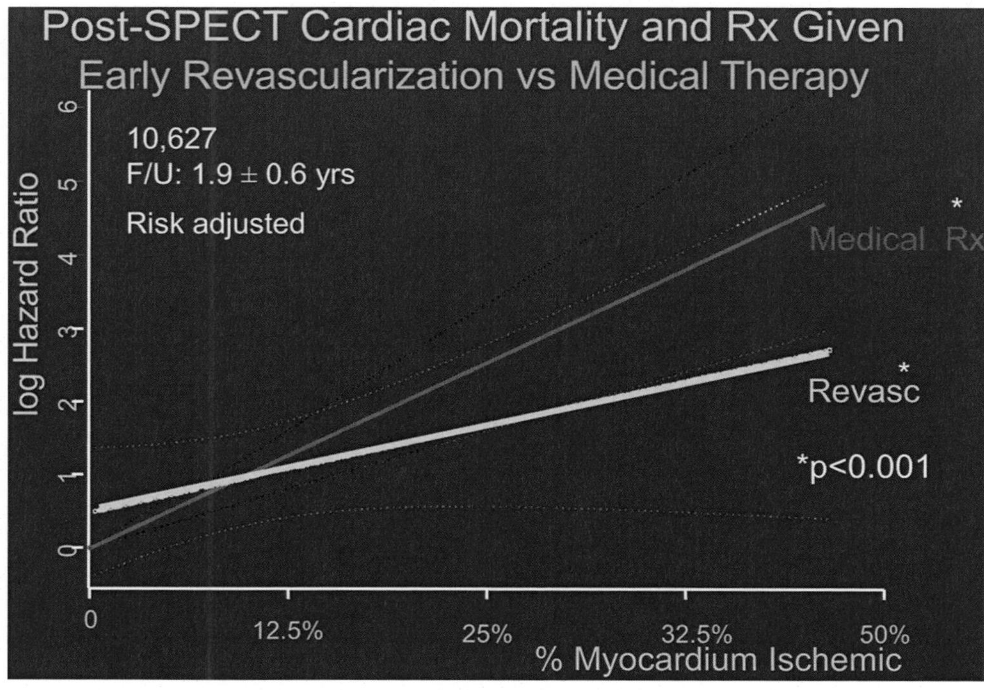

Fig. 20.24 Relationship between %myocardium ischemic and log of the hazard ratio in 10,647 patients treated either with medical therapy (*dashed line*) or early revascularization (<60 days post-SPECT MPS; *solid line*) based on multivariable modeling. In the setting of little or no ischemia, medical therapy is associated with superior survival; with increasing amounts of ischemia a progressive survival benefit with revascularization over medical therapy is present. 95 % confidence intervals are shown by the closely *dotted lines* (*Indicates p <0.001.) (Adapted from Hachamovitch et al. [101] with permission from Wolters Kluwer Health, Inc)

revascularization than with medical therapy. The “cross-over point” at which myocardial ischemia tipped the balance towards myocardial revascularization appeared to be more than 10 % ischemic myocardium. Thus, this study provided insight into a potential linkage between cardiac imaging results, patient treatment, and patient clinical outcomes. This linkage was further examined in higher-risk patient subsets including those with prior revascularization or small prior MI [102], elderly [103], and high risk diabetic patients by a recent study [104]. In long-term follow-up of 5200 elderly patients (≥75 years old) undergoing MPI, over 25 % of whom had prior MI, the threshold for benefit from revascularization appeared 15 % myocardium ischemic [103]. In another long-term follow-up study of 13,969 patients from the same registry, those with moderately to severely extensive ischemia appeared to benefit from revascularization even in the presence of known CAD or prior revascularization, providing they did not have extensive prior MI (>10 % fixed defect by MPI) [102]. The threshold for this apparent benefit was between 10 and 15 % myocardium ischemic (Fig. 20.25).

A small but provocative study has suggested that addition of quantitative myocardial blood flow reserve measurements may be associated with cardiac events independently and may modify prediction of benefit from early revascularization. In a study of 329 patients referred for invasive coronary angiography after PET scanning with CFR measurements, Taqueti et al. evaluated the relationship between CFR and observed benefit from revascularization. Patients were studied for the interaction between CFR findings and whether or not the patients were revascularized with respect to cardiovascular death or heart failure over a follow up of 3.1 years. Overall, only patients with reduced CFR had a significant improvement with revascularization. Further, a significant interaction between CFR and early CABG was noted, but not with PCI, such that patients with reduced CFR who underwent CABG had much greater freedom from event rate than patients those with low CFR who underwent PCI (Fig. 20.26) [105]. Gould et al. have recently expanded on the concepts suggested by the results of this small study [106], noting the importance of diffuse CAD in increasing the risk of myocardial infarction and decreasing the likelihood that stent placement across individual lesions will prevent MI. They further note that diffuse CAD can be assessed with CFR measurements by PET but are not assessed by FFR and conclude that consideration of CFR might improve selection of patients for revascularization.

While registry data suggests a benefit of revascularization in patients with moderate to severe ischemia, this benefit has not yet been validated in a randomized controlled trial. Whether an ischemia guided approach in SIHD improves outcomes is currently being evaluated in the ISCHEMIA trial (the International Study of Comparative Health Effectiveness with Medical and Invasive Approaches). This study is randomizing patients with moderate-to-severe ischemia based on the 10 % ischemia criterion suggested from the Cedars-Sinai data—as the entry criterion. Patients with left main CAD—assessed by blinded CCTA—are excluded. The remaining patients are being randomized to an invasive approach of catheterization with intent for ischemia guided revascularization + optimal medical therapy (OMT) vs a no catheterization approach with OMT alone.

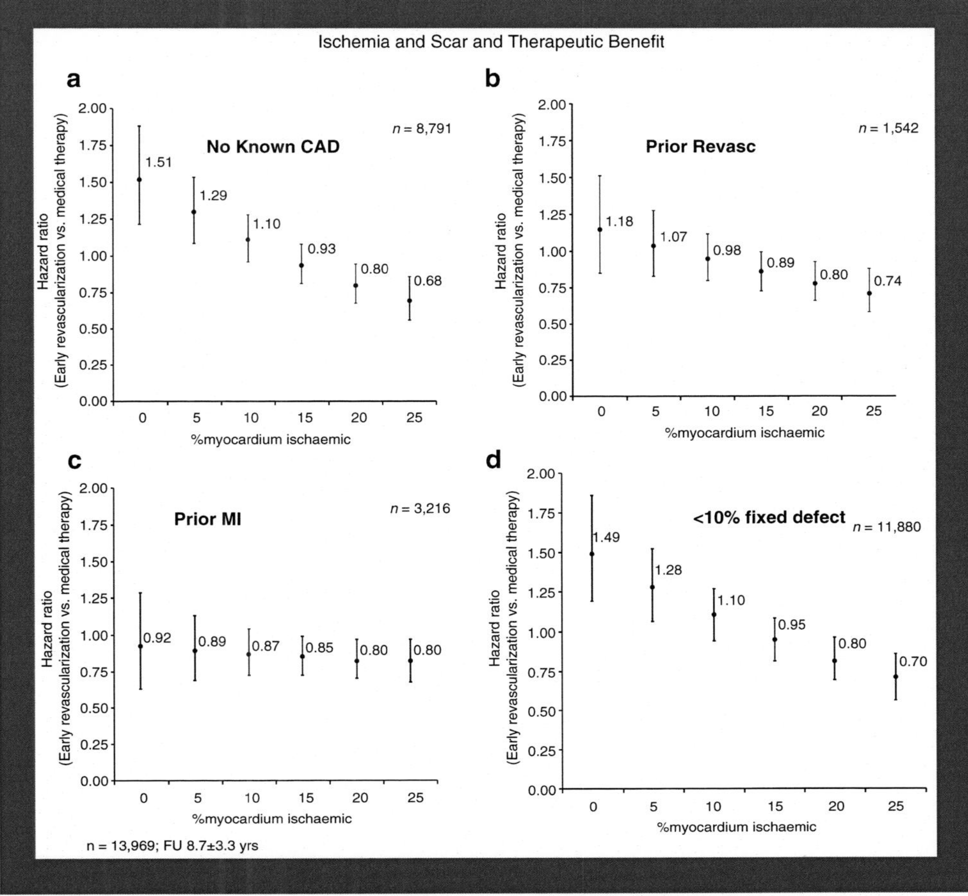

Fig. 20.25 Hazard ratio associated with early revascularization compared with medical therapy at specific values of %myocardium ischemic. (**a**) patients with no prior coronary artery disease, (**b**) patients with prior revascularization but no prior myocardial infarction, (**c**) patients with prior MI, and (**d**) patients with <10 % fixed defect. *P*-values as per Cox proportional hazards model (Adapted from Hachamovitch et al. [102] with permission from Oxford University Press)

Value of Ischemia Testing in the Patient with a High Likelihood of or Known CAD

A reasonable hypothesis is that the value of ischemia testing will depend on the pre-test risk (Fig. 20.27). If the ischemia guided management approach is confirmed in randomized clinical trials, there will be an opportunity for the value of ischemia testing to be shown; however, this value would likely be strongly dependent on the pre-test risk. If the pre-test risk is sufficiently high, ischemia testing might lead to improved outcomes by appropriately guided revascularization. Costs might be decreased compared to an approach without ischemia testing—such as that of using coronary CTA to guide the decision for proceeding to catheterization in this high risk group—since the use of CCTA alone might be associated with an excessive number of catheterizations and revascularizations as discussed above. As noted above, the use of CT perfusion of FFR_{CT} measurement in conjunction with CCTA might provide a means by which CCTA as the initial test could be of value in this patient group.

If used in a population of low risk, however, the ischemia testing is likely not to be of value. In this regard, there is an indication that the risk of patients currently undergoing testing may be too low for the testing to be of value. In a study of 39,515 patients referred for SPECT-MPI to the Cedars-Sinai laboratories, Rozanski et al. have shown that there has been a dramatic reduction in the frequency of abnormal test results over time [107]. Whereas in 1991 approximately 40 % of patients referred for testing had ischemia by SPECT-MPI, by 2009 this rate was less than 10 % (Fig. 20.28). Similar findings have now been reported from other centers.

What could be the explanation of the very low observed prevalence of abnormal SPECT-MPI studies? One answer is that the widely used Diamond-Forrester criteria for determining pre-test likelihood of angiographically significant CAD may not be applicable in the types of patients currently being referred for noninvasive testing. Data from the CONFIRM registry are enlightening in this regard. Cheng et al. reported that the Diamond-Forrester criteria markedly overestimated pretest likelihood of CAD [108]. In 8106 patients in with nonanginal chest pain, atypical angina, or typical angina, the Diamond-Forrester pre-test likelihood of angiographically significant CAD was 51 %. However, the observed frequency of ≥50 % stenosis was 18 %. Based on the pooled data from CCTA studies, approximately 90 % of patients with CCTA stenosis have ICA stenosis. Based on the report by Tonino et al. from the FAME trial, only 57 % of lesions judged visually to have ≥50 % stenosis have ischemia by FFR [109]. Further, it a meta-analysis by Zhou et al.,

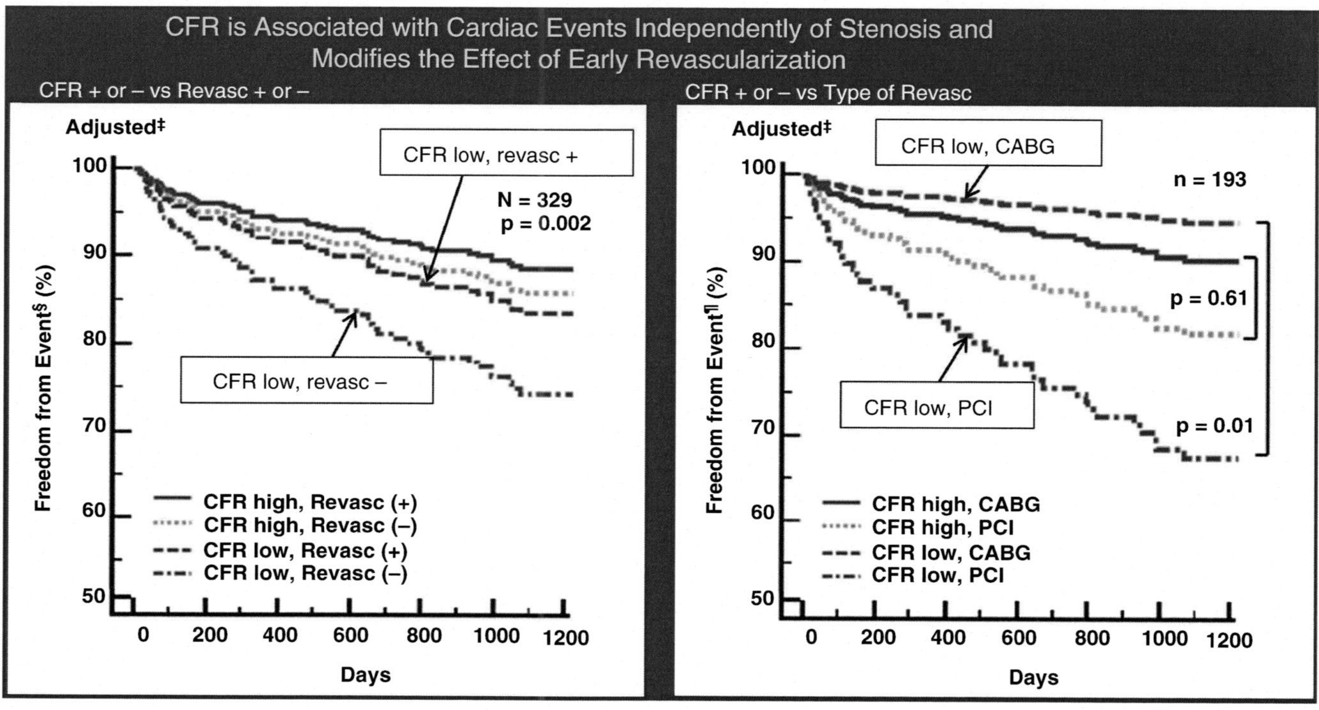

Fig. 20.26 Freedom from events according to coronary flow reserve (*CFR*) and early revascularization (*Revasc*) (*left*) and type of revascularization (revasc) right. Freedom from cardiovascular death or heart failure admission differed significantly among subgroups stratified by CFR and revascularization (*left*) (overall log-rank $P=0.03$; adjusted $P=0.002$) Patients with high CFR, independently of revascularization, experienced lower rates of events, whereas those with low CFR who did not undergo revascularization experienced the highest rate of events. In the subgroup of patients who underwent revascularization (*right*), there was no difference in event-free survival among those with high CFR (log-rank $P=0.76$; adjusted $P=0.61$), but in those with low CFR, only those who also underwent coronary artery bypass grafting (CABG), vs percutaneous coronary intervention (*PCI*), experienced lower rates of events (log-rank $P=0.02$; adjusted $P=0.01$) (Adapted from Taqueti et al. [105] with permission from Wolters Kluwer Health, Inc)

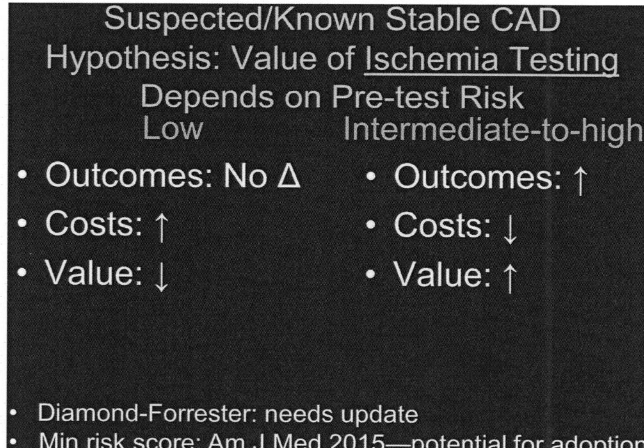

Fig. 20.27 Hypothesized value of using SPECT- or PET-MPI (ischemia testing) in symptomatic patients with suspected stable ischemic heart disease (SIHD)

it has been shown that only 77 % of patients with ischemia by FFR have ischemia by SPECT-MPI [110]. Multiplying these rates together, the result is that if the patients sent for testing have an intermediate pre-test likelihood of CAD by Diamond-Forrester criteria, it would be expected that 8.6 % would have ischemia by SPECT—very similar to what was reported by Rozanski et al. [107]. The results of the PROMISE trial confirm these calculations. While the pretest likelihood of CAD using the Diamond-Forrester criteria was 53.3 %, only 11.7 % had stenosis by CCTA and only 10.7 % had abnormal functional studies [83].

An updated approach to assessment of the pretest likelihood of CAD as well as of risk—the "CONFIRM Risk Score" in patients referred to noninvasive testing has recently been described based on an analysis of the CONFIRM data [111] with validation in the Cedars-Sinai nuclear cardiology database. The simple to implement score is illustrated in Fig. 20.29. An intuitive number is assigned for age (e.g., 4 for 40–49 years, 7 for >70 years), and 1 or 0 are assigned based on sex, angina, diabetes, hypertension, family history of premature CAD, and smoking. With a simple table the number converts to a risk of death or MI or a pre-test likelihood of CAD. The CONFIRM risk score was better calibrated than the Framingham Risk Score or the Diamond-Forrester pre-test likelihood calculations. Use of the CONFIRM risk score could lead to a more effective decision as to whether to use an imaging test in a given patient and which test to choose, and, ultimately, to a greater opportunity of noninvasive testing to demonstrate value.

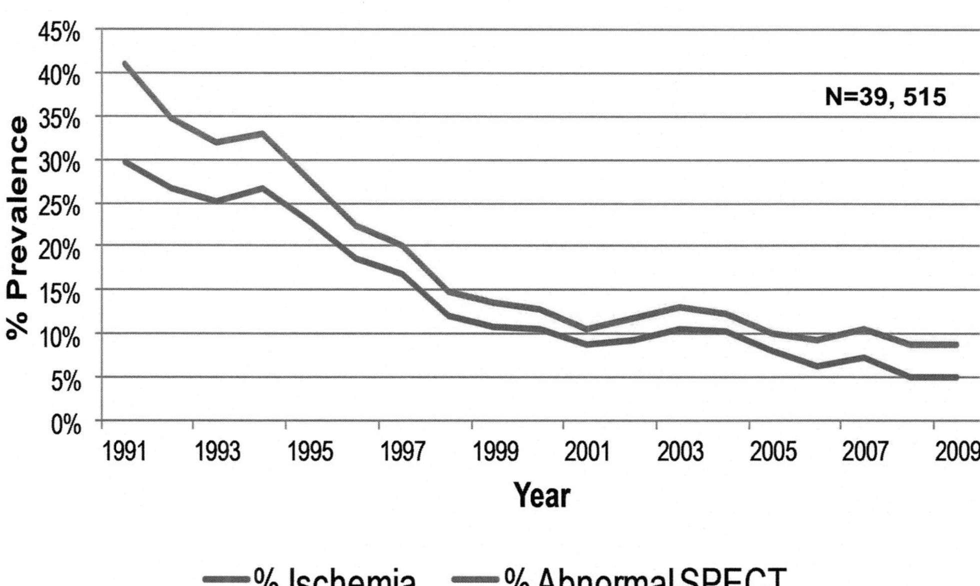

Fig. 20.28 Year by year prevalence of abnormal and ischemic SPECT-MPI studies between 1991 and 2009 among 39,515 diagnostic patients tested at Cedars-Sinai Medical Center (Adapted from Rozanskiet al. [107] with permission from Elsevier)

Assessment of Patients with Heart Failure and Known or Suspected CAD

At the end of the spectrum of patients with CAD who are referred for testing are the patients with heart failure. In this population, CCTA has a limited role—predominantly being to rule out ischemic cardiomyopathy in patients presenting with heart failure of unknown cause and in whom the likelihood if CAD is considered to be relatively low [112]. In the patient with an ischemic cardiomyopathy, myocardial viability imaging (PET or CMR) would be more likely than CCTA to be of value in guiding the decision for revascularization or transplantation.

Value of Imaging Depends on the Effect of Imaging on Patient Management

The fundamental value equation is quality divided by cost. Test quality ultimately rests in beneficial patient outcomes. Costs relate not only to the cost of testing but also to all of the costs resulting from the test. In consideration of the value of noninvasive imaging, there can be no value if the test does not improve the relationship between outcomes and costs, and this is dependent on the manner in which test results change patient management. The test itself has no effect. Unfortunately, there is evidence that often this last link-the link between the test and treatment change-is not as strong as it needs to be.

The SPARC (Study of Myocardial Perfusion and Coronary Anatomy Imaging Roles in Coronary Artery Disease) addressed these issues by evaluating 90-day post-test rates of catheterization and medication changes in a prospective registry of 1703 patients without a documented history of coronary artery disease and an intermediate to high likelihood of CAD undergoing cardiac SPECT- or PET-MPI or CCTA [113]. These results were classified as normal (or nonobstructive for CCTA), mildly abnormal, and moderately or severely abnormal. Baseline medication use was relatively infrequent. At 90 days, 9.6 % of patients underwent catheterization. While the rates of catheterization and medication changes increased in proportion to test abnormality findings, among patients with the most severe test result findings, 38–61 % were not referred to catheterization, 20–30 % were not receiving aspirin, and 20–25 % were not receiving a lipid-lowering agent at 90 days after the index test. Risk-adjusted analyses revealed that changes in use of aspirin and lipid lowering agent were greater after CCTA. The authors concluded that overall, noninvasive testing had only a modest impact on clinical management of patients referred for clinical testing. Although post-imaging use of cardiac catheterization and medical therapy increased in proportion to the degree of abnormality findings, the frequency of catheterization and medication change suggests possible under-treatment of higher risk patients. Even in the severely abnormal group, only 27 % had no catheterization or medication change.

As noted above, in the Scot-Heart trial, changes in treatment after CCTA testing compared to the non-imaging arm were clear, with 18 vs 4 % of patients being placed on preventive therapy in the CCTA and control arms, respectively. As noted, there was also a trend toward improved hard outcomes in the CCTA arm of the study. The effects of the CCTA vs functional testing in the PROMISE trial regarding changes in therapy have not yet been reported. The results of the FACTOR-64 study provide promising results regarding the

CONFIRM Risk Score

Prospective CONFIRM registry
N=14,004
Endpoint: 3 year death/MI

Risk Factor	Category	Points
Age	18-39	
	40-49	
	50-59	
	60-69	6
	>70	
Sex	Male	1
	Female	
Typical Angina	Yes	
	No	0
Diabetes	Yes	
	No	0
Hypertension	Yes	1
	No	
Family History	Yes	
	No	0
Smoking	Yes	1
	No	

Points	Risk of Death or MI (%)*	Likelihood of CAD
3	0.25	0
4	0.46	1.4
5	0.76	3.4
6	1.26	5.5
7	2.53	13.2
8	4.53	21.3
9	8.03	31.0
10	15.13	43.2
11	23.29	52.5
12	34.95	82.4
13	53.81	

Fig. 20.29 Table illustrating the CONFIRM risk score. Illustrated is scoring for a 65 year old male with a history of hypertension and smoking. The CONFIRM risk score (*) is 9, which would predict an 8.02 risk of death or MI and a 31 % likelihood of CAD (≥ 50% stenosis) (Reprinted from Min et al. [111] with permission from Elsevier)

influence of test results on patient therapy and possibly on hard outcomes; however, it should be noted, that changes in therapy in this study based on test results were part of the study design. The principal manner in which SPECT-MPI or PET-MPI studies alter patient management is principally in guiding decisions to consider revascularization. Regarding institution of preventive management measures after testing, the combined use of CAC with SPECT- or PET-MPI could allow similar effects as observed with CCTA with the use of MPI. Whether the ability of PET-MPI to assess myocardial blood flow reserve, with its prognostic implications, and potential added information regarding benefit from revascularization, will affect changes in patient management has yet to be examined.

The ability of a test to affect outcomes is dependent on and degree to which the test to the manner in which test results change therapy. The steps involved in this potential of testing to affect outcomes are well exemplified by the PARR-2 study (Fig. 20.30), which involved FDG PET scanning [114]. In this study, 430 patients in 9 centers with heart failure, known or suspected CAD and LVEF ≤35 % were randomized to a management plan assisted by FDG PET (n=218) or standard care (n=212), with specific recommendations regarding the use of FDG PET information for revascularization decisions. The outcome was a composite of cardiac death, myocardial infarction, and recurrent hospital stay for cardiac cause within 1 year. In the overall trial, there was no significant difference in the hazard ratio for the composite outcome in the PET vs SOC arm (p=0.15). For patients in whom the PET recommendations were followed, the hazard ratio was significant (p=0.019), illustrating that a test results can have a beneficial effect on outcome only if the test appropriately changes therapy. The further reliance of the outcome benefit of testing was subsequently illustrated in this study when expertise in performance and clinical use of the testing is present. A post-hoc analysis was performed comparing a subgroup of patients studied in five hospitals

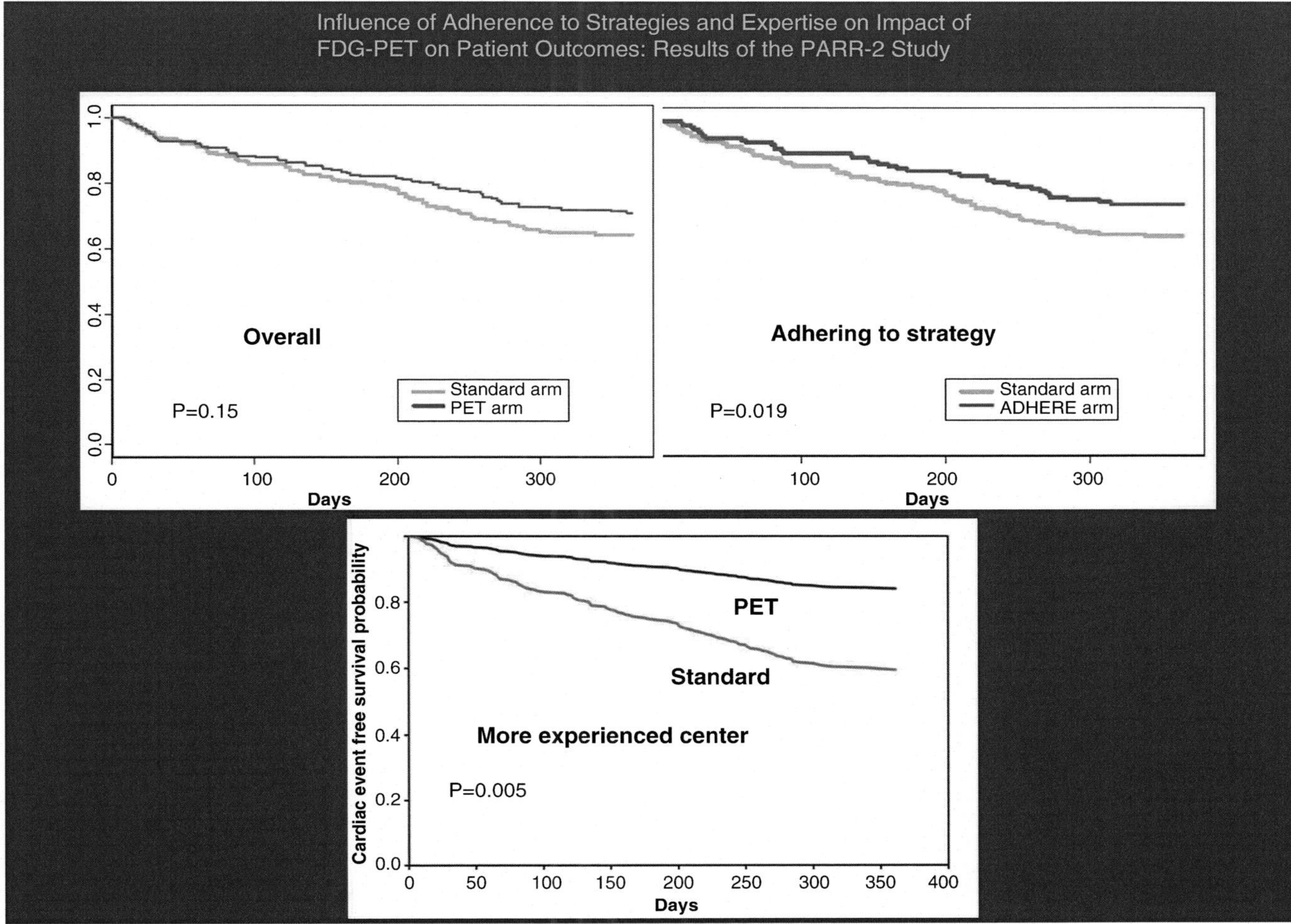

Fig. 20.30 Influence of adherence to strategies and expertise on impact of FDG-PET on patient outcomes as shown in two publications from the PARR-2 Trial. The *top two illustrations* illustrate composite outcome of cardiac death, myocardial infarction, recurrent hospital stay for cardiac cause within 1 year. *Green* PET arm, *Orange* Standard arm. In the overall trial (*left*), no survival benefit was shown. In the subset in whom the planned therapeutic strategy of the trial based on PET viability results was followed (*right*), a significant survival benefit in the PET arm was seen. When patients who were tested in a center with greater experience with FDG-PET were assessed (*lower* illustration), an even greater survival benefit in the PET arm was shown (*Top two panels*: (Adapted from Beanlands et al. [114] with permission from Elsevier))

with greater experience in and access to the use of the PET assisted strategy in the PARR-2 trial [115]. There was a significant reduction in cardiac events in the patient population studied at the five sites with expertise (p = 0.005) that had not been seen in the overall trial.

Conclusion

Technology cardiac CT and nuclear cardiology is constantly improving, such that the information provided be each form of testing is expanded, potentially decreasing the need for layered testing. The value of cardiac imaging depends on impact on outcomes and all costs related to performance of a test. In clinical applications, the potential value of the modalities is related to the setting in which they are employed. For prevention, data is strong in that CAC scanning can provide value by improving outcomes. In the patient with acute chest pain, CCTA appears to be able to shorten time in the hospital and reduce costs. In patients with suspected SIHD and an intermediate pre-test likelihood of CAD, the use of CCTA appears to be valuable. In patients who have known CAD or in whom a non-diagnostic CCTA is likely, improvement in outcomes is less likely and testing for ischemia may be preferred. In patients with a very high likelihood of CAD or known CAD, registry data suggests that ischemia testing, such as that provided by SPECT- or PET-MPI studies, may improve outcomes by improving selection of patients for revascularization. The ISCHEMIA trial will test whether a strategy basing decisions for revascularization on noninvasive assessment of ischemia is improves outcomes. In patients with heart failure, the use of CCTA is primarily to rule out ischemic cardiomyopathy. As with any form of testing, assessing the pre-test likelihood of disease is of paramount importance in determining the need for a test which could be of value. Recent data show that the pretest likelihood of

CAD and pretest risk is markedly overestimated by traditional approaches, most likely explaining a marked increase in frequency of normal stress SPECT-MPI studies. Updated methods for assessment of pre-test risk may lead to improved utilization of cardiac imaging procedures. In selected heart failure patients, of myocardial viability using PET or MRI may prove to provide value. In all of the applications of noninvasive imaging, value can only be achieved if the appropriate patients are selected for testing and if the test result changes therapy, such that cost savings or improved outcomes can follow the testing strategy.

Acknowledgement Supported in part by the Adelson Family Foundation and the Diane and Guilford Glazer Foundation

References

1. Mahmarian JJ, Cerqueira MD, Iskandrian AE, Bateman TM, Thomas GS, Hendel RC, Moye LA, Olmsted AW. Regadenoson induces comparable left ventricular perfusion defects as adenosine: a quantitative analysis from the advance MPI 2 trial. JACC Cardiovasc Imaging. 2009;2:959–68.
2. Xu Y, Hayes S, Ali I, Ruddy TD, Wells RG, Berman DS, Germano G, Slomka PJ. Automatic and visual reproducibility of perfusion and function measures for myocardial perfusion SPECT. J Nucl Cardiol. 2010;17:1050–7.
3. Berman DS, Kang X, Gransar H, Gerlach J, Friedman JD, Hayes SW, Thomson LE, Hachamovitch R, Shaw LJ, Slomka PJ, Yang LD, Germano G. Quantitative assessment of myocardial perfusion abnormality on SPECT myocardial perfusion imaging is more reproducible than expert visual analysis. J Nucl Cardiol. 2009;16:45–53.
4. Arsanjani R, Xu Y, Dey D, Vahistha V, Shalev A, Nakanishi R, Hayes S, Fish M, Berman D, Germano G, Slomka PJ. Improved accuracy of myocardial perfusion SPECT for detection of coronary artery disease by machine learning in a large population. J Nucl Cardiol. 2013;20:553–62.
5. Slomka PJ, Pan T, Berman DS, Germano G. Advances in SPECT and pet hardware. Prog Cardiovasc Dis. 2015;57:566–78.
6. Sharir T, Slomka PJ, Hayes SW, DiCarli MF, Ziffer JA, Martin WH, Dickman D, Ben-Haim S, Berman DS. Multicenter trial of high-speed versus conventional single-photon emission computed tomography imaging: quantitative results of myocardial perfusion and left ventricular function. J Am Coll Cardiol. 2010;55: 1965–74.
7. Nakazato R, Berman DS, Hayes SW, Fish M, Padgett R, Xu Y, Lemley M, Baavour R, Roth N, Slomka PJ. Myocardial perfusion imaging with a solid-state camera: simulation of a very low dose imaging protocol. J Nucl Med. 2013;54:373–9.
8. Einstein AJ, Blankstein R, Andrews H, Fish M, Padgett R, Hayes SW, Friedman JD, Qureshi M, Rakotoarivelo H, Slomka P, Nakazato R, Bokhari S, Di Carli M, Berman DS. Comparison of image quality, myocardial perfusion, and left ventricular function between standard imaging and single-injection ultra-low-dose imaging using a high-efficiency spect camera: the Millisievert study. J Nucl Med. 2014;55:1430–7.
9. Nakazato R, Slomka PJ, Fish M, Schwartz RG, Hayes SW, Thomson LE, Friedman JD, Lemley Jr M, Mackin ML, Peterson B, Schwartz AM, Doran JA, Germano G, Berman DS. Quantitative high-efficiency cadmium-zinc-telluride SPECT with dedicated parallel-hole collimation system in obese patients: results of a multi-center study. J Nucl Cardiol. 2015;22:266–75.
10. Slomka PJ, Dey D, Duvall WL, Henzlova MJ, Berman DS, Germano G. Advances in nuclear cardiac instrumentation with a view towards reduced radiation exposure. Curr Cardiol Rep. 2012;14:208–16.
11. Dey D, Slomka PJ, Berman DS. Achieving very-low-dose radiation exposure in cardiac computed tomography, single-photon emission computed tomography, and positron emission tomography. Circ Cardiovasc Imaging. 2014;7:723–34.
12. Arsanjani R, Hayes SW, Fish M, Shalev A, Nakanishi R, Thomson LE, Friedman JD, Germano G, Berman DS, Slomka P. Two-position supine/prone myocardial perfusion SPECT imaging improves visual inter-observer correlation and agreement. J Nucl Cardiol. 2014;21:703–11.
13. Slomka PJ, Nishina H, Abidov A, Hayes SW, Friedman JD, Berman DS, Germano G. Combined quantitative supine-prone myocardial perfusion SPECT improves detection of coronary artery disease and normalcy rates in women. J Nucl Cardiol. 2007;14:44–52.
14. Chang SM, Nabi F, Xu J, Raza U, Mahmarian JJ. Normal stress-only versus standard stress/rest myocardial perfusion imaging: similar patient mortality with reduced radiation exposure. J Am Coll Cardiol. 2010;55:221–30.
15. Duvall WL, Wijetunga MN, Klein TM, Razzouk L, Godbold J, Croft LB, Henzlova MJ. The prognosis of a normal stress-only Tc-99m myocardial perfusion imaging study. J Nucl Cardiol. 2010;17:370–7.
16. Dekemp RA, Declerck J, Klein R, Pan XB, Nakazato R, Tonge C, Arumugam P, Berman DS, Germano G, Beanlands RS, Slomka PJ. Multisoftware reproducibility study of stress and rest myocardial blood flow assessed with 3d dynamic PET/CT and a 1-tissue-compartment model of 82-Rb kinetics. J Nucl Med. 2013;54: 571–7.
17. Slomka PJ, Alexanderson E, Jacome R, Jimenez M, Romero E, Meave A, Le Meunier L, Dalhbom M, Berman DS, Germano G, Schelbert H. Comparison of clinical tools for measurements of regional stress and rest myocardial blood flow assessed with 13N-ammonia PET/CT. J Nucl Med. 2012;53:171–81.
18. Murthy VL, Naya M, Foster CR, Hainer J, Gaber M, Di Carli G, Blankstein R, Dorbala S, Sitek A, Pencina MJ, Di Carli MF. Improved cardiac risk assessment with noninvasive measures of coronary flow reserve. Circulation. 2011;124:2215–24.
19. Ziadi MC, Dekemp RA, Williams KA, Guo A, Chow BJ, Renaud JM, Ruddy TD, Sarveswaran N, Tee RE, Beanlands RS. Impaired myocardial flow reserve on rubidium-82 positron emission tomography imaging predicts adverse outcomes in patients assessed for myocardial ischemia. J Am Coll Cardiol. 2011;58:740–8.
20. Gould KL, Johnson NP. Physiologic stenosis severity, binary thinking, revascularization, and "hidden reality". Circ Cardiov Imag. 2015;8:e002970.
21. Gould KL, Johnson NP, Bateman TM, Beanlands RS, Bengel FM, Bober R, Camici PG, Cerqueira MD, Chow BJ, Di Carli MF, Dorbala S, Gewirtz H, Gropler RJ, Kaufmann PA, Knaapen P, Knuuti J, Merhige ME, Rentrop KP, Ruddy TD, Schelbert HR, Schindler TH, Schwaiger M, Sdringola S, Vitarello J, Williams Sr KA, Gordon D, Dilsizian V, Narula J. Anatomic versus physiologic assessment of coronary artery disease. Role of coronary flow reserve, fractional flow reserve, and positron emission tomography imaging in revascularization decision-making. J Am Coll Cardiol. 2013;62:1639–53.
22. Yu M, Guaraldi MT, Mistry M, Kagan M, McDonald JL, Drew K, Radeke H, Azure M, Purohit A, Casebier DS, Robinson SP. Bms-747158-02: a novel PET myocardial perfusion imaging agent. J Nucl Cardiol. 2007;14:789–98.
23. Maddahi J. Properties of an ideal PET perfusion tracer: new PET tracer cases and data. J Nucl Cardiol. 2012;19 Suppl 1:S30–7.
24. Berman DS, Maddahi J, Tamarappoo BK, Czernin J, Taillefer R, Udelson JE, Gibson CM, Devine M, Lazewatsky J, Bhat G, Washburn D. Phase II safety and clinical comparison with single-photon emission computed tomography myocardial perfusion

imaging for detection of coronary artery disease: Flurpiridaz f 18 positron emission tomography. J Am Coll Cardiol. 2013;61:469–77.
25. Berman DS, Wong ND, Gransar H, Miranda-Peats R, Dahlbeck J, Hayes SW, Friedman JD, Kang X, Polk D, Hachamovitch R, Shaw L, Rozanski A. Relationship between stress-induced myocardial ischemia and atherosclerosis measured by coronary calcium tomography. J Am Coll Cardiol. 2004;44:923–30.
26. Berman DS, Hachamovitch R, Shaw LJ, Friedman JD, Hayes SW, Thomson L, Fieno DS, Germano G, Slomka P, Wong ND, Kang X, Rozanski A. Roles of nuclear cardiology, cardiac computed tomography, and cardiac magnetic resonance: assessment of patients with suspected coronary artery disease. J Nucl Med. 2006;47:74–82.
27. Schenker MP, Dorbala S, Hong EC, Rybicki FJ, Hachamovitch R, Kwong RY, Di Carli MF. Interrelation of coronary calcification, myocardial ischemia, and outcomes in patients with intermediate likelihood of coronary artery disease: a combined positron emission tomography/computed tomography study. Circulation. 2008;117:1693–700.
28. Berman DS. Fourth annual Mario s. Verani, md memorial lecture: noninvasive imaging in coronary artery disease: changing roles, changing players. J Nucl Cardiol. 2006;13:457–73.
29. Rudd JH, Warburton EA, Fryer TD, Jones HA, Clark JC, Antoun N, Johnstrom P, Davenport AP, Kirkpatrick PJ, Arch BN, Pickard JD, Weissberg PL. Imaging atherosclerotic plaque inflammation with [18f]-fluorodeoxyglucose positron emission tomography. Circulation. 2002;105:2708–11.
30. Rudd JH, Myers KS, Bansilal S, Machac J, Rafique A, Farkouh M, Fuster V, Fayad ZA. 18-fluorodeoxyglucose positron emission tomography imaging of atherosclerotic plaque inflammation is highly reproducible: implications for atherosclerosis therapy trials. J Am Coll Cardiol. 2007;50:892–6.
31. Tawakol A, Fayad ZA, Mogg R, Alon A, Klimas MT, Dansky H, Subramanian SS, Abdelbaky A, Rudd JH, Farkouh ME, Nunes IO, Beals CR, Shankar SS. Intensification of statin therapy results in a rapid reduction in atherosclerotic inflammation: results of a multicenter fluorodeoxyglucose-positron emission tomography/computed tomography feasibility study. J Am Coll Cardiol. 2013;62:909–17.
32. Burke AP, Farb A, Malcom GT, Liang Y, Smialek JE, Virmani R. Plaque rupture and sudden death related to exertion in men with coronary artery disease. JAMA. 1999;281:921–6.
33. Moreno PR, Narula J. Thinking outside the lumen: fractional flow reserve versus intravascular imaging for major adverse cardiac event prediction. J Am Coll Cardiol. 2014;63:1141–4.
34. Dweck MR, Chow MW, Joshi NV, Williams MC, Jones C, Fletcher AM, Richardson H, White A, McKillop G, van Beek EJ, Boon NA, Rudd JH, Newby DE. Coronary arterial 18F-sodium fluoride uptake: a novel marker of plaque biology. J Am Coll Cardiol. 2012;59:1539–48.
35. Joshi NV, Vesey AT, Williams MC, Shah AS, Calvert PA, Craighead FH, Yeoh SE, Wallace W, Salter D, Fletcher AM, van Beek EJ, Flapan AD, Uren NG, Behan MW, Cruden NL, Mills NL, Fox KA, Rudd JH, Dweck MR, Newby DE. 18F-fluoride positron emission tomography for identification of ruptured and high-risk coronary atherosclerotic plaques: a prospective clinical trial. Lancet. 2014;383:705–13.
36. Motoyama S, Kondo T, Sarai M, Sugiura A, Harigaya H, Sato T, Inoue K, Okumura M, Ishii J, Anno H, Virmani R, Ozaki Y, Hishida H, Narula J. Multislice computed tomographic characteristics of coronary lesions in acute coronary syndromes. J Am Coll Cardiol. 2007;50:319–26.
37. Motoyama S, Sarai M, Harigaya H, Anno H, Inoue K, Hara T, Naruse H, Ishii J, Hishida H, Wong ND, Virmani R, Kondo T, Ozaki Y, Narula J. Computed tomographic angiography characteristics of atherosclerotic plaques subsequently resulting in acute coronary syndrome. J Am Coll Cardiol. 2009;54:49–57.
38. Shmilovich H, Cheng VY, Tamarappoo BK, Dey D, Nakazato R, Gransar H, Thomson LE, Hayes SW, Friedman JD, Germano G, Slomka PJ, Berman DS. Vulnerable plaque features on coronary CT angiography as markers of inducible regional myocardial hypoperfusion from severe coronary artery stenoses. Atherosclerosis. 2011;219:588–95.
39. Nakazato R, Shalev A, Doh JH, Koo BK, Gransar H, Gomez MJ, Leipsic J, Park HB, Berman DS, Min JK. Aggregate plaque volume by coronary computed tomography angiography is superior and incremental to luminal narrowing for diagnosis of ischemic lesions of intermediate stenosis severity. J Am Coll Cardiol. 2013;62:460–7.
40. Park HB, Heo R, o Hartaigh B, Cho I, Gransar H, Nakazato R, Leipsic J, Mancini GB, Koo BK, Otake H, Budoff MJ, Berman DS, Erglis A, Chang HJ, Min JK. Atherosclerotic plaque characteristics by CT angiography identify coronary lesions that cause ischemia: a direct comparison to fractional flow reserve. JACC Cardiovasc Imaging. 2015;8:1–10.
41. Dey D, Schepis T, Marwan M, Slomka PJ, Berman DS, Achenbach S. Automated three-dimensional quantification of noncalcified coronary plaque from coronary CT angiography: comparison with intravascular us. Radiology. 2010;257:516–22.
42. Diaz-Zamudio M, Dey D, Schuhbaeck A, Nakazato R, Gransar H, Slomka PJ, Narula J, Berman DS, Achenbach S, Min JK, Doh JH, Koo BK. Automated quantitative plaque burden from coronary CT angiography noninvasively predicts hemodynamic significance by using fractional flow reserve in intermediate coronary lesions. Radiology. 2015;276(2):408–15.
43. Rochitte CE, George RT, Chen MY, Arbab-Zadeh A, Dewey M, Miller JM, Niinuma H, Yoshioka K, Kitagawa K, Nakamori S, Laham R, Vavere AL, Cerci RJ, Mehra VC, Nomura C, Kofoed KF, Jinzaki M, Kuribayashi S, de Roos A, Laule M, Tan SY, Hoe J, Paul N, Rybicki FJ, Brinker JA, Arai AE, Cox C, Clouse ME, Di Carli MF, Lima JA. Computed tomography angiography and perfusion to assess coronary artery stenosis causing perfusion defects by single photon emission computed tomography: the core320 study. Eur Heart J. 2014;35:1120–30.
44. Cury RC, Kitt TM, Feaheny K, Blankstein R, Ghoshhajra BB, Budoff MJ, Leipsic J, Min JK, Akin J, George RT. A randomized, multicenter, multivendor study of myocardial perfusion imaging with regadenoson CT perfusion vs single photon emission CT. J Cardiovasc Comput Tomogr. 2015;9:103–12.e101–2.
45. Min JK, Leipsic J, Pencina MJ, Berman DS, Koo BK, van Mieghem C, Erglis A, Lin FY, Dunning AM, Apruzzese P, Budoff MJ, Cole JH, Jaffer FA, Leon MB, Malpeso J, Mancini GB, Park SJ, Schwartz RS, Shaw LJ, Mauri L. Diagnostic accuracy of fractional flow reserve from anatomic CT angiography. JAMA. 2012;308:1237–45.
46. Koo BK, Erglis A, Doh JH, Daniels DV, Jegere S, Kim HS, Dunning A, DeFrance T, Lansky A, Leipsic J, Min JK. Diagnosis of ischemia-causing coronary stenoses by noninvasive fractional flow reserve computed from coronary computed tomographic angiograms. Results from the prospective multicenter discover-flow (diagnosis of ischemia-causing stenoses obtained via noninvasive fractional flow reserve) study. J Am Coll Cardiol. 2011;58:1989–97.
47. Nørgaard BL, Leipsic J, Gaur S, Seneviratne S, Ko BS, Ito H, Jensen JM, Mauri L, De Bruyne B, Bezerra H, Osawa K, Marwan M, Naber C, Erglis A, Park SJ, Christiansen EH, Kaltoft A, Lassen JF, Bøtker HE, Achenbach S, NXT Trial Study Group. Diagnostic performance of non-invasive fractional flow reserve derived from coronary ct angiography in suspected coronary artery disease: the nxt trial. J Am Coll Cardiol. 2014;63(12):1145–55.
48. Stone NJ, Robinson JG, Lichtenstein AH, Bairey Merz CN, Blum CB, Eckel RH, Goldberg AC, Gordon D, Levy D, Lloyd-Jones DM, McBride P, Schwartz JS, Shero ST, Smith Jr SC, Watson K, Wilson PW. 2013 ACC/AHA guideline on the treatment of blood cholesterol to reduce atherosclerotic cardiovascular risk in adults:

a report of the American College of Cardiology/American Heart Assocication task force on practice guidelines. J Am Coll Cardiol. 2014;63:2889–934.

49. Kavousi M, Leening MJ, Nanchen D, Greenland P, Graham IM, Steyerberg EW, Ikram MA, Stricker BH, Hofman A, Franco OH. Comparison of application of the ACC/AHA guidelines, adult treatment panel iii guidelines, and European Society of Cardiology guidelines for cardiovascular disease prevention in a European cohort. JAMA. 2014;311:1416–23.
50. DeFilippis AP, Young R, Carrubba CJ, McEvoy JW, Budoff MJ, Blumenthal RS, Kronmal RA, McClelland RL, Nasir K, Blaha MJ. An analysis of calibration and discrimination among multiple cardiovascular risk scores in a modern multiethnic cohort. Ann Intern Med. 2015;162:266–75.
51. Detrano R, Guerci AD, Carr JJ, Bild DE, Burke G, Folsom AR, Liu K, Shea S, Szklo M, Bluemke DA, O'Leary DH, Tracy R, Watson K, Wong ND, Kronmal RA. Coronary calcium as a predictor of coronary events in four racial or ethnic groups. N Engl J Med. 2008;358:1336–45.
52. Erbel R, Möhlenkamp S, Moebus S, Schmermund A, Lehmann N, Stang A, Dragano N, Grönemeyer D, Seibel R, Kälsch H, Bröcker-Preuss M, Mann K, Siegrist J, Jöckel KH, Group HNRSI. Coronary risk stratification, discrimination, and reclassification improvement based on quantification of subclinical coronary atherosclerosis: the Heinz Nixdorf recall study. J Am Coll Cardiol. 2010;56:1397–406.
53. Yeboah J, McClelland RL, Polonsky TS, Burke GL, Sibley CT, O'Leary D, Carr JJ, Goff DC, Greenland P, Herrington DM. Comparison of novel risk markers for improvement in cardiovascular risk assessment in intermediate-risk individuals. JAMA. 2012;308:788–95.
54. Miedema MD, Duprez DA, Misialek JR, Blaha MJ, Nasir K, Silverman MG, Blankstein R, Budoff MJ, Greenland P, Folsom AR. Use of coronary artery calcium testing to guide aspirin utilization for primary prevention: estimates from the multi-ethnic study of atherosclerosis. Circ Cardiovasc Qual Outcomes. 2014;7:453–60.
55. Roberts ET, Horne A, Martin SS, Blaha MJ, Blankstein R, Budoff MJ, Sibley C, Polak JF, Frick KD, Blumenthal RS, Nasir K. Cost-effectiveness of coronary artery calcium testing for coronary heart and cardiovascular disease risk prediction to guide statin allocation: the multi-ethnic study of atherosclerosis (mesa). PLoS One. 2015;10:e0116377.
56. Rozanski A, Gransar H, Shaw LJ, Kim J, Miranda-Peats L, Wong ND, Rana JS, Orakzai R, Hayes SW, Friedman JD, Thomson LE, Polk D, Min J, Budoff MJ, Berman DS. Impact of coronary artery calcium scanning on coronary risk factors and downstream testing the eisner (early identification of subclinical atherosclerosis by noninvasive imaging research) prospective randomized trial. J Am Coll Cardiol. 2011;57:1622–32.
57. Nasir K, McClelland RL, Blumenthal RS, Goff Jr DC, Hoffmann U, Psaty BM, Greenland P, Kronmal RA, Budoff MJ. Coronary artery calcium in relation to initiation and continuation of cardiovascular preventive medications: the multi-ethnic study of atherosclerosis (mesa). Circ Cardiovasc Qual Outcomes. 2010;3:228–35.
58. Orakzai RH, Nasir K, Orakzai SH, Kalia N, Gopal A, Musunuru K, Blumenthal RS, Budoff MJ. Effect of patient visualization of coronary calcium by electron beam computed tomography on changes in beneficial lifestyle behaviors. Am J Cardiol. 2008;101:999–1002.
59. Taylor AJ, Bindeman J, Feuerstein I, Le T, Bauer K, Byrd C, Wu H, O'Malley PG. Community-based provision of statin and aspirin after the detection of coronary artery calcium within a community-based screening cohort. J Am Coll Cardiol. 2008;51:1337–41.
60. Ahmed HM, Blaha MJ, Nasir K, Jones SR, Rivera JJ, Agatston A, Blankstein R, Wong ND, Lakoski S, Budoff MJ, Burke GL, Sibley CT, Ouyang P, Blumenthal RS. Low-risk lifestyle, coronary calcium, cardiovascular events, and mortality: results from mesa. Am J Epidemiol. 2013;178:12–21.
61. Malik S, Budoff MJ, Katz R, Blumenthal RS, Bertoni AG, Nasir K, Szklo M, Barr RG, Wong ND. Impact of subclinical atherosclerosis on cardiovascular disease events in individuals with metabolic syndrome and diabetes: the multi-ethnic study of atherosclerosis. Diabetes Care. 2011;34:2285–90.
62. Wackers FJ, Young LH, Inzucchi SE, Chyun DA, Davey JA, Barrett EJ, Taillefer R, Wittlin SD, Heller GV, Filipchuk N, Engel S, Ratner RE, Iskandrian AE. Detection of silent myocardial ischemia in asymptomatic diabetic subjects: the diad study. Diabetes Care. 2004;27:1954–61.
63. Zellweger MJ, Maraun M, Osterhues HH, Keller U, Muller-Brand J, Jeger R, Pfister O, Burkard T, Eckstein F, von Felten S, Osswald S, Pfisterer M. Progression to overt or silent cad in asymptomatic patients with diabetes mellitus at high coronary risk: main findings of the prospective multicenter bardot trial with a pilot randomized treatment substudy. JACC Cardiovasc Imaging. 2014;7:1001–10.
64. Muhlestein JB, Lappe DL, Lima JA, Rosen BD, May HT, Knight S, Bluemke DA, Towner SR, Le V, Bair TL, Vavere AL, Anderson JL. Effect of screening for coronary artery disease using CT angiography on mortality and cardiac events in high-risk patients with diabetes: the factor-64 randomized clinical trial. JAMA. 2014;312:2234–43.
65. Budoff MJ, Dowe D, Jollis JG, Gitter M, Sutherland J, Halamert E, Scherer M, Bellinger R, Martin A, Benton R, Delago A, Min JK. Diagnostic performance of 64-multidetector row coronary computed tomographic angiography for evaluation of coronary artery stenosis in individuals without known coronary artery disease: results from the prospective multicenter accuracy (assessment by coronary computed tomographic angiography of individuals undergoing invasive coronary angiography) trial. J Am Coll Cardiol. 2008;52:1724–32.
66. Meijboom WB, Meijs MF, Schuijf JD, Cramer MJ, Mollet NR, van Mieghem CA, Nieman K, van Werkhoven JM, Pundziute G, Weustink AC, de Vos AM, Pugliese F, Rensing B, Jukema JW, Bax JJ, Prokop M, Doevendans PA, Hunink MG, Krestin GP, de Feyter PJ. Diagnostic accuracy of 64-slice computed tomography coronary angiography: a prospective, multicenter, multivendor study. J Am Coll Cardiol. 2008;52:2135–44.
67. Miller JM, Rochitte CE, Dewey M, Arbab-Zadeh A, Niinuma H, Gottlieb I, Paul N, Clouse ME, Shapiro EP, Hoe J, Lardo AC, Bush DE, de Roos A, Cox C, Brinker J, Lima JA. Diagnostic performance of coronary angiography by 64-row CT. N Engl J Med. 2008;359:2324–36.
68. Neglia D, Rovai D, Caselli C, Pietila M, Teresinska A, Aguade-Bruix S, Pizzi MN, Todiere G, Gimelli A, Schroeder S, Drosch T, Poddighe R, Casolo G, Anagnostopoulos C, Pugliese F, Rouzet F, Le Guludec D, Cappelli F, Valente S, Gensini GF, Zawaideh C, Capitanio S, Sambuceti G, Marsico F, Perrone Filardi P, Fernandez-Golfin C, Rincon LM, Graner FP, de Graaf MA, Fiechter M, Stehli J, Gaemperli O, Reyes E, Nkomo S, Maki M, Lorenzoni V, Turchetti G, Carpeggiani C, Marinelli M, Puzzuoli S, Mangione M, Marcheschi P, Mariani F, Giannessi D, Nekolla S, Lombardi M, Sicari R, Scholte AJ, Zamorano JL, Kaufmann PA, Underwood SR, Knuuti J. Detection of significant coronary artery disease by noninvasive anatomical and functional imaging. Circ Cardio Imag. 2015;8:e002179.
69. Amsterdam EA, Kirk JD, Bluemke DA, Diercks D, Farkouh ME, Garvey JL, Kontos MC, McCord J, Miller TD, Morise A, Newby LK, Ruberg FL, Scordo KA, Thompson PD. Testing of low-risk patients presenting to the emergency department with chest pain: a scientific statement from the American heart association. Circulation. 2010;122:1756–76.
70. Pope JH, Aufderheide TP, Ruthazer R, Woolard RH, Feldman JA, Beshansky JR, Griffith JL, Selker HP. Missed diagnoses of acute cardiac ischemia in the emergency department. N Engl J Med. 2000;342:1163–70.

71. Udelson JE, Beshansky JR, Ballin DS, Feldman JA, Griffith JL, Handler J, Heller GV, Hendel RC, Pope JH, Ruthazer R, Spiegler EJ, Woolard RH, Selker HP. Myocardial perfusion imaging for evaluation and triage of patients with suspected acute cardiac ischemia: a randomized controlled trial. JAMA. 2002;288:2693–700.
72. Duvall WL, Savino JA, Levine EJ, Baber U, Lin JT, Einstein AJ, Hermann LK, Henzlova MJ. A comparison of coronary cta and stress testing using high-efficiency spect MPI for the evaluation of chest pain in the emergency department. J Nucl Cardiol. 2014;21:305–18.
73. Goldstein JA, Chinnaiyan KM, Abidov A, Achenbach S, Berman DS, Hayes SW, Hoffmann U, Lesser JR, Mikati IA, O'Neil BJ, Shaw LJ, Shen MY, Valeti US, Raff GL. The CT-STAT (coronary computed tomographic angiography for systematic triage of acute chest pain patients to treatment) trial. J Am Coll Cardiol. 2011;58:1414–22.
74. Litt HI, Gatsonis C, Snyder B, Singh H, Miller CD, Entrikin DW, Leaming JM, Gavin LJ, Pacella CB, Hollander JE. CT angiography for safe discharge of patients with possible acute coronary syndromes. N Engl J Med. 2012;366:1393–403.
75. Hoffmann U, Truong QA, Schoenfeld DA, Chou ET, Woodard PK, Nagurney JT, Pope JH, Hauser TH, White CS, Weiner SG, Kalanjian S, Mullins ME, Mikati I, Peacock WF, Zakroysky P, Hayden D, Goehler A, Lee H, Gazelle GS, Wiviott SD, Fleg JL, Udelson JE. Coronary CT angiography versus standard evaluation in acute chest pain. N Engl J Med. 2012;367:299–308.
76. Hamilton-Craig C, Fifoot A, Hansen M, Pincus M, Chan J, Walters DL, Branch KR. Diagnostic performance and cost of CT angiography versus stress ECG – a randomized prospective study of suspected acute coronary syndrome chest pain in the emergency department (ct-compare). Int J Cardiol. 2014;177:867–73.
77. Anthem. Coronary artery imaging: contrast-enhanced Coronary Computed Tomography Angiography (CCTA), Coronary Magnetic Resonance Angiography (MRA) and Cardiac Magnetic Resonance Imaging (MRI). Medical Policy #: RAD 00035; Current Effective Date: 04/077/2015; Last Review Date: 02/05/2015.
78. Min JK, Dunning A, Lin FY, Achenbach S, Al-Mallah M, Budoff MJ, Cademartiri F, Callister TQ, Chang HJ, Cheng V, Chinnaiyan K, Chow BJ, Delago A, Hadamitzky M, Hausleiter J, Kaufmann P, Maffei E, Raff G, Shaw LJ, Villines T, Berman DS, Investigators C. Age- and sex-related differences in all-cause mortality risk based on coronary computed tomography angiography findings results from the international multicenter confirm (coronary ct angiography evaluation for clinical outcomes: an international multicenter registry) of 23,854 patients without known coronary artery disease. J Am Coll Cardiol. 2011;58:849–60.
79. Leipsic J, Taylor CM, Grunau G, Heilbron BG, Mancini GB, Achenbach S, Al-Mallah M, Berman DS, Budoff MJ, Cademartiri F, Callister TQ, Chang HJ, Cheng VY, Chinnaiyan K, Chow BJ, Delago A, Hadamitzky M, Hausleiter J, Cury R, Feuchtner G, Kim YJ, Kaufmann PA, Lin FY, Maffei E, Raff G, Shaw LJ, Villines TC, Min JK. Cardiovascular risk among stable individuals suspected of having coronary artery disease with no modifiable risk factors: results from an international multicenter study of 5262 patients. Radiology. 2013;267:718–26.
80. Arsanjani R, Berman DS, Gransar H, Cheng VY, Dunning A, Lin FY, Achenbach S, Al-Mallah M, Budoff MJ, Callister TQ, Chang HJ, Cademartiri F, Chinnaiyan KM, Chow BJ, DeLago A, Hadamitzky M, Hausleiter J, Kaufmann P, LaBounty TM, Leipsic J, Raff G, Shaw LJ, Villines TC, Cury RC, Feuchtner G, Kim YJ, Min JK. Left ventricular function and volume with coronary ct angiography improves risk stratification and identification of patients at risk for incident mortality: results from 7758 patients in the prospective multinational confirm observational cohort study. Radiology. 2014;273:70–7.
81. Nakazato R, Arsanjani R, Achenbach S, Gransar H, Cheng VY, Dunning A, Lin FY, Al-Mallah M, Budoff MJ, Callister TQ, Chang HJ, Cademartiri F, Chinnaiyan K, Chow BJ, Delago A, Hadamitzky M, Hausleiter J, Kaufmann P, Raff G, Shaw LJ, Villines T, Cury RC, Feuchtner G, Kim YJ, Leipsic J, Berman DS, Min JK. Age-related risk of major adverse cardiac event risk and coronary artery disease extent and severity by coronary ct angiography: results from 15 187 patients from the international multisite CONFIRM study. Eur Heart J Cardiovasc Imag. 2014;15: 586–94.
82. The SCOT-HEART Investigators. CT coronary angiography in patients with suspected angina due to coronary heart disease (SCOT-HEART): an open-label, parallel-group, multicentre trial. Lancet. 2015;385:2383–91.
83. Douglas PS, Hoffmann U, Patel MR, Mark DB, Al-Khalidi HR, Cavanaugh B, Cole J, Dolor RJ, Fordyce CB, Huang M, Khan MA, Kosinski AS, Krucoff MW, Malhotra V, Picard MH, Udelson JE, Velazquez EJ, Yow E, Cooper LS, Lee KL. Outcomes of anatomical versus functional testing for coronary artery disease. N Engl J Med. 2015;372:1291–300.
84. Schuijf JD, Jukema JW, van der Wall EE, Bax JJ. The current status of multislice computed tomography in the diagnosis and prognosis of coronary artery disease. J Nucl Cardiol. 2007;14(4): 604–12.
85. Zeb I, Abbas N, Nasir K, Budoff MJ. Coronary computed tomography as a cost-effective test strategy for coronary artery disease assessment – a systematic review. Atherosclerosis. 2014; 234:426–35.
86. Abidov A, Gallagher MJ, Chinnaiyan KM, Mehta LS, Wegner JH, Raff GL. Clinical effectiveness of coronary computed tomographic angiography in the triage of patients to cardiac catheterization and revascularization after inconclusive stress testing: results of a 2-year prospective trial. J Nucl Cardiol. 2009;16:701–13.
87. Rozanski A, Cohen R, Uretsky S. The coronary calcium treadmill test: a new approach to the initial workup of patients with suspected coronary artery disease. J Nucl Cardiol. 2013;20: 719–30.
88. Cremer P, Hachamovitch R. Assessing the prognostic implications of myocardial perfusion studies: identification of patients at risk vs patients who may benefit from intervention? Curr Cardiol Rep. 2014;16:472.
89. Shaw LJ, Hage FG, Berman DS, Hachamovitch R, Iskandrian A. Prognosis in the era of comparative effectiveness research: where is nuclear cardiology now and where should it be? J Nucl Cardiol. 2012;19:1026–43.
90. Bourque JM, Beller GA. Stress myocardial perfusion imaging for assessing prognosis: an update. JACC Cardiovasc Imaging. 2011;4:1305–19.
91. Dorbala S, Di Carli MF, Beanlands RS, Merhige ME, Williams BA, Veledar E, Chow BJ, Min JK, Pencina MJ, Berman DS, Shaw LJ. Prognostic value of stress myocardial perfusion positron emission tomography: results from a multicenter observational registry. J Am Coll Cardiol. 2013;61:176–84.
92. Berman DS, Shaw LJ, Min JK, Hachamovitch R, Abidov A, Germano G, Hayes SW, Friedman JD, Thomson LE, Kang X, Slomka P, Rozanski A. SPECT/PET myocardial perfusion imaging versus coronary ct angiography in patients with known or suspected CAD. Q J Nucl Med Mol Imaging. 2010;54: 177–200.
93. Berman DS, Hachamovitch R, Shaw LJ, Hayes SW, Germano G. Nuclear cardiology. In: Fuster VAR, O'Rourke RA, Roberts R, King SB, Wellens HJJ, editors. Hurst's the heart. New York: McGraw-Hill Companies; 2004. p. 563–97.
94. Boden WE, O'Rourke RA, Teo KK, Hartigan PM, Maron DJ, Kostuk WJ, Knudtson M, Dada M, Casperson P, Harris CL, Chaitman BR, Shaw L, Gosselin G, Nawaz S, Title LM, Gau G, Blaustein AS, Booth DC, Bates ER, Spertus JA, Berman DS, Mancini GB, Weintraub WS. Optimal medical therapy with or without PCI for stable coronary disease. N Engl J Med. 2007; 356:1503–16.

95. Frye RL, August P, Brooks MM, Hardison RM, Kelsey SF, MacGregor JM, Orchard TJ, Chaitman BR, Genuth SM, Goldberg SH, Hlatky MA, Jones TL, Molitch ME, Nesto RW, Sako EY, Sobel BE, Group BDS. A randomized trial of therapies for type 2 diabetes and coronary artery disease. N Engl J Med. 2009;360: 2503–15.
96. Tonino PA, De Bruyne B, Pijls NH, Siebert U, Ikeno F, van' t Veer M, Klauss V, Manoharan G, Engstrøm T, Oldroyd KG, Ver Lee PN, MacCarthy PA, Fearon WF, FAME Study Investigators. Fractional flow reserve versus angiography for guiding percutaneous coronary intervention. N Engl J Med. 2009;360:213–24.
97. Pijls NH, Fearon WF, Tonino PA, Siebert U, Ikeno F, Bornschein B, van't Veer M, Klauss V, Manoharan G, Engstrøm T, Oldroyd KG, Ver Lee PN, MacCarthy PA, De Bruyne B, Investigators FS. Fractional flow reserve versus angiography for guiding percutaneous coronary intervention in patients with multivessel coronary artery disease: 2-year follow-up of the fame (fractional flow reserve versus angiography for multivessel evaluation) study. J Am Coll Cardiol. 2010;56:177–84.
98. De Bruyne B, Pijls NH, Kalesan B, Barbato E, Tonino PA, Piroth Z, Jagic N, Mobius-Winkler S, Rioufol G, Witt N, Kala P, MacCarthy P, Engstrom T, Oldroyd KG, Mavromatis K, Manoharan G, Verlee P, Frobert O, Curzen N, Johnson JB, Juni P, Fearon WF. Fractional flow reserve-guided pci versus medical therapy in stable coronary disease. N Engl J Med. 2012;367:991–1001.
99. Li J, Elrashidi MY, Flammer AJ, Lennon RJ, Bell MR, Holmes DR, Bresnahan JF, Rihal CS, Lerman LO, Lerman A. Long-term outcomes of fractional flow reserve-guided vs. Angiography-guided percutaneous coronary intervention in contemporary practice. Eur Heart J. 2013;34:1375–83.
100. Hachamovitch R, Berman DS, Shaw LJ, Kiat H, Cohen I, Cabico JA, Friedman J, Diamond GA. Incremental prognostic value of myocardial perfusion single photon emission computed tomography for the prediction of cardiac death: differential stratification for risk of cardiac death and myocardial infarction. Circulation. 1998;97:535–43.
101. Hachamovitch R, Hayes SW, Friedman JD, Cohen I, Berman DS. Comparison of the short-term survival benefit associated with revascularization compared with medical therapy in patients with no prior coronary artery disease undergoing stress myocardial perfusion single photon emission computed tomography. Circulation. 2003;107:2900–7.
102. Hachamovitch R, Rozanski A, Shaw LJ, Stone GW, Thomson LE, Friedman JD, Hayes SW, Cohen I, Germano G, Berman DS. Impact of ischaemia and scar on the therapeutic benefit derived from myocardial revascularization vs. Medical therapy among patients undergoing stress-rest myocardial perfusion scintigraphy. Eur Heart J. 2011;32:1012–24.
103. Hachamovitch R, Kang X, Amanullah AM, Abidov A, Hayes SW, Friedman JD, Cohen I, Thomson LE, Germano G, Berman DS. Prognostic implications of myocardial perfusion single-photon emission computed tomography in the elderly. Circulation. 2009;120:2197–206.
104. Sorajja P, Chareonthaitawee P, Rajagopalan N, Miller TD, Frye RL, Hodge DO, Gibbons RJ. Improved survival in asymptomatic diabetic patients with high-risk SPECT imaging treated with coronary artery bypass grafting. Circulation. 2005;112:I311–6.
105. Taqueti VR, Hachamovitch R, Murthy VL, Naya M, Foster CR, Hainer J, Dorbala S, Blankstein R, Di Carli MF. Global coronary flow reserve is associated with adverse cardiovascular events independently of luminal angiographic severity and modifies the effect of early revascularization. Circulation. 2015;131:19–27.
106. Gould KL, Johnson NP, Kaul S, Kirkeeide RL, Mintz GS, Rentrop KP, Sdringola S, Virmani R, Narula J. Patient selection for elective revascularization to reduce myocardial infarction and mortality: new lessons from randomized trials, coronary physiology, and statistics. Circ Cardio Imag. 2015;8:e003099.
107. Rozanski A, Gransar H, Hayes SW, Min J, Friedman JD, Thomson LE, Berman DS. Temporal trends in the frequency of inducible myocardial ischemia during cardiac stress testing: 1991 to 2009. J Am Coll Cardiol. 2013;61:1054–65.
108. Cheng VY, Berman DS, Rozanski A, Dunning AM, Achenbach S, Al-Mallah M, Budoff MJ, Cademartiri F, Callister TQ, Chang HJ, Chinnaiyan K, Chow BJ, Delago A, Gomez M, Hadamitzky M, Hausleiter J, Karlsberg RP, Kaufmann P, Lin FY, Maffei E, Raff GL, Villines TC, Shaw LJ, Min JK. Performance of the traditional age, sex, and angina typicality-based approach for estimating pretest probability of angiographically significant coronary artery disease in patients undergoing coronary computed tomographic angiography: results from the multinational coronary ct angiography evaluation for clinical outcomes: an international multicenter registry (CONFIRM). Circulation. 2011;124:2423–32.
109. Tonino PA, Fearon WF, De Bruyne B, Oldroyd KG, Leesar MA, Ver Lee PN, MacCarthy PA, Van't Veer M, Pijls NH. Angiographic versus functional severity of coronary artery stenoses in the FAME study: fractional flow reserve versus angiography in multivessel evaluation. J Am Coll Cardiol. 2010;55(25):2816–21.
110. Zhou T, Yang LF, Zhai JL, Li J, Wang QM, Zhang RJ, Wang S, Peng ZH, Li M, Sun G. SPECT myocardial perfusion versus fractional flow reserve for evaluation of functional ischemia: a meta analysis. Eur J Radiol. 2014;83:951–6.
111. Min JK, Dunning A, Gransar H, Achenbach S, Lin FY, Al-Mallah M, Budoff MJ, Callister TQ, Chang HJ, Cademartiri F, Maffei E, Chinnaiyan K, Chow BJ, D'Agostino R, DeLago A, Friedman J, Hadamitzky M, Hausleiter J, Hayes SW, Kaufmann P, Raff GL, Shaw LJ, Thomson L, Villines T, Cury RC, Feuchtner G, Kim YJ, Leipsic J, Berman DS, Pencina M. Medical history for prognostic risk assessment and diagnosis of stable patients with suspected coronary artery disease. Am J Med. 2015;128(8):871–8.
112. Levine A, Hecht HS. Cardiac CT angiography in congestive heart failure. J Nucl Med. 2015;56 Suppl 4:46s–51.
113. Hachamovitch R, Nutter B, Hlatky MA, Shaw LJ, Ridner ML, Dorbala S, Beanlands RS, Chow BJ, Branscomb E, Chareonthaitawee P, Weigold WG, Voros S, Abbara S, Yasuda T, Jacobs JE, Lesser J, Berman DS, Thomson LE, Raman S, Heller GV, Schussheim A, Brunken R, Williams KA, Farkas S, Delbeke D, Schoepf UJ, Reichek N, Rabinowitz S, Sigman SR, Patterson R, Corn CR, White R, Kazerooni E, Corbett J, Bokhari S, Machac J, Guarneri E, Borges-Neto S, Millstine JW, Caldwell J, Arrighi J, Hoffmann U, Budoff M, Lima J, Johnson JR, Johnson B, Gaber M, Williams JA, Foster C, Hainer J, Di Carli MF, SPARC Investigators. Patient management after noninvasive cardiac imaging results from sparc (study of myocardial perfusion and coronary anatomy imaging roles in coronary artery disease). J Am Coll Cardiol. 2012;59:462–74.
114. Beanlands RS, Nichol G, Huszti E, Humen D, Racine N, Freeman M, Gulenchyn KY, Garrard L, de Kemp R, Guo A, Ruddy TD, Benard F, Lamy A, Iwanochko RM. F-18-fluorodeoxyglucose positron emission tomography imaging-assisted management of patients with severe left ventricular dysfunction and suspected coronary disease: a randomized, controlled trial (parr-2). J Am Coll Cardiol. 2007;50:2002–12.
115. Abraham A, Nichol G, Williams KA, Guo A, deKemp RA, Garrard L, Davies RA, Duchesne L, Haddad H, Chow B, DaSilva J, Beanlands RS. 18F-FDG pet imaging of myocardial viability in an experienced center with access to 18f-fdg and integration with clinical management teams: the Ottawa-five substudy of the parr 2 trial. J Nucl Med. 2010;51:567–74.

Coronary Computed Tomographic Angiography for Detection of Coronary Artery Disease: Analysis of Large-Scale Multicenter Trials and Registries

21

Leslee J. Shaw

Abstract

The field of coronary computed tomographic angiography (CCTA) has evolved dramatically with an ever increasing and robust evidence base to support its clinical utility in terms of an unparalleled diagnostic accuracy and effective risk stratification rivaling the more commonly applied, comparative stress imaging procedures. This chapter seeks to highlight the available high quality effectiveness evidence, including large observational and randomized trial data, that support the utility of CCTA as a valuable tool in the diagnosis of coronary artery disease.

Keywords

Quality Research • Effectiveness Research • Multicenter Trial • Randomized Trials

Introduction

The field of coronary computed tomographic angiography (CCTA) has evolved dramatically with an ever increasing and robust evidence base to support its clinical utility in terms of an unparalleled diagnostic accuracy and effective risk stratification rivaling the more commonly applied, comparative stress imaging procedures. It is difficult to fathom but, in 2005, 64-slice CCTA was introduced and, in less than a decade, all of our knowledge base on the strengths and limitations of this noninvasive, anatomic procedure have been revealed. The CCTA community, including combined expertise in cardiology and radiology, has strategically sought to answer both technical and clinical questions with regards to the accuracy and effectiveness of this procedure to guide optimal patient care strategies.

In this chapter, we will highlight the current high quality evidence based on the clinical utility of CCTA. Importantly, given the enormity of this task, we cannot be all inclusive but hope to provide readers with a smattering of the available evidence within selective indications which strongly support CCTA as clinically effective and enhancing patient care. Moreover, we will highlight specific leadership on the part of CCTA investigators to provide a clinically effective tool while enhancing radiation safety profiles.

Coverage with Evidence Development

In 2008, the Centers for Medicaid and Medicare Services reviewed the available evidence with CCTA and recommended that there be no national coverage determination due to a paucity of evidence in certain indications. Although one may argue that none of the other competitive and commonly-employed models were held to such a high standard, these new standards reflect our current state of affairs for payer policies. In today's challenging healthcare environment, coverage policies are garnered by a sufficiently high level of evidence noting that an imaging modality is capable of improving clinical outcomes of patients. This new standard has been termed patient-centered imaging and places the core aims of imaging aligned with each patient and the

L.J. Shaw, PhD
Department of Medicine, Emory Clinical Cardiovascular Research Institute, Emory University School of Medicine, 1462 Clifton Rd NE, Rm 529, Atlanta 30324, GA, USA
e-mail: lshaw3@emory.edu

M.J. Budoff, J.S. Shinbane (eds.), *Cardiac CT Imaging: Diagnosis of Cardiovascular Disease*,
DOI 10.1007/978-3-319-28219-0_21

ultimate goal of improved quality or quantity of life as initiated based on anatomic markers identified during the CCTA procedure. Given this new standard, where are we today in evidence for clinical indications?

Growth in CCTA Research

Since 2005, there has been an explosion in published research on CCTA. Based on statistics from Thomson Reuters' Web of Knowledge which collects data on all published manuscripts, approximately 30 peer-reviewed manuscripts were published in 2004 and this number has grown to over 180 for 2013. This is dramatic growth and reflects the fact that, in 2013, CCTA articles were cited over 3500 times. This acceleration in the published literature, as we will highlight, reflects not only the expansiveness of the evidence but also high quality evidence supporting CCTA as a highly effective diagnostic test procedure.

Specific Clinical Indications for CCTA with High Level Evidence Supporting Clinical Effectiveness

In this chapter, we will highlight specific evidence on three specific clinical indications for the use of CCTA including:

1. Diagnostic Testing for the Detection of High Risk Patients with Coronary Artery Calcium (CAC) Scoring
2. Acute Evaluation of Low Risk Chest Pain in the Emergency Department (ED)
3. Diagnosis and Risk Stratification of Patients with Stable Chest Pain

Detecting High Risk Patients with CAC Scoring

Let us begin our review of the CCTA evidence by focusing on the available and high quality evidence on screening of apparently healthy individuals. In 2010, the American College of Cardiology published a thorough review of the available evidence across all cardiovascular screening modalities [1]. We will highlight the results of this guideline but also discuss more recent publications which have extended these findings on the use of CAC screening. Although numerous reports were published using patient series, the National Institutes of Health – National Heart, Lung, and Blood Institute-sponsored Multi-Ethnic Study of Atherosclerosis (MESA) published 5-year outcome data following CAC scoring in 6724 asymptomatic apparently healthy people ages 45–84 years [2]. The evidence from this population cohort revealed that CAC scoring was independently predictive and highly effective at risk stratification of major adverse cardiac events (MACE) (i.e., cardiac death or nonfatal myocardial infarction). These results were confirmatory of prior findings noting a directly proportional relationship between CAC scores and MACE risk. That is, there is a very low risk of MACE in patients with no CAC or a zero score. As the CAC score increases (i.e., becomes more extensive), the overall MACE risk increases; such that for patients with a CAC score of 300–400 or higher, the MACE risk is at least 10 % over 5 years [2]. This risk is exceedingly high for asymptomatic individuals and has been consistently reported across numerous patient and population cohorts [3, 4].

One may actually quantify the added contribution to risk estimation using the net reclassification improvement (NRI) statistic [5]. Two reports have been published on the calculation of the NRI using the MESA population registry [6, 7]. In the first of these series, the NRI was 0.25 revealing that CAC findings improve the detection of lower or higher risk status for 1 in 4 individuals when compared to risk estimation using the Framingham risk score [6]. This NRI statistic for CAC is much higher than for other markers, such as high sensitivity C-reactive protein (CRP) [8]. An updated report from MESA, in intermediate risk individuals, compared the NRI for CAC as compared to other markers such as a family history of premature coronary heart disease, CRP, ankle brachial index, and carotid intima-media thickness (Fig. 21.1) [7]. If one examines the NRI results for a prognostic model estimating 7-year incidence of MACE (defined as myocardial infarction, coronary heart disease death, resuscitated cardiac arrest, or angina followed by coronary revascularization), the statistic for CAC was 0.66 and at least 6-fold higher than for many of the other risk markers [7].

A limitation with the available CAC evidence is the lack of randomized trials noting improved outcomes. Despite this there are several additional publications that are relevant to answering this question. In a related secondary analysis from the MESA registry, Blaha and colleagues reported on the number needed to treat (NNT) to save a life if CAC screening was employed to target treatment with statin therapy (in this case, 20 mg of rosuvastatin) [9]. This result revealed that if all patients with a 0 CAC score were treated with statins, the NNT would be over 500. However, if only patients with a CAC score of 100 or higher were targeted, then the NNT would be dramatically reduced to 24 [9].

There have been several intermediate outcome trials which have randomized patients to CAC scanning versus no scanning with primary outcomes of change in the Framingham risk score [10, 11]. In the Early Identification of Subclinical Atherosclerosis by Noninvasive Imaging Research (EISNER) trial, a 2:1 randomization had 1311 patients receiving CAC scanning and 623 did not receive CAC scanning [10]. The primary findings from this trial revealed that CAC scanning resulted in minimal change in the Framingham risk score (0.002 %) by comparison there was a marked worsening of this risk score in patients not

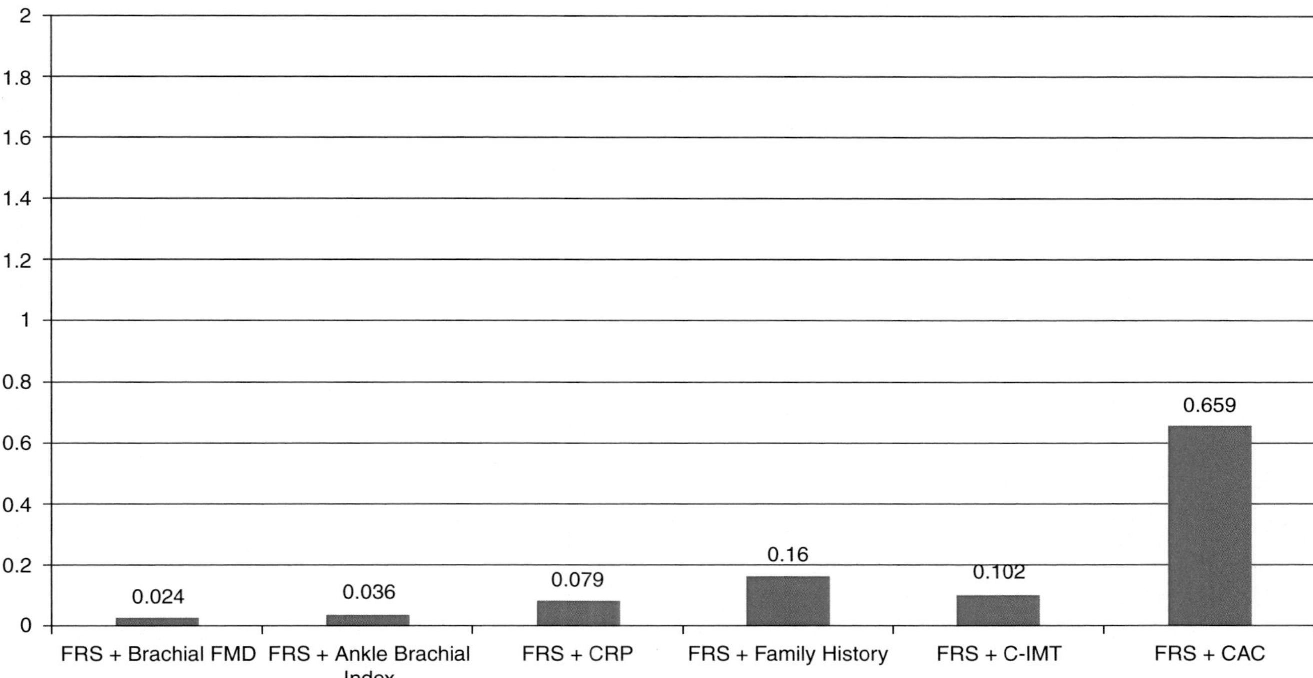

Fig. 21.1 Net reclassification improvement (NRI) results form the NIH-NHLBI-sponsored MESA registry including intermediate Framingham risk score (*FRS*) patients. The results indicate the NRI based on an array of screening tests including brachial flow mediate dilation (*FMD*), high sensitivity C-reactive protein (*CRP*), carotid intima media thickness (*C-IMT*), and coronary artery calcium (*CAC*). The NRI compares the added value of each of the sreening tests when compared to the FRS alone. The endpoint for this analysis is 7-year myocardial infarction, coronary heart disease death, resuscitated cardiac arrest, or angina followed by coronary revascularization

receiving the CAC scan (0.7 %, p=0.0003). As well, patients randomized to receive the CAC scan showed net favorable changes in systolic blood pressure (p=0.02), LDL cholesterol (p=0.04), and for improvements in waist circumference for those with an increased abdominal girth (p=0.01) [10].

The compilation of evidence is quite strong and does reveal that CAC scoring is highly effective at identifying high risk patients. Yet, to date, this body of evidence has not been compelling to support universal coverage for CAC scoring. Medicare covers CAC for asymptomatic persons in 17 states, however, most current Medicare policies are based on treatment for illness and not screening of the well. All screening coverage policies, such as mammography, must be legislated. To date, there is a lack of trial evidence, similar to that recently reported for lung cancer, which demonstrates improved outcomes for patients randomized to CAC scoring as compared to those without CAC scanning.

Efficiency of CCTA in the Acute Evaluation of Low Risk Chest Pain in the Emergency Department (ED)

As we turn to the available evidence in symptomatic patients, our initial review of the evidence is on the use of CCTA for the evaluation of low risk chest pain in the ED. This would largely include patients with a low risk Thrombolysis in Myocardial Ischemia (TIMI) risk score whose index troponin level was negative. For this indication, there are three relatively large randomized clinical trials which have been published and include a total of 3069 patients [12–14]. Each of the trials compared a CCTA-driven strategy as compared to the current standard of care (SOC); with this largely including some form of stress testing [12–14]. The most prominent finding from all 3 trials has been the time to diagnosis, length of stay, and the proportion of patients that were discharged from the ED [12–14]. For all trials, time efficiency was demonstrably superior with CCTA as compared to the SOC. For example, from one trial, 47 % of patients in the CCTA arm were discharged from the ED as compared to only 12 % of the SOC arm [12]. Thus, CCTA reduced the overall length of stay in the ED by 7.6 h [14]. Figure 21.2 depicts the proportional rate of discharge across the length of time spent in the ED [12].

The longer length of stay in those receiving the SOC led to higher costs of care for one trial (on average $1321 cost savings with CCTA) but in another trial, the CCTA arm led to more intensive care and resulted in similar ED costs (p=0.7) [13, 14]. To this extent, it remains uncertain as to whether the CCTA-guided diagnostic efficiency can lead to economic savings for the healthcare system. Moreover, we may learn that the prevalence of CAD identified by CCTA in

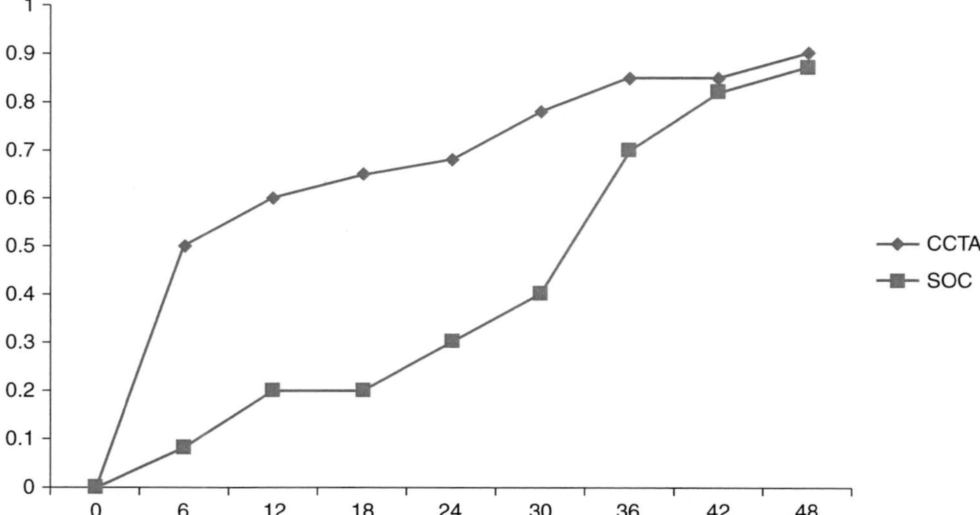

Fig. 21.2 An approximation of the proportion of patients discharged from the ED for those patients randomized to CCTA as compared with SOC. The medianlength of stay was 8.6 h for patients receiving CCTA as compared to 26.7 h for those within the SOC arm of the ROMICAT II trial

the ED may be the key factor in defining cost savings. That is, should the likelihood of CAD be elevated, the higher prevalence of CAD may require more intensive follow-up including invasive angiography or stress imaging studies that increase the overall costs of care. By comparison, should we be able to define patients with largely negative CCTA findings, then the lack of anatomic findings may prove to impact on cost savings to a greater extent when compared to higher risk populations. Of course, with this latter statement, one has to take care not to employ CCTA in too low risk patients where the radiation exposure would be unwarranted. Suffice it to say that additional explorations of the potential for cost minimization in the ED by selectively employing CCTA remains an area of active exploration.

An additional challenge with the current evidence base is the lack of longterm data on clinical effectiveness of randomization to CCTA versus SOC. The randomized trials employed thus far have largely examined near-term outcomes of 1–6 months [12–14]. From the ACRIN-PA trial, none of the 640 patients with a negative CCTA died or had a nonfatal myocardial infarction within one month of discharge from the ED [13]. The UK's National Health Service technology assessment supported the use of CCTA in the ED as a cost effective strategy for troponin negative patients [15]. A recent meta-analysis revealed that the near-term odds of readmission for an acute coronary syndrome were non-significant with an odds ratio of 1.2 (95 % confidence intervals: 0.7–2.2) [16]. In one recent report examining long-term (i.e., ~4 years follow-up) of 506 discharged patients without plaque and patients with nonobstructive plaque, only 1 % were readmitted for chest pain and none of the patients underwent revascularization, died, or had an acute coronary syndrome [17]. Data such as this on the long-term consequences of CCTA-guided discharge will surely help to ensure confidence and define the warranty period of the index diagnosis as to the presence and extent of CAD.

Despite the limitations, this robust body of evidence is superior to the stress imaging data. For example, there is but one large clinical trial on the impact of stress nuclear in the (ER Assessment of Sestamibi for Evaluation of Chest Pain [ERASE] Trial). The ERASE trial enrolled a total of 2127 patients who were randomized to receive an index resting nuclear scan as compared to usual care [18]. In 2127 patients, a total of 52 % of the usual care arm were discharged as compared to 42 % of those randomized to the nuclear scan arm (odds ratio: 0.68, 95 % confidence intervals = 0.57–0.82) [18]. Similar to CCTA, the extent to which patients have prior CAD which impacts on resting perfusion abnormalities are likely the critical factor in early discharge for patients presenting with acute chest pain. Despite this, the differential in discharge appears greater for CCTA as compared to that of the ERASE trial.

A point worth making in this discussion is the extent to which identification of an obstructive lesion is the source of the presenting symptoms. Despite a stenosis, the presence of collateral flow or the distal site of the stenosis may not prompt presenting symptoms and this remains an important consideration and challenge for CCTA. However, issues related to soft tissue attenuation with stress nuclear can result in a false positive rate of follow-up angiography that is unacceptably high [19]. The incorporation of CT fractional flow reserve (CT-FFR) calculations in conjunction with the anatomic findings may prove optimal for guiding patient care in the acute evaluation of chest pain [20]. The addition of FFR improves the diagnostic accuracy of anatomy defined by CCTA but is limited by the length of time required for the complex calculations and remote calculation of the FFR measurement. Despite this, improvements in the technology and the addition of this FFR measurement in the near-term post-discharge may prove optimal for long-term effectiveness of a CCTA-guided strategy following acute evaluation of chest pain in the ED.

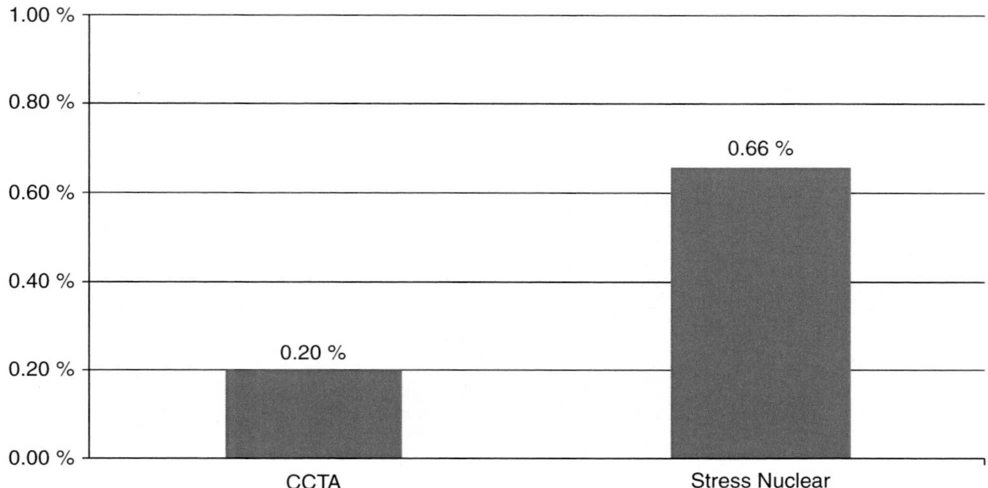

Fig. 21.3 Annual rate of major CAD events for patients with a negative CCTA and stress nuclear result

We highlighted the high quality of evidence on the use of CCTA in the ED and it is worth noting that the depth of evidence far exceeds that of other modalities. Likely, when additional clinical practice guidelines are updated on acute coronary syndrome care that CCTA will garner a high level recommendation based on these three randomized trials [12–14].

Diagnostic and Prognostic Value of CCTA in Multicenter Trials and Registries

Our next set of indications is to examine the available evidence supporting the use of CCTA in the evaluation of patients with stable chest pain. Notably, the evidence with CCTA is largely based on large, multicenter registries and several controlled clinical trials. If we start with the early evidence that examined the correlation of findings between CCTA and invasive coronary angiography, there are three controlled clinical trials that have been published [21–23]. These trials represented pivotal evidence that the anatomic findings that we commonly observe with invasive angiography were concordant with the newly introduced CCTA anatomic findings. In fact, the results revealed a high degree of accuracy for CCTA when compared to invasive anatomic findings. From one cohort with a low-intermediate risk of CAD, the diagnostic sensitivity and specificity for obstructive CAD on invasive angiography was 94 and 83 % [3]. From the CorE64 trial, the diagnostic sensitivity and specificity was 85 and 90 % [22]. As well, from one meta-analysis of the data on 64 slice CCTA, the diagnostic sensitivity and specificity was 94 and 85 % [24]. These data reveal an overall higher diagnostic accuracy for CCTA in the detection of obstructive CAD when compared to that of stress imaging [25].

Extending beyond these trials, there have been numerous reports on the prognostic relationship between obstructive and nonobstructive CAD findings on CCTA [26–31]. The largest of the registry data is that from the COronary CTA EvaluatioN For Clinical Outcomes: An InteRnational Multicenter (CONFIRM) multicenter and multinational registry enrolling more than 30,000 patients who have been followed for approximately 3–5 years for the occurrence of death from all-causes and nonfatal myocardial infarction [32]. Several important findings have been revealed by examining risk stratification data in a diverse and expansive group of patients. First, in all of these reports, CCTA findings of the extent and severity of CAD provide effective means to risk stratify patients [28]. Reports have been published across an array of age and gender subsets of diverse race/ethnicity [28, 33, 34], in the diabetic [35, 36], post-coronary bypass surgery [37], in patients with a family history of CAD [38], to name a few. The extensiveness of this evidence and its rapid accrual is a testimony to the CCTA's community of investigators who are eager to define the strengths and limitations of CCTA as an index diagnostic procedure.

Secondly, from this evidence base, multiple reports from diverse countries now report that patients with a normal CCTA have a very low rate of CAD events [28, 39–41]. A synthesis of this evidence examining follow-up through 7 years reveals that the major CAD event rate is approximately 0.2 % per year (Fig. 21.3) [28, 39–41]; similar to that of the general population. For stress echocardiography and nuclear imaging, the annual rate of major CAD event rates is generally <1 % per year but exceeds that for CCTA; generally in the range of 0.4–0.9 % [25, 42].

Third, several reports now reveal that the presence of mild but nonobstructive CAD is associated with an elevated hazard for death above and beyond that of patients with a normal CCTA [26–28, 31]. From one series of 2583 symptomatic patients with <50 % stenosis on CCTA and followed for approximately 3 years, the mortality hazard for all-cause death was elevated 2- to 6-fold for patients with 1–3 vessel

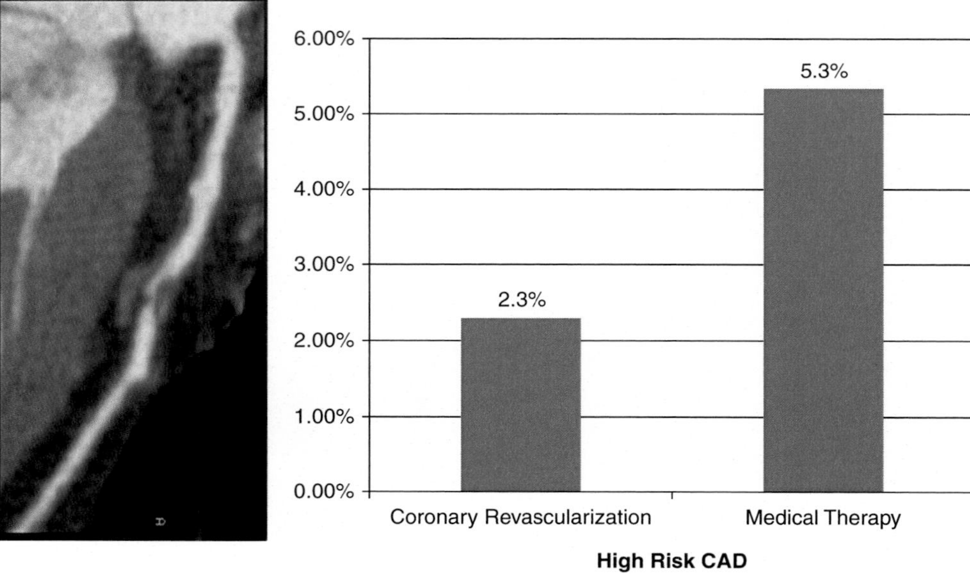

Fig. 21.4 Observational evidence on the impact of coronary revascularization based on CCTA-defined high risk CAD

nonobstructive CAD [31]. In ground-breaking work by Motoyama and Narula [26, 27], the presence of high risk plaque, defined as positive arterial remodeling and low attenuation plaque, was associated with a very high risk of incident acute coronary syndromes. In patients without any high risk plaque, the acute coronary syndrome rate was 0.5 % at 4-years of follow-up. By comparison, for patients with both positive remodeling and low attenuation plaque, the acute coronary syndrome rate was an astonishing 22 % at 4-years of follow-up. These data, as exploratory as they are, represent very exciting findings that we are only beginning to unfold. If we can further define and more reliably measure the burden of nonobstructive plaque and its relationship to acute coronary events, then this could revolutionize the field of diagnostic testing. We await further explorations from these groups that will help to improve risk detection of symptomatic patients.

A fourth important finding on the use of CCTA in the index evaluation of symptomatic patients is the identification of severe CAD, including multivessel and left main CAD, and the associated high risk status of these anatomic subsets. In patients with multivessel CAD, the annualized CAD event rates often are in the range of 8–10 % or higher [43]. Important observational findings from CONFIRM reveal that patients with high risk CAD receive a proportional risk reduction with coronary revascularization as compared to medical therapy [43]. Over 2 years of follow-up, the all-cause mortality rate for patients with high risk CAD was 5.3 % for those treated medically as compared to 2.3 % for those undergoing coronary revascularization (Fig. 21.4, p=0.0075). Additional data are required from a randomized trial setting to further unfurl the possibilities for therapeutic risk reduction based on CCTA findings. This latter point should also entail the initiation and intensification of preventive therapies and their impact on outcome among patients with nonobstructive CAD.

2012 Stable Ischemic Heart Disease Clinical Practice Guidelines: Indications for CCTA

Recently, a culmination of evidence among patients with stable chest pain was published in the 2012 American College of Cardiology's Stable Ischemic Heart Disease clinical practice guideline [44]. Based on this sizeable evidence base with CCTA, there are now 6 indications for CCTA in low-intermediate probability patients. There has been confusion on the part of readers of this guideline because the indications for CCTA mirror that of stress imaging. Despite this, all of the indications are Class IIa – IIb levels of evidence and the result of this strong body of evidence highlighted above.

Stable Ischemic Heart Disease Trials

There are a number of stable ischemic heart disease trials which have recently been completed and provide high quality evidence for CCTA (Table 21.1). One of these trials is the NIH-NHLBI-sponsored PROspective Multicenter Imaging Study for Evaluation of Chest Pain (PROMISE) Trial which has enrolled 10,000 patients who were followed for ~2.5 years. The PROMISE trial randomized patients to CCTA as compared to functional testing including stress electrocardiography, echocardiography, and nuclear imaging. Results from the PROMISE trial revealed no difference in the primary endpoint of death, acute coronary syndrome or major procedural complications, with a hazard ratio of 1.04 (95% confidence interval: 0.83–1.29, p=0.75) [48]. The challenge with the PROMISE trial was the enrollment of low risk patients with few reported events and including a population with the majority of patients having atypical chest pain symptoms. From a second trial, similar non-significant but trending results were reported in the SCOT-Heart trial with a hazard for coronary heart disease death or nonfatal myocardial infarction of 0.62 (95% confidence interval: 0.38–1.01, p=0.053). Based on the SCOT-Heart trial, there appears to be a trend toward improve outcomes for CCTA and this requires further exploration but may be due to the greater reported initiation of preventive medications that is frequently observed. Both of these trials establish CCTA as equally effective as functional imaging (Fig. 21.5) [49]. A second NIH-NHLBI-sponsored trial in patients with CCTA-defined CAD is the International Study of Comparative Health Effectiveness with Medical & Invasive Approaches Trial which will enroll 8000 patients who will be randomized to invasive coronary angiography-guided treatment as compared to prompt medical therapy (without invasive coronary angiography). These trials will and have demonstrably improved the quality of evidence and provide important information to guide selection of candidates and those who may or may not receive a benefit from testing with CCTA.

Conclusions

The evidence base on the clinical utility of CCTA has grown substantially over the past few years. This evidence emulates an important development and will be a path to rationally guiding healthcare coverage decisions using quality evidence from large registries and clinical trials.

Table 21.1 Stable ischemia heart disease trials

	Sponsor	Trial	N=	Endpoint	
Suspected CAD	AHRQ	Randomized evaluation of patients with stable angina comparing utilization of diagnostic examinations	4300	CAD death, MI, & revascularization	RAN[a] vs. MPI
	NIH-NHLBI	PROspective multicenter imaging study for evaluation of chest pain trial	10,000	2.5 years death, ACS, complications	RAN[a] vs. functional testing
Known CAD	NIH-NHLBI	International study of comparative health effectiveness with medical & invasive approaches trial	8000	4–6 years CV death or MI	Blinded CCTA to r/o LM & normal coronaries Completion: 7/19

Source: www.rescuetrial.org, www.promisetrial.org, www.ischemiatrial.org [45–47]
[a]*RAN* Randomization

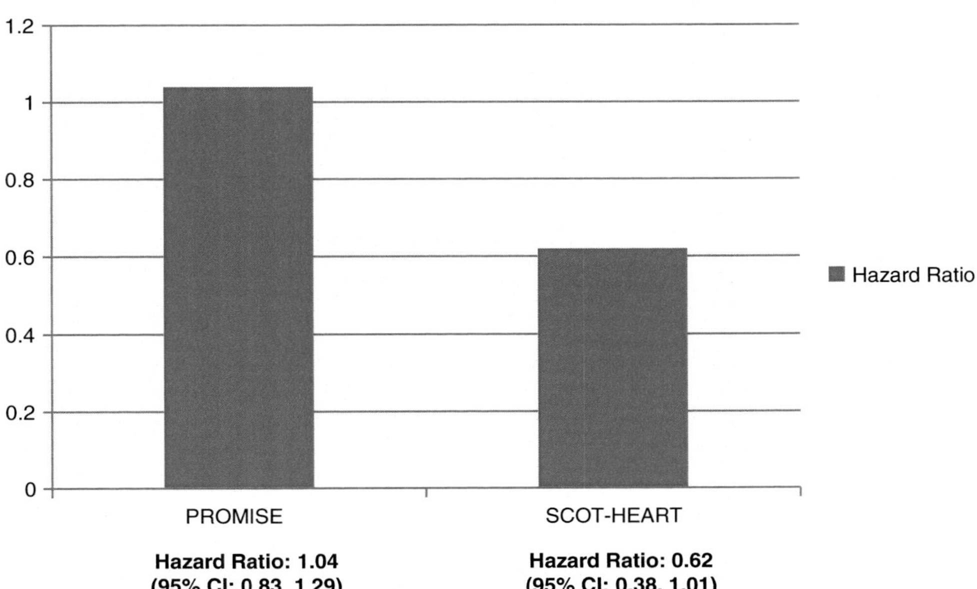

Fig. 21.5 Primary results from the PROMISE and SCOT-HEART trials revealing that CCTA was equally effective at near-term clinical outcomes

Table 21.2 A synopsis of the available evidence with CCTA for multicenter registries and from randomized or controlled clinical trials

		Randomized clinical or controlled clinical trials	
High quality:	**Multicenter registries**	**Near-term outcomes**	**Long-term outcomes**
Diagnostic accuracy	****	***	
Risk assessment	*****		*****
ED		*****	

A total of 5 stars are available for this ranking

The upcoming large clinical trials can further refine our evidence on the clinical utility of CCTA. The public and private payer community has largely been unresponsive to this evidence base and it may be that the evidence has been amassed so rapidly and that their ability to maintain current knowledge base has been slow to respond. Despite this, certainly the evidence supports a re-evaluation of the national and private payer policies for CCTA. This author's opinion on the quality of evidence with CCTA is reported in Table 21.2.

References

1. Greenland P, Alpert JS, Beller GA, Benjamin EJ, Budoff MJ, Fayad ZA, Foster E, Hlatky MA, Hodgson JM, Kushner FG, Lauer MS, Shaw LJ, Smith Jr SC, Taylor AJ, Weintraub WS, Wenger NK, Jacobs AK, Smith Jr SC, Anderson JL, Albert N, Buller CE, Creager MA, Ettinger SM, Guyton RA, Halperin JL, Hochman JS, Kushner FG, Nishimura R, Ohman EM, Page RL, Stevenson WG, Tarkington LG, Yancy CW, American College of Cardiology Foundation/American Heart Association Task Force on Practice Guidelines. 2010 ACCF/AHA guideline for assessment of cardiovascular risk in asymptomatic adults: a report of the American College of Cardiology Foundation/American Heart Association Task Force on practice guidelines. J Am Coll Cardiol. 2010;56:e50–103.
2. Detrano R, Guerci AD, Carr JJ, Bild DE, Burke G, Folsom AR, Liu K, Shea S, Szklo M, Bluemke DA, O'Leary DH, Tracy R, Watson K, Wong ND, Kronmal RA. Coronary calcium as a predictor of coronary events in four racial or ethnic groups. N Engl J Med. 2008;358:1336–45.
3. Budoff MJ, Shaw LJ, Liu ST, Weinstein SR, Mosler TP, Tseng PH, Flores FR, Callister TQ, Raggi P, Berman DS. Long-term prognosis associated with coronary calcification: observations from a registry of 25,253 patients. J Am Coll Cardiol. 2007;49:1860–70.
4. Erbel R, Mohlenkamp S, Moebus S, Schmermund A, Lehmann N, Stang A, Dragano N, Gronemeyer D, Seibel R, Kalsch H, Brocker-Preuss M, Mann K, Siegrist J, Jockel KH, Heinz Nixdorf Recall Study Investigative Group. Coronary risk stratification, discrimination, and reclassification improvement based on quantification of subclinical coronary atherosclerosis: the Heinz Nixdorf Recall study. J Am Coll Cardiol. 2010;56:1397–406.
5. Pencina MJ, D'Agostino Sr RB, D'Agostino Jr RB, Vasan RS. Evaluating the added predictive ability of a new marker: from area under the ROC curve to reclassification and beyond. Stat Med. 2008;27:157–72; discussion 207–12.
6. Polonsky TS, McClelland RL, Jorgensen NW, Bild DE, Burke GL, Guerci AD, Greenland P. Coronary artery calcium score and risk classification for coronary heart disease prediction. JAMA. 2010; 303:1610–6.
7. Yeboah J, McClelland RL, Polonsky TS, Burke GL, Sibley CT, O'Leary D, Carr JJ, Goff DC, Greenland P, Herrington DM. Comparison of novel risk markers for improvement in cardiovascular risk assessment in intermediate-risk individuals. JAMA. 2012; 308:788–95.
8. Wilson PW, Pencina M, Jacques P, Selhub J, D'Agostino Sr R, O'Donnell CJ. C-reactive protein and reclassification of cardiovascular risk in the Framingham Heart Study. Circ Cardiovasc Qual Outcomes. 2008;1:92–7.
9. Blaha MJ, Budoff MJ, DeFilippis AP, Blankstein R, Rivera JJ, Agatston A, O'Leary DH, Lima J, Blumenthal RS, Nasir K. Associations between C-reactive protein, coronary artery calcium, and cardiovascular events: implications for the JUPITER population from MESA, a population-based cohort study. Lancet. 2011; 378:684–92.
10. Rozanski A, Gransar H, Shaw LJ, Kim J, Miranda-Peats L, Wong ND, Rana JS, Orakzai R, Hayes SW, Friedman JD, Thomson LE, Polk D, Min J, Budoff MJ, Berman DS. Impact of coronary artery calcium scanning on coronary risk factors and downstream testing the EISNER (Early Identification of Subclinical Atherosclerosis by Noninvasive Imaging Research) prospective randomized trial. J Am Coll Cardiol. 2011;57:1622–32.
11. O'Malley PG, Feuerstein IM, Taylor AJ. Impact of electron beam tomography, with or without case management, on motivation, behavioral change, and cardiovascular risk profile: a randomized controlled trial. JAMA. 2003;289:2215–23.
12. Hoffmann U, Truong QA, Schoenfeld DA, Chou ET, Woodard PK, Nagurney JT, Pope JH, Hauser TH, White CS, Weiner SG, Kalanjian S, Mullins ME, Mikati I, Peacock WF, Zakroysky P, Hayden D, Goehler A, Lee H, Gazelle GS, Wiviott SD, Fleg JL, Udelson JE, Investigators R-I. Coronary CT angiography versus standard evaluation in acute chest pain. N Engl J Med. 2012;367:299–308.
13. Litt HI, Gatsonis C, Snyder B, Singh H, Miller CD, Entrikin DW, Leaming JM, Gavin LJ, Pacella CB, Hollander JE. CT angiography for safe discharge of patients with possible acute coronary syndromes. N Engl J Med. 2012;366:1393–403.
14. Goldstein JA, Chinnaiyan KM, Abidov A, Achenbach S, Berman DS, Hayes SW, Hoffmann U, Lesser JR, Mikati IA, O'Neil BJ, Shaw LJ, Shen MY, Valeti US, Raff GL, Investigators C-S. The CT-STAT (coronary computed tomographic angiography for systematic triage of acute chest pain patients to treatment) trial. J Am Coll Cardiol. 2011;58:1414–22.
15. Goodacre S, Thokala P, Carroll C, Stevens JW, Leaviss J, Al Khalaf M, Collinson P, Morris F, Evans P, Wang J. Systematic review, meta-analysis and economic modelling of diagnostic strategies for suspected acute coronary syndrome. Health Technol Assess. 2013;17:v–vi, 1–188.
16. D'Ascenzo F, Cerrato E, Biondi-Zoccai G, Omede P, Sciuto F, Presutti DG, Quadri G, Raff GL, Goldstein JA, Litt H, Frati G, Reed MJ, Moretti C, Gaita F. Coronary computed tomographic angiography for detection of coronary artery disease in patients presenting to the emergency department with chest pain: a meta-analysis of randomized clinical trials. Eur Heart J Cardiovasc Imaging. 2013;14:782–9.
17. Nasis A, Meredith IT, Sud PS, Cameron JD, Troupis JM, Seneviratne SK. Long-term outcome after CT angiography in patients with possible acute coronary syndrome. Radiology. 2014; 132680.

18. Udelson JE, Beshansky JR, Ballin DS, Feldman JA, Griffith JL, Handler J, Heller GV, Hendel RC, Pope JH, Ruthazer R, Spiegler EJ, Woolard RH, Selker HP. Myocardial perfusion imaging for evaluation and triage of patients with suspected acute cardiac ischemia: a randomized controlled trial. JAMA. 2002;288: 2693–700.
19. Patel MR, Peterson ED, Dai D, Brennan JM, Redberg RF, Anderson HV, Brindis RG, Douglas PS. Low diagnostic yield of elective coronary angiography. N Engl J Med. 2010;362:886–95.
20. Min JK, Leipsic J, Pencina MJ, Berman DS, Koo BK, van Mieghem C, Erglis A, Lin FY, Dunning AM, Apruzzese P, Budoff MJ, Cole JH, Jaffer FA, Leon MB, Malpeso J, Mancini GB, Park SJ, Schwartz RS, Shaw LJ, Mauri L. Diagnostic accuracy of fractional flow reserve from anatomic CT angiography. JAMA. 2012;308:1237–45.
21. Budoff MJ, Dowe D, Jollis JG, Gitter M, Sutherland J, Halamert E, Scherer M, Bellinger R, Martin A, Benton R, Delago A, Min JK. Diagnostic performance of 64-multidetector row coronary computed tomographic angiography for evaluation of coronary artery stenosis in individuals without known coronary artery disease: results from the prospective multicenter ACCURACY (Assessment by Coronary Computed Tomographic Angiography of Individuals Undergoing Invasive Coronary Angiography) trial. J Am Coll Cardiol. 2008;52:1724–32.
22. Miller JM, Rochitte CE, Dewey M, Arbab-Zadeh A, Niinuma H, Gottlieb I, Paul N, Clouse ME, Shapiro EP, Hoe J, Lardo AC, Bush DE, de Roos A, Cox C, Brinker J, Lima JA. Diagnostic performance of coronary angiography by 64-row CT. N Engl J Med. 2008;359: 2324–36.
23. Meijboom WB, van Mieghem CA, Mollet NR, Pugliese F, Weustink AC, van Pelt N, Cademartiri F, Nieman K, Boersma E, de Jaegere P, Krestin GP, de Feyter PJ. 64-slice computed tomography coronary angiography in patients with high, intermediate, or low pretest probability of significant coronary artery disease. J Am Coll Cardiol. 2007;50:1469–75.
24. Janne d'Othee B, Siebert U, Cury R, Jadvar H, Dunn EJ, Hoffmann U. A systematic review on diagnostic accuracy of CT-based detection of significant coronary artery disease. Eur J Radiol. 2008;65: 449–61.
25. Shaw LJ, Hage FG, Berman DS, Hachamovitch R, Iskandrian A. Prognosis in the era of comparative effectiveness research: where is nuclear cardiology now and where should it be? J Nucl Cardiol. 2012;19:1026–43.
26. Motoyama S, Kondo T, Sarai M, Sugiura A, Harigaya H, Sato T, Inoue K, Okumura M, Ishii J, Anno H, Virmani R, Ozaki Y, Hishida H, Narula J. Multislice computed tomographic characteristics of coronary lesions in acute coronary syndromes. J Am Coll Cardiol. 2007;50:319–26.
27. Motoyama S, Sarai M, Harigaya H, Anno H, Inoue K, Hara T, Naruse H, Ishii J, Hishida H, Wong ND, Virmani R, Kondo T, Ozaki Y, Narula J. Computed tomographic angiography characteristics of atherosclerotic plaques subsequently resulting in acute coronary syndrome. J Am Coll Cardiol. 2009;54:49–57.
28. Min JK, Dunning A, Lin FY, Achenbach S, Al-Mallah M, Budoff MJ, Cademartiri F, Callister TQ, Chang HJ, Cheng V, Chinnaiyan K, Chow BJ, Delago A, Hadamitzky M, Hausleiter J, Kaufmann P, Maffei E, Raff G, Shaw LJ, Villines T, Berman DS, CONFIRM Investigators. Age- and sex-related differences in all-cause mortality risk based on coronary computed tomography angiography findings results from the International Multicenter CONFIRM (Coronary CT Angiography Evaluation for Clinical Outcomes: an International Multicenter Registry) of 23,854 patients without known coronary artery disease. J Am Coll Cardiol. 2011;58:849–60.
29. Small GR, Yam Y, Chen L, Ahmed O, Al-Mallah M, Berman DS, Cheng VY, Chinnaiyan K, Raff G, Villines TC, Achenbach S, Budoff MJ, Cademartiri F, Callister TQ, Chang HJ, Delago A, Dunning A, Hadamitzky M, Hausleiter J, Kaufmann P, Lin F, Maffei E, Min JK, Shaw LJ, Chow BJ. Prognostic assessment of coronary artery bypass patients with 64-slice computed tomography angiography: anatomical information is incremental to clinical risk prediction. J Am Coll Cardiol. 2011;58:2389–95.
30. Hadamitzky M, Achenbach S, Al-Mallah M, Berman D, Budoff M, Cademartiri F, Callister T, Chang HJ, Cheng V, Chinnaiyan K, Chow BJ, Cury R, Delago A, Dunning A, Feuchtner G, Gomez M, Kaufmann P, Kim YJ, Leipsic J, Lin FY, Maffei E, Min JK, Raff G, Shaw LJ, Villines TC, Hausleiter J, CONFIRM Investigators. Optimized prognostic score for coronary computed tomographic angiography: results from the CONFIRM registry (COronary CT Angiography EvaluatioN For Clinical Outcomes: an InteRnational Multicenter Registry). J Am Coll Cardiol. 2013;62:468–76.
31. Lin FY, Shaw LJ, Dunning AM, Labounty TM, Choi JH, Weinsaft JW, Koduru S, Gomez MJ, Delago AJ, Callister TQ, Berman DS, Min JK. Mortality risk in symptomatic patients with nonobstructive coronary artery disease: a prospective 2-center study of 2,583 patients undergoing 64-detector row coronary computed tomographic angiography. J Am Coll Cardiol. 2011;58:510–9.
32. Min JK, Dunning A, Lin FY, Achenbach S, Al-Mallah MH, Berman DS, Budoff MJ, Cademartiri F, Callister TQ, Chang HJ, Cheng V, Chinnaiyan KM, Chow B, Delago A, Hadamitzky M, Hausleiter J, Karlsberg RP, Kaufmann P, Maffei E, Nasir K, Pencina MJ, Raff GL, Shaw LJ, Villines TC. Rationale and design of the CONFIRM (COronary CT Angiography EvaluatioN For Clinical Outcomes: an InteRnational Multicenter) Registry. J Cardiovasc Comput Tomogr. 2011;5:84–92.
33. Leipsic J, Taylor CM, Gransar H, Shaw LJ, Ahmadi A, Thompson A, Humphries K, Berman DS, Hausleiter J, Achenbach S, Al-Mallah M, Budoff MJ, Cademartiri F, Callister TQ, Chang HJ, Chow BJ, Cury RC, Delago AJ, Dunning AL, Feuchtner GM, Hadamitzky M, Kaufmann PA, Lin FY, Chinnaiyan KM, Maffei E, Raff GL, Villines TC, Gomez MJ, Min JK. Sex-based prognostic implications of nonobstructive coronary artery disease: results from the International Multicenter CONFIRM Study. Radiology. 2014:140269.
34. Hulten E, Villines TC, Cheezum MK, Berman DS, Dunning A, Achenbach S, Al-Mallah M, Budoff MJ, Cademartiri F, Callister TQ, Chang HJ, Cheng VY, Chinnaiyan K, Chow BJ, Cury RC, Delago A, Feuchtner G, Hadamitzky M, Hausleiter J, Kaufmann PA, Karlsberg RP, Kim YJ, Leipsic J, Lin FY, Maffei E, Plank F, Raff GL, Labounty TM, Shaw LJ, Min JK, CONFIRM Investigators. Usefulness of coronary computed tomography angiography to predict mortality and myocardial infarction among Caucasian, African and East Asian ethnicities (from the CONFIRM [Coronary CT Angiography Evaluation for Clinical Outcomes: an International Multicenter] Registry). Am J Cardiol. 2013;111:479–85.
35. Min JK, Labounty TM, Gomez MJ, Achenbach S, Al-Mallah M, Budoff MJ, Cademartiri F, Callister TQ, Chang HJ, Cheng V, Chinnaiyan KM, Chow B, Cury R, Delago A, Dunning A, Feuchtner G, Hadamitzky M, Hausleiter J, Kaufmann P, Kim YJ, Leipsic J, Lin FY, Maffei E, Raff G, Shaw LJ, Villines TC, Berman DS. Incremental prognostic value of coronary computed tomographic angiography over coronary artery calcium score for risk prediction of major adverse cardiac events in asymptomatic diabetic individuals. Atherosclerosis. 2014;232:298–304.
36. Rana JS, Dunning A, Achenbach S, Al-Mallah M, Budoff MJ, Cademartiri F, Callister TQ, Chang HJ, Cheng VY, Chinnaiyan K, Chow BJ, Cury R, Delago A, Feuchtner G, Hadamitzky M, Hausleiter J, Kaufmann P, Karlsberg RP, Kim YJ, Leipsic J, Labounty TM, Lin FY, Maffei E, Raff G, Villines TC, Shaw LJ, Berman DS, Min JK. Differences in prevalence, extent, severity, and prognosis of coronary artery disease among patients with and without diabetes undergoing coronary computed tomography angiography: results from 10,110 individuals from the CONFIRM (COronary CT Angiography

EvaluatioN For Clinical Outcomes): an InteRnational Multicenter Registry. Diabetes Care. 2012;35:1787–94.

37. Chow BJ, Ahmed O, Small G, Alghamdi AA, Yam Y, Chen L, Wells GA. Prognostic value of CT angiography in coronary bypass patients. JACC Cardiovasc Imaging. 2011;4:496–502.
38. Otaki Y, Gransar H, Berman DS, Cheng VY, Dey D, Lin FY, Achenbach S, Al-Mallah M, Budoff MJ, Cademartiri F, Callister TQ, Chang HJ, Chinnaiyan K, Chow BJ, Delago A, Hadamitzky M, Hausleiter J, Kaufmann P, Maffei E, Raff G, Shaw LJ, Villines TC, Dunning A, Min JK. Impact of family history of coronary artery disease in young individuals (from the CONFIRM registry). Am J Cardiol. 2013;111:1081–6.
39. Hadamitzky M, Taubert S, Deseive S, Byrne RA, Martinoff S, Schomig A, Hausleiter J. Prognostic value of coronary computed tomography angiography during 5 years of follow-up in patients with suspected coronary artery disease. Eur Heart J. 2013;34:3277–85.
40. Ostrom MP, Gopal A, Ahmadi N, Nasir K, Yang E, Kakadiaris I, Flores F, Mao SS, Budoff MJ. Mortality incidence and the severity of coronary atherosclerosis assessed by computed tomography angiography. J Am Coll Cardiol. 2008;52:1335–43.
41. Andreini D, Pontone G, Mushtaq S, Bartorelli AL, Bertella E, Antonioli L, Formenti A, Cortinovis S, Veglia F, Annoni A, Agostoni P, Montorsi P, Ballerini G, Fiorentini C, Pepi M. A long-term prognostic value of coronary CT angiography in suspected coronary artery disease. JACC Cardiovasc Imaging. 2012;5:690–701.
42. Metz LD, Beattie M, Hom R, Redberg RF, Grady D, Fleischmann KE. The prognostic value of normal exercise myocardial perfusion imaging and exercise echocardiography: a meta-analysis. J Am Coll Cardiol. 2007;49:227–37.
43. Min JK, Berman DS, Dunning A, Achenbach S, Al-Mallah M, Budoff MJ, Cademartiri F, Callister TQ, Chang HJ, Cheng V, Chinnaiyan K, Chow BJ, Cury R, Delago A, Feuchtner G, Hadamitzky M, Hausleiter J, Kaufmann P, Karlsberg RP, Kim YJ, Leipsic J, Lin FY, Maffei E, Plank F, Raff G, Villines T, Labounty TM, Shaw LJ. All-cause mortality benefit of coronary revascularization vs. medical therapy in patients without known coronary artery disease undergoing coronary computed tomographic angiography: results from CONFIRM (COronary CT Angiography EvaluatioN For Clinical Outcomes: an InteRnational Multicenter Registry). Eur Heart J. 2012;33:3088–97.
44. Fihn SD, Gardin JM, Abrams J, Berra K, Blankenship JC, Dallas AP, Douglas PS, Foody JM, Gerber TC, Hinderliter AL, King 3rd SB, Kligfield PD, Krumholz HM, Kwong RY, Lim MJ, Linderbaum JA, Mack MJ, Munger MA, Prager RL, Sabik JF, Shaw LJ, Sikkema JD, Smith Jr CR, Smith Jr SC, Spertus JA, Williams SV, American College of Cardiology Foundation, American Heart Association Task Force on Practice Group, American College of Physicians, American Association for Thoracic Surgery, Preventive Cardiovascular Nurses Association, Society for Cardiovascular Angiography and Interventions, and Society of Thoracic Surgeons. 2012 ACCF/AHA/ACP/AATS/PCNA/SCAI/STS guideline for the diagnosis and management of patients with stable ischemic heart disease: a report of the American College of Cardiology Foundation/American Heart Association Task Force on Practice Guidelines, and the American College of Physicians, American Association for Thoracic Surgery, Preventive Cardiovascular Nurses Association, Society for Cardiovascular Angiography and Interventions, and Society of Thoracic Surgeons. J Am Coll Cardiol. 2012;60:e44–164.
45. American College of Radiology Imaging Network. Rescue: an ACRIN cardiovascular clinical trial. A study for patients with stable angina-comparing two methods of evaluating coronary artery disease [Internet] Accessed 11 Nov 2014. Available at: www.rescue-trial.org.
46. PROMISE: prospective multicenter imagining study for evaluation of chest pain. [Internet] Accessed 11 Nov 2014. Available at: https://www.promisetrial.org/.
47. ISCHMIA Study. [Internet]. Available at: https://www.ischemiatrial.org/. Accessed 11 Nov 2014.
48. Douglas PS, Hoffmann U. Anatomical versus functional testing for coronary artery disease. The New England Journal of Medicine. 2015;373:91.
49. Investigators S-H. CT coronary angiography in patients with suspected angina due to coronary heart disease (SCOT-HEART): an open-label, parallel-group, multicentre trial. Lancet. 2015; 385:2383–91.

22 Cardiothoracic Surgery Applications: Virtual CT Imaging Approaches to Procedural Planning

Jerold S. Shinbane, Craig J. Baker, Mark J. Cunningham, and Vaughn A. Starnes

Abstract

Cardiovascular computed tomographic angiography (CCTA) has led to a paradigm shift in planning and performance of cardiothoracic surgical procedures, providing information essential to decisions regarding surgical intervention. As the operating room and interventional cardiology laboratory have evolved, merging into a hybrid space, CCTA has assumed an essential role in determination of the optimal therapeutic modality and path of approach for percutaneous, minimally invasive robotic and open surgical approaches in this setting. CCTA has particular significance to planning of reoperation for coronary artery disease, valvular heart disease, pericardial disease, congenital heart disease, cardiac masses, and advanced heart failure. Communication of the data beyond the written report can be achieved through images relevant for orientation and interventional approach. Review of these virtual views with the multidisciplinary team is important for maximal application and impact of this technology.

Keywords

Anomalous Coronary Arteries • Aortic Surgery • Cardiovascular Computed Tomographic Angiography • Cardiothoracic Surgery • Computed Tomography • Congenital Heart Disease • Coronary Artery Bypass Graft Surgery • Minimally Invasive Robotic Surgery • Percutaneous Pulmonary Valve Replacement • Transcatheter Aortic Valve Implantation

Introduction

Cardiovascular computed tomographic angiography (CCTA) has led to a paradigm shift in planning and performance of cardiothoracic surgical procedures, providing information essential to decisions regarding proceeding with surgical intervention, facilitation of pre-surgical planning, and assessment for surgical efficacy and sequelae. CCTA provides a digitalized and individualized "Netter" illustration of the relationships between thoracic skeletal, vascular, visceral, and cardiac structures (Fig. 22.1, Video 1). Full field 3-D reconstructions utilizing editing software enable visualization of multidimensional planes. Assessment of these views is important for planning surgical access to target structures while avoiding important vascular and visceral thoracic structures which may be in close proximity to the incisional plane.

Electronic supplementary material The online version of this chapter (doi:10.1007/978-3-319-28219-0_22) contains supplementary material, which is available to authorized users.

J.S. Shinbane, MD, FACC, FHRS, FSCCT (✉)
Division of Cardiovascular Medicine, Department of Internal Medicine, Keck School of Medicine of the University of Southern California, 1520 San Pablo Suite 300, Los Angeles, CA 90033, USA
e-mail: shinbane@usc.edu

C.J. Baker, MD, FACS • M.J. Cunningham, MD
Department of Surgery, Keck School of Medicine of the University of Southern California, Los Angeles, CA USA

V.A. Starnes, MD
Cardiovascular Thoracic Institute, Department of Surgery, Keck School of Medicine of the University of Southern California, Los Angeles, CA USA

M.J. Budoff, J.S. Shinbane (eds.), *Cardiac CT Imaging: Diagnosis of Cardiovascular Disease*, DOI 10.1007/978-3-319-28219-0_22

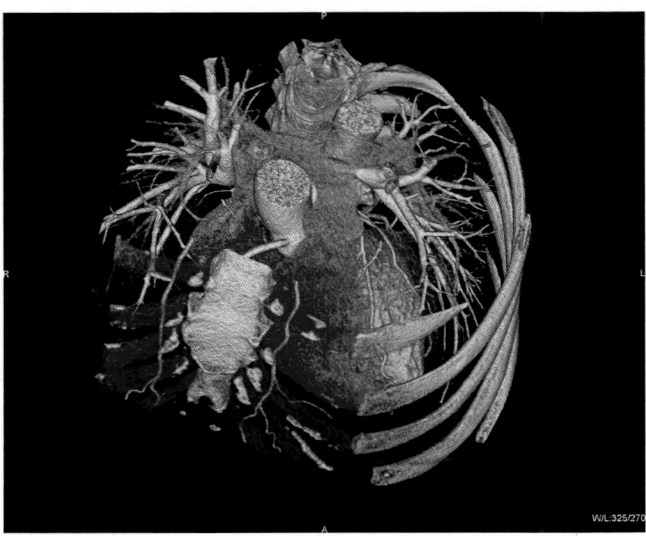

Fig. 22.1 A 3-D reconstruction demonstrating the relationships between thoracic skeletal, vascular, visceral, and cardiac structures

The operating room and interventional cardiology laboratory have evolved, merging into a hybrid space utilized by a multidisciplinary team of surgeons, interventional cardiologists and imagers. CCTA plays an essential role in decisions and guidance for determination of the optimal therapeutic modality and path of approach for percutaneous, minimally invasive robotic and open surgical approaches in this setting. Communication of the data beyond the written report can be achieved through images relevant for orientation and interventional approach. Review of these virtual views with the multidisciplinary team is important for maximal application and impact of this technology.

Imaging Related to Surgery for Coronary Artery Disease

CCTA has particular significance to planning of re-operation for coronary artery disease, as the number of prior operations incrementally increases risk. At re-operation, the majority of adverse events occur during sternotomy or pre-bypass dissection due to injury to bypass grafts and great vessels [1, 2]. CCTA can visualize high risk sternotomy anatomy through demonstration of structures coursing immediately posterior to the sternum which may require special precautions (Figs. 22.2 and 22.3). High risk features on CCTA include the right ventricle or aorta less than 1 cm from chest wall and coronary artery bypass grafts coursing across the midline less than 1 cm from the sternum [3]. Pre-operative CCTA assessment of the relationship of cardiovascular structures to the sternum has been used to plan alternate approaches in patients with high risk sternotomy anatomy, including: cancellation of surgery, non-sternotomy incisional approach, deep hypothermic cardiac arrest, initiation of peripheral cardiopulmonary bypass, and peripheral vascular dissection and exposure prior to midline sternotomy [3, 4]. Skeletal defects, traumatic injury, metastatic disease, abscess, and osteomyelitis in the sternum can also be identified (Figs. 22.4 and 22.5).

In the setting of initial surgery as well as re-operation for obstructive coronary artery disease, the use of CCTA to define native coronary anatomy has limitations due to calcification of native coronary arteries and inability to define collateral flow; therefore invasive coronary arteriography remains the gold standard. CCTA can be useful in assessing graft location and graft patency (Fig. 22.6). CCTA may be useful prior to recurrent coronary artery bypass graft surgery in situations where cardiac catheterization was unable to completely define graft anatomy, particularly as to whether a graft was occluded versus unable to be cannulated at cardiac catheterization. CCTA in unoperated as well as previously operated settings can define the location and patency of the left and right internal mammary arteries (Fig. 22.7). Depending on the field of view, CCTA can assess for subclavian artery stenoses. Surgical clip artifacts may make assessment of grafts more challenging, particularly at the anastomosis site with the native coronary artery (Fig. 22.8). Aortic characteristics, such as profound calcification/porcelain aorta, are important for surgical approaches requiring cross-clamping of the aorta or implantation of saphenous vein grafts into the aorta.

Imaging Related to Surgery for Valvular Disease

CCTA for Surgical Versus Percutaneous Approach to Aortic Valve Disease

CCTA has become essential to decision-making and preplanning related to transcatheter aortic valve implantation (TAVI), minimally invasive robotic or open surgical approaches for aortic valve replacement. Percutaneous approaches employ TAVI balloon-expandable and self-expanding valves [5–7]. CCTA provides data for decisions as to the feasibility of versus contraindication to TAVI access routes for percutaneous valve deployment including transfemoral, transapical subclavian artery, or direct aortic approaches [8, 9]. CCTA imaged anatomy limiting a transfemoral or aortic route include peripheral arterial diameter limitations based on catheter size, aortic tortuousity, high risk atheromas, severe vascular calcification, chronic dissections and aneurysms. CCTA related factors and potential limitations for consideration of a transapical approach to TAVI include the morphology and location of the left ventricular apex, alignment of the left ventricular axis to the left ventricular outflow tract, significant septal hypertrophy and presence of ventricular thrombi.

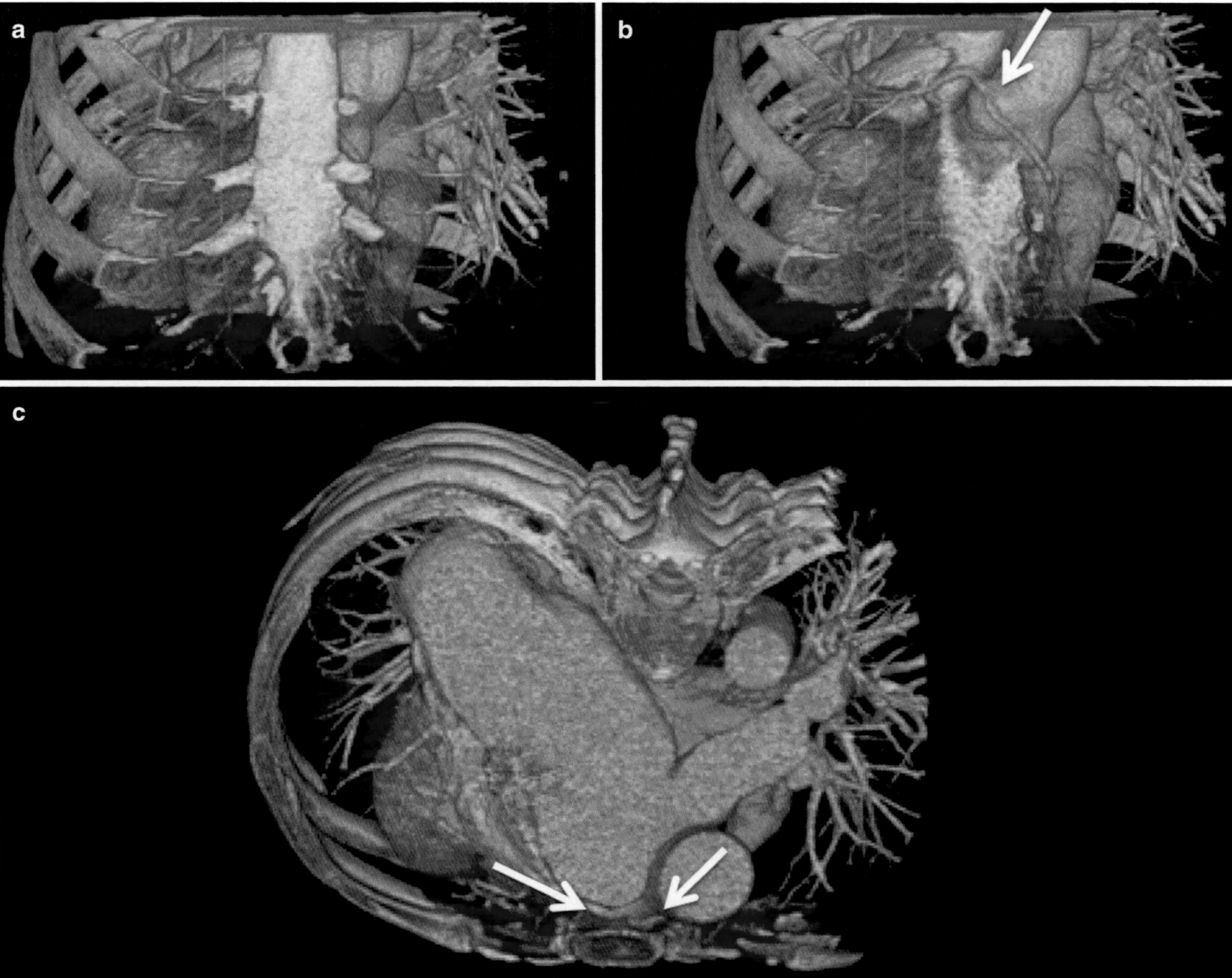

Fig. 22.2 Anomalous coronary arteries coursing in close proximity to the sternum. Panel (**a**) A 3-D volume rendered view demonstrating the sternum. Panel (**b**) A 3-D volume rendered view with the sternum partially edited to demonstrate the anomalous coronary circulation (*arrow*). Panel (**c**) A 3-D volume rendered view demonstrating the relationship of the anomalous coronary arteries (*arrows*) to the sternum

Aortic annulus characteristics can also limit use of TAVI and therefore require operative approaches in patients who are otherwise candidates for surgery. CCTA is the gold standard for annular geometry, measurements and physiology for assessment of valve sizing and potential contraindication to a TAVI approach based on annulus size and morphology (Fig. 22.9). The annulus is often ovoid rather than circular in shape, and can have variation in cusp length, height and relation to the coronary artery ostia. Annular dynamic morphologic changes occur throughout the cardiac cycle with assessment for the largest diameter preferable [10]. Potential annular eccentricity and elasticity therefore make detailed coaxial characterization and measurement of the annulus essential for decisions as to a percutaneous versus surgical approach and appropriate sizing of valves when TAVI is an option. In plane aligned aortic annular measurements of maximum and minimum diameter, area, and circumference at the attachments of all three aortic cusps, "hinge points" in a "virtual ring", are essential for accurate assessment and provide virtual orientation for the TAVI team. The optimal fluoroscopic view for coaxial deployment should be noted by the RAO/LAO and cranial/caudal viewing angle of the "virtual ring" created by these "hinge points" [9, 11].

Detailed CCTA annular characterization and measurements are essential to avoid undersizing or oversizing of the valve relative to the annulus and avoidance of issues related to the coronary artery ostia. Valve undersizing can lead to valve embolization or perivalvular leak. CCTA characteristics, including the relationship of valve diameter relative to average annular diameter, degree of aortic root calcification, angulation between the left ventricular outflow tract and the ascending aorta, and eccentricity of the annulus, are factors potentially predictive of post-procedure regurgitation [12–14]. CCTA aortic annular sizing algorithms developed to modestly oversize the implanted valve have led to reduction of perivalvular regurgitation [15]. Differences in individual TAVI device characteristics and available sizes are also important to decisions based on CCTA dimensions in order to avoid significant oversizing [16]. Valve oversizing can lead to annular rupture. Additionally, moderate to severe sub-annular left ventricular outflow tract calcium predicts rupture [17].

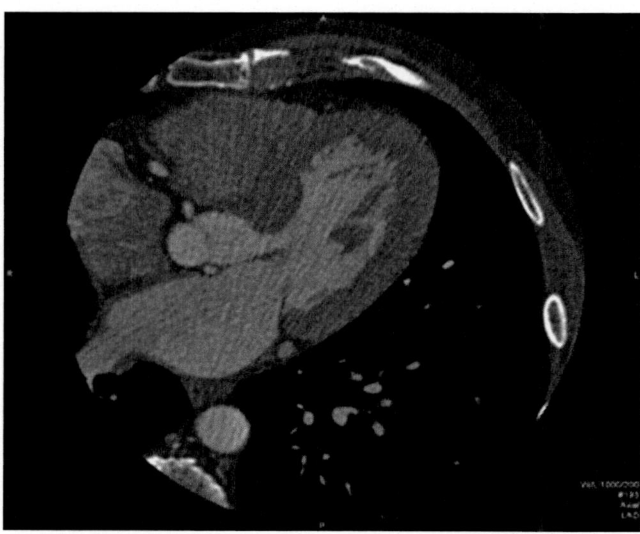

Fig. 22.3 A 2-D axial view showing the right ventricle coursing immediately posterior to the sternum

Relationships and characteristics of the annulus in relation to the coronary artery ostia must be taken into account with CCTA analysis. Definition of the quantitative relationship between the aortic annulus, aortic sinuses, sinotubular junction and the coronary artery ostia are important in order to avoid coronary artery compromise due to the device or atherosclerotic plaque with valve deployment. If the annular to ostial height is too small, the ostia could be covered by the device. The extent and morphology of annular and sub-annular calcification is important, as this atherosclerotic plaque can embolize into or partially or completely obstruct the coronary artery ostium [18–22]. Given the possibility of these complications, CCTA cardiovascular relationships to the sternum need to be noted for TAVI candidates, as the need for emergent conversion to an open sternotomy surgical approach is a potential scenario. TAVI can also lead to conduction abnormalities including high grade atrioventricular block. CCTA findings of deep valve placement relative to the annulus, severe calcification of the landing site, and prosthesis/patient mismatch have been associated with left bundle branch block and high grade atrioventricular block [23–28].

Multiple factors make CCTA assessment of the coronary arteries challenging in severe to critical aortic stenosis patients. Given the advanced age of many patients being considered for TAVI, as well as the underlying pathophysiology of calcific aortic stenosis, significant calcification of the coronary arteries is often present. From a CCTA image acquisition standpoint, acute beta blockade and sublingual nitroglycerin may be contraindicated as part of the CCTA imaging protocol in patients with severe to critical aortic

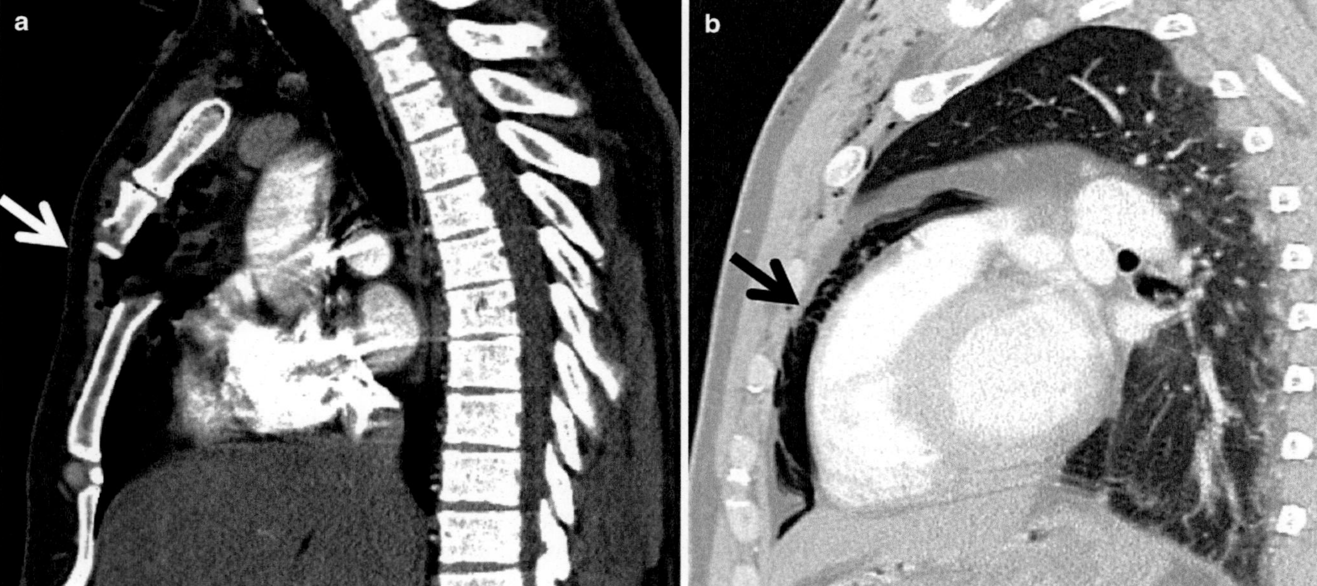

Fig. 22.4 Sagittal views demonstrating traumatic injury to the chest. Panel (**a**) Demonstration of sternal fracture (*arrow*). Panel (**b**) Demonstration of pneumopericardium (*arrow*)

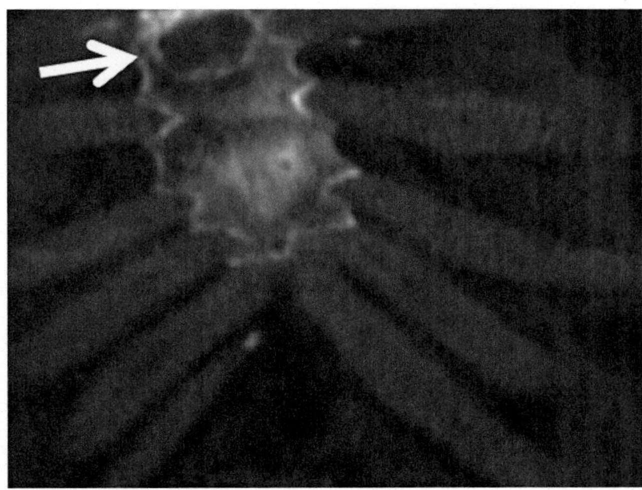

Fig. 22.5 Sternal metastasis in a patient with aortic dissection

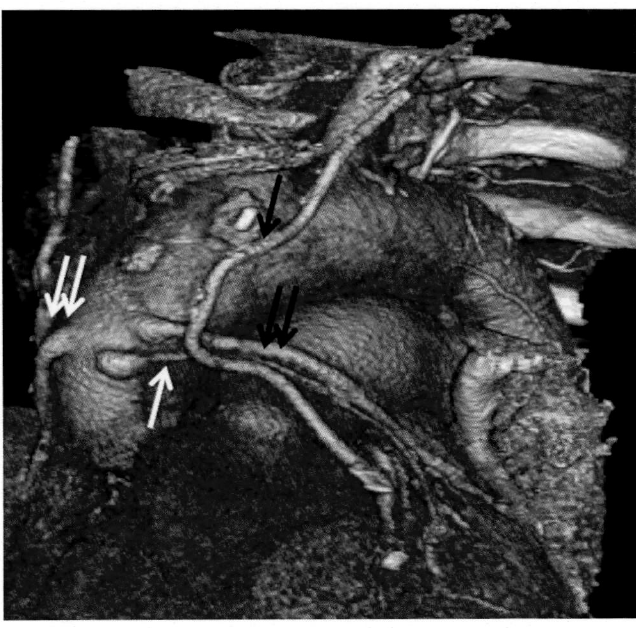

Fig. 22.6 A 3-D view showing a left internal mammary artery graft to the left anterior descending coronary artery (*black arrow*), saphenous vein graft to an obtuse marginal branch (*double black arrow*), saphenous vein graft to a diagonal artery (*white arrow*), and saphenous vein graft to the posterior descending artery (*double white arrow*)

stenosis, further limiting the ability to assess the coronary arteries. In other aortic valve scenarios, such as chronic severe aortic regurgitation, CCTA may be useful as an alternative to invasive cardiac catheterization prior to aortic valve surgery in patients with low to intermediate risk of coronary artery disease [29].

Endocarditis involving the aortic valve and aortic root can potentially lead to a higher risk of complications with invasive cardiac catheterization due to large aortic vegetations, aortic pseudo-aneurysms, and aortic root abscesses. CCTA can define the extent of infection through visualization of abscesses, pseudo- aneurysms, fistulas, the relationship of the coronary arteries to these structures, and presence of coronary artery disease (Figs. 22.10, 22.11, 22.12, and 22.13, Video 2) [30]. As these patients are sometimes critically ill, heart rate control may be difficult, but images may still be diagnostic. Prosthetic valve function can be viewed similarly to fluoroscopic views in order to assess mechanical valve motion as well as the presence of thrombus/vegetation (Fig. 22.14).

CCTA for Surgical Versus Percutaneous Approach to Pulmonary Valve Disease

With the advent of percutaneous pulmonary valve replacement, surgical decision-making for pulmonary valve disease must include assessment for the feasibility, risks and benefits of each approach [31–34]. CCTA can be useful in imaging many important decision-making factors including the size and degree of calcification of the pulmonary annulus, the presence of anomalous coronary arteries, and the 3-D relationship of the coronary arteries to the pulmonary annulus (Fig. 22.15) [35]. These factors are important to avoid complications such as compression of the coronary arteries with valve deployment, pulmonary regurgitation due to undersizing of the valve relative to the annulus, or conduit/annulus rupture due to oversizing of the valve relative to the annulus. The close proximity of anomalous coronary arteries or enlarged right heart structures to the sternum are important to identify in case emergent open surgical intervention is required.

CCTA for Surgical Versus Percutaneous Approach to Mitral Valve Disease

Research and clinical approaches to mitral valve disease include a spectrum of options including percutaneous clipping of valve leaflets, percutaneous mitral annuloplasty, transcatheter mitral valve replacement, minimally invasive robotic mitral valve repair or replacement, and open sternotomy mitral valve repair or replacement. Anatomic definition of the valve leaflets, annulus, subvalvular apparatus, relationship of the coronary arteries and cardiac veins to the left atrioventricular groove, and presence or absence of coronary artery disease are important components of CCTA analyses for decision-making and planning. Mitral annular size and geometry factors including valve tenting, height and tethering of the mitral leaflets variability in number of heads and insertions of the posterior papillary muscle, interpapillary muscle distance, mitral valve sphericity index, intercommissural and septolateral distance , and anterior and posterior circumference of the mitral annulus can be

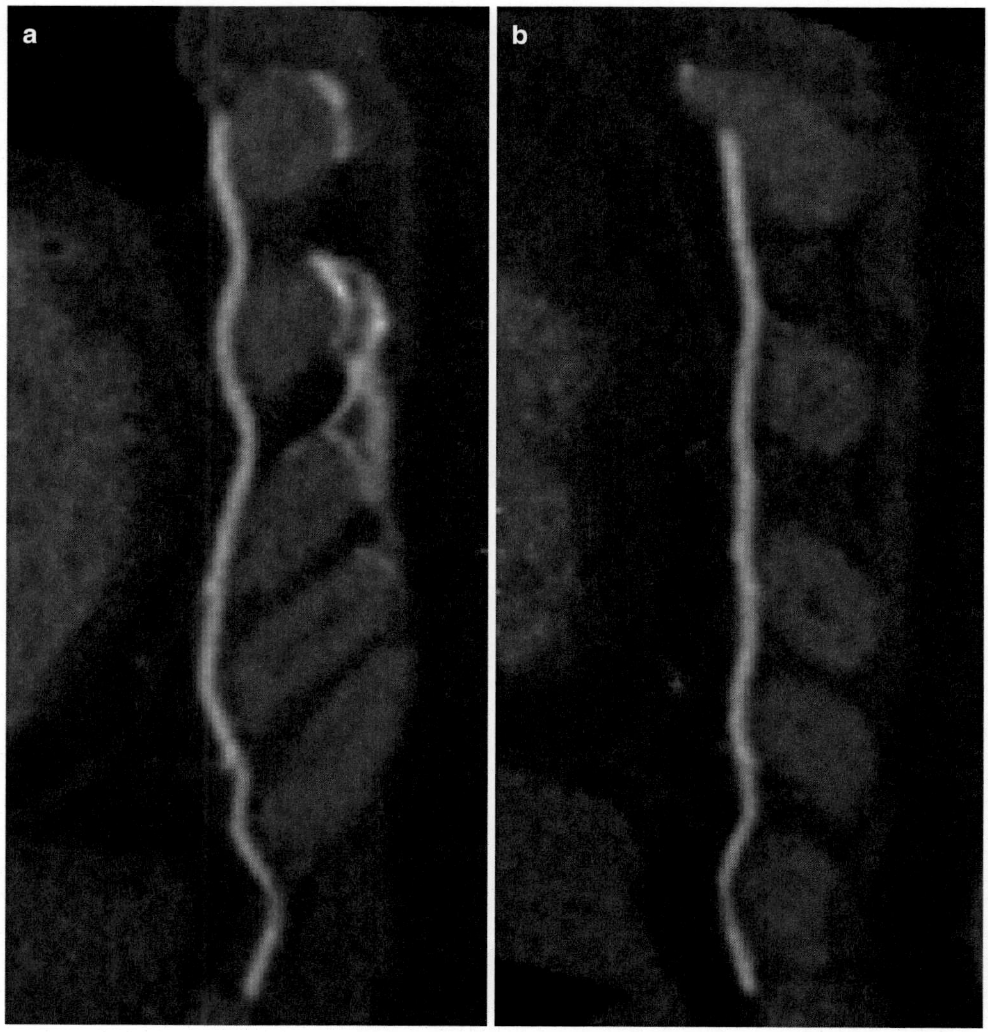

Fig. 22.7 CCTA visualization of the left (**a**) and right (**b**) internal mammary arteries

assessed [36–38]. Mitral annular contour has a complex 3-D non-planar saddle-shaped morphology. More simplified, planar measurements may be important to annular sizing for valve implantation [39].

The presence of significant aorto-iliac disease limiting peripheral cardiopulmonary bypass as well as the extent and location of mitral calcification can limit minimally invasive surgical approaches to mitral valve disease. CCTA can be useful to determine a right thoracotomy robotic versus sternotomy approach based on the degree of mitral valve calcification as well as the degree of aorto-iliac disease [40, 41]. CCTA is also useful as an alternative to coronary artery catheterization in low to intermediate risk patients in preoperative decisions for robotic mitral valve repair [42].

Assessment of the 3-D spatial relationship of the circumflex coronary artery in the left atrioventricular groove and the mitral annulus are important to the placement of the sewing ring in mitral annuloplasty surgeries for mitral regurgitation (Fig. 22.16) [43]. CCTA can assess the relationship of the coronary sinus / great cardiac vein, circumflex coronary artery and mitral annulus for novel percutaneous mitral annuloplasty procedures utilizing the cardiac vein system. There is great variability in these relationships, and segments where the circumflex coronary artery courses between the coronary sinus/great cardiac vein and the annulus can potentially compress the circumflex coronary artery [44–48].

Imaging Related to Surgery for Congenital Heart Disease

In congenital heart disease, the multitude of individual anomalies in the native state as well as palliative and corrective repairs in the operated state make the characterization of complete individualized anatomy in relation to the thorax important for hybrid lab interventional, minimally robotic and open surgical approaches. Decisions regarding

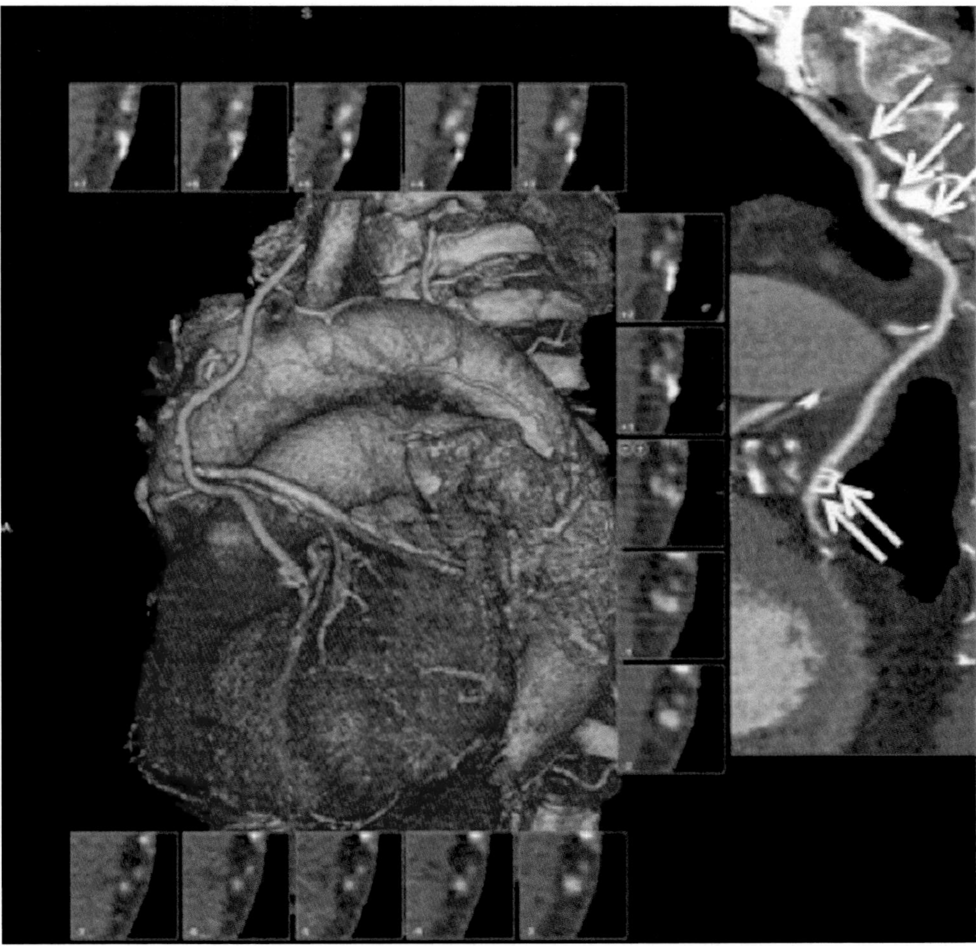

Fig. 22.8 Surgical clip artifacts (*white arrows*) with a clip (*double white arrow*) obscuring the anastomosis of the left internal mammary artery graft to the left anterior descending coronary artery

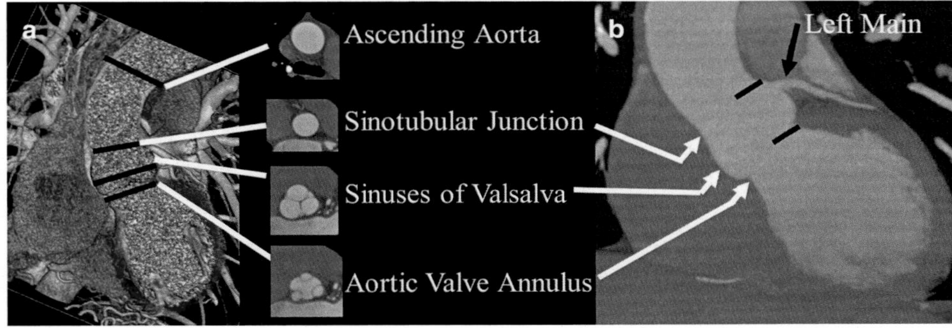

Fig. 22.9 Panel (**a**) A 3-D view of the aortic root demonstrating coaxial 2-D double oblique views of the aortic annulus, sinuses of Valsalva, sinotubular junction and ascending aorta. Panel (**b**) A 2-D double oblique maximal intensity projection demonstrating the distance from the left main coronary artery to the aortic valve annulus

the use of CCTA versus CMR depend on multiple factors, including the age of the patient, need for assessment of coronary anatomy, and presence of pacemakers or ICDs. CCTA is useful for determining anatomy and physiology important to surgical planning, particularly in patients with non-MR conditional pacemakers and implantable cardiac defibrillators as CMR can be limited in use in these settings [49–51]. The associated radiation with CCTA is a major issue, although techniques to minimize dose are being advanced [52–55].

Image definition of thoracic and abdominal situs, rotational abnormalities of thoracic vasculature, atrial and ventricular septal defects, shunts and fistulas, and anomalous large and small vessel anatomy can be achieved and defined in one 3-D data set (Figs. 22.17, 22.18, 22.19, 22.20, 22.21, and 22.22, Videos 3, 4, 5 and 6). CCTA is useful for specific questions that other imaging modalities are unable to answer as well as for creation of comprehensive roadmaps, particularly when the previous history of anatomy and previous surgical interventions are not known or well-defined. Innovations

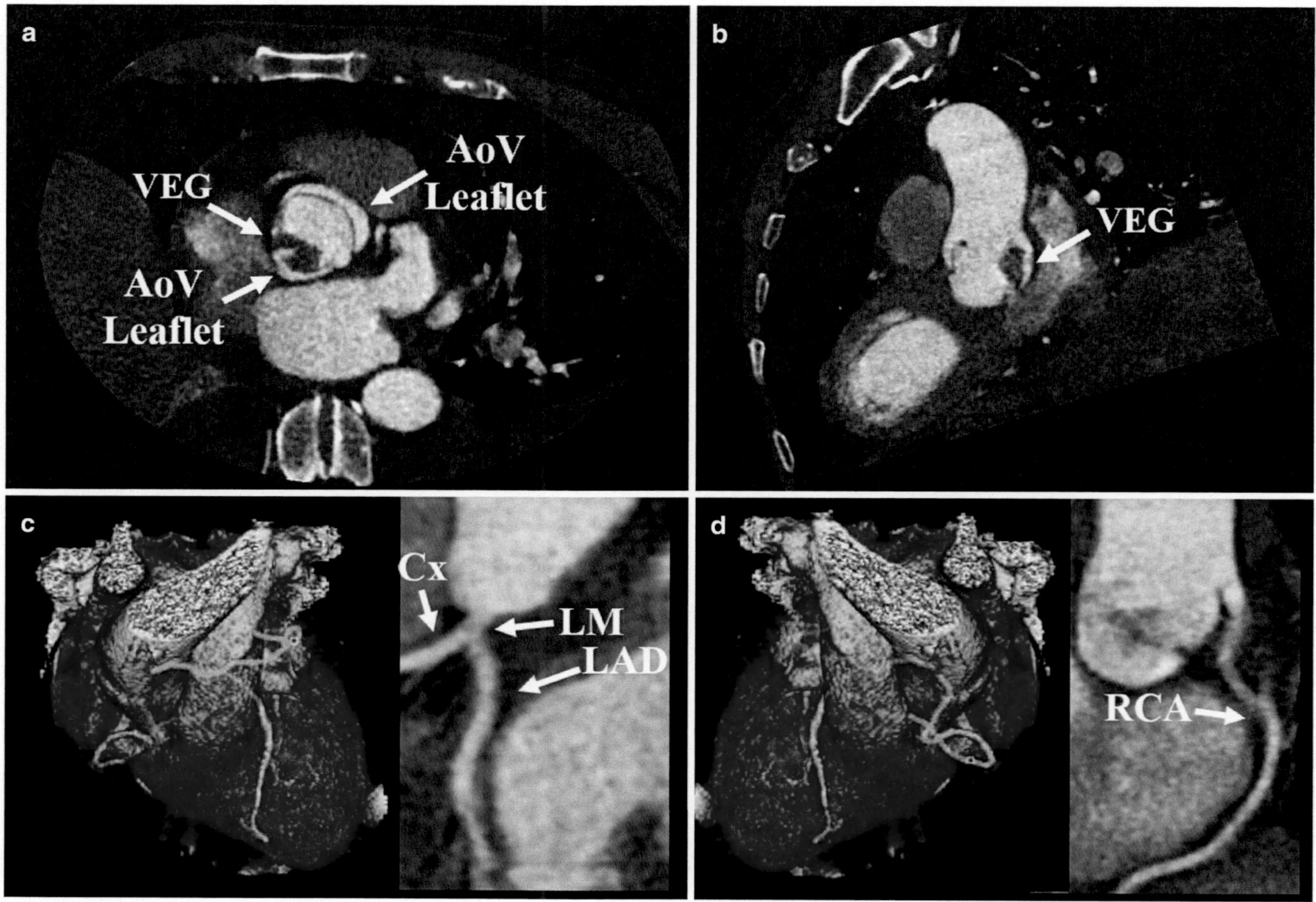

Fig. 22.10 Bicuspid aortic valve endocarditis with arterial emboli. Due to high risk of invasive coronary artery angiography in this scenario, CCTA was performed prior to aortic valve replacement. The study demonstrated no evidence of aortic root abscess, aortic pseudoaneurysm, or obstructive coronary artery disease. Panel (**a**) A 2-D double oblique view demonstrating a large, friable, vegetation on bicuspid aortic valve leaflet. Panel (**b**) A 2-D double oblique image of the aortic root viewed in long axis showing the vegetation to be in close proximity to the sinuses of Valsalva. Panel (**c**) A curved multiplanar reformatted view and corresponding 3-D reconstruction showing a patent left coronary artery circulation. Panel (**d**) A curved multiplanar reformatted view and corresponding 3-D reconstruction showing a patent right coronary artery. *AoV* aortic valve, *Cx* circumflex coronary artery, *LAD* left anterior descending coronary artery, *LM* left main coronary artery, *VEG* vegetation, *RCA* right coronary artery

in scanner hardware and software have lowered the radiation doses allowing for imaging in infants and children with congenital heart disease [54, 55, 57].

Post-surgical Sequelae: Tetralogy of Fallot, Single Ventricle Physiology and Transposition of the Great Arteries

In complex congenital heart disease, such as tetralogy of Fallot, single ventricle physiology and transposition of the great arteries, CCTA can provide assessment of the unoperated state as well as for sequelae of operative palliation or repair. In the pre-operative state, CCTA is useful for characterizing anomalous coronary artery anatomy for surgical planning [58]. In the post-operative setting of reconstructed right ventricular outflow tract with pulmonary valve regurgitation, cardiovascular magnetic resonance imaging (CMR) is a gold standard of measurement for assessment of right ventricular size, right ventricular function, and pulmonary valve fractional regurgitation. Some of these patients, though, have cardiac devices, potentially limiting the use of CMR. In comparison to CMR, CCTA assessment of right ventricular function and pulmonary regurgitant fraction, calculated by the difference between biventricular systolic volume difference, can be achieved with the caveats that right ventricular volume can be overestimated and pulmonic regurgitant fraction underestimated using CMR as a gold standard [59]. CCTA can characterize the anatomy of the reconstructed pulmonary outflow tract and pulmonary vasculature for pulmonary artery stenosis or enlargement/aneurysm (Videos 7 and 8).

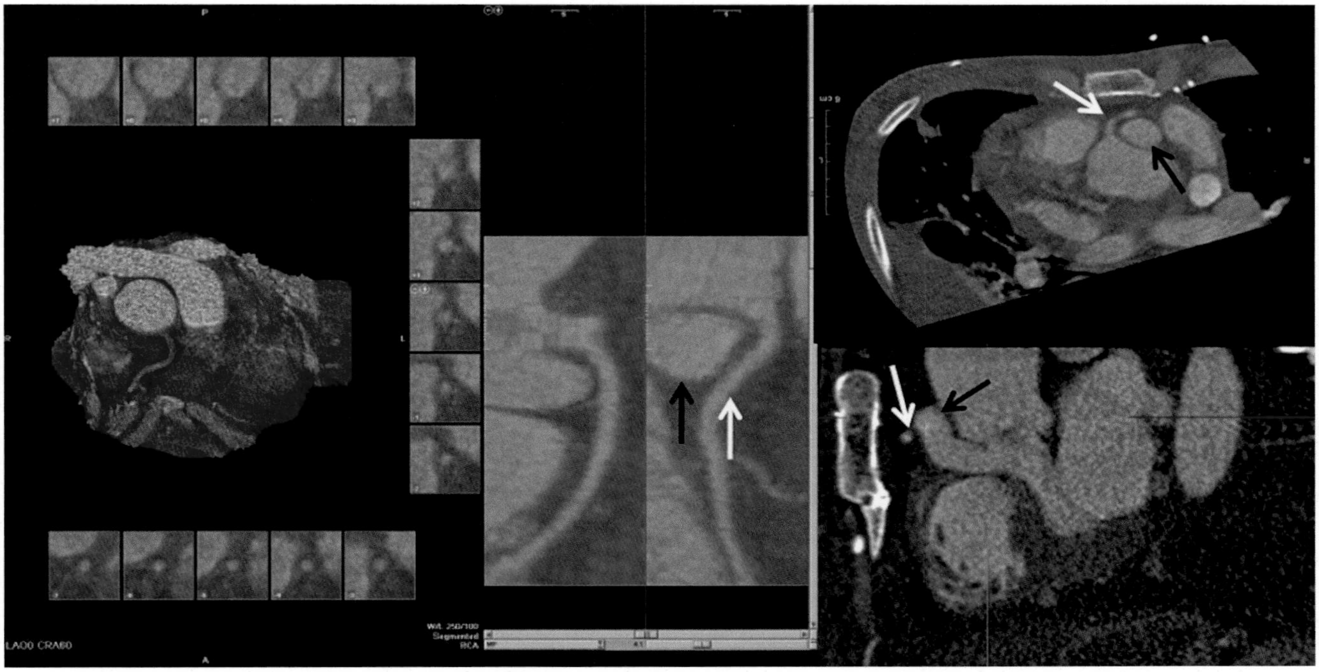

Fig. 22.11 Multiplane views showing the relationship of an aortic pseudoaneurysm (*black arrows*) to the right coronary artery (*white arrows*) in a patient with aortic valve endocarditis

For patients with surgical repair for single ventricle physiology, opacification of the complete Fontan circuit can require specialized injection protocols, with venous injection from two sites (upper and lower extremity) or delayed timing of imaging relative to injection in order to fully opacify the Fontan and pulmonary vasculature [60]. In surgically treated transposition of the great arteries, CCTA can provide assessment of stents and baffles, re-implanted coronary arteries, and assessment of ventricular function [61–64].

Atrial and ventricular sepal defects can occur as single anomalies or in association with additional complex anatomy. CCTA can characterize defects, providing such details as double-oblique assessment of coaxial defect size and rim characteristics as well as providing preoperative assessment for other cardiovascular anomalies which may need to be addressed at the time of surgical repair. In patients with septal defects with identified complex additional anomalies, CCTA provides information important to surgical decision-making and planning [56, 65–68].

Patent Ductus Arteriosus

In patients with patent ductus arteriosus, CCTA provides important information for deciding between surgical and percutaneous closure approach through precise characterization of morphology and size and assessment for other associated cardiothoracic anomalies facilitating appropriate sizing of ductus occlusion devices (Fig. 22.23). Options for surgical versus percutaneous closure are dependent on patent ductus arteriosus size, morphology, and location and orifice size of the aortic and pulmonary artery insertions. A percutaneous approach may be preferable for a ductal size of less than 3 mm in diameter (coil occlusion) and 3–14 mm (coil or device occlusion) [69]. Ductal size of greater than 14 mm and those with complex morphology are associated with increased risk of complications with percutaneous closure and surgical closure is usually performed, although in certain situations in high risk surgical patients, percutaneous closure has been employed [70].

Anomalous Coronary Arteries

Specific morphologies of anomalous coronary arteries can lead to ischemia, infarction, and sudden cardiac death. Decisions regarding potential surgical therapy for correction depend on identification of high risk anatomy in the appropriate clinical scenario. The CT imager should have an understanding of how these anatomic details affect surgical decision-making, planning and performance of procedures. CCTA can characterize detailed anatomy for surgical decisions relating to anomalous coronary arteries. Anatomic details include individual coronary artery presence or absence, origin, ostial characteristics, course, termination, presence of coronary artery disease or aneurysm, and 3-D

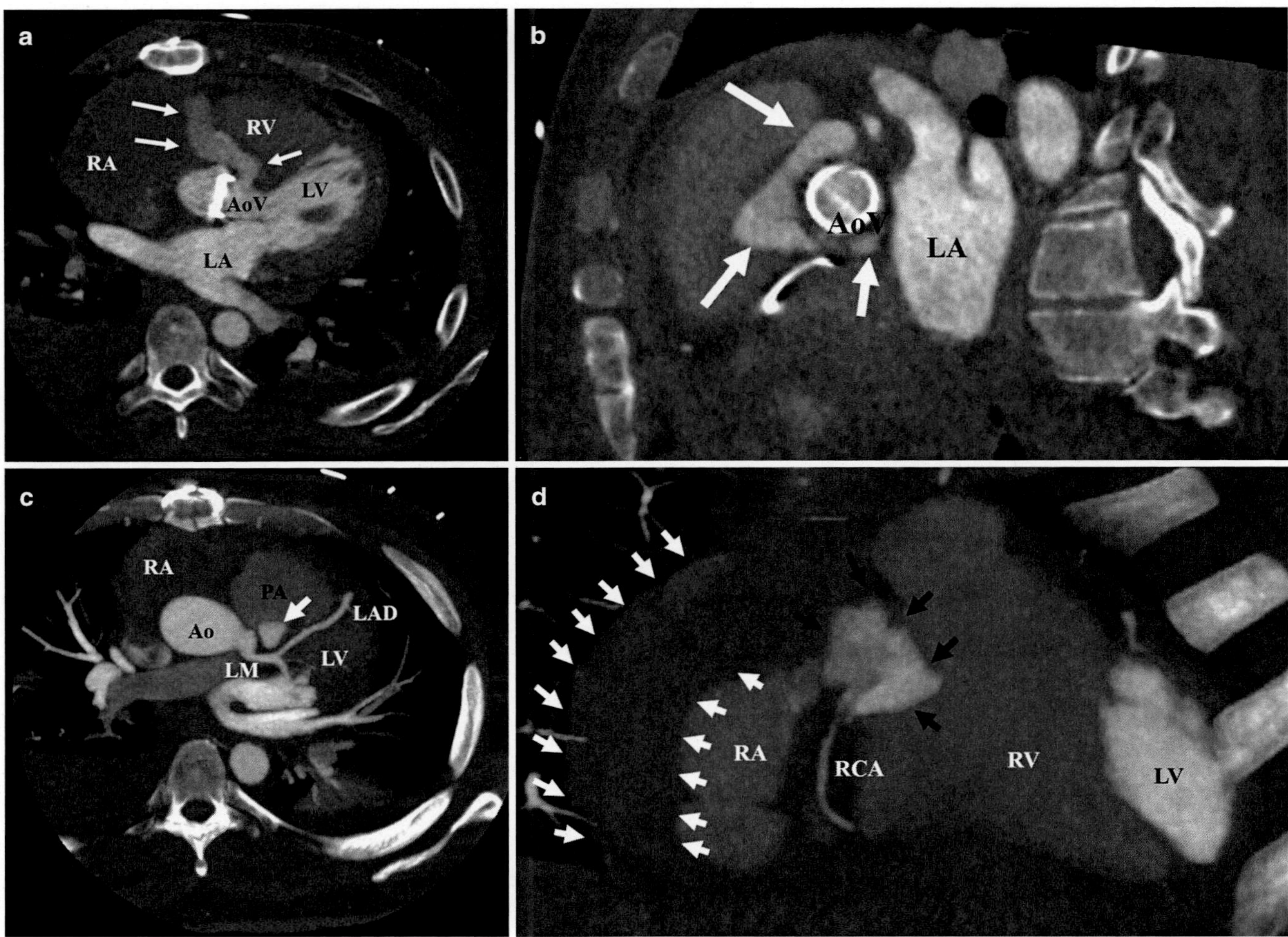

Fig. 22.12 Aortic valve endocarditis involving a mechanical valve with paravalvular pseudoaneurysm/contained rupture. Panels (**a–c**) Multiple 2-D double oblique views demonstrate the aortic valve pseudoaneurysm/contained rupture (*white arrows*) extending along the superior aspect of the right atrioventricular groove. Panel (**d**) A 2-D double oblique view demonstrating the pseudoaneurysm/contained rupture (*black arrows*) causing narrowing of the proximal right coronary artery, which subsequently courses into the pericardial sac with right atrial hemopericardium/hematoma (*white arrows*) causing severe right atrial compression. *AoV* aortic valve, *LA* left atrium, *LAD* left anterior descending coronary artery, *LM* left main coronary artery, *LV* left ventricle, *PA* pulmonary artery, *RA* right atrium, *RCA* right coronary artery, *RV* right ventricle

relationship to other cardiovascular structures (Figs. 22.24, 22.25, 22.26, 22.27, 22.28, 22.29, 22.30, 22.31, 22.32, 22.33, 22.34, 22.35, 22.36, 22.37, and 22.38, Videos 9 and 10). In regard to the origin, the coronary artery can arise from the aortic sinuses, other locations on the aorta or other vascular structures. Viewing the aortic sinuses as a clock face in the axial plane, the normal coronary artery origins are at approximately 11 o'clock for right coronary artery and 4 o'clock for left main. Ostial morphology can include a separate ostium, a shared ostium with another coronary artery, or an ostium off of another coronary artery. Ostial morphologies include presence of a slit-like ostium, and for retrospectively gated studies, dynamic ostial compression due to adjacent vascular structures. For coronary arteries arising from the contralateral sinus, there are four main pathways for the anomalous artery to course back to its usual myocardial distribution: pre- pulmonic, inter-arterial, trans-septal, or retro-aortic. The termination of an anomalous coronary artery can be into a capillary distribution usual for a given coronary artery, the capillary distribution in another myocardial segment, a cardiac chamber, or another arterial or venous vascular structure. The lumen can have no evidence of coronary atherosclerosis, non-obstructive coronary atherosclerosis, obstructive coronary artery disease, or aneurysmal dilatation.

High risk features for cardiovascular events include absence of a coronary artery with inadequate compensatory arterial supply to a myocardial distribution, coronary artery take-off from the contralateral sinus with a slit-like ostium and inter- arterial course, or an anomalous coronary artery

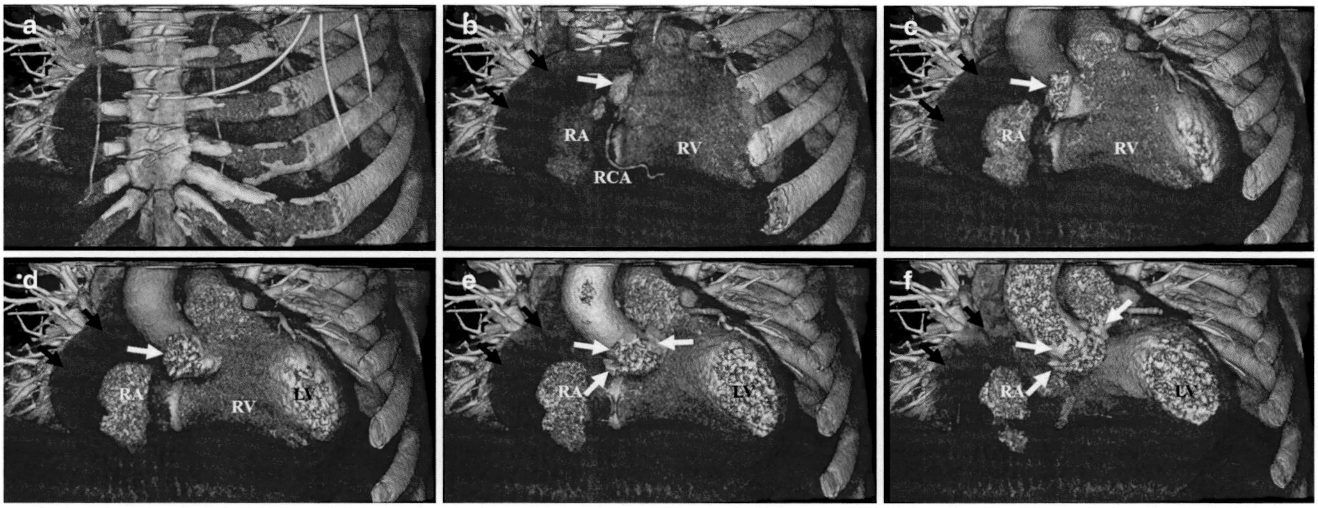

Fig. 22.13 Mechanical aortic valve endocarditis (same case as Fig. 22.12). Serial virtual sternotomy 3-D reconstructions demonstrating the anatomy from anterior to posterior (**a**–**f**). The pseudoaneurysm/contained rupture (*white arrows*) extends along the superior aspect of the right atrioventricular groove, causing narrowing of the proximal right coronary artery. The pseudoaneurysm/contained rupture subsequently courses into the pericardial sac with right atrial hemopericardium/ hematoma (*black arrows*). *RA* Right atrium, *RCA* right coronary artery, *RV* right ventricle

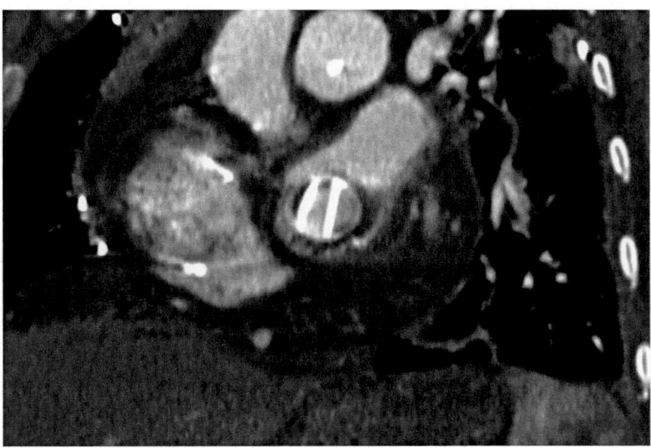

Fig. 22.14 Images demonstrating an immobile thrombus on the anterior leaflet of a mechanical prosthetic mitral valve which caused the leaflet to be immobile

arising from another structure such as the pulmonary artery. Pre-pulmonic, intra-septal and retro-aortic courses are usually low risk morphologies [35, 71]. For high risk anatomy in the appropriate clinical situation, detailed characterization of the anomalous coronary anatomy defines the available surgical approaches including reimplantation of a coronary artery, unroofing of a coronary artery, bypass of a coronary artery, or translocation of other cardiovascular structures impeding flow to a coronary artery [69, 72]. Scenarios of bypass of a coronary artery require significant stenosis of the artery as otherwise competitive flow can lead to poor maturation or closure of the bypass graft. The surgical approach to a coronary artery off of the pulmonary artery is reimplantation of the coronary artery. Surgical approaches to an interarterial course depend on the location and characteristics of the anomalous coronary artery ostium. For an intramural aortic course with a slit-like ostium above the sinotubular junction, the coronary artery can be unroofed, whereas, below the sinotubular junction the artery can be fenestrated. For a separate ostium without an intramural aortic course, the artery can be reimplanted. For a shared ostium without an intramural course, unroofing or reimplantation would not be feasible, and therefore the pulmonary artery can be translocated. In anomalous coronary arteries with obstructive coronary artery disease, coronary artery bypass grafting can be performed. This is not feasible in the other scenarios as there would be competitive flow due to the lack of coronary artery disease. In regard to abnormal termination of a coronary artery into a venous structure, either percutaneous or surgical occlusion can be performed depending on the caliber and tortuosity of the vessel.

CCTA Imaging Related to Surgery for Advanced Heart Failure

In the setting of coronary artery disease associated with severe ischemic cardiomyopathy, challenging decisions relate to transplant versus high risk coronary artery bypass surgery, often with additional decisions as to valvular repair or replacement and ventricular aneurysmectomy. Assessment of myocardial viability has become important to the pre-procedure decision-making process. CMR has played an important role due to the ability to assess for infarct related fibrosis as well as regional contractility (Fig. 22.39) [73–76]. These images can also be used for decision-making regarding viability and ventricular dimensions for planning of

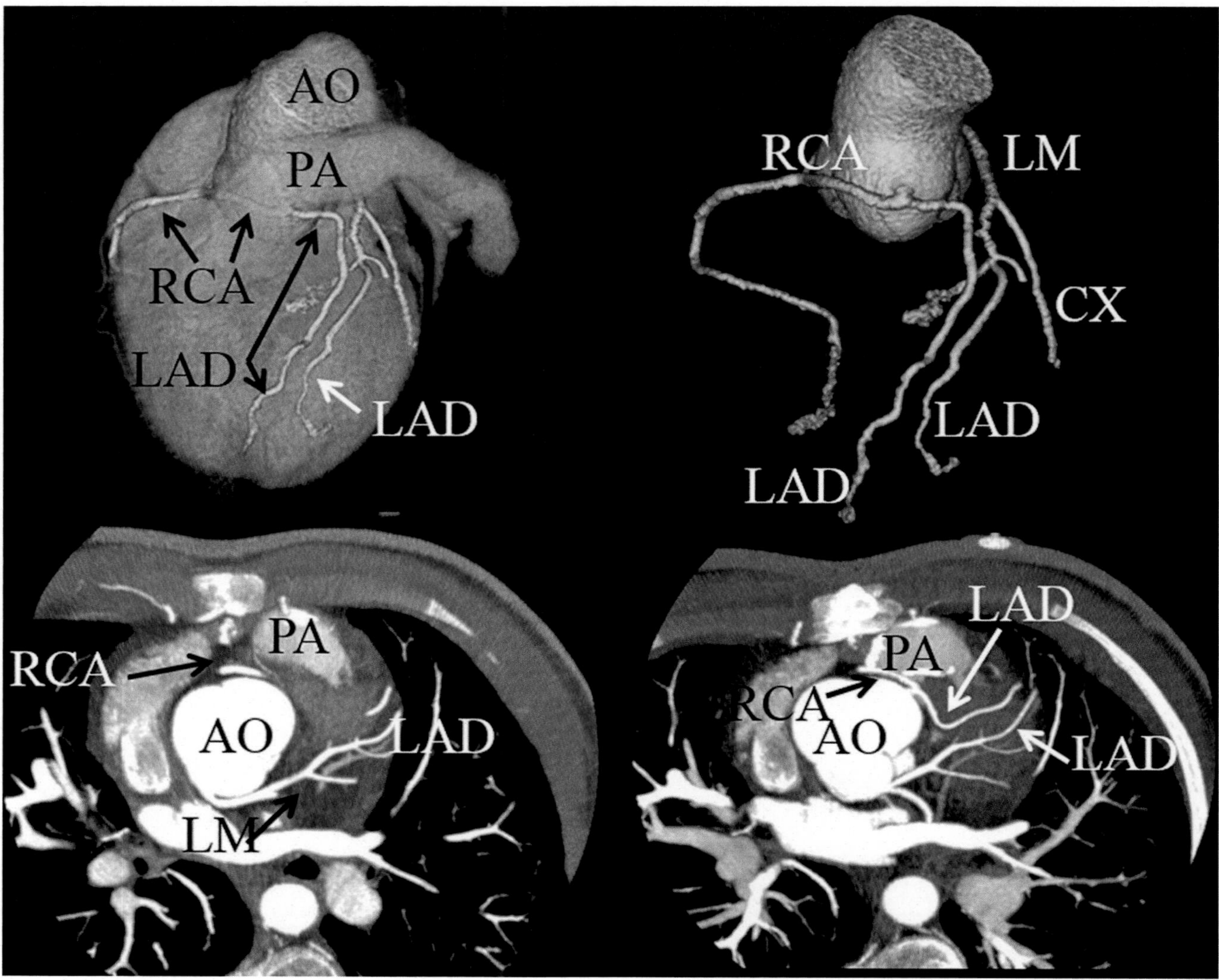

Fig. 22.15 Repaired Tetralogy of Fallot with a retroaortic left main and duplication of arterial supply to the left anterior descending coronary artery distribution from left and right coronary arteries in the setting of stenosis of the pulmonary valve conduit. 3-D reconstructions (*upper panels*) demonstrate a long left main arising from the left coronary sinus which courses retroaortic between the aorta and the left atrium and subsequently gives off a left anterior descending coronary artery and circumflex coronary artery. The right coronary sinus gives off a single short ostium which subsequently gives off a right coronary artery that traverses anteriorly between the aorta and a heavily calcified pulmonary conduit, and a branch which courses within the vascular distribution of the left ventricular anterior wall and septum. There is therefore duplication of arterial supply to the left ventricular anterior wall distribution. 2-D thick maximum intensity projection views (*lower panels*) show the coronary sinuses are rotated clockwise. Consequently, the left main coronary artery originates more posterior than usual, at approximately the 7 o'clock location on the aortic clock face in the axial view. The right coronary artery origin is likewise rotated clockwise, with the ostium at the 2 o'clock location. Percutaneous intervention for repair of the homograft stenosis was inadvisable due to the close proximity of the right coronary artery to the pulmonary conduit. Given the close proximity of cardiovascular structures to the sternum, the patient was placed on cardiopulmonary bypass via right groin vessels prior to redo sternotomy in order to decompress the right ventricle. Revision of the right ventricular outflow tract, and pulmonary valve replacement were performed. During conduit/homograft resection, the posterior layer of the conduit was left intact in order to avoid injury to the anomalous right coronary artery. *Ao* aorta, *CX* circumflex coronary artery, *LAD* left anterior descending coronary artery, *LM* left main coronary artery, *PA* pulmonary artery, *RCA* right coronary artery, *RV* right ventricle (Reprinted from Shinbane et al. [35] with permission from SAGE Publications)

revascularization. More recently, CCTA delayed enhancement imaging has been shown to reliably demonstrate fibrosis associated with myocardial infarction. In animal models, delayed contrast imaging has been shown to correlate with acute and chronic infarct shape and transmurality including assessment for necrosis in the acute setting [77]. This technique requires re-imaging 10–15 min after administration of iodinated contrast and therefore requires additional radiation. The technique has been demonstrated to correlate with thallium SPECT assessment of viability [78]. In the setting of acute myocardial infarction, CCTA delayed enhancement correlates with CMR assessment of viability [79]. Delayed

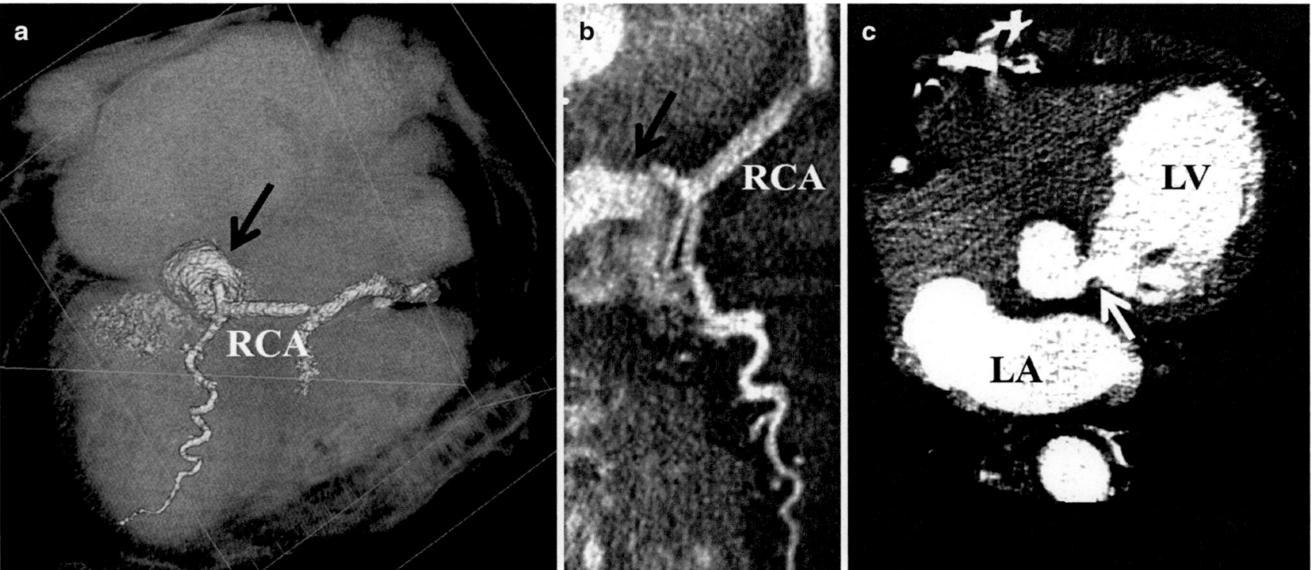

Fig. 22.16 Distal right coronary artery fistula to the left ventricle at level of mitral annulus in patient with a previous history of mitral valve surgery. Panel (**a**) 3-D view demonstrating the distal the aneurysmal distal right coronary artery (*arrow*). Panel (**b**) Curved multiplanar reformatted view of the distal the aneurysmal distal right coronary artery (*arrow*). Panel (**c**) A 2-D double oblique view of the fistulous connection of the aneurysmal distal right coronary artery to the left ventricle at the level of the mitral annulus (*arrow*). *LV* left ventricle, *RV* right ventricle, *LA* left atrium, *LV* left ventricle, *RCA* right coronary artery

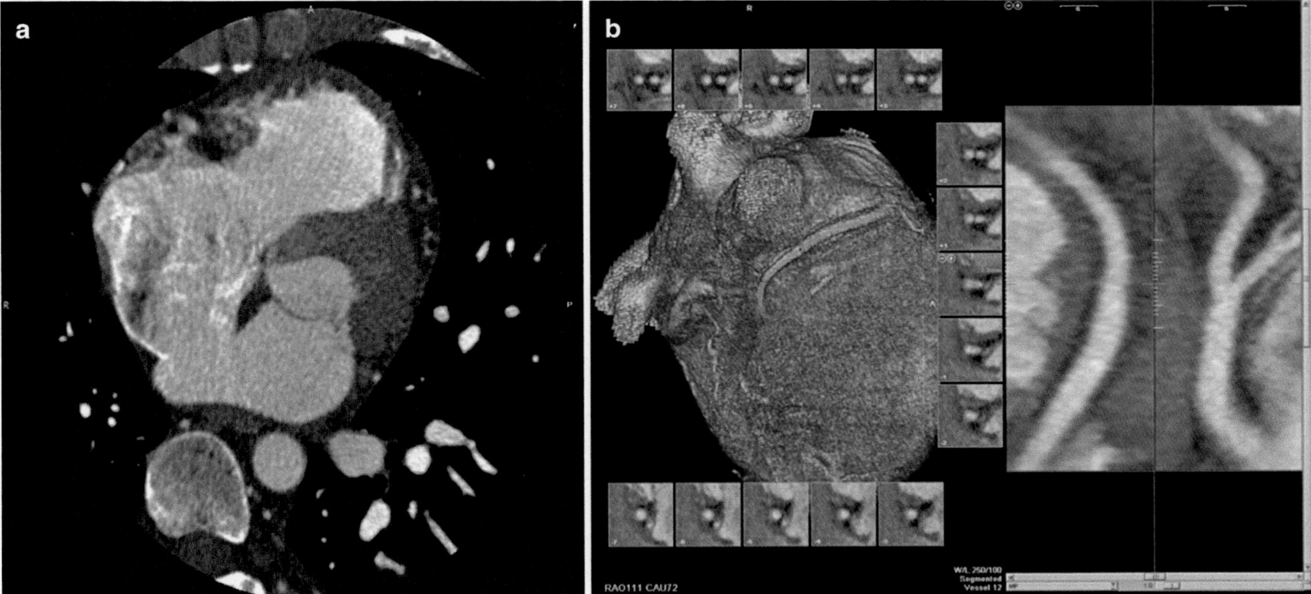

Fig. 22.17 Presurgical assessment for repair of atrial septal defect. (**a**) 2-D axial view showing a large secundum atrial septal defect. (**b**) Curved multiplanar reformat demonstrating no evidence of obstructive coronary artery disease in the right coronary artery segment shown

enhancement imaging can also be performed immediately after cardiac catheterization without contrast reinjection (Fig. 22.40). In preliminary studies in this setting, the degree of CCTA delayed enhancement was associated with increased subsequent heart failure admissions, correlated with low dose dobutamine assessment of viability, was an independent predictor of future cardiovascular events, and correlated with angiographic and clinical assessment of reperfusion with percutaneous coronary intervention [80–84]. As techniques evolve, CCTA delayed enhancement imaging may ultimately serve in a similar capacity to CMR for preoperative decision-making and planning.

Ventricular assist devices have become an integral part of advanced heart failure management as bridges to cardiac

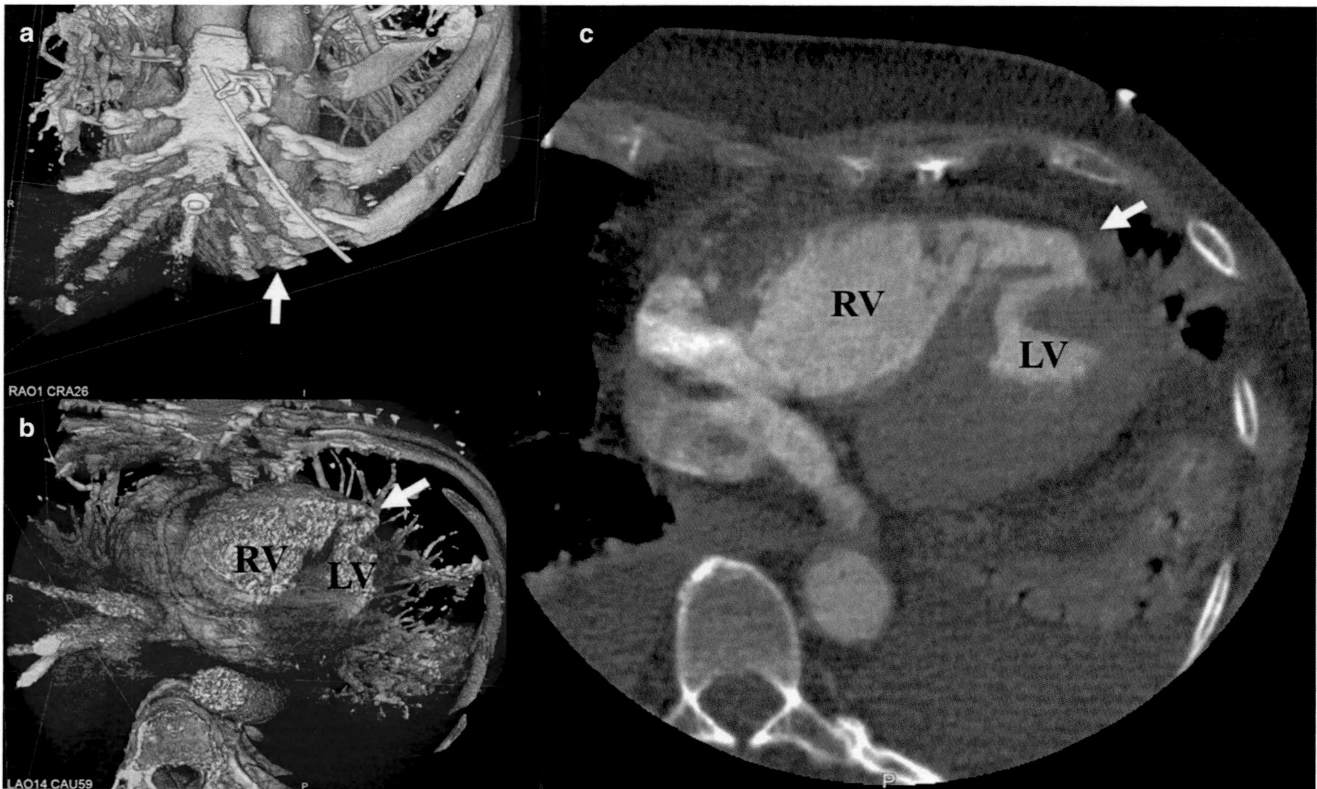

Fig. 22.18 A restrictive apical muscular ventricular septal defect with a circuitous course. The defect is oriented anteroposterior on the left ventricular side septum but courses laterally on the right ventricular side. The presence of prominent right ventricular apical muscle bands also contributes to the circuitous course of the ventricular septal defect. Panel (**a**) A 3-D coronal reconstruction demonstrating the level of the level of the ventricular septal defect (*arrow*). Panel (**b**) A 3-D axial reconstruction demonstrating the ventricular septal defect (*arrow*). Panel (**c**) A 2-D double oblique view of the ventricular septal defect (*arrow*)

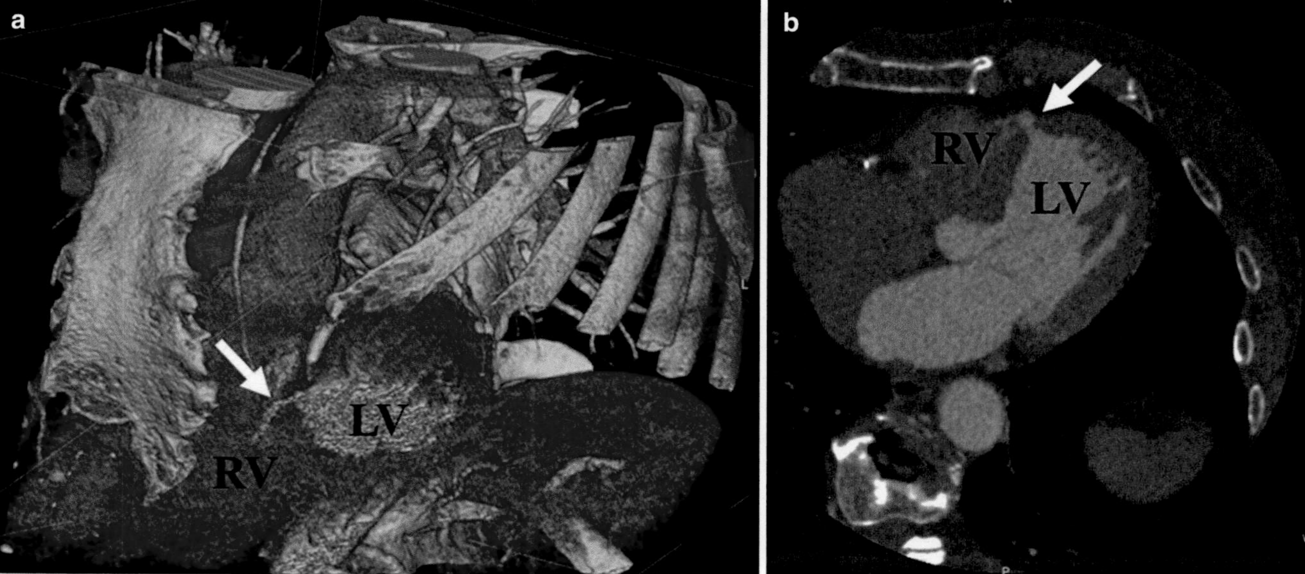

Fig. 22.19 Restrictive mid anteroseptal ventricular septal defect due to old anterior myocardial infarction with myocardial wall thinning and contrast evidence of left to right flow. Panel (**a**) A 3-D reconstruction demonstrating the ventricular septal defect (*arrow*). Panel (**b**) A 2-D double oblique view of the ventricular septal defect (*arrow*). *LV* left ventricle, *RV* right ventricle

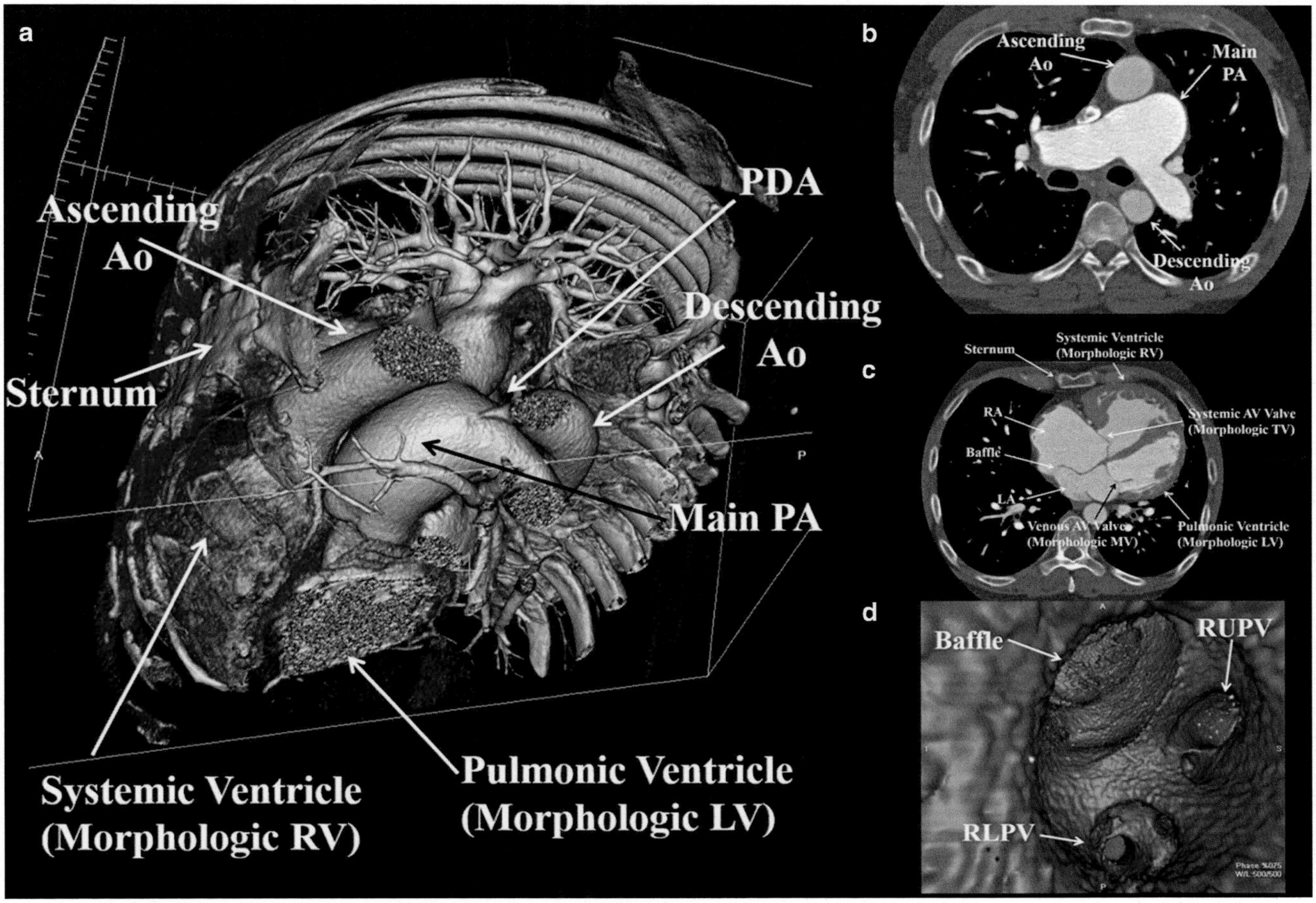

Fig. 22.20 CCTA demonstrating D Transposition of great arteries, status post previous interatrial baffle, with additional finding of patent ductus arteriosus. Panel (**a**) A 3-D reconstruction. Panel (**b**) A 2-D axial view demonstrating the aorta to be anterior and slightly rightward of the enlarged main pulmonary artery. Panel (**c**) A 2-D axial view demonstrating the anatomic positions and physiologic relationships of the ventricles. The systemic ventricle (morphologic right ventricle) is in close proximity to the sternum. Panel (**d**) Virtual endovascular view of the patent baffle as it enters the left atrium. *Ao* aorta, *LV* left ventricle, *PA* pulmonary artery, *PDA* patent ductus arteriosus, *RLPV* right lower pulmonary vein, *RUPV* right upper pulmonary vein, *RV* right ventricle

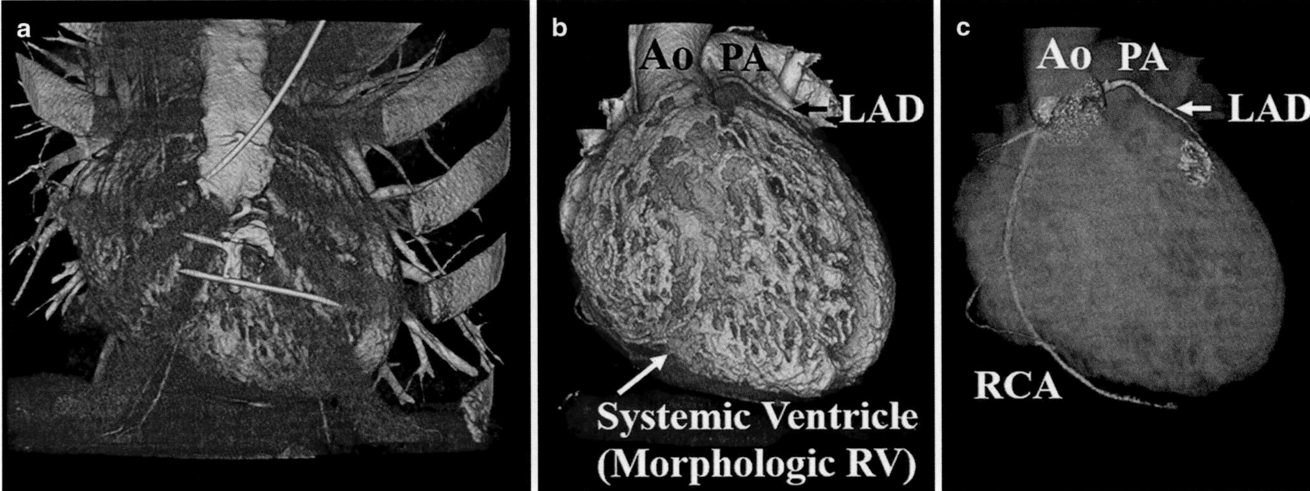

Fig. 22.21 CCTA showing D transposition of the great arteries, status post interatrial baffle. Panel (**a**) A 3-D reconstruction coronal view with skeletal structure. Panel (**b**) A 3-D reconstruction coronal view with skeletal structure removed. Panel (**c**) A 3-D reconstruction coronal view highlighting the coronary artery anatomy. There is mirror image location of the right coronary artery which arises posteriorly on the aortic sinus and supplies the pulmonary ventricle (morphologic left ventricle). *Ao* aorta, *LAD* left anterior descending coronary artery, *PA* pulmonary artery, *RCA* right coronary artery, *RV* right ventricle

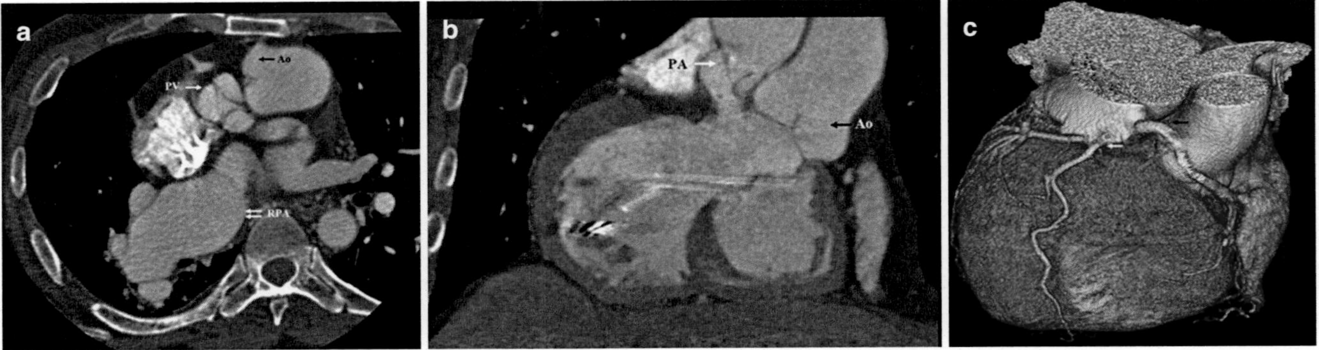

Fig. 22.22 Unoperated congenitally corrected transposition of the great arteries, dextrocardia, nonrestrictive ventricular septal defect, pulmonary stenosis and anomalous coronary arteries. Panels (**a**, **b**) Axial (**a**) and coronal (**b**) CCTA demonstrates the aorta (*black arrow*) arising anterior and leftward of the main pulmonary artery (*white arrow*). Pulmonary stenosis is present. On this diastolic image, the open pulmonary valve represents insufficiency. The right pulmonary artery demonstrates poststenotic dilatation (*double white arrows* on **a**). Panel (**c**) 3-D volume rendered CCTA views demonstrate that the left (*black arrow*) and right (*white arrow*) coronary arteries arise from the most anterior cusp of the aorta and follow their respective morphologic ventricles. *Ao* aorta, *PV* pulmonary valve, *RPA* right pulmonary artery (Reprinted from Shinbane et al. [56] with permission from SAGE Publications)

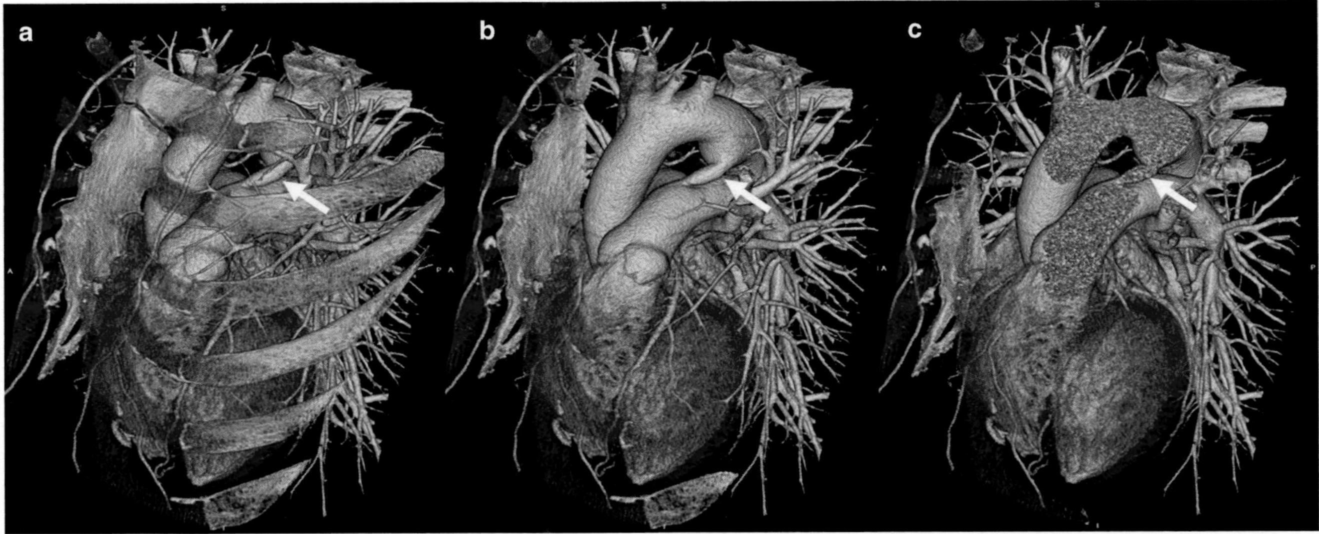

Fig. 22.23 CCTA demonstration of a tubular patent ductus arteriosus measuring 2.2 cm in length arising from a prominent aortic ductus diverticulum and communicating with the superior portion of the main pulmonary artery (*arrow*). Given the size and characteristics, a percutaneous ductal occluder device closure rather than surgical closure was performed. Panel (**a**) A 3-D reconstruction in context of skeletal structures. Panel (**b**) A 3-D reconstruction with skeletal structures removed. Panel (**c**) A 3-D reconstruction with editing plane demonstrating the lumen of the patent ductus arteriosus

transplant as well as destination devices for those patients who are not candidates for transplant. CCTA can be helpful in assessment of feasibility of ventricular assist device implantation in children and small adults, as well as to identify potential obstacles to sternotomy incision for placement (Fig. 22.41, Video 11). In patients with implanted ventricular assist devices, CCTA can identify components of the system to assess for etiologies of ventricular assist device malfunction (Fig. 22.42). In patients with pulsatile devices, electrocardiographic-gating can be utilized, while in those continuous-flow devices peripheral pulse-gating can be used to assess for etiologies of low output and low flow states [85]. CCTA can assess for issues throughout the system, including: inflow obstruction by papillary muscle, inflow cannula malposition, thrombus, air in the cannula, outflow cannula kinking or malposition, and aortic root thrombus [85–89].

In heart transplant patients, CCTA has been preliminarily studied to assess coronary arteries for chronic allograft vasculopathy. The high negative predictive value of CCTA may potentially be useful in this setting [90–93]. Limitations in assessment of coronary branch vessels less than 1.5 mm for chronic allograft vasculopathy, nephrotoxic effects of iodinated contrast, and issues of timing and frequency of assessment leading to potential cumulative effects of radiation in

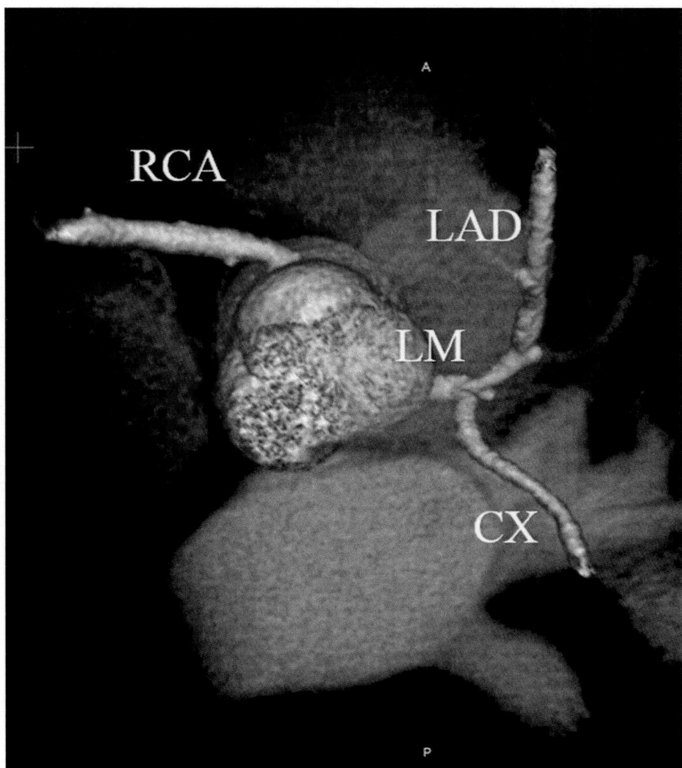

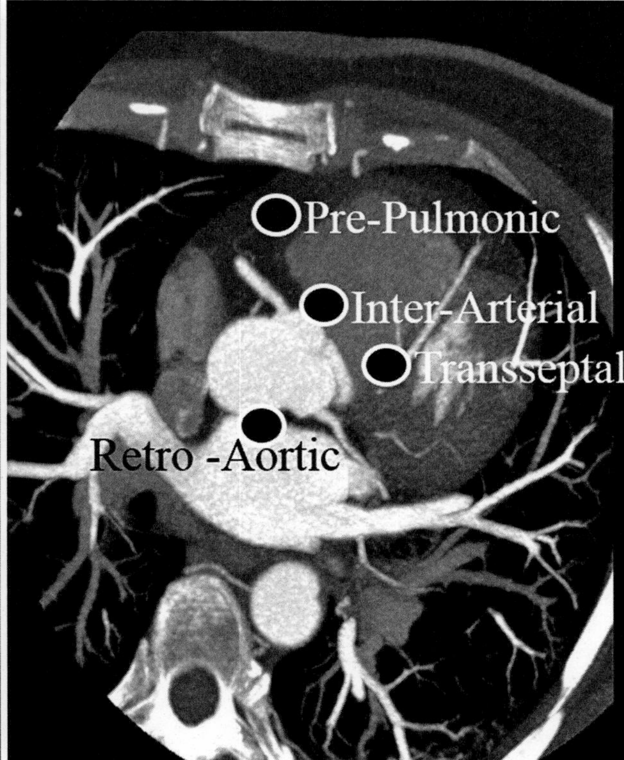

Fig. 22.24 Normal coronary artery origins and anomalous coronary artery courses. 3-D axial view reconstruction (*left panel*) demonstrates normal coronary artery origins with the right coronary artery origin at 11 o'clock and the left main coronary artery origin at 3:30 on the aortic clock face. Thick maximum intensity projection in the axial view shows the four primary courses (*black circles*) for anomalous coronary arteries arising from the contralateral sinus. *CX* circumflex coronary artery, *LAD* left anterior descending coronary artery, *LM* left main coronary artery, *RCA* right coronary artery (Reprinted from Shinbane et al. [35] with permission from SAGE Publications)

this immunosuppressed population, necessitates further investigation of the role of CCTA post-transplant [94, 95].

CCTA Imaging Related to Surgery for Cardiac Masses

While definitive diagnosis of cardiac tumors requires pathologic examination of the mass histology, CCTA can be used to characterize masses and associated findings important to diagnosis and pre-surgical work-up and planning (Fig. 22.43) [96, 97]. CCTA can define morphology including 3-D shape, single versus multiple masses, and wide-based versus narrow-based connection to the myocardium. Tissue characteristics, including attenuation of the mass, homogeneity versus heterogeneity of attenuation in different areas within the mass, presence and pattern of calcification, and presence and pattern of vascularity, can be defined with CCTA. Descriptive features of the location of the mass in relation to cardiovascular and thoracic structure should be noted, including: intracameral, intramyocardial epicardial or pericardial location of the mass, invasion or involvement of other cardiac or thoracic structures by the mass from its primary location, relationship of the mass to the coronary arteries, pericardial studding or effusion, and presence of lymphadenopathy or other thoracic masses within the field of view. CCTA can also provide coronary artery assessment for obstructive coronary artery disease prior to surgery. All of these factors are important to decisions as to resectability and surgical approach once a histologic tissue diagnosis is made.

CCTA Imaging Related to Surgery for Pericardial Disease

Assessment for constrictive pericarditis is challenging and often involves multiple modalities of imaging including echocardiography as well as invasive cardiac catheterization to assess hemodynamic elements. CCTA can be helpful in assessing pericardial thickness by cardiac region as well as by the degree of calcification [98–100]. Surgical complications can occur due to vascular damage related to dissecting the pericardium away from the coronary arteries. CCTA can define the relationship between the pericardium and coronary arteries, including areas of pericardial thickening, pericardial calcification, as well as tethering of coronary arteries on dynamic images (Fig. 22.44).

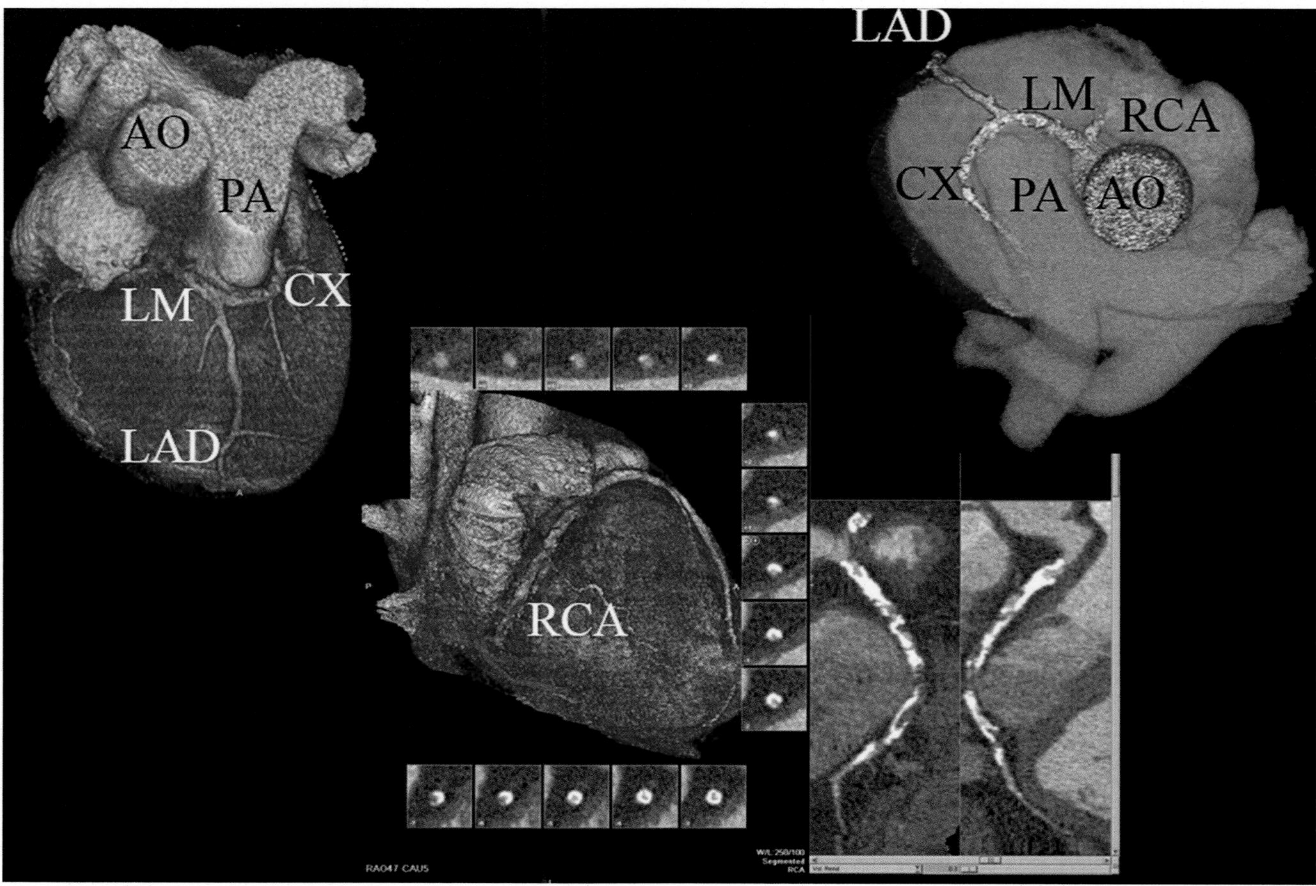

Fig. 22.25 Left coronary artery arising from a shared ostium on the right coronary sinus with a prepulmonic course and single-vessel right coronary artery coronary artery disease. 3-D reconstructions (*upper and lower left panels*) demonstrate a left coronary artery arising from a separate ostium on the right coronary sinus with a prepulmonic course. A curved multiplanar reformat (*lower right panel*) shows significant atherosclerotic disease of the right coronary artery. Cardiac catheterization demonstrated proximal occlusion of the right coronary artery with left to right collaterals. In this case, medical management of the diseased single vessel was chosen. *AO* aorta, *CX* circumflex coronary artery, *LAD* left anterior descending coronary artery, *LM* left main coronary artery, *PA* pulmonary artery, *RCA* right coronary artery (Reprinted from Shinbane et al. [35] with permission from SAGE Publications)

Decisions regarding percutaneous versus surgical approaches to drain pericardial fluid collections can be facilitated by CT assessment of the location, extent, and tissue characteristics of the pericardial effusion [101]. A percutaneous approach may be limited by the complexity of the effusion due to loculation of the effusion or effusion tissue attenuation consistent with blood, proteinaceous material, or thrombus. Accessibility by a sub-xiphoid approach can be determined by the relation of the effusion to skeletal and thoracic structures (Fig. 22.45). For posterior effusions, particularly in the setting of post cardiothoracic surgery, a sub-xiphoid approach may not be feasible, while a CT guided drainage may be achievable.

CCTA Imaging for Aortic Surgery

CCTA and CMR diagnosis of acute and chronic aortic disease is well-established. These technologies can visualize dissection, intramural hematoma, penetrating ulcer, aortic aneurysm, and aortic rupture. Details of a dissection flap entry and exit site, location and extent of true and false lumen, dissection into branch vessels, involvement of the sinuses of Valsalva, dissection into the coronary arteries, and dissection into the pericardium can be defined (Figs. 22.46 and 22.47) [102–104]. CCTA can assess coronary artery anatomy when cardiac catheterization is high risk or unachievable due to aortic pathology, such as severe atherosclerotic disease with large atheromas, thrombi, aneurysms, or dissections. Similarly, in emergency department settings, when rapid assessment for thoracic and coronary artery traumatic abnormalities are crucial and time dependent, CCTA may be useful [105–107]. CCTA provides assessment of vascular dimensions for endograft sizing and placement important to endovascular aneurysm repair [108]. The presence and degree of atherosclerosis, calcification, and thrombus can be important to cross clamp decisions related to multiple types of cardiothoracic procedures. CCTA can also be useful in the assessment of infected aortic aneurysms, with findings including saccular structure, contiguous soft tissue masses,

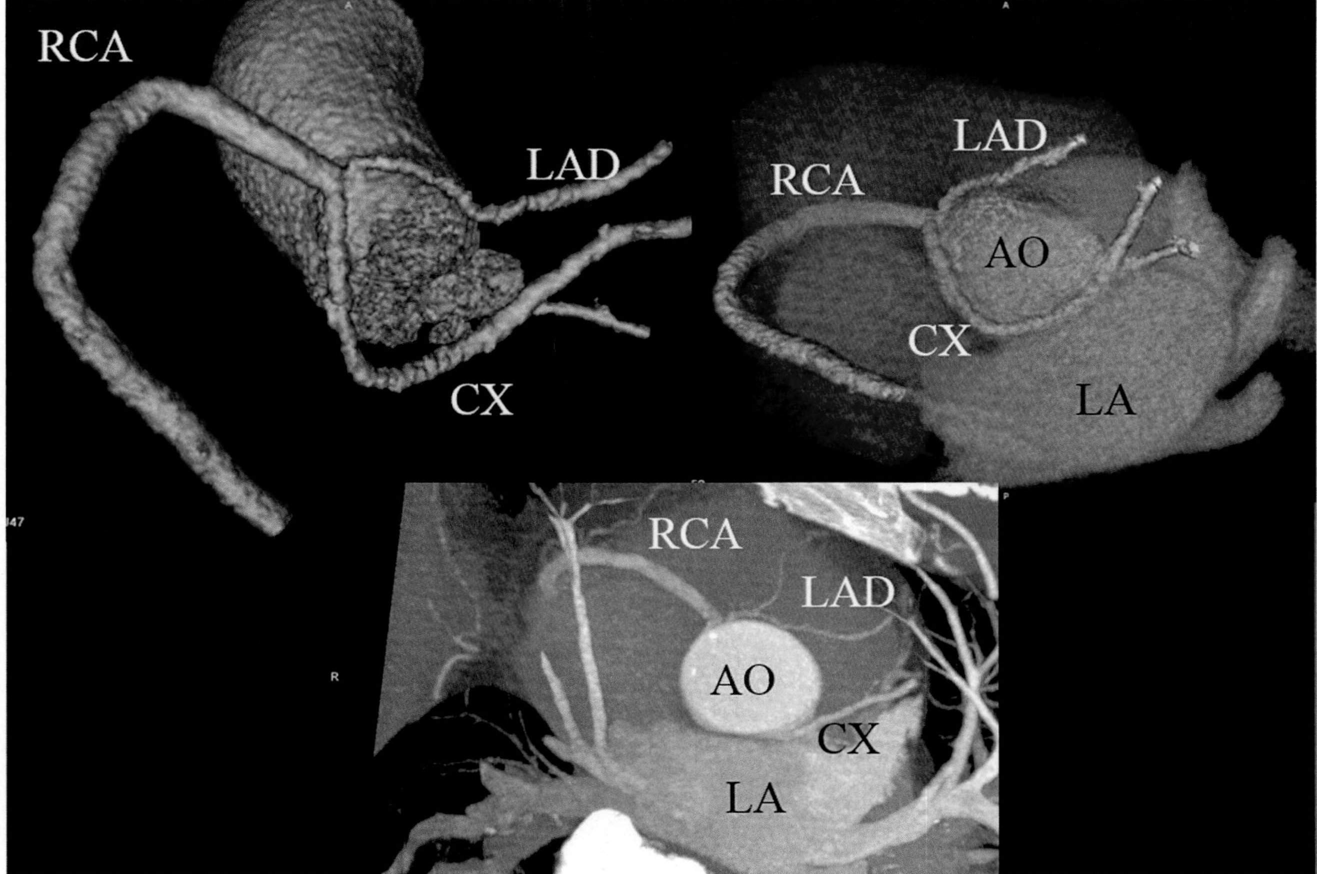

Fig. 22.26 Left coronary artery branches arising from the right coronary sinus with a prepulmonic left anterior descending coronary artery arising from a separate ostium with a subsequent intramyocardial course and a retroaortic circumflex arising off of the coronary artery. 3-D reconstructions (*upper panels*) demonstrate the left anterior descending coronary artery arising just anterior and cranial to the right coronary artery arising from a separate ostium off of the right coronary sinus. The circumflex coronary artery arises off of the right coronary artery and courses retroaortic, terminating in obtuse marginal branches. 2-D double oblique thick maximum intensity projection (*lower panel*) shows the separate right sinus ostium giving off a conus branch coursing anterior to the right ventricular outflow tract with the diminutive left anterior descending coronary artery coursing intramyocardially via a transseptal course as well as the retroaortic circumflex. Surgery was not required due to lower risk anatomic features, and due to the lack of obstructive coronary artery disease. *AO* aorta, *CX* circumflex coronary artery, *LAD* left anterior descending coronary artery, *LA* left atrium, *LM* left main coronary artery, *RCA* right coronary artery (Reprinted from Shinbane et al. [35] with permission from SAGE Publications)

contrast enhancement, fluid, gas, and adjoining bone destruction [109]. For other aortic abnormalities, such as coarctation of the aorta, CCTA is useful for decision-making related to percutaneous or surgical intervention. Characterization of coarctation location, size, calcification, collateral circulation, as well as associated congenital anomalies, can be achieved.

Conclusions

The spectrum of cardiothoracic surgical options continues to expand. CCTA can facilitate surgical procedures and requires continued investigation to define optimal procedural approaches to coronary artery, valvular, and aortic pathology. Although the cardiothoracic surgeon may not necessarily be the CCTA reading physician, detailed knowledge of the images and workstation software capabilities are essential in order to attain a 3-D understanding of an individual patient's pre-surgical cardiothoracic anatomy. Viewing modalities and presentations intuitive to the surgical approach are being advanced with 3-D printing of individualized heart models from CCTA data for surgical planning [110–114]. A close working relationship between the imager, interventional cardiologist and surgeon and presentation of relevant pre- surgical images to the multidisciplinary team are import to the comprehensive utilization of data to define approaches to particular cardiovascular disease processes.

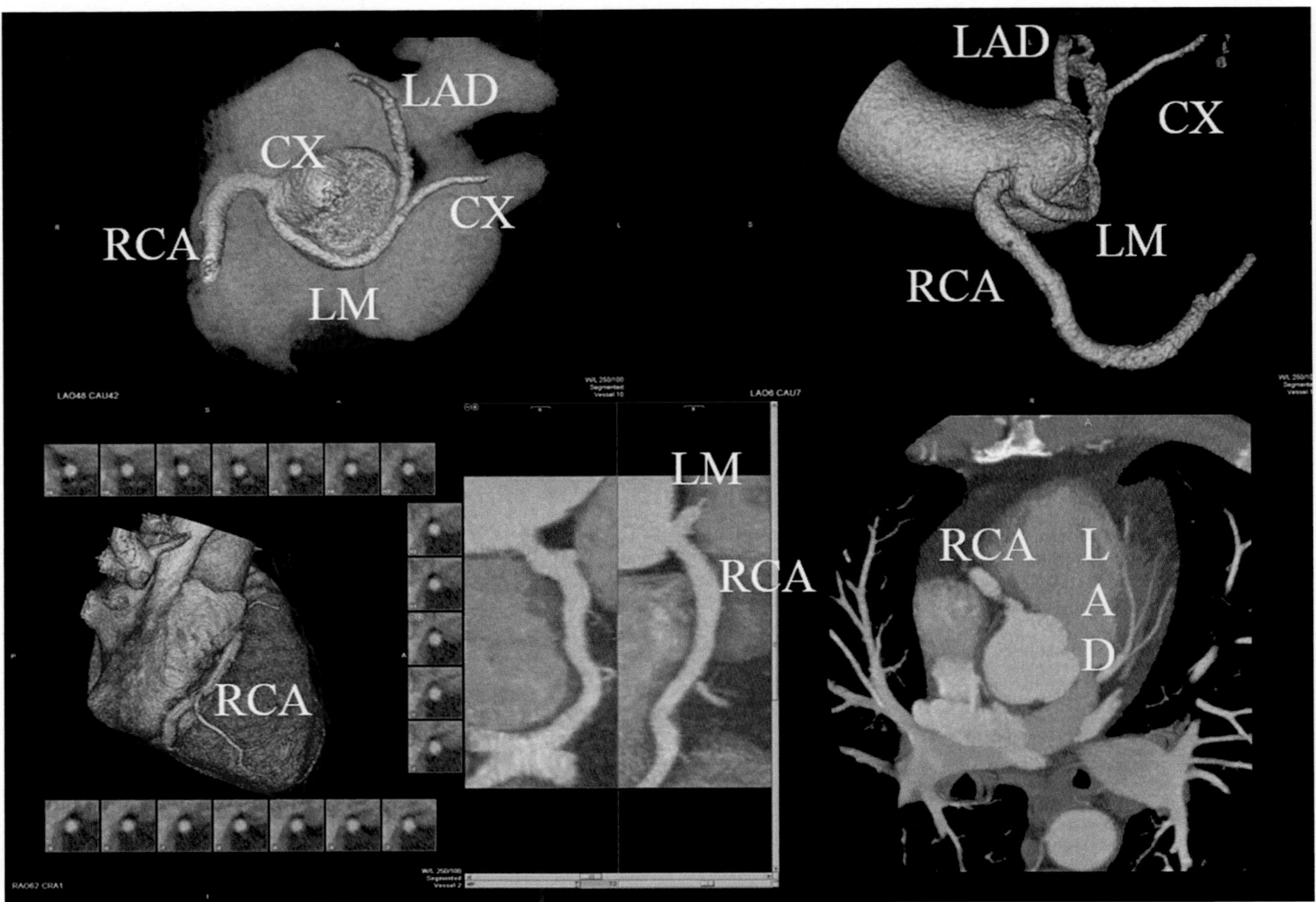

Fig. 22.27 Left coronary artery arising from a shared ostium on the right coronary sinus with a retroaortic course and myocardial bridging of the left anterior descending coronary artery. 3-D reconstructions (*upper panels*) demonstrate anomalous origin of the left main coronary artery off of its own ostium of the right coronary sinus taking a retrograde aortic course between the aorta and the left atrium. A curved multiplanar reformat (*lower left panel*) shows the separate ostia of the left main and right coronary artery. A 2-D double oblique thick maximum intensity projection view (*lower right panel*) shows myocardial bridging of the left anterior descending coronary artery. Given the lower risk anatomy and lack of obstructive coronary artery disease, surgical intervention was not required. *CX* circumflex coronary artery, *LAD* left anterior descending coronary artery, *LM* left main coronary artery, *RCA* right coronary artery (Reprinted from Shinbane et al. [35] with permission from SAGE Publications.)

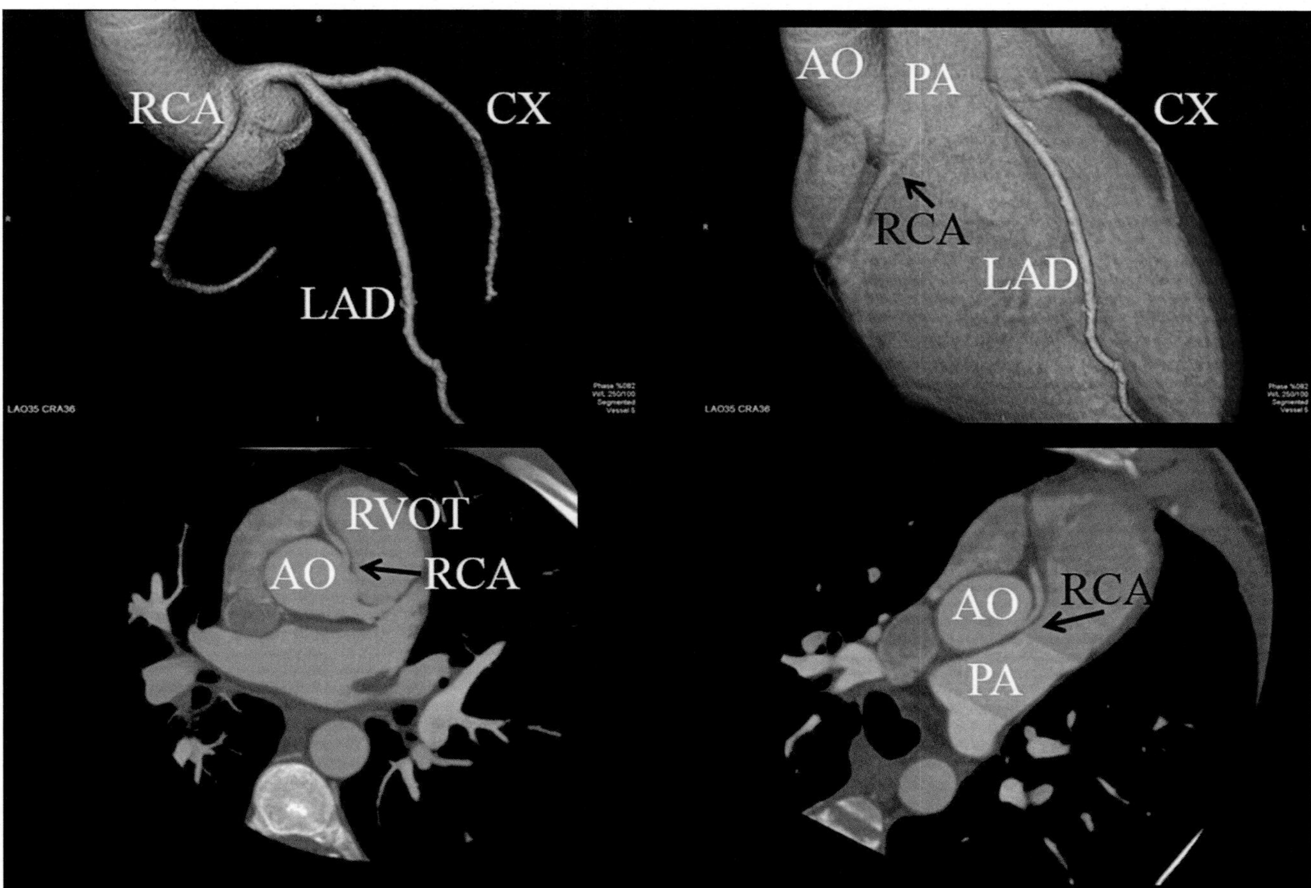

Fig. 22.28 Right coronary artery arising with a high takeoff from a separate ostium on the left coronary sinus with an interarterial course. 3-D reconstructions (*upper panels*) demonstrate anomalous takeoff of the right coronary artery from the superior portion of the left coronary sinus with an interarterial course between the aorta and the pulmonary artery. Two-D double oblique thick maximum intensity projection views (*lower panels*) show the interarterial course and the slit-like orifice of the right coronary artery. Due to symptoms of exertional syncope and high risk anatomy, surgical treatment was recommended. A minimally invasive unroofing of the artery was performed, with the aorta opened in an oblique fashion and incised following the track of the right coronary artery as it coursed through the intramural portion of the aorta for 1.5 cm, allowing correction of the slit like orifice and rerouting of the interarterial course without the need for sternotomy in an athlete. *AO* aorta, *CX* circumflex coronary artery, *LAD* left anterior descending coronary artery, *LM* left main coronary artery, *PA* pulmonary artery, *RCA* right coronary artery, *RVOT* right ventricular outflow tract (Reprinted from Shinbane et al. [35] with permission from SAGE Publications)

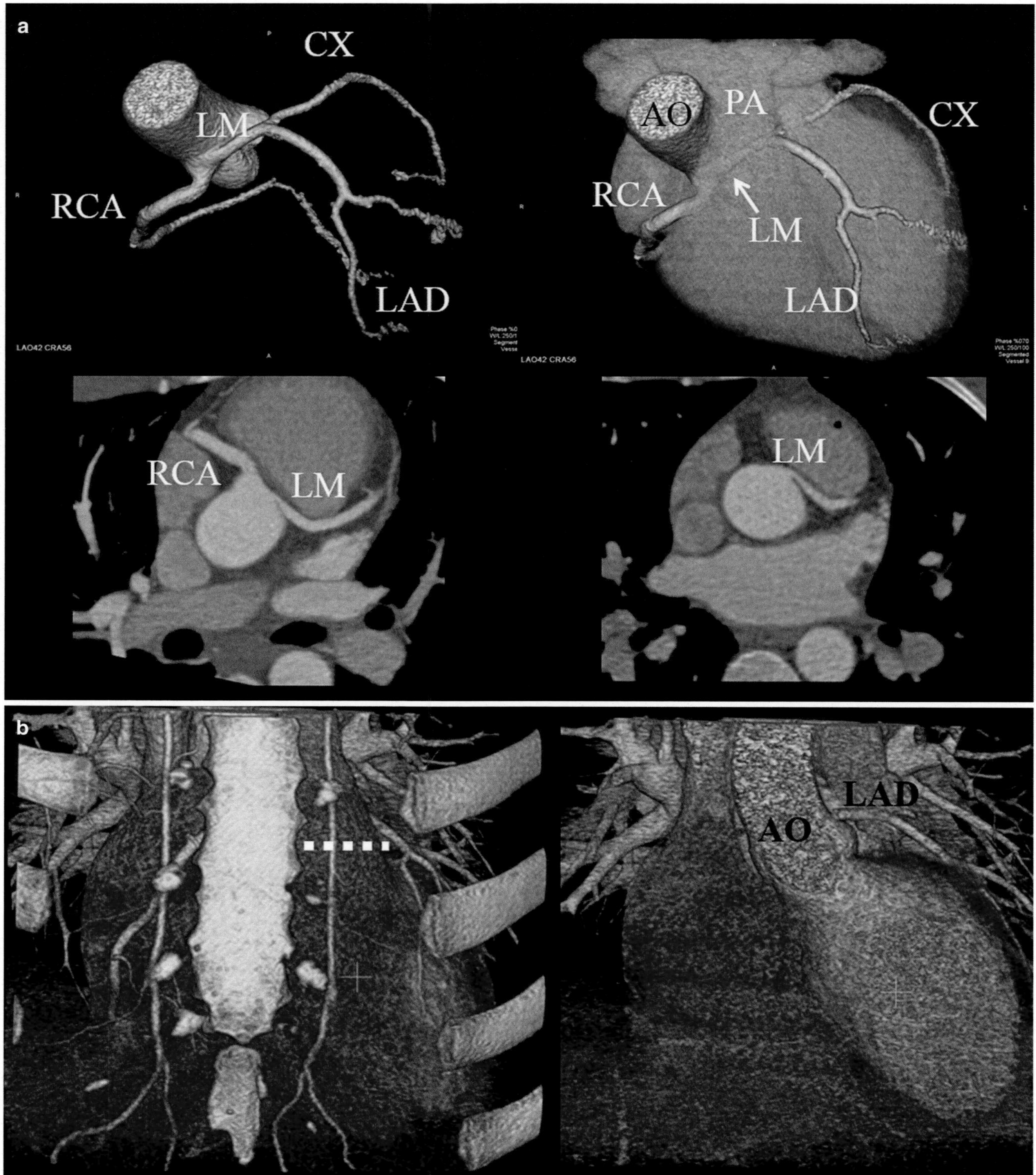

Fig. 22.29 Panel (**a**) Left main coronary artery arising from a separate ostium within the right coronary sinus with an interarterial course. 3-D reconstructions (*upper panels*) demonstrate an anomalous takeoff of the left main coronary artery from its own ostium within the right coronary sinus with an interarterial course between the aorta and the pulmonary artery. 2-D double oblique thick maximum intensity projection views (*lower panels*) show the intraarterial course and left main coronary artery with a slit-like orifice. Due to symptoms of exertional chest pain, positive cardiac enzymes and high risk anatomy, surgical treatment was recommended. A minimally invasive approach through a small 2nd intercostal space incision was used in order to avoid sternotomy. As the slit-like ostium had an extremely short course, re-implantation of the LM was performed. Panel (**b**) The 3D views show the minimally invasive surgical approach (*white dotted line*) through a small second intercostal space incision perpendicular to sternum. *AO* aorta, *CX* circumflex coronary artery, *LAD* left anterior descending coronary artery, *LM* left main coronary artery, *PA* pulmonary artery, *RCA* right coronary artery (Reprinted from Shinbane et al. [35] with permission from SAGE Publications)

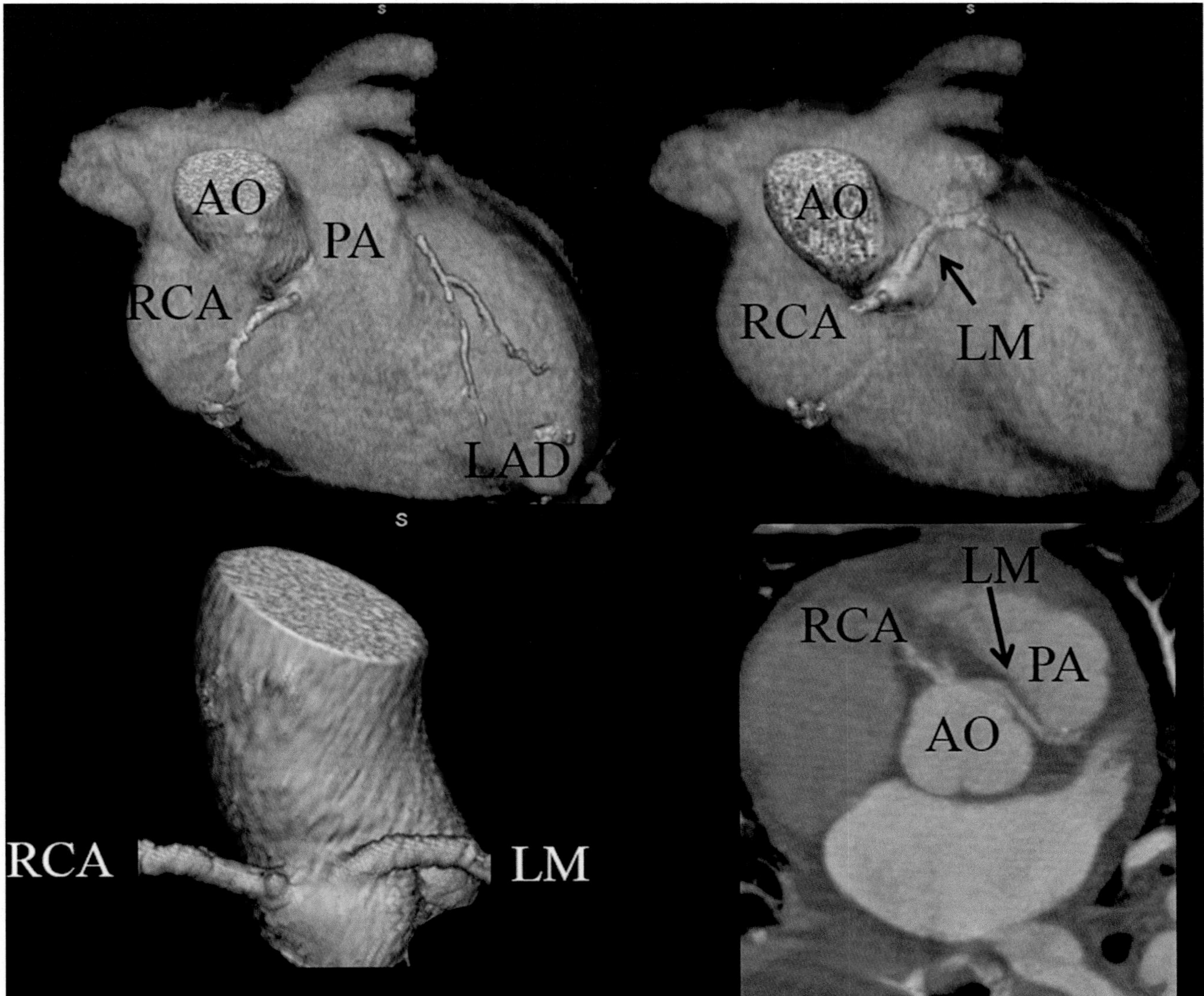

Fig. 22.30 Left main coronary artery (*LM*) arising from a separate ostium within the right coronary sinus with an interarterial course and multivessel coronary artery disease. 3-D reconstructions (*upper panels, lower left panel*) demonstrate an anomalous takeoff of the LM from its own ostium within the right coronary sinus with an interarterial course between the aorta and the pulmonary artery. 2-D double oblique thick maximum intensity projection view (*lower right panel*) shows the intra-arterial course of the LM with a slit-like orifice. Due to presentation with cardiogenic shock, intraaortic balloon pump placement and cardiac catheterization had been performed with subsequent CCTA to further characterize anomalous coronary anatomy. Given the presence of multivessel coronary artery disease, standard coronary artery bypass surgery was performed. *AO* aorta, *LAD* left anterior descending coronary artery, *LM* left main coronary artery, *PA* pulmonary artery, *RCA* right coronary artery (Reprinted from Shinbane et al. [35] with permission from SAGE Publications)

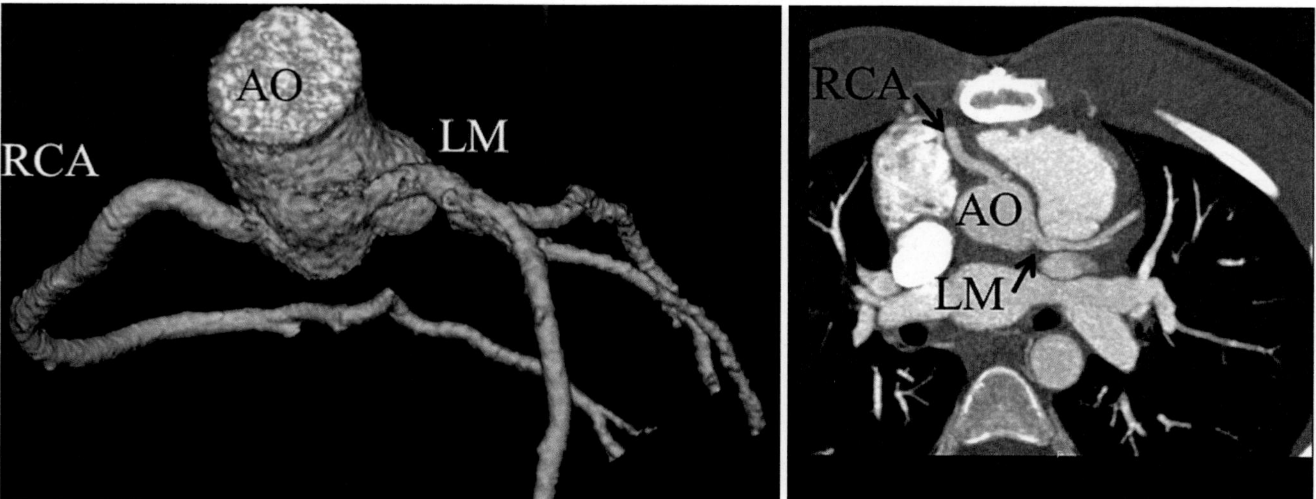

Fig. 22.31 Left coronary artery arising from a separate ostium on the right coronary sinus with an interarterial course with previous surgical unroofing. 3-D reconstruction (*left panel*) demonstrates the left coronary artery with the left main coronary artery originating from its own ostium off of the right coronary sinus. There has been previous unroofing of the interarterial left main course with surgical widening and extension to the commissure between the left and right coronary sinuses. 2-D double oblique thick maximum intensity projection views (*right panel*) show the ostium has been surgically widened and extended to the commissure between the left and the right coronary sinus. There was no obstructive coronary artery disease within any of these vessels. No further intervention was necessary. *AO* aorta, *LM* left main coronary artery, *RCA* right coronary artery (Reprinted from Shinbane et al. [35] with permission from SAGE Publications)

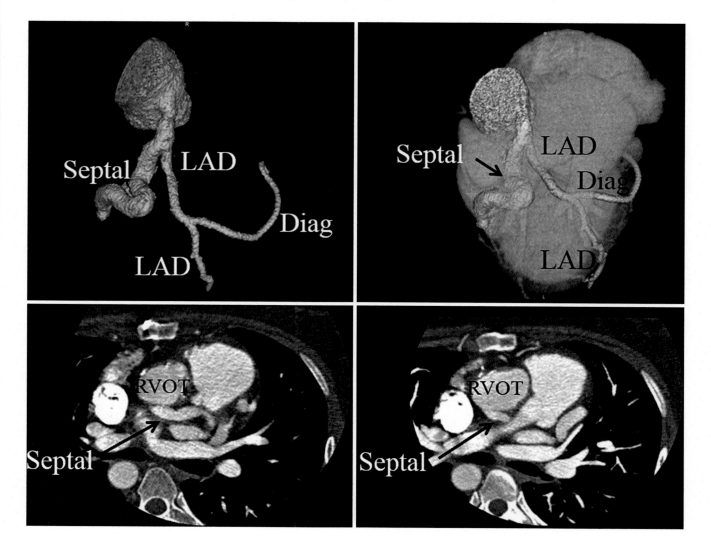

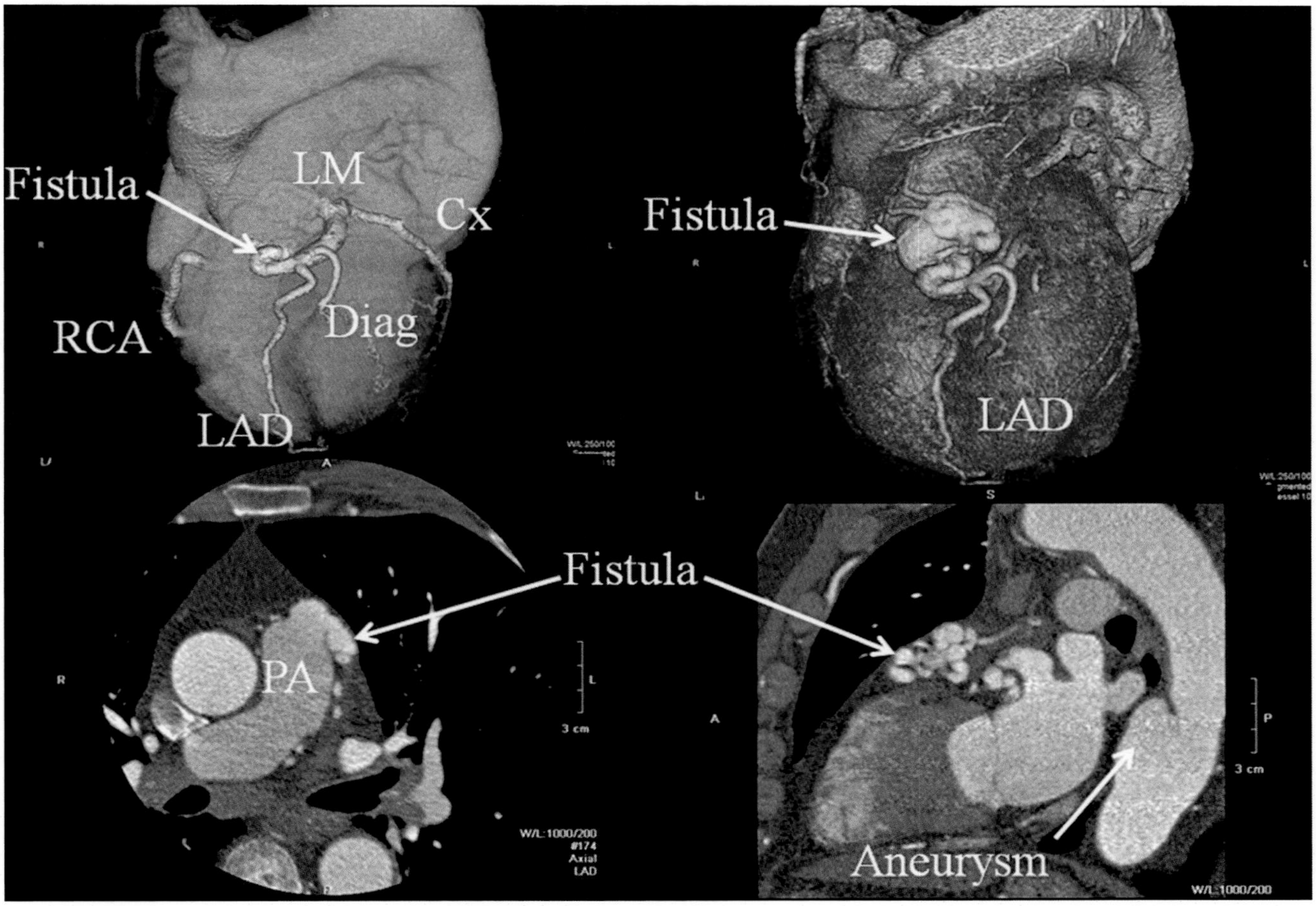

Fig. 22.33 Anomalous coronary artery termination with a serpiginous coronary artery fistula from the proximal left anterior descending coronary artery to the main pulmonary artery. 3-D reconstructions (*upper panels*) demonstrate an extremely serpiginous fistula extended from the proximal left anterior descending coronary artery to the main pulmonary artery. 2-D double oblique thick maximum intensity projection views (*lower panels*) demonstrate the termination of the fistula into the left anterolateral aspect of the main pulmonary artery just distal to the pulmonic valve. The remainder of the left anterior descending artery followed a normal course without evidence of stenosis. The coronary artery origins were normal. There was no evidence of obstructive coronary artery disease. An incidental wide-mouthed saccular aneurysm of the descending thoracic aorta at the level of the left atrium is seen in the *lower right panel*. Given the size and profound tortuosity of the fistula in the setting of exertional chest pain, surgical ligation of the fistula via a median sternotomy approach was performed. *CX* circumflex coronary artery, *Diag* diagonal branch, *LAD* left anterior descending coronary artery, *LM* left main coronary artery, *PA* pulmonary artery, *RCA* right coronary artery (Reprinted from Shinbane et al. [35] with permission from SAGE Publications)

Fig. 22.32 Anomalous termination of a coronary artery with coronary artery fistula from the first septal perforating branch of the left anterior descending coronary artery to the right ventricular outflow tract with history of Tetralogy of Fallot repair. 3-D reconstructions (*upper panels*) show a large caliber and tortuous left main coronary artery with a posterior and cranial takeoff. A fistula from a septal branch of the left anterior descending coronary artery terminates in the right ventricular infundibulum. After takeoff of the fistula, the left anterior descending coronary artery continues as a normal caliber vessel along the anterior interventricular groove. 2-D double oblique thick maximum intensity projection views (*lower panels*) demonstrate the termination of the fistula into the posterior aspect of the right ventricular outflow tract. Portions of the right coronary artery coursed immediately posterior to the sternum. No significant stenoses of the coronary arteries were present. Other findings included a prosthetic aortic valve with normal leaflet motion, a right-sided aortic arch and descending aorta, and evidence of a prior repair of a ventricular septal defect. Given these findings, a percutaneous left anterior descending coronary artery to right ventricular outflow tract fistula occlusion with a 4-mm vascular plug was performed. *Diag* diagonal branch, *LAD* left anterior descending coronary artery, *RVOT* right ventricular outflow tract (Reprinted from Shinbane et al. [35] with permission from SAGE Publications)

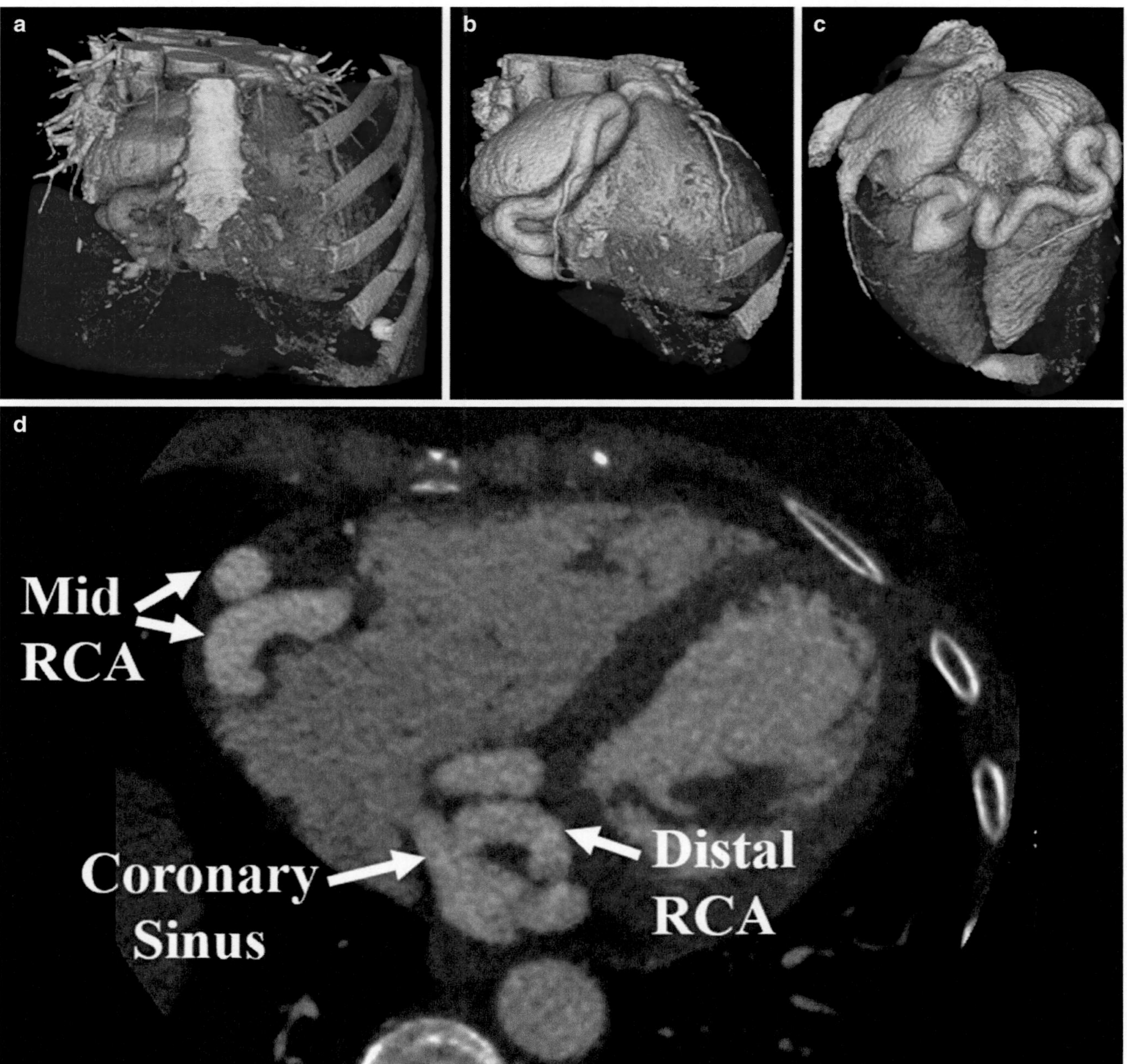

Fig. 22.34 Arteriovenous fistula due to anomalous right coronary artery termination into the coronary sinus. The right coronary artery is dilated throughout its course with a maximum dimension of 1.6 × 1.6 cm and serpiginous in morphology. Panel (**a**) A 3-D reconstruction with skeletal structure. Panel (**b**) A 3-D reconstruction with skeletal structure removed. Panel (**c**) Posterior rotation of 3-D reconstruction. Panel (**d**) A 2-D double oblique view demonstrating the abnormal termination of the right coronary artery with an arteriovenous connection to the coronary sinus, with the connection approximately 7 mm cm distal to the coronary sinus ostium. Surgical closure was performed. *RCA* right coronary artery

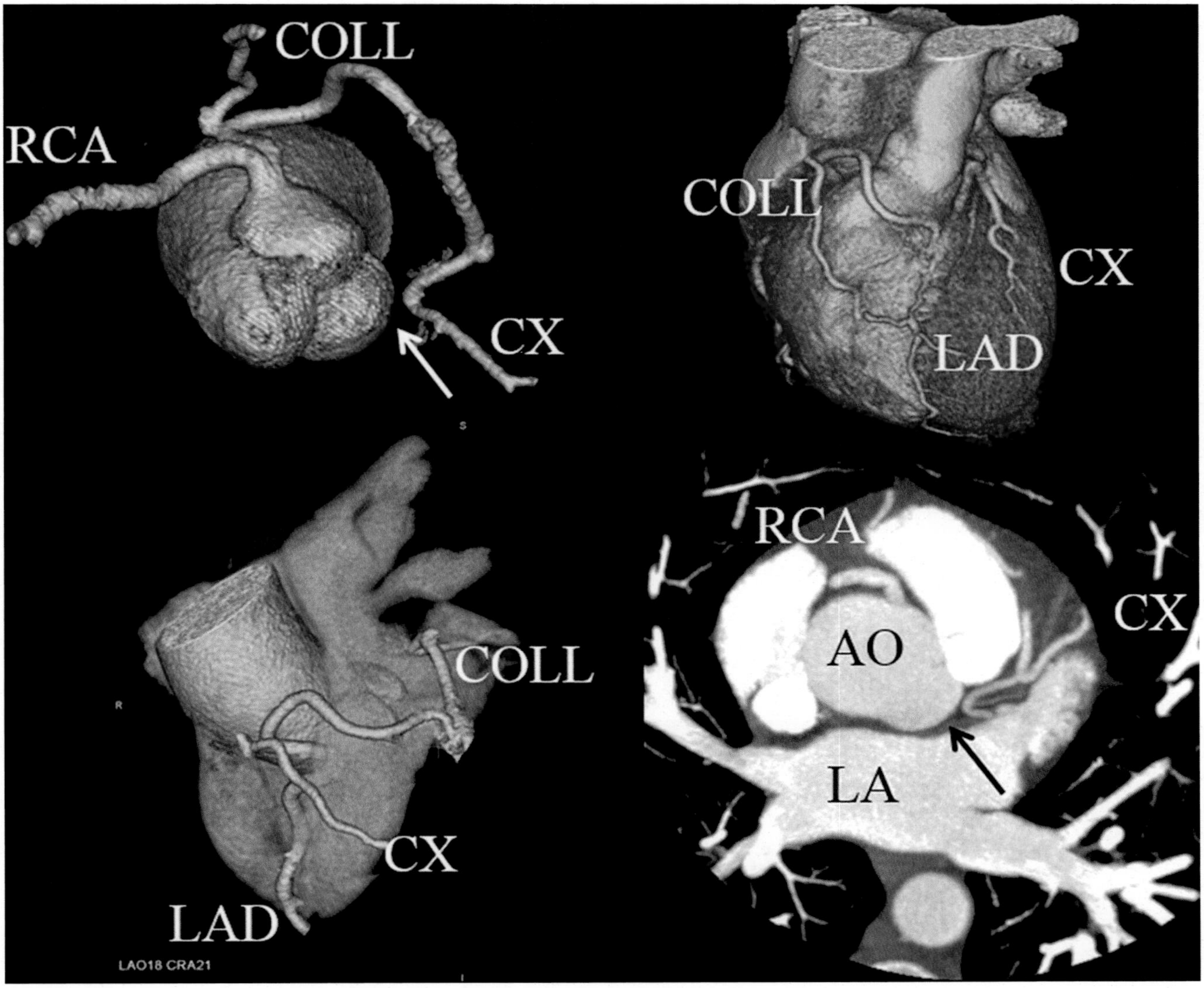

Fig. 22.35 Congenital atresia of the left main coronary artery. 3-D reconstructions (*upper and lower left panel*) demonstrate absence of left main coronary artery with a single coronary artery ostium off of the right coronary sinus. This single ostium gives off a right coronary artery right coronary artery and immediately after the ostium gives off a vessel which courses prepulmonic branching into a conus branch as well as two large collateral branches supplying a diminutive left coronary system with an underdeveloped left anterior descending coronary artery and circumflex. A 2-D double oblique thick maximum intensity projection view (*lower right panel*) shows lack of connection between the left anterior descending coronary artery and circumflex and the left coronary sinus. This single ostium gave off the right coronary artery that provided large collateral branches supplying a diminutive left coronary system with an underdeveloped left anterior descending coronary artery and circumflex. Cardiac catheterization demonstrated other small right-to-left collaterals to the diminutive left anterior descending coronary artery and circumflex. Surgical management was challenging since the left anterior descending coronary artery and circumflex were underdeveloped. Coronary artery bypass was performed off pump with a free left internal mammary artery anastomosed distally to a diagonal branch and anastomosed proximally to the aorta. *AO* aorta, *COLL* collateral, *CX* circumflex coronary artery, *LAD* left anterior descending coronary artery, *LA* left atrium, *LM* left main coronary artery, *RCA* right coronary artery (Reprinted from Shinbane et al. [35] with permission from SAGE Publications)

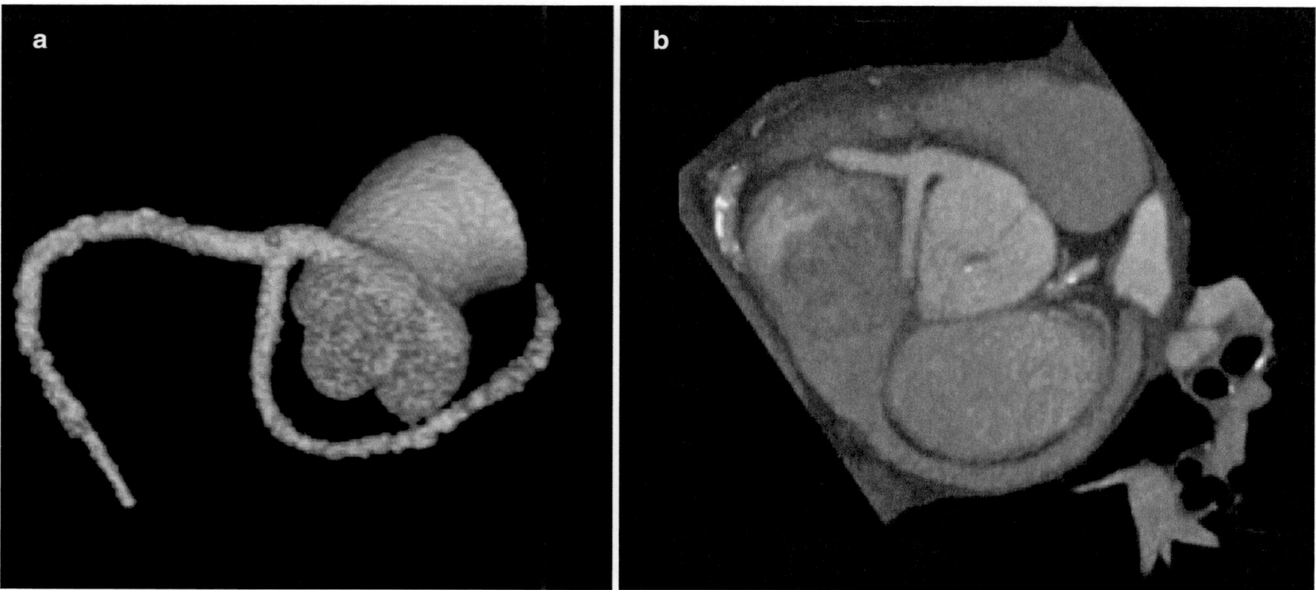

Fig. 22.36 Anomalous coronary artery anatomy with a single coronary ostium arising from the right coronary sinus giving off a left main taking a retroaortic course and a right coronary artery. (**a**) 3-D reconstruction of the coronary arteries. (**b**) Double-oblique maximal intensity projection

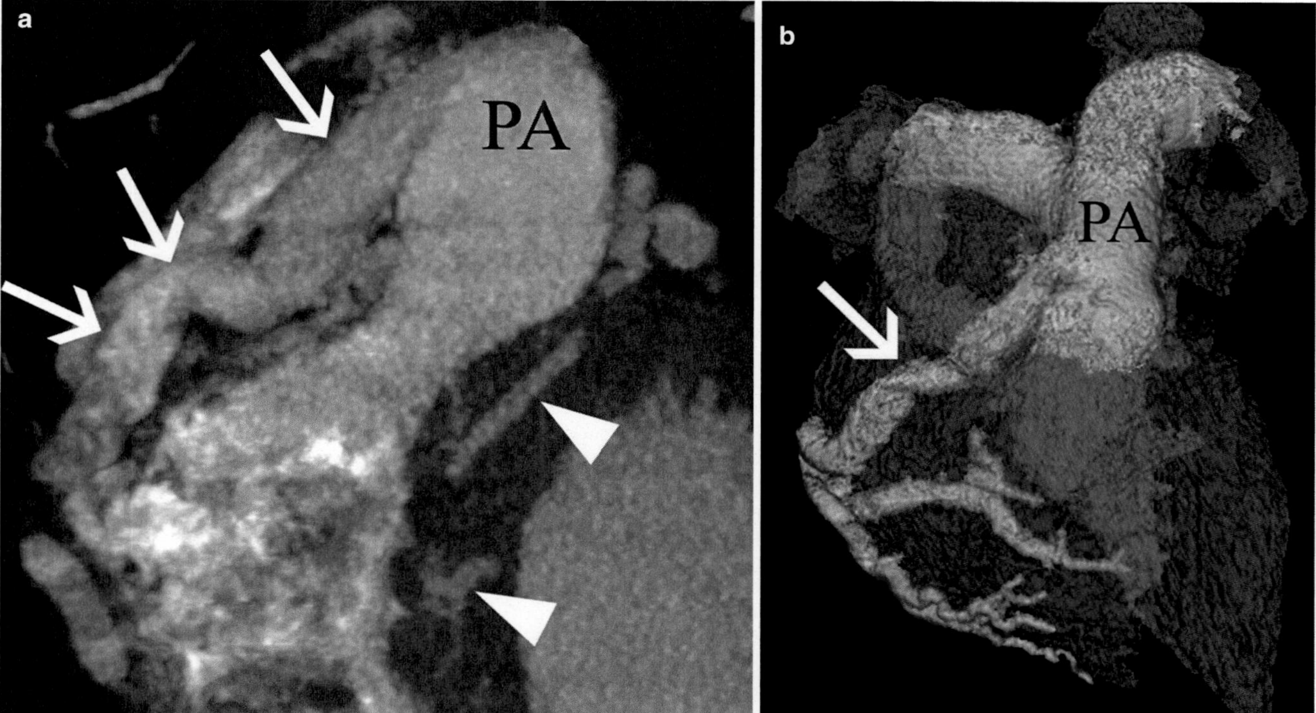

Fig. 22.37 Origin of the right coronary artery from the pulmonary artery in a 38-year-old man with chest pain and anomalous anatomy at cardiac catheterization. Oblique coronal CCTA image (Panel **a**) and volume rendered image (Panel **b**) show origin of the right coronary artery (*arrows*) from the main pulmonary artery. Note the dilated vessels in the septum (*arrowheads* in **a**), which likely represent dilated left-to-right collateral arteries that formed due to increased flow. Usually, the left main coronary artery is the more common anomalous coronary artery originating from the pulmonary artery. The patient's presentation in adulthood was also unusual. *PA* pulmonary artery (Reprinted from Shriki et al. [71]; Reproduced with permission from the Radiological Society of North America, RSNA®.)

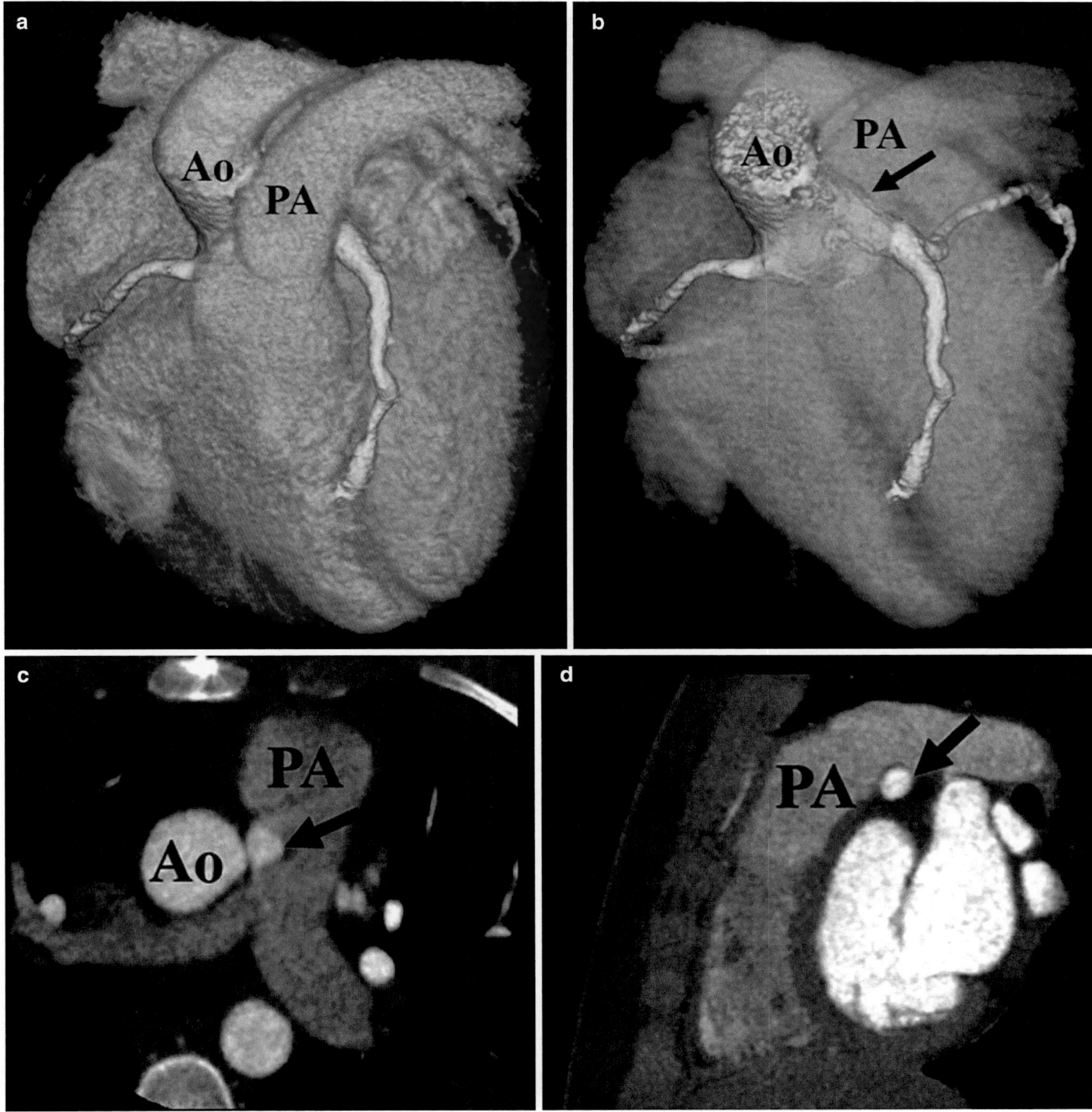

Fig. 22.38 Takeuchi repair of anomalous left coronary artery from the pulmonary artery with an aortopulmonary window with an intrapulmonary tunnel baffling aortic flow to the left coronary artery. Panel (**a**) A 3-D reconstruction demonstrating the relationship of the aorta and pulmonary artery to the coronary artery. Panel (**b**) A 3-D reconstruction with the pulmonary artery made more translucent demonstrating the aortic baffle to the left coronary artery. Panels (**c**, **d**) 2-D double oblique views demonstrating the baffling of aortic flow (*black arrows*) to the left coronary artery tunneled through the pulmonary artery. *Ao* aorta, *PA* pulmonary artery

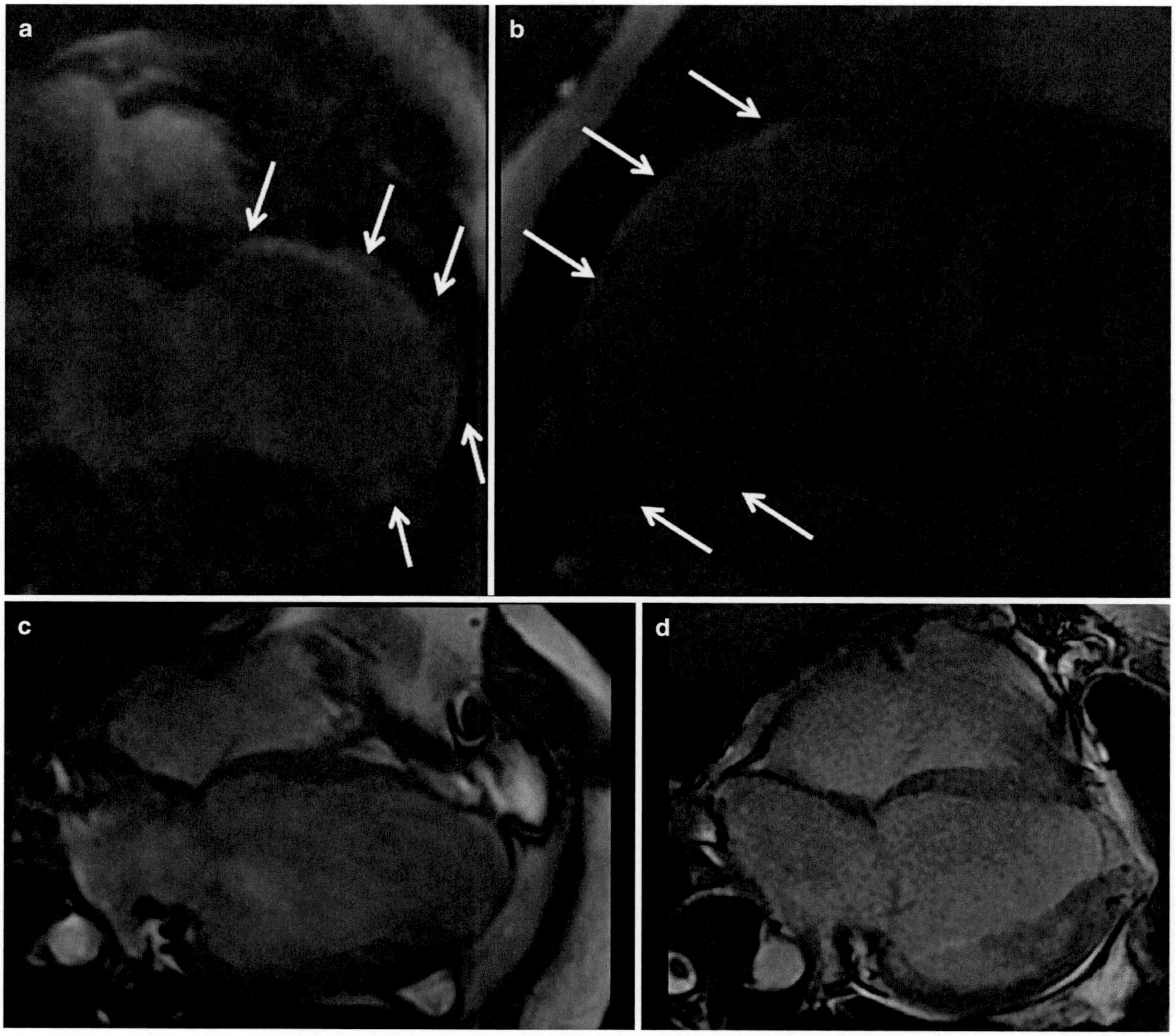

Fig. 22.39 Magnetic resonance imaging assessment in a patient with ischemic cardiomyopathy showing transmural mid to distal anterior and inferior wall myocardial infarctions (*arrows*) on delayed gadolinium enhancement views with viability of basal segments of these walls and of the lateral territory. Panel (**a**) 4 chamber delayed gadolinium enhanced view. Panel (**b**) 2 chamber delayed gadolinium enhanced view. The patient underwent coronary artery bypass graft surgery and ventricular aneurysmectomy. Panel (**c**) Pre-surgical steady state free precession 4 chamber view. Panel (**d**) Post-surgical steady state free precession 4 chamber view

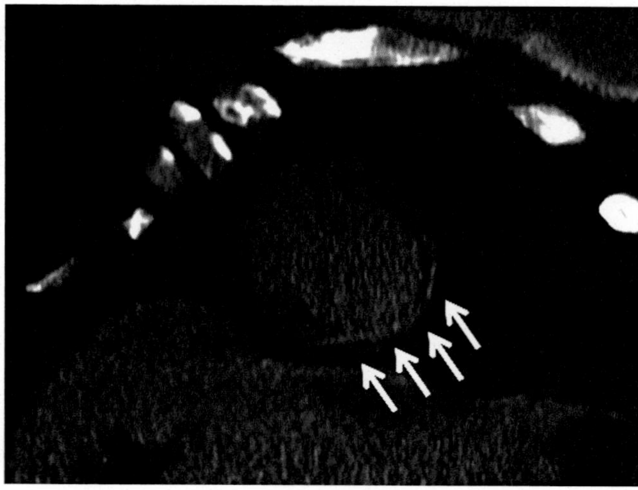

Fig. 22.40 Delayed CT contrast enhancement imaging performed immediately after cardiac catheterization without contrast reinjection demonstrating inferior and inferolateral delayed enhancement (*arrows*) on a short axis view

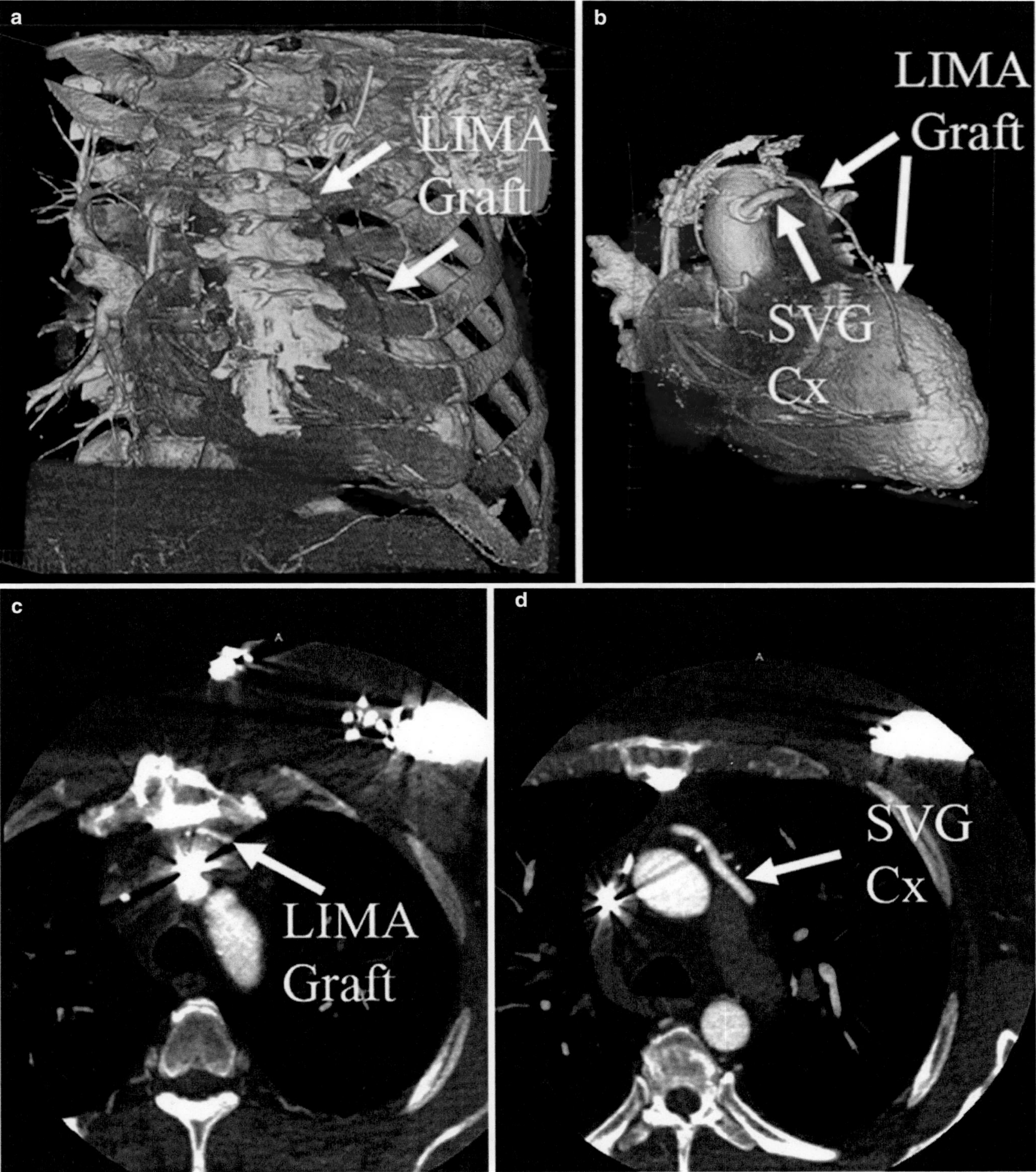

Fig. 22.41 CCTA for pre-surgical planning prior to left ventricular assist device placement. Panel (**a**) A 3-D reconstruction in the context of skeletal structure. Panel (**b**) A 3-D reconstruction with skeletal structures removed. Panel (**c**) 2-D axial view demonstrating the location of the left internal mammary artery graft to the left anterior descending coronary artery in relation to the sternum. Panel (**d**) 2-D axial view demonstrating the location of a saphenous vein graft to the circumflex coronary artery in relation to the sternum. *Cx* circumflex coronary artery, *LIMA* left internal mammary artery, *SVG* saphenous vein graft

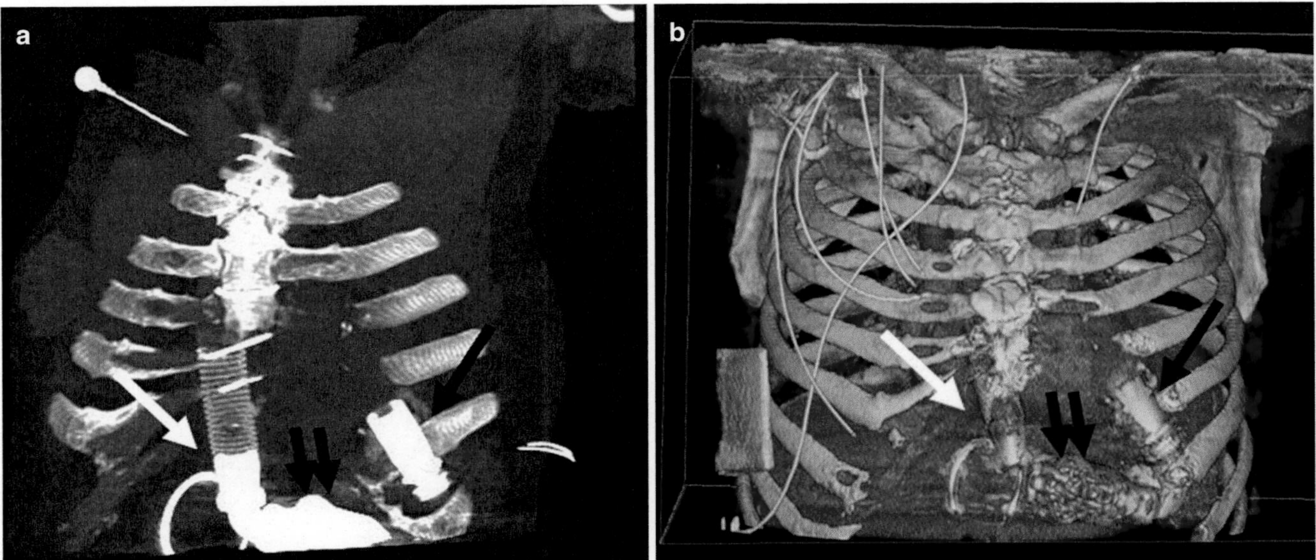

Fig. 22.42 Left ventricular assist device for advanced heart failure. Panel (**a**) A 2-D double oblique thick maximum intensity projection view demonstrating inflow conduit/valve (*back arrow*) to the pump, left ventricular assist device pump (*black double arrow*), and outflow conduit from the pump (*white arrow*). Panel (**b**). 3-D reconstruction in context of skeletal structures demonstrating inflow conduit/valve (*back arrow*) to the pump, left ventricular assist device pump (*black double arrow*), and outflow conduit from the pump (*white arrow*)

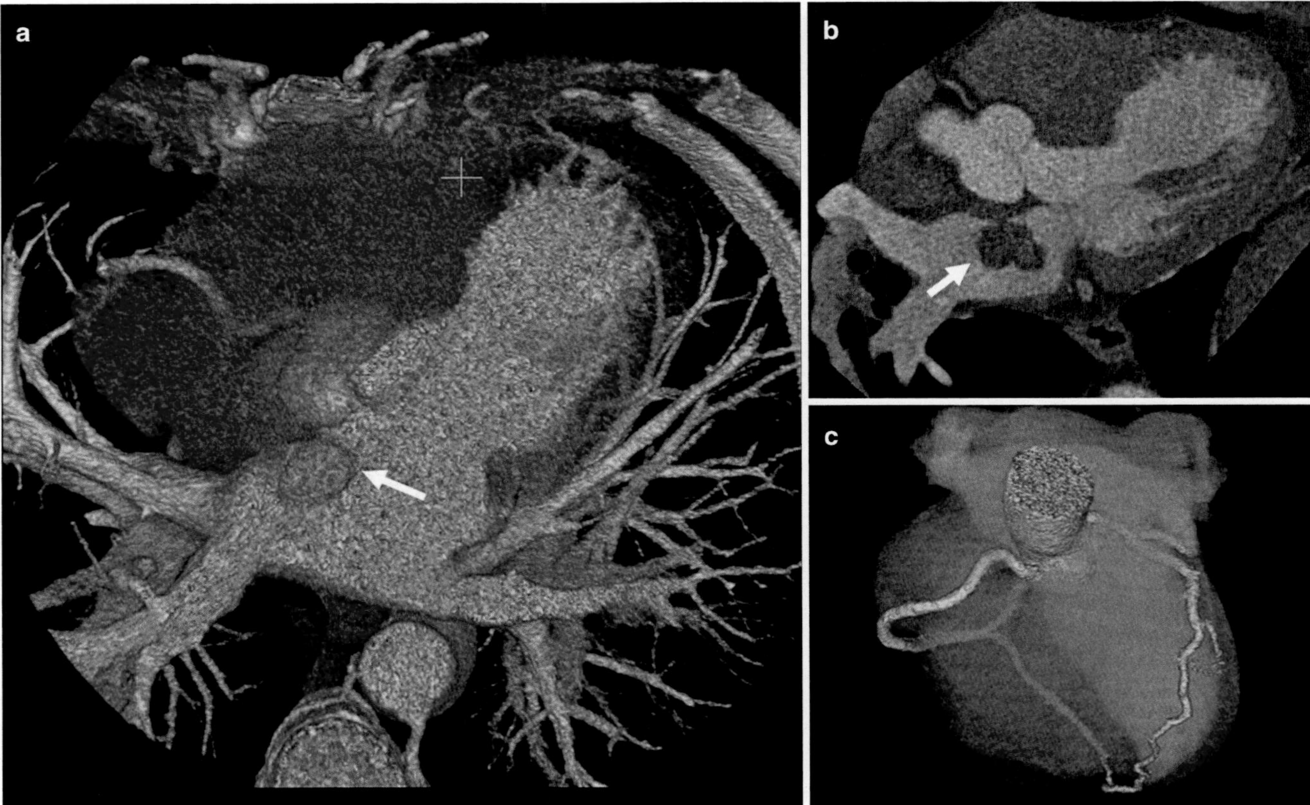

Fig. 22.43 CCTA demonstrating a solitary low attenuation lobulated left atrial mass measuring 2.4 cm (craniocaudal) with a narrow stalk attached to the interatrial septum near the fossa ovalis. There were hyperlucent areas and heterogeneous enhancement with contrast as well as areas of calcification. There was no involvement of other cardiac structures. Surgical excision was performed with histologic diagnosis of left atrial myxoma with organizing thrombus formation. Panel (**a**) 3-D reconstruction demonstrating the left atrial mass (*arrow*). Panel (**b**) 2-D double oblique view demonstrating characteristics of the mass (*arrow*), including lobulation, a narrow stalk attached to the interatrial septum near the fossa ovalis, and heterogeneity with hyperlucent areas and heterogeneous enhancement with contrast. Panel (**c**) 3-D reconstruction of the coronary arteries demonstrating no evidence of coronary artery disease

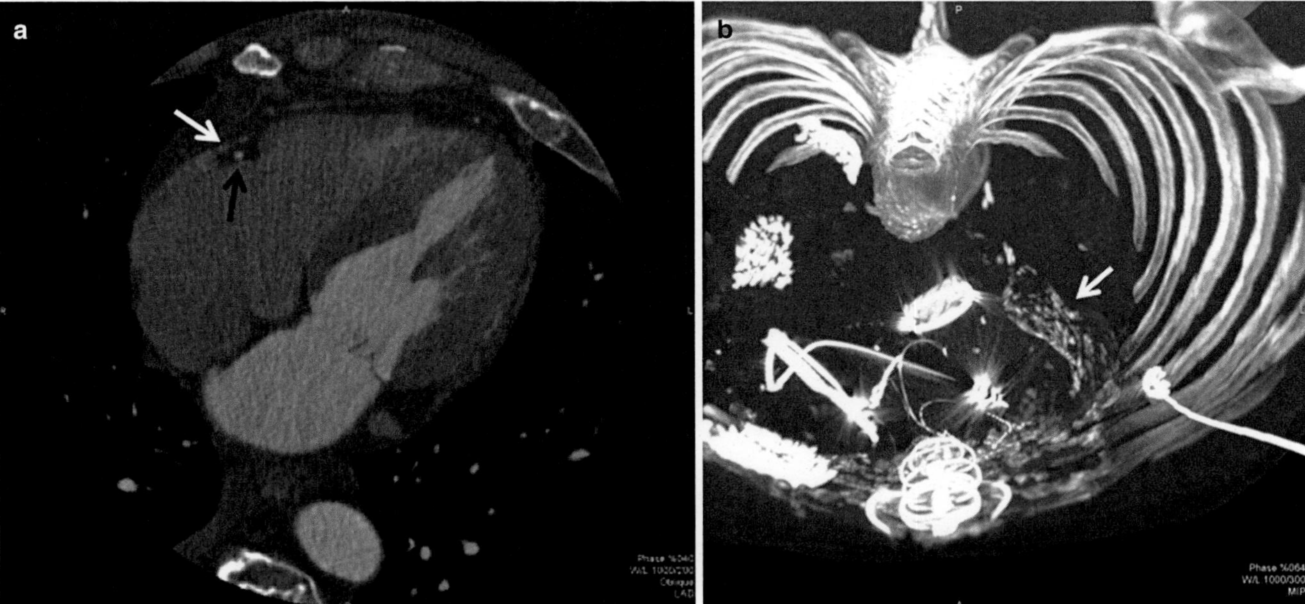

Fig. 22.44 Panel (**a**) Oblique 2-D image demonstrating the relationship of the right coronary artery (*black arrow*) to thickened pericardium (*white arrow*) prior to pericardiectomy in a patient with constrictive pericarditis. Panel (**b**) Calcific constrictive pericarditis (*white arrow*) in a patient with rheumatic heard disease, mitral valve replacement, and a dual chamber pacemaker

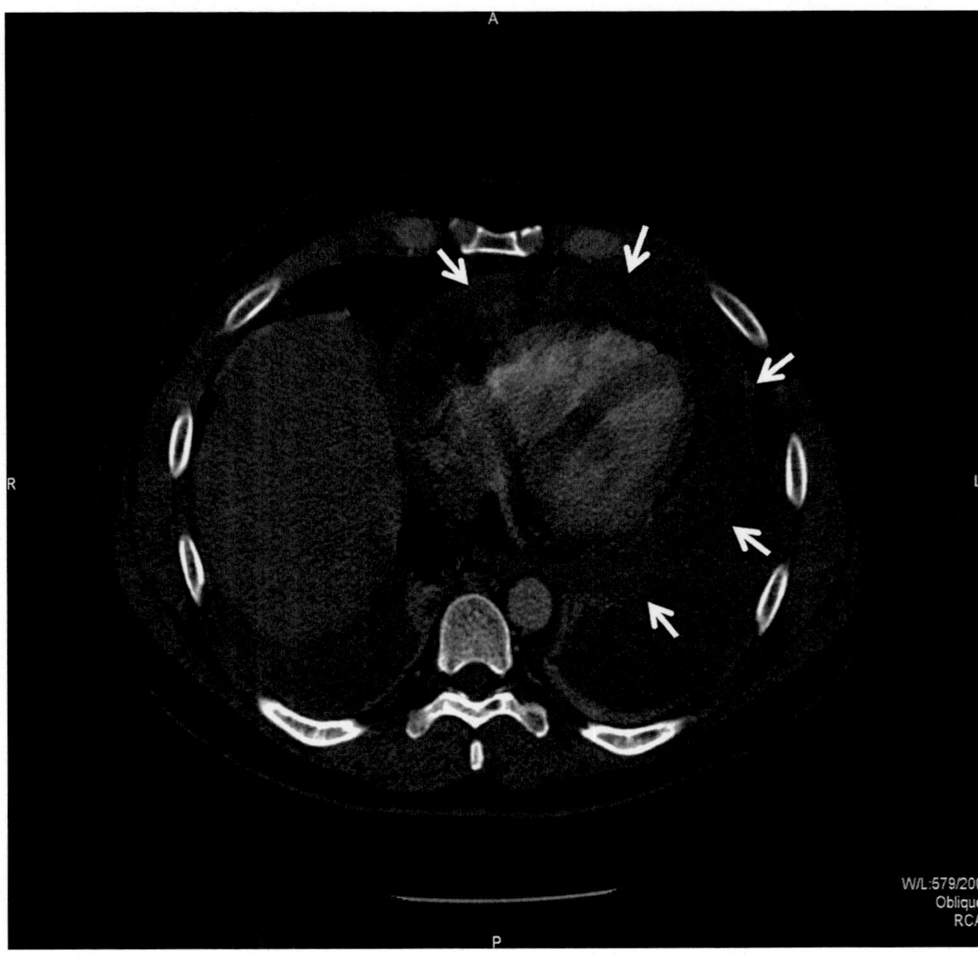

Fig. 22.45 A large circumferential effusion (*arrows*) with tissue attenuation, consistent proteinaceous material, and complexity of structure which required open surgical dissection

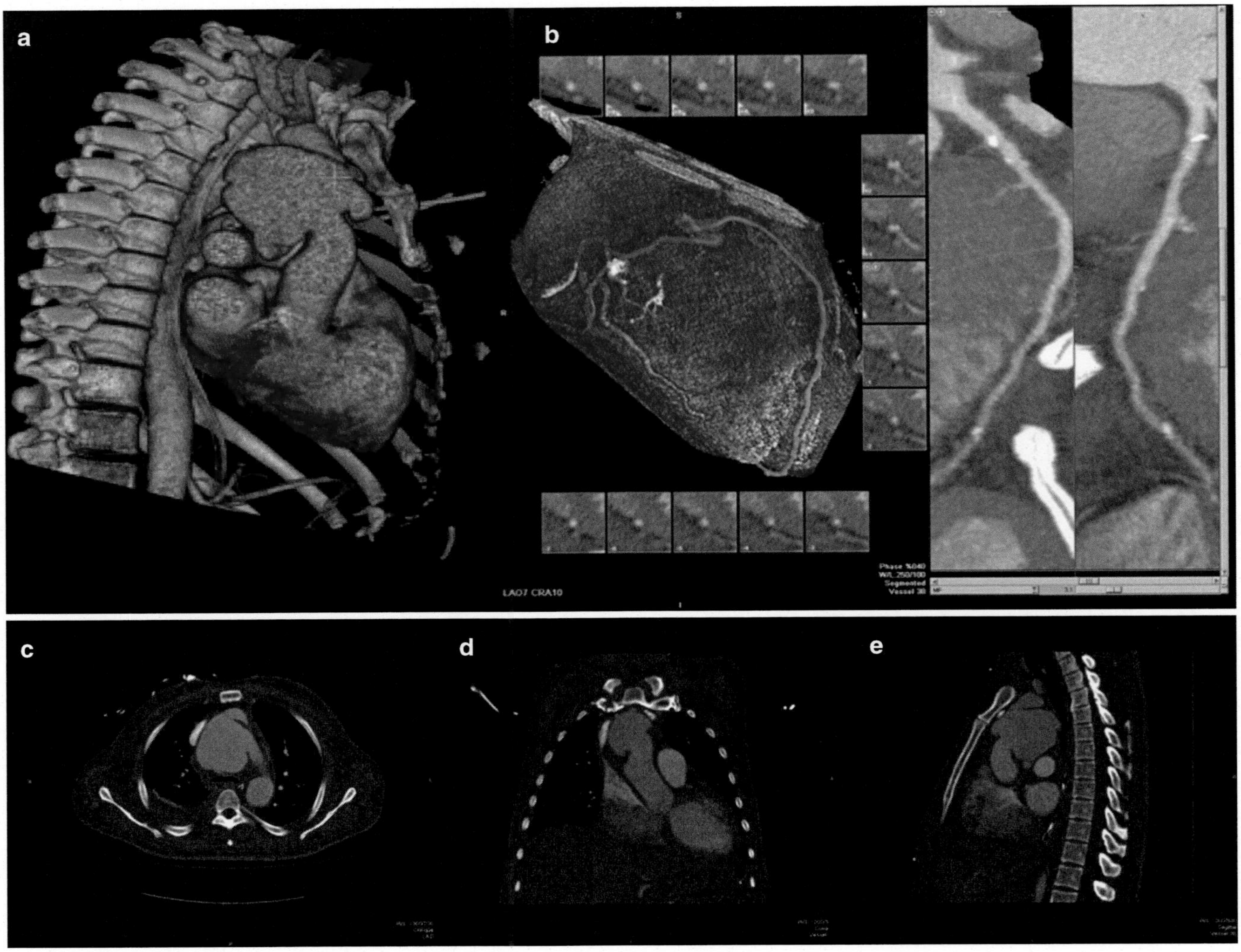

Fig. 22.46 A large aortic aneurysm which may impede invasive cardiac catheterization, with multimodal views including Panel (**a**) 3-D view; Panel (**b**) Curved multiplanar reformat view visualizing the left anterior descending coronary artery; Panel (**c**) Axial view; Panel (**d**) Coronal view; Panel (**e**) Sagittal view

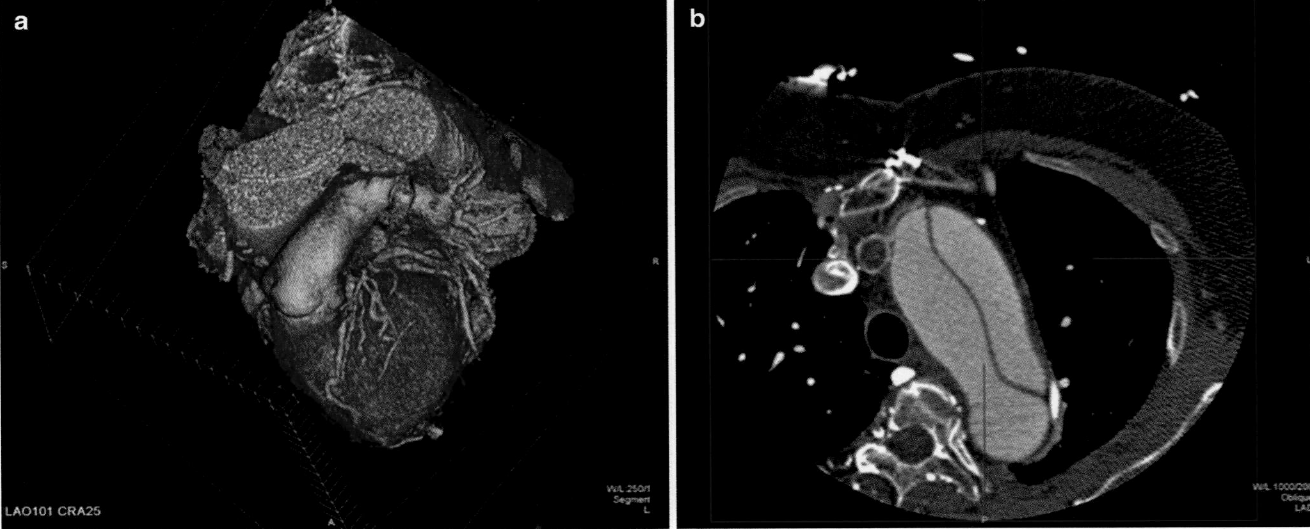

Fig. 22.47 Aortic dissection making cardiac catheterization challenging for assessment for coronary artery disease. Panel (**a**) 3-D view. Panel (**b**) double oblique 2-D view of an aortic dissection

References

1. Roselli EE, Pettersson GB, Blackstone EH, Brizzio ME, Houghtaling PL, Hauck R, et al. Adverse events during reoperative cardiac surgery: frequency, characterization, and rescue. J Thorac Cardiovasc Surg. 2008;135(2):316–23, 23 e1–6.
2. Sabik 3rd JF, Blackstone EH, Houghtaling PL, Walts PA, Lytle BW. Is reoperation still a risk factor in coronary artery bypass surgery? Ann Thorac Surg. 2005;80(5):1719–27.
3. Kamdar AR, Meadows TA, Roselli EE, Gorodeski EZ, Curtin RJ, Sabik JF, et al. Multidetector computed tomographic angiography in planning of reoperative cardiothoracic surgery. Ann Thorac Surg. 2008;85(4):1239–45.
4. Gasparovic H, Rybicki FJ, Millstine J, Unic D, Byrne JG, Yucel K, et al. Three dimensional computed tomographic imaging in planning the surgical approach for redo cardiac surgery after coronary revascularization. Eur J CardioThorac Surg. 2005; 28(2):244–9.
5. Mack MJ, Leon MB, Smith CR, Miller DC, Moses JW, Tuzcu EM, et al. 5-year outcomes of transcatheter aortic valve replacement or surgical aortic valve replacement for high surgical risk patients with aortic stenosis (PARTNER 1): a randomised controlled trial. Lancet. 2015;385(9986):2477–84.
6. Kapadia SR, Leon MB, Makkar RR, Tuzcu EM, Svensson LG, Kodali S, et al. 5-year outcomes of transcatheter aortic valve replacement compared with standard treatment for patients with inoperable aortic stenosis (PARTNER 1): a randomised controlled trial. Lancet. 2015;385(9986):2485–91.
7. Chieffo A, Buchanan GL, Van Mieghem NM, Tchetche D, Dumonteil N, Latib A, et al. Transcatheter aortic valve implantation with the Edwards SAPIEN versus the Medtronic CoreValve Revalving system devices: a multicenter collaborative study: the PRAGMATIC Plus Initiative (Pooled-RotterdAm-Milano-Toulouse In Collaboration). J Am Coll Cardiol. 2013; 61(8):830–6.
8. Kurra V, Schoenhagen P, Roselli EE, Kapadia SR, Tuzcu EM, Greenberg R, et al. Prevalence of significant peripheral artery disease in patients evaluated for percutaneous aortic valve insertion: preprocedural assessment with multidetector computed tomography. J Thorac Cardiovasc Surg. 2009;137(5):1258–64.
9. Achenbach S, Delgado V, Hausleiter J, Schoenhagen P, Min JK, Leipsic JA. SCCT expert consensus document on computed tomography imaging before transcatheter aortic valve implantation (TAVI)/transcatheter aortic valve replacement (TAVR). J Cardiovasc Comput Tomogr. 2012;6(6):366–80.
10. Blanke P, Russe M, Leipsic J, Reinohl J, Ebersberger U, Suranyi P, et al. Conformational pulsatile changes of the aortic annulus: impact on prosthesis sizing by computed tomography for transcatheter aortic valve replacement. JACC Cardiovasc Interv. 2012;5(9):984–94.
11. Blanke P, Schoepf UJ, Leipsic JA. CT in transcatheter aortic valve replacement. Radiology. 2013;269(3):650–69.
12. Watanabe Y, Lefevre T, Arai T, Hayashida K, Bouvier E, Hovasse T, et al. Can we predict post-procedural paravalvular leak after Edwards Sapien transcatheter aortic valve implantation? Catheter Cardiovasc Interv. 2015;86(1):144–51.
13. Azzalini L, Ghoshhajra BB, Elmariah S, Passeri JJ, Inglessis I, Palacios IF, et al. The aortic valve calcium nodule score (AVCNS) independently predicts paravalvular regurgitation after transcatheter aortic valve replacement (TAVR). J Cardiovasc Comput Tomogr. 2014;8(2):131–40.
14. Anger T, Bauer V, Plachtzik C, Geisler T, Gawaz M, Oberhoff M, et al. Non-invasive and invasive predictors of paravalvular regurgitation post CoreValve(R) stent prosthesis implantation in aortic valves. J Interv Cardiol. 2014;27(3):275–83.
15. Binder RK, Webb JG, Willson AB, Urena M, Hansson NC, Norgaard BL, et al. The impact of integration of a multidetector computed tomography annulus area sizing algorithm on outcomes of transcatheter aortic valve replacement: a prospective, multicenter, controlled trial. J Am Coll Cardiol. 2013;62(5):431–8.
16. Dvir D, Webb JG, Piazza N, Blanke P, Barbanti M, Bleiziffer S, et al. Multicenter evaluation of transcatheter aortic valve replacement using either SAPIEN XT or CoreValve: degree of device oversizing by computed-tomography and clinical outcomes. Catheteriz Cardiovasc Interv. 2015;86:508–15.
17. Barbanti M, Yang TH, Rodes Cabau J, Tamburino C, Wood DA, Jilaihawi H, et al. Anatomical and procedural features associated with aortic root rupture during balloon-expandable transcatheter aortic valve replacement. Circulation. 2013;128(3):244–53.
18. Tops LF, Wood DA, Delgado V, Schuijf JD, Mayo JR, Pasupati S, et al. Noninvasive evaluation of the aortic root with multislice computed tomography implications for transcatheter aortic valve replacement. JACC Cardiovasc Imaging. 2008;1(3):321–30.
19. Akhtar M, Tuzcu EM, Kapadia SR, Svensson LG, Greenberg RK, Roselli EE, et al. Aortic root morphology in patients undergoing percutaneous aortic valve replacement: evidence of aortic root remodeling. J Thorac Cardiovasc Surg. 2009;137(4):950–6.
20. Wood DA, Tops LF, Mayo JR, Pasupati S, Schalij MJ, Humphries K, et al. Role of multislice computed tomography in transcatheter aortic valve replacement. Am J Cardiol. 2009;103(9):1295–301.
21. Masson JB, Kovac J, Schuler G, Ye J, Cheung A, Kapadia S, et al. Transcatheter aortic valve implantation: review of the nature, management, and avoidance of procedural complications. JACC Cardiovasc Interv. 2009;2(9):811–20.
22. Stabile E, Sorropago G, Cioppa A, Cota L, Agrusta M, Lucchetti V, et al. Acute left main obstructions following TAVI. EuroIntervention. 2010;6(1):100–5.
23. Testa L, Latib A, De Marco F, De Carlo M, Agnifili M, Latini RA, et al. Clinical impact of persistent left bundle-branch block after transcatheter aortic valve implantation with CoreValve Revalving System. Circulation. 2013;127(12):1300–7.
24. Latsios G, Gerckens U, Buellesfeld L, Mueller R, John D, Yuecel S, et al. "Device landing zone" calcification, assessed by MSCT, as a predictive factor for pacemaker implantation after TAVI. Catheter Cardiovasc Interv. 2010;76(3):431–9.
25. Guetta V, Goldenberg G, Segev A, Dvir D, Kornowski R, Finckelstein A, et al. Predictors and course of high-degree atrioventricular block after transcatheter aortic valve implantation using the CoreValve Revalving System. Am J Cardiol. 2011;108(11):1600–5.
26. Freeman M, Webb JG, Willson AB, Wheeler M, Blanke P, Moss RR, et al. Multidetector CT predictors of prosthesis-patient mismatch in transcatheter aortic valve replacement. J Cardiovasc Comput Tomogr. 2013;7(4):248–55.
27. Nazif TM, Dizon JM, Hahn RT, Xu K, Babaliaros V, Douglas PS, et al. Predictors and clinical outcomes of permanent pacemaker implantation after transcatheter aortic valve replacement: the PARTNER (Placement of AoRtic TraNscathetER Valves) trial and registry. JACC Cardiovasc Interv. 2015;8(1 Pt A):60–9.
28. Binder RK, Webb JG, Toggweiler S, Freeman M, Barbanti M, Willson AB, et al. Impact of post-implant SAPIEN XT geometry and position on conduction disturbances, hemodynamic performance, and paravalvular regurgitation. JACC Cardiovasc Interv. 2013;6(5):462–8.
29. Scheffel H, Leschka S, Plass A, Vachenauer R, Gaemperli O, Garzoli E, et al. Accuracy of 64-slice computed tomography for the preoperative detection of coronary artery disease in patients with chronic aortic regurgitation. Am J Cardiol. 2007; 100(4):701–6.
30. Feuchtner GM, Stolzmann P, Dichtl W, Schertler T, Bonatti J, Scheffel H, et al. Multislice computed tomography in infective endocarditis: comparison with transesophageal echocardiography and intraoperative findings. J Am Coll Cardiol. 2009;53(5): 436–44.

31. McElhinney DB, Hellenbrand WE, Zahn EM, Jones TK, Cheatham JP, Lock JE, et al. Short- and medium-term outcomes after transcatheter pulmonary valve placement in the expanded multicenter US melody valve trial. Circulation. 2010;122(5):507–16.
32. Zahn EM, Hellenbrand WE, Lock JE, McElhinney DB. Implantation of the melody transcatheter pulmonary valve in patients with a dysfunctional right ventricular outflow tract conduit early results from the u.s. Clinical trial. J Am Coll Cardiol. 2009;54(18):1722–9.
33. Armstrong AK, Balzer DT, Cabalka AK, Gray RG, Javois AJ, Moore JW, et al. One-year follow-up of the Melody transcatheter pulmonary valve multicenter post-approval study. JACC Cardiovasc Interv. 2014;7(11):1254–62.
34. Meadows JJ, Moore PM, Berman DP, Cheatham JP, Cheatham SL, Porras D, et al. Use and performance of the Melody Transcatheter Pulmonary Valve in native and postsurgical, nonconduit right ventricular outflow tracts. Circ Cardiovasc Interv. 2014;7(3):374–80.
35. Shinbane JS, Shriki J, Fleischman F, Hindoyan A, Withey J, Lee C, et al. Anomalous coronary arteries: cardiovascular computed tomographic angiography for surgical decisions and planning. World J Pediatr Congenital Heart Surg. 2013;4(2):142–54.
36. Delgado V, Tops LF, Schuijf JD, de Roos A, Brugada J, Schalij MJ, et al. Assessment of mitral valve anatomy and geometry with multislice computed tomography. JACC Cardiovasc Imaging. 2009;2(5):556–65.
37. Shudo Y, Matsumiya G, Sakaguchi T, Miyagawa S, Yoshikawa Y, Yamauchi T, et al. Assessment of changes in mitral valve configuration with multidetector computed tomography: impact of papillary muscle imbrication and ring annuloplasty. Circulation. 2010;122(11 Suppl):S29–36.
38. Gordic S, Nguyen-Kim TD, Manka R, Sundermann S, Frauenfelder T, Maisano F, et al. Sizing the mitral annulus in healthy subjects and patients with mitral regurgitation: 2D versus 3D measurements from cardiac CT. Int J Cardiovasc Imaging. 2014;30(2):389–98.
39. Blanke P, Dvir D, Cheung A, Ye J, Levine RA, Precious B, et al. A simplified D-shaped model of the mitral annulus to facilitate CT-based sizing before transcatheter mitral valve implantation. J Cardiovasc Comput Tomogr. 2014;8(6):459–67.
40. Moodley S, Schoenhagen P, Gillinov AM, Mihaljevic T, Flamm SD, Griffin BP, et al. Preoperative multidetector computed tomograpy angiography for planning of minimally invasive robotic mitral valve surgery: impact on decision making. J Thorac Cardiovasc Surg. 2013;146(2):262–8 e1.
41. Higgins J, Mayo J, Skarsgard P. Cardiac computed tomography facilitates operative planning in patients with mitral calcification. Ann Thorac Surg. 2013;95(1):e9–11.
42. Morris MF, Suri RM, Akhtar NJ, Young PM, Gruden JF, Burkhart HM, et al. Computed tomography as an alternative to catheter angiography prior to robotic mitral valve repair. Ann Thorac Surg. 2013;95(4):1354–9.
43. Ghersin N, Abadi S, Sabbag A, Lamash Y, Anderson RH, Wolfson H, et al. The three-dimensional geometric relationship between the mitral valvar annulus and the coronary arteries as seen from the perspective of the cardiac surgeon using cardiac computed tomography. Eur J CardioThorac Surg. 2013;44(6):1123–30.
44. Mao S, Shinbane JS, Girsky MJ, Child J, Carson S, Oudiz RJ, et al. Coronary venous imaging with electron beam computed tomographic angiography: three-dimensional mapping and relationship with coronary arteries. Am Heart J. 2005;150(2):315–22.
45. Choure AJ, Garcia MJ, Hesse B, Sevensma M, Maly G, Greenberg NL, et al. In vivo analysis of the anatomical relationship of coronary sinus to mitral annulus and left circumflex coronary artery using cardiac multidetector computed tomography: implications for percutaneous coronary sinus mitral annuloplasty. J Am Coll Cardiol. 2006;48(10):1938–45.
46. Feldman T, Kar S, Rinaldi M, Fail P, Hermiller J, Smalling R, et al. Percutaneous mitral repair with the MitraClip system: safety and midterm durability in the initial EVEREST (Endovascular Valve Edge-to-Edge REpair Study) cohort. J Am Coll Cardiol. 2009;54(8):686–94.
47. Feldman T, Young A. Percutaneous approaches to valve repair for mitral regurgitation. J Am Coll Cardiol. 2014;63(20):2057–68.
48. Attizzani GF, Ohno Y, Capodanno D, Cannata S, Dipasqua F, Imme S, et al. Extended use of percutaneous edge-to-edge mitral valve repair beyond EVEREST (Endovascular Valve Edge-to-Edge Repair) criteria: 30-day and 12-month clinical and echocardiographic outcomes from the GRASP (Getting Reduction of Mitral Insufficiency by Percutaneous Clip Implantation) registry. JACC Cardiovasc Interv. 2015;8(1 Pt A):74–82.
49. Cook SC, Dyke 2nd PC, Raman SV. Management of adults with congenital heart disease with cardiovascular computed tomography. J Cardiovasc Comput Tomogr. 2008;2(1):12–22.
50. Shinbane JS, Colletti PM, Shellock FG. MR imaging in patients with pacemakers and other devices: engineering the future. JACC Cardiovasc Imaging. 2012;5(3):332–3.
51. Shinbane JS, Colletti PM, Shellock FG. Magnetic resonance imaging in patients with cardiac pacemakers: era of "MR Conditional" designs. J Cardiovasc Magn Reson. 2011;13:63.
52. Hoffmann A, Engelfriet P, Mulder B. Radiation exposure during follow-up of adults with congenital heart disease. Int J Cardiol. 2007;118(2):151–3.
53. Ben Saad M, Rohnean A, Sigal-Cinqualbre A, Adler G, Paul JF. Evaluation of image quality and radiation dose of thoracic and coronary dual-source CT in 110 infants with congenital heart disease. Pediatr Radiol. 2009;39(7):668–76.
54. Huang MP, Liang CH, Zhao ZJ, Liu H, Li JL, Zhang JE, et al. Evaluation of image quality and radiation dose at prospective ECG-triggered axial 256-slice multi-detector CT in infants with congenital heart disease. Pediatr Radiol. 2011;41(7):858–66.
55. Paul JF, Rohnean A, Elfassy E, Sigal-Cinqualbre A. Radiation dose for thoracic and coronary step-and-shoot CT using a 128-slice dual-source machine in infants and small children with congenital heart disease. Pediatr Radiol. 2011;41(2):244–9.
56. Shinbane JS, Shriki J, Hindoyan A, Ghosh B, Chang P, Farvid A, et al. Unoperated congenitally corrected transposition of the great arteries, nonrestrictive ventricular septal defect, and pulmonary stenosis in middle adulthood: do multiple wrongs make a right? World J Pediatr Congenital Heart Surg. 2012;3(1):123–9.
57. Ihlenburg S, Rompel O, Rueffer A, Purbojo A, Cesnjevar R, Dittrich S, et al. Dual source computed tomography in patients with congenital heart disease. Thorac Cardiovasc Surg. 2014;62(3):203–10.
58. Vastel-Amzallag C, Le Bret E, Paul JF, Lambert V, Rohnean A, El Fassy E, et al. Diagnostic accuracy of dual-source multislice computed tomographic analysis for the preoperative detection of coronary artery anomalies in 100 patients with tetralogy of Fallot. J Thorac Cardiovasc Surg. 2011;142(1):120–6.
59. Yamasaki Y, Nagao M, Yamamura K, Yonezawa M, Matsuo Y, Kawanami S, et al. Quantitative assessment of right ventricular function and pulmonary regurgitation in surgically repaired tetralogy of Fallot using 256-slice CT: comparison with 3-Tesla MRI. Eur Radiol. 2014;24(12):3289–99.
60. Park EA, Lee W, Chung SY, Yin YH, Chung JW, Park JH. Optimal scan timing and intravenous route for contrast-enhanced computed tomography in patients after Fontan operation. J Comput Assist Tomogr. 2010;34(1):75–81.
61. Cook SC, McCarthy M, Daniels CJ, Cheatham JP, Raman SV. Usefulness of multislice computed tomography angiography

to evaluate intravascular stents and transcatheter occlusion devices in patients with d-transposition of the great arteries after mustard repair. Am J Cardiol. 2004;94(7):967–9.

62. Oztunc F, Baris S, Adaletli I, Onol NO, Olgun DC, Guzeltas A, et al. Coronary events and anatomy after arterial switch operation for transposition of the great arteries: detection by 16-row multislice computed tomography angiography in pediatric patients. Cardiovasc Intervent Radiol. 2009;32(2):206–12.
63. Ou P, Celermajer DS, Marini D, Agnoletti G, Vouhe P, Brunelle F, et al. Safety and accuracy of 64-slice computed tomography coronary angiography in children after the arterial switch operation for transposition of the great arteries. JACC Cardiovasc Imaging. 2008;1(3):331–9.
64. Raman SV, Cook SC, McCarthy B, Ferketich AK. Usefulness of multidetector row computed tomography to quantify right ventricular size and function in adults with either tetralogy of Fallot or transposition of the great arteries. Am J Cardiol. 2005; 95(5):683–6.
65. Quaife RA, Chen MY, Kim M, Klein AJ, Jehle A, Kay J, et al. Pre-procedural planning for percutaneous atrial septal defect closure: transesophageal echocardiography compared with cardiac computed tomographic angiography. J Cardiovasc Comput Tomogr. 2010;4(5):330–8.
66. Kivisto S, Hanninen H, Holmstrom M. Partial anomalous pulmonary venous return and atrial septal defect in adult patients detected with 128-slice multidetector computed tomography. J Cardiothorac Surg. 2011;6:126.
67. Rajiah P, Kanne JP. Computed tomography of septal defects. J Cardiovasc Comput Tomogr. 2010;4(4):231–45.
68. Amat F, Le Bret E, Sigal-Cinqualbre A, Coblence M, Lambert V, Rohnean A, et al. Diagnostic accuracy of multidetector spiral computed tomography for preoperative assessment of sinus venosus atrial septal defects in children. Interact Cardiovasc Thorac Surg. 2011;12(2):179–82.
69. Warnes CA, Williams RG, Bashore TM, Child JS, Connolly HM, Dearani JA, et al. ACC/AHA 2008 Guidelines for the Management of Adults with Congenital Heart Disease: a report of the American College of Cardiology/American Heart Association Task Force on Practice Guidelines (writing committee to develop guidelines on the management of adults with congenital heart disease). Circulation. 2008;118(23):e714–833.
70. Garcia-Montes JA, Camacho-Castro A, Sandoval-Jones JP, Buendia-Hernandez A, Calderon-Colmenero J, Patino-Bahena E, et al. Closure of large patent ductus arteriosus using the Amplatzer Septal Occluder. Cardiol Young. 2015;25(3):491–5.
71. Shriki JE, Shinbane JS, Rashid MA, Hindoyan A, Withey JG, DeFrance A, et al. Identifying, characterizing, and classifying congenital anomalies of the coronary arteries. Radiographics. 2012;32(2):453–68.
72. Mainwaring RD, Reddy VM, Reinhartz O, Petrossian E, MacDonald M, Nasirov T, et al. Anomalous aortic origin of a coronary artery: medium-term results after surgical repair in 50 patients. Ann Thorac Surg. 2011;92(2):691–7.
73. Kim RJ, Wu E, Rafael A, Chen EL, Parker MA, Simonetti O, et al. The use of contrast-enhanced magnetic resonance imaging to identify reversible myocardial dysfunction. N Engl J Med. 2000;343(20):1445–53.
74. Klein C, Nekolla SG, Bengel FM, Momose M, Sammer A, Haas F, et al. Assessment of myocardial viability with contrast-enhanced magnetic resonance imaging: comparison with positron emission tomography. Circulation. 2002;105(2):162–7.
75. Kuhl HP, Beek AM, van der Weerdt AP, Hofman MB, Visser CA, Lammertsma AA, et al. Myocardial viability in chronic ischemic heart disease: comparison of contrast-enhanced magnetic resonance imaging with (18)F-fluorodeoxyglucose positron emission tomography. J Am Coll Cardiol. 2003;41(8):1341–8.
76. Selvanayagam JB, Kardos A, Francis JM, Wiesmann F, Petersen SE, Taggart DP, et al. Value of delayed-enhancement cardiovascular magnetic resonance imaging in predicting myocardial viability after surgical revascularization. Circulation. 2004;110(12): 1535–41.
77. Lardo AC, Cordeiro MA, Silva C, Amado LC, George RT, Saliaris AP, et al. Contrast-enhanced multidetector computed tomography viability imaging after myocardial infarction: characterization of myocyte death, microvascular obstruction, and chronic scar. Circulation. 2006;113(3):394–404.
78. Chiou KR, Liu CP, Peng NJ, Huang WC, Hsiao SH, Huang YL, et al. Identification and viability assessment of infarcted myocardium with late enhancement multidetector computed tomography: comparison with thallium single photon emission computed tomography and echocardiography. Am Heart J. 2008;155(4): 738–45.
79. Mahnken AH, Koos R, Katoh M, Wildberger JE, Spuentrup E, Buecker A, et al. Assessment of myocardial viability in reperfused acute myocardial infarction using 16-slice computed tomography in comparison to magnetic resonance imaging. J Am Coll Cardiol. 2005;45(12):2042–7.
80. Sato A, Hiroe M, Nozato T, Hikita H, Ito Y, Ohigashi H, et al. Early validation study of 64-slice multidetector computed tomography for the assessment of myocardial viability and the prediction of left ventricular remodelling after acute myocardial infarction. Eur Heart J. 2008;29(4):490–8.
81. Habis M, Capderou A, Ghostine S, Daoud B, Caussin C, Riou JY, et al. Acute myocardial infarction early viability assessment by 64-slice computed tomography immediately after coronary angiography: comparison with low-dose dobutamine echocardiography. J Am Coll Cardiol. 2007;49(11):1178–85.
82. Habis M, Capderou A, Sigal-Cinqualbre A, Ghostine S, Rahal S, Riou JY, et al. Comparison of delayed enhancement patterns on multislice computed tomography immediately after coronary angiography and cardiac magnetic resonance imaging in acute myocardial infarction. Heart. 2009;95(8):624–9.
83. Sato A, Nozato T, Hikita H, Akiyama D, Nishina H, Hoshi T, et al. Prognostic value of myocardial contrast delayed enhancement with 64-slice multidetector computed tomography after acute myocardial infarction. J Am Coll Cardiol. 2012;59(8):730–8.
84. Rodriguez-Granillo GA, Rosales MA, Baum S, Rennes P, Rodriguez-Pagani C, Curotto V, et al. Early assessment of myocardial viability by the use of delayed enhancement computed tomography after primary percutaneous coronary intervention. JACC Cardiovasc Imaging. 2009;2(9):1072–81.
85. Raman SV, Sahu A, Merchant AZ, Louis LB, Firstenberg MS, Sun B. Noninvasive assessment of left ventricular assist devices with cardiovascular computed tomography and impact on management. J Heart Lung Transpl. 2010;29(1):79–85.
86. Boruah PK, Baruah D, Mahr C, Gaglianello N, Shahir K. Intermittent left ventricular assist device inflow tract obstruction by prolapsing papillary muscle detected by multi-detector computed tomography (MDCT). Int J Cardiol. 2014;176(1): e13–4.
87. Bolen MA, Popovic ZB, Gonzalez-Stawinski G, Schoenhagen P. Left ventricular assist device malposition interrogated by 4-D cine computed tomography. J Cardiovasc Comput Tomogr. 2011;5(3):186–8.
88. Sorensen EN, Hiivala NJ, Jeudy J, Rajagopal K, Griffith BP. Computed tomography correlates of inflow cannula malposition in a continuous-flow ventricular-assist device. J Heart Lung Transpl. 2013;32(6):654–7.
89. Mishkin JD, Enriquez JR, Meyer DM, Bethea BT, Thibodeau JT, Patel PC, et al. Utilization of cardiac computed tomography angiography for the diagnosis of left ventricular assist device thrombosis. Circ Heart Fail. 2012;5(2):e27–9.

90. von Ziegler F, Leber AW, Becker A, Kaczmarek I, Schonermarck U, Raps C, et al. Detection of significant coronary artery stenosis with 64-slice computed tomography in heart transplant recipients: a comparative study with conventional coronary angiography. Int J Cardiovasc Imaging. 2009;25(1):91–100.
91. von Ziegler F, Rummler J, Kaczmarek I, Greif M, Schenzle J, Helbig S, et al. Detection of significant coronary artery stenosis with cardiac dual-source computed tomography angiography in heart transplant recipients. Transplant Int. 2012;25(10):1065–71.
92. Barthelemy O, Toledano D, Varnous S, Fernandez F, Boutekadjirt R, Ricci F, et al. Multislice computed tomography to rule out coronary allograft vasculopathy in heart transplant patients. J Heart Lung Transpl. 2012;31(12):1262–8.
93. Wever-Pinzon O, Romero J, Kelesidis I, Wever-Pinzon J, Manrique C, Budge D, et al. Coronary computed tomography angiography for the detection of cardiac allograft vasculopathy: a meta-analysis of prospective trials. J Am Coll Cardiol. 2014;63(19):1992–2004.
94. Rohnean A, Houyel L, Sigal-Cinqualbre A, To NT, Elfassy E, Paul JF. Heart transplant patient outcomes: 5-year mean follow-up by coronary computed tomography angiography. Transplantation. 2011;91(5):583–8.
95. Kobashigawa J. Coronary computed tomography angiography: is it time to replace the conventional coronary angiogram in heart transplant patients? J Am Coll Cardiol. 2014;63(19):2005–6.
96. Hoey ET, Mankad K, Puppala S, Gopalan D, Sivananthan MU. MRI and CT appearances of cardiac tumours in adults. Clin Radiol. 2009;64(12):1214–30.
97. Rajiah P, Kanne JP, Kalahasti V, Schoenhagen P. Computed tomography of cardiac and pericardiac masses. J Cardiovasc Comput Tomogr. 2011;5(1):16–29.
98. Suh SY, Rha SW, Kim JW, Park CG, Seo HS, Oh DJ, et al. The usefulness of three-dimensional multidetector computed tomography to delineate pericardial calcification in constrictive pericarditis. Int J Cardiol. 2006;113(3):414–6.
99. von Erffa J, Daniel WG, Achenbach S. Three-dimensional visualization of severe pericardial calcification in constrictive pericarditis using multidetector-row computed tomography. Eur Heart J. 2006;27(3):275.
100. Kameda Y, Funabashi N, Kawakubo M, Uehara M, Hasegawa H, Kobayashi Y, et al. Heart in an eggshell – eggshell appearance calcified constrictive pericarditis demonstrated by three-dimensional images of multislice computed tomography. Int J Cardiol. 2007;120(2):269–72.
101. Rifkin RD, Mernoff DB. Noninvasive evaluation of pericardial effusion composition by computed tomography. Am Heart J. 2005;149(6):1120–7.
102. Hayter RG, Rhea JT, Small A, Tafazoli FS, Novelline RA. Suspected aortic dissection and other aortic disorders: multidetector row CT in 373 cases in the emergency setting. Radiology. 2006;238(3):841–52.
103. Yoshida S, Akiba H, Tamakawa M, Yama N, Hareyama M, Morishita K, et al. Thoracic involvement of type A aortic dissection and intramural hematoma: diagnostic accuracy – comparison of emergency helical CT and surgical findings. Radiology. 2003;228(2):430–5.
104. Yoshikai M, Ikeda K, Itoh M, Noguchi R. Detection of coronary artery disease in acute aortic dissection: the efficacy of 64-row multidetector computed tomography. J Card Surg. 2008; 23(3):277–9.
105. Smayra T, Noun R, Tohme-Noun C. Left anterior descending coronary artery dissection after blunt chest trauma: assessment by multi-detector row computed tomography. J Thorac Cardiovasc Surg. 2007;133(3):811–2.
106. Sato Y, Matsumoto N, Komatsu S, Matsuo S, Kunimasa T, Yoda S, et al. Coronary artery dissection after blunt chest trauma: depiction at multidetector-row computed tomography. Int J Cardiol. 2007;118(1):108–10.
107. Scaglione M, Pinto A, Pinto F, Romano L, Ragozzino A, Grassi R. Role of contrast-enhanced helical CT in the evaluation of acute thoracic aortic injuries after blunt chest trauma. Eur Radiol. 2001;11(12):2444–8.
108. Higashiura W, Sakaguchi S, Tabayashi N, Taniguchi S, Kichikawa K. Impact of 3-dimensional-computed tomography workstation for precise planning of endovascular aneurysm repair. Circulation J. 2008;72(12):2028–34.
109. Lin MP, Chang SC, Wu RH, Chou CK, Tzeng WS. A comparison of computed tomography, magnetic resonance imaging, and digital subtraction angiography findings in the diagnosis of infected aortic aneurysm. J Comput Assist Tomogr. 2008;32(4): 616–20.
110. Sodian R, Schmauss D, Markert M, Weber S, Nikolaou K, Haeberle S, et al. Three-dimensional printing creates models for surgical planning of aortic valve replacement after previous coronary bypass grafting. Ann Thorac Surg. 2008;85(6): 2105–8.
111. Schmauss D, Schmitz C, Bigdeli AK, Weber S, Gerber N, Beiras-Fernandez A, et al. Three-dimensional printing of models for preoperative planning and simulation of transcatheter valve replacement. Ann Thorac Surg. 2012;93(2):e31–3.
112. Schmauss D, Gerber N, Sodian R. Three-dimensional printing of models for surgical planning in patients with primary cardiac tumors. J Thorac Cardiovasc Surg. 2013;145(5):1407–8.
113. Schmauss D, Juchem G, Weber S, Gerber N, Hagl C, Sodian R. Three-dimensional printing for perioperative planning of complex aortic arch surgery. Ann Thorac Surg. 2014;97(6): 2160–3.
114. Ma XJ, Tao L, Chen X, Li W, Peng ZY, Chen Y, et al. Clinical application of three-dimensional reconstruction and rapid prototyping technology of multislice spiral computed tomography angiography for the repair of ventricular septal defect of tetralogy of Fallot. Genet Molecul Res. 2015;14(1):1301–9.

Computed Tomographic Angiography in the Assessment of Congenital Heart Disease and Coronary Artery Anomalies

23

Priya Pillutla and Stephen C. Cook

Abstract

Advances in medical and surgical care have significantly increased the numbers of children and adults living with congenital heart disease (CHD). This chapter will discuss anatomical and imaging considerations for the major CHD lesions. Additionally, the role of computed tomography in the planning of percutaneous and surgical repairs will be addressed, as well as the use of this modality to monitor for possible post-intervention complications. Finally, clinically significant coronary anomalies will be reviewed.

Keywords

Congenital heart disease • Cardiac computed tomography • Coronary anomalies

Introduction

Congenital heart disease (CHD) is the most common congenital disorder in newborns [1–3]. Approximately 6 per 1000 live births in the United States are affected by complex CHD and as many as 75 per 1000 live births have simple lesions such as ventricular septal defects [4]. Improved medical and surgical care in addition to evolving percutaneous methods of intervention have decreased early and late mortality. As a result, mortality in infants and children with CHD dropped 31 % between 1987 and 2005 [5] and the adult population has undergone rapid growth. As of 2000, there were nearly equal numbers of adults and children with severe CHD [6]. Currently, it is estimated there are approximately 800,000 adults with CHD in the United States [7] with a prevalence in the adult population of 3000 per million [8].

P. Pillutla, MD (✉)
Adult Congenital Heart Disease Program, Harbor-UCLA Medical Center, 1124 W. Carson Street, RB2, Torrance, CA 90502, USA
e-mail: ppillutla@labiomed.org

S.C. Cook, MD, FACC
Adult Congenital Heart Disease Center, Heart Institute, Children's Hospital of Pittsburgh of UPMC, Pittsburgh, PA, USA

Prior to the introduction of cardiovascular magnetic resonance (CMR) imaging and cardiovascular computed tomographic angiography (CCTA), transthoracic echocardiography (TTE) and cardiac catheterization were the primary imaging modalities in the diagnosis and evaluation of the patient with complex CHD [9]. Advances in TTE imaging and its widespread availability have allowed it to largely replace cardiac catheterization as the predominant imaging modality for CHD in children in most centers and the use of diagnostic cardiac catheterization in CHD appears to have declined [10]. In the hands of a skilled technologist, TTE provides non-invasive information regarding complex CHD while avoiding radiation and intravenous contrast exposure associated with serial cardiac catheterizations. It also can be performed rapidly, provides important hemodynamic data and is relatively inexpensive.

Both TTE and catheterization have disadvantages with regards to imaging the adult with CHD. Anatomic windows for ultrasound may be limited by chest wall deformities (e.g., pectus deformities, spinal abnormalities) and post-surgical changes. Transesophageal echocardiography can circumvent some of these pitfalls but it requires an experienced operator and carries the risks of any invasive procedure including conscious sedation. Additionally, it has limited use in the assessment of anterior structures such as conduits.

M.J. Budoff, J.S. Shinbane (eds.), *Cardiac CT Imaging: Diagnosis of Cardiovascular Disease*,
DOI 10.1007/978-3-319-28219-0_23

CMR allows for three-dimensional structural and functional assessment of the heart as well as delineation of extra-cardiac structures without ionizing radiation. The benefits of CMR in the evaluation of the adult CHD patient are diverse including quantification of both left and right ventricular size and systolic function, shunt quantification, evaluation and quantification of valvar disease, and assessment of myocardial perfusion and fibrosis [11]. Despite these numerous applications and advantages, CMR has several limitations including prolonged acquisition time, signal void artifact due to prior transcatheter interventions [12], claustrophobia, high acquisition costs and the inability to perform CMR in patients with implantable cardioverter defibrillators or pacemakers.

Concurrently, there have been numerous advances (e.g., reduced scan times; higher spatial/temporal resolution) in the field of cardiovascular CT [13]. Consequently, CCTA provides a suitable alternative to CMR. It yields an accurate assessment of intra- and extra-cardiac anatomy for patients with both simple and complex CHD while overcoming the limitations of CMR. Furthermore, CCTA can provide accurate quantification of volume and function comparable to CMR although such protocols typically require higher radiation doses [14]. In contrast to CMR, acquisition time is brief. Therefore, this technique should be strongly considered in patients with poor echocardiographic windows and contraindications to CMR.

Unfortunately, CCTA is not without disadvantages. This technique still requires exposure to ionizing radiation as well as nephrotoxic contrast. Importantly, patients with CHD have many potential sources of ongoing radiation exposure that often begin in infancy and continue throughout life. Serial chest radiography, nuclear scans, computed tomography scans and diagnostic/therapeutic catheterizations are frequently performed in the setting of prior corrective or palliative interventions [15]. Therefore, physicians who perform and/or refer patients for this procedure should be familiar with radiation exposure and techniques available to reduce radiation exposure at the time of CCTA examination. Fortunately, there are now a number of low-radiation protocols that can be employed to significantly reduce the radiation exposure including reduction of tube voltage (for example to 80 kVp when feasible), adequate heart rate control, use of prospectively triggered scanning, iterative reconstruction and spectral detectors [16–25].

CT Imaging Protocol

Methodical pre-study planning is of critical importance in the patient with CHD. Repeating a study due to suboptimal technique exposes the patient to excessive contrast and radiation exposure. Furthermore, crucial structures may be missed on a "standard" study. Collaboration with a specialist in adult CHD may avoid many potential pitfalls. Prior to commencing a study, the following should be described if possible: the diagnostic indication, the original anatomic defects, operative repairs if any and post-surgical anatomic and hemodynamic changes. Thus, the study can be tailored for the individual patient to provide the appropriate extent of anatomic coverage, proper timing of contrast administration, selection of the best image acquisition protocol and special attention to the structures of interest.

Cardiac Anatomy: A Sequential Approach

CHD is highly variable in its complexity and anatomic arrangements. Attempts to adequately describe complicated lesions have led to a nuanced taxonomy of eponyms, synonymous and near-synonymous terms. For instance, even the basic terms of "left" and "right" can lead to confusion. By convention, they refer to morphologic characteristics of a cardiac chamber rather than position within the chest.

To reduce clinical confusion and facilitate academic study, various systematic schemata have been developed. Van Praagh's "segmental approach" [26] describes each of the three main segments of cardiac anatomy (the atria, ventricles and great arteries) in series. This is analogous to the construction of a home, where each segment builds off the prior with the atria serving as the foundation. The sequence is often abbreviated by a sequence of three letters (X, Y, Z) where the first letter describes visceral-atrial situs, the second ventricular looping and the third the relationships of the great arteries. This analysis is often helpful, particularly for the evaluation of those with complex CHD, as it provides a systematic and standardized approach that can be applied to any patient.

Atrial Situs

Atrial situs most often follows the positioning of the unpaired abdominal viscera. For instance, the normal arrangement is *situs solitus* (**S**, _, _), in which the morphologic right atrium, systemic venous return and liver are on the right side of the patient. The morphologic left atrium, pulmonary venous return, stomach and spleen are on the left side. The morphology of the atrial appendage provides important clues regarding right or left-sidedness (See Fig. 23.1).

The mirror image of this arrangement (with the morphologic right atrium and liver on the patient's left and the morphologic left atrium, stomach and spleen on the patient's right) is *situs inversus* (**I**, _, _). Cases of both atria having characteristics of either the left or right atrium (atrial isomerism) are described as *situs ambiguus* (**A**, _, _), also known as the heterotaxy syndrome.

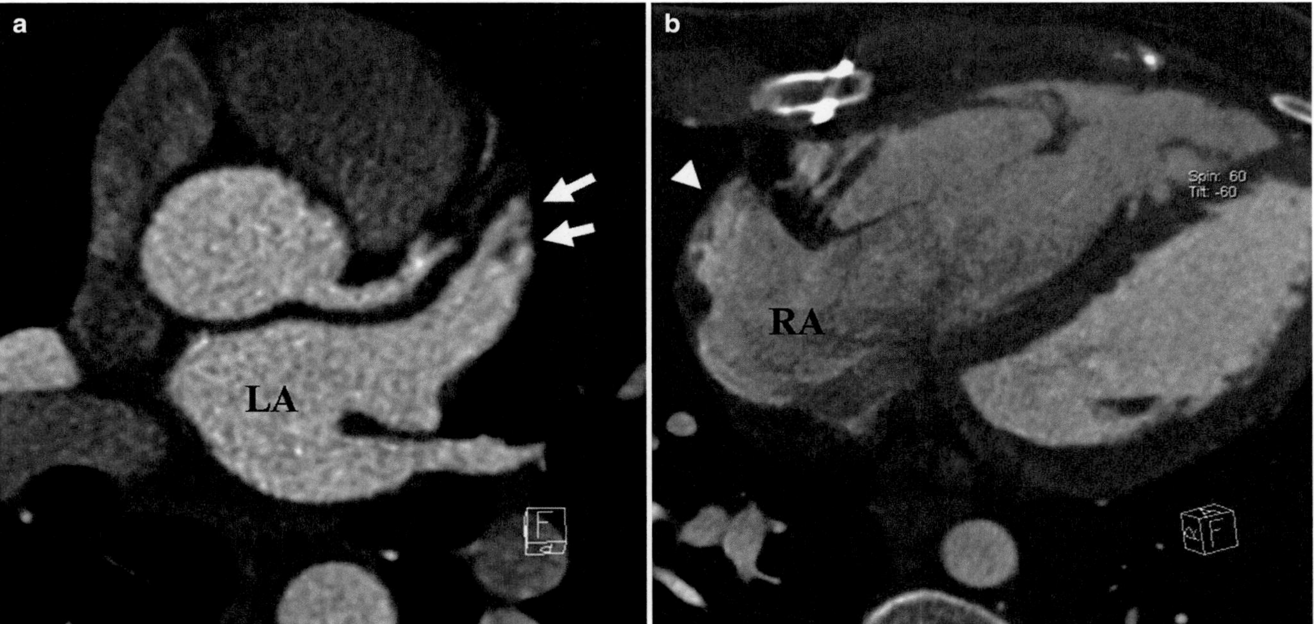

Fig. 23.1 Oblique axial view (**a**) demonstrates the features of a morphologic left atrium (*LA*), including its finger-like appearance and pectinate muscles (*arrows*). In contrast, the oblique coronal view (**b**) demonstrates a broad-based triangular appendage (*arrowhead*) suggestive of a right atrial appendage. *RA* right atrium

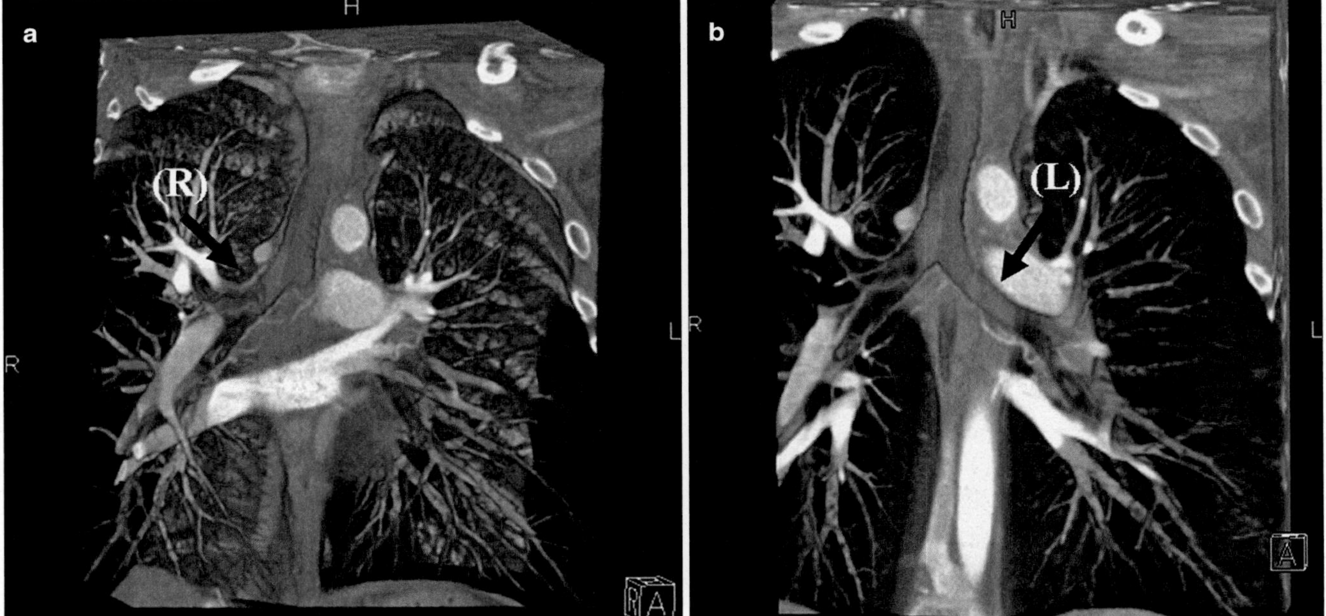

Fig. 23.2 Volume-rendered three-dimensional reconstructions (**a**, **b**) demonstrating pulmonary situs solitus. The pulmonary artery of the morphologic right lung travels anteriorly to the bronchus (*R*). The pulmonary artery of the morphologic left lung (*L*) travels over its main bronchus and posterior to the upper lobe bronchus

Bronchial morphology may further assist in determining atrial situs as the two frequently correlate with one another. Normally, the first branch of the right mainstem bronchus courses above (eparterial) the right pulmonary artery whereas the first branch of the left mainstem bronchus courses below (hyparterial) the left pulmonary artery (See Fig. 23.2). This bronchial configuration indirectly suggests atrial situs solitis.

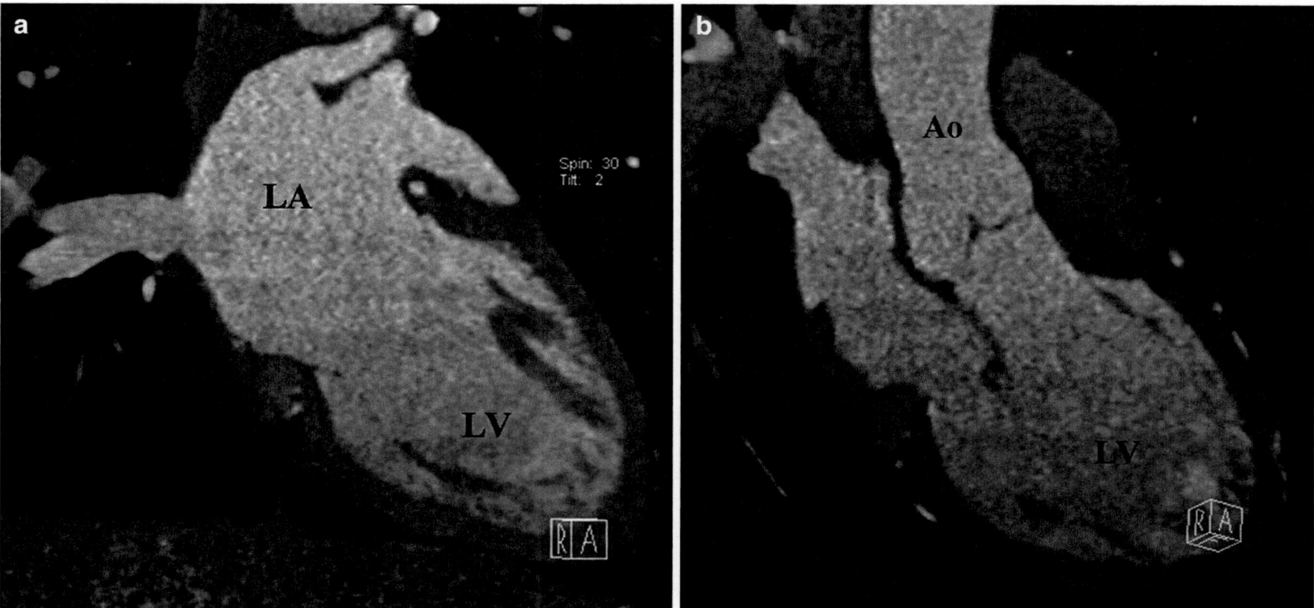

Fig. 23.3 Atrioventricular and ventriculoarterial concordance. The oblique coronal view (**a**) demonstrates atrioventricular concordance between the left atrium (*LA*) and left ventricle (*LV*). The oblique coronal view (**b**) demonstrates ventriculoarterial concordance between the LV and the aorta (*Ao*)

Atrial Isomerism

Atrial isomerism, commonly referred to as heterotaxy syndrome, is the result of duplication of the structures typical of either the left or right side of the body. This syndrome is associated with intestinal abnormalities, poorly functioning or absent splenic tissue, and complex CHD [27]. In right atrial isomerism, both atria have the broad based triangular atrial appendages typical of the right atrium and receive systemic venous return (superior vena cava or SVC, inferior vena cava or IVC, and coronary sinus). This is typically associated with bilateral trilobed lungs, a large liver which spans the abdomen and asplenia. Left atrial isomerism is characterized by both atria having narrow based atrial appendages and receiving the ipsilateral pulmonary veins. This is associated with bilateral bilobed lungs, interruption of the IVC, a midline liver and polysplenia.

Ventricular Looping

The normal anatomic position of the morphologic right ventricle is to the right and anterior of the left ventricle. This arrangement is called "*D-loop*" (_, **D**, _) and results from rightward or dextro-looping of the primitive heart early in fetal development. If the primitive heart developed in a leftward (levo-) fashion, it can result in the left ventricle anterior and rightward of the right ventricle or "*L-loop*" (_, **L**, _).

Features of the morphologic right ventricle include the presence of coarse trabeculae, a prominent moderator band, tricuspid valve attachments to the septum and free wall, and absence of fibrous continuity between the tricuspid valve and semilunar valve. Additionally, the tricuspid valve is normally located more apically within the right ventricle when compared to the mitral valve. In contrast, the morphologic left ventricle has a smooth septal surface and fibrous continuity between the mitral and semilunar valves.

Semilunar Valve Relationships

Van Praagh described six potential relationships of the aortic and pulmonary valves. Each variant is defined by the position of the aortic valve relative to the pulmonary valve. In the normal relationship, *solitus* (_, _, **S**), the aortic valve is rightward and posterior of the pulmonary valve. If the aortic valve is leftward and posterior, it is termed inversus (_, _, **I**). When the aortic valve is rightward and anterior, it is termed D-malposition (_, _, **D**), and when the aortic valve is leftward and anterior, it is L-malposition (_, _, **L**). Uncommonly, the aortic valve can lie directly *anterior* (_, _, **A**) or directly *posterior* (_, _, **P**) to the pulmonary valve.

Concordant/Discordant Relationships

Tynan and colleagues [28] proposed an alternate means of describing complicated CHD. Their approach places greater emphasis on the connections between the different segments. Segments can be *concordant* (normally related) or *discordant* (See Fig. 23.3). For instance, if the right atrium connects normally via a tricuspid valve to the right ventricle, there is *atrioventricular concordance*. If the right ventricle then gives rise to the pulmonary artery, there is *ventriculoarterial concordance*. In d-transposition of the great arteries (d-TGA), in which the right ventricle gives rise to the aorta, there is *ventriculoarterial discordance*. Atrioventricular connections may also be *absent* (e.g., tricuspid atresia) or *doubly-committed* (connected to both ventricles, either equally or unequally).

Congenital Heart Defects of Simple and Moderate Complexity

Venous Abnormalities

Systemic Venous Abnormalities

Systemic venous anomalies include bilateral SVC (which may or may not be connected via a bridging innominate vein), a unilateral left SVC (which most frequently drains into an enlarged coronary sinus, less commonly draining directly to the left atrium) and interrupted IVC (often with continuation via the azygous or hemiazygous veins).

Pulmonary Venous Abnormalities

Abnormal pulmonary venous return is described as being total or partial. In total anomalous venous return (TAPVR), all four pulmonary veins drain anomalously. There are four variants of TAPVR: supracardiac, cardiac, infracardiac and mixed. *Supracardiac*-type is the most common with the pulmonary veins connecting to the systemic venous circulation via the SVC, innominate vein or azygos vein. *Cardiac*-type describes the pulmonary veins draining to the coronary sinus or a similar vein into the right atrium. In patients with the *infracardiac*-type, the pulmonary veins drain into the portal or hepatic veins. *Mixed* is any combination of the above venous abnormalities. If any of these lesions are associated with any degree of obstruction, which is particularly common in the infracardiac-type, severe pulmonary congestion may result. In this setting, surgical palliation is usually required during the newborn period.

If at least one of the veins drains inappropriately, it is described as partial (PAPVR). There is a wide spectrum of anatomic malformations in PAPVR and many different types of connections between the systemic venous and pulmonary venous circulations have been reported [29–32]. PAPVR is often associated with a sinus venosus atrial septal defect (ASD). When the right-sided pulmonary veins drain anomalously to the IVC (typically near the diaphragm) and in the presence of right lung hypoplasia, this constellation is termed "scimitar syndrome" (from the resemblance of the curvilinear anomalous connection to a curved sword).

Late complications following surgical correction of either TAPVR or PAPVR include stenosis of the SVC, the anastomosis site or the pulmonary veins. CCTA, which is well characterized in the evaluation of the pulmonary veins prior to or following radiofrequency ablation [33] is ideally suited to evaluate the pulmonary venous anatomy in the adult CHD patient with native disease as well as the post-operative patient to determine the presence/absence of stenosis after prior palliative repair (See Fig. 23.4).

Cor Triatriatum

Cor triatriatum is caused when there is stenosis of the common pulmonary vein [34]. Hence, the pulmonary veins enter a "pulmonary venous" chamber which drains into the left atrium (cor triatriatum sinistrum) via an opening. It may alternatively communicate with the right atrium. This orifice may be imperforate, restrictive, multiple, or large and nonrestrictive. Cor triatiatrum dextrum is caused by persistence of the right valve of the sinus venosus and divides the right atrium into three chambers; it is far less common. Commonly associated defects include atrial septal defect or patent foramen ovale, PAPVR and persistent left SVC.

Without surgical correction, a highly restrictive communication between the pulmonary venous confluence and the left atrium is associated with high mortality during infancy. In contrast, the patient with mild or no obstruction may not present until later in adult life. CCTA provides excellent spatial resolution for defining pulmonary venous and pulmonary venous anatomy in this condition, both in the unrepaired and post-operative state.

Defects in Septation

Atrial Septal Defects

Atrial septal defects, or ASDs, are among the most common congenital heart defects. They are classified by their anatomic location. The two most common variants, secundum and primum, are true defects within the atrial septum. The sinus venous defect is not a true defect in the atrial septum but rather a deficiency in the wall separating the pulmonary veins from the right atrium. This results in a left-to-right shunt similar to the primum and secundum ASDs. The coronary sinus ASD shares a similar aberration and physiologic outcome. Here, there is a deficiency in the wall separating the coronary sinus from the left atrium (See Fig. 23.5).

Of these, ostium secundum defects or *secundum ASDs*, are the most common variant. Ostium primum defects or *primum ASDs* are the next most common. As the primum portion of the atrial septum is contiguous with the atrioventricular valves and intraventricular septum, primum ASDs are typically classified within the spectrum of atrioventricular septal defects (AVSDs or atrioventricular canal defects).

Sinus venous ASDs are uncommon and account for approximately 5–10 % of all ASDs [35]. They most often

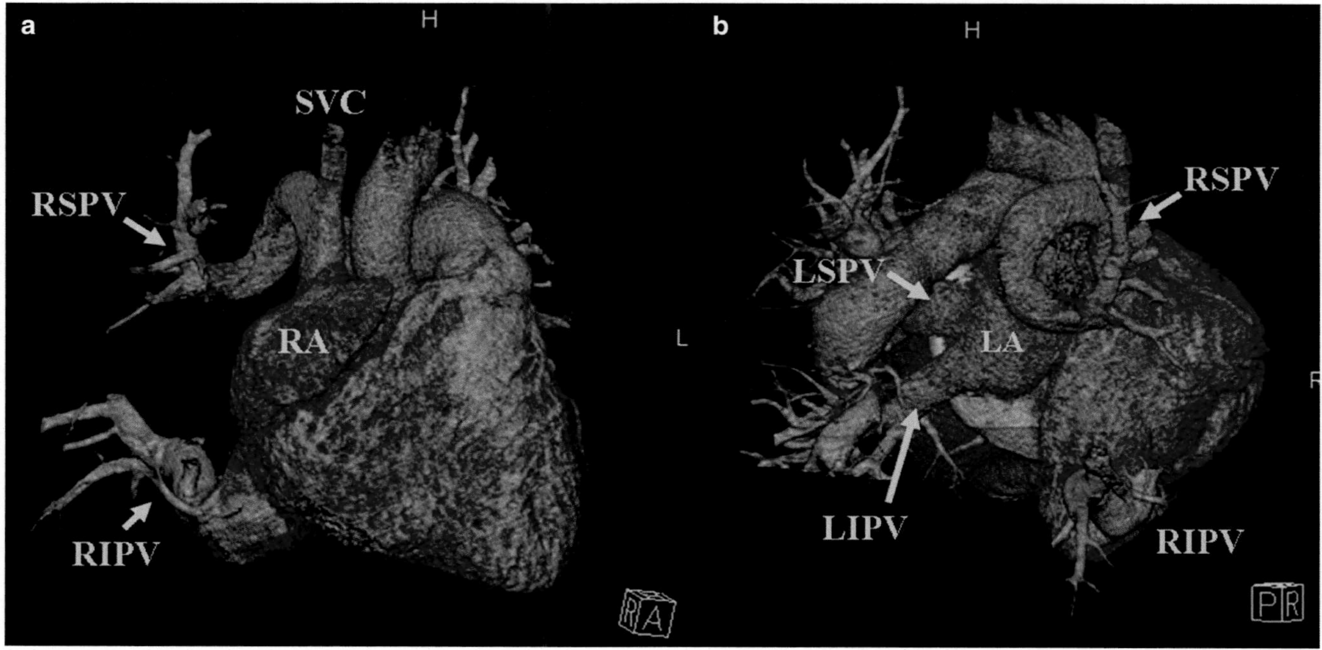

Fig. 23.4 Volume rendered three dimensional reconstructions demonstrate anomalous return of the right superior pulmonary vein (*RSPV*) to the superior vena cava (*SVC*) and right inferior pulmonary vein (*RIPV*) to the inferior vena cava (**a**). Note the normal return of the left pulmonary veins to the left atrium (**b**). *LA* left atrium, *LIPV* left inferior pulmonary vein, *LSPV* left superior pulmonary vein, *RA* right atrium

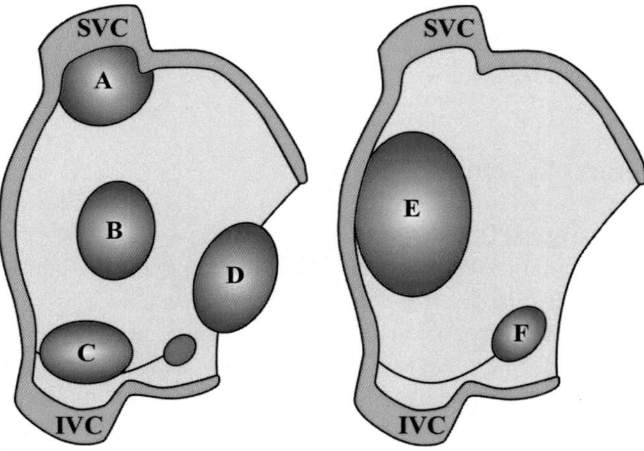

Fig. 23.5 Atrial septal defects: A indicates the superior sinus venosus atrial septal defect (*ASD*); *B* secundum ASD, *C* inferior sinus venosus ASD, *D* ostium primum ASD or partial atrioventricular septal defect, *E* secundum ASD without posterior septal rim, and *F* coronary sinus ASD. *SVC* superior vena cava, *IVC* inferior vena cava (Reprinted from Webb et al. [35] with permission of Wolters Kluwer)

occur at the junction of the SVC and the right atrium. A defect in this area creates a connection between the right upper pulmonary veins and the right atrium. Less commonly, they can involve the junction of the IVC and the right lower pulmonary veins. *Coronary sinus defects* are more rare and often described as an "unroofing" of the coronary sinus, allowing drainage from the coronary sinus into the left atrium. While these defects do not involve the atrial septum, they are physiologically similar.

Because of increased right atrial compliance, shunt flow across the ASD is left to right (in the presence of normal pulmonary vascular resistance). Significant shunts lead to volume overload and dilation of the right-sided cardiac chambers. Thus, closure of an ASD is indicated (either surgically or percutaneously) if right atrial or right ventricular enlargement are present, with or without symptoms [36]. In the presence of severe pulmonary hypertension, the shunt may reverse direction and flow from right to left (Eisenmenger physiology). The etiology of pulmonary hypertension in such patients is not clear and may not be solely due to a large left to right shunt over many decades [35]. ASD closure may be considered in patients with pulmonary hypertension provided there is a net left-to-right shunt and evidence of subsystemic pulmonary arterial pressure or evidence of pulmonary arterial vasoreactivity [36].

Prior to the advent of atrial septal occlusion devices performed in the cardiac catheterization laboratory [37], the treatment of choice had largely been surgical management. Currently, many secundum defects can now be managed percutaneously with fewer complications and shorter inpatient hospital stays when compared with conventional surgical management [38]. The success of percutaneous closure is determined by the presence of adequate rims of atrial tissue to secure the device.

The spatial resolution of multi-detector CT provides an excellent modality for pre-procedural planning in ASD

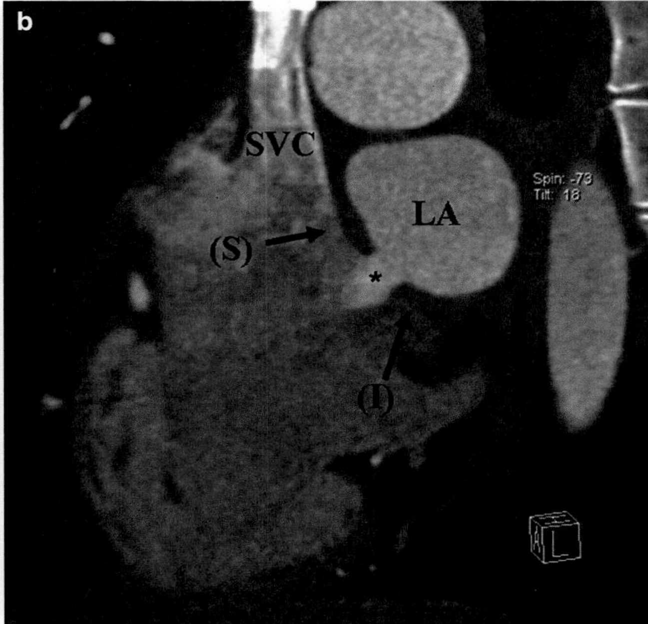

Fig. 23.6 Oblique axial (**a**) and sagittal (**b**) views demonstrate the anatomy of the atrial septal defect (*) as well as anatomic information regarding surrounding rims that are often helpful in the pre-interventional assessment to determine suitability for transcatheter closure. (*I*) inferior rim, *LA* left atrium, (*R*) retroaortic rim, (*S*) superior rim, *SVC* superior vena cava

closure, particularly if a percutaneous approach is planned [39]. Complete CT assessment prior to percutaneous closure of a secundum ASD should include assessment of pulmonary venous anatomy and exclusion of anomalous pulmonary venous return, the dimensions of the defect, presence of any fenstrations and characterization of the superior, inferior and retroaortic rims (See Fig. 23.6). Rims may be deficient or absent and are a key factor in choosing the appropriate closure strategy. Sinus venosus and primum ASDs should be specifically excluded. Additionally, depending upon the age of the patient, characterization of the coronary arteries may be necessary.

CCTA may be useful in the post-procedure patient, particularly if a percutaneous closure was performed. The study should include characterization of device seating, assessment to exclude tissue erosion from the device, impingement on surrounding structures such as the atrioventricular or semilunar valves, pulmonary venous obstruction, and pericardial effusion [40]. A residual shunt should also be excluded.

Ventricular Septal Defects

As with ASDs, ventricular septal defects (VSDs) are among the most common CHD lesions. They too are described by their position within the septum. The ventricular septum is divided into four regions: *inlet, membranous, outlet* and *muscular*. The *inlet* septum separates the mitral and tricuspid valves. The *muscular* septum extends from the inlet towards the apex of the heart. The *membranous* septum itself is small and extends from under the aortic valve towards the septal leaflet of the tricuspid valve; defects that cross into the muscular, inlet or outlet septum are termed *perimembranous. Outlet* or *supracristal* (other terms include infundibular, conal, subpulmonary or doubly committed subarterial) defects are in the smooth-walled septum, in continuity with the crista supraventricularis and the pulmonary valve.

The natural history and presentation of VSDs are variable. Small defects located in the muscular septum may undergo spontaneous closure. Occasionally, aneurysmal tissue from the tricuspid valve may result in spontaneous closure of a perimembranous VSD. Small, restrictive defects may be of little hemodynamic consequence. However, large nonrestrictive defects expose the right ventricle and pulmonary artery bed to the systemic pressure of the left ventricle. Over time, due to increased pulmonary blood flow, pulmonary vascular resistance will rise and ultimately lead to a reversal of the shunt (right-to-left) consistent with Eisenmenger physiology. Thus early surgical intervention is indicated for defects causing a significant left-to-right shunt and evidence of left-sided volume overload [36] in order to avoid progressive and irreversible changes of pulmonary vascular disease. Other considerations for surgical referral include secondary phenomena such as infective endocarditis or aortic regurgitation (often seen in the setting of a supracristal VSD).

Ongoing advances in transcatheter techniques now provide an alternative method to address defects located in the

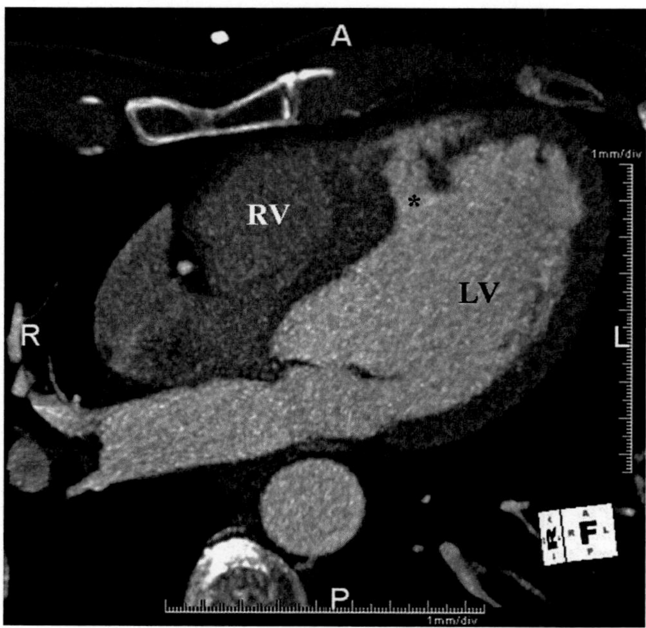

Fig. 23.7 An oblique axial image demonstrates a restrictive, muscular ventricular septal defect (VSD; *)

perimembranous and muscular portions of the interventricular septum in select cases [41, 42]. This technique has been demonstrated to be safe and effective when performed in experienced centers. The most significant late-onset complication in the perimembranous closure group is complete atrioventricular block, which requires careful serial follow-up.

Following either surgical or percutaneous device closure, CCTA has utility in assessing the adequacy of closure via the detection of residual defects (See Fig. 23.7). It is also useful in the pre-catheterization assessment to evaluate defect size as well as relationship of the defect to surrounding anatomic structures to determine suitability for percutaneous closure.

Atrioventricular Septal Defects

Atrioventricular septal defects (AVSD) include a range of anomalies which share defects within the atrioventricular (AV) septum and, often, defects of the AV valves [43]. Up to 45 % of patients with Down syndrome have CHD and, of these, approximately 45 % have an AVSD [44].

A number of terms are used to further classify the various anatomic features and "balance" of the ventricles associated with the AVSD. A *complete* AVSD has a single defect with a primum ASD and inlet VSD along with a common AV valve. A *partial* AVSD always includes a primum ASD and there are two distinct AV valves. A *transitional* AVSD is a partial AVSD accompanied by a small inlet VSD; there are often anomalous chordal attachments to the ventricular septum. A *balanced* AVSD occurs when the left and right ventricles are of equal size. Here, the common AV valve is symmetrically located over both ventricles. An *unbalanced* AVSD occurs when one of the ventricles is significantly smaller than the other. AVSDs are characterized by anterior displacement of the left ventricular outflow tract (LVOT), causing it to elongate and narrow. This "gooseneck" deformity can cause significant LVOT obstruction and may be worsened by abnormal attachments from the AV valves.

Thus, notable morphological features of AVSDs which may be seen on CT include the following: insertion of the AV valve leaflets at the same level at the crux of the heart (rather than the normal apical displacement of the tricuspid valve); any deficiency in the AV septum; anterior displacement and elongation of the LVOT and abnormal AV valves. The left AV valve is often cleft.

Most adult patients with this diagnosis will have undergone prior surgical palliation in infancy. Late complications associated with AVSDs include left or right AV valve regurgitation associated with a cleft or otherwise structurally abnormal valve, residual atrial or ventricular level shunt and LVOT obstruction.

Aortic Abnormalities

Patent Ductus Arteriosus

The ductus arteriosus is a fetal vascular channel connecting the main pulmonary trunk to the descending aorta and which is essential for fetal circulation. Before birth, the ductus arteriosus allows much of the oxygenated blood from the placenta to bypass the pulmonary vascular bed and supply the systemic circulation via the descending aorta. It typically closes spontaneously within a week following birth. Beyond this time, if the vessel remains patent, a shunt (patent ductus arteriosus or PDA) now exists between the systemic and pulmonary vascular beds.

This may be beneficial in certain congenital heart conditions such as pulmonary atresia or hypoplastic left heart syndrome, for which the PDA can provide a stable source of blood flow to either the pulmonary or systemic circulation. In an otherwise normal circulation, a PDA may have serious sequelae that are mainly determined by the size of the size of the ductus. As pulmonary vascular resistance falls following birth, the left-to-right shunt increases. Though a small PDA is often of little hemodynamic consequence, a large PDA can expose the pulmonary vascular bed to excess pulmonary blood flow, eventually causing increased pulmonary vascular resistance and pulmonary hypertension. Pulmonary hypertension may persist even after the duct is closed.

While surgical ligation of a ductus is a straightforward surgical procedure, catheter-based techniques have now become the procedure of choice for the majority of PDAs [45]. Pre-intervention CCTA is useful to characterize the

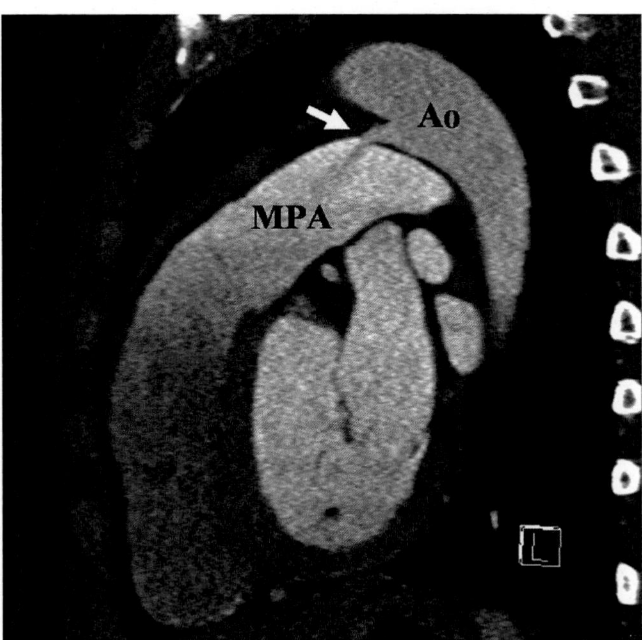

Fig. 23.8 Oblique sagittal view demonstrates a small patent ductus ateriosus (*arrow*). *Ao* Aorta, *MPA* main pulmonary artery

size, shape and course of the duct as well as its diameter at the pulmonary and aortic ends. These factors help determine the type of occluder device chosen at the time of intervention (See Fig. 23.8).

Aortopulmonary Window

The aortopulmonary (AP) window is a rare congenital defect defined as a direct communication between the pulmonary artery and the ascending aorta. While physiologically similar to a large PDA, most cases of AP window have a defect in the proximal portion of the AP septum, between the semilunar valves and the pulmonary bifurcation. Nearly half of affected patients have associated defects including aortic origin of the right pulmonary artery, interrupted aortic arch, tetralogy of Fallot or coronary anomalies [46–49].

Surgical closure is indicated for nearly all patients with AP window. A small AP window may present in adulthood with a continuous murmur and left heart enlargement. If the AP window is large and nonrestrictive, however, the patient will present with pulmonary hypertension, cyanosis and Eisenmenger physiology. In the patient with an unoperated AP window, CCTA should inspect and confirm not only the presence of a window but also associated lesions. For those with repaired AP windows, serial late CCTA should evaluate the aortic and pulmonary artery architecture.

Coarctation of the Aorta/Interrupted Aortic Arch

Coarctation of the aorta (CoA) is defined as a focal narrowing of the aorta. Most commonly the area of narrowing is just distal to the origin of the left subclavian artery at the insertion of the ductus arteriosus. This "juxtaductal" tissue of the aorta has characteristics similar to ductal tissue leading to further constriction in the post-natal period. This single theory does not fully explain the pathophysiology since there also exists a diffuse form of CoA characterized by hypoplasia of the transverse arch.

This malformation may occur in isolation (simple CoA) or in conjunction with other abnormalities (complex CoA). Complex CoA is often associated with a bicuspid aortic valve, subaortic stenosis, VSDs, mitral valve abnormalities such as parachute mitral valve, intracranial aneurysms or Turner syndrome.

When discovered in infancy, CoA is most often repaired surgically. Current surgical techniques include resection of the CoA with end-to-end anastomosis, subclavian flap aortoplasty, patch aortoplasty and interposition jump graft. Each technique has specific advantages, disadvantages and associated long-term complications. Native lesions identified in the adolescent or young adult are sometimes treated with balloon angioplasty but there may be residual stenosis, restenosis or aneurysm formation at the intervention site [50]. Stent implantation is a favorable approach for select patients with both native CoA and recoarctation and there are long-term studies demonstrating acceptable safety and efficacy [36, 51–55].

Complications in the patient with unoperated CoA are numerous and include systemic arterial hypertension, accelerated coronary artery disease, stroke, aortic dissection or rupture, congestive heart failure or intracranial hemorrhage [56]. Late complications in operated CoA include recoarctation, aortic dilation and aortic dissection. Thus, life-long followup and late postoperative imaging via CCTA or CMR are imperative for the patient with CoA, even in the setting of an acceptable surgical or percutaneous result.

CCTA offers significant advantages in the assessment of the patient with CoA who has previously undergone transcatheter therapy, particularly stenting. Many transcatheter devices including stents create significant signal void artifact precluding an accurate assessment of the anatomy of interest on CMR. In contrast, CCTA provides an accurate assessment of the lumen of the stented segment and surrounding anatomic structures without significant artifact.

The CCTA exam in a patient with native CoA or recoarctation should include the dimensions and anatomy (such as aneurysm and dissection) of the CoA segment, precise measurements of the entire aortic arch (which may be hypoplastic) and description of collateral vessels bypassing the region of stenosis [57]. Because of the risk of accelerated coronary artery disease, special attention should be paid to the coronary arteries. Finally, associated congenital cardiac lesions including other forms of left ventricular outflow tract obstruction (bicuspid aortic valve, subaortic stenosis) and mitral valve anomalies should be excluded.

Interruption of the aorta is defined as a complete separation between the ascending and descending aorta. There are multiple branching patterns but the morphology can be generally classified as Type A (interruption distal to the left subclavian artery), Type B (between the carotid and subclavian arteries) or Type C (between the carotid arteries) [58]. Aortic interruptions may be associated with other congenital anomalies including transposition of the great arteries, conotruncal anomalies with a VSD or subaortic stenosis. Surgical therapy is required to restore continuity of the aorta and concomitant defects. Late complications primarily involve restenosis at the site of prior surgical repair. CCTA may be used in this population for characterization of the aorta, arch anatomy and other cardiac defects as well as evaluation of post-operative complications and/or to assess the efficacy of prior interventions.

Congenital Valvar Disease

Bicuspid Aortic Valve/Valvar Aortic Stenosis

A bicuspid aortic valve (BAV) is one of the most common congenital heart abnormalities, affecting slightly more than 1 % of the general population [4]. The term "bicuspid" is a misnomer. The valve apparatus is typically composed of three cusps but two of the cusps are fused. The resulting valve is functionally bicuspid. Most commonly this fusion is along the left and right coronary cusps. Most congenitally malformed aortic valves are bicuspid but the aortic valve can be unicuspid, quadricuspid or simply dysplastic. The aortic annulus may be hypoplastic. Rheumatic heart disease accounts for a significant proportion of acquired aortic valve stenosis in the pediatric population.

BAV can lead to aortic stenosis, aortic regurgitation or mixed valvar disease with both stenosis and regurgitation. Importantly, BAV is associated with abnormalities in the aortic media which can cause dilation of the proximal ascending aorta and which are unrelated to the severity of valve disease [59]. Thus, BAV is a disease both of the aortic valve and of the aorta. BAV is also associated with an increased risk of coarctation, interrupted aortic arch [60] and coronary artery anomalies [61].

Transthoracic echocardiography is the primary non-invasive modality in the evaluation of aortic valvar disease. This technique provides an assessment of the valve (degree of stenosis/regurgitation), ventricular size/function and the proximal ascending aorta and arch. In patients with poor acoustic windows (e.g., obesity, pulmonary disease, chest wall deformities), CCTA provides an alternate method to assess valve morphology and dimensions. CCTA estimates of valve area correlate highly with TEE dimensions [62]. Importantly, particularly in the patient with BAV, CCTA permits for comprehensive imaging of the aorta in addition to the aortic valve. Complementary three-dimensional volume-rendered reconstructions performed with off-line analysis may provide important information about aortic dimensions that can guide management.

Subvalvar Aortic Stenosis

Subvalvar aortic stenosis (subAS) is most frequently caused by a fibrous membrane or ring of tissue although it can also assume a diffusely hypoplastic or focal tunnel-type obstruction. Although it can occur in isolation, more than half of cases are associated with another congenital defect such as VSD, CoA, Shone's complex, PDA, persistent left SVC or valvar aortic stenosis [63, 64]. There is also an association with mitral valve abnormalities [65, 66]. The degree of stenosis may remain stable but most tend progress over time. Additionally, subAS may be associated with aortic regurgitation. In contrast to valvar aortic stenosis, this lesion is not amenable to catheter-based interventions and the management is surgical when indicated. Unfortunately, there is a significant risk of recurrence despite surgical intervention. Thus, a history of subAS or associated defects should prompt close inspection of the left ventricular outflow tract in patients undergoing CCTA examinations (See Fig. 23.9).

Supravalvar Aortic Stenosis

Supravalvar aortic stenosis (supraAS) is defined as stenosis immediately above the sinuses of Valsalva. This is an uncommon occurrence in the general population but affects 30–50 % of individuals with Williams Syndrome (7q11.23 deletion syndrome) [67, 68]. Features of Williams syndrome include supraAS, peripheral pulmonary stenosis, a characteristic facial appearance, developmental delay and often a particularly cheerful and outgoing personality. Associated lesions include aortic valve abnormalities, Shone's complex and coronary artery abnormalities. Individuals with supraAS are thought to be at risk of premature atherosclerosis due to continuous exposure of the coronary arteries to supranormal pressures. The treatment of choice, due to the proximity to the coronary arteries, is surgical. CCTA may assist in the initial diagnosis of this defect and may furthermore provide insight into the coronary artery anatomy and late outcomes in this population that have not yet been well established.

Pulmonary Stenosis

Congenital pulmonary valvar stenosis (PS) is most often an isolated defect, but it may also occur in combination with subvalvar stenosis. A wide variety of malformations of the valve can be present including the classical form (a dome-shaped valve), a hypoplastic valve annulus, thickened or fused leaflets or even a dysplastic, myxomatous valve [69]. In cases of significant PS, the right ventricle and right ventricular outflow tract become hypertrophied and there is often dynamic subvalvar obstruction. Additionally, severe PS

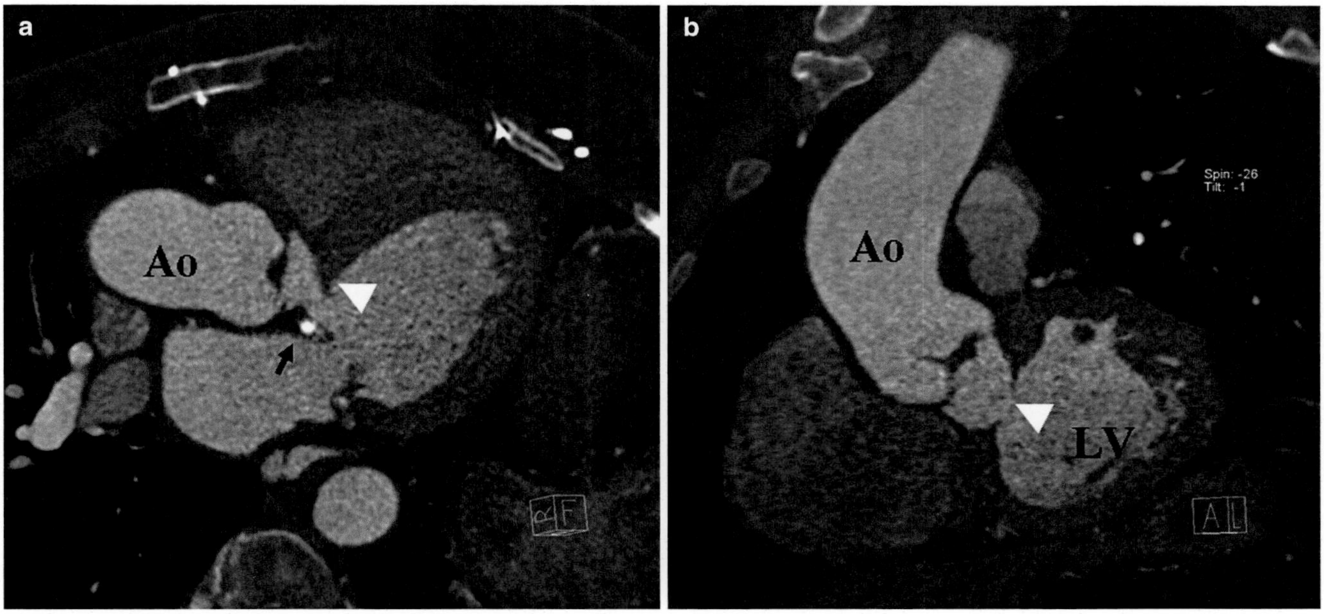

Fig. 23.9 Oblique axial (**a**) and sagittal (**b**) views demonstrating a discrete subaortic membrane (*arrowhead*) in a patient with a bicuspid aortic valve and coarctation of the aorta. Note the calcification of the anterior mitral valve leaflet (*arrow*). *Ao* aorta, *LV* left ventricle

is typically accompanied by poststenotic dilation of the main pulmonary artery. Valvar PS is encountered more frequently in individuals with Noonan syndrome [70–72].

Severe or critical PS diagnosed at any age is generally treated with balloon valvuloplasty. However, in complex cases (such as those with a hypoplastic pulmonary valve annulus, severe pulmonary insufficiency or subvalvar/supravalvar PS), surgery is usually the treatment of choice. Surgery is also reserved for patients with dysplastic valves that often do not respond to transcatheter therapy. An important late complication following either balloon valvuloplasty or surgical valvotomy is pulmonary regurgitation.

The anterior position of the pulmonary valve and the right ventricular outflow tract may preclude complete evaluation with echocardiography, particularly in the patient with prior surgery. CCTA is well suited to image this patient population for delineation of the right ventricular outflow tract, pulmonary valve annulus and distal structures including the branch pulmonary arteries. Pre-interventional assessment of pulmonary valve anatomy and dimensions may help predict suitability for balloon valvuloplasty. Lastly, CCTA can provide quantification of right ventricular size and function in patients following transcatheter or surgical intervention who have residual PS or regurgitation.

Other Lesions

Tetralogy of Fallot

Tetralogy of Fallot (TOF) is the most common cause of cyanotic CHD. It is comprised of the following: malalignment VSD, right ventricular outflow tract obstruction (RVOTO), overriding aorta and right ventricular hypertrophy secondary to RVOTO. Anterior and superior displacement of the outlet (infundibular) septum is the defining feature and accounts for the first three components of this defect. Right ventricular hypertrophy is a consequence of RVOTO. The degree of RVOTO varies and may include dysplastic pulmonary valve leaflets as well as subpulmonary or pulmonary arterial involvement.

TOF can be "syndromic" (associated with additional noncardiac congenital anomalies) or "nonsyndromic." Important syndromes associated with TOF include DiGeorge syndrome (22q11.2 microdeletion), Down syndrome (Trisomy 21), Edward syndrome (Trisomy 18) and Patau syndrome (Trisomy 13). TOF may be associated with other congenital cardiac abnormalities including ASDs, left SVC to coronary sinus or a right aortic arch. Approximately 5–10 % will have coronary anomalies [73–75] including the left anterior descending artery arising from the right coronary artery, circumflex artery arising from the right coronary artery, a large conus branch or a single coronary artery system.

The complete intracardiac repair of TOF includes relief of RVOTO and patch closure of the VSD. Operative repair of RVOTO may occur via a variety of techniques. Patients with a restrictive pulmonary valve annulus may require a longitudinal incision of the pulmonary valve with subsequent patch augmentation (transannular patch) and augmentation of the pulmonary arteries when indicated. In more severe forms (pulmonary atresia), a right ventricular-to-pulmonary artery conduit is performed to establish continuity between the right ventricle and pulmonary arteries.

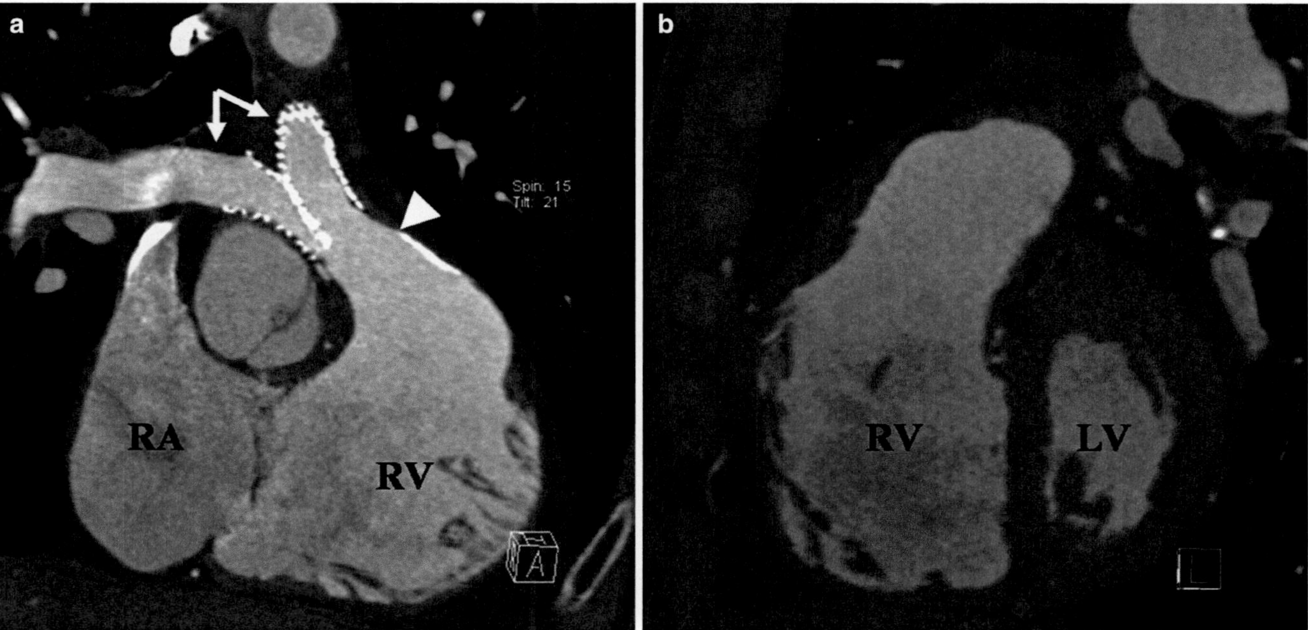

Fig. 23.10 The oblique coronal (**a**) and sagittal (**b**) views demonstrate the long-term complications associated with tetralogy of Fallot. Lifelong pulmonary insufficiency is a consequence associated with prior surgical palliations (*arrowhead*) that results in a dilated right ventricle (*RV*) when compared to the size of the left ventricle (*LV*). Prior palliative procedures often result in branch pulmonary artery stenosis often requiring transcatheter therapy (*arrows*). *RA* right atrium

Following these repairs, there may be significant residual pulmonary regurgitation. This is often well tolerated until adolescence and young adulthood, when progressive right ventricular enlargement and systolic dysfunction may cause dyspnea on exertion, chest pain, ventricular arrhythmias or even sudden cardiac death. Therefore, symptomatic patients with these findings should be considered for surgical pulmonary valve replacement. Novel transcatheter pulmonary valve implantation techniques are currently being used (such as the Melody® Transcatheter Pulmonary Valve, Medtronic, Fridley, MN and Edwards SAPIEN Pulmonic Transcatheter Heart Valve, Edwards LifeSciences LLC, Irvine, CA) to address pulmonary valve disease while avoiding the risks associated with multiple re-operations in this complex group of patients [76].

Non-invasive imaging studies obtained routinely or in anticipation of pulmonary valve replacement should assess right and left ventricular volumes and function, anatomy and size of the right ventricular outflow tract, presence/absence of residual VSD and anatomy of the proximal and distal branch pulmonary arteries (See Fig. 23.10). The distance between the coronary arteries and the sternum should be examined and, care should be taken to examine the course of the left anterior descending artery as it may cross over the right ventricular outflow tract. Finally, CCTA plays an important role in pre-procedure planning for transcatheter interventions. Particular attention should be paid to conduit or right ventricular outflow tract dimensions and the distance between the coronary arteries and the RVOT as cases of catastrophic coronary artery compression during transcatheter valve implantation have been reported [77, 78].

Lastly, progressive aortic root dilation is frequently demonstrated in the adult tetralogy of Fallot population despite adequate surgical repair [79]. This process may be due to an inherent aortopathy rather than a sequelae of the intracardiac defects [80]. Therefore, CCTA assessment of the adolescent or adult patient with TOF should include close inspection of the aortic anatomy at the time of examination. It can be helpful to index the aortic root size to body surface area and age using standard nomograms [81, 82].

Congenital Heart Defects of Great Complexity

Double Outlet Right Ventricle

Double outlet right ventricle (DORV) is a type of ventriculo-arterial discordance in which both great arteries arise 50 % or more from the right ventricle. DORV is not a single congenital defect, but rather a continuum of defects best understood by the relationship by the relationship between the great vessels and the position of the VSD. The location of the VSD further corresponds with each specific physiologic subtype [83].

The location of the VSD may be *subaortic, subpulmonic, doubly-committed* (a single defect lying inferior to both the aorta and pulmonary artery) or *remote* from the great arteries (in other words noncommitted). The relationship of the great arteries is defined by the position of the aorta relative to the

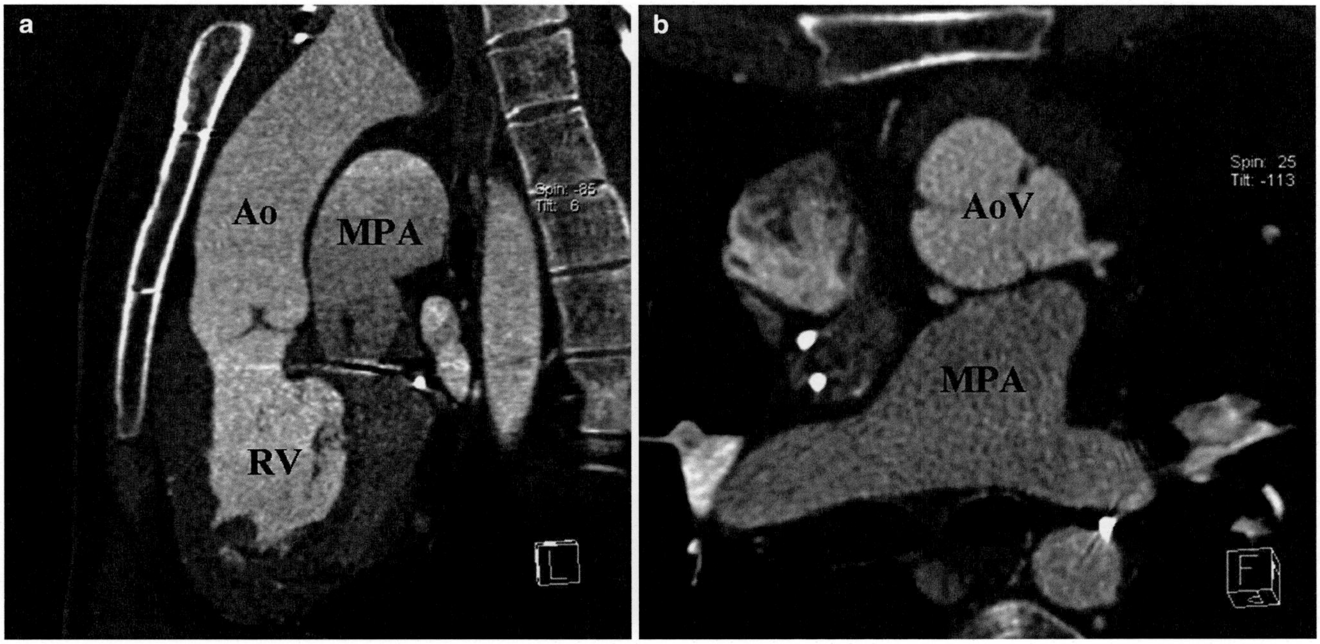

Fig. 23.11 An oblique saggital view (**a**) and oblique axial view (**b**) demonstrate the the key anatomic findings in d-transposition of the great arteries. The oblique saggital view demonstrates ventriculoarterial discordance between the right ventricle (*RV*) and the aorta (*AO*). The oblique axial view displays the anterior-posterior relationship of the great arteries. *MPA* main pulmonary artery, *AoV* aortic valve

pulmonary artery. Although normal relationships may exist, typically the aorta lies *rightward and posterior* to the pulmonary artery. Alternatively, the aorta may lie side by side or *rightward and anterior* to the pulmonary artery with the subpulmonic variant (d-TGA physiology) of DORV.

PS is commonly observed in DORV, occurring in over 50 % of cases [84–86]. Other associated anomalies include secundum ASDs, relative hypoplasia of the left ventricle, mitral valve anomalies (atrioventricular attachments to the septum), a persistent left SVC, and coronary artery anomalies. CoA or arch hypoplasia commonly occurs in the subpulmonary variant of DORV (Taussig-Bing anomaly). Although these associated defects are relatively uncommon, when present, they create a significant impact on the physiology of the underlying defect as well as surgical management options.

Given the variety of anatomic relationships and associated features, surgical palliative approaches to repair of DORV are diverse. Repairs often include closure of the VSD such that blood flow is routed ("tunneled") to restore continuity between the left ventricle and the aorta (subaortic DORV). An arterial switch procedure may be performed to restore left ventricular-aortic continuity in patients with DORV with subpulmonary VSD. Associated features such as ASDs and atrioventricular valve chordae are addressed simultaneously. In some cases, biventricular repair is not always possible, and a single ventricle palliation is performed (e.g., staged Fontan procedure). Occasionally a "one and one-half ventricle" repair may be chosen. In this scenario, a cavopulmonary anastomosis (usually a bidirectional Glenn shunt) partially unloads the right ventricle. Systemic venous return from the SVC will be via the Glenn to the pulmonary artery; the right ventricle will pump only IVC systemic venous return to the lungs.

Late outcomes of DORV are variable and are chiefly determined by the underlying anatomy and type of surgical palliation. Complications include obstruction of the right ventricular-to-pulmonary artery conduit, stenosis of interventricular tunnels, subaortic stenosis, and neo-aortic valve regurgitation or neo-aortic root dilation (in patients undergoing arterial switch). CCTA is suitable in the pre-operative assessment of this lesion as it accurately describes the three-dimensional relationship of the VSD to surrounding structures such as the great arteries and coronary arteries. Furthermore, it provides an accurate assessment of post-operative anatomic changes particularly to conduits and the neo-aorta.

D-Transposition of the Great Arteries

D-Transposition of the great arteries (TGA) is one of the most common severe congenital cardiac anomalies and is often lethal to affected infants if intervention is not performed. Although TGA may accompany other complex CHD (for example DORV), this term is most commonly used to describe isolated ventriculoarterial discordance. In other words, the right ventricle gives rise to the aorta and coronary arteries and the left ventricle gives rise to the pulmonary artery (See Fig. 23.11).

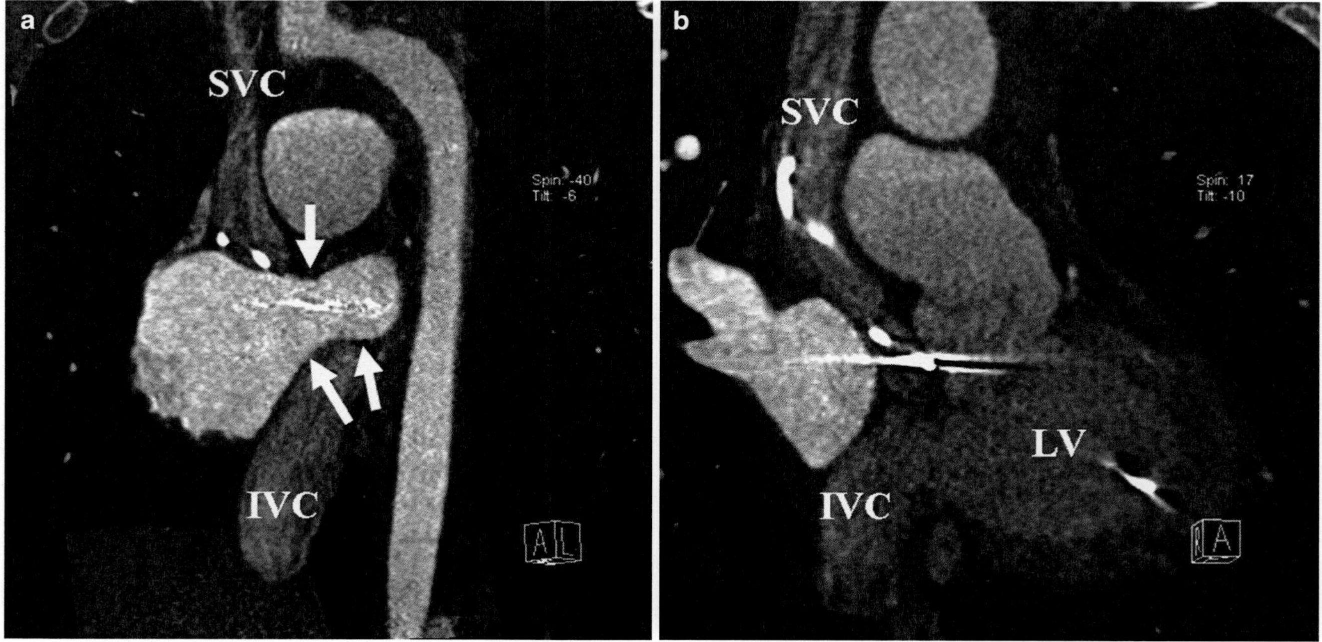

Fig. 23.12 An oblique saggital view (**a**) demonstrates the anatomic appearance of the pulmonary venous baffle (*arrows*) in this patient with d-transposition of the great arteries and an atrial switch (Mustard procedure). The coronal view (**b**) reveals the systemic venous baffle. Although pacing leads and contrast opacification in the systemic right ventricle impair image quality, systemic venous baffle obstruction can still be seen (*arrowhead*). Secondary findings such as a prominent azygous vein may suggest the presence of this anomaly

The name d-TGA arises from the most common anatomic relationship of the aortic and pulmonary valves resulting in this anatomic relationship. The aorta is transposed with pulmonary artery such that the aorta is anterior and rightward of the pulmonary artery. Recall that, the prefixes *d-* and *l-* describe only the anatomic position of the aortic and pulmonary valves and not the arrangement of the remaining segmental cardiac anatomy. Associated defects include VSD, left ventricular outflow tract obstruction, CoA and coronary artery abnormalities.

The physiology of d-TGA is often described as two circulations "in parallel" in contrast to the normal circulation, which occurs "in series." The systemic venous return passes from the right atrium into the right ventricle, then to the aorta and systemic arterial circulation without ever reaching the lungs. Similarly, the pulmonary venous return enters the left atrium and left ventricle only to return to the pulmonary arterial bed.

Without a substantial mixing lesion, this parallel circulation is not sustainable and can quickly result in death. Continuous prostaglandin infusion can maintain patency of the ductus arteriosus and facilitate mixing. In the absence of a significant ASD or VSD, a balloon atrial septostomy may be necessary to stabilize an infant until definitive surgical repair can be performed. Prior to the availability of balloon septostomy, a surgical excision of atrial tissue without cardio-pulmonary bypass was performed (the Blalock-Hanlon procedure).

Before the advent of improved coronary artery surgical techniques, redirecting blood at the atrial level was associated with lower mortality than attempting to switch the aorta and pulmonary arteries to their typical anatomic positions. The Mustard and the Senning procedures "baffle" pulmonary venous return to the right ventricle and systemic venous return to the left ventricle. This allows oxygen-rich blood to reach the systemic circulation via the morphologic right ventricle and oxygen-poor blood to reach the lungs via the morphologic left ventricle.

While the redirection of atrial blood flow restores a normal circulation, there are negative late sequelae. The superior and inferior systemic venous baffles that redirect venous return from the SVC and IVC (respectively) to the morphologic left ventricle can develop baffle leaks or stenosis. Similarly, the pulmonary venous baffle may develop stenosis as well. Finally, the morphologic right ventricle is not well suited to tolerate lifelong systemic blood pressure. This ultimately leads to hypertrophy, dilation and failure.

In the patient with a Mustard or Senning palliation, CCTA is valuable to assess not only the complex anatomy and associated post-operative changes encountered with this population, but also the late onset complications such as baffle obstruction and residual hemodynamic lesions (See Fig. 23.12). Although CMR is frequently performed to assess quantification of RV volumes and function, CCTA may be utilized to quantify this data in this population as well.

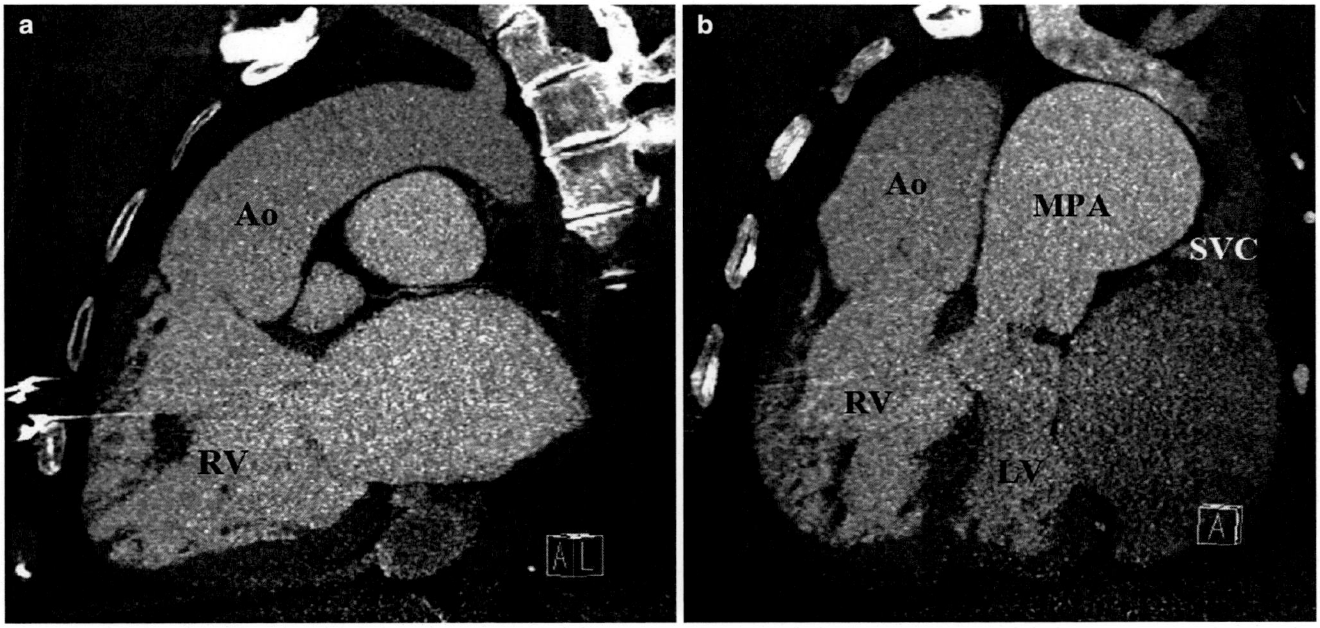

Fig. 23.13 The oblique saggital (**a**) and coronal (**b**) images display the underlying anatomy and demonstrate ventriculoarterial discordance in this patient with congenitally corrected transposition of the great arteries (CCTGA). Here, the systemic right ventricle (*RV*) is in communication with the aorta (*Ao*). Further, there is dilation of the main pulmonary artery (*MPA*) segment, suggesting right ventricular outflow tract (RVOT) obstruction. RVOT obstruction is often associated with a large ventricular septal defect. *LV* left ventricle, *SVC* superior vena cava

Contemporary surgical repair of d-TGA is the arterial switch procedure, in which the aorta and pulmonary arteries are switched to restore ventriculoarterial concordance. This requires excision and mobilization of the proximal coronary arteries and surrounding "buttons" of aortic tissue along with the Lecompte maneuver to bring the pulmonary artery to the anterior position. Late sequelae following the arterial switch include coronary artery abnormalities, myocardial ischemia, stenosis at the great artery anastomoses or arrhythmias. There may also be neo-aortic root dilation and neo-aortic valve regurgitation [87–90].

In the patient who has undergone an arterial switch procedure, CCTA is an ideal modality for assessment of the coronary arteries [91]. It also is extremely useful for examining the great artery anastomoses and neoaorta. In particular, one should carefully inspect the pulmonary arteries to exclude the presence of branch pulmonary artery stenosis as a result of the Lecompte maneuver.

Congenitally Corrected Transposition of the Great Arteries

In congenitally corrected transposition of the great arteries (CCTGA), both atrioventricular and ventriculoarterial discordance are present. Systemic venous return courses from the right atrium through the mitral valve and morphologic left ventricle, ultimately reaching the pulmonary arterial bed via the pulmonary valve. Similarly, pulmonary venous return courses from the left atrium through the tricuspid valve into a morphologic right ventricle and ultimately the systemic circulation via the aortic valve. In other words, "two wrongs make a right." Other terms for this condition include "l-TGA" or ventricular inversion.

Patients with CCTGA usually have a normal (levocardia) or midline (mesocardia) position of the heart within the chest. However, 20 % of patients have dextrocardia, in which the heart is on the right side of the chest and 5 % will have situs inversus [92–95].

Over 90 % have associated lesions, most commonly VSD, left ventricular outflow tract obstruction or abnormalities of the systemic atrioventricular valve (morphologic tricuspid valve) such as Ebstein-type malformations.

The most common late complications associated with this condition are systemic atrioventricular valve regurgitation and systemic (morphologic right) ventricular dysfunction and arrhythmias third degree atrioventricular (AV) block is particularly frequent [96, 97]. CCTA is helpful for defining the underlying anatomy and associated defects for patients with CCTGA (See Fig. 23.13). It also is an ideal tool for assessment of coronary venous anatomy to facilitate lead placement at the time of pacemaker implantation.

Truncus Arteriosus

In truncus arteriosus, a single great artery (rather than two, aorta and pulmonary artery) arises from the base of the heart. This single artery then gives rise to the coronary arteries, pulmonary arteries and aorta. The truncal valve is usually trileaflet (69 %) but regurgitation is not uncommon. The classification scheme presented here, Collett and Edwards, defines truncus arteriosus by the relationship of the pulmonary arteries [98]. A Type I truncus has a short common pulmonary arterial trunk which gives rise to both pulmonary arteries. Type II is defined by the absence of a main pulmonary artery segment. The left and right branch pulmonary arteries arise in close proximity to one another from the ascending truncal artery. In type III, there is no main pulmonary artery segment, and the left and right pulmonary arteries arise separately at a distance from one another. Type IV is defined by the absence of pulmonary arteries. Here, the lungs are supplied by aortopulmonary collateral vessels. This type is more accurately classified as pulmonary atresia and is no longer considered within the spectrum of truncus arteriosus.

Truncus arteriosus is usually an isolated phenomenon but has been reported in patients with DiGeorge syndrome (22q.11.2 microdeletion). Associated conditions include aortic arch anomalies including right aortic arch, coarctation of the aorta and interruption of the aorta. Other commonly associated defects include PDA, absence of a pulmonary artery and persistent left SVC.

This defect usually presents in the newborn period and, when diagnosed sufficiently early (before the development of severe pulmonary vascular disease), is treated by surgical palliation. Surgical repair of truncus typically utilizes a conduit from the right ventricle to either the main pulmonary artery segment (Type I) or the branch pulmonary arteries (Types II and III). The long-term survival following initial successful repair continues to improve and therefore the number of adolescents and adults with this complex lesion will continue to grow. For this reason, it is imperative to recognize late complications associated with this defect. CCTA evaluation should include close inspection of the right ventricle-pulmonary artery conduit to determine the presence/absence of stenosis or calcification, anatomy of the proximal and distal branch pulmonary arteries, neo-aortic root dilatation, and ventricular volumes and function.

Single Ventricle Lesions

Among the most complex congenital heart lesions are those with severe hypoplasia or atresia of the left or right ventricle. Consequently, these patients are reliant on a single ventricle to perfuse both the pulmonary and systemic vascular beds. The full spectrum of single ventricle lesions is beyond the scope of this text. Nonetheless, the most important variations are *tricuspid atresia* and *hypoplastic left heart syndrome.* Despite the wide variation in single ventricle pathology, the types of surgical palliations ultimately share a similar physiologic goal.

As its name suggests, tricuspid atresia is defined by the absence of a tricuspid valve. Initially, blood returning to the right atrium passes through an ASD to the left heart and mixes with pulmonary venous return. The right ventricle is usually atretic or hypoplastic; it receives blood from the left ventricle via a VSD. If there is ventriculoarterial concordance, the pulmonary arteries are often small and rely upon the duct for pulmonary blood flow. Alternatively, if there is ventriculoarterial discordance, the aorta arises from the rudimentary right ventricle, and, upon occasion, there may be aortic obstruction requiring ductal patency.

Hypoplastic left heart syndrome (HLHS) describes a spectrum of left-sided abnormalities that are insufficient to meet the demands of the systemic circulation. They are further qualified by stenosis or atresia of mitral and aortic valves. In other words: there may be mitral stenosis and aortic stenosis (MS/AS), mitral stenosis and aortic atresia (MS/AA) or mitral atresia and aortic atresia (MA/AA) [99]. If the ascending aorta is severely atretic, the carotid and coronary arteries rely upon retrograde ductal blood flow for adequate perfusion.

In most cases of single ventricle physiology, either the systemic or pulmonary bed relies upon patency of the ductal artery. If the ductal artery constricts or becomes stenotic, the results can be catastrophic. Ductal patency can be maintained with a continuous infusion of prostaglandin and more recently stents may be delivered via cardiac catheterization. Often a surgical shunt must be created to maintain a more stable blood supply.

Modern congenital heart surgery can be traced to 1944 with the creation of a systemic to pulmonary shunt conceived of by Helen Taussig and performed by Alfred Blalock with assistance from Vivian Thomas [100]. The original or *classic Blalock-Taussig shunt* (BT shunt) is a direct anastomosis of the subclavian artery to the ipsilateral pulmonary artery. Adaptations in this surgical technique led to the development of the *modified BT shunt* in which an artificial (e.g., Gore-Tex) graft connects the subclavian artery to the pulmonary artery without disrupting the integrity of the subclavian artery from the affected arm (See Fig. 23.14) [101]. Other systemic to pulmonary arterial shunts include the *Waterston shunt* (ascending aorta to right pulmonary artery), the *Potts shunt* (descending aorta to left pulmonary artery), and the *Cooley shunt* (proximal ascending aorta to right pulmonary artery within the pericardium). An alternative strategy used sometimes for the palliation of hypoplastic left heart syndrome is the *Sano shunt*, a conduit located between the right ventricle and the pulmonary artery. Contemporary *central shunts* utilize an artificial graft between the ascending aorta and the main pulmonary artery.

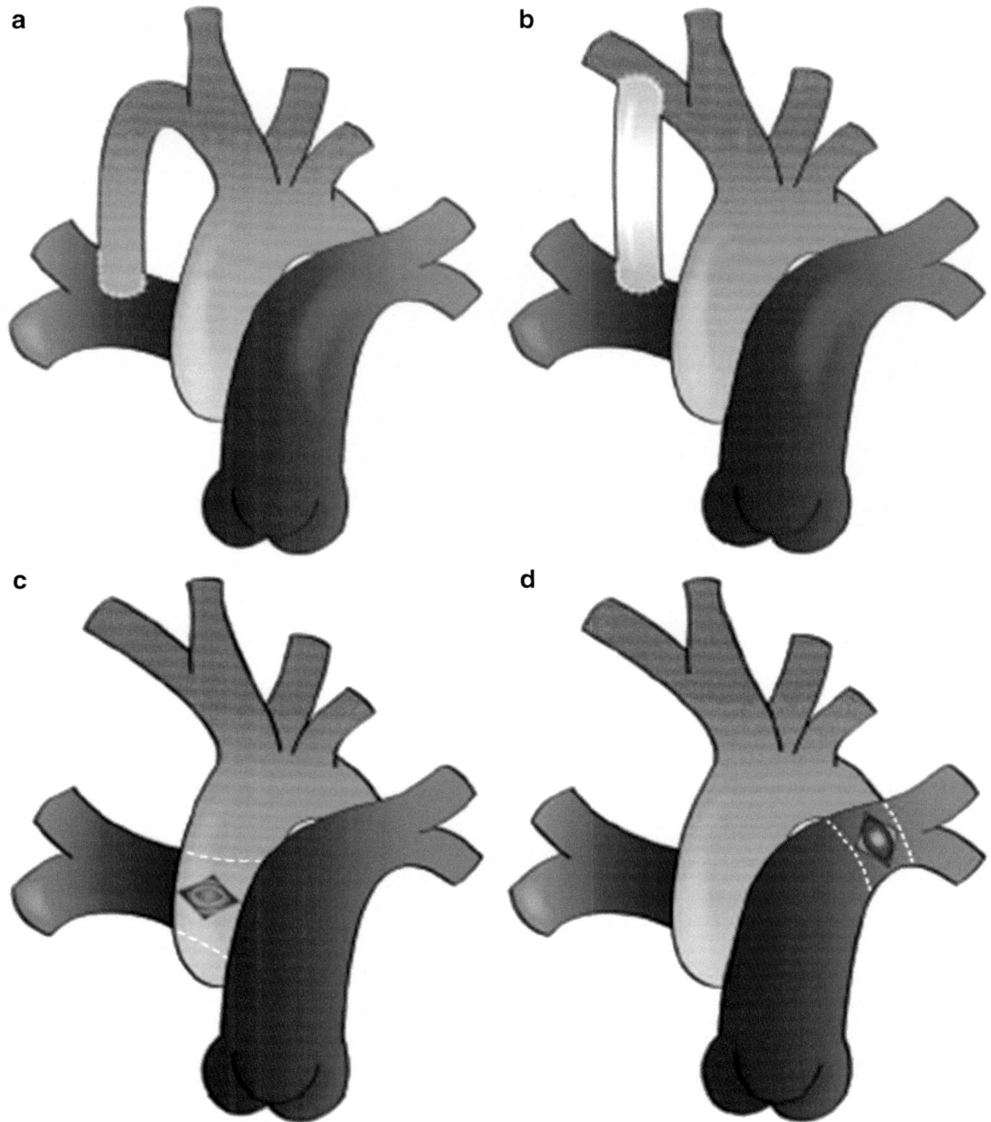

Fig. 23.14 Aortopulmonary shunts. (**a**) The classic Blalock-Taussig shunt, (**b**) a modified Blalock-Taussig shunt, (**c**) a Waterston shunt, and (**d**) the Potts shunt (Reprinted from Khairy et al. [101] with permission of Wolters Kluwer)

Although they are stable sources of pulmonary blood flow, systemic to pulmonary arterial shunts often lead to distortion of the pulmonary artery architecture because blood flow is often directed towards one pulmonary artery. As pulmonary vascular resistance decreases with age, congestive heart failure may develop as a result of excessive pulmonary blood flow. Pulmonary hypertension may develop. Most importantly, these shunts can become kinked, occluded, narrowed or thrombosed, compromising pulmonary blood supply.

In some circumstances, complete repair is not immediately feasible or must be delayed. Here, surgical banding of the pulmonary arteries is often utilized as an initial palliation. Restricting the diameter of the pulmonary arteries can protect the pulmonary vascular bed from excessive blood flow. Surgical bands can be placed around either the main pulmonary artery (MPA) or the proximal branch left and right branch pulmonary arteries. Unfortunately, banding can cause negative sequelae, particularly if the band was placed on a young patient who later outgrows the size of the band. Occasionally, the band may migrate distally, occluding one pulmonary artery and resulting in unopposed pulmonary arterial flow to the opposite branch. Post-stenotic dilation may result if the band that is placed too tightly. Structures proximal to this band gradient are also exposed to increased afterload, and, as a result, pulmonary valve regurgitation, right ventricular enlargement and dysfunction and tricuspid valve insufficiency may ensue.

As patients grow and pulmonary vascular resistance drops, BT shunts typically can no longer provide adequate pulmonary blood flow. The *Glenn shunt (bidirectional)* is an end-to-side anastomosis of the SVC to the undivided

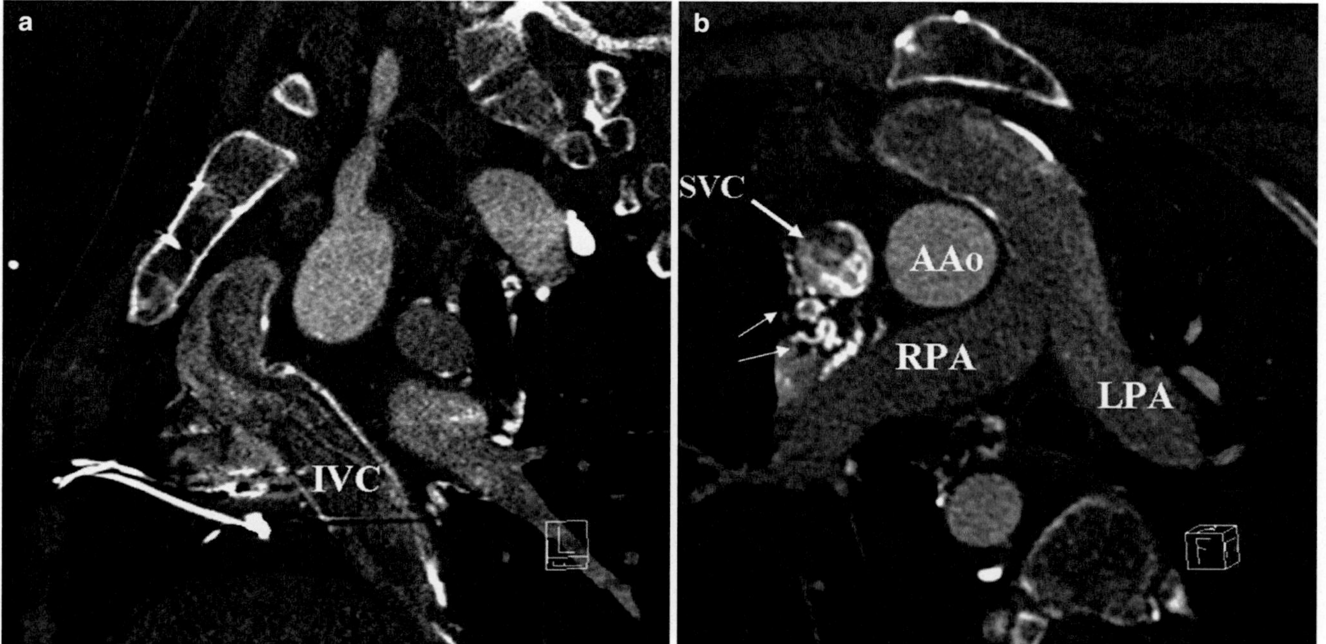

Fig. 23.15 Oblique sagittal (**a**) and axial (**b**) views demonstrate the challenges of accurately defining Fontan anatomy. Despite an accurate timing bolus, this is a low cardiac output state leading to accumulation of contrast in the superior vena cava (*SVC*) and poor opacification of desired anatomic structures. In addition, collaterals (*arrows*) may create a "steal phenomenon," resulting in poor contrast opacification. Further, incomplete opacification of the IVC diminishes diagnostic accuracy to assess for thombus in this segment of the cavopulmonary anastomosis. *AAo* ascending aorta, *LPA* left pulmonary artery, *RPA* right pulmonary artery

pulmonary artery. It is most often performed as the second stage in a series of staged palliations for single ventricle physiology. The third stage, the *Fontan procedure,* is the final palliative procedure which connects the IVC directly to the pulmonary artery. The Glenn and Fontan shunts cannot be safely performed in infancy as pulmonary vascular resistance must first fall substantially, allowing a small gradient between systemic venous pressure and pulmonary arterial pressure to drive forward flow.

The Fontan procedure has undergone significant evolution since its inception in 1971 [102]. Earlier techniques utilized an atriopulmonary (right atrial appendage-to-pulmonary artery) anastomosis. Late-onset complications including atrial arrhythmias, compression of the pulmonary veins and thrombus (as a result of severe atrial enlargement) prompted surgical revisions of this technique. Surgical techniques currently in use utilize conduits made of artificial or pericardial tissue to direct systemic venous return directly to the pulmonary arteries via either intracardiac (*lateral tunnel Fontan*) or extracardiac (*extracardiac Fontan*) routes. Occasionally, a fenestration is placed within the Fontan itself to serve as a "pop-off" for elevated systemic venous return (but at the cost of cyanosis). If pulmonary vascular resistance remains low post-operatively, such fenestrations can be later closed percutaneously. Collaterals (aortopulmonary or systemic venous) are frequent in this population [103–105].

CCTA imaging may be promising in the assessment of the single ventricle patient to assess late-onset complications including thrombus within the Fontan, fenestrations, collaterals and single ventricle function [106]. However, there are important limitations of this technique. The issues of low-cardiac output, frequent collaterals and asymmetric blood flow between the left and right lungs resulting from prior cavopulmonary anastomoses create technical challenges for an accurate gated CCTA examination (See Fig. 23.15). Simultaneous contrast injection from both an upper and lower extremity will allow dense and homogenous opacification of the entire circulation but can be technically challenging [107]. Due to these limitations, CMR is often the imaging modality of choice unless otherwise contraindicated.

Summary

Adults with CHD represent a large and diverse group of patients with both simple and complex disease. Physicians who care for patients with CHD challenged by the unique needs of this rapidly growing population, including the need for frequent non-invasive cardiovascular imaging. Although CMR has historically been recognized as the non-invasive imaging tool of choice in this patient population, advances in CCTA have allowed it to become an extremely powerful imaging modality as well. Due to the complexity of CHD, imaging specialists should understand the importance of proper patient and protocol selection for CCTA and, ideally, collaborate with adult congenital specialists to help plan and successfully execute the CCTA examination.

Coronary Artery Anomalies

Incidence and Definitions

Congenital coronary anomalies affect between 0.2 and 5.6 % of the general population [108–112]. The incidence varies considerably between studies due to a number of factors including referral bias, fewer autopsies being performed and absence of strict diagnostic criteria. In addition, coronary anomalies can vary widely in severity. The presenting symptom for some anomalies may be sudden cardiac death; others may be entirely benign and never diagnosed. Some authors have reported that coronary anomalies may cause anywhere between 12 and 19 % of deaths among young athletes [113–115].

In the normal coronary circulation, the left main coronary artery arises from the left ostium (located centrally within the left sinus of Valsalva) and gives rise to the left anterior descending artery and circumflex artery. The left anterior descending artery courses along the anterior interventricular groove, gives off septal perforators and supplies most of the septum, anterior wall and apex while the circumflex artery wraps posteriorly around the left atrioventricular groove. The right coronary artery arises from the right ostium (centrally located within the right sinus of Valsalva), giving off the marginal branch to the right ventricle and then curving posteriorly in the atrioventricular groove. Angelini and colleagues [116] suggest, in the context of known normal coronary anatomy, the following definitions: *normal* (seen in >1 % of the general population), *normal variant* (uncommon variant but seen in >1 % of the population) and *anomaly* (observed in <1 % of the population).

Clinical Significance

Congenital coronary anomalies have been reported as the cause of chest pain, arrhythmias, myocardial infarction and sudden cardiac death. Yamanaka and colleagues [108], in a survey of 126,595 angiograms, classified 80 % of anomalies as "benign" and 20 % as being potentially responsible for serious sequelae. The literature has consistently reported an association between certain coronary anomalies (such as anomalous left coronary artery from the pulmonary artery or origin of the left coronary artery from the right sinus of Valsalva) and adverse clinical outcomes. Such coronary variants may account for up to 15 % of sudden cardiac deaths in athletes [114, 116]. Outcomes in milder forms of coronary anomalies (i.e. "normal variants") are less well defined. Coronary artery anomalies may also occur in concert with congenital heart defects (discussed later in this chapter).

Selected Lesions

Abnormal Coronary Origins: ALCAPA and ARCAPA

Anomalous origin of the left coronary from the pulmonary artery (ALCAPA, also called the Bland-White-Garland syndrome) is a serious anomaly in which the left coronary artery arises from the pulmonary artery [117] (See Fig. 23.16). During fetal life, due to elevated pulmonary vascular resistance, myocardial perfusion is thought to be normal. However, upon birth, the pulmonary vascular resistance begins to fall, leading to insufficient perfusion of the left ventricle. Typically there is vigorous collateral formation from the right coronary artery but despite this, the majority present in infancy with symptoms of congestive heart failure. Others may never have symptoms and there are reports of patients reaching adulthood [118–121] though it appears to still confer a risk of sudden cardiac death.

Anomalous origin of the right coronary artery from the pulmonary artery (ARCAPA) is a much rarer anomaly which also has been associated with sudden cardiac death [122].

Coronary Artery Origin from the Improper Sinus Including Single Coronary Arteries

Coronary arteries may be seen to arise anomalously from the incorrect sinus, with an incidence of 0.92 % for origin of the right coronary artery from the left sinus and 0.15 % for left coronary artery from the right sinus [123]. Single coronary arteries are even rarer, occurring in approximately 0.024–0.066 % of the population [108, 124, 125]. Although single coronary arteries are an isolated finding in the majority of cases, they may be associated with other cardiac defects or cause sudden cardiac death [125, 126].

In broad terms, coronary arteries arising from the incorrect sinus (including single coronary arteries) may take a number of routes including retrocardiac, retroaortic, infraseptal (supracristal), pre-pulmonary (crossing the right ventricular outflow tract) or intra-aortic (between the aorta and pulmonary artery) [123] (See Figs. 23.17, 23.18, 23.19 and 23.20). Of these, the intra-aortic course has been most consistently implicated as a possible cause of sudden cardiac death. The ostium of the anomalously placed artery may be slit-like, possibly predisposing to compression between the great arteries [127–129]. Sudden cardiac death, when it occurs, is often precipitated by effort [129], which likely explains the increased incidence in athletes [113, 115, 130–133].

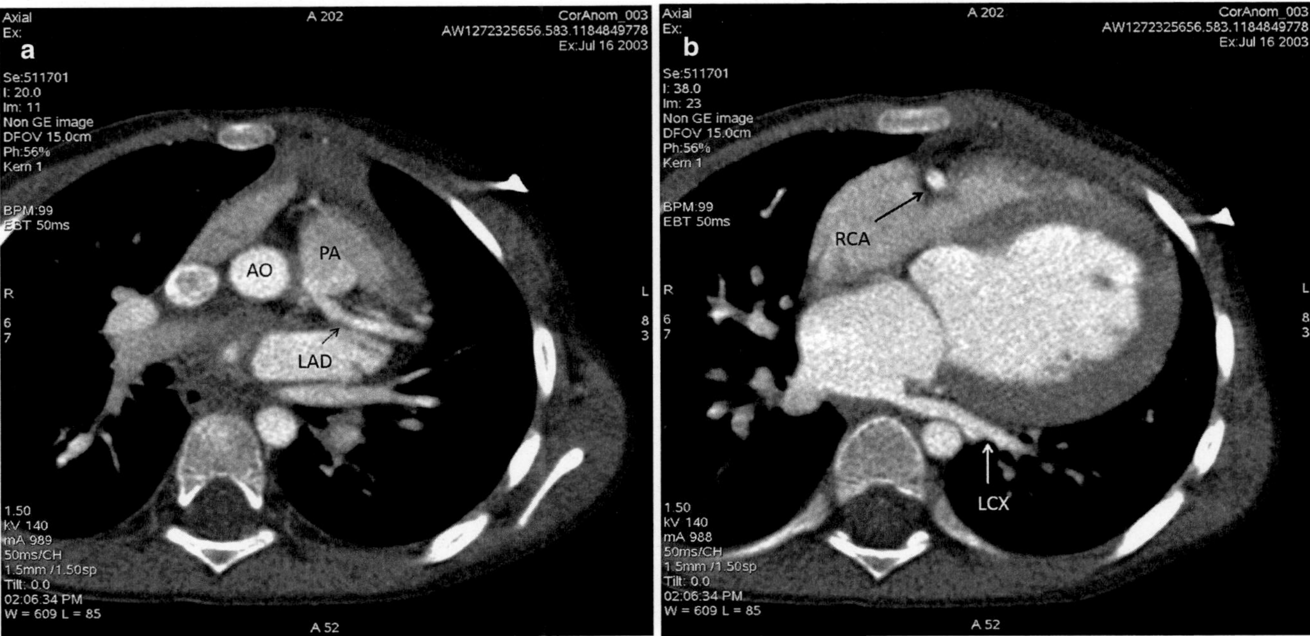

Fig. 23.16 A 2 month old infant presented with failure to thrive. Axial views (**a**) and (**b**) demonstrating the LAD arising from the pulmonary artery (anomalous left coronary artery arising from the pulmonary artery or ALCAPA) (Note that the LCX arises normally from the aorta (though its origin is posteriorly displaced) and the right coronary artery is dilated. *AO* aorta, *PA* pulmonary artery, *LAD* left anterior descending artery, *RCA* right coronary artery, *LCX* left circumflex artery

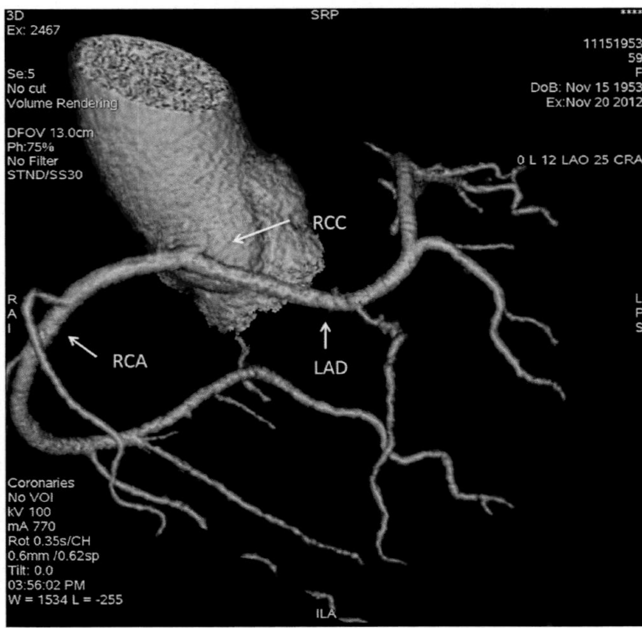

Fig. 23.17 This three-dimensional reconstruction demonstrates a single coronary artery, arising from the right coronary cusp. *RCC* right coronary cusp, *LAD* left anterior descending artery, *RCA* right coronary artery

Normal Variants and Minor Coronary Anomalies

Other coronary variants with minor or no significant clinical sequelae include intramural course (also known as "myocardial bridging"), "absent" left main (better described as dual origin of the left anterior descending and left circumflex arteries) and geographical variations of the coronary ostia within the appropriate sinus (See Fig. 23.21).

Coronary Anomalies in Congenital Heart Disease

Multiple coronary anomalies have been reported in patients with d-transposition of the great arteries (d-TGA) [134]. Most frequently, the left coronary artery arises from the "anterior facing" sinus and the right coronary artery arises from the "posterior facing" sinus. As in normal hearts, there may be single coronary arteries, multiple coronary ostia or coronary arteries arising from an improper cusp. In patients who have undergone the arterial switch procedure (in which the coronary arteries are re-implanted into the neo-aorta), coronary events are not infrequent with a prevalence of 2–11 % [135–140]. Thus, it is critically important to evaluate on CCTA the coronary arterial origins and course to exclude kinking, compression and intimal thickening [135, 141, 142].

Patients with tetralogy of Fallot also commonly have coronary anomalies including single coronary arteries in 5 %, coronary arteries with anomalous origins in 5 % and a large conus artery in anywhere from 20 to 40 % [73, 74, 143]. Of particular concern is the variant in which the left anterior descending artery arises from the right coronary artery, crossing the right ventricular outflow tract in the process. This can pose difficulties during surgery as the left anterior artery will be at risk when the chest is opened. Careful assessment for coronary anomalies in this population can

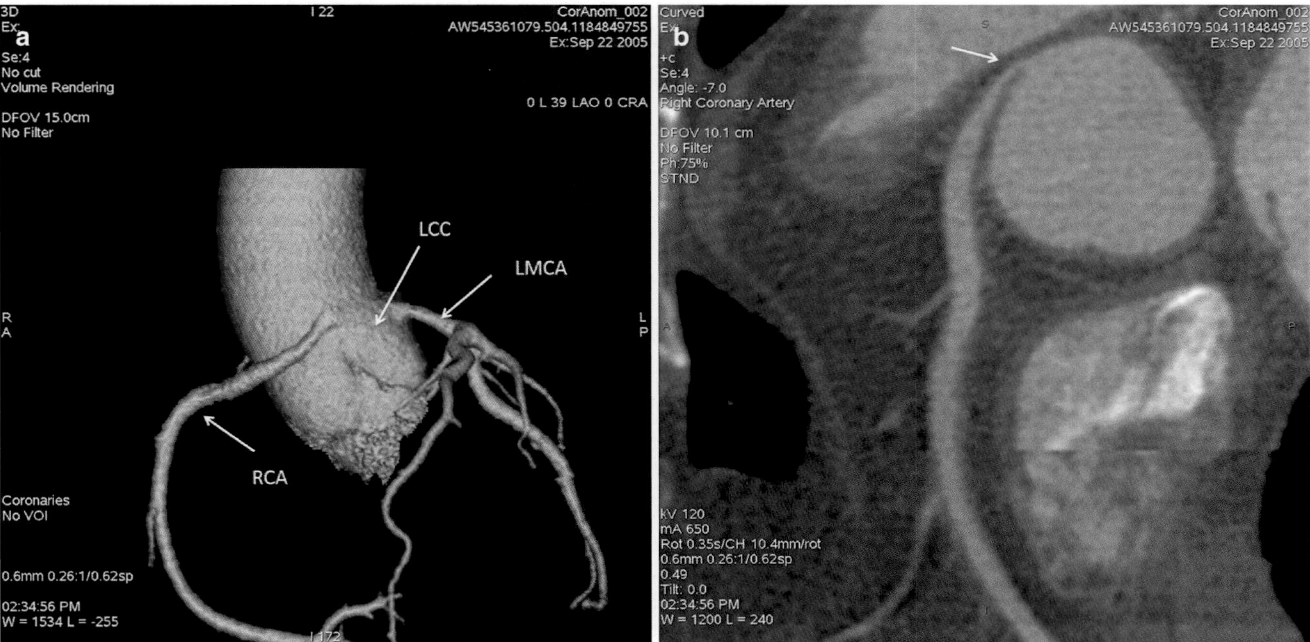

Fig. 23.18 (**a**, **b**) (**a**) Shown in this three-dimensional reconstruction is an anomalous right coronary artery originating from the left coronary cusp. (**b**) Curved multi-planar reconstruction demonstrates the slit-like origin (*arrow*) of the right coronary artery. *LCC* left coronary cusp, *LAD* left coronary artery, *RCA* right coronary artery

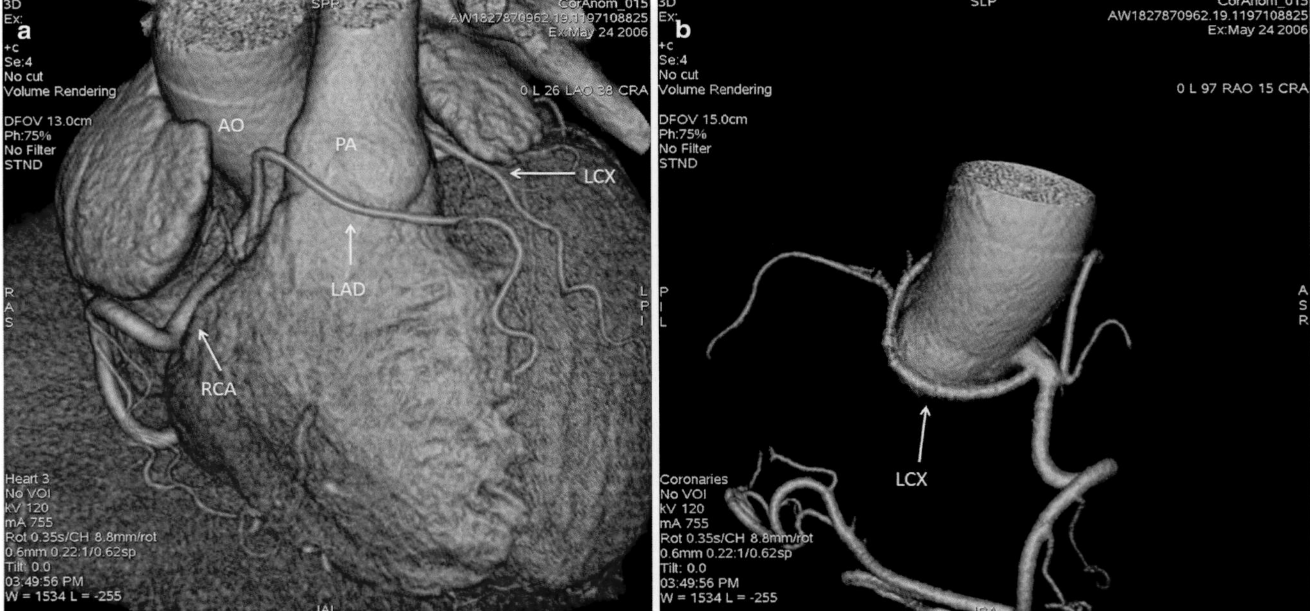

Fig. 23.19 (**a**, **b**) Three-dimensional reconstructions demonstrates a single coronary artery variant in which the left anterior descending artery courses anterior to the pulmonary artery and the circumflex artery travels behind the aorta. *AO* aorta, *PA* pulmonary artery, *LCX* left circumflex artery, *LAD* left coronary artery, *RCA* right coronary artery

help guide surgical repair [144] and should therefore be excluded prior to any intervention to the right ventricular outflow tract.

Congenitally corrected transposition (l-TGA) typically follows a similar pattern to d-TGA, in which the two main coronary ostia arise from the "facing" sinus. As the coronary arteries not infrequently arise from the improper sinus, it may be helpful to describe both the origin of the anomalous artery in addition to the territory supplied. The left coronary artery will, as in normal individuals, supply the

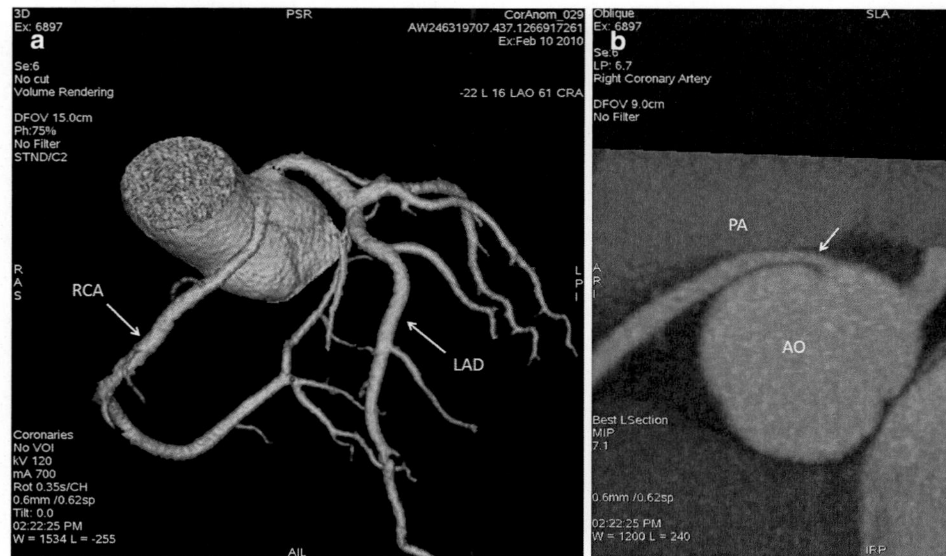

Fig. 23.20 (**a**, **b**) (**a**) Three-dimensional reconstruction shows an anomalous right coronary artery arising from the left coronary cusp, following an intra-arterial course. (**b**) Curved multiplanar reconstruction demonstrates the intraarterial course in addition to the slit-like orifice of the right coronary artery (*arrow*). *AO* aorta, *PA* pulmonary artery, *RCA* right coronary artery, *LAD* left anterior descending artery

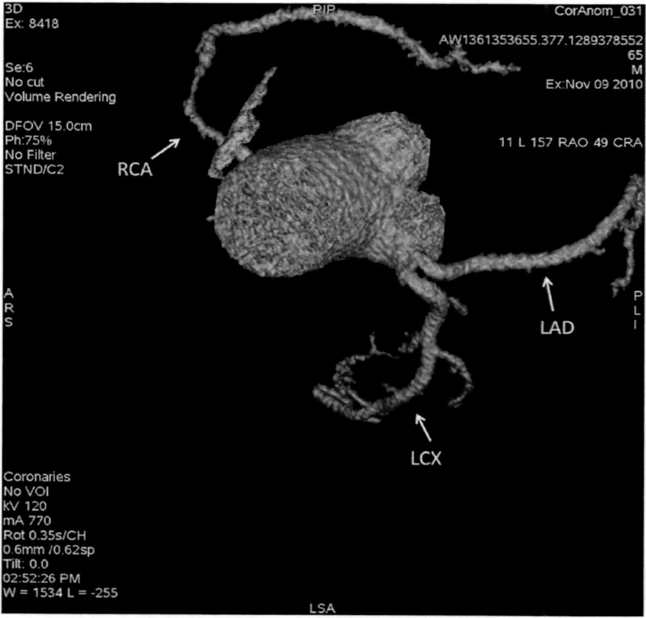

Fig. 23.21 Three-dimensional reconstruction demonstrates dual ostia for the left coronary artery and left circumflex artery ("absent left main"), a benign variant. *RCA* right coronary artery, *LAD* left anterior descending artery, *LCX* left circumflex artery

morphologic left ventricle but arises from the "right facing" sinus. The right coronary artery will supply the morphologic (systemic) right ventricle but arises from the "left facing" sinus [145].

References

1. Tennant PW, Pearce MS, Bythell M, Rankin J. 20-year survival of children born with congenital anomalies: a population-based study. The Lancet. 1920;375(9715):649–56.
2. Bird TM, Hobbs CA, Cleves MA, Tilford JM, Robbins JM. National rates of birth defects among hospitalized newborns. Birth Defects Res A Clin Mol Teratol. 2006;76(11):762–9.
3. Canfield MA, Honein MA, Yuskiv N, Xing J, Mai CT, Collins JS, et al. National estimates and race/ethnic-specific variation of selected birth defects in the United States, 1999–2001. Birth Defects Res A Clin Mol Teratol. 2006;76(11):747–56.
4. Hoffman JI, Kaplan S. The incidence of congenital heart disease. J Am Coll Cardiol. 2002;39(12):1890–900.
5. Khairy P, Ionescu-Ittu R, Mackie AS, Abrahamowicz M, Pilote L, Marelli AJ. Changing mortality in congenital heart disease. J Am Coll Cardiol. 2010;56(14):1149–57.
6. Marelli AJ, Mackie AS, Iwaki H, Rahme E, Pilote L. Congenital heart disease in the general population: changing prevalence and age distribution. Circulation. 2007;115:163–72.
7. Warnes CA, Liberthson R, Danielson GK, Dore A, Harris L, Hoffman JI, et al. Task force 1: the changing profile of congenital heart disease in adult life. J Am Coll Cardiol. 2001;37(5):1170–5.
8. van der Bom T, Bouma BJ, Meijboom FJ, Zwinderman AH, Mulder BJ. The prevalence of adult congenital heart disease, results from a systematic review and evidence based calculation. Am Heart J. 2012;164(4):568–75.
9. Ho VB. ACR appropriateness criteria on suspected congenital heart disease in adults. J Am Coll Radiol. 2008;5(2):97–104.
10. Han BK, Lesser AM, Vezmar M, Rosenthal K, Rutten-Ramos SLJ, Caye D, et al. Cardiovascular imaging trends in congenital heart disease: a single center experience. J Cardiovasc Comput Tomogr. 2013;7(6):361–6.
11. Knauth Meadows A, Ordovas K, Higgins CB, Reddy GP. Magnetic resonance imaging in the adult with congenital heart disease. Semin Roentgenol. 2008;43(3):246–58.

12. Cook SC, Raman SV. Multidetector computed tomography in the adolescent and young adult with congenital heart disease. J Cardiovasc Comput Tomogr. 2008;2(1):36–49.
13. Otero HJ, Steigner ML, Rybicki FJ. The "post-64" era of coronary CT angiography: understanding new technology from physical principles. Radiol Clin North Am. 2009;47(1):79–90.
14. Raman SV, Cook SC, McCarthy B, Ferketich AK. Usefulness of multidetector row computed tomography to quantify right ventricular size and function in adults with either tetralogy of Fallot or transposition of the great arteries. Am J Cardiol. 2005;95(5): 683–6.
15. Hoffmann A, Engelfriet P, Mulder B. Radiation exposure during follow-up of adults with congenital heart disease. Int J Cardiol. 2007;118(2):151–3.
16. Neefjes LA, Dharampal AS, Rossi A, Nieman K, Weustink AC, Dijkshoorn ML, et al. Image quality and radiation exposure using different low-dose scan protocols in dual-source CT coronary angiography: randomized study. Radiology. 2011;261(3):779–86.
17. Khan A, Khosa F, Nasir K, Yassin A, Clouse ME. Comparison of radiation dose and image quality: 320-MDCT versus 64-MDCT coronary angiography. AJR Am J Roentgenol. 2011;197(1):163.
18. Stolzmann P, Goetti R, Baumueller S, Plass A, Falk V, Scheffel H, et al. Prospective and retrospective ECG-gating for CT coronary angiography perform similarly accurate at low heart rates. Eur J Radiol. 2011;79(1):85–91.
19. Hosch W, Heye T, Schulz F, Lehrke S, Schlieter M, Giannitsis E, et al. Image quality and radiation dose in 256-slice cardiac computed tomography: comparison of prospective versus retrospective image acquisition protocols. Eur J Radiol. 2011;80(1): 127–35.
20. Choi TY, Malpeso J, Li D, Sourayanezhad S, Budoff MJ. Radiation dose reduction with increasing utilization of prospective gating in 64-multidetector cardiac computed tomography angiography. J Cardiovasc Comput Tomogr. 2011;5(4):264–70.
21. LaBounty TM, Leipsic J, Poulter R, Wood D, Johnson M, Srichai MB, et al. Coronary CT angiography of patients with a normal body mass index using 80 kVp versus 100 kVp: a prospective, multicenter, multivendor randomized trial. Am J Roentgenol. 2011;197(5):W860–7.
22. Leipsic J, LaBounty TM, Mancini GJ, Heilbron B, Taylor C, Johnson MA, et al. A prospective randomized controlled trial to assess the diagnostic performance of reduced tube voltage for coronary CT angiography. Am J Roentgenol. 2011;196(4): 801–6.
23. Zhang C, Zhang Z, Yan Z, Xu L, Yu W, Wang R. 320-row CT coronary angiography: effect of 100-kV tube voltages on image quality, contrast volume, and radiation dose. Int J Cardiovasc Imaging. 2011;27(7):1059–68.
24. Oda S, Utsunomiya D, Funama Y, Awai K, Katahira K, Nakaura T, et al. A low tube voltage technique reduces the radiation dose at retrospective ECG-gated cardiac computed tomography for anatomical and functional analyses. Acad Rradiol. 2011;18(8): 991–9.
25. Ghadri JR, Küest SM, Goetti R, Fiechter M, Pazhenkottil AP, Nkoulou RN, et al. Image quality and radiation dose comparison of prospectively triggered low-dose CCTA: 128-slice dual-source high-pitch spiral versus 64-slice single-source sequential acquisition. Int J Cardiovasc Imaging. 2012;28(5):1217–25.
26. Van Praagh R. Terminology of congenital heart disease. Glossary and commentary. Circulation. 1977;56(2):139–43.
27. Applegate KE, Goske MJ, Pierce G, Murphy D. Situs revisited: imaging of the heterotaxy syndrome 1. Radiographics. 1999;19(4): 837–52.
28. Tynan MJ, Becker AE, Macartney FJ, Jimenez MQ, Shinebourne EA, Anderson RH. Nomenclature and classification of congenital heart disease. Br Heart J. 1979;41(5):544–53.
29. Van Meter JC, LeBlanc JG, Culpepper 3rd WS, Ochsner JL. Partial anomalous pulmonary venous return. Circulation. 1990;82(5 Suppl):IV195–8.
30. Broy C, Bennett S. Partial anomalous pulmonary venous return. Mil Med. 2008;173(6):523–4.
31. Shumacker HB. Partial anomalous pulmonary venous return. Chest J. 1966;49(3):309–16.
32. Gustafson RA, Warden HE, Murray GF, Hill RC, Rozar GE. Partial anomalous pulmonary venous connection to the right side of the heart. J Thorac Cardiovasc Surg. 1989;98(5 Pt 2):861–8.
33. Lacomis JM, Wigginton W, Fuhrman C, Schwartzman D, Armfield DR, Pealer KM. Multi-detector row CT of the left atrium and pulmonary veins before radio-frequency catheter ablation for atrial fibrillation. Radiographics. 2003;23(suppl_1):S35–48.
34. Brown David W, Geva T. Anomalies of the pulmonary veins. In: Allen Hugh D, Driscoll DJ, Shaddy Robert E, Feltes Timothy F, editors. Moss and Adams' heart disease in infants, children and adolescents. 8th ed. Philadelphia: Lippincott Williams & Wilkins; 2013. p. 809–39.
35. Webb G, Gatzoulis MA. Atrial septal defects in the adult recent progress and overview. Circulation. 2006;114(15):1645–53.
36. Warnes CA, Williams RG, Bashore TM, Child JS, Connolly HM, Dearani JA, et al. ACC/AHA 2008 guidelines for the management of adults with congenital heart disease: a Report of the American College of Cardiology/American Heart Association Task Force on Practice Guidelines (Writing Committee to Develop Guidelines on the Management of Adults With Congenital Heart Disease) Developed in Collaboration With the American Society of Echocardiography, Heart Rhythm Society, International Society for Adult Congenital Heart Disease, Society for Cardiovascular Angiography and Interventions, and Society of Thoracic Surgeons. J Am Coll Cardiol. 2008;52(23):e143–263.
37. King TD, Thompson SL, Steiner C, Mills NL. Secundum atrial septal defect: nonoperative closure during cardiac catheterization. JAMA. 1976;235(23):2506–9.
38. Du ZD, Hijazi ZM, Kleinman CS, Silverman NH, Larntz K. Comparison between transcatheter and surgical closure of secundum atrial septal defect in children and adults: results of a multicenter nonrandomized trial. J Am Coll Cardiol. 2002;39(11):1836–44.
39. Gade CL, Bergman G, Naidu S, Weinsaft JW, Callister TQ, Min JK. Comprehensive evaluation of atrial septal defects in individuals undergoing percutaneous repair by 64-detector row computed tomography. Int J Cardiovasc Imaging. 2007;23(3):397–404.
40. Zaidi AN, Cheatham JP, Raman SV, Cook SC. Multislice computed tomographic findings in symptomatic patients after amplatzer septal occluder device implantation. J Interv Cardiol. 2009;22(1):92–7.
41. Butera G, Carminati M, Chessa M, Piazza L, Micheletti A, Negura DG, et al. Transcatheter closure of perimembranous ventricular septal defects: early and long-term results. J Am Coll Cardiol. 2007;50(12):1189–95.
42. Holzer R, Balzer D, Cao QL, Lock K, Hijazi ZM. Device closure of muscular ventricular septal defects using the amplatzer muscular ventricular septal defect occluder: immediate and mid-term results of a US registry. J Am Coll Cardiol. 2004; 43(7):1257–63.
43. Craig B. Atrioventricular septal defect: from fetus to adult. Heart. 2006;92(12):1879–85.
44. Freeman SB, Taft LF, Dooley KJ, Allran K, Sherman SL, Hassold TJ, et al. Population-based study of congenital heart defects in Down syndrome. Am J Med Genet. 1998;80(3):213–7.
45. Grifka R, Transcatheter PDA. Closure: equipment and technique. J Interv Cardiol. 2001;14(1):97–107.
46. Mori K, Ando M, Takao A, Ishikawa S, Imai Y. Distal type of aortopulmonary window. Report of 4 cases. Br Heart J. 1978; 40(6):681–9.

47. Berry TE, Bharati S, Muster AJ, Idriss FS, Santucci B, Lev M, et al. Distal aortopulmonary septal defect, aortic origin of the right pulmonary artery, intact ventricular septum, patent ductus arteriosus and hypoplasia of the aortic isthmus: a newly recognized syndrome. Am J Cardiol. 1982;49(1):108–16.
48. Bertolini A, Dalmonte P, Bava GL, Moretti R, Cervo G, Marasini M. Aortopulmonary septal defects. A review of the literature and report of ten cases. J Cardiovasc Surg (Torino). 1994;35(3): 207–13.
49. Blieden LC, Moller JH. Aorticopulmonary septal defect. An experience with 17 patients. Br Heart J. 1974;36(7):630.
50. Rao PS. Coarctation of the aorta. Curr Cardiol Rep. 2005;7(6): 425–34.
51. Hamdan MA, Maheshwari S, Fahey JT, Hellenbrand WE. Endovascular stents for coarctation of the aorta: initial results and immediate-term follow-up. J Am Coll Cardiol. 2001;38(5): 1518–23.
52. Chessa M, Carrozza M, Butera G, Pizza L, Negura DG, Bussadori C, et al. Results and mid-long-term follow-up of stent implantation for native and recurrent coarctation of the aorta. Eur Heart J. 2014;26(24):2728–32.
53. Forbes TJ, Moore P, Pedra CA, Zahn EM, Nykanen D, Amin Z, et al. Intermediate follow-up following intravascular stenting for treatment of coarctation of the aorta. Catheter Cardiovasc Interv. 2007;70(4):569–77.
54. Forbes TJ, Garekar S, Amin Z, Zahn EM, Nykanen D, Moore P, et al. Procedural results and acute complications in stenting native and recurrent coarctation of the aorta in patients over 4 years of age: a multi-institutional study. Catheter Cardiovasc Interv. 2007; 70(2):276–85.
55. Forbes TJ, Kim DW, Du W, Turner DR, Holzer R, Amin Z, et al. Comparison of surgical, stent, and balloon angioplasty treatment of native coarctation of the aorta: an observational study by the CCISC (Congenital Cardiovascular Interventional Study Consortium). J Am Coll Cardiol. 2011;58(25):2664–74.
56. Cohen MARC, Fuster V, Steele PM, Driscoll D, McGoon DC. Coarctation of the aorta. Long-term follow-up and prediction of outcome after surgical correction. Circulation. 1989;80(4): 840–5.
57. Sebastiá C, Quiroga S, Boyé R, Perez-Lafuente M, Castellà E, Alvarez-Castells A. Aortic stenosis: spectrum of diseases depicted at multisection CT. Radiographics. 2003;23(Suppl_1):S79–91.
58. Weinberg Paul M, Natarajan S, Rogers Lindsay S. Aortic arch and vascular anomalies. In: Allen Hugh D, Driscoll DJ, Shaddy Robert E, Feltes Timothy F, editors. Moss and Adams' heart disease in infants, children, and adolescents. 8th ed. Philadelphia: Lippincott Williams & Wilkins; 2013. p. 758–98.
59. Siu SC, Silversides CK. Bicuspid aortic valve disease. J Am Coll Cardiol. 2010;55(25):2789–800.
60. Duran AC, Frescura C, Sans-Coma V, Angelini A, Basso C, Thiene G. Bicuspid aortic valves in hearts with other congenital heart disease. J Heart Valve Dis. 1995;4(6):581–90.
61. Roberts WC. The congenitally bicuspid aortic valve: a study of 85 autopsy cases. Am J Cardiol. 1970;26(1):72–83.
62. Feuchtner GM, Müeller S, Bonatti J, Schachner T, Velik-Salchner C, Pachinger O, et al. Sixty-four slice CT evaluation of aortic stenosis using planimetry of the aortic valve area. Am J Roentgenol. 2007;189(1):197–203.
63. Newfeld EA, Muster AJ, Paul MH, Idriss FS, Riker WL. Discrete subvalvular aortic stenosis in childhood: study of 51 patients. Am J Cardiol. 1976;38(1):53–61.
64. Kelly DT, Wulfsberc E, ROWE RD. Discrete subaortic stenosis. Circulation. 1972;46(2):309–22.
65. Cohen L, Bennani R, Hulin S, Malergue MC, Yemets I, Kalangos A, et al. Mitral valvar anomalies and discrete subaortic stenosis. Cardiol Young. 2002;12(02):138–46.
66. Marasini M, Zannini L, Ussia GP, Pinto R, Moretti R, Lerzo F, et al. Discrete subaortic stenosis: incidence, morphology and surgical impact of associated subaortic anomalies. Ann Thorac Surg. 2003;75(6):1763–8.
67. Williams JCP, Barratt-Boyes BG, Lowe JB. Supravalvular aortic stenosis. Circulation. 1961;24(6):1311–8.
68. Beuren AJ, Schulze C, Eberle P, Harmjanz D, Apitz J. The syndrome of supravalvular aortic stenosis, peripheral pulmonary stenosis, mental retardation and similar facial appearance. Am J Cardiol. 1964;13(4):471–83.
69. Gikonyo BM, Lucas RV, Edwards JE. Anatomic features of congenital pulmonary valvar stenosis. Pediatr Cardiol. 1987;8(2): 109–16.
70. Noonan JA. Hypertelorism with Turner phenotype: a new syndrome with associated congenital heart disease. American Journal of Diseases of Children. 1968;116(4):373–80.
71. Mendez HM, Opitz JM, Reynolds JF. Noonan syndrome: a review. Am J Med Genet. 1985;21(3):493–506.
72. Burch M, Sharland M, Shinebourne E, Smith G, Patton M, McKenna W. Cardiologic abnormalities in Noonan syndrome: phenotypic diagnosis and echocardiographic assessment of 118 patients. J Am Coll Cardiol. 1993;22(4):1189–92.
73. Dabizzi RP, Caprioli G, Aiazzi L, Castelli C, Baldrighi G, Parenzan L, et al. Distribution and anomalies of coronary arteries in tetralogy of fallot. Circulation. 1980;61(1):95–102.
74. Fellows KE, Freed MD, Keane JF, Praagh R, Bernhard WF, Castaneda AC. Results of routine preoperative coronary angiography in tetralogy of Fallot. Circulation. 1975;51(3):561–6.
75. Hurwitz RA, Smith W, King H, Girod DA, Caldwell RL. Tetralogy of Fallot with abnormal coronary artery: 1967 to 1977. J Thorac Cardiovasc Surg. 1980;80(1):129–34.
76. Lurz P, Bonhoeffer P, Taylor AM. Percutaneous pulmonary valve implantation: an update. Expert Rev Cardiovasc Ther. 2009;7(7): 823–33.
77. Wittwer ED, Pulido JN, Gillespie SM, Cetta F, Dearani JA. Left main coronary artery compression following Melody pulmonary valve implantation: use of Impella support as rescue therapy and perioperative challenges with ECMO. Case Rep Crit Care 2014 (2014), Article ID 959704, 3 pages.
78. Morray BH, McElhinney DB, Cheatham JP, Zahn EM, Berman DP, Sullivan PM, et al. Risk of coronary artery compression among patients referred for transcatheter pulmonary valve implantation a multicenter experience. Circ Cardiovasc Interv. 2013;6(5):535–42.
79. Niwa K, Siu SC, Webb GD, Gatzoulis MA. Progressive aortic root dilatation in adults late after repair of tetralogy of fallot. Circulation. 2002;106(11):1374–8.
80. Tan JL, Davlouros PA, McCarthy KP, Gatzoulis MA, Ho SY. Intrinsic histological abnormalities of aortic root and ascending aorta in tetralogy of fallot: evidence of causative mechanism for aortic dilatation and aortopathy. Circulation. 2005;112(7):961–8.
81. Roman MJ, Devereux RB, Kramer-Fox R, O'Loughlin J. Two-dimensional echocardiographic aortic root dimensions in normal children and adults. Am J Cardiol. 1989;64(8):507–12.
82. Mongeon FP, Gurvitz MZ, Broberg CS, Aboulhosn J, Opotowsky AR, Kay JD, et al. Aortic root dilatation in adults with surgically repaired tetralogy of Fallot: a multicenter cross-sectional study. Circulation. 2013;127(2):172–9.
83. Bashore TM. Adult congenital heart disease right ventricular outflow tract lesions. Circulation. 2007;115(14):1933–47.
84. Van Praagh R, Pérez-Trevino C, Reynolds JL, Moes CAF, Keith JD, Roy DL, et al. Double outlet right ventricle {S, D, L} with subaortic ventricular septal defect and pulmonary stenosis: report of six cases. Am J Cardiol. 1975;35(1):42–53.
85. Sondheimer HM, Freedom RM, Olley PM. Double outlet right ventricle: clinical spectrum and prognosis. Am J Cardiol. 1977; 39(5):709–14.

86. Zamora R, Moller JH, Edwards JE. Double-outlet right ventricle anatomic types and associated anomalies. Chest J. 1975;68(5):672–7.
87. Losay J, Touchot A, Serraf A, Litvinova A, Lambert V, Piot JD, et al. Late outcome after arterial switch operation for transposition of the great arteries. Circulation. 2001;104 Suppl 1:I-121.
88. Kirklin JW, Blackstone EH, Tchervenkov CI, Castaneda AR. Clinical outcomes after the arterial switch operation for transposition. Patient, support, procedural, and institutional risk factors. Congenital Heart Surgeons Society. Circulation. 1992;86(5):1501–15.
89. Prifti E, Crucean A, Bonacchi M, Bernabei M, Murzi B, Luisi SV, et al. Early and long term outcome of the arterial switch operation for transposition of the great arteries: predictors and functional evaluation. Eur J Cardiothorac Surg. 2002;22(6):864–73.
90. Schwartz ML, Gauvreau K, del Nido P, Mayer JE, Colan SD. Long-term predictors of aortic root dilation and aortic regurgitation after arterial switch operation. Circulation. 2004;110(11 Suppl 1):II-128.
91. Ou P, Celermajer DS, Marini D, Agnoletti G, Vouhé P, Brunelle F, et al. Safety and accuracy of 64-slice computed tomography coronary angiography in children after the arterial switch operation for transposition of the great arteries. JACC Cardiovasc Imaging. 2008;1(3):331–9.
92. Allwork SP, Bentall HH, Becker AE, Cameron H, Gerlis LM, Wilkinson JL, et al. Congenitally corrected transposition of the great arteries: morphologic study of 32 cases. Am J Cardiol. 1976;38(7):910–23.
93. Schiebler GL, Edwards JE, Burchell HB, DuShane JW, Ongley PA, Wood EH. Congenital corrected transposition of the great vessels: a study of 33 cases. Pediatrics. 1961;27(5):851–88.
94. Bjarke BB, Kidd BSL. Congenitally corrected transposition of the great arteries a clinical study of 101 cases. Acta Paediatr. 1976;65(2):153–60.
95. Van Praagh R, Papagiannis J, Grünenfelder J, Bartram U, Martanovic P. Pathologic anatomy of corrected transposition of the great arteries: medical and surgical implications. Am Heart J. 1998;135(5):772–85.
96. Graham TP, Bernard YD, Mellen BG, Celermajer D, Baumgartner H, Cetta F, et al. Long-term outcome in congenitally corrected transposition of the great arteries: a multi-institutional study. J Am Coll Cardiol. 2000;36(1):255–61.
97. Presbitero P, Somerville J, Rabajoli F, Stone S, Conte MR. Corrected transposition of the great arteries without associated defects in adult patients: clinical profile and follow up. Br Heart J. 1995;74(1):57–9.
98. Collett RW, Edwards JE. Persistent truncus arteriosus; a classification according to anatomic types. Surg Clin North Am. 1949;29(4):1245.
99. Tchervenkov CI, Jacobs JP, Weinberg PM, Aiello VD, Béland MJ, Colan SD, et al. The nomenclature, definition and classification of hypoplastic left heart syndrome. Cardiol Young. 2006;16(04):339–68.
100. Blalock A, Taussig HB. The surgical treatment of malformations of the heart: in which there is pulmonary stenosis or pulmonary atresia. JAMA. 1945;128(3):189–202.
101. Khairy P, Poirier N, Mercier LAE. Univentricular heart. Circulation. 2007;115(6):800–12.
102. Fontan F, Baudet E. Surgical repair of tricuspid atresia. Thorax. 1971;26(3):240–8.
103. Grosse-Wortmann L, Al-Otay A, Yoo SJ. Aortopulmonary collaterals after bidirectional cavopulmonary connection or Fontan completion quantification with MRI. Circ Cardiovasc Imaging. 2009;2(3):219–25.
104. Triedman JK, Bridges ND, Mayer JE, Lock JE. Prevalence and risk factors for aortopulmonary collateral vessels after Fontan and bidirectional Glenn procedures. J Am Coll Cardiol. 1993;22(1):207–15.
105. McElhinney DB, Reddy VM, Hanley FL, Moore P. Systemic venous collateral channels causing desaturation after bidirectional cavopulmonary anastomosis: evaluation and management. J Am Coll Cardiol. 1997;30(3):817–24.
106. Spevak PJ, Johnson PT, Fishman EK. Surgically corrected congenital heart disease: utility of 64-MDCT. Am J Roentgenol. 2008;191(3):854–61.
107. Greenberg SB, Bhutta ST. A dual contrast injection technique for multidetector computed tomography angiography of Fontan procedures. Int J Cardiovasc Imaging. 2008;24(3):345–8.
108. Yamanaka O, Hobbs RE. Coronary artery anomalies in 126,595 patients undergoing coronary arteriography. Cathet Cardiovasc Diagn. 1990;21(1):28–40.
109. Click RL, Holmes DR, Vlietstra RE, Kosinski AS, Kronmal RA. Anomalous coronary arteries: location, degree of atherosclerosis and effect on survival: a report from the Coronary Artery Surgery Study. J Am Coll Cardiol. 1989;13(3):531–7.
110. Baitaxe HA, Wixson D. The incidence of congenital anomalies of the coronary arteries in the adult population 1. Radiology. 1977;122(1):47–52.
111. Engel HJ, Torres C, Page HL. Major variations in anatomical origin of the coronary arteries: angiographic observations in 4,250 patients without associated congenital heart disease. Cathet Cardiovasc Diagn. 1975;1(2):157–69.
112. Angelini P, Villason S, Chan AV, Diez JG. Normal and anomalous coronary arteries in humans. In: Angelini P, editor. Coronary artery anomalies: a comprehensive approach. Philadelphia: Lippincott Williams & Wilkins; 1999. p. 27–150.
113. Van Camp SP, Bloor CM, Mueller FO, Cantu RC, Olson HG. Nontraumatic sports death in high school and college athletes. Med Sci Sports Exerc. 1995;27(5):641–7.
114. Maron BJ, Thompson PD, Puffer JC, McGrew CA, Strong WB, Douglas PS, et al. Cardiovascular preparticipation screening of competitive athletes a statement for health professionals from the Sudden Death Committee (clinical cardiology) and Congenital Cardiac Defects Committee (cardiovascular disease in the young). American Heart Association. Circulation. 1996;94(4):850–6.
115. Burke AP, Farb A, Virmani R, Goodin J, Smialek JE. Sports-related and non-sports-related sudden cardiac death in young adults. Am Heart J. 1991;121(2):568–75.
116. Angelini P, Velasco JA, Flamm S. Coronary anomalies incidence, pathophysiology, and clinical relevance. Circulation. 2002;105(20):2449–54.
117. Bland EF, White PD, Garland J. Congenital anomalies of the coronary arteries: report of an unusual case associated with cardiac hypertrophy. Am Heart J. 1933;8(6):787–801.
118. Fierens C, Budts W, Denef B, Van de Werf F. A 72 year old woman with ALCAPA. Heart. 2000;83(1):e2.
119. Kristensen T, Kofoed KF, Helqvist S, Helvind M, Søndergaard L. Anomalous origin of the left coronary artery from the pulmonary artery (ALCAPA) presenting with ventricular fibrillation in an adult: a case report. J Cardiothorac Surg. 2008;3:33.
120. Selzman CH, Zimmerman MA, Campbell DN. ALCAPA in an adult with preserved left ventricular function. J Card Surg. 2003;18(1):25–8.
121. Kang WC, Chung WJ, Choi CH, Park KY, Jeong MJ, Ahn TH, et al. A rare case of anomalous left coronary artery from the pulmonary artery (ALCAPA) presenting congestive heart failure in an adult. Int J Cardiol. 2007;115(2):e63–7.
122. Williams IA, Gersony WM, Hellenbrand WE. Anomalous right coronary artery arising from the pulmonary artery: a report of 7 cases and a review of the literature. Am Heart J. 2006;152(5):1004.e9.
123. Angelini P. Coronary artery anomalies: an entity in search of an identity. Circulation. 2007;115:1296–305.

124. Lipton MJ, Barry WH, Obrez I, Silverman JF, Wexler L. Isolated single coronary artery: diagnosis, angiographic classification, and clinical significance 1. Radiology. 1979;130(1):39–47.
125. Desmet W, Vanhaecke J, Vrolix M, Van de Werf F, Piessens J, Willems J, et al. Isolated single coronary artery: a review of 50 000 consecutive coronary angiographies. Eur Heart J. 1992;13(12): 1637–40.
126. Sharbaugh AH, White RS. Single coronary artery: analysis of the anatomic variation, clinical importance, and report of five cases. JAMA. 1974;230(2):243–6.
127. Kragel AH, Roberts WC. Anomalous origin of either the right or left main coronary artery from the aorta with subsequent coursing between aorta and pulmonary trunk: analysis of 32 necropsy cases. Am J Cardiol. 1988;62(10):771–7.
128. Cheitlin MD, De Castro CM, McAllister HA. Sudden death as a complication of anomalous left coronary origin from the anterior sinus of Valsalva A not-so-minor congenital anomaly. Circulation. 1974;50(4):780–7.
129. Frescura C, Basso C, Thiene G, Corrado D, Pennelli T, Angelini A, et al. Anomalous origin of coronary arteries and risk of sudden death: a study based on an autopsy population of congenital heart disease. Hum Pathol. 1998;29(7):689–95.
130. Basso C, Maron BJ, Corrado D, Thiene G. Clinical profile of congenital coronary artery anomalies with origin from the wrong aortic sinus leading to sudden death in young competitive athletes. J Am Coll Cardiol. 2000;35(6):1493–501.
131. Taylor AJ, Rogan KM, Virmani R. Sudden cardiac death associated with isolated congenital coronary artery anomalies. J Am Coll Cardiol. 1992;20(3):640–7.
132. Eckart RE, Scoville SL, Campbell CL, Shry EA, Stajduhar KC, Potter RN, et al. Sudden death in young adults: a 25-year review of autopsies in military recruits. Ann Intern Med. 2004;141(11): 829–34.
133. Drory Y, Turetz Y, Hiss Y, Lev B, Fisman EZ, Pines A, et al. Sudden unexpected death in persons<40 years of age. Am J Cardiol. 1991;68(13):1388–92.
134. Wernovsky G, Sanders SP. Coronary artery anatomy and transposition of the great arteries. Coron Artery Dis. 1993;4(2): 148–58.
135. Legendre A, Losay J, Touchot-Kone A, Serraf A, Belli E, Piot JD, et al. Coronary events after arterial switch operation for transposition of the great arteries. Circulation. 2003;108(10 Suppl 1): II-186.
136. Brown JW, Park HJ, Turrentine MW. Arterial switch operation: factors impacting survival in the current era. Ann Thorac Surg. 2001;71(6):1978–84.
137. Yamaguchi M, Hosokawa Y, Imai Y, Kurosawa H, Yasui H, Yagihara T, et al. Early and midterm results of the arterial switch operation for transposition of the great arteries in Japan. J Thorac Cardiovasc Surg. 1990;100(2):261–9.
138. Prêtre R, Tamisier D, Bonhoeffer P, Mauriat P, Pouard P, Sidi D, et al. Results of the arterial switch operation in neonates with transposed great arteries. The Lancet. 2001;357(9271):1826–30.
139. Von Bernuth G. 25 years after the first arterial switch procedure: mid-term results. Thorac Cardiovasc Surg. 2000;48(04):228–32.
140. Mayer Jr JE, Sanders SP, Jonas RA, Castaneda AR, Wernovsky G. Coronary artery pattern and outcome of arterial switch operation for transposition of the great arteries. Circulation. 1990; 82(5 Suppl):IV139–45.
141. Tanel RE, Wernovsky G, Landzberg MJ, Perry SB, Burke RP. Coronary artery abnormalities detected at cardiac catheterization following the arterial switch operation for transposition of the great arteries. Am J Cardiol. 1995;76(3):153–7.
142. Hauser M, Bengel FM, Kühn A, Sauer U, Zylla S, Braun SL, et al. Myocardial blood flow and flow reserve after coronary reimplantation in patients after arterial switch and Ross operation. Circulation. 2001;103(14):1875–80.
143. Meng CCL, Eckner FAO, Lev M. Coronary artery distribution in tetralogy of Fallot. Arch Surg. 1965;90(3):363–6.
144. Humes RA, Driscoll DJ, Danielson GK, Puga FJ. Tetralogy of Fallot with anomalous origin of left anterior descending coronary artery. Surgical options. J Thorac Cardiovasc Surg. 1987;94(5): 784–7.
145. Scott LD, Paul MG. Congenital anomalies of the coronary vessels and the aortic root. In: Allen Hugh D, Driscoll DJ, Shaddy Robert E, Feltes Timothy F, editors. Moss and Adams' heart disease in infants, children and adolescents. 8th ed. Philadelphia: Lippincott Williams & Wilkins; 2013. p. 746–57.

CCTA Cardiac Electrophysiology Applications: Substrate Identification, Virtual Procedural Planning, and Procedural Facilitation

24

Jerold S. Shinbane, Leslie A. Saxon, Rahul N. Doshi, Philip M. Chang, and Matthew J. Budoff

Abstract

Cardiovascular computed tomographic angiography (CCTA) is a valuable adjunctive tool in the diagnosis and treatment of electrophysiologic disease. This modality provides visualization of anatomy important to arrhythmia substrate identification, as well as electrophysiology procedural planning, facilitation, and follow-up. Atrial fibrillation ablation requires a detailed understanding of an individual patient's presence and degree of atrial myopathy and 3-D characterization of the relationships between the left atrium, the surrounding cardiac and extracardiac thoracic structures. Electroanatomic mapping with CCTA image integration has revolutionized catheter–based therapies by allowing for electrical mapping and ablation to occur on a 3-D map of the patient's individual atrial anatomy. CCTA imaging has assumed an important role in decisions and planning of atrial appendage occlusion device procedures. Ventricular arrhythmias are associated with a spectrum of cardiovascular structural abnormalities which can be identified by CCTA. Cardiomyopathic substrates associated with ventricular arrhythmias can be identified, although fibrosis imaging is more evolved with cardiovascular magnetic resonance imaging. CCTA can visualize the coronary venous system providing roadmaps for lead placement when obstacles to standard approaches are identified. The role of CCTA will expand due to continued development of novel cardiac electrophysiology applications for arrhythmogenic substrate identification and procedural facilitation.

Keywords

Ablation • Atrial Fibrillation • Anomalous Coronary Arteries • Cardiac Electrophysiology • Cardiomyopathy • Cardiovascular Magnetic Resonance Imaging • Computed Tomography • Congenital Heart Disease • Electrophysiology • Ventricular Tachycardia

Electronic supplementary material The online version of this chapter (doi:10.1007/978-3-319-28219-0_24) contains supplementary material, which is available to authorized users.

J.S. Shinbane, MD, FACC, FHRS, FSCCT (✉)
Division of Cardiovascular Medicine, Department of Internal Medicine, Keck School of Medicine of the University of Southern California, 1520 San Pablo Suite 300, Los Angeles, CA 90033, USA
e-mail: shinbane@usc.edu

L.A. Saxon, MD, FACC, FHRS • R.N. Doshi, MD, FACC, FHRS
P.M. Chang, MD
Department of Medicine, Division of Cardiovascular Medicine, Department of Internal Medicine, Keck School of Medicine of the University of Southern California, Los Angeles, CA, USA

M.J. Budoff, MD
David Geffen School of Medicine at UCLA, Los Angeles Biomedical Research Institute, Torrance, CA, USA

M.J. Budoff, J.S. Shinbane (eds.), *Cardiac CT Imaging: Diagnosis of Cardiovascular Disease*,
DOI 10.1007/978-3-319-28219-0_24

Introduction

Cardiovascular computed tomographic angiography (CCTA) can comprehensively assess cardiovascular structure and function relevant to the assessment, treatment, and follow-up of patients with electrophysiologically-related disease processes. CCTA provides 3-D visualization of cardiac chambers, coronary vessels, and thoracic vasculature, including structures particularly important to cardiac electrophysiology such as the coronary veins, pulmonary veins, and left atrium. This comprehensive technology is extremely useful for the identification and characterization of cardiovascular substrates relevant to cardiac electrophysiology, and has great relevance to treatment of arrhythmias through pre-procedure planning, procedural facilitation, and procedural follow-up.

Technical Issues Related to Image Acquisition in Patients with Arrhythmias

There are a variety of approaches for imaging patients with arrhythmia issues based on indication for study, rate and rhythm at the time of study, presence of a pacemaker or ICD and programmed lower rate and mode, CT scanner, imaging and injection protocol, and editing software. Particular attention to details of patient preparation and image acquisition and processing is important to optimizing CCTA studies in patients who may have irregular rhythms due to premature atrial contractions, premature ventricular contractions, or other arrhythmias including atrial fibrillation and atrial flutter. Medications to control heart rate and rhythm as well as pacemaker reprogramming to regularize rhythms may be useful. Acquisition protocols which compensate for irregular beats through deletion of short R-R intervals and analysis of mid-diastolic phases of the R-R interval with an absolute rather than relative time from the preceding R wave can improve image quality [1].

The indication for the CCTA study is important to decisions regarding the correct field of view and target structures requiring maximum contrast opacification. The contrast circulation time and the injection protocol are important factors to take into account to achieve maximal opacification of the region or regions of interest. Assessment of right ventricular function as well as coronary venous anatomy requires protocols providing adequate contrast enhancement to these structures, while still opacifying other cardiac structures and coronary arterial anatomy. Multiphase injection protocols with varying amounts of contrast, diluted contrast, and/or saline can be administered at variable speeds of delivery to optimally opacify structures for various electrophysiology indications (Fig. 24.1).

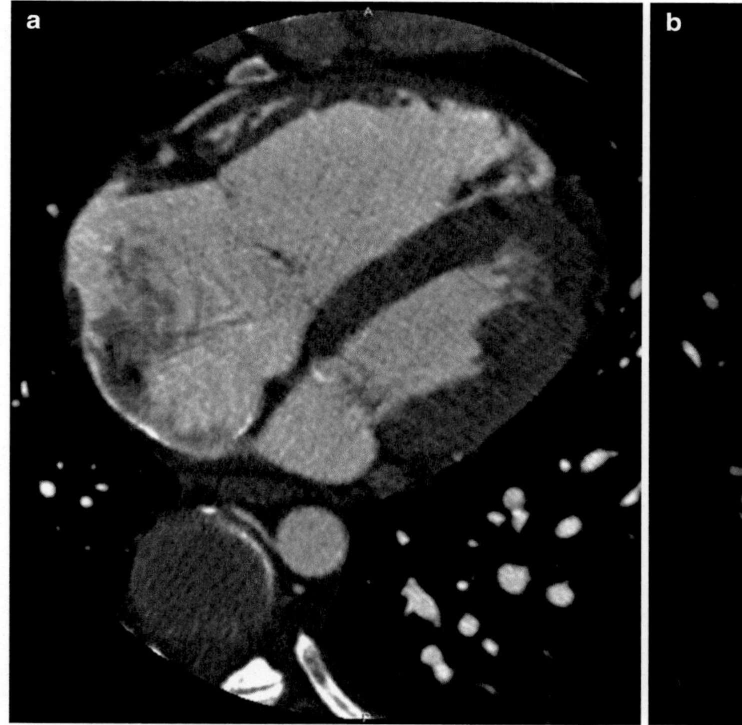

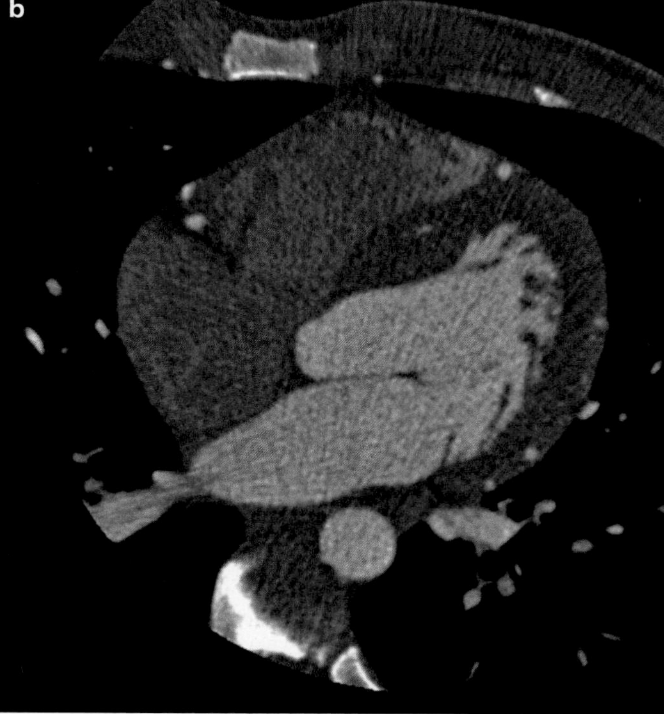

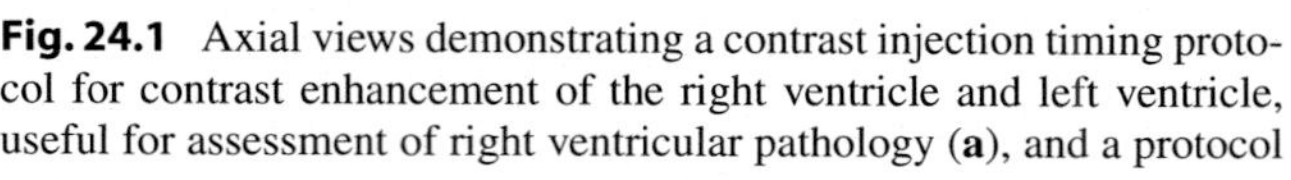

Fig. 24.1 Axial views demonstrating a contrast injection timing protocol for contrast enhancement of the right ventricle and left ventricle, useful for assessment of right ventricular pathology (**a**), and a protocol for contrast enhancement of the left ventricle, useful for coronary artery assessment without streak artifacts in the superior vena cava (**b**)

As patients having CCTA for arrhythmia applications often undergo electrophysiology procedures which may require fluoroscopy, techniques to limit radiation dose are extremely important. Dose reductions can be achieved through limitation of field of view to essential structures and use of dose limiting imaging protocols. Prospective gating techniques or retrospective gating with dose modulation can be used in some circumstances, but these techniques can be more limited in the setting of irregular rhythms.

Gated imaging can be problematic in the setting of the rhythm irregularity and elevated heart rate, but is feasible in some scenarios. Problems with irregularity can lead to "step ladder" artifact limiting the ability to obtain diagnostic assessment of segments of the coronary arteries [2, 3]. This artifact can be minimized using volume scanners which can image the field of view in a single heartbeat. With retrospective gating, cardiac structures including each coronary artery segment can be analyzed in the most optimal phase, but at the cost of an increased radiation dose. Assessment of the coronary arteries with retrospective gating is achievable in patients in atrial fibrillation prior to ablation [4]. With prospective gating, algorithms rejecting beats outside of a specified range have been developed for patients with irregular rhythms [5, 6]. In the setting of atrial fibrillation with higher average ventricular rate response, end-systole may be a more optimal phase of image reconstruction than end diastole [7, 8].

In patients with pacemakers and ICDs and higher programmed pacing rates the pacing rate can be transiently programmed down to the optimal rate for imaging, such as 60 bpm, if the patient's native underlying heart rate is below this value and the patient's underlying condition allows this change in programming. Reprogramming pacing function to a non-rate responsive modes can be helpful as the breath hold process can trigger a rate response with some devices. The presence of pacemakers or ICDs can also lead to beam hardening artifacts which can impact image quality.

Decisions as to the use of CCTA versus CMR in patients with pacemakers and ICDs depend on device specifics. The application of CMR for patients with cardiac pacemakers and ICDs has undergone evolution with the advent of MR conditional devices which allow for the use of MR imaging under specified conditions [9–12]. Even in scenarios where CMR can be performed, imaging artifacts can be problematic. Novel algorithms to decrease artifact are being developed [13, 14].

CCTA for Cardiovascular Diagnostic Assessment and Procedural Facilitation for Atrial Arrhythmias

Atrial Fibrillation Ablation

The potential mechanisms of initiation and perpetuation of atrial fibrillation are multiple, with their relative roles still being investigated. These potential mechanisms affecting arrhythmia initiation and perpetuation include premature atrial foci from the pulmonary veins and atria, autonomic influences, rotors defined by atrial anatomic and electrophysiologic substrate, and reentrant atrial flutter and atrial tachycardia circuits defined by regional electrophysiology, cardiac structure, and myocardial fibrosis. Given these multiple mechanisms, a variety of approaches to ablation target atrial anatomy and electrophysiology, including catheter-based segmental or complete circumferential electrical isolation of the pulmonary veins, ablation of ectopic atrial foci, long linear lesions providing pathways of preferential conduction, ablation of autonomic input, antral lesions targeting anatomy related to rotors, and ablation of reentrant circuits. Percutaneous catheter-based approaches are used to access the left atrium via either a single or double transseptal technique depending on the number and types of left atrial catheters employed.

The performance of atrial fibrillation ablation requires definition of an individual patient's presence and degree of atrial myopathy as well as characterization of the relationships between the left atrium and the surrounding cardiac and thoracic structures. A pre-procedure study serves multiple purposes, acting as a means to decide whether to proceed with ablation based on the degree of atrial myopathy, a roadmap for procedural planning, a 3-D data set for intra-procedure electroanatomic mapping and ablation, and a template for comparison to future potential studies assessing for complications such pulmonary vein stenosis. CCTA characterization of the left atrium and pulmonary veins is achieved through multiple modalities of evaluation including multiplane 2-D views, volumetric quantification of the atria, 3-D reconstructions, and virtual endovascular atrial views.

Left Atrial Myopathy: Left Atrial Size, Morphology and Function

Atrial morphology is complex and therefore characterization of the presence and degree of atrial myopathy based on volumetric assessment of size and function is of paramount importance. Left atrial volume is an important predictor of procedural success with atrial fibrillation ablation, as recurrence of atrial fibrillation is associated with an increased left atrial volume (Fig. 24.2) [15, 16].

CCTA left atrial indexed volume reference values have been reported [17–19]. In patients in sinus rhythm at the time of the CCTA, atrial ejection fraction can be calculated with retrospective gating (Fig. 24.3) [20]. CCTA left atrial volumes correlate with CMR volumes [21]. Preprocedure assessment of left atrial size and pulmonary vein anatomy and size are similar for CMR and CCTA, although cumulative radiation dose is decreased with CMR for image guided ablation [22]. Variation in pulmonary vein anatomy branching patterns can be characterized [23]. Assessment of atrial

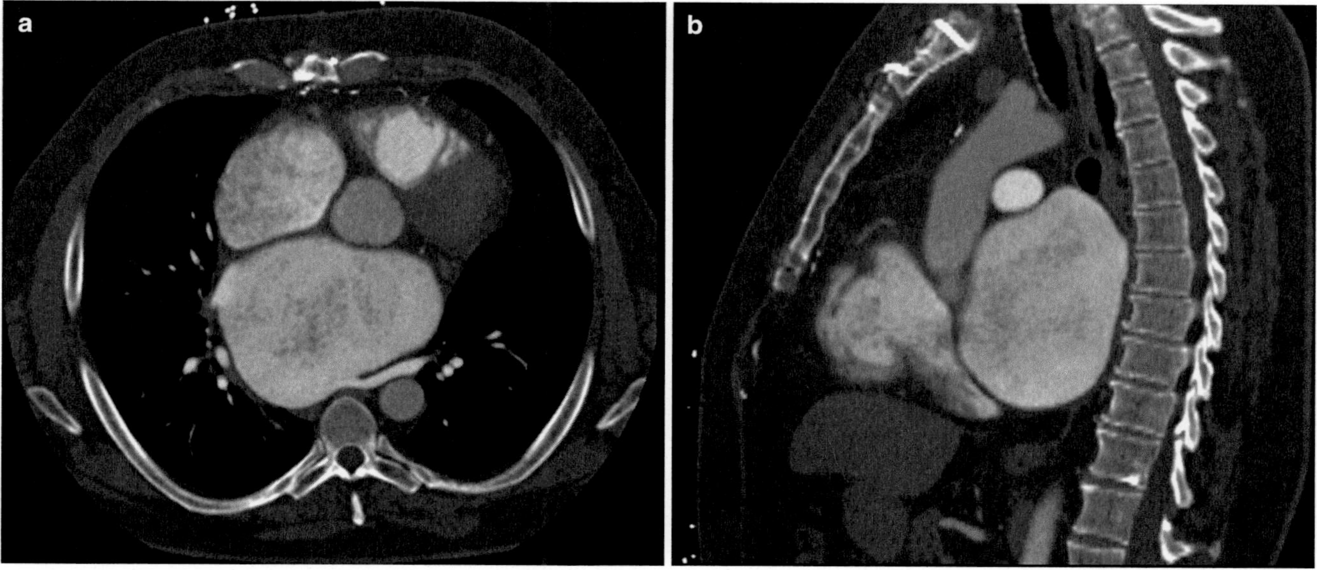

Fig. 24.2 Axial (**a**) and sagittal (**b**) views demonstrating profound atrial enlargement in a patient with atrial fibrillation. The left atrial volume was greater than 450 cc

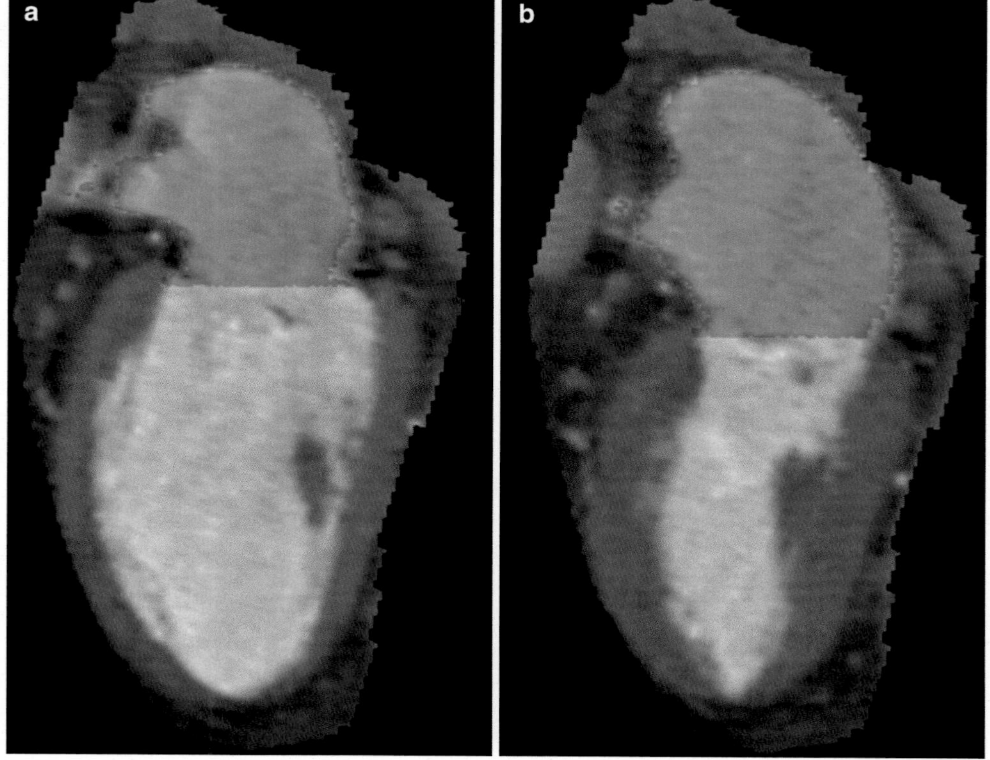

Fig. 24.3 Assessment of left atrial volume during atrial systole (**a**) and diastole (**b**)

wall thickness can be performed at multiple relevant locations including at the pulmonary veins, left pulmonary vein/ left atrial appendage ridge and posterior left atrium [24, 25]. Thicker left pulmonary vein/left atrial appendage ridges as assessed by CCTA are associated with a higher rate of atrial fibrillation recurrence and therefore have potential implications for ablation approach to this anatomy (Fig. 24.4) [25, 26]. CCTA provides volumetric evidence of reverse remodeling with successful atrial fibrillation ablation [27]. Successful ablation is associated

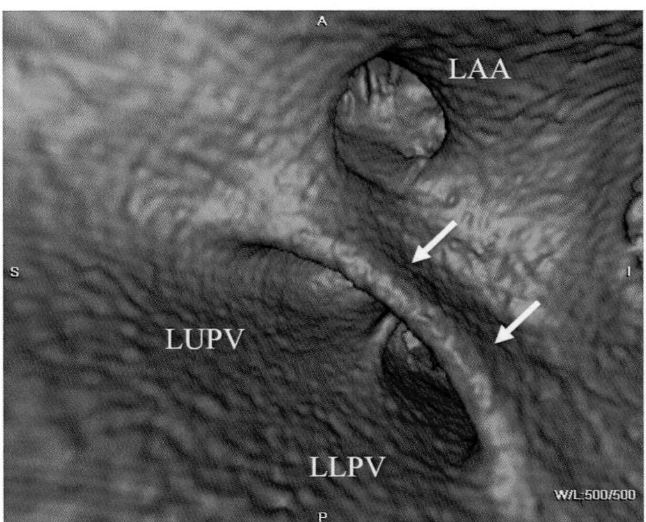

Fig. 24.4 Endovascular view showing a prominent ridge (*arrows*) between the left atrial appendage and left upper pulmonary vein. *LAA* left atrial appendage, *LUPV* left upper pulmonary vein, *LLPV* left lower pulmonary vein

with changes in atrial morphology with reversal of spherical remodeling [28]. In patients with paroxysmal atrial fibrillation, reverse remodeling with improvement of atrial transport function has been demonstrated by CCTA with successful ablation [29].

In addition to atrial size and function, the visualization of atrial fibrosis is important to assessment for atrial myopathy. CMR has been the primary imaging modality for this assessment through characterization of focal fibrosis with late gadolinium enhancement and diffuse fibrosis with T1 mapping. Challenges exist though as left atrial wall thickness is at the limit of the spatial resolution of CMR. Atrial fibrosis can be characterized by CMR delayed gadolinium enhancement [30]. The degree of left atrial fibrosis has been associated with sick sinus syndrome, history of stroke, and decreased atrial pump function [31–33]. The degree of preablation late gadolinium enhancement fibrosis has been associated with arrhythmia recurrence [34–36]. Post ablation left atria have increased scar density compared to preablation native fibrosis [37]. Delayed gadolinium enhancement can assess the adequacy of lesion sets associated with pulmonary vein isolation. Identification of gaps in lesion sets may be the substrate post ablation arrhythmias and therefore serve as targets for subsequent ablation therapy [38]. The completeness of pulmonary vein isolation as well as posterior and septal wall debulking lesions as assessed by CMR are markers of greater ablation success, particularly in the setting of higher pre- ablation scar burden [39, 40]. Patients diagnosed with "lone" atrial fibrillation have evidence of atrial fibrosis on CMR and procedural outcome of atrial fibrillation ablation for "lone" atrial fibrillation demonstrated similar ablation results to those with comorbidities, with the degree of fibrosis being the determining factor of success [41]. Post contrast T1 assessment of diffuse fibrosis correlates with decreased tissue voltage, and presence of atrial fibrillation. It also predicts success of ablation [42]. CCTA first pass attenuation can identify areas of atrial low voltage areas, but requires further investigation [43].

Left Atrial Anatomy Relevant to Atrial Fibrillation Ablation

Pulmonary venous anatomy demonstrates great variability regarding vein number, location, size, shape, and ostial complexity. CCTA can visualize these pulmonary vein characteristics and can define the relationship between veins as well as between the left upper pulmonary vein and left atrial appendage (Figs. 24.5, 24.6, and 24.7, Video 1). Workstation software can be used to quantify characteristics of the pulmonary vein ostia, including area, maximum diameter, minimum diameter, and eccentricity. Key to these measurements is identification of the left atrial/pulmonary vein interface, determination of the long axis of the vein at the ostium, and recognition that the vein ostium is often an ovoid rather than circular shape (Fig. 24.8). Three-D reconstructions can serve as a roadmaps for ablation as well as templates for post ablation changes [44, 45]. In relation to other modalities, CCTA and CMR offer similar ability to assess pulmonary vein morphology [46]. CCTA in comparison to invasive venography, intracardiac echo, and transesophageal echo performed during the procedure was superior to all of these other modalities in identifying veins. CCTA and intracardiac echo provided comparable assessment of pulmonary vein diameter, while diameters were larger based on venography and smaller based on transesophageal echo [47, 48].

Pulmonary vein stenosis is a potential complication of atrial fibrillation ablation [49, 50]. The reported incidence is dependent on imaging technique, definition of a significant stenosis, and degree of surveillance [51]. As techniques have evolved with recognition of the need to ablate in the atrium outside of the pulmonary veins, the incidence of pulmonary vein stenosis has significantly decreased. Stenosis can occur when ablation lesions are applied directly to the pulmonary veins [52]. Imaging technologies which can visualize the atrial/pulmonary vein interface are therefore important to ablation lesion application within the atria rather than the pulmonary veins. CCTA integration with catheter-based mapping has also been shown to decrease the incidence of pulmonary vein stenosis [53]. As pulmonary vein stenosis can preexist ablation due to either extrinsic compression by other thoracic structures or due to a congenital etiology, the preprocedure study serves as a

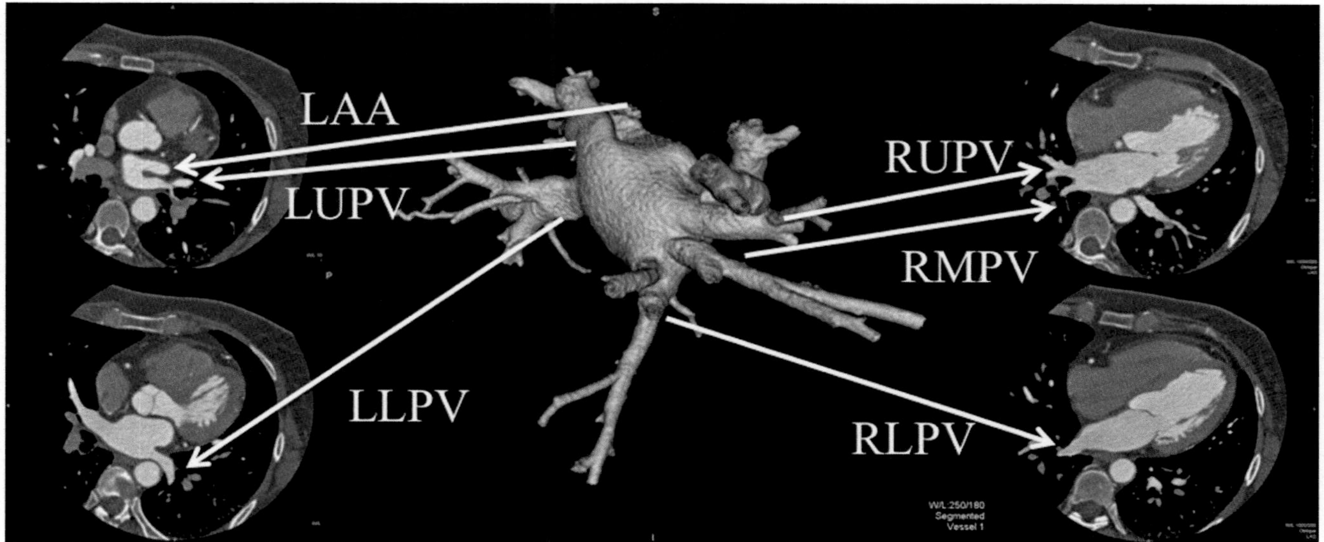

Fig. 24.5 Characterization of the left atrium and pulmonary veins demonstrated through 2-D axial views and 3-D volumetric reconstruction, demonstrating 2 left-sided pulmonary veins and variant anatomy with 3-right sided pulmonary veins. *LAA* left atrial appendage, *LUPV* left upper pulmonary vein, *LLPV* left lower pulmonary vein, *RUPV* right upper pulmonary vein, *RMPV* right middle pulmonary vein, and *RLPV* right lower pulmonary vein

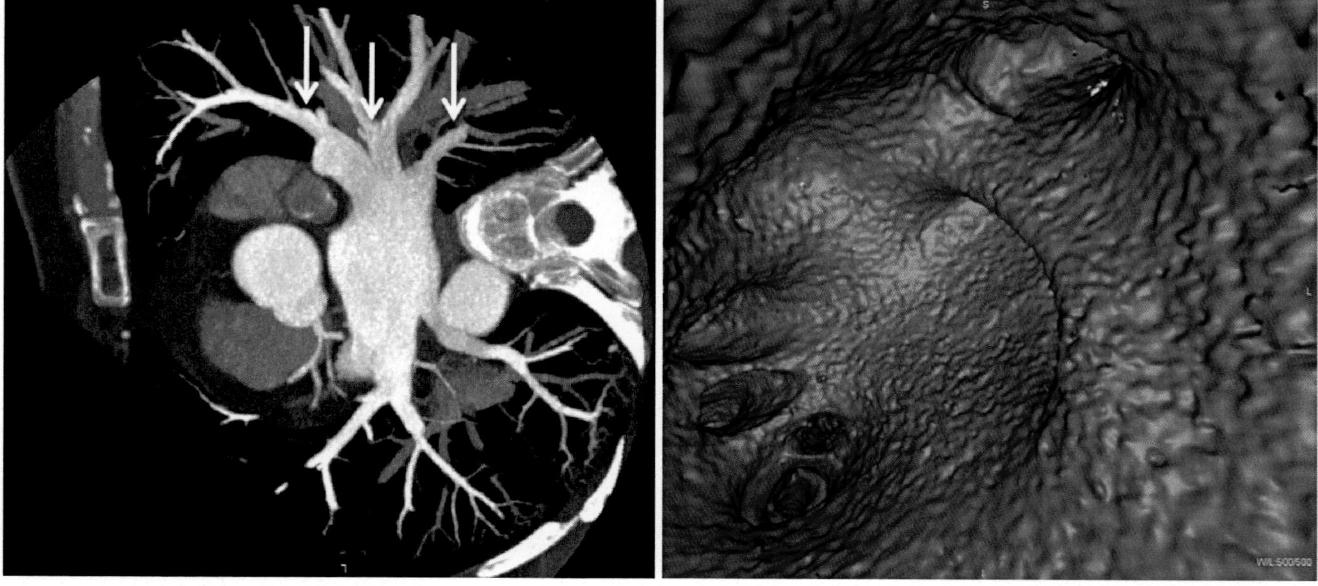

Fig. 24.6 Characterization of the left atrium and pulmonary veins demonstrated through double oblique thick MIP (*left panel*), and a 3-D endocardial view demonstrating 3-right sided pulmonary veins (*right panel*)

template appropriate interpretation of pulmonary vein findings post ablation [54]. Although CCTA is superior for pulmonary vein identification, transesophageal echo can be a complementary modality for assessment of the pathophysiologic significance of stenosis [52]. The incidence of pulmonary vein stenosis is decreasing, but establishment of screening algorithms and guidelines to assess the true current incidence and time course of the development of pulmonary vein stenosis after atrial fibrillation ablation is necessary [55]. CCTA is useful for the recognition of the anatomic degree of pulmonary vein stenosis (Fig. 24.9) [56]. In scenarios with moderate stenosis, the functional significance of the pulmonary vein stenosis can be assessed by transesophageal echo and lung perfusion via assessment with V/Q scan [57]. CCTA integration with fluoroscopy can also facilitate procedural performance of pulmonary vein stenting [58]. The patency of pulmonary vein stents can also be visualized with CCTA (Fig. 24.10).

Atrial anatomy other than the pulmonary veins important to facilitation of atrial fibrillation ablation can be defined by CCTA. Atrial septal characteristics important to transseptal puncture include definition of the location and size of the fossa ovalis, presence of a patent foramen ovale, and presence and degree of lipomatous hypertrophy of the atrial septum (Fig. 24.11). Atrial masses and thrombi can be identified, which could contraindicate transseptal catheterization. CCTA can display the location of and wall thickness of left atrial diverticulae (Fig. 24.12, Video 2). CCTA has shown these structures to have thinner walls than atrial myocardium with frequent location near pulmonary veins and atrial appendage ostia [59]. Atrial diverticulae could potentially complicate catheter placement and manipulation if they are mistaken for the orifices of pulmonary veins. Definition of anatomy of the mitral isthmus is important as ablation lines are sometimes applied to this region. The 3-D relationship of the circumflex coronary artery, coronary sinus/great cardiac vein in relation to the left atrium and mitral annulus can be defined by CCTA [60]. Given these anatomic relationships, there is the potential for coronary artery damage with the application of ablation lesions in this area, potentially leading to myocardial infarction with the need for emergent stenting. Additionally, sinus node dysfunction may occur as a left sinus node artery can course in this space [61]. Bachmann's bundle is an interatrial muscle band providing a pathway of preferential conduction between the atria. This bundle and its vascular supply can be visualized with CCTA and could potentially be in the path of a left atrial ablation roof line [62].

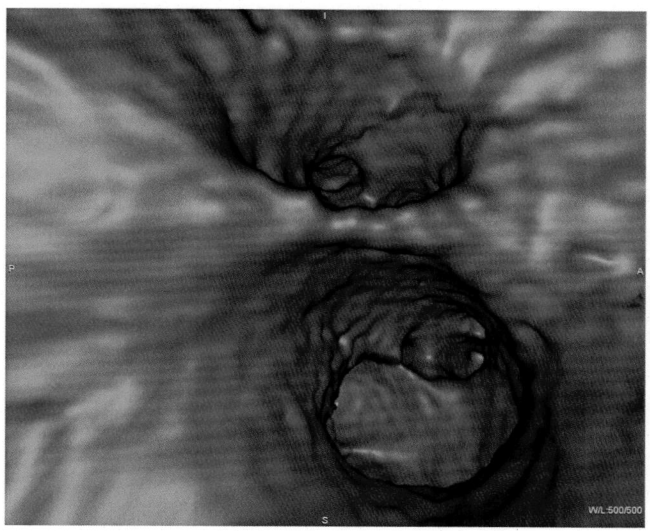

Fig. 24.7 Characterization of the relationship between and ostial characteristics of a right upper and right middle pulmonary vein on a 3-D endocardial view

Thoracic Anatomy Relevant to Atrial Fibrillation Ablation

Thoracic anatomy relevant to ablation includes the relationship of the esophagus and aorta to the posterior left atrium and pulmonary veins. Left atrial-esophageal fistula has been reported as a fatal complication of atrial fibrillation ablation [63]. The relationship between the thin wall of the posterior left atrium, pulmonary veins, esophagus and aorta can be visualized prior to ablation (Figs. 24.13 and 24.14). There is variability of the course of the esophagus and degree of contact between the posterior left atrium/pulmonary veins, esophagus and aorta [64, 65]. Barium swallow at the time of CT has been used to opacify the esophagus for electroanatomic image integration with ablation procedures [66]. Esophageal motility, change of the position of the esophagus with respiration, and patient position, can change the spatial relationship of the esophagus to the posterior left atrium from the CCTA to the procedure as well as during the ablation procedure [67, 68].Additionally a variable layer of a

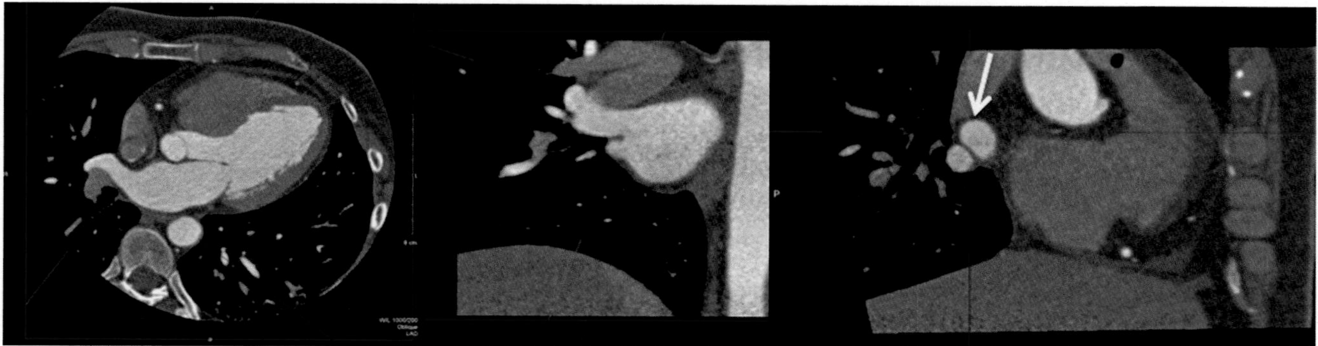

Fig. 24.8 Identification the left atrial/pulmonary vein interface, determination of the long axis of the vein at the os, and en face visualization of an ovoid pulmonary vein os.

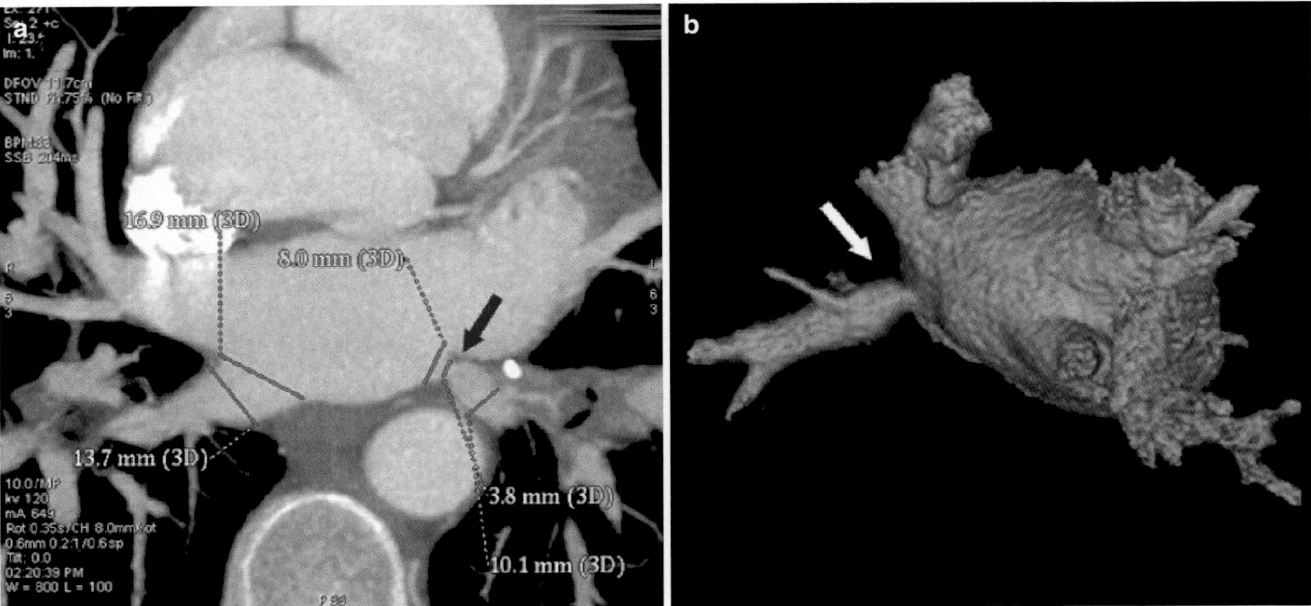

Fig. 24.9 2-D (**a**) and 3-D (**b**) volume rendered images demonstrating significant pulmonary vein stenosis (*arrow*) of a left lower pulmonary vein (Courtesy of Dr. Jeffrey Schussler, Baylor University Medical Center, Dallas, Texas)

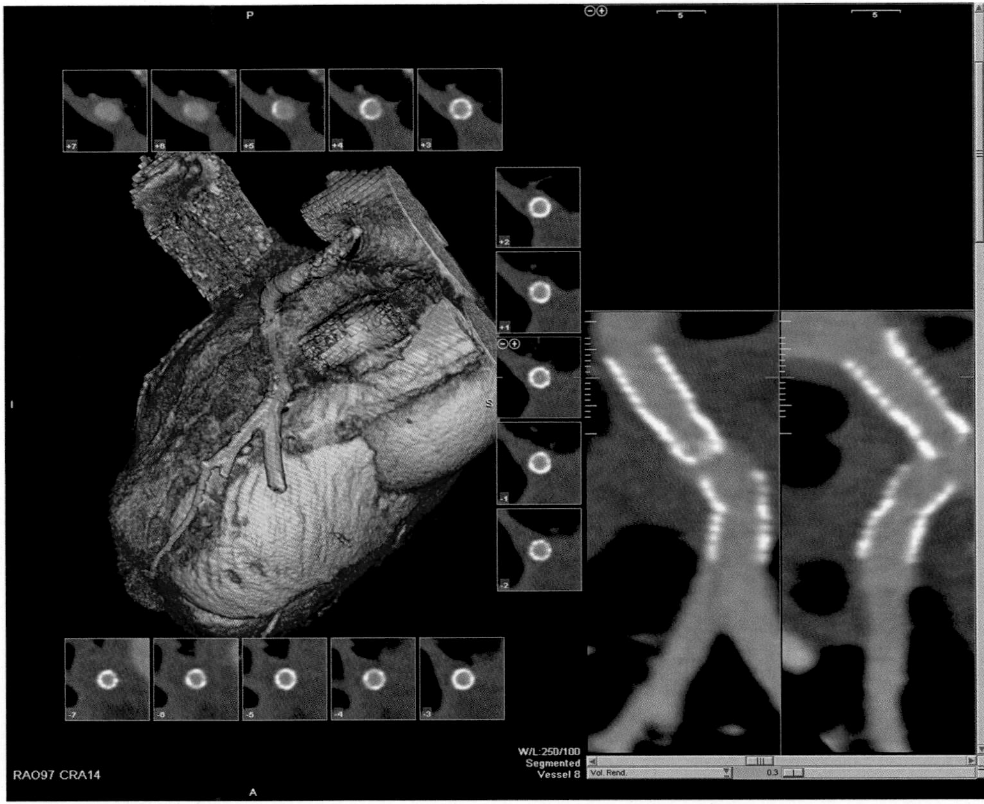

Fig. 24.10 Curved multiplanar views of pulmonary vein stents

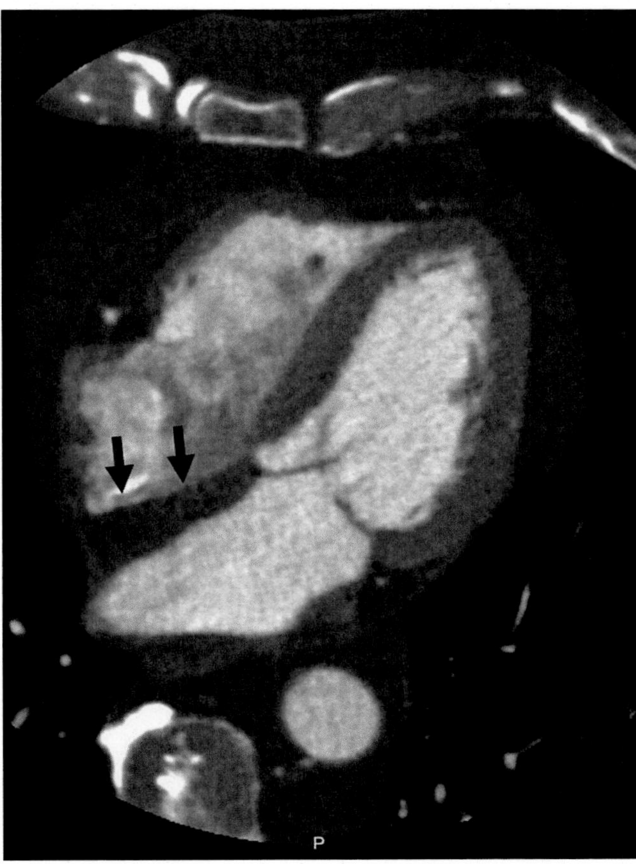

Fig. 24.11 3-D double oblique view demonstrating lipomatous hypertrophy of ther inter-atrail septum (*arrows*)

pericardial fat pad can be visualized around the pulmonary veins and posterior left atrium with CT which could conceivably provide some insulation to the esophagus with application of ablation lesions in the left atrium [64, 69]. CCTA identification of the coronary venous system is important for catheter placement, mapping, and for ablation lines [70]. The relationship between the upper pulmonary veins and the bronchi can be characterized by CCTA and is important to understand in order to avoid the rare but possible complication of atrio-bronchial fistula with ablation [71–73]. The phrenic nerve has been visualized with CCTA, which can be important to avoid diaphragmatic paralysis with atrial fibrillation ablation [74]. Epicardial adipose tissue can be quantified and has been associated with atrial fibrillation [75]. Incidental thoracic findings visualized on CCTA have also been demonstrated to influence decisions regarding proceeding with atrial fibrillation ablation [76].

CCTA Image Integration for Procedural Facilitation of Atrial Fibrillation Ablation

Electroanatomic mapping with CCTA image integration has revolutionized catheter–based therapies by allowing for electrical mapping and ablation to occur on a 3-D map of the patient's individual endocardial left atrial anatomy (Figs. 24.15, 24.16, 24.17, and 24.18, Videos 3, 4, 5, 6). The process involves importation of the unprocessed DICOM images into the electrophysiology mapping system, use of

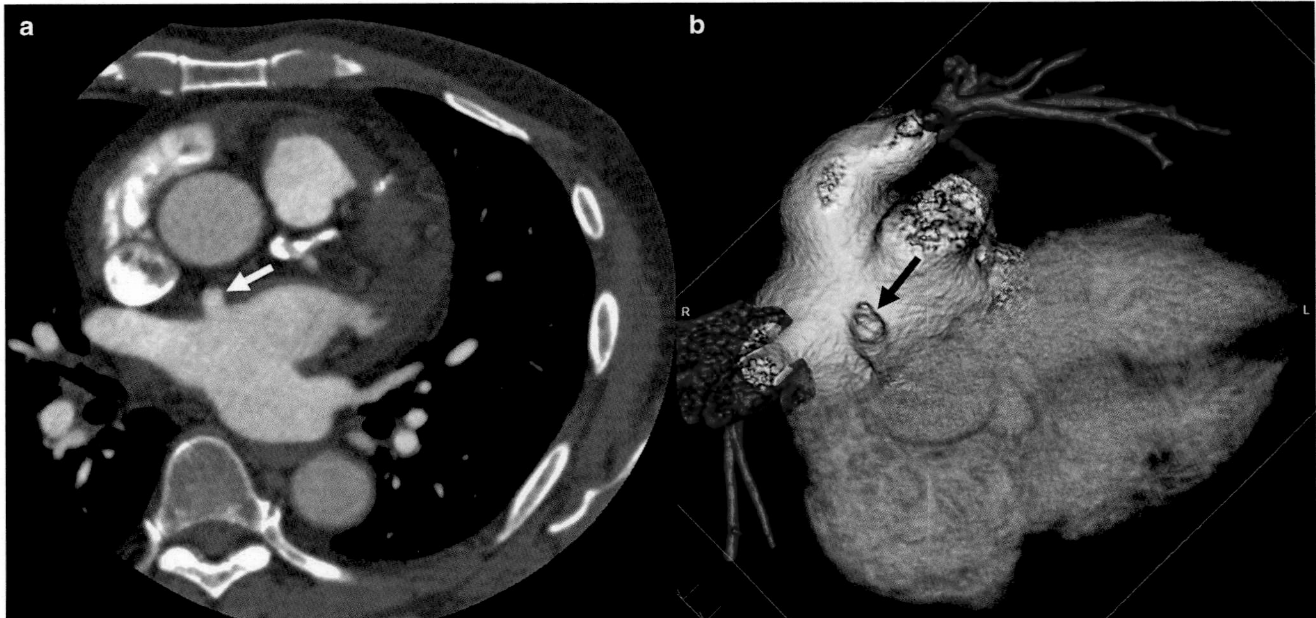

Fig. 24.12 2-D double oblique (**a**) and 3-D (**b**) views demonstrating an atrial diverticulum (*arrows*) located on the anterior superior portion of the left atrium

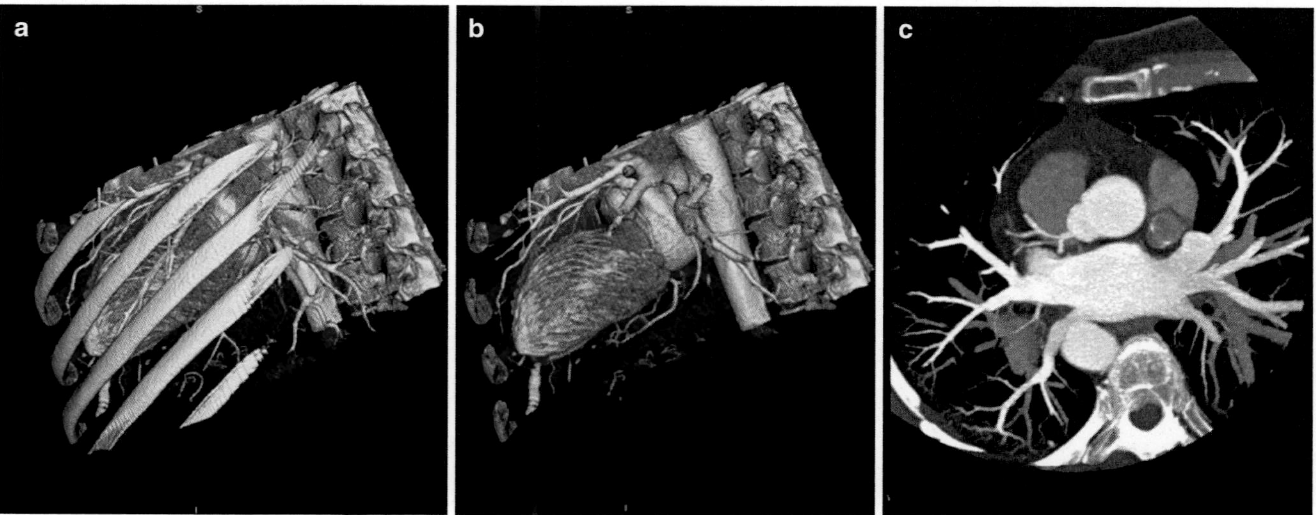

Fig. 24.13 3-D reconstructions (**a** and **b**) demonstrating the relationship of the aorta to the posterior left atrium and left lower pulmonary vein. A double oblique view (**c**) demonstrating the relationship of the esophagus and aorta to the posterior left atrium and pulmonary veins

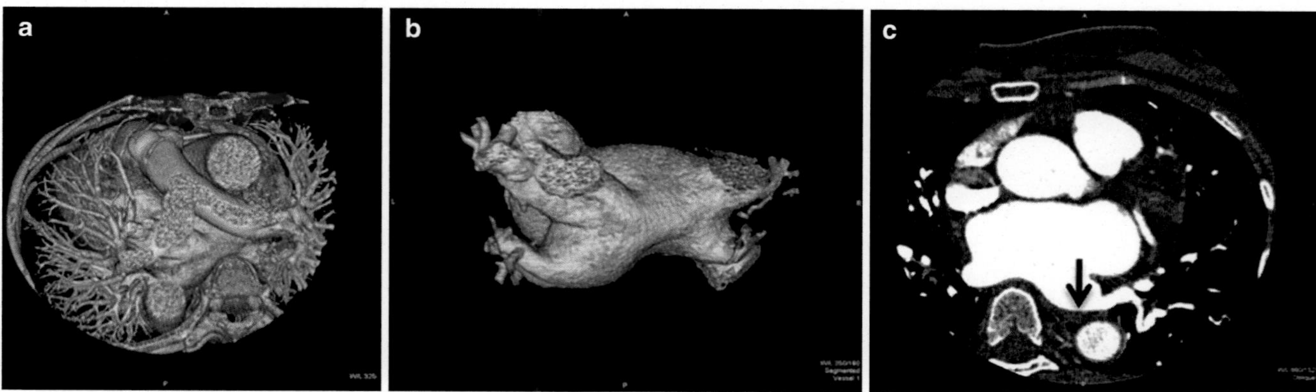

Fig. 24.14 3-D reconstructions (**a** and **b**) demonstrating the relationship of the aorta to the posterior left atrium and left lower pulmonary vein. A 2-D axial view (**c**) demonstrates the relationship of the esophagus and aorta to the posterior left atrium and pulmonary veins. In this case, the esophagus (*arrow*) is "sandwiched" between spine and aorta at the level of the left lower pulmonary vein.

edge detection software to delineate and edit down to relevant cardiac and vascular structures including the left atrium and in some electrophysiology laboratories the aorta and esophagus. Subsequently, a separate catheter-based anatomic map is created using fiduciary landmark points in the left atrium followed by registration of surface points defining the endocardial boundaries of the left atrium. The anatomic catheter-based map is then integrated with the CCTA images with assessment of markers of successful integration defined by an acceptable catheter to endocardium distances which have been demonstrated to be accurate [77, 78]. If registration is inadequate, catheter based points are edited and new points registered to ensure that the atrial endocardial surface has been adequately mapped. Atrial size is important to integration techniques as greater misregistration occurs with larger dimensions [79].

Electroanatomic mapping with image integration allows for arrhythmia activation and propagation, voltage maps, catheter position, and ablation lesion set location to be displayed on the 3-D CCTA reconstruction. Ablation guided by integration of pre-procedure CCTA with real time catheter-based electroanatomic maps can increase the efficacy of and decrease complications associated with atrial fibrillation ablation. This technique has been shown to be helpful in increasing restoration of sinus rhythm and decreasing recurrence of atrial fibrillation compared to electroanatomic mapping alone [53, 80]. Clinical outcome though is still dependent on achieving successful pulmonary vein isolation [81]. The localization of the ablation catheter tip on the endocardial left atrial reconstruction can help to ensure that radiofrequency

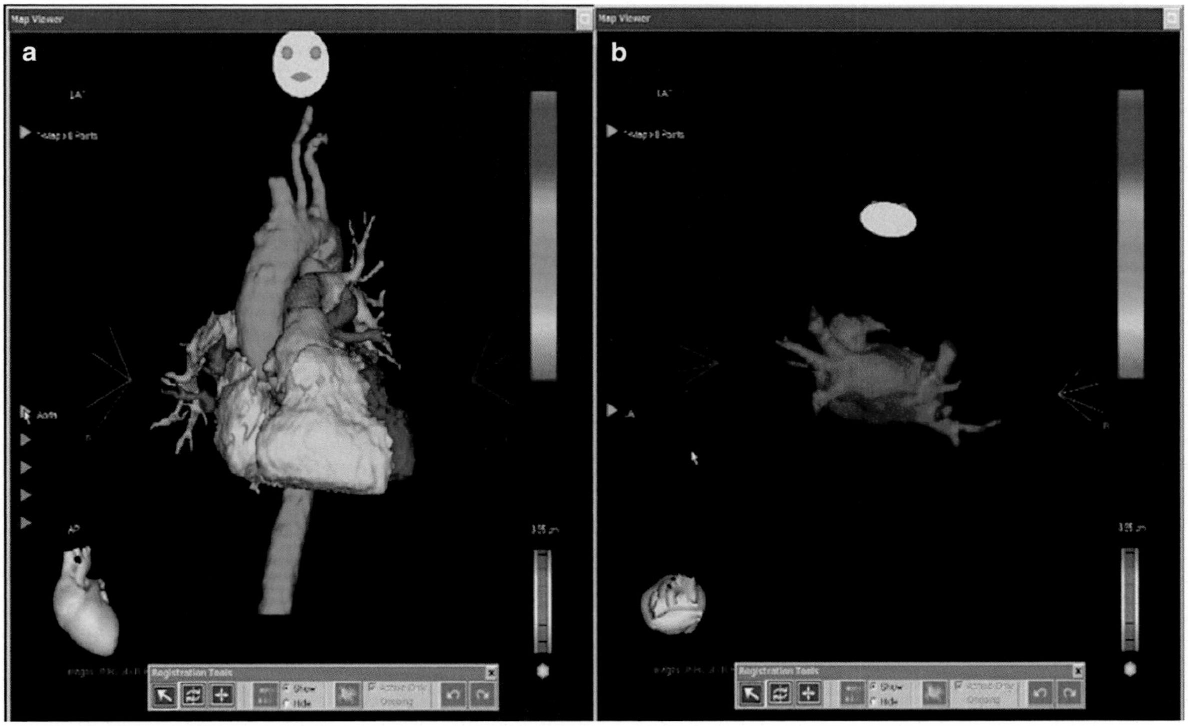

Fig. 24.15 Initial image processing for electroanatomic mapping with CCTA image integration showing segmentation of vascular structures (**a**) with the aorta (*green*), pulmonary arteries (*orange*), right atrium and right ventricle (*yellow*) edited out, with the left atrium (*purple*) subsequently rotated to demonstrate the posterior left atrium (**b**)

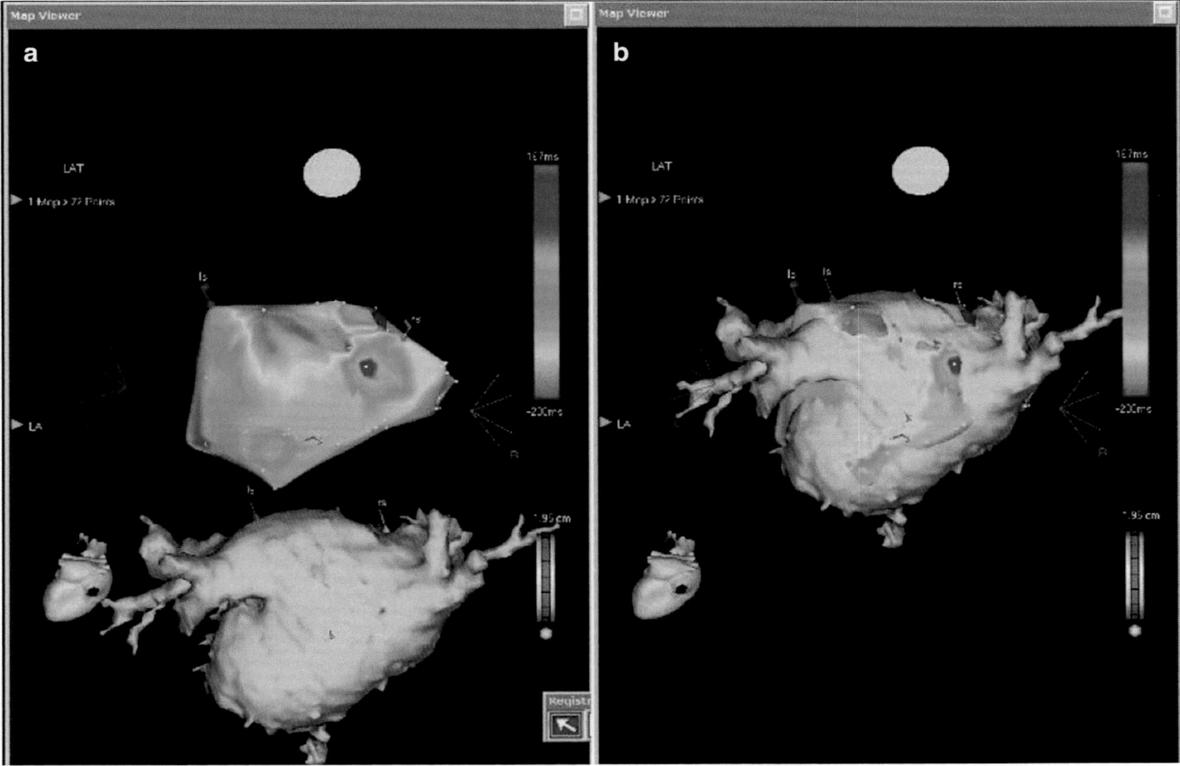

Fig. 24.16 Image processing for electroanatomic mapping with CCTA image integration with a catheter-based anatomic map of the left atrium (**a**, *upper image*) and the 3-D volume rendered CT image of the left atrium (**a**, *lower image*) with integration of these images (**b**)

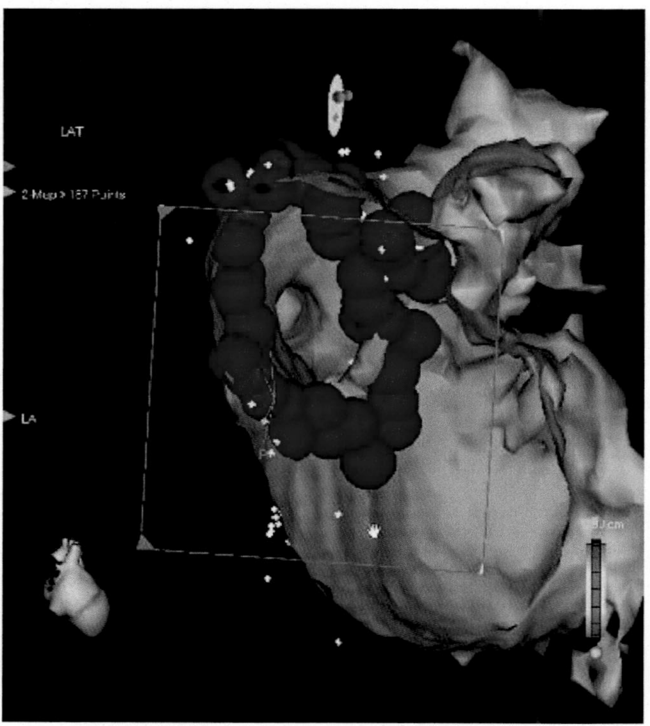

Fig. 24.17 Electroanatomic mapping with image integration demonstrating an endocardial view of the left upper pulmonary vein after radiofrequency catheter isolation of the vein with encircling radiofrequency energy applications (*red spheres*)

applications are placed in the atrium and not in the pulmonary veins or ostia to avoid pulmonary vein stenosis. Subsequent to ablation, mapping using this system can be performed to ensure electrical isolation of the pulmonary veins.

Placement of uninterrupted ablation lines around pulmonary veins and as long linear lesions within the atrium are important to the performance of atrial fibrillation ablation, as gaps within these lesion lines can lead to unsuccessful procedures. Gaps within ablation lines can also serve as a substrate for post-ablation atrial flutter reentry [82, 83]. Image integration allows for registration of the position of ablation lesions, therefore facilitating placement of lesion sets to create continuous lines.

CCTA or CMR image integration with catheter-based intracardiac maps can be additionally merged with intracardiac echocardiography, providing real time visualization of the esophagus, visualization of transseptal puncture, appendage thrombi, ablation catheter contact and lesion depth, pulmonary vein stenosis, and pericardial effusion (Figs. 24.19 and 24.20) [84–89]. Multimodal imaging with integration of CCTA images and real-time fluoroscopy is also being preliminarily investigated [90]. The integration of cone beam CT obtained at the time of ablation with electroanatomic mapping has also been performed [91].

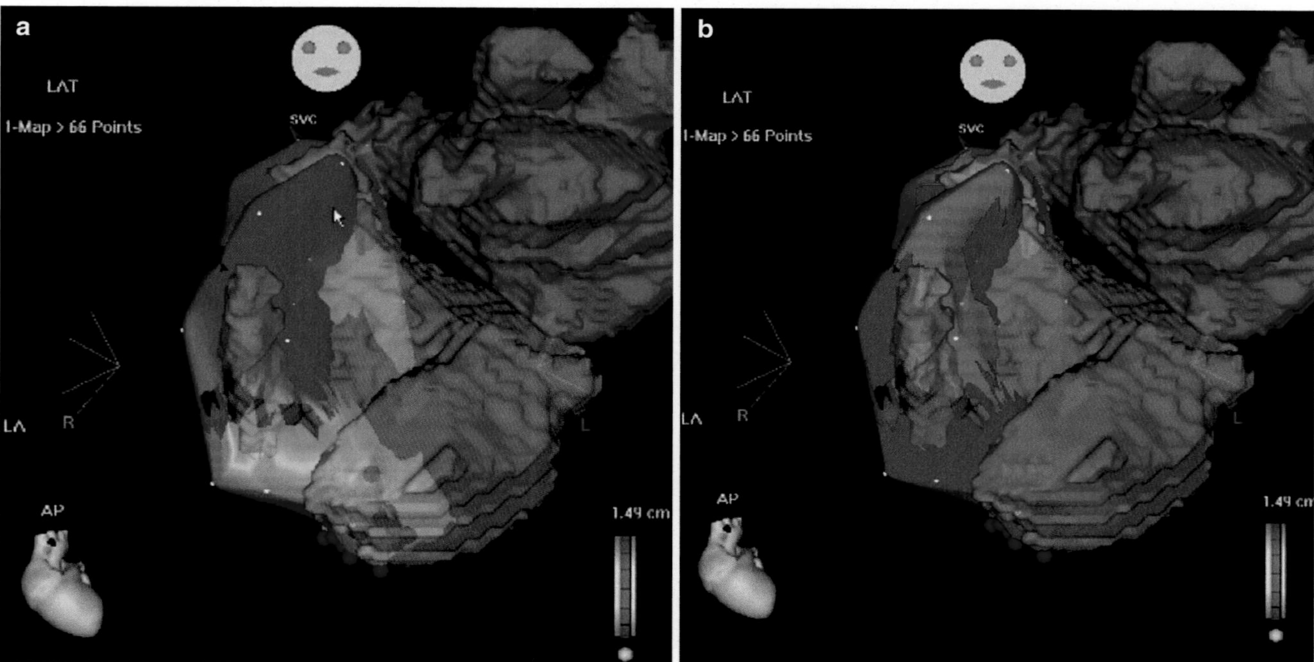

Fig. 24.18 Electroanatomic mapping with image integration demonstrating mapping of arrhythmia electrical activation (**a**) and arrhythmia wavefront propagation (**b**)

Atrial Appendage Thrombus Assessment

The recognition of atrial thrombi is extremely important prior to consideration of atrial fibrillation ablation. The left atrial appendage is a complicated potentially multi-lobed tube-like structure with an intricate array of pectinate muscles (Fig. 24.21). Contractile function of the appendage in the setting of atrial myopathy and atrial fibrillation is depressed with concomitant decreased flow velocity. These factors make it difficult to analyze for thrombi, as filling defects can be due to inadequate contrast filling of the appendage [92–94].

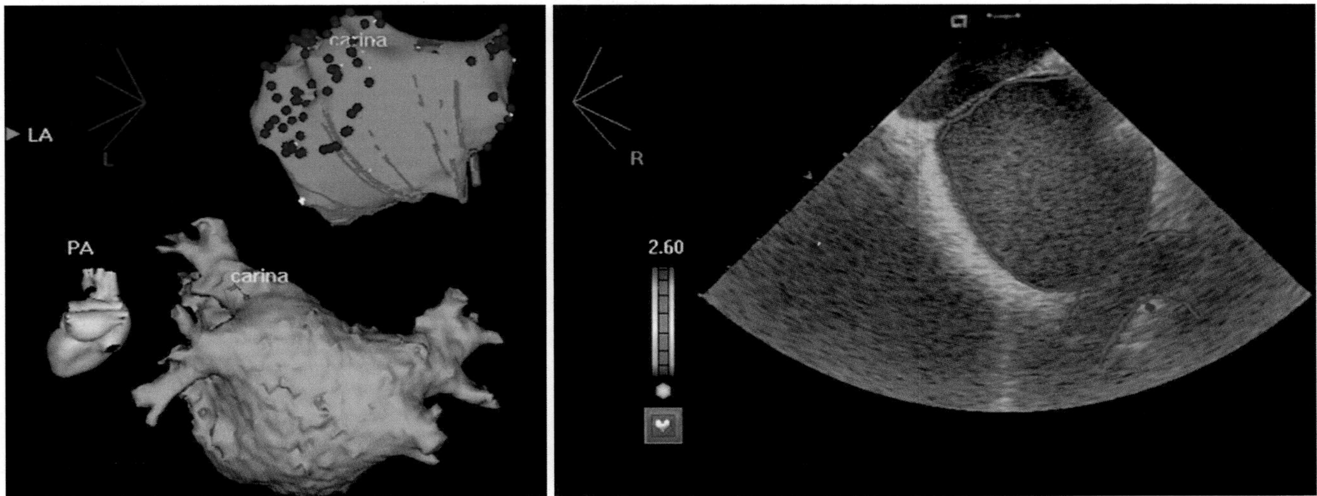

Fig. 24.19 Components of electroanatomic mapping with CCTA and intracardiac echo image integration, with a catheter-based anatomic map (*upper left image*), CCTA (*lower left image*), and intracardiac echo (*right image*)

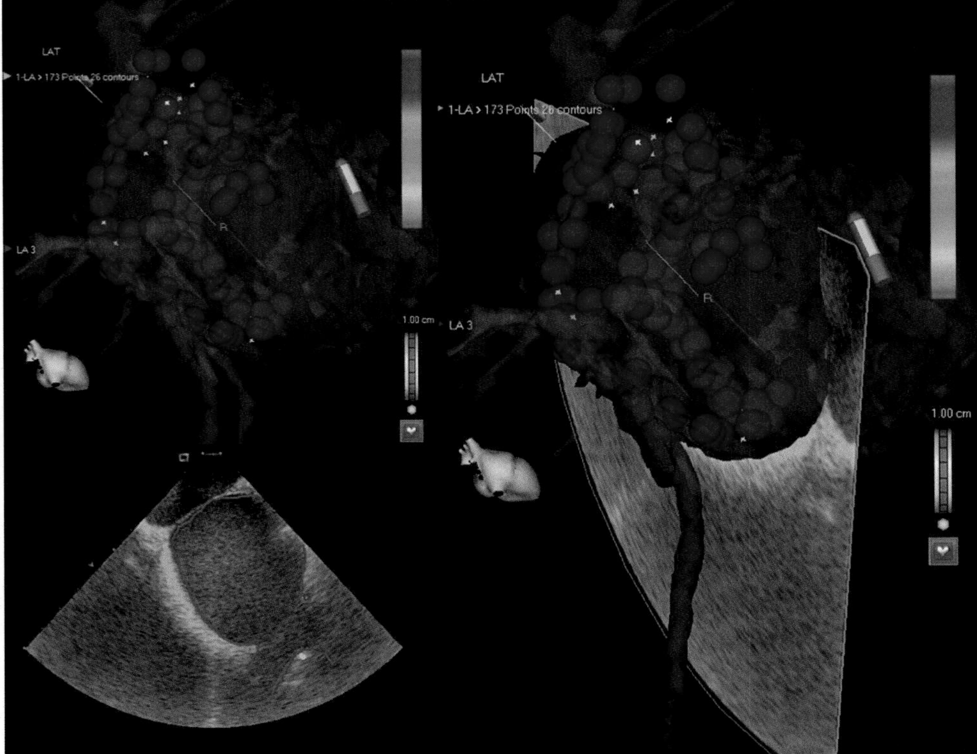

Fig. 24.20 Electroanatomic mapping with CCTA and intracardiac echo image integration demonstrating an endocardial view after radiofrequency catheter pulmonary vein isolation with encircling radiofrequency energy applications (*red spheres*)

Transesophageal echo is the gold standard for the assessment of left atrial appendage thrombi. In patients with pre-procedure non-gated CCTA prior to atrial fibrillation ablation, the sensitivity is high for ruling out thrombus, especially in lower risk patients (age <52 and CHADS2 score <1), but specificity, positive predictive value, and inter-observer consensus remains more limited (Fig. 24.22) [95–101]. The degree of pseudofilling defects correlate with the degree of left atrial emptying abnormality in patients with chronic atrial fibrillation as assessed by CCTA volumetric analysis [102]. Delayed CCTA images allow more time for left atrial appendage filling, improving detection of pseudofilling defects (Fig. 24.23) [103–105]. These images can be performed with a more restricted field of view to limit radiation exposure with delayed imaging. Imaging in the prone position may decrease false positive results [106]. The left atrial appendage/ascending aorta Hounsfield Unit ratio is inversely related to the degree of spontaneous echo contrast and presence of thrombi [107]. This ratio may be useful as there are limitations to the visual assessment of the left atrial appendage for thrombus [99]. Definition of the optimal left atrial appendage/ascending aorta Hounsfield Unit ratio is dependent on whether the ratio is

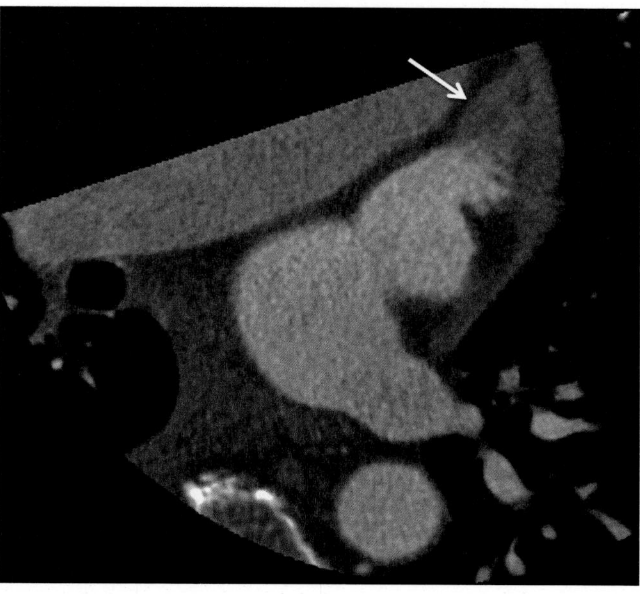

Fig. 24.22 Double oblique 2-D view demonstrating a filling defect (*arrow*) in the tip of the left atrial appendage with a differential diagnosis of incomplete filling of the appendage versus thrombus

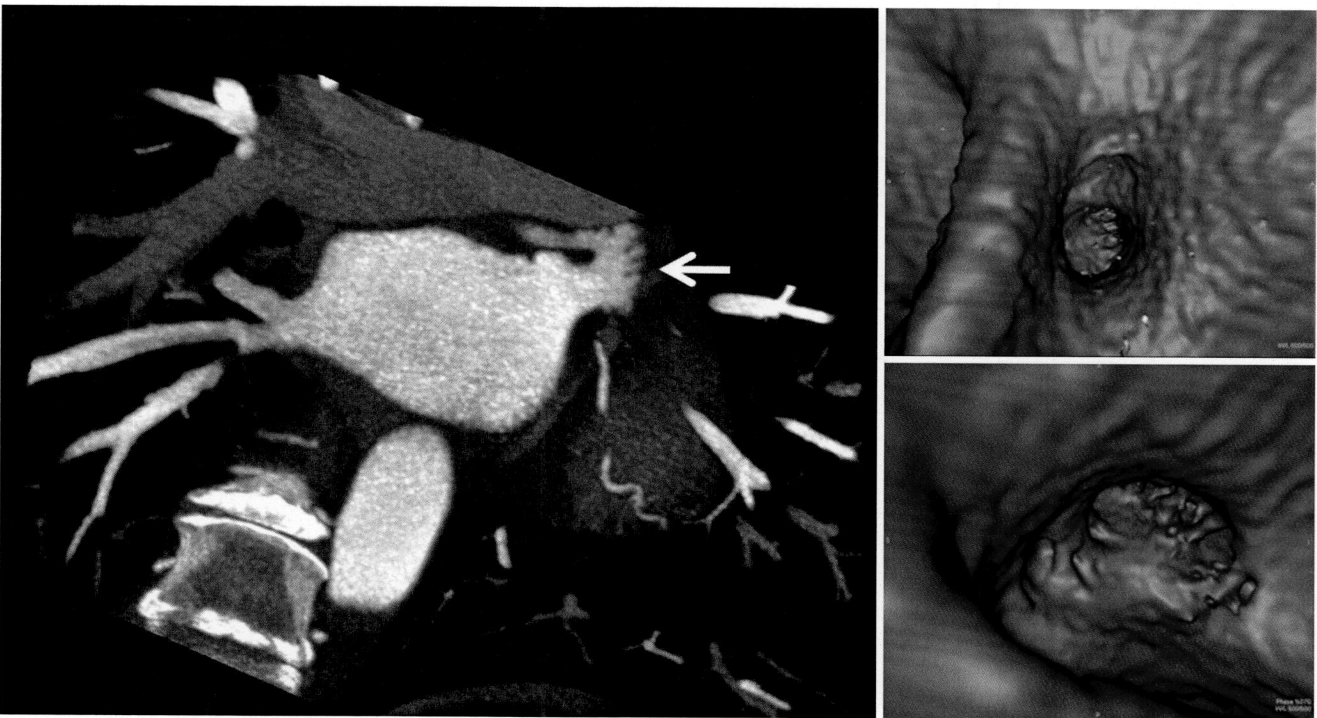

Fig. 24.21 Double oblique 2-D view (*left panel*) showing the complex anatomy of the left atrial appendage (*arrow*) with a multi-lobed tube-like structure with an intricate array of pectinate muscles. Endocardial views (*right panels*) show the shape of the left atrial appendage ostium and ridge separating it from the left upper pulmonary vein

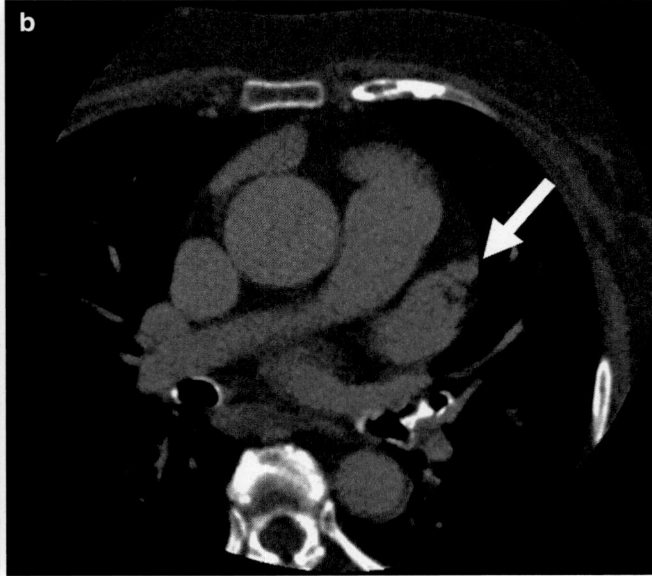

Fig. 24.23 2-D double oblique views of the left atrial appendage showing a filling defect (*arrow*) on first pass imaging (**a**) and complete opacification (*arrow*) of the appendage on a delayed image (**b**)

assessed during standard left atrial opacification or delayed images and whether the focus is on sensitivity and negative predictive values or specificity and positive predictive value. With these techniques the sensitivity and negative predictive value are excellent with some limitations to positive predictive value and specificity [99, 108–110].

Left Atrial Appendage Occlusion Devices for Stroke Prevention with Atrial Fibrillation/Atrial Flutter

Devices have been developed for left atrial appendage occlusion to decrease thromboembolic risk associated with atrial fibrillation and atrial flutter [111, 112]. Classification systems defining left atrial appendage morphology are evolving as multiple shapes and geometries exist [113]. These morphologies can be defined by the left atrial appendage ostial size, morphology and location, the length of the main body, the number, length, angulation and degree of trabeculation of lobes, and the relationship of the appendage to other structures (Figs. 24.24, 24.25, 24.26, 24.27, and 24.28, Videos 7, 8, 9, 10, 11, 12). CCTA defined left atrial appendage morphology has become important to decisions to whether to proceed with closure, the choice of closure approach, and the specific type of closure device [114, 115]. The methods for left atrial appendage occlusion include endovascular occlusion via a transseptal route, minimally invasive catheter-based epicardial occlusion, and minimally invasive or open surgical appendectomy. CCTA can provide virtual procedural images defining the path and possible obstacles to transseptal, subxiphoid transcatheter, minimally invasive surgical or open surgical approaches (Figs. 24.29 and 24.30). Stroke risk based on left atrial appendage morphology requires further study due to variability in results [116–122].

CCTA in Other Supraventricular Tachycardias

CCTA definition of atrial structures is important to the spectrum of supraventricular tachycardia ablation. CCTA has been used to define anatomic characteristics important to ablation of cavotricuspid isthmus dependent atrial flutter. Visualization of characteristics including steep angulation of a thick-walled cavotricuspid isthmus and prominence of the Eustachian ridge distinguished challenging cases and determined successful approach to this anatomy [123]. CCTA with image integration and electroanatomic mapping is useful for ablation of complex atrial tachycardia circuits [124].

For ablation of accessory pathways in Wolff-Parkinson-White syndrome, issues related to the coronary sinus/great cardiac vein have ramifications for mapping. The coronary sinus/great cardiac vein has a variable location in relation to the mitral annulus often coursing above the annulus rather

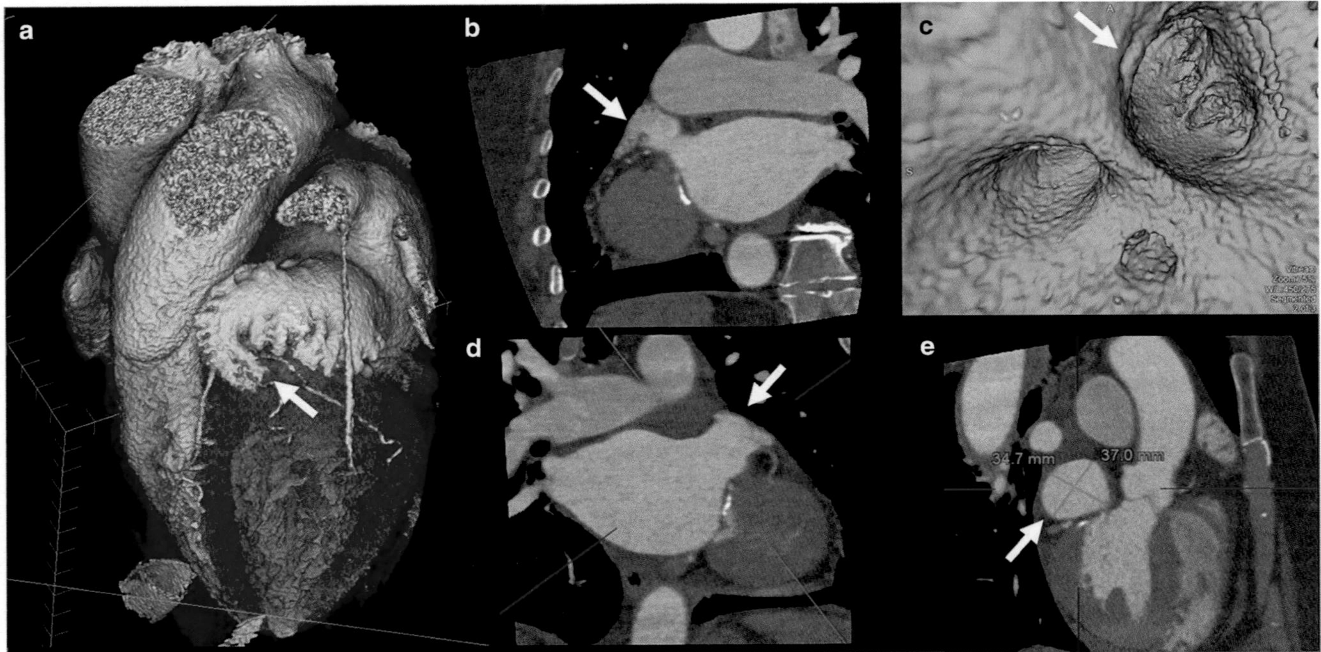

Fig. 24.24 Multimodal views demonstrating a "chicken-wing" morphology left atrial appendage (*arrows*) with a long main lobe which subsequently has an acute angulation. Views include: 3-D (**a**), 2-D double oblique (**b**), endovascular (**c**), and 2-D double oblique aligned along long axis (**d**) and short axis (**e**) of the appendage ostium

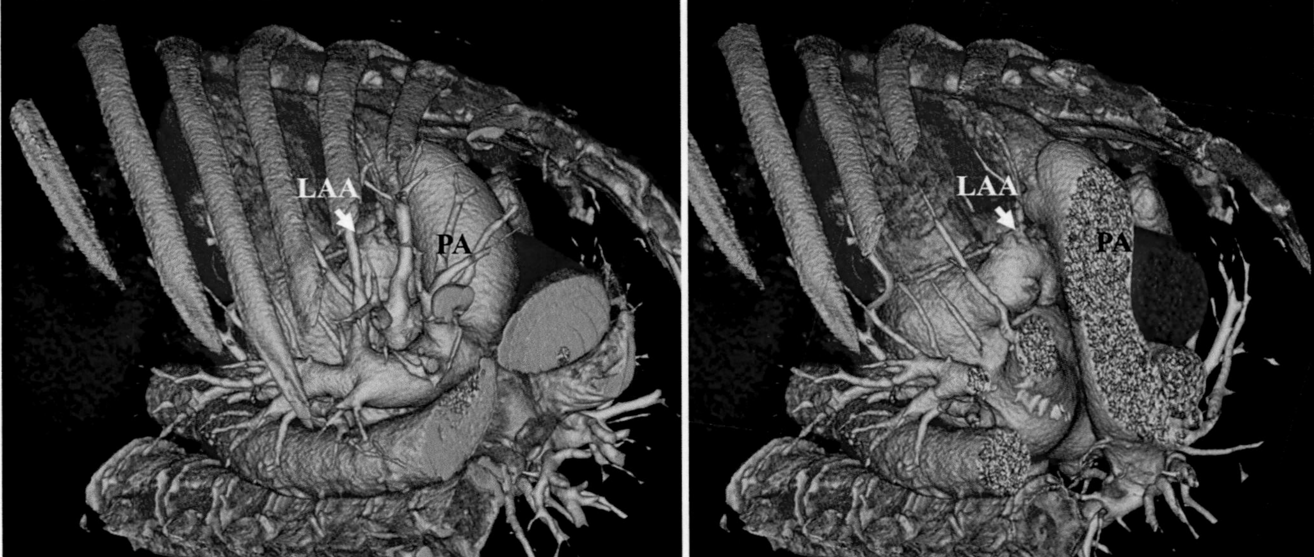

Fig. 24.25 Left lateral 3-D views demonstrating the relationship of a "chicken wing" morphology left atrial appendage to an aneurysmal pulmonary artery. *LAA* left atrial appendage, *PA* main pulmonary artery

than at the annular level. In these anatomic scenarios, coronary sinus catheters record the atrial insertion of an accessory pathway rather than providing a true annular signal [125]. CCTA can define the individual relationship between the coronary sinus/great cardiac vein and the annulus important to interpretation of coronary sinus lead electrograms. In regard to ablation in the coronary sinus, knowledge of the relationship of the coronary sinus to the circumflex coronary artery is important in order to avoid complications. CCTA can define areas of crossing and overlap between these structures (Fig. 24.31) [60, 126]. CCTA can also define anatomic findings important to catheter placement and mapping of certain accessory pathway substrates. The presence of a coronary sinus diverticulum or isolated unroofed coronary sinus can be visualized [127, 128].

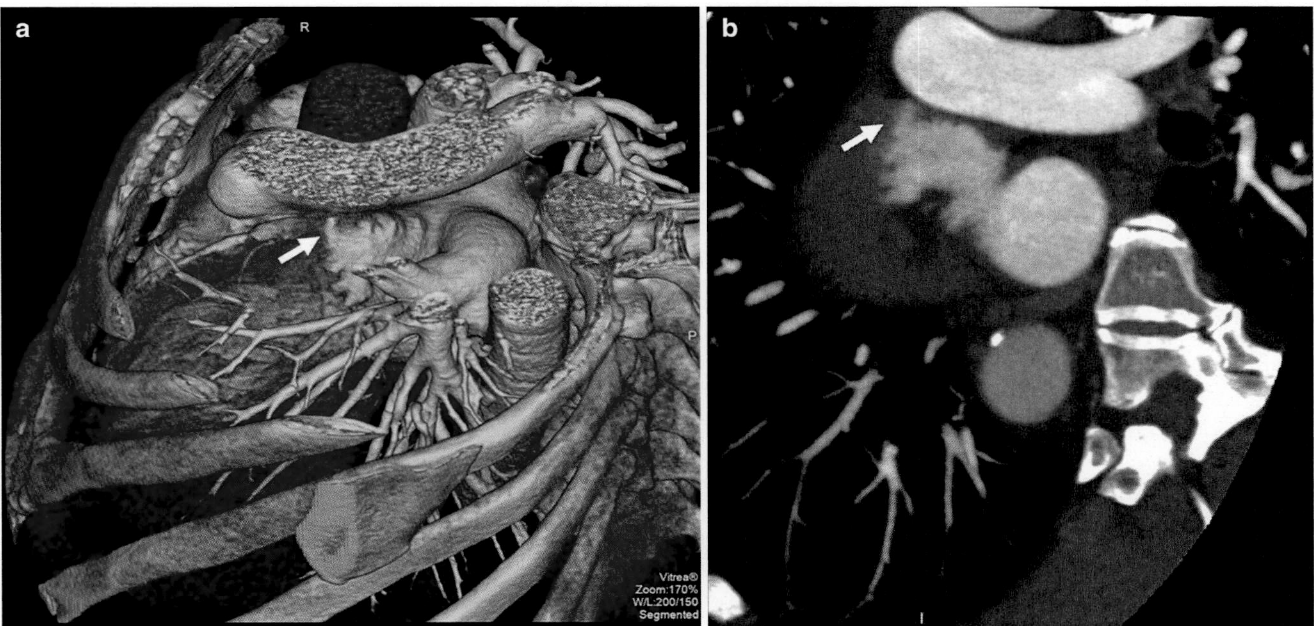

Fig. 24.26 3-D (**a**) and 2-D double oblique (**b**) views demonstrating the morphology of the left atrial appendage to be "cauliflower" shaped (*arrow*) with a single short lobe

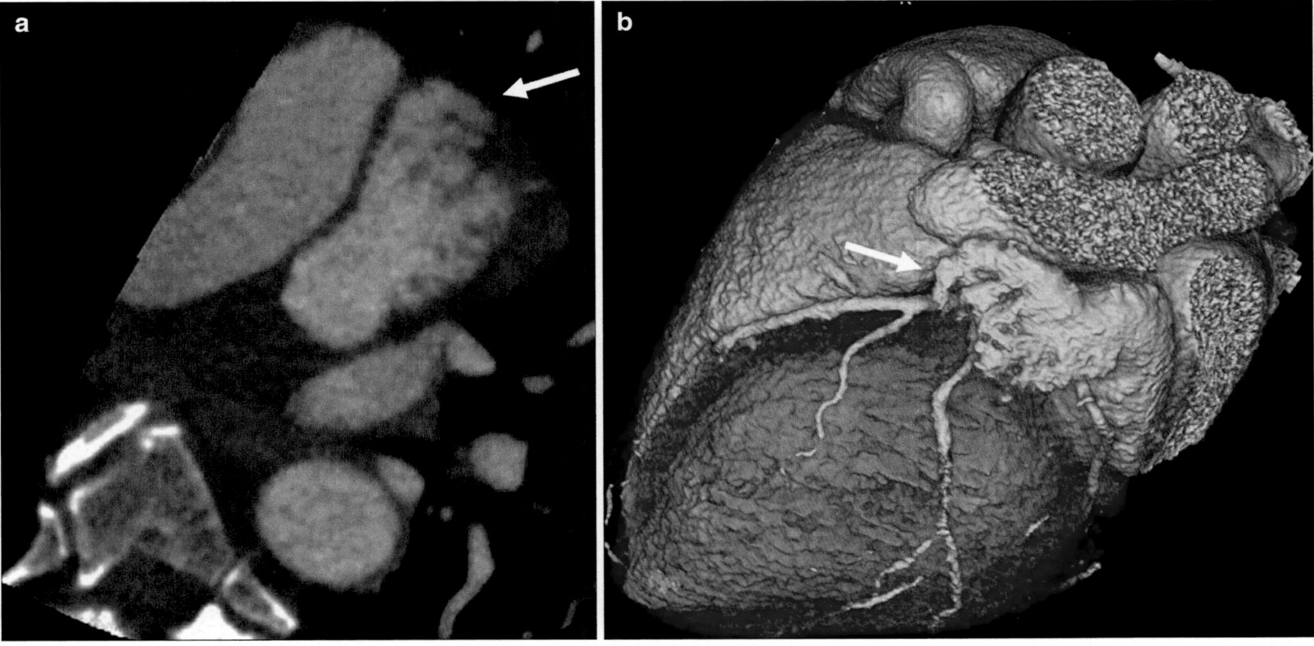

Fig. 24.27 3-D (**a**) and 2-D double oblique (**b**) views demonstrating the morphology of the left atrial appendage to be "cactus" shaped (*arrow*) with a long main lobe followed by several branching lobes

Assessment of Anatomic Substrates Associated with Ventricular Arrhythmias and Sudden Cardiac Death

Ventricular arrhythmias are associated with a spectrum of cardiovascular structural or primary electrophysiologic abnormalities, often with the first manifestation of disease being sudden death. Vascular and valvular anatomies associated with sudden cardiac death due to hemodynamic compromise or ventricular arrhythmias can be identified by CCTA, and include anomalous coronary arteries, severe coronary artery disease, critical aortic stenosis, and aortic

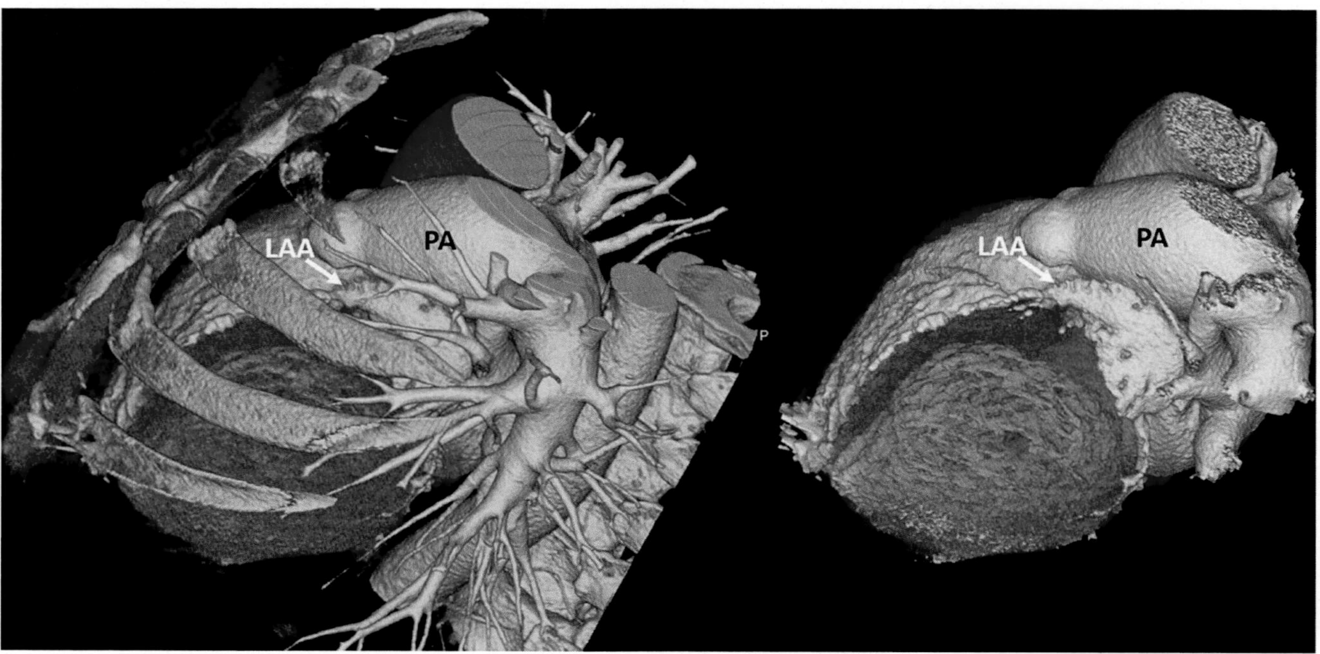

Fig. 24.28 Left lateral 3-D views demonstrating the anterior angulation of the left atrial appendage. *LAA* left atrial appendage, *PA* main pulmonary artery

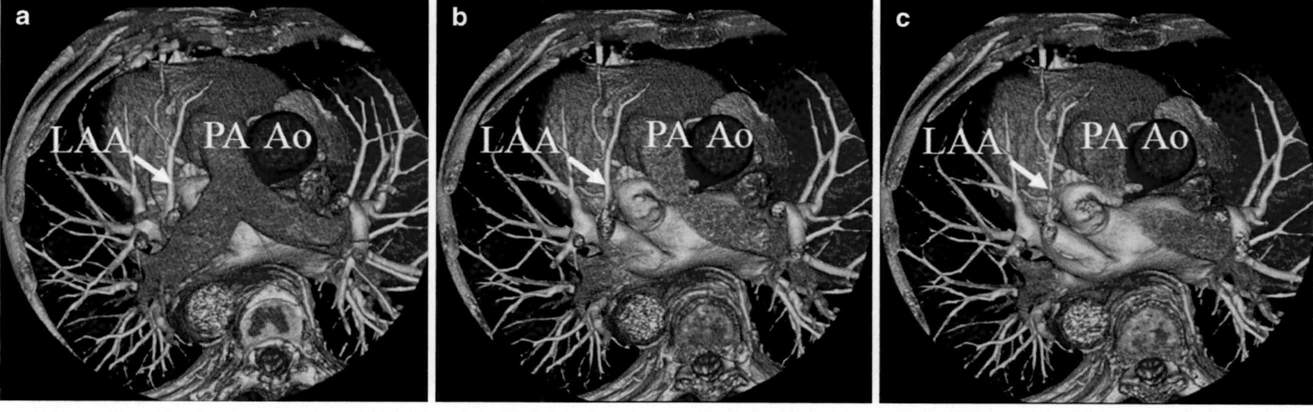

Fig. 24.29 Serial cranial to caudal 3-D axial views (**a–c**) demonstrating the anatomic relationship between a "chicken-wing" morphology left atrial appendage and the main pulmonary artery. *Ao* aorta, *LAA* left atrial appendage, *PA* main pulmonary artery

aneurysm and dissection. High risk anomalous coronary artery anatomies include coronary artery off of the contralateral sinus with an interarterial course and slit-like ostium, coronary artery origin from the pulmonary artery, and left main coronary atresia, all of which can be visualized by CCTA [129–132].

Cardiomyopathic substrates associated with sudden cardiac death due to hemodynamic compromise or ventricular arrhythmias can be identified by CCTA. Cine-CCTA can characterize cardiomyopathic substrates through reproducible volumetric measurement of ventricular volumes and ejection fraction, ventricular wall thickness, and ventricular regional wall motion. Direct visualization of the coronary arteries with CCTA may facilitate differentiation between ischemic and non-ischemic cardiomyopathy [133–135].

The visualization of myocardial fibrosis is important to the differential diagnosis and prognosis of cardiomyopathic states. CMR delayed gadolinium enhancement has played a primary role in fibrosis imaging. CMR delayed contrast enhancement has the ability to visualize myocardial infarct scar and its anatomic relationship to viable myocardium [136–139]. In ischemic cardiomyopathy, delayed contrast enhancement can be used to localize myocardial segments with scar, determine the morphology, transmurality and complexity of scar, and define the total percentage of myo-

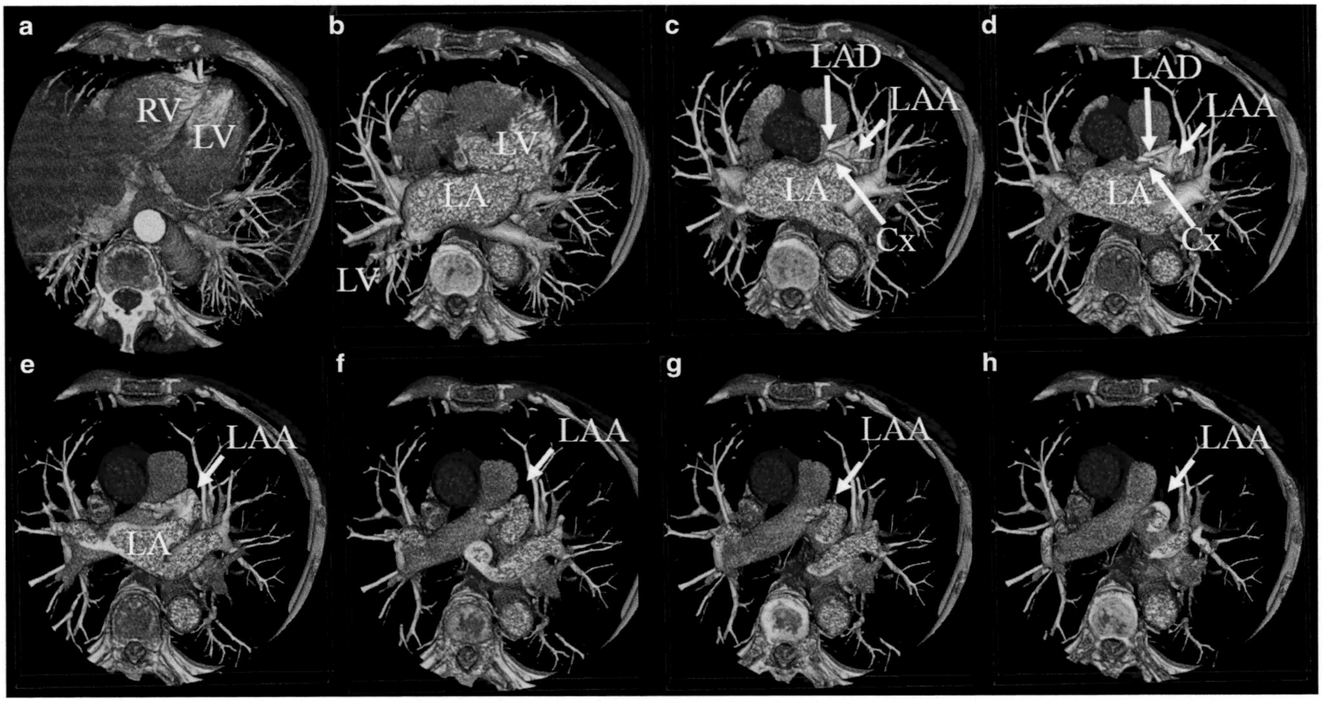

Fig. 24.30 Serial caudal to cranial (**a**–**h**) 3-D axial views demonstrating a virtual subxiphoid approach to a "chicken-wing" morphology left atrial appendage. *Cx* circumflex coronary artery, *LAD* left anterior descending coronary artery, *LA* left atrium, *LAA* left atrial appendage, *LV* left ventricle, and *RV* right ventricle

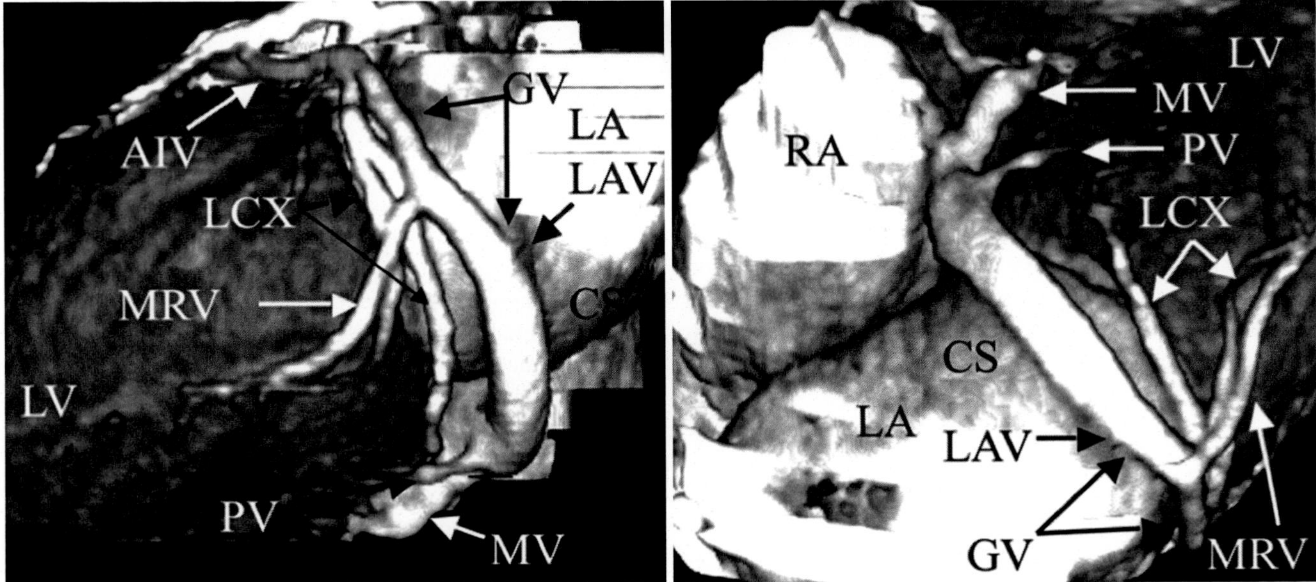

Fig. 24.31 The left-lateral view (*left panel*) and diaphragmatic view (*right panel*) of the heart. The left circumflex coronary artery and coronary veins are clearly displayed. The great cardiac vein is seen overlying the left circumflex coronary artery for a short (<30 mm) segment. The marginal vein is dominant, and the posterior vein is small in size. *AIV* anterior interventricular vein, *CS* coronary sinus, *GV* great cardiac vein, *LA* left atrium, *LAV* left atrial vein, *LCX* left circumflex coronary artery, *LV* left ventricle, *MV* middle cardiac vein, *MRV* marginal vein, *PV* posterior vein (Reprinted from Mao et al. [60] with permission from Elsevier)

cardium infarcted. The presence and degree of delayed contrast enhancement is associated with increased ventricular arrhythmias and worse prognosis in ischemic cardiomyopathy [140–142], nonischemic dilated cardiomyopathy [142–147], hypertrophic cardiomyopathy [148–154], and arrhythmogenic right ventricular cardiomyopathy [155, 156]. CMR derived 3-D location, transmurality, heterogeneity and complexity of the scar, presence of an anatomic isthmus, and relation of the fibrosis to the atrioventricular annuli can assist in the planning and performance of ventricular tachycardia ablation. These imaging factors can help to delineate whether an epicardial approach is required to reach a ventricular tachycardia circuit, whether ablation lines should be extended to an atrioventricular annulus, and where the location of a potential critical isthmus areas for ablation [157–162]. Integration of 3-D fibrosis reconstruction from late gadolinium enhancement CMR with electroanatomic catheter mapping in the EP laboratory can further facilitate ventricular tachycardia ablation [157].

The presence of a non-MR conditional implantable device continues to limit the application of CMR imaging. Additional limitation is related to quality of image acquisition in patients with devices. In settings where delayed gadolinium enhancement CMR has been utilized in patients with ICDs, artifact can potentially limit image quality, but techniques to minimize these artifacts are being investigated [14]. CCTA delayed contrast enhancement imaging is particularly useful in the assessment of patients with preexisting non-MR conditional cardiac devices. Delayed enhancement imaging with CCTA can image fibrosis associated with myocardial infarction [163–165]. Lipomatous metaplasia of areas of chronic myocardial infarction can be identified with CT [166]. CCTA delayed contrast enhancement can characterize dense areas of fibrosis in hypertrophic cardiomyopathy [167].

The diagnosis of arrhythmogenic right ventricular cardiomyopathy/dysplasia involves criteria including clinical and family history, electrophysiologic findings, and right ventricular structural, functional and tissue pathology abnormalities [168, 169]. Although CMR imaging has been the diagnostic imaging modality of choice, CCTA can also visualize the anatomic features associated with arrhythmogenic right ventricular cardiomyopathy/dysplasia, such as epicardial and myocardial fat, low-attenuation trabeculations, right ventricular free wall scalloping, right ventricular enlargement, and global and regional right ventricular wall motion abnormalities (Fig. 24.32) [170, 171]. Biventricular involvement in arrhythmogenic right ventricular cardiomyopathy/dysplasia by CCTA has also been seen [172].

Ventricular Tachycardia Ablation

CCTA can be useful in the planning and performance of ablation for ventricular tachycardia. CT can define areas of wall thinning which correlate with areas of low voltage and abnormal ventricular activity important to ventricular tachycardia circuits [173]. CT defined areas of lipomatous metaplasia in regions of chronic myocardial infarction can be defined and may have relevance to critical sites of ventricular tachycardia circuits [174]. The combined integration of CMR assessment of fibrosis and CCTA derived wall thinning and location of the coronary arteries with electroanatomic mapping is feasible and provides important features for ventricular tachycardia ablation [175]. Multiple techniques have been used to integrate CCTA images into modalities for mapping and ablation of ventricular tachycardia circuits. CCTA delayed contrast enhancement imaging of infarct scar has been used to facilitate epicardial ablation of a ventricular tachycardia circuit in the setting of an ICD [176]. Myocardial infarct scar related ventricular tachycardia circuits have been ablated in sinus rhythm, facilitated by integration of single-photon emission CT, CCTA, and electroanatomic mapping [177]. Facilitation of ventricular tachycardia ablation through fusion imaging of delayed enhancement CMR, CCTA and electroanatomic mapping for ablation of ventricular tachycardia has been performed [178]. CCTA has also demonstrated evidence of microvascular obstruction after radiofrequency ablation of ventricular tachycardia as evidenced by wall motion abnormalities, first pass hypoenhancement and delayed contrast hyperenhancement correlating with CMR [179].

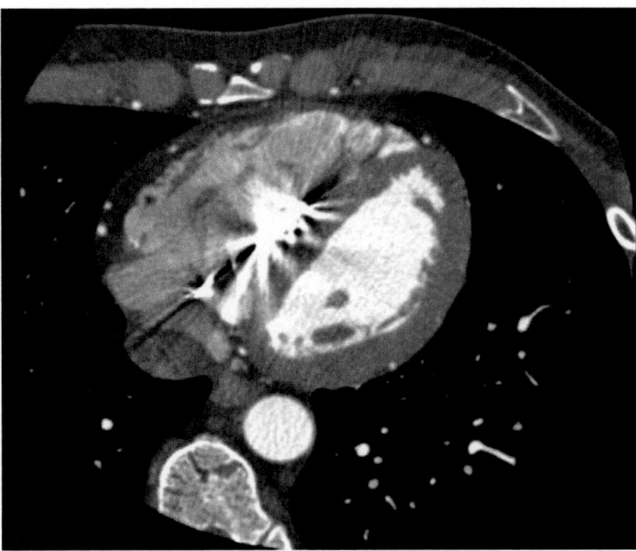

Fig. 24.32 CCTA axial view demonstrating fibrofatty replacement of right ventricular myocardium, low-attenuation trabeculations, and right ventricular free wall scalloping in arrhythmogenic right ventricular cardiomyopathy. A right ventricular defibrillation lead is present with beam hardening artifact.

For patients with congenital heart disease undergoing supraventricular and ventricular tachycardia ablation, CMR also characterizes important anatomy for procedural planning. Important findings on CMR include ventricular septal defects, ventricular thrombus, baffle pathways to the ventricles, and myocardial fibrosis. Pressure and volume overload from unrepaired and repaired congenital lesions as well as atrial and ventricular surgical incisions lead to fibrosis and therefore arrhythmia substrate [180–185]. Challenges of ventricular tachycardia ablation include mapping during ventricular arrhythmias with attendant risk of hemodynamic instability. Characterization of critical isthmuses based on advanced cardiac imaging are useful to ablation of ventricular tachycardia circuits while the patient is in sinus rhythm. Ventricular tachycardia incisional reentry isthmuses in operated congenital heart disease can be defined and ablated in sinus rhythm by spanning isthmuses between annuli and scar/patch [186]. The combination of remote magnetic navigation, 3-D image integration, and electroanatomic mapping has facilitated safe and feasible ablation in patients with complex congenital anomalies [187].

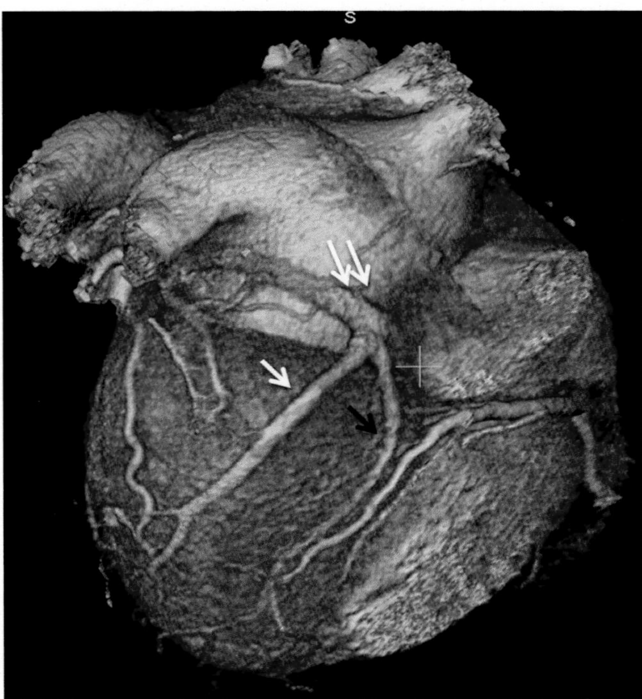

Fig. 24.33 3-D volume rendered image demonstrating visualization of the coronary venous system including the coronary sinus (*double white arrow*), a middle cardiac vein (*black arrow*), and a posterolateral vein (*single white arrow*)

CCTA for Device Therapies

CCTA can visualize the coronary venous system and may potentially play an important role in cardiac resynchronization therapy (CRT) [60, 188]. CRT is used to optimize cardiac function through resynchronization of ventricular contraction in patients with dilated ischemic and non-ischemic cardiomyopathy, ventricular conduction abnormalities, and moderate to severe heart failure. With CRT, a pacing lead is placed in a branch vessel of the coronary venous system to achieve left ventricular pacing. As opposed to the right atrial and right ventricular leads, which can be actively fixated in many positions in their respective chambers with relative ease, placement of the coronary venous lead can be challenging, as lead position is limited by the individual confines and variation of the existing coronary venous anatomy.

CCTA coronary venous imaging can provide roadmaps for lead placement, with potential avoidance of a percutaneous approach in the setting of inadequate anatomy. Detailed assessment of the coronary venous anatomy includes coronary sinus diameter, 3-D location of branch vessels relative to the left ventricle myocardial segments , branch vessel diameter and angulation off of the coronary sinus/great cardiac vein (Figs. 24.33 and 24.34, Videos 13 and 14) [60]. CCTA can also visualize structures which could complicate access to the coronary venous system, such as a prominent Thebesian valve covering the coronary sinus ostium (Fig. 24.35) [189]. Other abnormalities, such as coronary sinus diverticulae, left superior vena cava to coronary sinus connections, and unroofed coronary sinuses can also be identified (Figs. 24.36 and 24.37). Visualization of the phrenic nerve and its relation to the coronary venous anatomy may be important to lead placement in order to avoid diaphragmatic pacing (Fig. 24.38) [190]. CCTA is deemed appropriate for the assessment of coronary venous imaging for CRT [191–193].

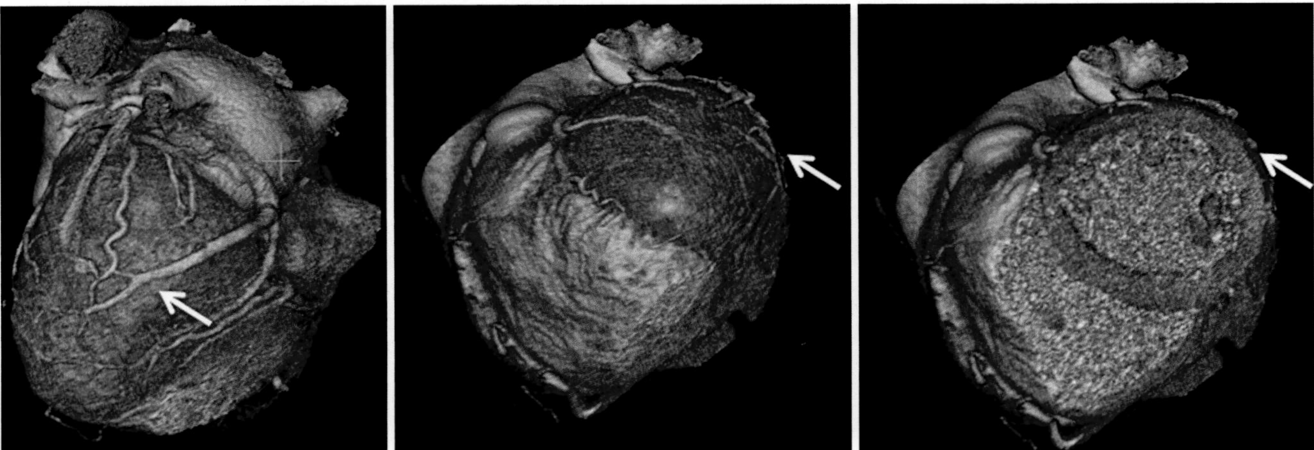

Fig. 24.34 CCTA 3-D views demonstrating localization of the myocardial segment associated with the distal portion of the posterolateral vein (*arrows*)

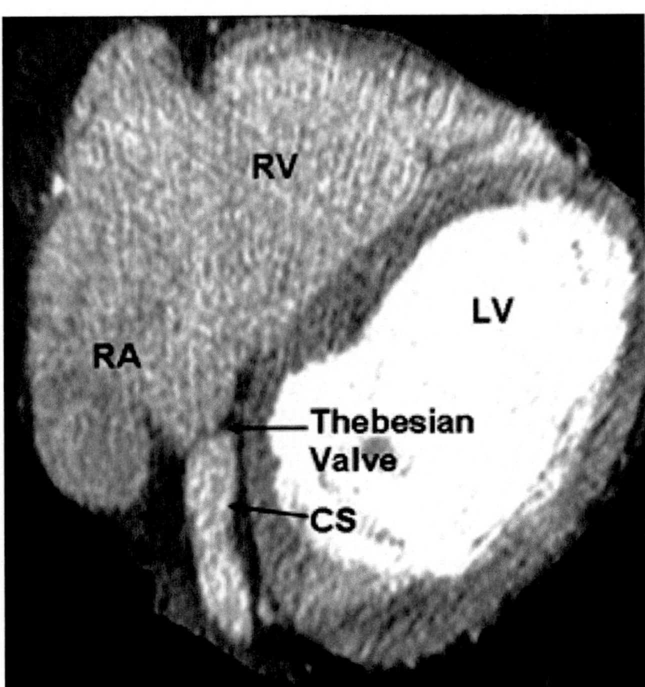

Fig. 24.35 Axial images at the coronary sinus os level demonstrating a prominent Thebesian valve. *CS* coronary sinus, *RA* right atrium, *RV* right ventricle, and *LV* left ventricle (Reprinted from Shinbane et al. [189] with permission from John Wiley and Sons)

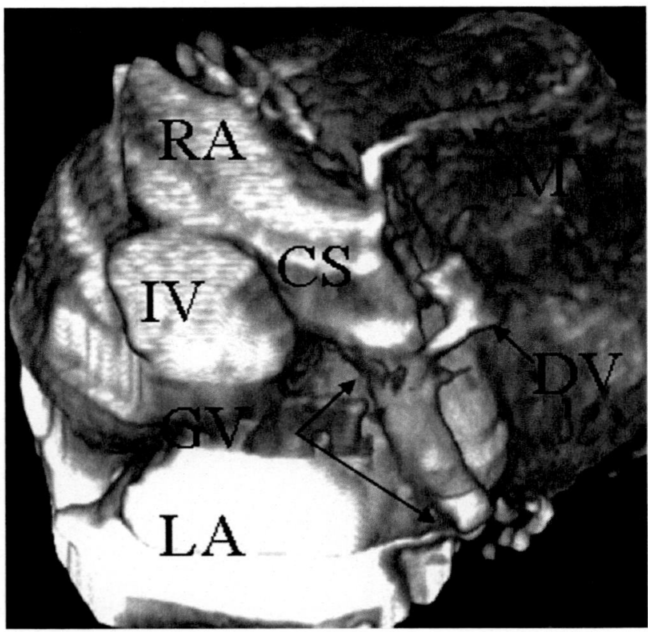

Fig. 24.36 CCTA demonstrating a coronary sinus diverticulum (*arrow*). *CS* coronary sinus, *DV* diverticulum, *GV* great cardiac vein, *IV* inferior vena cava, *LA* left atrium, *MV* marginal vein, and *RA* right atrium

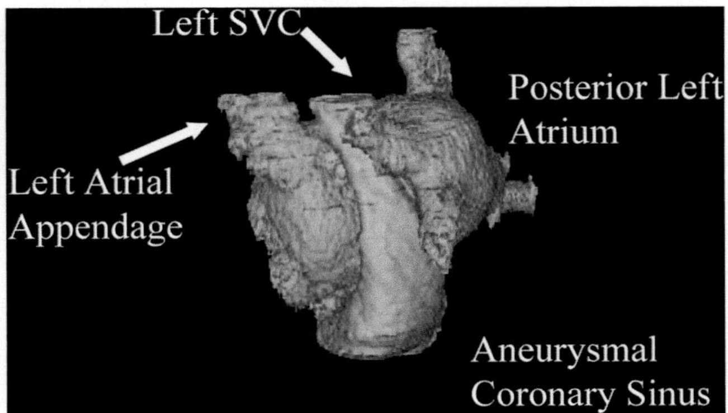

Fig. 24.37 3-D volume rendered view demonstrating a left superior vena cava with connection to an aneurysmal coronary sinus. A right-sided superior vena cava was not present

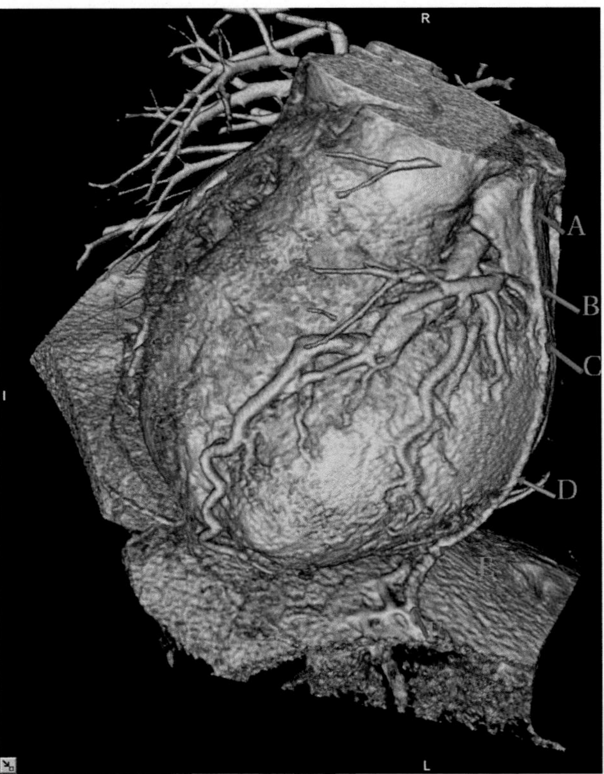

Fig. 24.38 3-D volume rendered image showing visualization of the course (*a–e*) of the left phrenic nerve (Reprinted from Matsumoto et al. [190] with permission from Elsevier)

Preliminary data suggest that pre-procedure knowledge of the 3-D coronary venous anatomy can facilitate procedures through decreased procedure time and utilization of guide catheters [194]. CCTA fusion with fluoroscopy has been performed preliminarily with accurate fusion of structures [195]. CCTA can be used to plan CRT approach when obstacles to standard approaches are identified. CCTA delineation of ostial abnormalities limiting access to the coronary sinus ostium have permitted procedural planning and facilitation of alternate approaches to endovascular access rather than proceeding to epicardial lead placement (Fig. 24.39) [196]. CCTA defined assessment of the location of the coronary

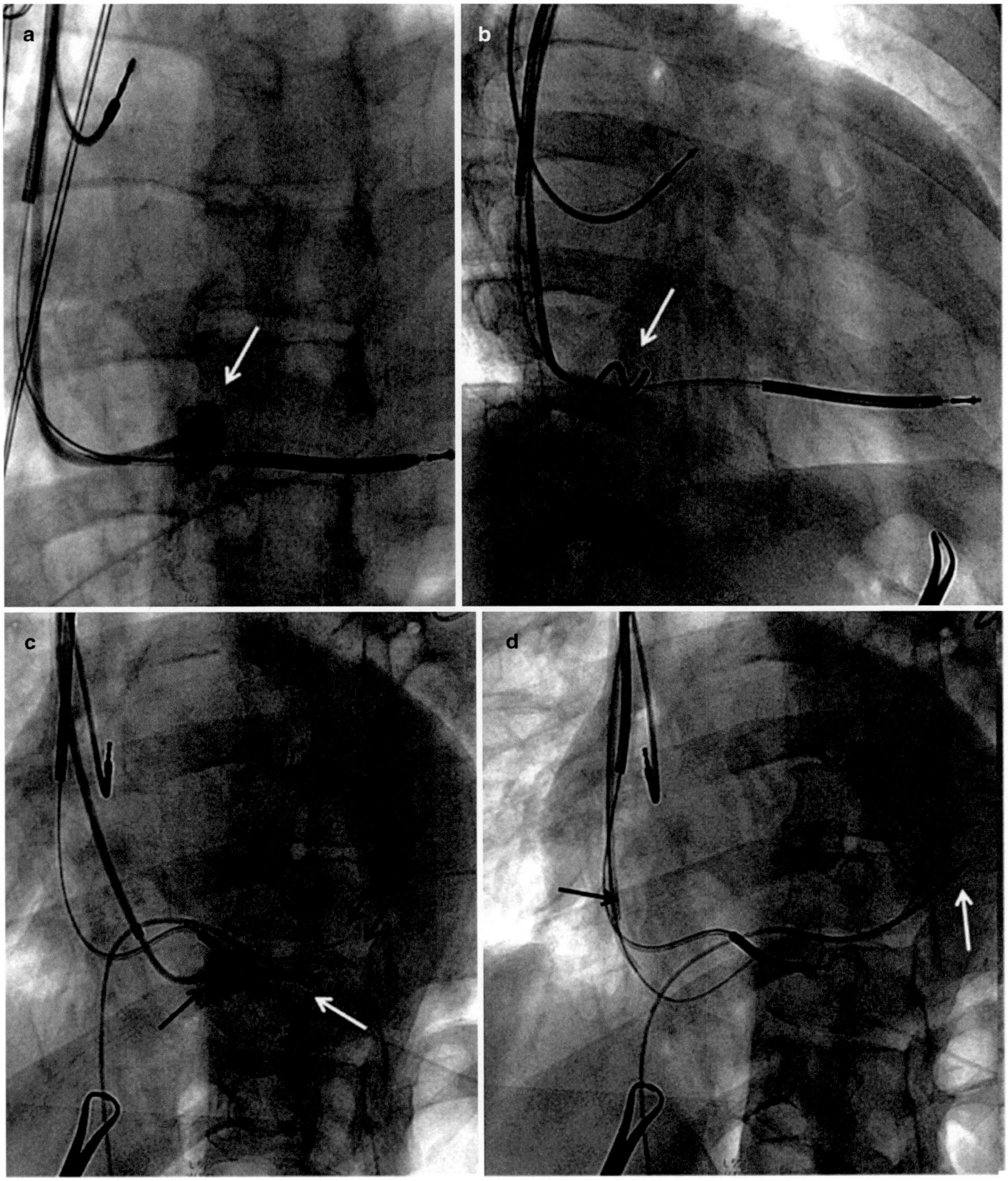

Fig. 24.39 Double cannulation approach to coronary venous lead placement in the setting of a prominent Thebesian valve. Panel (**a**): 2-D axial view (**a**) demonstrating a well-formed and prominent Thebesian valve (*black arrow*) covering the coronary sinus ostium. Serial intraprocedure fluoroscopy images showing the sequential stages of coronary sinus cannulation and coronary venous left ventricular lead placement. Panel (**b**): placement of 7 French steerable decapolar coronary sinus catheter (*white arrow*) from a right femoral vein into the coronary sinus ostium (right anterior oblique [RAO] view). Panels (**c** and **d**): coaxial alignment of both 7-French multipurpose sheath with the inner sheath engaged in the coronary sinus ostium (*black arrow*) with a torque wire extending into the great cardiac vein (*double black arrow*) and 7-French steerable decapolar coronary sinus catheter from the right femoral vein (*white arrow*) (RAO view). Panel (**d**): 7-French multipurpose outer and inner sheath have been pulled back to the mid right atrium (*black arrow*). The torque wire from left subclavian approach (*double black arrow*) and 7-French steerable decapolar coronary sinus catheter from the right femoral vein (*white arrow*) have been advanced further into the great cardiac vein (RAO view) (Reprinted from Cao et al. [196] with permission from John Wiley and Sons)

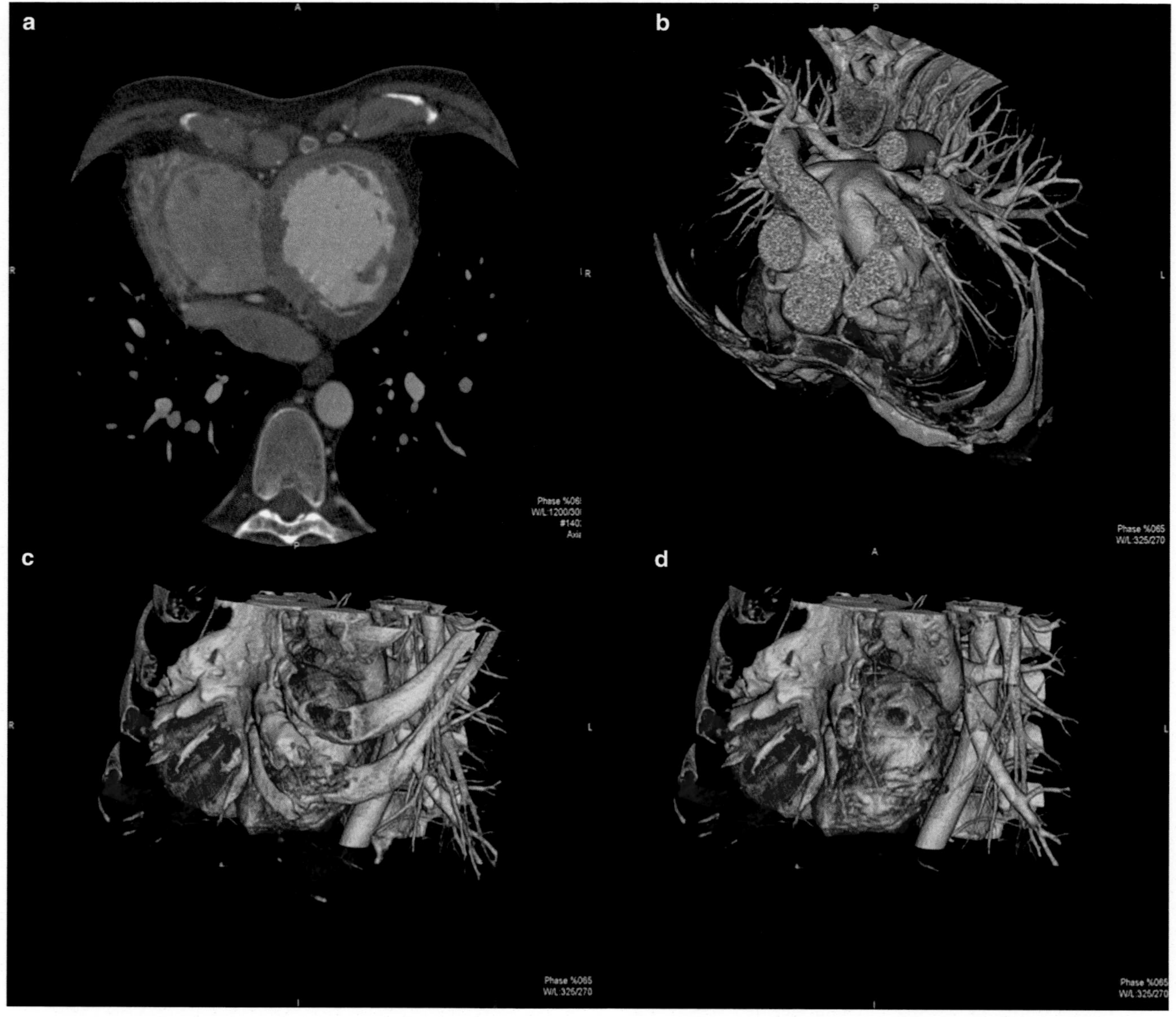

Fig. 24.40 2-D (**a**) and 3-D (**b–d**) views demonstrating anterior rotation of the left ventricle and relation to skeletal structures useful to planning a minimally invasive approach to epicardial left ventricular lead placement in a patient with coronary venous anatomy not amenable to a percutaneous approach to cardiac resynchronization therapy

sinus ostium in relation to the floor of the right atrium has been identified as a factor leading to challenging CRT coronary venous lead placement with a high coronary sinus ostium [197]. In cases where the coronary venous anatomy is not amenable to a venous approach to left ventricular lead placement, CCTA can facilitate planning of approach to epicardial lead placement (Fig. 24.40). Postprocedurally, CCTA is useful for 3-D assessment of pacemaker and ICD lead placement. With CRT, postprocedure CT was more accurate than fluoroscopy and chest x-ray for documentation of exact lead position [198, 199]. CCTA can detect lead perforation as evidenced by a lead tip visualized beyond the epicardium and can also demonstrate the presence of pericardial effusion [200–203].

Non-response is an issue in approximately one third of patients undergoing CRT. The correlation between CCTA visualized sites of coronary venous branch veins and echo derived area of latest mechanical activation has been associated with acute response to CRT, with lack of response associated with disparity in location between these sites [204]. The CMR literature has shown that the amount and location of myocardial infarct scar is important to CRT response. The percent total scar derived from delayed gadolinium enhancement imaging has predicted response to

CRT, with greater response in patients with less than 15 % percent total scar and poor response in patients with posterolateral scar [205–207]. CCTA delayed contrast enhancement imaging for assessment of non-response requires study. Comprehensive analysis of factors important to response to CRT including coronary venous anatomy, 3-D global and regional ventricular function, and delayed enhancement require further assessment for CRT planning and facilitation to maximize response.

Conclusions

CCTA provides extensive imaging data important to the diagnosis and treatment of electrophysiologically-relevant cardiovascular disease. Advanced cardiac imaging has furthered the field of cardiac electrophysiology and will continue to have an impact through application to a greater spectrum of arrhythmogenic substrates as well as ablation and device procedures.

References

1. Matsutani H, Sano T, Kondo T, Morita H, Arai T, Sekine T, et al. ECG-edit function in multidetector-row computed tomography coronary arteriography for patients with arrhythmias. Circ J Off J Jpn Circ Soc. 2008;72(7):1071–8.
2. Shinbane JS. Cardiovascular computed tomographic angiography in patients with atrial fibrillation: challenges of anatomy, physiology, and electrophysiology. J Cardiovasc Comput Tomogr. 2008;2(3):181–2.
3. Tsiflikas I, Drosch T, Brodoefel H, Thomas C, Reimann A, Till A, et al. Diagnostic accuracy and image quality of cardiac dual-source computed tomography in patients with arrhythmia. Int J Cardiol. 2010;143(1):79–85.
4. Sohns C, Kruse S, Vollmann D, Luthje L, Dorenkamp M, Seegers J, et al. Accuracy of 64-multidetector computed tomography coronary angiography in patients with symptomatic atrial fibrillation prior to pulmonary vein isolation. Eur Heart J Cardiovasc Imaging. 2012;13(3):263–70.
5. Lee AM, Engel LC, Shah B, Liew G, Sidhu MS, Kalra M, et al. Coronary computed tomography angiography during arrhythmia: radiation dose reduction with prospectively ECG-triggered axial and retrospectively ECG-gated helical 128-slice dual-source CT. J Cardiovasc Comput Tomogr. 2012;6(3):172–83.e2.
6. Sidhu MS, Venkatesh V, Hoffmann U, Ghoshhajra BB. Advanced adaptive axial-sequential prospectively electrocardiogram-triggered dual-source coronary computed tomographic angiography in a patient with atrial fibrillation. J Comput Assist Tomogr. 2011;35(6):747–8.
7. Rist C, Johnson TR, Muller-Starck J, Arnoldi E, Saam T, Becker A, et al. Noninvasive coronary angiography using dual-source computed tomography in patients with atrial fibrillation. Invest Radiol. 2009;44(3):159–67.
8. Oda S, Honda K, Yoshimura A, Katahira K, Noda K, Oshima S, et al. 256-Slice coronary computed tomographic angiography in patients with atrial fibrillation: optimal reconstruction phase and image quality. Eur Radiol. 2016;26(1):55–63.
9. Shinbane JS, Colletti PM, Shellock FG. MR in patients with pacemakers and ICDs: defining the issues. J Cardiovasc Magn Reson Off J Soc Cardiovasc Magnetic Reson. 2007;9(1):5–13.
10. Shinbane JS, Colletti PM, Shellock FG. Magnetic resonance imaging in patients with cardiac pacemakers: era of "MR Conditional" designs. J Cardiovasc Magn Reson Off J Soc Cardiovasc Magn Reson. 2011;13:63.
11. Shinbane JS, Colletti PM, Shellock FG. MR imaging in patients with pacemakers and other devices: engineering the future. JACC Cardiovasc Imaging. 2012;5(3):332–3.
12. Wilkoff BL, Bello D, Taborsky M, Vymazal J, Kanal E, Heuer H, et al. Magnetic resonance imaging in patients with a pacemaker system designed for the magnetic resonance environment. Heart Rhythm Off J Heart Rhythm Soc. 2011;8(1):65–73.
13. Gupta A, Subhas N, Primak AN, Nittka M, Liu K. Metal artifact reduction: standard and advanced magnetic resonance and computed tomography techniques. Radiol Clin North Am. 2015; 53(3):531–47.
14. Stevens SM, Tung R, Rashid S, Gima J, Cote S, Pavez G, et al. Device artifact reduction for magnetic resonance imaging of patients with implantable cardioverter-defibrillators and ventricular tachycardia: late gadolinium enhancement correlation with electroanatomic mapping. Heart Rhythm Off J Heart Rhythm Soc. 2014;11(2):289–98.
15. Abecasis J, Dourado R, Ferreira A, Saraiva C, Cavaco D, Santos KR, et al. Left atrial volume calculated by multi-detector computed tomography may predict successful pulmonary vein isolation in catheter ablation of atrial fibrillation. Europace Eur Pacing Arrhythmias Cardiac Electrophysiol J Working Groups Cardiac Pacing Arrhythmias Cardiac Cell Electrophysiol Eur Soc Cardiol. 2009;11(10):1289–94.
16. Helms AS, West JJ, Patel A, Lipinski MJ, Mangrum JM, Mounsey JP, et al. Relation of left atrial volume from three-dimensional computed tomography to atrial fibrillation recurrence following ablation. Am J Cardiol. 2009;103(7):989–93.
17. Lin FY, Devereux RB, Roman MJ, Meng J, Jow VM, Jacobs A, et al. Cardiac chamber volumes, function, and mass as determined by 64-multidetector row computed tomography: mean values among healthy adults free of hypertension and obesity. JACC Cardiovasc Imaging. 2008;1(6):782–6.
18. Mahabadi AA, Samy B, Seneviratne SK, Toepker MH, Bamberg F, Hoffmann U, et al. Quantitative assessment of left atrial volume by electrocardiographic-gated contrast-enhanced multidetector computed tomography. J Cardiovasc Comput Tomogr. 2009;3(2):80–7.
19. Christiaens L, Varroud-Vial N, Ardilouze P, Ragot S, Mergy J, Bonnet B, et al. Real three-dimensional assessment of left atrial and left atrial appendage volumes by 64-slice spiral computed tomography in individuals with or without cardiovascular disease. Int J Cardiol. 2010;140(2):189–96.
20. Wolf F, Ourednicek P, Loewe C, Richter B, Gossinger HD, Gwechenberger M, et al. Evaluation of left atrial function by multidetector computed tomography before left atrial radiofrequency-catheter ablation: comparison of a manual and automated 3D volume segmentation method. Eur J Radiol. 2010;75(2):e141–6.
21. Agner BF, Kuhl JT, Linde JJ, Kofoed KF, Akeson P, Rasmussen BV, et al. Assessment of left atrial volume and function in patients with permanent atrial fibrillation: comparison of cardiac magnetic resonance imaging, 320-slice multi-detector computed tomography, and transthoracic echocardiography. Eur Heart J Cardiovasc Imaging. 2014;15(5):532–40.
22. Pontone G, Andreini D, Bertella E, Petulla M, Russo E, Innocenti E, et al. Comparison of cardiac computed tomography versus cardiac magnetic resonance for characterization of left atrium anatomy before radiofrequency catheter ablation of atrial fibrillation. Int J Cardiol. 2015;179:114–21.
23. Kaseno K, Tada H, Koyama K, Jingu M, Hiramatsu S, Yokokawa M, et al. Prevalence and characterization of pulmonary vein variants in patients with atrial fibrillation determined using 3-dimensional computed tomography. Am J Cardiol. 2008;101(11):1638–42.
24. Dewland TA, Wintermark M, Vaysman A, Smith LM, Tong E, Vittinghoff E, et al. Use of computed tomography to identify atrial

fibrillation associated differences in left atrial wall thickness and density. Pacing Clin Electrophysiol PACE. 2013;36(1):55–62.
25. Suenari K, Nakano Y, Hirai Y, Ogi H, Oda N, Makita Y, et al. Left atrial thickness under the catheter ablation lines in patients with paroxysmal atrial fibrillation: insights from 64-slice multidetector computed tomography. Heart Vessels. 2013;28(3):360–8.
26. Makita Y, Nakano Y, Oda N, Suenari K, Sairaku A, Kajihara K, et al. Use of preprocedural multidetector computed tomography to decrease atrial fibrillation recurrence following extensive encircling circumferential pulmonary vein isolation. J Cardiol. 2012;60(3): 236–41.
27. Hanazawa K, Kaitani K, Hayama Y, Onishi N, Tamaki Y, Miyake M, et al. Effect of radiofrequency catheter ablation of persistent atrial fibrillation on the left atrial function: assessment by 320-row multislice computed tomography. Int J Cardiol. 2015;179:449–54.
28. Bisbal F, Guiu E, Cabanas P, Calvo N, Berruezo A, Tolosana JM, et al. Reversal of spherical remodelling of the left atrium after pulmonary vein isolation: incidence and predictors. Europace Eur Pacing Arrhythmias Cardiac Electrophysiol J Working Groups Cardiac Pacing Arrhythmias Cardiac Cell Electrophysiol Eur Soc Cardiol. 2014;16(6):840–7.
29. Tsao HM, Hu WC, Wu MH, Tai CT, Chang SL, Lin YJ, et al. The impact of catheter ablation on the dynamic function of the left atrium in patients with atrial fibrillation: insights from four-dimensional computed tomographic images. J Cardiovasc Electrophysiol. 2010;21(3):270–7.
30. Oakes RS, Badger TJ, Kholmovski EG, Akoum N, Burgon NS, Fish EN, et al. Detection and quantification of left atrial structural remodeling with delayed-enhancement magnetic resonance imaging in patients with atrial fibrillation. Circulation. 2009;119(13): 1758–67.
31. Akoum N, McGann C, Vergara G, Badger T, Ranjan R, Mahnkopf C, et al. Atrial fibrosis quantified using late gadolinium enhancement MRI is associated with sinus node dysfunction requiring pacemaker implant. J Cardiovasc Electrophysiol. 2012;23(1): 44–50.
32. Daccarett M, Badger TJ, Akoum N, Burgon NS, Mahnkopf C, Vergara G, et al. Association of left atrial fibrosis detected by delayed-enhancement magnetic resonance imaging and the risk of stroke in patients with atrial fibrillation. J Am Coll Cardiol. 2011;57(7):831–8.
33. Habibi M, Lima JA, Khurram IM, Zimmerman SL, Zipunnikov V, Fukumoto K, et al. Association of left atrial function and left atrial enhancement in patients with atrial fibrillation: cardiac magnetic resonance study. Circ Cardiovasc Imaging. 2015;8(2), e002769.
34. Marrouche NF, Wilber D, Hindricks G, Jais P, Akoum N, Marchlinski F, et al. Association of atrial tissue fibrosis identified by delayed enhancement MRI and atrial fibrillation catheter ablation: the DECAAF study. JAMA. 2014;311(5):498–506.
35. Akoum N, Wilber D, Hindricks G, Jais P, Cates J, Marchlinski F, et al. MRI assessment of ablation-induced scarring in atrial fibrillation: analysis from the DECAAF study. J Cardiovasc Electrophysiol. 2015;26(5):473–80.
36. McGann C, Akoum N, Patel A, Kholmovski E, Revelo P, Damal K, et al. Atrial fibrillation ablation outcome is predicted by left atrial remodeling on MRI. Circ Arrhythm Electrophysiol. 2014;7(1): 23–30.
37. Fukumoto K, Habibi M, Gucuk Ipek E, Khurram IM, Zimmerman SL, Zipunnikov V, et al. Comparison of preexisting and ablation-induced late gadolinium enhancement on left atrial magnetic resonance imaging. Heart Rhythm Off J Heart Rhythm Soc. 2015;12(4):668–72.
38. Badger TJ, Daccarett M, Akoum NW, Adjei-Poku YA, Burgon NS, Haslam TS, et al. Evaluation of left atrial lesions after initial and repeat atrial fibrillation ablation: lessons learned from delayed-enhancement MRI in repeat ablation procedures. Circ Arrhythm Electrophysiol. 2010;3(3):249–59.
39. Segerson NM, Daccarett M, Badger TJ, Shabaan A, Akoum N, Fish EN, et al. Magnetic resonance imaging-confirmed ablative debulking of the left atrial posterior wall and septum for treatment of persistent atrial fibrillation: rationale and initial experience. J Cardiovasc Electrophysiol. 2010;21(2):126–32.
40. Akoum N, Daccarett M, McGann C, Segerson N, Vergara G, Kuppahally S, et al. Atrial fibrosis helps select the appropriate patient and strategy in catheter ablation of atrial fibrillation: a DE-MRI guided approach. J Cardiovasc Electrophysiol. 2011;22(1):16–22.
41. Mahnkopf C, Badger TJ, Burgon NS, Daccarett M, Haslam TS, Badger CT, et al. Evaluation of the left atrial substrate in patients with lone atrial fibrillation using delayed-enhanced MRI: implications for disease progression and response to catheter ablation. Heart Rhythm Off J Heart Rhythm Soc. 2010;7(10): 1475–81.
42. Ling LH, McLellan AJ, Taylor AJ, Iles LM, Ellims AH, Kumar S, et al. Magnetic resonance post-contrast T1 mapping in the human atrium: validation and impact on clinical outcome after catheter ablation for atrial fibrillation. Heart Rhythm Off J Heart Rhythm Soc. 2014;11(9):1551–9.
43. Ling Z, McManigle J, Zipunnikov V, Pashakhanloo F, Khurram IM, Zimmerman SL, et al. The association of left atrial low-voltage regions on electroanatomic mapping with low attenuation regions on cardiac computed tomography perfusion imaging in patients with atrial fibrillation. Heart Rhythm Off J Heart Rhythm Soc. 2015;12(5):857–64.
44. Scharf C, Sneider M, Case I, Chugh A, Lai SW, Pelosi Jr F, et al. Anatomy of the pulmonary veins in patients with atrial fibrillation and effects of segmental ostial ablation analyzed by computed tomography. J Cardiovasc Electrophysiol. 2003;14(2):150–5.
45. Jongbloed MR, Dirksen MS, Bax JJ, Boersma E, Geleijns K, Lamb HJ, et al. Atrial fibrillation: multi-detector row CT of pulmonary vein anatomy prior to radiofrequency catheter ablation–initial experience. Radiology. 2005;234(3):702–9.
46. Hamdan A, Charalampos K, Roettgen R, Wellnhofer E, Gebker R, Paetsch I, et al. Magnetic resonance imaging versus computed tomography for characterization of pulmonary vein morphology before radiofrequency catheter ablation of atrial fibrillation. Am J Cardiol. 2009;104(11):1540–6.
47. Wood MA, Wittkamp M, Henry D, Martin R, Nixon JV, Shepard RK, et al. A comparison of pulmonary vein ostial anatomy by computerized tomography, echocardiography, and venography in patients with atrial fibrillation having radiofrequency catheter ablation. Am J Cardiol. 2004;93(1):49–53.
48. To AC, Gabriel RS, Park M, Lowe BS, Curtin RJ, Sigurdsson G, et al. Role of transesophageal echocardiography compared to computed tomography in evaluation of pulmonary vein ablation for atrial fibrillation (ROTEA study). J Am Soc Echocardiogr Off Publ Am Soc Echocardiogr. 2011;24(9):1046–55.
49. Robbins IM, Colvin EV, Doyle TP, Kemp WE, Loyd JE, McMahon WS, et al. Pulmonary vein stenosis after catheter ablation of atrial fibrillation. Circulation. 1998;98(17):1769–75.
50. Packer DL, Keelan P, Munger TM, Breen JF, Asirvatham S, Peterson LA, et al. Clinical presentation, investigation, and management of pulmonary vein stenosis complicating ablation for atrial fibrillation. Circulation. 2005;111(5):546–54.
51. Dong J, Vasamreddy CR, Jayam V, Dalal D, Dickfeld T, Eldadah Z, et al. Incidence and predictors of pulmonary vein stenosis following catheter ablation of atrial fibrillation using the anatomic pulmonary vein ablation approach: results from paired magnetic resonance imaging. J Cardiovasc Electrophysiol. 2005;16(8): 845–52.
52. Sigurdsson G, Troughton RW, Xu XF, Salazar HP, Wazni OM, Grimm RA, et al. Detection of pulmonary vein stenosis by transesophageal echocardiography: comparison with multidetector computed tomography. Am Heart J. 2007;153(5):800–6.

53. Martinek M, Nesser HJ, Aichinger J, Boehm G, Purerfellner H. Impact of integration of multislice computed tomography imaging into three-dimensional electroanatomic mapping on clinical outcomes, safety, and efficacy using radiofrequency ablation for atrial fibrillation. Pacing Clin Electrophysiol PACE. 2007; 30(10):1215–23.
54. Wongcharoen W, Tsao HM, Wu MH, Tai CT, Chang SL, Lin YJ, et al. Preexisting pulmonary vein stenosis in patients undergoing atrial fibrillation ablation: a report of five cases. J Cardiovasc Electrophysiol. 2006;17(4):423–5.
55. Rostamian A, Narayan SM, Thomson L, Fishbein M, Siegel RJ. The incidence, diagnosis, and management of pulmonary vein stenosis as a complication of atrial fibrillation ablation. J Interv Cardiac Electrophysiol Int J Arrhythmias Pacing. 2014;40(1):63–74.
56. Saad EB, Marrouche NF, Saad CP, Ha E, Bash D, White RD, et al. Pulmonary vein stenosis after catheter ablation of atrial fibrillation: emergence of a new clinical syndrome. Ann Intern Med. 2003;138(8):634–8.
57. Saad EB, Rossillo A, Saad CP, Martin DO, Bhargava M, Erciyes D, et al. Pulmonary vein stenosis after radiofrequency ablation of atrial fibrillation: functional characterization, evolution, and influence of the ablation strategy. Circulation. 2003;108(25):3102–7.
58. Krishnaswamy A, Tuzcu EM, Kapadia SR. Integration of MDCT and fluoroscopy using C-arm computed tomography to guide structural cardiac interventions in the cardiac catheterization laboratory. Catheter Cardiovasc Interv Off J Soc Cardiac Angiogr Interv. 2015;85(1):139–47.
59. Peng LQ, Yu JQ, Yang ZG, Wu D, Xu JJ, Chu ZG, et al. Left atrial diverticula in patients referred for radiofrequency ablation of atrial fibrillation: assessment of prevalence and morphologic characteristics by dual-source computed tomography. Circ Arrhythm Electrophysiol. 2012;5(2):345–50.
60. Mao S, Shinbane JS, Girsky MJ, Child J, Carson S, Oudiz RJ, et al. Coronary venous imaging with electron beam computed tomographic angiography: three-dimensional mapping and relationship with coronary arteries. Am Heart J. 2005;150(2):315–22.
61. Chugh A, Makkar A, Yen Ho S, Yokokawa M, Sundaram B, Pelosi F, et al. Manifestations of coronary arterial injury during catheter ablation of atrial fibrillation and related arrhythmias. Heart Rhythm Off J Heart Rhythm Soc. 2013;10(11):1638–45.
62. Saremi F, Channual S, Krishnan S, Gurudevan SV, Narula J, Abolhoda A. Bachmann Bundle and its arterial supply: imaging with multidetector CT–implications for interatrial conduction abnormalities and arrhythmias. Radiology. 2008;248(2):447–57.
63. Pappone C, Oral H, Santinelli V, Vicedomini G, Lang CC, Manguso F, et al. Atrio-esophageal fistula as a complication of percutaneous transcatheter ablation of atrial fibrillation. Circulation. 2004;109(22):2724–6.
64. Lemola K, Sneider M, Desjardins B, Case I, Han J, Good E, et al. Computed tomographic analysis of the anatomy of the left atrium and the esophagus: implications for left atrial catheter ablation. Circulation. 2004;110(24):3655–60.
65. Cury RC, Abbara S, Schmidt S, Malchano ZJ, Neuzil P, Weichet J, et al. Relationship of the esophagus and aorta to the left atrium and pulmonary veins: implications for catheter ablation of atrial fibrillation. Heart Rhythm Off J Heart Rhythm Soc. 2005;2(12):1317–23.
66. Piorkowski C, Hindricks G, Schreiber D, Tanner H, Weise W, Koch A, et al. Electroanatomic reconstruction of the left atrium, pulmonary veins, and esophagus compared with the "true anatomy" on multislice computed tomography in patients undergoing catheter ablation of atrial fibrillation. Heart Rhythm Off J Heart Rhythm Soc. 2006;3(3):317–27.
67. Good E, Oral H, Lemola K, Han J, Tamirisa K, Igic P, et al. Movement of the esophagus during left atrial catheter ablation for atrial fibrillation. J Am Coll Cardiol. 2005;46(11):2107–10.
68. Gavin AR, Singleton CB, McGavigan AD. Assessment of oesophageal position by direct visualization with luminal contrast compared with segmentation from pre-acquired computed tomography scan-implications for ablation strategy. Europace Eur Pacing Arrhythmias Cardiac Electrophysiol J Working Groups Cardiac Pacing Arrhythmias Cardiac Cell Electrophysiol Eur Soc Cardiol. 2014;16(9):1304–8.
69. Jang SW, Kwon BJ, Choi MS, Kim DB, Shin WS, Cho EJ, et al. Computed tomographic analysis of the esophagus, left atrium, and pulmonary veins: implications for catheter ablation of atrial fibrillation. J Interv Cardiac Electrophysiol Int J Arrhythmias Pacing. 2011;32(1):1–6.
70. Lemola K, Mueller G, Desjardins B, Sneider M, Case I, Good E, et al. Topographic analysis of the coronary sinus and major cardiac veins by computed tomography. Heart Rhythm Off J Heart Rhythm Soc. 2005;2(7):694–9.
71. Wu MH, Wongcharoen W, Tsao HM, Tai CT, Chang SL, Lin YJ, et al. Close relationship between the bronchi and pulmonary veins: implications for the prevention of atriobronchial fistula after atrial fibrillation ablation. J Cardiovasc Electrophysiol. 2007;18(10):1056–9.
72. Li YG, Yang M, Li Y, Wang Q, Yu L, Sun J. Spatial relationship between left atrial roof or superior pulmonary veins and bronchi or pulmonary arteries by dual-source computed tomography: implication for preventing injury of bronchi and pulmonary arteries during atrial fibrillation ablation. Europace Eur Pacing Arrhythmias Cardiac Electrophysiol J Working Groups Cardiac Pacing Arrhythmias Cardiac Cell Electrophysiol Eur Soc Cardiol. 2011;13(6):809–14.
73. Desai AK, Osahan DS, Undavia MB, Nair GB. Bronchial injury post-cryoablation for atrial fibrillation. Ann Am Thorac Soc. 2015;12(7):1103–4.
74. Squara F, Desjardins B, Marchlinski FE, Supple GE. Prospective 3-dimensional computed tomography segmentation of the pericardiac right phrenic nerve in the setting of atrial fibrillation ablation. Circ Arrhythm Electrophysiol. 2014;7(3):561–2.
75. Opolski MP, Staruch AD, Kusmierczyk M, Witkowski A, Kwiecinska S, Kosek M, et al. Computed tomography angiography for prediction of atrial fibrillation after coronary artery bypass grafting: proof of concept. J Cardiol. 2015;65(4):285–92.
76. Wissner E, Wellnitz CV, Srivathsan K, Scott LR, Altemose GT. Value of multislice computed tomography angiography of the thorax in preparation for catheter ablation for the treatment of atrial fibrillation: the impact of unexpected cardiac and extracardiac findings on patient care. Eur J Radiol. 2009;72(2):284–8.
77. Kistler PM, Earley MJ, Harris S, Abrams D, Ellis S, Sporton SC, et al. Validation of three-dimensional cardiac image integration: use of integrated CT image into electroanatomic mapping system to perform catheter ablation of atrial fibrillation. J Cardiovasc Electrophysiol. 2006;17(4):341–8.
78. Sra J, Krum D, Hare J, Okerlund D, Thompson H, Vass M, et al. Feasibility and validation of registration of three-dimensional left atrial models derived from computed tomography with a noncontact cardiac mapping system. Heart Rhythm Off J Heart Rhythm Soc. 2005;2(1):55–63.
79. Heist EK, Chevalier J, Holmvang G, Singh JP, Ellinor PT, Milan DJ, et al. Factors affecting error in integration of electroanatomic mapping with CT and MR imaging during catheter ablation of atrial fibrillation. J Interv Cardiac Electrophysiol Int J Arrhythmias Pacing. 2006;17(1):21–7.
80. Kistler PM, Rajappan K, Jahngir M, Earley MJ, Harris S, Abrams D, et al. The impact of CT image integration into an electroanatomic mapping system on clinical outcomes of catheter ablation of atrial fibrillation. J Cardiovasc Electrophysiol. 2006;17(10): 1093–101.
81. Kistler PM, Rajappan K, Harris S, Earley MJ, Richmond L, Sporton SC, et al. The impact of image integration on catheter ablation of atrial fibrillation using electroanatomic mapping: a prospective randomized study. Eur Heart J. 2008;29(24):3029–36.

82. Haissaguerre M, Hocini M, Sanders P, Sacher F, Rotter M, Takahashi Y, et al. Catheter ablation of long-lasting persistent atrial fibrillation: clinical outcome and mechanisms of subsequent arrhythmias. J Cardiovasc Electrophysiol. 2005;16(11):1138–47.
83. Chae S, Oral H, Good E, Dey S, Wimmer A, Crawford T, et al. Atrial tachycardia after circumferential pulmonary vein ablation of atrial fibrillation: mechanistic insights, results of catheter ablation, and risk factors for recurrence. J Am Coll Cardiol. 2007;50(18):1781–7.
84. Aleong R, Heist EK, Ruskin JN, Mansour M. Integration of intracardiac echocardiography with magnetic resonance imaging allows visualization of the esophagus during catheter ablation of atrial fibrillation. Heart Rhythm Off J Heart Rhythm Soc. 2008;5(7):1088.
85. Jongbloed MR, Bax JJ, van der Wall EE, Schalij MJ. Thrombus in the left atrial appendage detected by intracardiac echocardiography. Int J Cardiovasc Imaging. 2004;20(2):113–6.
86. Lakkireddy D, Rangisetty U, Prasad S, Verma A, Biria M, Berenbom L, et al. Intracardiac echo-guided radiofrequency catheter ablation of atrial fibrillation in patients with atrial septal defect or patent foramen ovale repair: a feasibility, safety, and efficacy study. J Cardiovasc Electrophysiol. 2008;19(11):1137–42.
87. den Uijl DW, Tops LF, Tolosana JM, Schuijf JD, Trines SA, Zeppenfeld K, et al. Real-time integration of intracardiac echocardiography and multislice computed tomography to guide radiofrequency catheter ablation for atrial fibrillation. Heart Rhythm Off J Heart Rhythm Soc. 2008;5(10):1403–10.
88. Ren JF, Marchlinski FE, Callans DJ. Left atrial thrombus associated with ablation for atrial fibrillation: identification with intracardiac echocardiography. J Am Coll Cardiol. 2004;43(10):1861–7.
89. Saliba W, Thomas J. Intracardiac echocardiography during catheter ablation of atrial fibrillation. Europace Eur Pacing Arrhythmias Cardiac Electrophysiol J Working Groups Cardiac Pacing Arrhythmias Cardiac Cell Electrophysiol Eur Soc Cardiol. 2008;10 Suppl 3:iii42–7.
90. Knecht S, Skali H, O'Neill MD, Wright M, Matsuo S, Chaudhry GM, et al. Computed tomography-fluoroscopy overlay evaluation during catheter ablation of left atrial arrhythmia. Europace Eur Pacing Arrhythmias Cardiac Electrophysiol J Working Groups Cardiac Pacing Arrhythmias Cardiac Cell Electrophysiol Eur Soc Cardiol. 2008;10(8):931–8.
91. Ejima K, Shoda M, Yagishita D, Futagawa K, Yashiro B, Sato T, et al. Image integration of three-dimensional cone-beam computed tomography angiogram into electroanatomical mapping system to guide catheter ablation of atrial fibrillation. Europace Eur Pacing Arrhythmias Cardiac Electrophysiol J Working Groups Cardiac Pacing Arrhythmias Cardiac Cell Electrophysiol Eur Soc Cardiol. 2010;12(1):45–51.
92. Qamruddin S, Shinbane J, Shriki J, Naqvi TZ. Left atrial appendage: structure, function, imaging modalities and therapeutic options. Expert Rev Cardiovasc Ther. 2010;8(1):65–75.
93. Garcia MJ. Detection of left atrial appendage thrombus by cardiac computed tomography: a word of caution. JACC Cardiovasc Imaging. 2009;2(1):77–9.
94. Saremi F, Channual S, Gurudevan SV, Narula J, Abolhoda A. Prevalence of left atrial appendage pseudothrombus filling defects in patients with atrial fibrillation undergoing coronary computed tomography angiography. J Cardiovasc Comput Tomogr. 2008;2(3):164–71.
95. Martinez MW, Kirsch J, Williamson EE, Syed IS, Feng D, Ommen S, et al. Utility of nongated multidetector computed tomography for detection of left atrial thrombus in patients undergoing catheter ablation of atrial fibrillation. JACC Cardiovasc Imaging. 2009;2(1):69–76.
96. Achenbach S, Sacher D, Ropers D, Pohle K, Nixdorff U, Hoffmann U, et al. Electron beam computed tomography for the detection of left atrial thrombi in patients with atrial fibrillation. Heart. 2004;90(12):1477–8.
97. Shapiro MD, Neilan TG, Jassal DS, Samy B, Nasir K, Hoffmann U, et al. Multidetector computed tomography for the detection of left atrial appendage thrombus: a comparative study with transesophageal echocardiography. J Comput Assist Tomogr. 2007;31(6):905–9.
98. Hur J, Kim YJ, Nam JE, Choe KO, Choi EY, Shim CY, et al. Thrombus in the left atrial appendage in stroke patients: detection with cardiac CT angiography--a preliminary report. Radiology. 2008;249(1):81–7.
99. Patel A, Au E, Donegan K, Kim RJ, Lin FY, Stein KM, et al. Multidetector row computed tomography for identification of left atrial appendage filling defects in patients undergoing pulmonary vein isolation for treatment of atrial fibrillation: comparison with transesophageal echocardiography. Heart Rhythm Off J Heart Rhythm Soc. 2008;5(2):253–60.
100. Tang RB, Dong JZ, Zhang ZQ, Li ZA, Liu XP, Kang JP, et al. Comparison of contrast enhanced 64-slice computed tomography and transesophageal echocardiography in detection of left atrial thrombus in patients with atrial fibrillation. J Interv Cardiac Electrophysiol Int J Arrhythmias Pacing. 2008;22(3):199–203.
101. Gottlieb I, Pinheiro A, Brinker JA, Corretti MC, Mayer SA, Bluemke DA, et al. Diagnostic accuracy of arterial phase 64-slice multidetector CT angiography for left atrial appendage thrombus in patients undergoing atrial fibrillation ablation. J Cardiovasc Electrophysiol. 2008;19(3):247–51.
102. Ishiyama M, Akaike G, Matsusako M, Ueda T, Makidono A, Ohde S, et al. Severity of pseudofilling defect in the left atrial appendage on cardiac computed tomography is a simple predictor of the degree of left atrial emptying dysfunction in patients with chronic atrial fibrillation. J Comput Assist Tomogr. 2012;36(4):450–4.
103. Hur J, Kim YJ, Lee HJ, Ha JW, Heo JH, Choi EY, et al. Left atrial appendage thrombi in stroke patients: detection with two-phase cardiac CT angiography versus transesophageal echocardiography. Radiology. 2009;251(3):683–90.
104. Sawit ST, Garcia-Alvarez A, Suri B, Gaztanaga J, Fernandez-Friera L, Mirelis JG, et al. Usefulness of cardiac computed tomographic delayed contrast enhancement of the left atrial appendage before pulmonary vein ablation. Am J Cardiol. 2012;109(5):677–84.
105. Romero J, Husain SA, Kelesidis I, Sanz J, Medina HM, Garcia MJ. Detection of left atrial appendage thrombus by cardiac computed tomography in patients with atrial fibrillation: a meta-analysis. Circ Cardiovasc Imaging. 2013;6(2):185–94.
106. Tani T, Yamakami S, Matsushita T, Okamoto M, Toyama J, Suzuki S, et al. Usefulness of electron beam tomography in the prone position for detecting atrial thrombi in chronic atrial fibrillation. J Comput Assist Tomogr. 2003;27(1):78–84.
107. Kim YY, Klein AL, Halliburton SS, Popovic ZB, Kuzmiak SA, Sola S, et al. Left atrial appendage filling defects identified by multidetector computed tomography in patients undergoing radiofrequency pulmonary vein antral isolation: a comparison with transesophageal echocardiography. Am Heart J. 2007;154(6):1199–205.
108. Choi BH, Ko SM, Hwang HK, Song MG, Shin JK, Kang WS, et al. Detection of left atrial thrombus in patients with mitral stenosis and atrial fibrillation: retrospective comparison of two-phase computed tomography, transoesophageal echocardiography and surgical findings. Eur Radiol. 2013;23(11):2944–53.
109. Hur J, Pak HN, Kim YJ, Lee HJ, Chang HJ, Hong YJ, et al. Dual-enhancement cardiac computed tomography for assessing left atrial thrombus and pulmonary veins before radiofrequency catheter ablation for atrial fibrillation. Am J Cardiol. 2013;112(2):238–44.
110. Budoff MJ, Shittu A, Hacioglu Y, Gang E, Li D, Bhatia H, et al. Comparison of transesophageal echocardiography versus

computed tomography for detection of left atrial appendage filling defect (thrombus). Am J Cardiol. 2014;113(1):173–7.
111. Meier B, Blaauw Y, Khattab AA, Lewalter T, Sievert H, Tondo C, et al. EHRA/EAPCI expert consensus statement on catheter-based left atrial appendage occlusion. Europace Eur Pacing Arrhythmias Cardiac Electrophysiol J Working Groups Cardiac Pacing Arrhythmias Cardiac Cell Electrophysiol Eur Soc Cardiol. 2014;16(10):1397–416.
112. Masoudi FA, Calkins H, Kavinsky CJ, Drozda Jr JP, Gainsley P, Slotwiner DJ, et al. ACC/HRS/SCAI left atrial appendage occlusion device societal overview: a professional societal overview from the American College of Cardiology, Heart Rhythm Society, and Society for Cardiovascular Angiography and Interventions. J Am Coll Cardiol. 2015;2015.
113. Koplay M, Erol C, Paksoy Y, Kivrak AS, Ozbek S. An investigation of the anatomical variations of left atrial appendage by multidetector computed tomographic coronary angiography. Eur J Radiol. 2012;81(7):1575–80.
114. van Rosendael PJ, Katsanos S, van den Brink OW, Scholte AJ, Trines SA, Bax JJ, et al. Geometry of left atrial appendage assessed with multidetector-row computed tomography: implications for transcatheter closure devices. EuroIntervJ EuroPCR Collab Working Group Interv Cardiol Eur Soc Cardiol. 2014;10(3):364–71.
115. Freixa X, Tzikas A, Basmadjian A, Garceau P, Ibrahim R. The chicken-wing morphology: an anatomical challenge for left atrial appendage occlusion. J Interv Cardiol. 2013; 26(5):509–14.
116. Di Biase L, Santangeli P, Anselmino M, Mohanty P, Salvetti I, Gili S, et al. Does the left atrial appendage morphology correlate with the risk of stroke in patients with atrial fibrillation? Results from a multicenter study. J Am Coll Cardiol. 2012;60(6):531–8.
117. Fukushima K, Fukushima N, Kato K, Ejima K, Sato H, Fukushima K, et al. Correlation between left atrial appendage morphology and flow velocity in patients with paroxysmal atrial fibrillation. Eur Heart J Cardiovasc Imaging. 2016;17(1):59–66.
118. Petersen M, Roehrich A, Balzer J, Shin DI, Meyer C, Kelm M, et al. Left atrial appendage morphology is closely associated with specific echocardiographic flow pattern in patients with atrial fibrillation. Europace Eur Pacing Arrhythmias Cardiac Electrophysiol J Working Groups Cardiac Pacing Arrhythmias Cardiac Cell Electrophysiol Eur Soc Cardiol. 2015;17(4):539–45.
119. Nedios S, Kornej J, Koutalas E, Bertagnolli L, Kosiuk J, Rolf S, et al. Left atrial appendage morphology and thromboembolic risk after catheter ablation for atrial fibrillation. Heart Rhythm Off J Heart Rhythm Soc. 2014;11(12):2239–46.
120. Kosiuk J, Nedios S, Kornej J, Koutalas E, Bertagnolli L, Rolf S, et al. Impact of left atrial appendage morphology on peri-interventional thromboembolic risk during catheter ablation of atrial fibrillation. Heart Rhythm Off J Heart Rhythm Soc. 2014;11(9):1522–7.
121. Anselmino M, Scaglione M, Di Biase L, Gili S, Santangeli P, Corsinovi L, et al. Left atrial appendage morphology and silent cerebral ischemia in patients with atrial fibrillation. Heart Rhythm Off J Heart Rhythm Soc. 2014;11(1):2–7.
122. Lee JM, Seo J, Uhm JS, Kim YJ, Lee HJ, Kim JY, et al. Why is left atrial appendage morphology related to strokes? An analysis of the flow velocity and orifice size of the left atrial appendage. J Cardiovasc Electrophysiol. 2015;26(9):922–27.
123. Kajihara K, Nakano Y, Hirai Y, Ogi H, Oda N, Suenari K, et al. Variable procedural strategies adapted to anatomical characteristics in catheter ablation of the cavotricuspid isthmus using a preoperative multidetector computed tomography analysis. J Cardiovasc Electrophysiol. 2013;24(12):1344–51.
124. Sommer P, Piorkowski C, Arya A, Hindricks G. Successful integration of a computed tomography-based left atrial three-dimensional model in an electroanatomically reconstructed right atrium for ablation of biatrial tachycardia. Heart Rhythm Off J Heart Rhythm Soc. 2011;8(1):152–3.
125. Shinbane JS, Lesh MD, Stevenson WG, Klitzner TS, Natterson PD, Wiener I, et al. Anatomic and electrophysiologic relation between the coronary sinus and mitral annulus: implications for ablation of left-sided accessory pathways. Am Heart J. 1998;135(1): 93–8.
126. Gopal A, Shah A, Shareghi S, Bansal N, Nasir K, Gopal D, et al. The role of cardiovascular computed tomographic angiography for coronary sinus mitral annuloplasty. J Invasive Cardiol. 2010;22(2):67–73.
127. Morin DP, Parker H, Khatib S, Dinshaw H. Computed tomography of a coronary sinus diverticulum associated with Wolff-Parkinson-White syndrome. Heart Rhythm Off J Heart Rhythm Soc. 2012;9(8):1338–9.
128. Miyahara Y, Kataoka K, Kawada M. Isolated unroofed coronary sinus on three-dimensional computed tomographic imaging. Ann Thorac Surg. 2012;93(6):2072.
129. Shinbane JS, Shriki J, Fleischman F, Hindoyan A, Withey J, Lee C, et al. Anomalous coronary arteries: cardiovascular computed tomographic angiography for surgical decisions and planning. World J Pediatr Congenit Heart Surg. 2013;4(2): 142–54.
130. Shriki JE, Shinbane JS, Rashid MA, Hindoyan A, Withey JG, DeFrance A, et al. Identifying, characterizing, and classifying congenital anomalies of the coronary arteries. Radiogr Rev Publ Radiol Soc N Am Inc. 2012;32(2):453–68.
131. Levisman J, Budoff M, Karlsberg R. Congenital atresia of the left main coronary artery: cardiac CT. Cathete Cardiovasc Interv Off J Soc Cardiac Angiogr Interv. 2009;74(3):465–7.
132. Opolski MP, Pregowski J, Kruk M, Witkowski A, Kwiecinska S, Lubienska E, et al. Prevalence and characteristics of coronary anomalies originating from the opposite sinus of Valsalva in 8,522 patients referred for coronary computed tomography angiography. Am J Cardiol. 2013;111(9):1361–7.
133. Andreini D, Pontone G, Pepi M, Ballerini G, Bartorelli AL, Magini A, et al. Diagnostic accuracy of multidetector computed tomography coronary angiography in patients with dilated cardiomyopathy. J Am Coll Cardiol. 2007;49(20):2044–50.
134. Andreini D, Pontone G, Bartorelli AL, Agostoni P, Mushtaq S, Bertella E, et al. Sixty-four-slice multidetector computed tomography: an accurate imaging modality for the evaluation of coronary arteries in dilated cardiomyopathy of unknown etiology. Circ Cardiovasc Imaging. 2009;2(3):199–205.
135. Bhatti S, Hakeem A, Yousuf MA, Al-Khalidi HR, Mazur W, Shizukuda Y. Diagnostic performance of computed tomography angiography for differentiating ischemic vs nonischemic cardiomyopathy. J Nucl Cardiol Off Publ Am Soc Nucl Cardiol. 2011;18(3):407–20.
136. Kim RJ, Wu E, Rafael A, Chen EL, Parker MA, Simonetti O, et al. The use of contrast-enhanced magnetic resonance imaging to identify reversible myocardial dysfunction. N Engl J Med. 2000;343(20):1445–53.
137. Klein C, Nekolla SG, Bengel FM, Momose M, Sammer A, Haas F, et al. Assessment of myocardial viability with contrast-enhanced magnetic resonance imaging: comparison with positron emission tomography. Circulation. 2002;105(2):162–7.
138. Kuhl HP, Beek AM, van der Weerdt AP, Hofman MB, Visser CA, Lammertsma AA, et al. Myocardial viability in chronic ischemic heart disease: comparison of contrast-enhanced magnetic resonance imaging with (18)F-fluorodeoxyglucose positron emission tomography. J Am Coll Cardiol. 2003;41(8):1341–8.
139. Selvanayagam JB, Kardos A, Francis JM, Wiesmann F, Petersen SE, Taggart DP, et al. Value of delayed-enhancement cardiovascular magnetic resonance imaging in predicting myo-

cardial viability after surgical revascularization. Circulation. 2004;110(12):1535–41.
140. Bello D, Fieno DS, Kim RJ, Pereles FS, Passman R, Song G, et al. Infarct morphology identifies patients with substrate for sustained ventricular tachycardia. J Am Coll Cardiol. 2005;45(7):1104–8.
141. Bello D, Einhorn A, Kaushal R, Kenchaiah S, Raney A, Fieno D, et al. Cardiac magnetic resonance imaging: infarct size is an independent predictor of mortality in patients with coronary artery disease. Magn Reson Imaging. 2011;29(1):50–6.
142. Gao P, Yee R, Gula L, Krahn AD, Skanes A, Leong-Sit P, et al. Prediction of arrhythmic events in ischemic and dilated cardiomyopathy patients referred for implantable cardiac defibrillator: evaluation of multiple scar quantification measures for late gadolinium enhancement magnetic resonance imaging. Circ Cardiovasc Imaging. 2012;5(4):448–56.
143. Nazarian S, Bluemke DA, Lardo AC, Zviman MM, Watkins SP, Dickfeld TL, et al. Magnetic resonance assessment of the substrate for inducible ventricular tachycardia in nonischemic cardiomyopathy. Circulation. 2005;112(18):2821–5.
144. Assomull RG, Prasad SK, Lyne J, Smith G, Burman ED, Khan M, et al. Cardiovascular magnetic resonance, fibrosis, and prognosis in dilated cardiomyopathy. J Am Coll Cardiol. 2006;48(10):1977–85.
145. Wu KC, Weiss RG, Thiemann DR, Kitagawa K, Schmidt A, Dalal D, et al. Late gadolinium enhancement by cardiovascular magnetic resonance heralds an adverse prognosis in nonischemic cardiomyopathy. J Am Coll Cardiol. 2008; 51(25):2414–21.
146. Cho JR, Park S, Choi BW, Kang SM, Ha JW, Chung N, et al. Delayed enhancement magnetic resonance imaging is a significant prognostic factor in patients with non-ischemic cardiomyopathy. Circ J Off J Jpn Circ Soc. 2010;74(3):476–83.
147. Lehrke S, Lossnitzer D, Schob M, Steen H, Merten C, Kemmling H, et al. Use of cardiovascular magnetic resonance for risk stratification in chronic heart failure: prognostic value of late gadolinium enhancement in patients with non-ischaemic dilated cardiomyopathy. Heart. 2011;97(9):727–32.
148. Matoh F, Satoh H, Shiraki K, Saitoh T, Urushida T, Katoh H, et al. Usefulness of delayed enhancement magnetic resonance imaging to differentiate dilated phase of hypertrophic cardiomyopathy and dilated cardiomyopathy. J Card Fail. 2007;13(5):372–9.
149. Suk T, Edwards C, Hart H, Christiansen JP. Myocardial scar detected by contrast-enhanced cardiac magnetic resonance imaging is associated with ventricular tachycardia in hypertrophic cardiomyopathy patients. Heart Lung Circ. 2008;17(5):370–4.
150. Adabag AS, Maron BJ, Appelbaum E, Harrigan CJ, Buros JL, Gibson CM, et al. Occurrence and frequency of arrhythmias in hypertrophic cardiomyopathy in relation to delayed enhancement on cardiovascular magnetic resonance. J Am Coll Cardiol. 2008;51(14):1369–74.
151. Oka K, Tsujino T, Nakao S, Lee-Kawabata M, Ezumi A, Masai M, et al. Symptomatic ventricular tachyarrhythmia is associated with delayed gadolinium enhancement in cardiac magnetic resonance imaging and with elevated plasma brain natriuretic peptide level in hypertrophic cardiomyopathy. J Cardiol. 2008;52(2):146–53.
152. Kwon DH, Smedira NG, Rodriguez ER, Tan C, Setser R, Thamilarasan M, et al. Cardiac magnetic resonance detection of myocardial scarring in hypertrophic cardiomyopathy: correlation with histopathology and prevalence of ventricular tachycardia. J Am Coll Cardiol. 2009;54(3):242–9.
153. Fluechter S, Kuschyk J, Wolpert C, Doesch C, Veltmann C, Haghi D, et al. Extent of late gadolinium enhancement detected by cardiovascular magnetic resonance correlates with the inducibility of ventricular tachyarrhythmia in hypertrophic cardiomyopathy. J Cardiovasc Mag Reson Off J Soc Cardiovasc Magn Reson. 2010;12:30.
154. Green JJ, Berger JS, Kramer CM, Salerno M. Prognostic value of late gadolinium enhancement in clinical outcomes for hypertrophic cardiomyopathy. JACC Cardiovasc Imaging. 2012;5(4):370–7.
155. Casolo G, Di Cesare E, Molinari G, Knoll P, Midiri M, Fedele F, et al. Diagnostic work up of arrhythmogenic right ventricular cardiomyopathy by cardiovascular magnetic resonance (CMR). Consensus statement La Radiologia Medica. 2004;108(1–2):39–55.
156. Tandri H, Saranathan M, Rodriguez ER, Martinez C, Bomma C, Nasir K, et al. Noninvasive detection of myocardial fibrosis in arrhythmogenic right ventricular cardiomyopathy using delayed-enhancement magnetic resonance imaging. J Am Coll Cardiol. 2005;45(1):98–103.
157. Dickfeld T, Tian J, Ahmad G, Jimenez A, Turgeman A, Kuk R, et al. MRI-Guided ventricular tachycardia ablation: integration of late gadolinium-enhanced 3D scar in patients with implantable cardioverter-defibrillators. Circ Arrhythm Electrophysiol. 2011;4(2):172–84.
158. Yokokawa M, Tada H, Koyama K, Naito S, Oshima S, Taniguchi K. Nontransmural scar detected by magnetic resonance imaging and origin of ventricular tachycardia in structural heart disease. Pacing Clin Electrophysiol PACE. 2009;32 Suppl 1:S52–6.
159. Ashikaga H, Sasano T, Dong J, Zviman MM, Evers R, Hopenfeld B, et al. Magnetic resonance-based anatomical analysis of scar-related ventricular tachycardia: implications for catheter ablation. Circ Res. 2007;101(9):939–47.
160. Schmidt A, Azevedo CF, Cheng A, Gupta SN, Bluemke DA, Foo TK, et al. Infarct tissue heterogeneity by magnetic resonance imaging identifies enhanced cardiac arrhythmia susceptibility in patients with left ventricular dysfunction. Circulation. 2007;115(15):2006–14.
161. Bogun FM, Desjardins B, Good E, Gupta S, Crawford T, Oral H, et al. Delayed-enhanced magnetic resonance imaging in nonischemic cardiomyopathy: utility for identifying the ventricular arrhythmia substrate. J Am Coll Cardiol. 2009;53(13):1138–45.
162. Heidary S, Patel H, Chung J, Yokota H, Gupta SN, Bennett MV, et al. Quantitative tissue characterization of infarct core and border zone in patients with ischemic cardiomyopathy by magnetic resonance is associated with future cardiovascular events. J Am Coll Cardiol. 2010;55(24):2762–8.
163. Mahnken AH, Koos R, Katoh M, Wildberger JE, Spuentrup E, Buecker A, et al. Assessment of myocardial viability in reperfused acute myocardial infarction using 16-slice computed tomography in comparison to magnetic resonance imaging. J Am Coll Cardiol. 2005;45(12):2042–7.
164. Chiou KR, Liu CP, Peng NJ, Huang WC, Hsiao SH, Huang YL, et al. Identification and viability assessment of infarcted myocardium with late enhancement multidetector computed tomography: comparison with thallium single photon emission computed tomography and echocardiography. Am Heart J. 2008;155(4):738–45.
165. Sato A, Hiroe M, Nozato T, Hikita H, Ito Y, Ohigashi H, et al. Early validation study of 64-slice multidetector computed tomography for the assessment of myocardial viability and the prediction of left ventricular remodelling after acute myocardial infarction. Eur Heart J. 2008;29(4):490–8.
166. Shriki JE, Shinbane J, Lee C, Khan AR, Burns N, Hindoyan A, et al. Incidental myocardial infarct on conventional nongated CT: a review of the spectrum of findings with gated CT and cardiac MRI correlation. AJR Am J Roentgenol. 2012;198(3):496–504.
167. Zhao L, Ma X, Feuchtner GM, Zhang C, Fan Z. Quantification of myocardial delayed enhancement and wall thickness in hypertrophic cardiomyopathy: multidetector computed tomography versus magnetic resonance imaging. Eur J Radiol. 2014;83(10):1778–85.
168. McKenna WJ, Thiene G, Nava A, Fontaliran F, Blomstrom-Lundqvist C, Fontaine G, et al. Diagnosis of arrhythmogenic right ventricular dysplasia/cardiomyopathy. Task Force of the Working Group Myocardial and Pericardial Disease of the

European Society of Cardiology and of the Scientific Council on Cardiomyopathies of the International Society and Federation of Cardiology. Br Heart J. 1994;71(3):215–8.

169. Marcus FI, McKenna WJ, Sherrill D, Basso C, Bauce B, Bluemke DA, et al. Diagnosis of arrhythmogenic right ventricular cardiomyopathy/dysplasia: proposed modification of the task force criteria. Circulation. 2010;121(13):1533–41.
170. Wu YW, Tadamura E, Kanao S, Yamamuro M, Nishiyama K, Kimura T, et al. Structural and functional assessment of arrhythmogenic right ventricular dysplasia/cardiomyopathy by multislice computed tomography: comparison with cardiovascular magnetic resonance. Int J Cardiol. 2007;115(3):e118–21.
171. Bomma C, Dalal D, Tandri H, Prakasa K, Nasir K, Roguin A, et al. Evolving role of multidetector computed tomography in evaluation of arrhythmogenic right ventricular dysplasia/cardiomyopathy. Am J Cardiol. 2007;100(1):99–105.
172. Matsuo S, Sato Y, Nakae I, Masuda D, Yomota M, Ashihara T, et al. Left ventricular involvement in arrhythmogenic right ventricular cardiomyopathy demonstrated by multidetector-row computed tomography. Int J Cardiol. 2007;115(3):e129–31.
173. Komatsu Y, Cochet H, Jadidi A, Sacher F, Shah A, Derval N, et al. Regional myocardial wall thinning at multidetector computed tomography correlates to arrhythmogenic substrate in postinfarction ventricular tachycardia: assessment of structural and electrical substrate. Circ Arrhythm Electrophysiol. 2013;6(2):342–50.
174. Sasaki T, Calkins H, Miller CF, Zviman MM, Zipunnikov V, Arai T, et al. New insight into scar-related ventricular tachycardia circuits in ischemic cardiomyopathy: fat deposition after myocardial infarction on computed tomography–A pilot study. Heart Rhythm Off J Heart Rhythm Soc. 2015;12(7):1508–18.
175. Cochet H, Komatsu Y, Sacher F, Jadidi AS, Scherr D, Riffaud M, et al. Integration of merged delayed-enhanced magnetic resonance imaging and multidetector computed tomography for the guidance of ventricular tachycardia ablation: a pilot study. J Cardiovasc Electrophysiol. 2013;24(4):419–26.
176. Cesario DA, Shinbane JS, Cao M, Saxon LA, Cunningham M, Essilfie G. Use of CT delayed enhancement imaging and a ventricular assist device in ablation of recurrent ventricular tachycardia. Innov Cardiac Rhythm Manag. 2010;1:54–8.
177. Friehling M, Menon PG, Ludwig DR, Schwartzman D. Single-photon emission computed tomographic-multidetector computed tomographic fusion image integration: a potential aid to left ventricular substrate ablation. Europace Euro Pacing Arrhythmias Cardiac Electrophysiol J Working Groups Cardiac Pacing Arrhythmias Cardiac Cell Electrophysiol Eur Soc Cardiol. 2014;16(12):1860–3.
178. Akutsu Y, Kaneko K, Kodama Y, Li HL, Suyama J, Watanabe N, et al. Stratified three-dimensional fusion imaging of delayed enhancement magnetic resonance and multi-detector computed tomography to identify a ventricular tachycardia focus. Int J Cardiovasc Imaging. 2013;29(8):1705–6.
179. Estornell-Erill J, Ridocci-Soriano F, Quesada-Dorador A, Federico-Zaragoza P, Fabregat-Andres O, Palanca-Gil V, et al. Images in cardiology. Microvascular obstruction after radiofrequency ablation of ventricular tachycardia: comprehensive evaluation by magnetic resonance imaging and computed tomography. J Am Coll Cardiol. 2010;56(13):e25.
180. Rathod RH, Prakash A, Powell AJ, Geva T. Myocardial fibrosis identified by cardiac magnetic resonance late gadolinium enhancement is associated with adverse ventricular mechanics and ventricular tachycardia late after Fontan operation. J Am Coll Cardiol. 2010;55(16):1721–8.
181. Teh AW, Medi C, Lee G, Rosso R, Sparks PB, Morton JB, et al. Long-term outcome following ablation of atrial flutter occurring late after atrial septal defect repair. Pacing Clin Electrophysiol PACE. 2011;34(4):431–5.
182. Yap SC, Harris L, Downar E, Nanthakumar K, Silversides CK, Chauhan VS. Evolving electroanatomic substrate and intra-atrial reentrant tachycardia late after Fontan surgery. J Cardiovasc Electrophysiol. 2012;23(4):339–45.
183. Valente AM, Gauvreau K, Assenza GE, Babu-Narayan SV, Schreier J, Gatzoulis MA, et al. Contemporary predictors of death and sustained ventricular tachycardia in patients with repaired tetralogy of Fallot enrolled in the INDICATOR cohort. Heart. 2014;100(3):247–53.
184. Oosterhof T, Mulder BJ, Vliegen HW, de Roos A. Corrected tetralogy of Fallot: delayed enhancement in right ventricular outflow tract. Radiology. 2005;237(3):868–71.
185. Harris MA, Johnson TR, Weinberg PM, Fogel MA. Delayed-enhancement cardiovascular magnetic resonance identifies fibrous tissue in children after surgery for congenital heart disease. J Thorac Cardiovasc Surg. 2007;133(3):676–81.
186. Zeppenfeld K, Schalij MJ, Bartelings MM, Tedrow UB, Koplan BA, Soejima K, et al. Catheter ablation of ventricular tachycardia after repair of congenital heart disease: electroanatomic identification of the critical right ventricular isthmus. Circulation. 2007;116(20):2241–52.
187. Ueda A, Suman-Horduna I, Mantziari L, Gujic M, Marchese P, Ho SY, et al. Contemporary outcomes of supraventricular tachycardia ablation in congenital heart disease: a single-center experience in 116 patients. Circ Arrhythm Electrophysiol. 2013;6(3):606–13.
188. Jongbloed MR, Lamb HJ, Bax JJ, Schuijf JD, de Roos A, van der Wall EE, et al. Noninvasive visualization of the cardiac venous system using multislice computed tomography. J Am Coll Cardiol. 2005;45(5):749–53.
189. Shinbane JS, Girsky MJ, Mao S, Budoff MJ. Thebesian valve imaging with electron beam CT angiography: implications for resynchronization therapy. Pacing Clin Electrophysiol PACE. 2004;27(9):1331–2.
190. Matsumoto Y, Krishnan S, Fowler SJ, Saremi F, Kondo T, Ahsan C, et al. Detection of phrenic nerves and their relation to cardiac anatomy using 64-slice multidetector computed tomography. Am J Cardiol. 2007;100(1):133–7.
191. Carbonaro S, Villines TC, Hausleiter J, Devine PJ, Gerber TC, Taylor AJ. International, multidisciplinary update of the 2006 Appropriateness Criteria for cardiac computed tomography. J Cardiovasc Comput Tomogr. 2009;3(4):224–32.
192. Hendel RC, Patel MR, Kramer CM, Poon M, Hendel RC, Carr JC, et al. ACCF/ACR/SCCT/SCMR/ASNC/NASCI/SCAI/SIR 2006 appropriateness criteria for cardiac computed tomography and cardiac magnetic resonance imaging: a report of the American College of Cardiology Foundation Quality Strategic Directions Committee Appropriateness Criteria Working Group, American College of Radiology, Society of Cardiovascular Computed Tomography, Society for Cardiovascular Magnetic Resonance, American Society of Nuclear Cardiology, North American Society for Cardiac Imaging, Society for Cardiovascular Angiography and Interventions, and Society of Interventional Radiology. J Am Coll Cardiol. 2006;48(7):1475–97.
193. European Heart Rhythm A, European Society of C, Heart Rhythm S, Heart Failure Society of A, American Society of E, American Heart A, et al. 2012 EHRA/HRS expert consensus statement on cardiac resynchronization therapy in heart failure: implant and follow-up recommendations and management. Heart Rhythm: Off J Heart Rhythm Soc. 2012;9(9):1524–76.
194. Girsky MJ, Shinbane JS, Ahmadi N, Mao S, Flores F, Budoff MJ. Prospective randomized trial of venous cardiac computed tomographic angiography for facilitation of cardiac resynchronization therapy. Pacing Clin Electrophysiol PACE. 2010;33(10):1182–7.
195. Auricchio A, Sorgente A, Soubelet E, Regoli F, Spinucci G, Vaillant R, et al. Accuracy and usefulness of fusion imaging between

three-dimensional coronary sinus and coronary veins computed tomographic images with projection images obtained using fluoroscopy. Europace Euro Pacing Arrhythmias Cardiac Electrophysiol J Working Groups Cardiac Pacing Arrhythmias Cardiac Cell Electrophysiol Eur Soc Cardiol. 2009;11(11):1483–90.

196. Cao M, Chang P, Garon B, Shinbane JS. Cardiac resynchronization therapy: double cannulation approach to coronary venous lead placement via a prominent thebesian valve. Pacing Clin Electrophysiol PACE. 2013;36(3):e70–3.

197. Da Costa A, Gate-Martinet A, Rouffiange P, Cerisier A, Nadrouss A, Bisch L, et al. Anatomical factors involved in difficult cardiac resynchronization therapy procedure: a non-invasive study using dual-source 64-multi-slice computed tomography. Europace Eur Pacing Arrhythmias Cardiac Electrophysiol J Working Groups Cardiac Pacing Arrhythmias Cardiac Cell Electrophysiol Eur Soc Cardiol. 2012;14(6):833–40.

198. Sommer A, Kronborg MB, Norgaard BL, Gerdes C, Mortensen PT, Nielsen JC. Left and right ventricular lead positions are imprecisely determined by fluoroscopy in cardiac resynchronization therapy: a comparison with cardiac computed tomography. Europace Eur Pacing Arrhythmias Cardiac Electrophysiol J Working Groups Cardiac Pacing Arrhythmias Cardiac Cell Electrophysiol Eur Soc Cardiol. 2014;16(9):1334–41.

199. Rickard J, Ingelmo C, Sraow D, Wilkoff BL, Grimm RA, Schoenhagen P, et al. Chest radiography is a poor predictor of left ventricular lead position in patients undergoing cardiac resynchronization therapy: comparison with multidetector computed tomography. J Interv Cardiac Electrophysiol Int J Arrhythmias Pacing. 2011;32(1):59–65.

200. Pang BJ, Lui EH, Joshi SB, Tacey MA, Alison J, Seneviratne SK, et al. Pacing and implantable cardioverter defibrillator lead perforation as assessed by multiplanar reformatted ECG-gated cardiac computed tomography and clinical correlates. Pacing Clin Electrophysiol PACE. 2014;37(5):537–45.

201. Yavari A, Khawaja ZO, Krishnamoorthy S, McWilliams ET. Perforation of right ventricular free wall by pacemaker lead detected by multidetector computed tomography. Europace Eur Pacing Arrhythmias Cardiac Electrophysiol J Working Groups Cardiac Pacing Arrhythmias Cardiac Cell Electrophysiol Eur Soc Cardiol. 2009;11(2):252–4.

202. Kim YS, Oh S, Park KW, Ree Cho K, Choi YS. Uncomplicated right ventricular lead perforation diagnosed with computed tomography after permanent pacemaker implantation. Clin Cardiol. 2009;32(7):E54.

203. der Maur AC, Hoffmann A, Brink T, Erne P. Cardiac computed tomography for the diagnosis of right ventricular implantable cardioverter-defibrillator lead perforation. Eur Heart J. 2009;30(7):869.

204. Van de Veire NR, Marsan NA, Schuijf JD, Bleeker GB, Wijffels MC, van Erven L, et al. Noninvasive imaging of cardiac venous anatomy with 64-slice multi-slice computed tomography and noninvasive assessment of left ventricular dyssynchrony by 3-dimensional tissue synchronization imaging in patients with heart failure scheduled for cardiac resynchronization therapy. Am J Cardiol. 2008;101(7):1023–9.

205. White JA, Yee R, Yuan X, Krahn A, Skanes A, Parker M, et al. Delayed enhancement magnetic resonance imaging predicts response to cardiac resynchronization therapy in patients with intraventricular dyssynchrony. J Am Coll Cardiol. 2006; 48(10):1953–60.

206. Bleeker GB, Kaandorp TA, Lamb HJ, Boersma E, Steendijk P, de Roos A, et al. Effect of posterolateral scar tissue on clinical and echocardiographic improvement after cardiac resynchronization therapy. Circulation. 2006;113(7):969–76.

207. Chalil S, Stegemann B, Muhyaldeen SA, Khadjooi K, Foley PW, Smith RE, et al. Effect of posterolateral left ventricular scar on mortality and morbidity following cardiac resynchronization therapy. Pacing Clin Electrophysiol PACE. 2007;30(10):1201–9.

Cardiovascular CT: Interventional Cardiology Applications

25

Jeffrey M. Schussler

Abstract

Interventional cardiologists should embrace cardiac CT as a helpful additional to their armamentarium in the treatment of cardiovascular disease. CCTA can improve the discrimination of patients for whom invasive evaluation and treatment will be most helpful. It can be used in lieu of invasive evaluation after coronary and cardiac intervention, and is now mandatory in the evaluation of the structural heart disease patient.

Keywords

CCTA • Coronary CTA • CTCA • Coronary angiography • Percutaneous coronary intervention • PCI • Non-invasive Angiography

Introduction

With its high specificity, coronary computed tomographic angiography (CCTA) can be an extremely helpful test in determining which patients do not require cardiac catheterization. Given this fact, it seems somewhat counterintuitive that this technology would be embraced by interventional cardiologists. One would theorize that a strong non-invasive angiography program would reduce volume and divert patients away from the catheterization lab. In fact, centers where CCTA is available do not appear to have led to a reduction in invasive volumes [1].

Prior to invasive catheterization, CCTA can also help interventionalists plan percutaneous coronary intervention (PCI) strategies by alerting them to the presence of left main, ostial, or multivessel disease, length and severity of lesions, presence and amount of calcification, tortuosity, coronary variants, and anomalies. It can also be used to guide strategies for approaching chronic total occlusions. After percutaneous revascularization, CCTA has utility in evaluation of stent patency, and after coronary artery bypass grafting (CABG) to evaluate graft patency. In the arena of structural heart disease, it can be used for planning for transcatheter aortic valve replacement, atrial septal defect closure, as well as planning of other cardiac interventional procedures. In addition, given the climate of scrutiny regarding appropriateness of interventions, CCTA can be used to reduce unnecessary diagnostic cardiac catheterization volume.

Invasive Cardiac Catheterization

Invasive cardiac catheterization, the "gold standard" diagnostic technique for the evaluation of coronary artery disease (CAD), has been used for clinical evaluation of coronary stenosis since the 1960s [2–4]. However, it has several well-known drawbacks. There is a certain degree of inter-observer variation when describing degree of stenosis [5]. Quantitative coronary angiography, which is not used routinely in clinical practice, is helpful but does not eliminate this error [6, 7].

J.M. Schussler, MD, FACC, FSCAI, FSCCT, FACP
Division of Cardiology, Department of Internal Medicine, Baylor University Medical Center, Dallas, TX/Jack and Jane Hamilton Heart and Vascular Hospital, 621 N. Hall St. Suite 400, Dallas, TX 75226, USA

Division of Cardiology, Department of Medicine, Texas A&M College of Medicine, Dallas, TX, USA
e-mail: Jeffrey.Schussler@Baylorhealth.edu

M.J. Budoff, J.S. Shinbane (eds.), *Cardiac CT Imaging: Diagnosis of Cardiovascular Disease*,
DOI 10.1007/978-3-319-28219-0_25

Invasive coronary angiography allows only for the definition of the lumen of the coronary. The plaque protruding into the lumen of the coronary artery remains non-visualized unless intravascular ultrasound is used [8, 9]. This may lead to under-identification of the presence of disease in patients with minimal angiographic disease, and can contribute to underestimation of plaque burden due to compensatory expansion of the coronary arteries [10–13]. These non-flow-limiting stenoses can be the cause of future acute coronary syndromes and myocardial infarction [14].

There is a small but inherent risk of complication associated with invasive evaluation of the coronary arteries. This is due to the need to directly instrument the coronary arteries, as well as the obligate arterial access. The risk of major complications such as death are approximately 0.1 % [15, 16], with a combined risk of all major complications, such as stroke, renal failure, or major bleeding, of ≤2 % [17, 18]. Minor complications, such as local pain, ecchymosis, or hematoma at the access site, can be higher, and are frequently a source of delayed discharge and patient dissatisfaction [19].

Invasive coronary angiography is considered the "gold standard" for definitive cardiac evaluation in patients with chest pain [20]. As it is such a powerful tool, invasive angiography has even been suggested as the test of choice in inpatients with chest pain [21]. Angiography has been shown to be better able to detect the presence of atherosclerotic coronary disease than functional tests, reduces early returns to the emergency department, and has an overall higher level of patient satisfaction [22]. Invasive angiography has even been suggested as the screening test of choice in the primary prevention of CAD [23]. However, due to the aforementioned risks, it often is used as a second line study in patients who have low-to-moderate presumed risk or after performing functional testing [24].

CT Coronary Evaluation Prior to Invasive Coronary Evaluation

Determination of Coronary Atherosclerosis Prior to Invasive Evaluation or Intervention

While traditional invasive angiography may be highly accurate, less than 40 % of those patients who have invasive angiography ultimately are found to have significant coronary disease [25]. With its high specificity and negative predictive value, CCTA has the ability to accurately evaluate those patients who have no significant coronary disease, obviating the need for further evaluation [26].

In patients with chest pain who have no observable coronary disease by CCTA, there is a nearly 100 % chance that they will not require further cardiac evaluation, and will have no cardiac events for several years (Fig. 25.1) [27]. Accuracy is high enough to determine whether coronary arteries have high-grade lesions, and which have minimal disease (Fig. 25.2), and can accurately exclude left main or multi-vessel coronary disease prior to catheterization [28–32]. This can mean the difference between planning an intervention on a single proximal vessel or on the expectation of a difficult multiple vessel intervention [33, 34].

CCTA may also allow for improved planning of antiplatelet loading prior to catheterization. If suspected surgical disease is discovered on CCTA, a "loading dose" of clopidogrel may be withheld, reducing a delay in surgical revascularization (Fig. 25.3). While still not standard of care, newer studies suggest that it may be feasible in the future to send patients directly to coronary artery bypass graft surgery without invasive angiography, relying on CCTA alone to guide surgical decision-making [35]. Once lesions are found, CCTA can also act as a "preview" of the coronary anatomy for planning of stent placement, including stent sizing prior to invasive coronary angiography (Fig. 25.4) [36].

Visualization of Coronary Ostia

Visualization of the ostia of the coronaries may help an interventionalist in several ways. Anomalous coronary arteries are better seen with CT, and can be helpful in planning catheter selection prior to invasive angiography [37]. Even in cases where true anomalies are not present, it can be helpful to know that a patient has an "anterior takeoff" of a right coronary or a "posterior takeoff" of a left main, as this may lead to use of specific types of catheters for the engagement of that artery (Fig. 25.5). Coronary CT is superior to invasive angiography in evaluating location and severity of ostial stenosis (Fig. 25.6), and does not induce coronary spasm, which can mimic ostial disease [38].

Chronic Total Occlusions

Since the bolus of contrast reaches the arteries simultaneously, it is difficult to distinguish high-grade lesions from totally occluded coronaries. Newer data suggest that when occlusions are found, CCTA may be helpful in defining the length of stenosis, complexity of the plaque, and therefore give insight into the potential ease or difficulty in undertaking complex percutaneous revascularization of these lesions (Fig. 25.7) [39–42].

Left Main Disease

The presence of severe left main disease is potentially dangerous if not known prior to diagnostic angiography. Placement

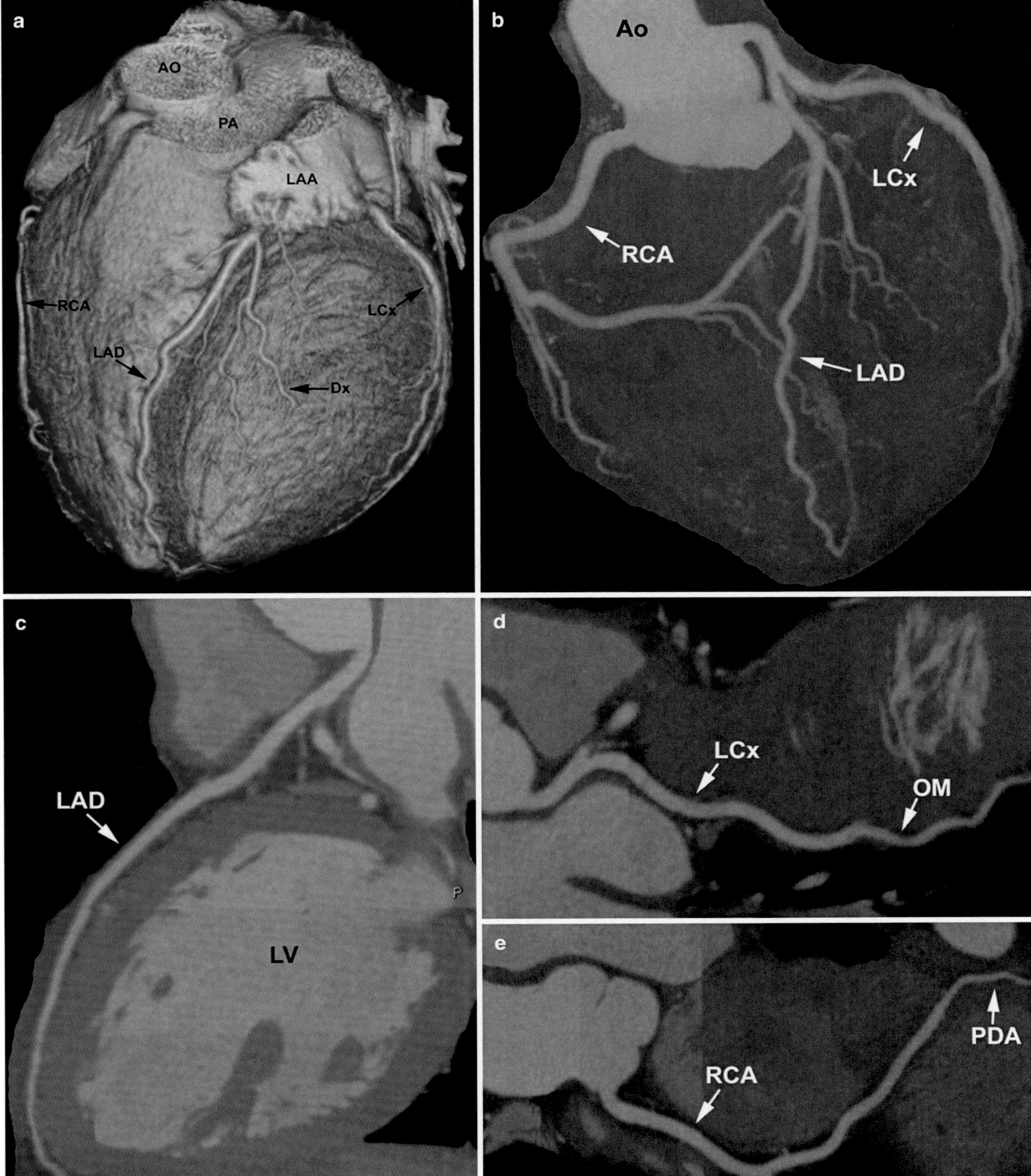

Fig. 25.1 Normal CCTA in a patient with risk factors for coronary disease and chest pain. A 3-D view (**a**) and maximum intensity projection (**b**) of the coronary anatomy demonstrates a right dominant system without coronary anomalies. Individual curved reformatted images of the left anterior descending (**c**), left circumflex (**d**), and right coronary artery (**e**) demonstrate no plaque in any of the arterial tree. *Ao* aorta, *LAA* left atrial appendage, *LAD* left anterior descending, *Dx* diagonal, *LCx* left circumflex, *RCA* right coronary artery, *PA* pulmonary artery, *LV* left ventricle, *OM* obtuse marginal, *PDA* posterior descending artery

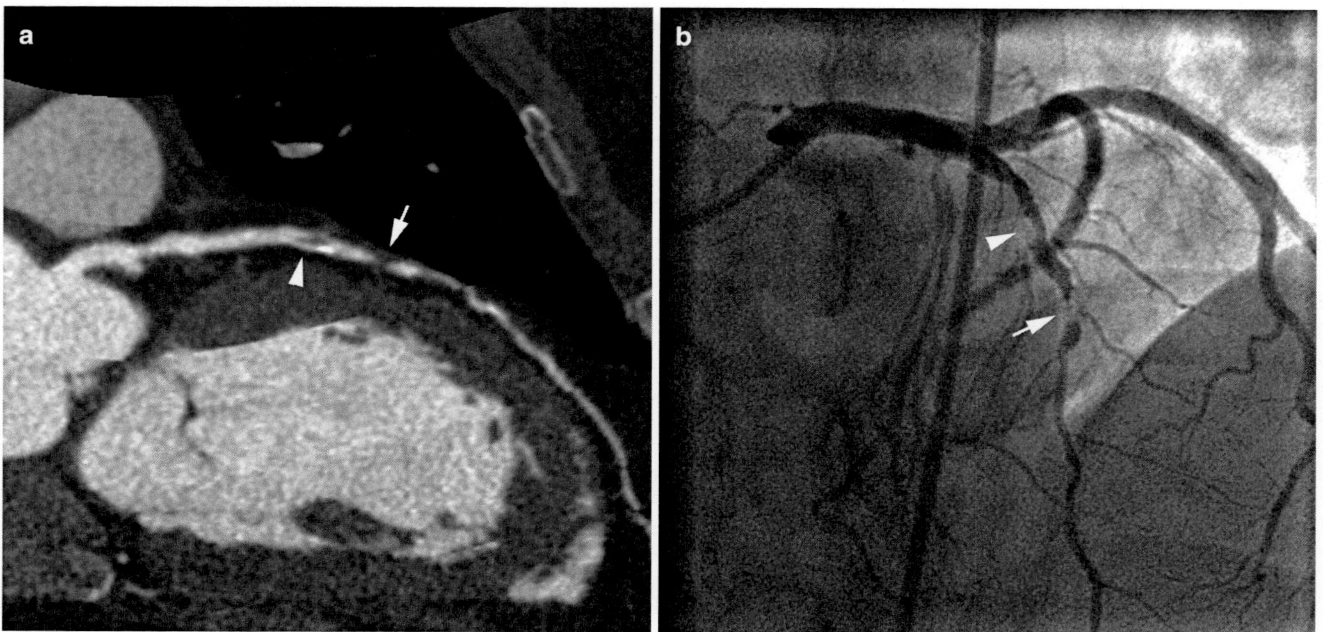

Fig. 25.2 Patient with chest pain referred for CCTA. On CT images, a high-grade lesion is seen in the mid left anterior descending (**a**, *arrow*). More moderate plaque is noted proximal to the lesion (**a**, *arrowhead*). The same lesions are seen on the follow-up invasive angiogram (**b**)

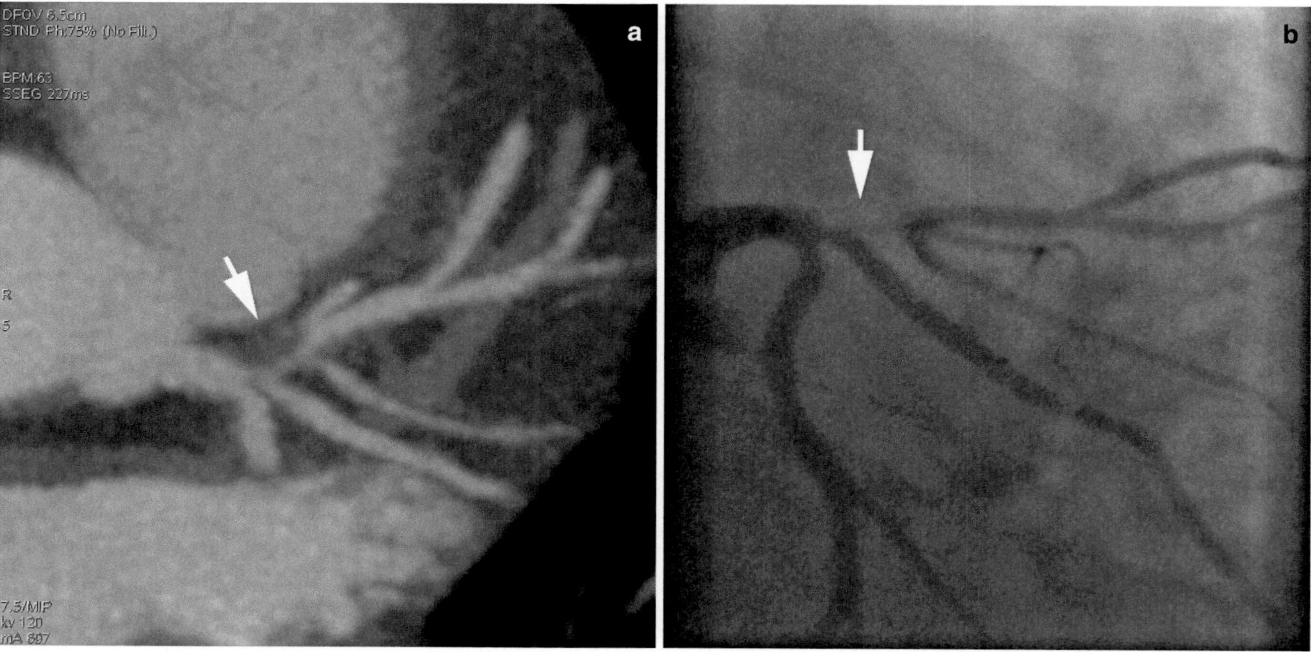

Fig. 25.3 A CCTA demonstrating a high-grade non-calcified plaque involving the ostium of the left anterior descending (LAD) and distal left main (**a**, *arrow*). The invasive angiogram (**b**) is shown for comparison. Based on the findings of the CCTA scan, it was felt that the location of the plaque was unfavorable for PCI as there would be a high risk for compromise of the left circumflex, ramus intermedius (RI), and first diagonal branches. This was less apparent on invasive angiography. A surgical consultation was obtained, and the patient went on to successful bypass of the LAD, diagonal, and RI

of a catheter into a diseased left main coronary artery can cause dramatic reduction of coronary blood flow, and can even result in death during diagnostic angiography [43, 44]. In a situation where left main disease is discovered on the CCTA, plans can be made to use smaller diagnostic catheters, or even have an intra-aortic balloon pump stationed close at hand.

Left main disease identified on the CCTA allows preparation for the potential hemodynamic compromise of

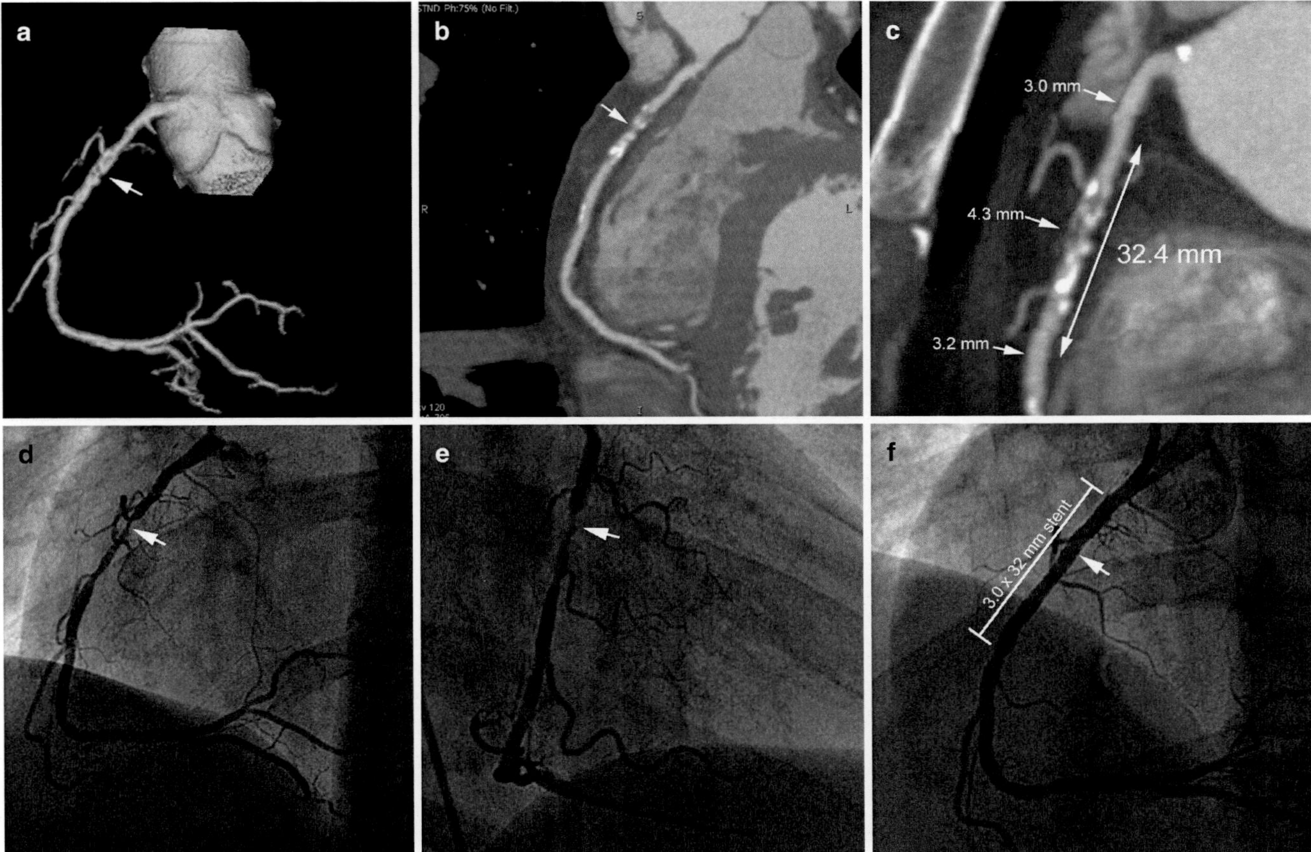

Fig. 25.4 CCTA of a patient with cardiac risk factors and chest pain. A CCTA (**a**, **b**, *arrows*) demonstrated a high grade lesion in the proximal right coronary artery. The severity is suggested by the complex nature of the plaque, with both soft and calcific portions, as well as the compensatory expansion of the artery within the most severe area (**c**). The length and the extent of plaque were evident from the CCTA (**d**). Invasive coronary angiogram confirmed the high grade lesion in the right coronary artery. A stent was selected (**e**) to cover not only the high grade area (*arrow*), but also the more moderate plaque proximal and distal to the most severe portions of the lesion (**f**) (Reprinted from Bhella et al. [36]. With permission from Bhella et al., Baylor University Medical Center Proceedings)

engaging a catheter in a severely diseased left main coronary artery. It is important to remember that CCTA cannot provide hemodynamic information. It is prudent to proceed to invasive evaluation if non-invasive angiography suggests significant left main stenosis (Fig. 25.8). Now that left main coronary intervention has become more commonplace, CTCA is a useful tool in pre-PCI planning for left main coronary intervention. It allows for accurate sizing of vessels, and gives additional insight into plaque burden, calcification and geometry of the major epicardial branches [46–48].

Fractional Flow Reserve and Myocardial Perfusion Using Computed Tomography

As with invasive angiography, CT coronary angiography provides an anatomic assessment of coronary artery stenoses. It is clear that CCTA is at least as good, if not better, than perfusion assessment in evaluating for the presence and significance of coronary disease [49, 50]. Functional assessment of coronary lesions, especially when combined with anatomic assessment, allows for improved discrimination of flow limiting versus non-flow limiting stenosis [51]. Proving functional significance prior to PCI leads to enduring clinical benefit [52, 53]. Newer techniques combining non-invasive coronary angiography with either myocardial perfusion (CT-MPI) or fractional flow reserve (FFRCT) may allow for both anatomic as well as functional evaluation using CT [54, 55].

Plaque Evaluation

Comparison of CTCA with Intravascular Ultrasound

CCTA, like intravascular ultrasound (IVUS), has the ability to visualize plaque and to roughly quantify its amount [56–58]. It is well known that patients with minimal CAD may still

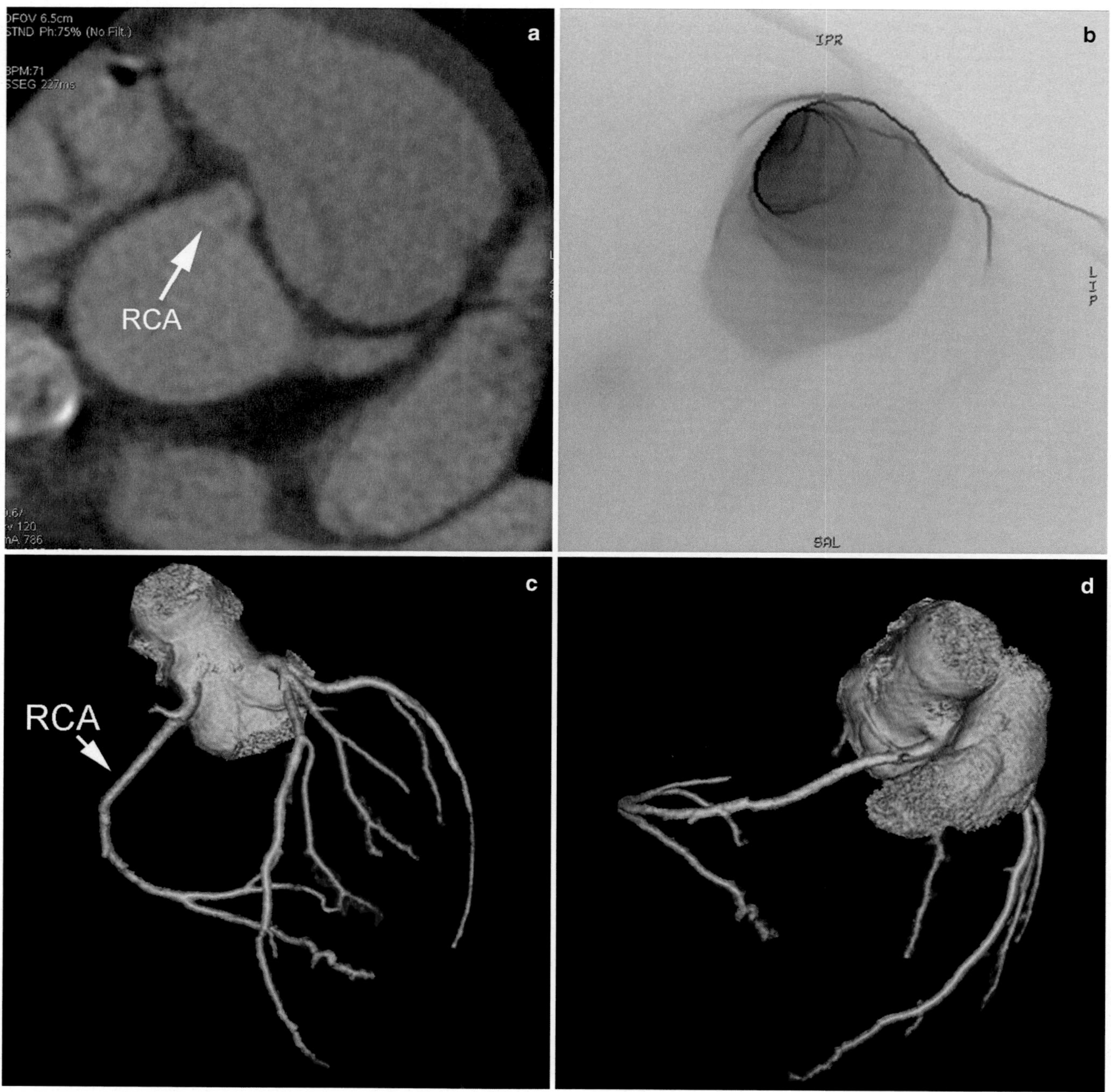

Fig. 25.5 CCTA of a patient with an "anterior" takeoff of the right coronary artery (RCA). The axial image (**a**) demonstrates the ostium of the right coronary artery slightly higher and more anterior than normally seen. The location on the axial "clock-face" of the aortic root is approximately "1 o'clock" rather than the normal "10 to 12 o'clock" location of a typical RCA ostium. This RCA location is not truly anomalous and has no impact on the function of the artery. The ostium, seen on the 3-D reconstructed image (**b**), has a normal round orifice. Three dimensional views (**c**) show the high-anterior takeoff in relation to the cusp and the left main. The pulmonary outflow (**d**) does not impinge on the artery. This artery would be best catheterized using a modified Amplatz-type catheter rather than a typical Judkins-right catheter

have events due to plaque which is not fully defined by invasive coronary angiography. These types of non-stenotic plaques are detectable by CCTA, and there is ongoing research in the evaluation of plaque-stability using CCTA (Fig. 25.9) [59–62].

Coronary Remodeling

Unless IVUS is used, Glagov remodeling of coronary atherosclerotic lesions can be appreciated on CCTA better than with invasive angiography (Fig. 25.10) [63]. As

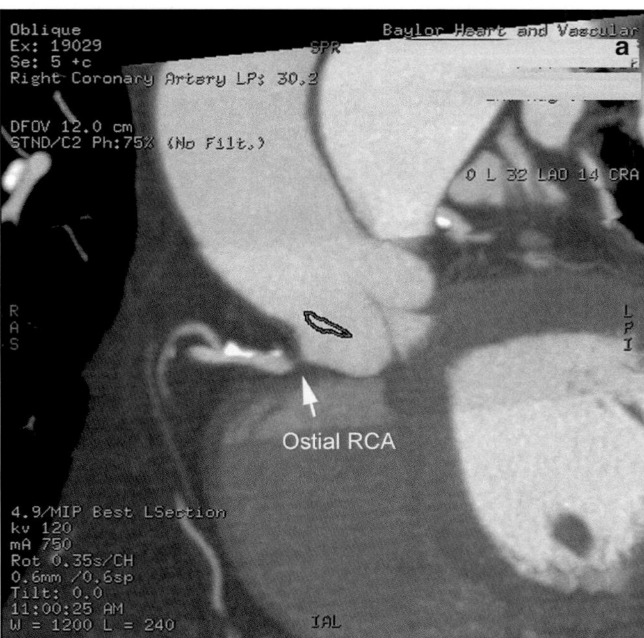

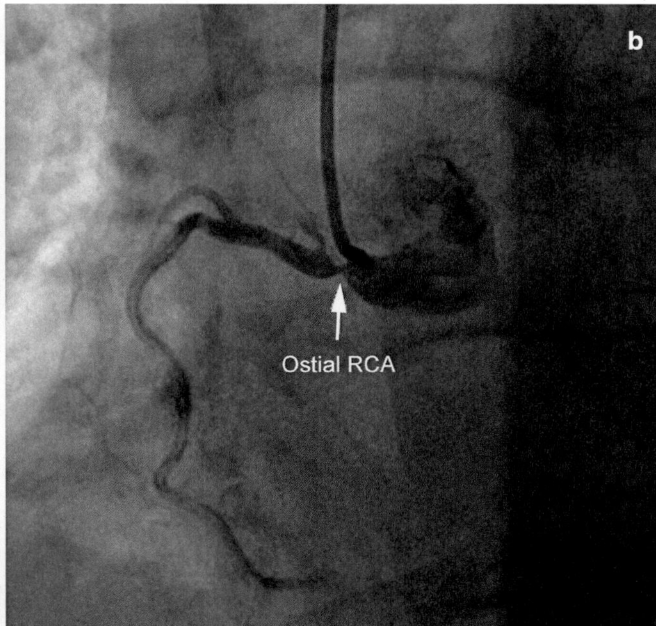

Fig. 25.6 Oblique reconstructed views of the right coronary artery (RCA) demonstrate a focal, high-grade ostial lesion (**a** – *arrow*). Corresponding invasive angiogram (**b** – *arrow*) confirms location and severity of this blockage. Given the CCTA, care was taken with the diagnostic angiogram not to aggressively "seat" the catheter inside the artery. Foreknowledge of the anatomy allowed for planning of guide selection, as well as pre-loading with dual antiplatelet therapy, as there was no suggest of surgical disease

the plaque intrudes on the lumen of the artery, compensatory arterial expansion occurs, which is seen on CCTA, but not by conventional angiography [64, 65]. Outward coronary remodeling is often a clue that the plaque is unstable, or that the stenosis seen by CCTA is severe (Fig. 25.11) [66, 67].

Post Intervention Evaluation by CTCA

Post-PCI Evaluation

While technically more challenging, CCTA can be used for coronary evaluation after stent placement. Imaging through stents, especially in smaller caliber arteries, can be problematic due to a significant amount of beam hardening artifact due to the scatter of x-rays by the metallic stents. It is important to use appropriate window and threshold levels to obtain adequate images, and techniques are available to assist in reducing artifact. In-stent restenosis, a process that occurs through smooth muscle cell migration and neointimal hyperplasia, has also been successfully evaluated by CCTA (Fig. 25.12) [68, 69]. Patients who have had ostial stents placed can be evaluated for geographic "miss" of stenoses, in preparation for repeat coronary angiography or intervention [70, 71].

Post-bypass Evaluation

There is excellent data to support the use of CCTA in the evaluation of CABG patients [72–74]. In some respects, the imaging of bypass grafts is easier than native arteries, as there is less movement of the grafts and greater contrast between the contrast in the grafts and the surrounding tissue. Visualization of graft patency is often more easily performed using 3-D views rather than axial or even MPR views. For many newer post-bypass studies, CCTA has become the test of choice to evaluate graft patency rather than traditional invasive evaluation [75–79] (Fig. 25.13).

In post CABG patients, it is important to alert the technologist that the study is to be performed with the intention of looking at aorta-coronary bypass grafts, so that more of the ascending aorta is visualized. Slice thickness may be increased to reduce radiation. Imaging can be performed on conduits with metallic proximal connectors, but there may be some hardening artifact when many metallic clips are present [77, 80, 81].

Patients are sometimes referred for invasive catheterization with a history of CABG surgery, without information regarding the types of grafts or which arteries were bypassed. It can then be a challenging and time-consuming task to find all of the grafts at cardiac catheterization. CCTA can be helpful, not only by delineating which grafts are patent, but by providing a "roadmap" as to the number of grafts, their

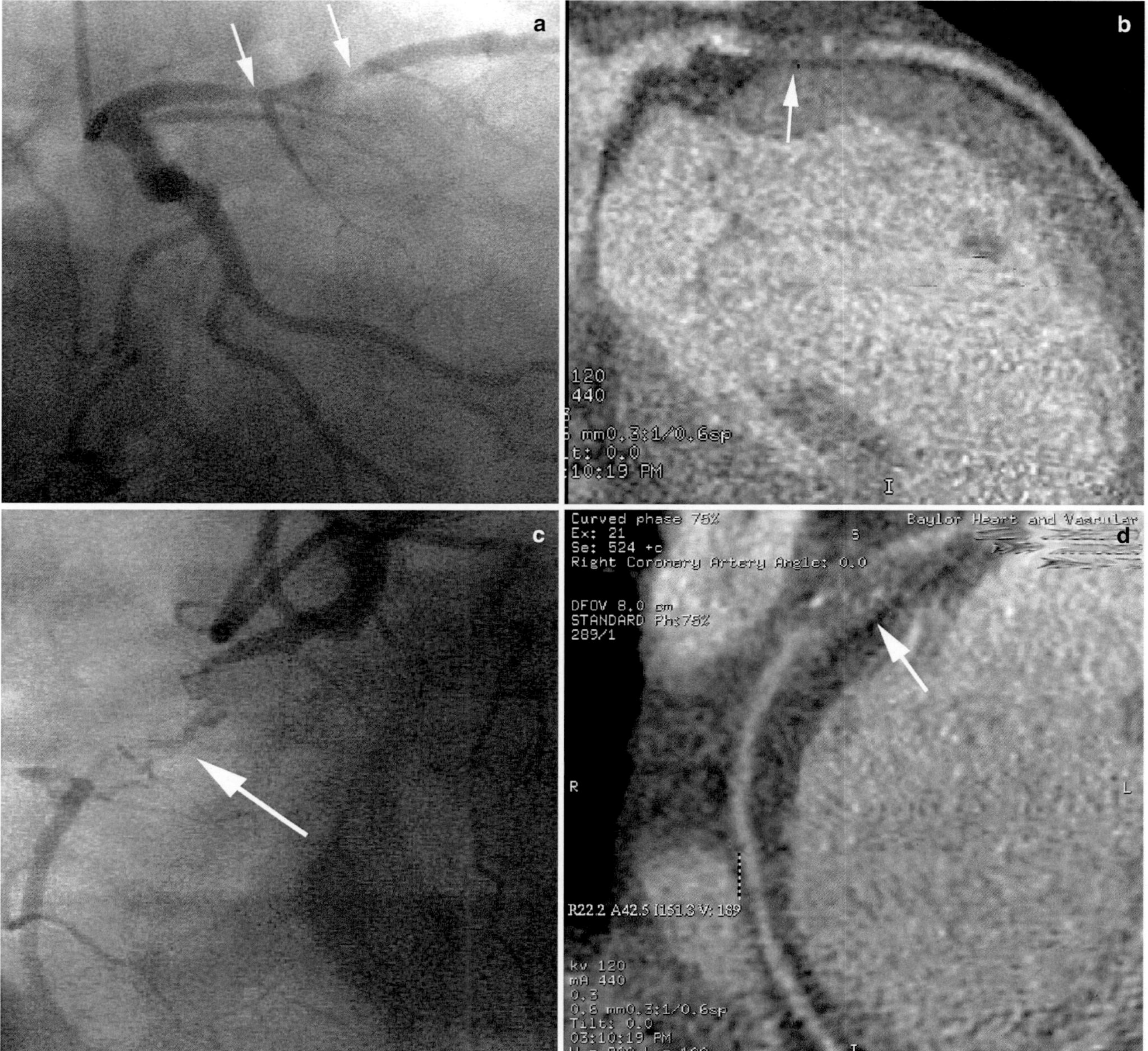

Fig. 25.7 A patient with multivessel coronary disease: A high-grade lesion is shown in the left anterior descending, demonstrated by invasive angiography (**a**) and CCTA (**b**). The lesion has the same CCTA characteristics as a complete occlusion with bridging collaterals (**c**, **d** – *arrow*). Severity of stenosis is suggested by the paucity of contrast, compensatory expansion, and a large plaque burden in the artery. Complete occlusions cannot be easily distinguished from very high-grade stenoses based on CCTA characteristics

origins, as well as the location of the anastomoses with native vessels prior to invasive angiography.

Even though evaluation of bypass grafts is relatively straightforward with CCTA, it has to be kept in mind that in most cases the clinical situation will warrant evaluating not only the status of the patient's bypass grafts, but also that of the native coronary arteries either distal to the bypass insertion site or of those coronary arteries that did not receive a bypass graft. Frequently, evaluation of native arteries in patients with bypass grafts tends to be difficult or even impossible with CCTA because of the often pronounced calcification that exists in the native coronary arteries of CABG patients [82, 83].

Evaluation of the Non-coronary Cardiac Surgery Patient

There is growing literature to support a strategy of non-invasive coronary angiography in patients with only low or moderate risk for coronary disease, prior to non-coronary cardiac surgery [84]. In patients with valvular disease, such

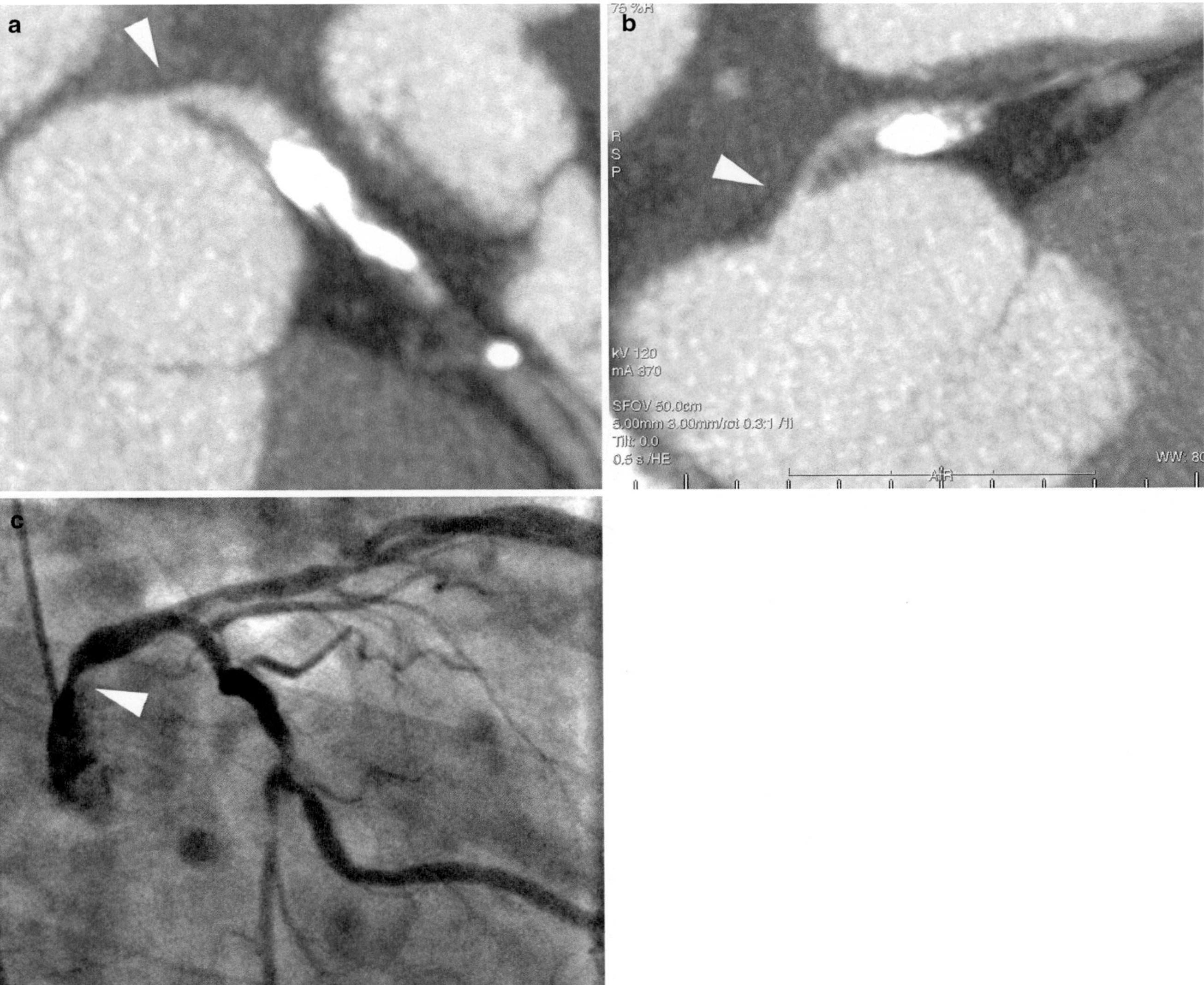

Fig. 25.8 A high-grade stenosis of the left main coronary artery seen by CCTA (**a**, **b**, *arrowhead*). The corresponding invasive coronary angiogram is seen (**c**, *arrowhead*), demonstrating a severe angiographic stenosis. There was immediate "damping" of the pressure tracing upon engagement of a 4-French diagnostic catheter. The noninvasive study was so dramatically abnormal that it prompted the operator to deliberately choose a smaller French-sized catheter than normal, and have an intra-aortic balloon pump in the room prior to catheterization (Reprinted from Schussler et al. [45]. With permission from Schussler et al., Baylor University Medical Center Proceedings)

as aortic valve stenosis or regurgitation, it is feasible to exclude concomitant coronary stenosis prior to aortic valve surgery or even TAVR [85–87]. With congenital heart disease, coronary anomalies, or cardiac masses, it may actually be more advantageous to perform a CCTA, as it gives additional structural information which is relevant to the case [37, 88–90]. Technology is now at the point where many decisions to proceed with cardiac surgery can proceed without any invasive tests being performed (Fig. 25.14).

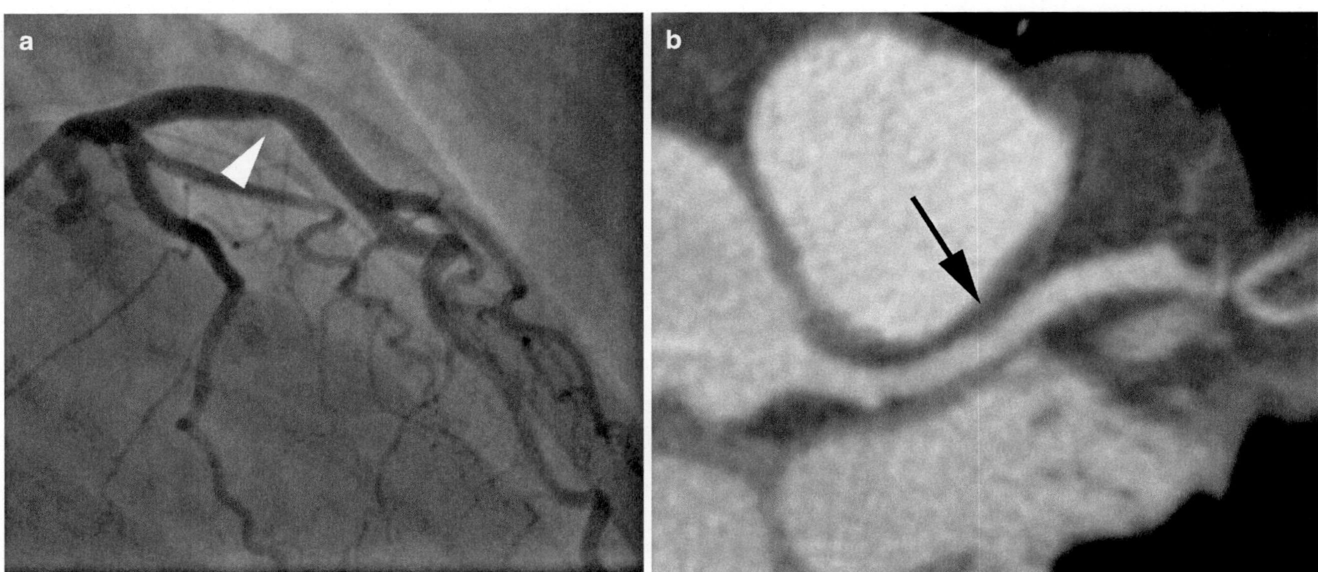

Fig. 25.9 Essentially "normal" coronary angiogram in a 33-year-old woman. A "luminal irregularity" (**a**, *white arrowhead*) in the left anterior descending artery corresponds to a non-calcified plaque (**b**, *black arrow*) seen by CCTA. It is possible that by defining asymptomatic, subclinical plaque in younger patients, they may be prescribed statin therapy long before they would otherwise have been treated, which may change their long-term clinical course

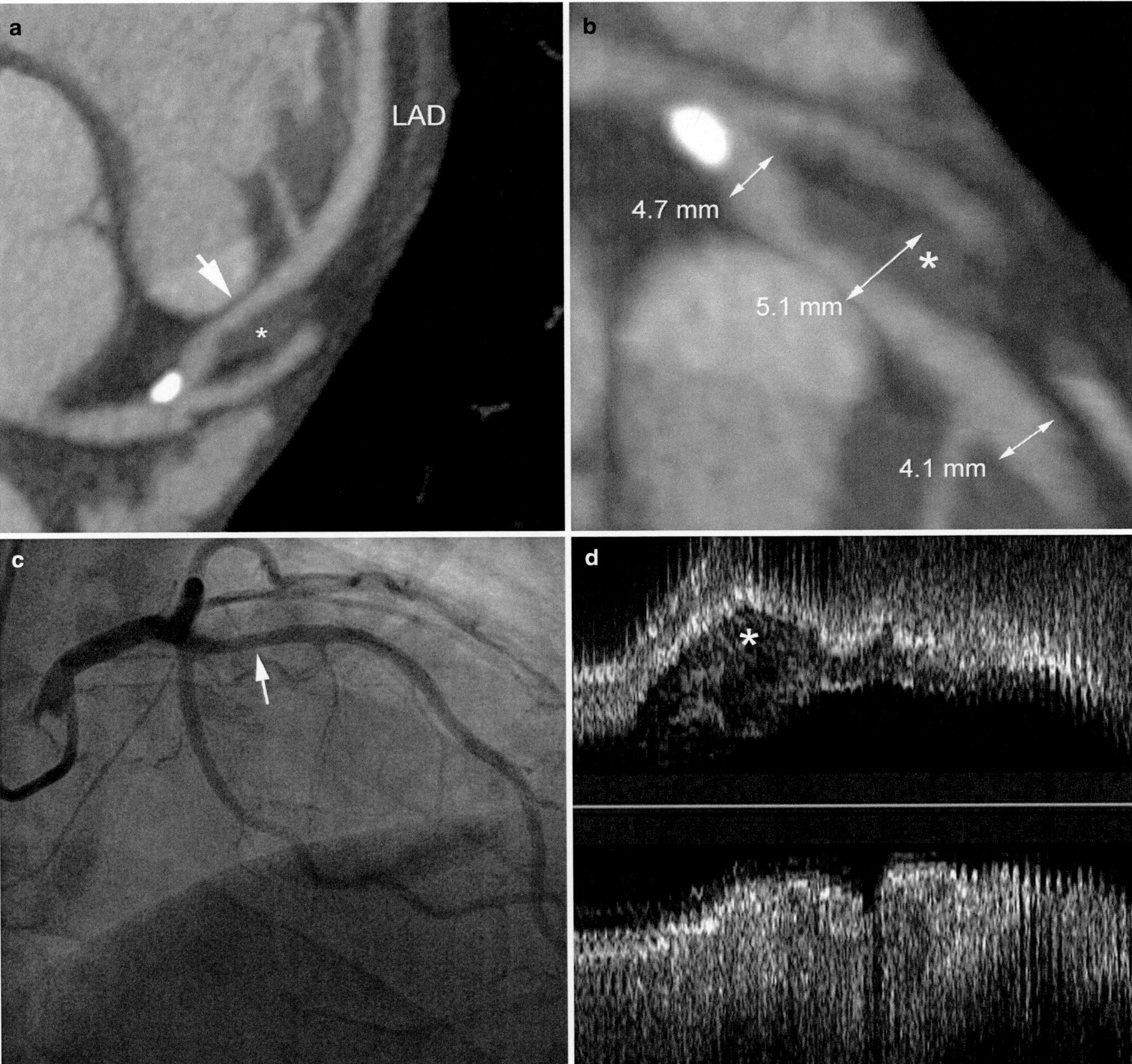

Fig. 25.10 CCTA of a patient with unstable angina demonstrating a large plaque burden impinging on the lumen of the proximal LAD (**a**, *arrow, asterisk*). The area of highest plaque burden (**b**) shows compensatory arterial expansion (*asterisk*), compared to the artery proximal and distal to the plaque. Coronary angiography (**c**) is unable to demonstrate the severity of plaque burden as accurately, but intravascular ultrasound (IVUS) (**d**, *asterisk*) confirms the CCTA findings. IVUS tends to more accurately correspond to CCTA findings, as it shows both intraluminal plaque as well as plaque morphology in the wall of the artery

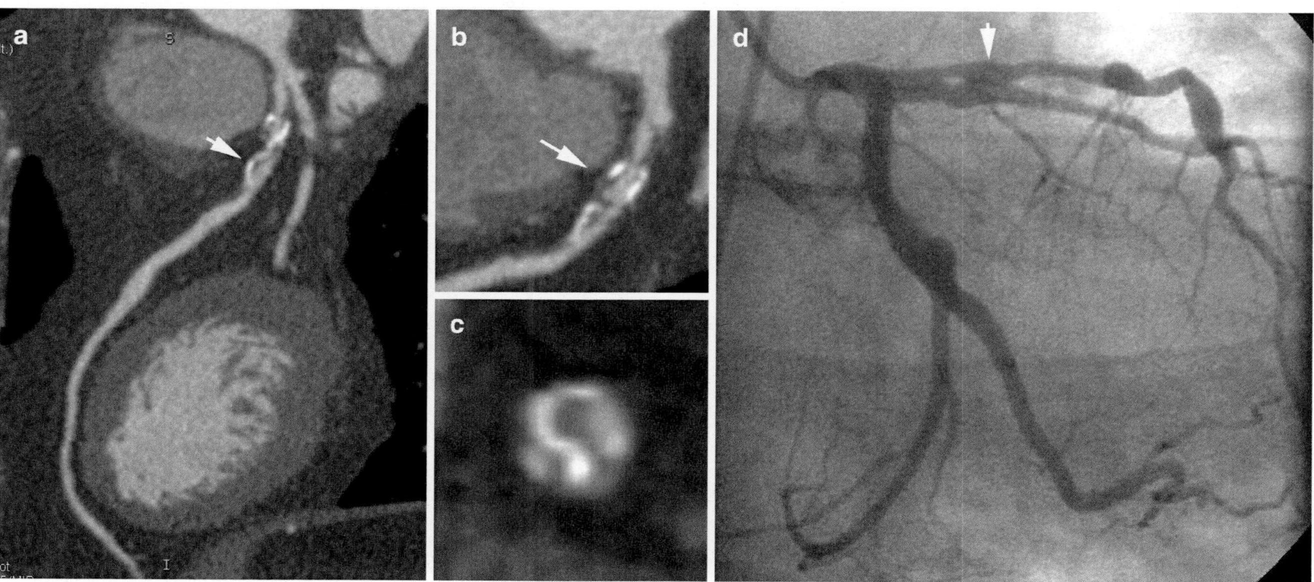

Fig. 25.11 CCTA and invasive angiogram in a man with chest pain: The proximal LAD has a complex, high-grade stenosis (**a**, *arrow*). Closer and cross-sectional views of the plaque (**b**, *arrow*; **c**) show that it is made up of soft and calcified plaque, and there is expansion of the artery when compared to more proximal reference sections. Invasive angiography (**d**, *arrow*) may not as accurately demonstrate the severity of plaque burden due to the compensatory expansion and lack of arterial wall visualization

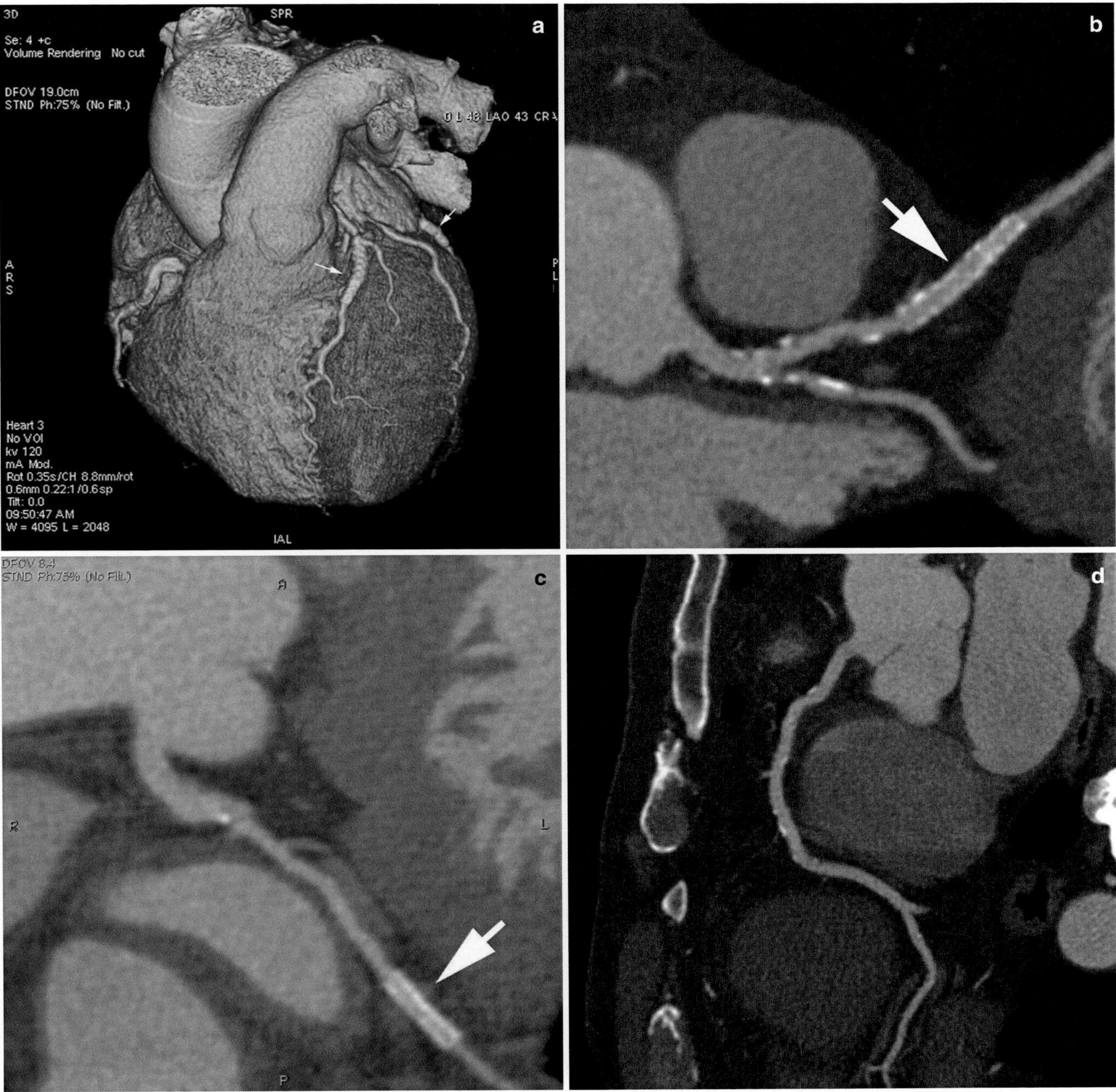

Fig. 25.12 A CCTA of a patient with previous stents placed in the left anterior descending (LAD) and left circumflex (LCx), now having chest pain. Three dimensional image (**a**) show the location of the stents (*arrows*). The curved reformatted CT images demonstrate patency of the LAD stent (**b**, *arrow*) and the LCx stent (**c**, *arrow*). The right coronary artery has only minimal disease (**d**). No further cardiac testing was needed with this patient

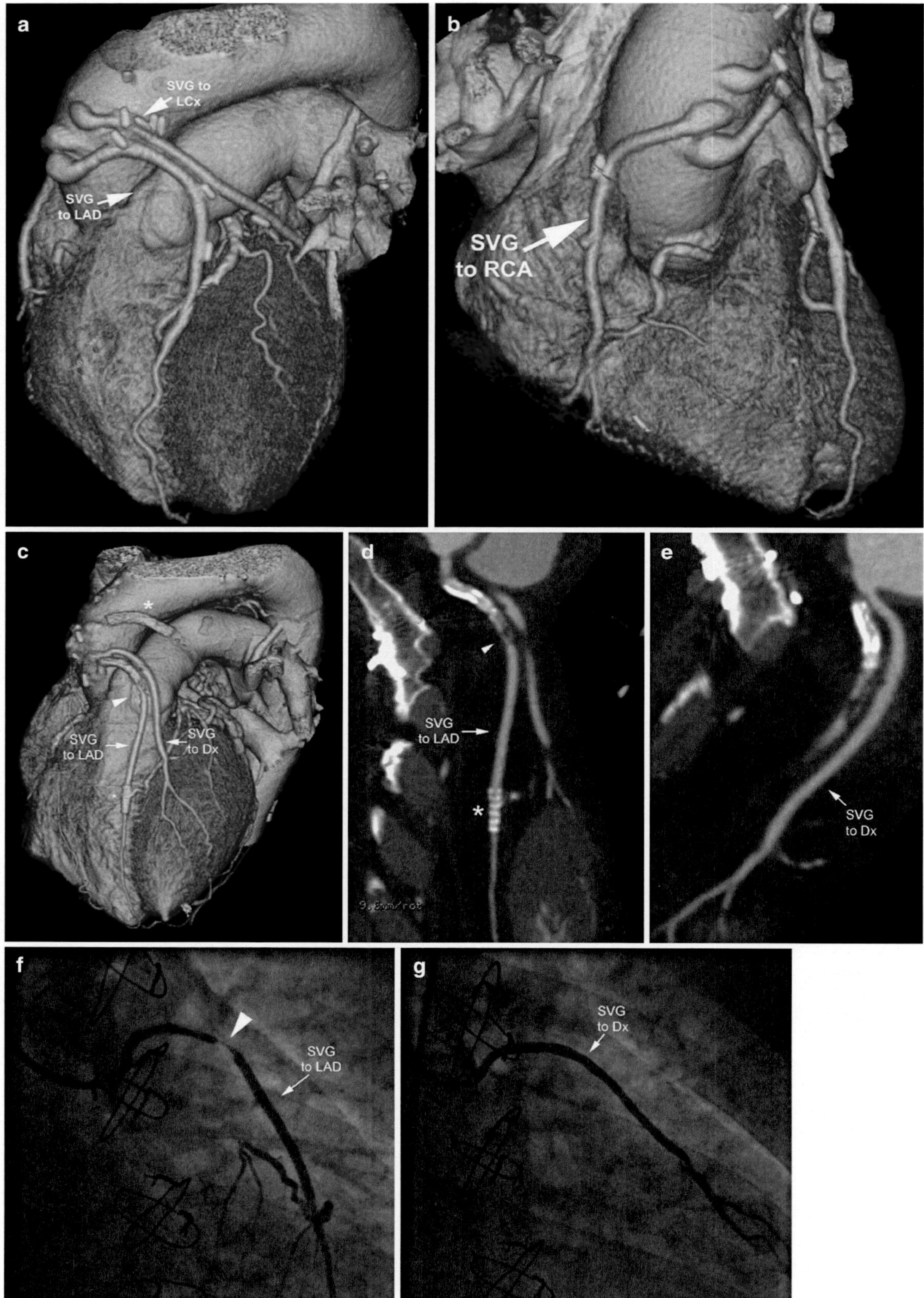

Fig. 25.13 Cardiac CTA (3D images) of a patient with patent coronary bypasses is seen in panels **a** and **b**. Three-dimensional imaging is quite adequate in visualizing patent saphenous vein grafts (SVG), and multiplanar reformatted (MPR) images are unnecessary. A patient with diseased coronary bypasses is seen using 3-D imaging (**c**). The graft to the diagonal (Dx) is patent, which is confirmed on MPR imaging (**e**) as well as invasive angiography (**g**). The SVG to the left anterior descending (LAD) has a high grade lesion (**d**, *arrowhead*), which is seen on invasive angiography (**f**). An occluded SVG with previous stent is seen on the 3D images (**c**, *asterisk*)

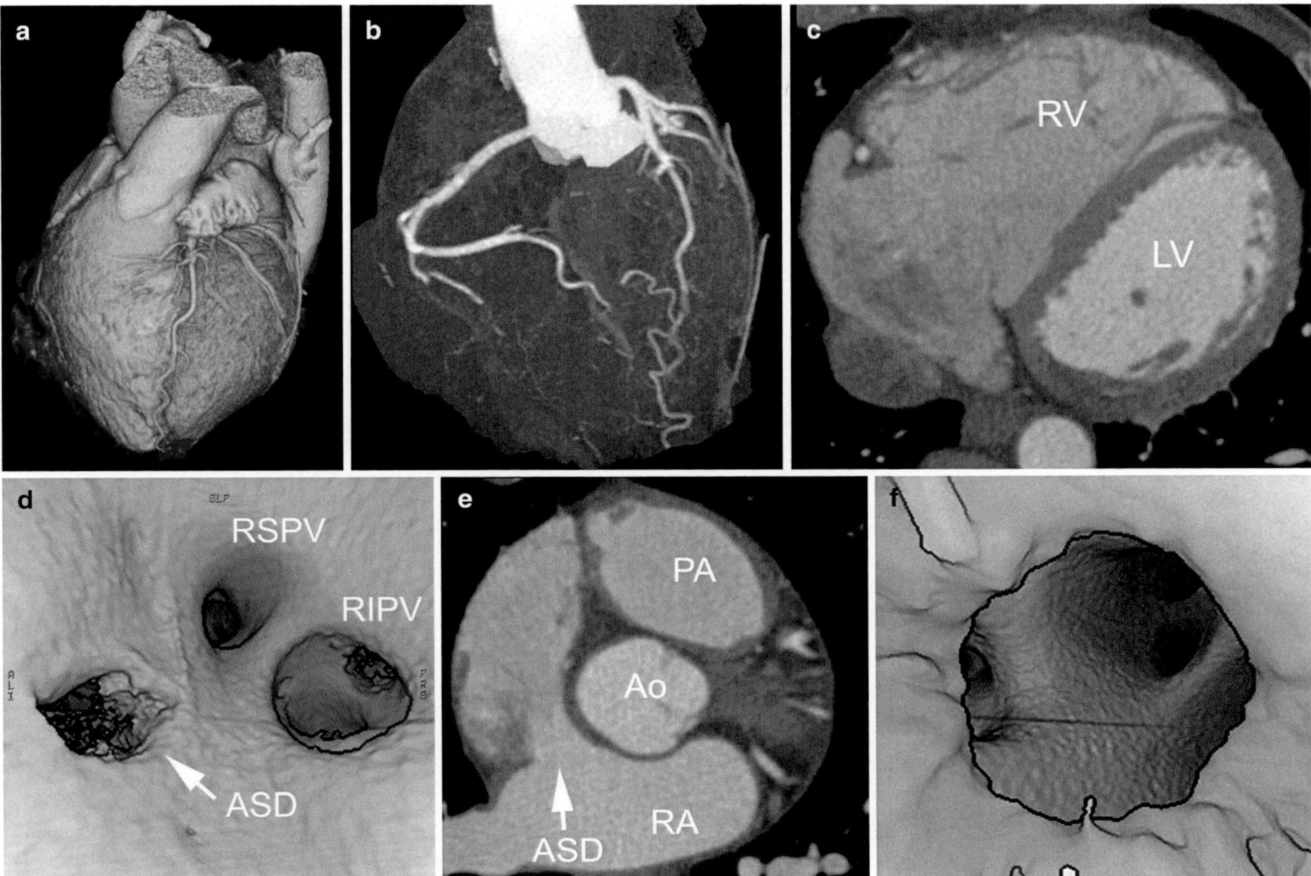

Fig. 25.14 CCTA performed in a young patient who is to undergo atrial septal defect (ASD) closure. The 3-D and MIP views (**a**, **b**) show no significant coronary disease. This was confirmed with review of the axial and reformatted images (not pictured). Axial image of the heart (**c**) clearly shows enlargement of the right ventricle (RV) compared to the left ventricle (LV), which is a sign of the chronicity of the volume overload of the right heart from the ASD. The ASD is shown from an "internal" view (**d**, *arrow*). This also allows for the evaluation of the size and location of the pulmonary veins (*RSPV* right superior pulmonary vein, *RIPV* right inferior pulmonary vein), which can alter management from percutaneous to surgical closure. Axial view (**e**) shows relation of the pulmonary artery (PA) to the aorta (Ao) as well as the clear conduit from the left atrium (LA) to the right atrium. An "internal" view of the ASD as seen from the right atrium shows the location of the left sided pulmonary veins across the left atrium (**f**) (Reprinted from Reese et al. [90]. With permission from Baylor Health Care System. ©Baylor Health Care System)

Conclusion

Interventional cardiologists should embrace CCTA as a helpful addition to their armamentarium to diagnose and treat cardiovascular disease. There are many situations in which the use of CCTA is not only complementary, but an improvement on its invasive counterpart in the evaluation of the cardiac patient. It can be an enormous aid in the planning of complex interventional procedures, and can give additional information which invasive angiography cannot. Further reductions in radiation dosage, improvements in resolution, and more rapid acquisition time will increase the interventionalist's usage of cardiac CT.

References

1. Auseon AJ, Advani SS, Bush CA, Raman SV. Impact of 64-slice multidetector computed tomography on other diagnostic studies for coronary artery disease. Am J Med. 2009;122(4):387–91. Epub 2009/04/01.
2. Selinger H. Selective coronary cine-angiography. W V Med J. 1966;62(10):336–7.
3. Spellberg RD, Unger I. The percutaneous femoral artery approach to selective coronary arteriography. Circulation. 1967;36(5):730–3.
4. Weidner W, MacAlpin R, Hanafee W, Kattus A. Percutaneous transaxillary selective coronary angiography. Radiology. 1965;85(4):652–7.
5. Banerjee S, Crook AM, Dawson JR, Timmis AD, Hemingway H. Magnitude and consequences of error in coronary angiography interpretation (the ACRE study). Am J Cardiol. 2000;85(3): 309–14.
6. Goldberg RK, Kleiman NS, Minor ST, Abukhalil J, Raizner AE. Comparison of quantitative coronary angiography to visual estimates of lesion severity pre and post PTCA. Am Heart J. 1990; 119(1):178–84.
7. Herrington DM, Siebes M, Walford GD. Sources of error in quantitative coronary angiography. Cathet Cardiovasc Diagn. 1993;29(4): 314–21.
8. Nissen SE, Gurley JC. Application of intravascular ultrasound for detection and quantitation of coronary atherosclerosis. Int J Card Imaging. 1991;6(3-4):165–77.
9. Topol EJ, Nissen SE. Our preoccupation with coronary luminology. The dissociation between clinical and angiographic findings in ischemic heart disease. Circulation. 1995;92(8):2333–42.
10. Arnett EN, Isner JM, Redwood DR, Kent KM, Baker WP, Ackerstein H, et al. Coronary artery narrowing in coronary heart disease: comparison of cineangiographic and necropsy findings. Ann Intern Med. 1979;91(3):350–6.
11. Glagov S, Weisenberg E, Zarins CK, Stankunavicius R, Kolettis GJ. Compensatory enlargement of human atherosclerotic coronary arteries. N Engl J Med. 1987;316(22):1371–5.
12. Stiel GM, Stiel LS, Schofer J, Donath K, Mathey DG. Impact of compensatory enlargement of atherosclerotic coronary arteries on angiographic assessment of coronary artery disease. Circulation. 1989;80(6):1603–9.
13. Yamashita T, Colombo A, Tobis JM. Limitations of coronary angiography compared with intravascular ultrasound: implications for coronary interventions. Prog Cardiovasc Dis. 1999;42(2):91–138.
14. Macieira-Coelho E, Cantinho G, da Costa BB, Garcia-Alves M, Lacerda AP, Dionisio I, et al. Minimal residual coronary obstructions in patients who suffered a first myocardial infarction. A prospective study comparing coronary angiography and exercise thallium scintigraphy. Clin Cardiol. 1993;16(12):879–82.
15. Kennedy JW, Baxley WA, Bunnel IL, Gensini GG, Messer JV, Mudd JG, et al. Mortality related to cardiac catheterization and angiography. Cathet Cardiovasc Diagn. 1982;8(4):323–40.
16. Noto Jr TJ, Johnson LW, Krone R, Weaver WF, Clark DA, Kramer Jr JR, et al. Cardiac catheterization 1990: a report of the Registry of the Society for Cardiac Angiography and Interventions (SCA&I). Cathet Cardiovasc Diagn. 1991;24(2):75–83.
17. Scanlon PJ, Faxon DP, Audet AM, Carabello B, Dehmer GJ, Eagle KA, et al. ACC/AHA guidelines for coronary angiography. A report of the American College of Cardiology/American Heart Association Task Force on practice guidelines (Committee on Coronary Angiography). Developed in collaboration with the Society for Cardiac Angiography and Interventions. J Am Coll Cardiol. 1999;33(6):1756–824.
18. Heuser RR. Outpatient coronary angiography: indications, safety, and complication rates. Herz. 1998;23(1):21–6.
19. Ammann P, Brunner-La Rocca HP, Angehrn W, Roelli H, Sagmeister M, Rickli H. Procedural complications following diagnostic coronary angiography are related to the operator's experience and the catheter size. Catheter Cardiovasc Interv. 2003;59(1):13–8.
20. Patel MR, Bailey SR, Bonow RO, Chambers CE, Chan PS, Dehmer GJ, et al. ACCF/SCAI/AATS/AHA/ASE/ASNC/HFSA/HRS/SCCM/SCCT/SCMR/STS 2012 appropriate use criteria for diagnostic catheterization: a report of the American College of Cardiology Foundation Appropriate Use Criteria Task Force, Society for Cardiovascular Angiography and Interventions, American Association for Thoracic Surgery, American Heart Association, American Society of Echocardiography, American Society of Nuclear Cardiology, Heart Failure Society of America, Heart Rhythm Society, Society of Critical Care Medicine, Society of Cardiovascular Computed Tomography, Society for Cardiovascular Magnetic Resonance, and Society of Thoracic Surgeons. J Am Coll Cardiol. 2012;59(22):1995–2027. Epub 2012/05/15.
21. deFilippi CR, Rosanio S, Tocchi M, Parmar RJ, Potter MA, Uretsky BF, et al. Randomized comparison of a strategy of predischarge coronary angiography versus exercise testing in low-risk patients in a chest pain unit: in-hospital and long-term outcomes. J Am Coll Cardiol. 2001;37(8):2042–9.
22. Wyer PC. Predischarge coronary angiography was better than exercise testing for reducing hospital use after low-risk chest pain. ACP J Club. 2002;136(1):8.
23. Gandelman G, Bodenheimer MM. Screening coronary arteriography in the primary prevention of coronary artery disease. Heart Dis. 2003;5(5):335–44.
24. Patel MR, Dehmer GJ, Hirshfeld JW, Smith PK, Spertus JA. ACCF/SCAI/STS/AATS/AHA/ASNC, 2009 Appropriateness Criteria for Coronary Revascularization: a report by the American College of Cardiology Foundation Appropriateness Criteria Task Force, Society for Cardiovascular Angiography and Interventions, Society of Thoracic Surgeons, American Association for Thoracic Surgery, American Heart Association, and the American Society of Nuclear Cardiology Endorsed by the American Society of Echocardiography, the Heart Failure Society of America, and the Society of Cardiovascular Computed Tomography. J Am Coll Cardiol. 2009;53(6):530–53. Epub 2009/02/07.
25. Patel MR, Peterson ED, Dai D, Brennan JM, Redberg RF, Anderson HV, et al. Low diagnostic yield of elective coronary angiography. N Engl J Med. 2010;362(10):886–95. Epub 2010/03/12.
26. Ravipati G, Aronow WS, Lai H, Shao J, DeLuca AJ, Weiss MB, et al. Comparison of sensitivity, specificity, positive predictive value, and negative predictive value of stress testing versus 64-multislice coronary computed tomography angiography in predicting obstructive coronary artery disease diagnosed by coronary angiography. Am J Cardiol. 2008;101(6):774–5. Epub 2008/03/11.

27. Fazel P, Peterman MA, Schussler JM. Three-year outcomes and cost analysis in patients receiving 64-slice computed tomographic coronary angiography for chest pain. Am J Cardiol. 2009;104(4): 498–500.
28. Budoff MJ, Dowe D, Jollis JG, Gitter M, Sutherland J, Halamert E, et al. Diagnostic performance of 64-multidetector row coronary computed tomographic angiography for evaluation of coronary artery stenosis in individuals without known coronary artery disease: results from the prospective multicenter ACCURACY (Assessment by Coronary Computed Tomographic Angiography of Individuals Undergoing Invasive Coronary Angiography) trial. J Am Coll Cardiol. 2008;52(21):1724–32. Epub 2008/11/15.
29. Meijboom WB, Meijs MF, Schuijf JD, Cramer MJ, Mollet NR, van Mieghem CA, et al. Diagnostic accuracy of 64-slice computed tomography coronary angiography: a prospective, multicenter, multivendor study. J Am Coll Cardiol. 2008;52(25):2135–44. Epub 2008/12/20.
30. Mowatt G, Cook JA, Hillis GS, Walker S, Fraser C, Jia X, et al. 64-Slice computed tomography angiography in the diagnosis and assessment of coronary artery disease: systematic review and meta-analysis. Heart. 2008;94(11):1386–93. Epub 2008/08/02.
31. Stein JH, Uretz EF, Parrillo JE, Barron JT. Cost and appropriateness of radionuclide exercise stress testing by cardiologists and non-cardiologists. Am J Cardiol. 1996;77(2):139–42. Epub 1996/01/15.
32. Dharampal AS, Papadopoulou SL, Rossi A, Meijboom WB, Weustink A, Dijkshoorn M, et al. Diagnostic performance of computed tomography coronary angiography to detect and exclude left main and/or three-vessel coronary artery disease. Eur Radiol. 2013;23(11):2934–43. Epub 2013/07/03.
33. Otsuka M, Bruining N, Van Pelt NC, Mollet NR, Ligthart JM, Vourvouri E, et al. Quantification of coronary plaque by 64-slice computed tomography: a comparison with quantitative intracoronary ultrasound. Invest Radiol. 2008;43(5):314–21. Epub 2008/04/22.
34. Van Mieghem CA, Thury A, Meijboom WB, Cademartiri F, Mollet NR, Weustink AC, et al. Detection and characterization of coronary bifurcation lesions with 64-slice computed tomography coronary angiography. Eur Heart J. 2007;28(16):1968–76. Epub 2007/07/12.
35. Kim SY, Lee HJ, Kim YJ, Hur J, Hong YJ, Yoo KJ, et al. Coronary computed tomography angiography for selecting coronary artery bypass graft surgery candidates. Ann Thorac Surg. 2013;95(4):1340–6. Epub 2013/03/07.
36. Bhella PS, Hassan Y, Schussler JM. Usefulness of 64-slice coronary computed tomographic angiography in the planning of percutaneous coronary intervention. Proc (Bayl Univ Med Cent). 2010;23(1):27–8. Epub 2010/02/17.
37. Berbarie RF, Dockery WD, Johnson KB, Rosenthal RL, Stoler RC, Schussler JM. Use of multislice computed tomographic coronary angiography for the diagnosis of anomalous coronary arteries. Am J Cardiol. 2006;98(3):402–6. Epub 2006/07/25.
38. Pflederer T, Marwan M, Ropers D, Daniel WG, Achenbach S. CT angiography unmasking catheter-induced spasm as a reason for left main coronary artery stenosis. J Cardiovasc Comput Tomogr. 2008;2(6):406–7. Epub 2008/12/17.
39. Mollet NR, Hoye A, Lemos PA, Cademartiri F, Sianos G, McFadden EP, et al. Value of preprocedure multislice computed tomographic coronary angiography to predict the outcome of percutaneous recanalization of chronic total occlusions. Am J Cardiol. 2005;95(2):240–3. Epub 2005/01/12.
40. Van Mieghem CA, van der Ent M, de Feyter PJ. Percutaneous coronary intervention for chronic total occlusions: value of preprocedural multislice CT guidance. Heart. 2007;93(11):1492. Epub 2007/10/16.
41. Singh S, Singh N, Gulati GS, Ramakrishnan S, Kumar G, Sharma S, et al. Dual-source computed tomography for chronic total occlusion of coronary arteries. Catheter Cardiovasc Interv. 2014. doi:10.1002/ccd.25516.
42. Li P, Gai LY, Yang X, Sun ZJ, Jin QH. Computed tomography angiography-guided percutaneous coronary intervention in chronic total occlusion. J Zhejiang Univ Sci B. 2010;11(8):568–74. Epub 2010/07/30.
43. Curtis MJ, Traboulsi M, Knudtson ML, Lester WM. Left main coronary artery dissection during cardiac catheterization. Can J Cardiol. 1992;8(7):725–8. Epub 1992/09/01.
44. Devlin G, Lazzam L, Schwartz L. Mortality related to diagnostic cardiac catheterization. The importance of left main coronary disease and catheter induced trauma. Int J Card Imaging. 1997;13(5):379–84. discussion 85-6. Epub 1997/11/14.
45. Schussler JM, Dockery WD, Johnson KB, Rosenthal RL, Stoler RC. Critical left main coronary artery stenosis diagnosed by computed tomographic coronary angiography. Proc (Bayl Univ Med Cent). 2005;18(5):407.
46. Morice MC, Serruys PW, Kappetein AP, Feldman TE, Stahle E, Colombo A, et al. Five-year outcomes in patients with left main disease treated with either percutaneous coronary intervention or coronary artery bypass grafting in the synergy between percutaneous coronary intervention with taxus and cardiac surgery trial. Circulation. 2014;129(23):2388–94. Epub 2014/04/05.
47. Ko BS, Crossett M, Seneviratne SK. Pre-procedural combined coronary angiography and stress myocardial perfusion imaging using 320-detector CT in unprotected left main and ostial left anterior descending artery intervention. Cardiovascular intervention and therapeutics. 2014. Epub 2014/08/02.
48. Gauss S, Pflederer T, Marwan M, Daniel WG, Achenbach S. Analysis of left main coronary artery and branching geometry by coronary CT angiography. Int J Cardiol. 2011;146(3):469–70. Epub 2010/12/15.
49. Budoff MJ, Rasouli ML, Shavelle DM, Gopal A, Gul KM, Mao SS, et al. Cardiac CT angiography (CTA) and nuclear myocardial perfusion imaging (MPI)-a comparison in detecting significant coronary artery disease. Acad Radiol. 2007;14(3):252–7. Epub 2007/02/20.
50. Gupta G, Anwar A, Brophey MD, Schussler JM. Complementary utility of multislice computed tomographic coronary angiography for detection of high-grade lesions in patients with negative stress myocardial perfusion imaging. Proc (Bayl Univ Med Cent). 2008;21(4):389–91. Epub 2008/11/05.
51. Tonino PA, De Bruyne B, Pijls NH, Siebert U, Ikeno F, van' t Veer M, et al. Fractional flow reserve versus angiography for guiding percutaneous coronary intervention. N Engl J Med. 2009; 360(3):213–24. Epub 2009/01/16.
52. Pijls NH, Fearon WF, Tonino PA, Siebert U, Ikeno F, Bornschein B, et al. Fractional flow reserve versus angiography for guiding percutaneous coronary intervention in patients with multivessel coronary artery disease: 2-year follow-up of the FAME (Fractional Flow Reserve Versus Angiography for Multivessel Evaluation) study. J Am Coll Cardiol. 2010;56(3):177–84. Epub 2010/06/12.
53. Tonino PA, Fearon WF, De Bruyne B, Oldroyd KG, Leesar MA, Ver Lee PN, et al. Angiographic versus functional severity of coronary artery stenoses in the FAME study fractional flow reserve versus angiography in multivessel evaluation. J Am Coll Cardiol. 2010;55(25):2816–21. Epub 2010/06/29.
54. Choi AD, Joly JM, Chen MY, Weigold WG. Physiologic evaluation of ischemia using cardiac CT: Current status of CT myocardial perfusion and CT fractional flow reserve. J Cardiovasc Comput Tomogr. 2014;8(4):272–81. Epub 2014/08/26.
55. Ko BS, Cameron JD, Leung M, Meredith IT, Leong DP, Antonis PR, et al. Combined CT coronary angiography and stress myocardial perfusion imaging for hemodynamically significant stenoses in patients with suspected coronary artery disease: a comparison with fractional flow reserve. JACC Cardiovasc Imaging. 2012;5(11):1097–111. Epub 2012/11/17.
56. Andreini D, Pontone G, Bartorelli AL, Trabattoni D, Mushtaq S, Bertella E, et al. Comparison of feasibility and diagnostic accuracy

of 64-slice multidetector computed tomographic coronary angiography versus invasive coronary angiography versus intravascular ultrasound for evaluation of in-stent restenosis. Am J Cardiol. 2009;103(10):1349–58. Epub 2009/05/12.
57. Wijpkema JS, Tio RA, Zijlstra F. Quantification of coronary lesions by 64-slice computed tomography compared with quantitative coronary angiography and intravascular ultrasound. J Am Coll Cardiol. 2006;47(4):891; author reply -2. Epub 2006/02/21.
58. Hammer-Hansen S, Kofoed KF, Kelbaek H, Kristensen T, Kuhl JT, Thune JJ, et al. Volumetric evaluation of coronary plaque in patients presenting with acute myocardial infarction or stable angina pectoris-a multislice computerized tomography study. Am Heart J. 2009;157(3):481–7. Epub 2009/03/03.
59. Inoue F, Sato Y, Matsumoto N, Tani S, Uchiyama T. Evaluation of plaque texture by means of multislice computed tomography in patients with acute coronary syndrome and stable angina. Circ J. 2004;68(9):840–4. Epub 2004/08/27.
60. Kunimasa T, Sato Y, Sugi K, Moroi M. Evaluation by multislice computed tomography of atherosclerotic coronary artery plaques in non-culprit, remote coronary arteries of patients with acute coronary syndrome. Circ J. 2005;69(11):1346–51. Epub 2005/10/26.
61. Kunita E, Fujii T, Urabe Y, Tsujiyama S, Maeda K, Tasaki N, et al. Coronary plaque stabilization followed by color code plaque(TM) analysis with 64-slice multidetector row computed tomography. Circ J. 2008. Epub 2008/12/17.
62. Yang QH, Chen YJ, Liu QQ, Dong M, Wen L, Song X, et al. Comparison of 320-row computed tomography coronary angiography with conventional angiography for the assessment of coronary artery disease with different atherosclerotic plaque characteristics. J Comput Assist Tomogr. 2012;36(6):646–53. Epub 2012/11/30.
63. Schwartz BG, Schussler JM, Rosenthal RL. Tumor-like coronary atheroma: a modern coronary evaluation with a historical perspective. Texas Heart Institute journal / from the Texas Heart Institute of St Luke's Episcopal Hospital, Texas Children's Hospital. 2011;38(3):275–8. Epub 2011/07/02.
64. Funabashi N, Asano M, Komuro I. Non-calcified plaques of coronary arteries with obvious outward remodeling demonstrated by multislice computed tomography. Int J Cardiol. 2006;109(2):264. Epub 2006/04/29.
65. Tanaka M, Tomiyasu KI, Fukui M, Akabame S, Kobayashi-Takenaka Y, Nakano K, et al. Evaluation of characteristics and degree of remodeling in coronary atherosclerotic lesions by 64-detector multislice computed tomography (MSCT). Atherosclerosis. 2008. Epub 2008/09/09.
66. Pedrazzini GB, D'Angeli I, Vassalli G, Faletra FF, Klersy C, Pasotti E, et al. Assessment of coronary stenosis, plaque burden and remodeling by multidetector computed tomography in patients referred for suspected coronary artery disease. J Cardiovasc Med (Hagerstown). 2011;12(2):122–30. Epub 2010/11/04.
67. Kroner ES, van Velzen JE, Boogers MJ, Siebelink HM, Schalij MJ, Kroft LJ, et al. Positive remodeling on coronary computed tomography as a marker for plaque vulnerability on virtual histology intravascular ultrasound. Am J Cardiol. 2011;107(12):1725–9. Epub 2011/04/13.
68. Hang CL, Lee YW, Guo GB, Youssef AA, Yip HK, Liu CF, et al. Evaluation of coronary artery stent patency by using 64-slice multi-detector computed tomography and conventional coronary angiography: a comparison with intravascular ultrasonography. Int J Cardiol. 2013;166(1):90–5. Epub 2011/11/08.
69. Abdelkarim MJ, Ahmadi N, Gopal A, Hamirani Y, Karlsberg RP, Budoff MJ. Noninvasive quantitative evaluation of coronary artery stent patency using 64-row multidetector computed tomography. J Cardiovasc Comput Tomogr. 2010;4(1):29–37. Epub 2010/02/18.
70. Rubinshtein R, Ben-Dov N, Halon DA, Lavi I, Finkelstein A, Lewis BS, et al. Geographic miss with aorto-ostial coronary stent implantation: insights from high-resolution coronary computed tomography angiography. EuroIntervention. 2014. Epub 2014/04/04.
71. Dehghani P, Marcuzzi D, Cheema AN. Use of multislice CT coronary angiography to assess degree of left main stent overhang into the aorta. Heart. 2009;95(9):708. Epub 2009/04/16.
72. Jabara R, Chronos N, Klein L, Eisenberg S, Allen R, Bradford S, et al. Comparison of multidetector 64-slice computed tomographic angiography to coronary angiography to assess the patency of coronary artery bypass grafts. Am J Cardiol. 2007;99(11):1529–34. Epub 2007/05/29.
73. Chiurlia E, Menozzi M, Ratti C, Romagnoli R, Modena MG. Follow-up of coronary artery bypass graft patency by multislice computed tomography. Am J Cardiol. 2005;95(9):1094–7. Epub 2005/04/22.
74. Meyer TS, Martinoff S, Hadamitzky M, Will A, Kastrati A, Schomig A, et al. Improved noninvasive assessment of coronary artery bypass grafts with 64-slice computed tomographic angiography in an unselected patient population. J Am Coll Cardiol. 2007;49(9):946–50. Epub 2007/03/06.
75. Gao C, Liu Z, Li B, Xiao C, Wu Y, Wang G, et al. Comparison of graft patency for off-pump and conventional coronary arterial bypass grafting using 64-slice multidetector spiral computed tomography angiography. Interact Cardiovasc Thorac Surg. 2009;8(3):325–9. Epub 2008/12/11.
76. Marini D, Agnoletti G, Brunelle F, Sidi D, Bonnet D, Ou P. Cardiac CT angiography after coronary artery surgery in children using 64-slice CT scan. Eur J Radiol. 2008. Epub 2008/07/16.
77. Schussler JM, White CH, Fontes MA, Master SA, Hamman BL. Spyder proximal coronary vein graft patency over time: the SPPOT study. Heart Surg Forum. 2009;12(1):E49–53. Epub 2009/02/24.
78. Schachner T, Feuchtner GM, Bonatti J, Bonaros N, Oehlinger A, Gassner E, et al. Evaluation of robotic coronary surgery with intraoperative graft angiography and postoperative multislice computed tomography. Ann Thorac Surg. 2007;83(4):1361–7. Epub 2007/03/27.
79. Gorantla R, Murthy JS, Muralidharan TR, Mandava R, Dev B, Chandaga H, et al. Diagnostic accuracy of 64-slice multidetector computed tomography in evaluation of post-coronary artery bypass grafts in correlation with invasive coronary angiography. Indian Heart J. 2012;64(3):254–60. Epub 2012/06/06.
80. Peterman MA, Hamman BL, Schussler JM. 64-Slice CT angiography of saphenous vein graft anastomoses fashioned with interrupted nitinol clips. Ann Thorac Surg. 2007;83(3):1204. Epub 2007/02/20.
81. Schussler JM, Hamman BL. Multislice cardiac computed tomography of symmetry bypass connector. Heart. 2004;90(12):1480. Epub 2004/11/18.
82. Malagutti P, Nieman K, Meijboom WB, van Mieghem CA, Pugliese F, Cademartiri F, et al. Use of 64-slice CT in symptomatic patients after coronary bypass surgery: evaluation of grafts and coronary arteries. Eur Heart J. 2007;28(15):1879–85. Epub 2006/07/19.
83. Nazeri I, Shahabi P, Tehrai M, Sharif-Kashani B, Nazeri A. Assessment of patients after coronary artery bypass grafting using 64-slice computed tomography. Am J Cardiol. 2009;103(5):667–73. Epub 2009/02/24.
84. Berbarie RF, Aslam MK, Kuiper JJ, Matter GJ, Martin AW, Roberts WC, et al. Preoperative exclusion of significant coronary artery disease by 64-slice CT coronary angiography in a patient with a left atrial myxoma. Proc (Bayl Univ Med Cent). 2006;19((2):121. Epub 2006/04/13.
85. Gilard M, Cornily JC, Pennec PY, Joret C, Le Gal G, Mansourati J, et al. Accuracy of multislice computed tomography in the preoperative assessment of coronary disease in patients with aortic valve stenosis. J Am Coll Cardiol. 2006;47(10):2020–4. Epub 2006/05/16.
86. Scheffel H, Leschka S, Plass A, Vachenauer R, Gaemperli O, Garzoli E, et al. Accuracy of 64-slice computed tomography for the preoperative detection of coronary artery disease in patients with chronic aortic regurgitation. Am J Cardiol. 2007;100(4):701–6. Epub 2007/08/19.

87. Andreini D, Pontone G, Mushtaq S, Bartorelli AL, Ballerini G, Bertella E, et al. Diagnostic accuracy of multidetector computed tomography coronary angiography in 325 consecutive patients referred for transcatheter aortic valve replacement. Am Heart J. 2014;168(3):332–9. Epub 2014/09/01.
88. Gibbs WN, Hamman BL, Roberts WC, Schussler JM. Diagnosis of congenital unicuspid aortic valve by 64-slice cardiac computed tomography. Proc (Bayl Univ Med Cent). 2008;21((2):139. Epub 2008/04/03.
89. Tandon A, Allison RB, Grayburn PA, Hamman BL, Schussler JM. Preoperative visualization of a muscular ventricular septal defect by 64-slice cardiac computed tomography. Proc (Bayl Univ Med Cent). 2008;21(3):281. Epub 2008/07/17.
90. Reese EA, Graybum PA, Hebeler RF, Rothstein JM, Schussler JM. Preoperative visualization of an atrial septal defect by 64-slice cardiac computed tomography. Proc (Bayl Univ Med Cent). 2009;22(3):234–5. Epub 2009/07/28.

Cardiovascular Magnetic Resonance Imaging: Overview of Clinical Applications in the Context of Cardiovascular CT

26

Jerold S. Shinbane, Jabi E. Shriki, Antreas Hindoyan, and Patrick M. Colletti

Abstract

CMR can evaluate myocardial contractility, volumetry, strain, flow, perfusion, viability, and vascular anatomy without ionizing radiation or iodinated contrast agents. Multiple pulse sequences are acquired in different orientations to the heart and relevant vasculature, some of which require gadolinium-based contrast agents. A strength of CMR is the ability to determine tissue characteristics including edema, hemorrhage, iron content, inflammation, and diffuse and focal fibrosis useful for the diagnosis of cardiomyopathic processes, pericardial disease, and cardiac masses. CMR assessment of cardiovascular structure, function, hemodynamics, extracardiac vasculature and thoracic structure, makes it a useful adjunct to echocardiography in patients with congenital heart disease and valvular disease. Although imaging of the coronary arteries is feasible with CMR, CCTA is the gold standard for non-invasive coronary angiography providing detailed visualization of the entire coronary artery tree. Decisions related to performing CMR versus CCTA require information patient profile and strengths and limitations of each modality in relation to the posed clinical question.

Keywords

Anomalous Coronary Arteries • Cardiomyopathy • Cardiovascular Computed Tomographic Angiography • Cardiovascular Magnetic Resonance Imaging • CMR • Computed Tomography • Congenital Heart Disease • Gadolinium • T1 • T2

Introduction

Technologic advances in cardiovascular magnetic resonance imaging (CMR) and cardiovascular computed tomography angiography (CCTA) allow these modalities to comprehensively visualize cardiovascular structures and function. The decision to perform CMR versus CCTA requires knowledge of the individual strengths and limitations of these imaging techniques, the specific details of a patient's medical history, and the clinical questions which need to be answered. In many clinical scenarios, echocardiography is performed as the initial

Electronic supplementary material The online version of this chapter (doi:10.1007/978-3-319-28219-0_26) contains supplementary material, which is available to authorized users.

J.S. Shinbane, MD, FACC, FHRS, FSCCT (✉)
Division of Cardiovascular Medicine, Department of Internal Medicine, Keck School of Medicine of the University of Southern California, 1520 San Pablo Suite 300, Los Angeles, CA 90033, USA
e-mail: shinbane@usc.edu

J.E. Shriki, MD
Department of Radiology, Puget VA Health System, University of Washington, Seattle, WA, USA
e-mail: shriki@uw.edu

A. Hindoyan, MD
Division of Cardiovascular Medicine, Department of Internal Medicine, Keck School of Medicine of the University of Southern California, Los Angeles, CA, USA

P.M. Colletti, MD
Department of Radiology, Keck School of Medicine of the University of Southern California, Los Angeles, CA, USA
e-mail: colletti@usc.edu

M.J. Budoff, J.S. Shinbane (eds.), *Cardiac CT Imaging: Diagnosis of Cardiovascular Disease*,
DOI 10.1007/978-3-319-28219-0_26

study to assess cardiovascular substrates, with CMR or CCTA performed when further cardiovascular characterization is necessary and a noninvasive approach is preferable. Given the rapid evolution of CMR, appropriateness criteria have been developed for specific cardiovascular indications [1, 2].

Principles of CMR in Comparison to CCTA

CT creates a 3-D spatial x-ray transmission electron density map of the tissues within an imaging slice or volume. With the use of currently available multidetector and dual source CT scanners, this may be performed within seconds with acquisition of a data cube with subsequent multiplanar and 3-D image analysis. CMR can evaluate myocardial contractility, volumetry, strain, flow, perfusion, viability, and vascular anatomy without ionizing radiation or iodinated contrast agents. Multiple pulse sequences are acquired in different orientations to the heart and relevant vasculature, some of which require gadolinium-based contrast agents. These modalities include: steady state free precession for volumes and function, T2 black blood imaging without and with fat saturation for anatomy and edema, pre contrast T1 mapping for diffuse fibrosis, T2* assessment of iron content, velocity-encoded imaging for hemodynamics and flow, tagging for strain, MR contrast angiography, first pass perfusion, post contrast T1 mapping for diffuse fibrosis and delayed gadolinium enhancement for inflammation and fibrosis.

CMR generally requires a system with components including a cardiac specific multi-element receiver coil for coverage with preservation of resolution and for parallel (simultaneous) data acquisitions, cardiac triggering hardware and software, and a cardiac processing workstation with appropriate software. Advances in acquisition efficiency may allow for non-gated real time cardiac imaging for localization and for applications in investigational protocols.

Strengths and Limitations of CMR Versus CCTA

Strengths of CMR include evaluation of myocardial tissue characteristics, myocardial perfusion, ventricular function, myocardial metabolism, viability, shunts, valvular function, flow velocities, and peripheral vasculature without the need for iodinated contrast media or x-ray irradiation. Paramagnetic contrast agents have greatly expanded the applications of CMR. The paramagnetic element gadolinium, when attached to a chelating agent like DTPA, provides a means for contrast enhancement, allowing assessment of perfusion and delayed enhancement to detect acutely infarcted myocardium and chronic myocardial scar. CMR spectroscopy provides non-invasive assessment of myocardial metabolism, providing a mechanistic understanding of myocardial function when using ^{31}P to depict the high energy phosphates, phosphocreatine and ATP, and inorganic phosphate to evaluate intracellular pH.

In comparisons to CMR, the strengths of CCTA technologies currently include a greater ability to characterize details of coronary vasculature, shorter study times, and the ability to image patients with non-MR conditional devices. As opposed to data acquisition with CCTA as one axial imaging sequence leading to one comprehensive 3-D data cube, CMR requires multiple views and MR imaging sequences. CT also allows quantification of coronary artery calcium for risk stratification. Both CCTA and CMR technologies are advancing rapidly, and therefore future applications may change comparative strengths and limitations.

Patient Selection and Preparation

While there is considerable effort focused on reducing the radiation exposure with CCTA techniques, the lack of ionizing radiation is an important strength of CMR. This issue is especially important in young patients, who may be at increased long term risk of malignancy [3]. As opposed to iodinated contrast agents used in CCTA, which enhance vascular structures by increasing CT Hounsfield Units, gadolinium-based contrast agents are paramagnetic and change the magnetic properties of water in close proximity to the contrast agent.

The relative safety of gadolinium-based contrast agents is a significant strength of MR. Iodinated contrast agents are associated with a significant incidence of acute side effects including allergic reaction, hypotension, bronchospasm, and pulmonary edema along with acute and chronic nephropathy. Gadolinium-based contrast agents though have been rarely associated with both worsening renal function and in patients with moderate to severe renal dysfunction, particularly those on dialysis, nephrogenic systemic fibrosis, prompting guidelines for use of these agents [4–6]. CMR techniques such as black blood imaging and bright blood imaging allow for differentiation of vasculature without the injection of a contrast agent.

CMR imaging sequences and technology continue to rapidly evolve with 3-D real time acquisition and increased field strengths to 3 Tesla with attendant increased signal to noise ratio, but can be limited by field inhomogeneity and specific absorption rate limits [7–9]. The effects, safety, and imaging characteristics of field strengths greater than 3 Tesla require further investigation [10–12].

Patient size and body habitus are also important in deciding which imaging modality to employ. Image quality can be compromised in patients with an increased body mass index with CCTA and may require increased radiation exposure for adequate imaging [13]. This limitation is less significant with CMR, although there are limitations in MR access due to extreme patient size related to magnet bore diameter and table weight limits.

Prior to CMR, patients require a complete history for ferromagnetic prosthetic implants, devices, or depositions.

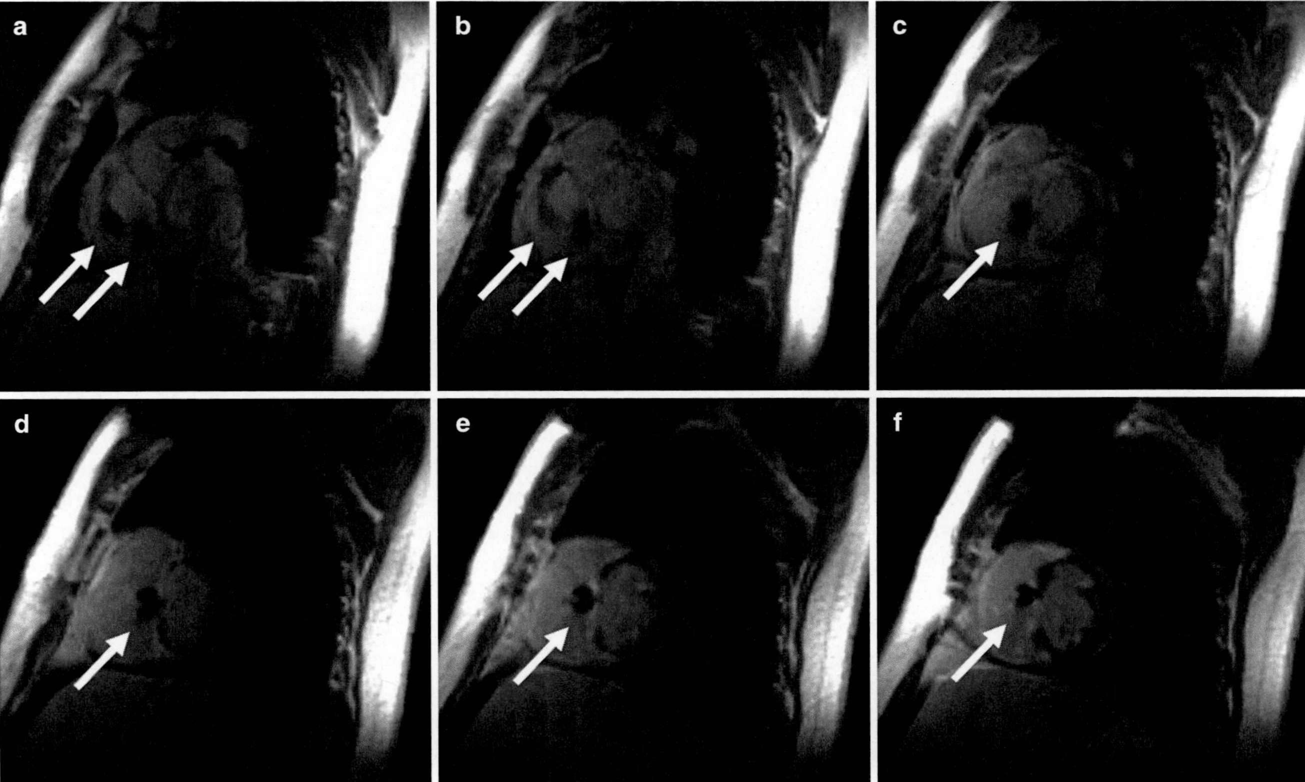

Fig. 26.1 Artifact caused by pacemaker leads (*arrows*) on serial short axis delayed gadolinium enhancement images in the setting of an MR conditional pacemaker. Panels (**a**–**f**) Serial slices base to mid ventricle

These may have relative or absolute contraindications to MR imaging. It is important to ensure that patients with susceptible devices are not exposed to the MR environment. Most prosthetic heart valves and annuloplasty rings can be safely scanned, but specific details of compatibility need to be assessed individually prior to patient study [14]. There has been evolution in the scanning of patients with cardiac devices such as pacemakers and implantable cardiac defibrillators over time. Initially considered absolute contraindications for MRI, some preliminary data suggested that imaging may not be absolutely contraindicated in this setting with specification of certain device and scanning conditions [15, 16]. Detailed knowledge of patient, device, scanner, scanning protocol, alternative imaging techniques and importance of the clinical question are important factors in determination of individualized risk versus benefit of performance of an MR study [17, 18]. Some cardiac device technologies have now been engineered to be MR conditional [18–23]. Even in the setting of scanning patients with MR conditional devices, artifacts caused by leads and generators can affect image quality (Fig. 26.1).

Although study times for CMR have decreased due to advances in technology as well as efficiency of imaging centers in performing protocols, studies are still significantly longer than those achieved with CCTA which have scanning times on the order of seconds. The patient's ability to lie still in a supine position and comply with breath hold commands is important to both technologies, but can be more easily achieved with CCTA given the short study times. Claustrophobia is a common consideration in imaging some patients, although, with appropriate premedication, this is seldom a cause for premature termination of an examination [24, 25]. Larger bore magnets, open magnets, and visual devices allowing patients to see out of the magnet may make this even less of an issue in the future.

During image acquisition, special attention needs to be focused on electrocardiographic recording for monitoring and gating, as the MR environment can interfere with sensing of the QRS complex. Attention to skin prep, lead placement, and ECG vector can improve the ability to perform ECG gating, which is especially important when stress imaging is being considered [26, 27]. Due to acoustic noise associated with scanning, auditory protection with ear plugs is necessary [28].

Coronary Artery Visualization

CMR techniques can visualize coronary arteries for the assessment of coronary artery disease [29–33]. Additionally, CMR can assess patency and stenoses of coronary artery bypass grafts [34]. Advances in technique have improved the ability to visualize coronary arteries with respiratory gating, but there are issues of cardiac, coronary artery, and respiratory motion as well as problems with assessment of small caliber vessels [35–37]. Whole heart imaging with respiratory gating has improved the ability to visualize the coronary arteries [31–33]. Although imaging of the coronary arteries is feasible with CMR, CCTA is the gold standard for noninvasive coronary angiography providing detailed visualization of the entire coronary artery tree. An additional strength of CCTA is fractional flow reserve based on using computational fluid dynamics to assess for the significance of coronary artery stenoses [38–42].

Since myocardial infarction can occur due to plaque rupture and thrombosis in coronary arteries without obstructive disease, there is a need for techniques to characterize plaques potentially at higher risk for rupture [43, 44]. Both CCTA and CMR can assess tissue characteristics of coronary artery plaque, but identification of vulnerable plaques requires further study [45]. CMR can assess tissue characteristics of vessel wall and atheromas through assessment of fibrous tissue, fat, and calcified lesion components, but requires continued investigation to identify characteristics of vulnerable plaques [46, 47]. CMR can assess for vascular remodeling with changes in wall thickness and lumen size [48]. Non-calcified plaque detection and quantification between CMR and CT have been comparable, but CMR provides greater information on tissue characteristics associated with plaques and vascular injury [49, 50].

Anomalous coronary arteries can be diagnosed with CMR [29, 51]. In addition to definition of anatomy of anomalous coronary artery origin, CMR can also assess functional significance through perfusion imaging [52]. CCTA can more comprehensively assess the characteristics of anomalous coronary arteries including ostial location and morphology, course, termination, and 3-D relationship to thoracic vascular and nonvascular structure [53, 54].

CMR is also useful in the assessment and understanding of microvascular coronary artery disease. Phosphorus-31 nuclear magnetic resonance spectroscopy has provided a window into understanding myocardial metabolism through assessment of myocardial high-energy phosphates. This tool has allowed insight into mechanisms of chest pain in the absence of obstructive coronary artery disease [55]. Studies have demonstrated direct evidence of metabolic abnormalities consistent with ischemia in women with chest pain without obstructive coronary artery disease, and proven essential in forwarding the understanding of microvascular coronary artery disease [56].

Assessment for Ventricular Myopathy

Ischemic Cardiomyopathy

CMR can characterize cardiac structures and function by reproducibly assessing right and left ventricular volumes, ejection fraction, wall thickness, and wall motion [57–62]. The ability to comprehensively assess ejection fraction, wall motion, perfusion, and viability is a great strength of CMR in the characterization of myocardial substrates associated with coronary artery disease. Multimodal assessment with components including coronary anatomy, ventricular function, perfusion with pharmacologic stress, and assessment of fibrosis provides comprehensive evaluation of ischemic heart disease with high accuracy and predictive value [30, 63–66].

The performance of rest and stress first pass imaging as well as delayed enhancement imaging are practical strengths of CMR important to characterization of ischemia, myocardial infarction, and ischemic cardiomyopathy (Figs. 26.2, 26.3, 26.4, 26.5, 26.6 and 26.7, Video 1). First-pass perfusion images of the heart, acquired immediately after injection of gadolinium can be obtained with CMR and are useful in evaluation of perfusion abnormalities at rest and during pharmacologic stress [67–70]. CMR perfusion correlates with invasive fractional flow reserve and offers prognostic information important to risk stratification [68, 71–74]. Quantitative perfusion analysis and 3-D myocardial perfusion providing whole heart coverage are being investigated [65, 75]. Preliminary comparison of a CCTA protocol including coronary angiography and stress/rest perfusion versus CMR perfusion demonstrated similar accuracy using invasive catheterization with fractional flow reserve as a gold standard [76].

The advent of CCTA fractional flow reserve allows for the assessment of hemodynamic significance of coronary artery stenoses. CCTA fractional flow reserve can be obtained from standard images using computational fluid dynamics to assess for significance of coronary artery stenoses. Specialized computational programs may be applied to good quality CCTA datasets to track the longitudinal enhanced coronary artery attenuation in search of relative differential drop-off that may be associated with reduced fractional flow reserve. In initial studies, the use of CCTA coupled with CT fractional flow reserve has increased the diagnostic accuracy of studies over traditional stress imaging modalities using invasive fractional flow reserve as a gold standard [38–42]. Further innovation, with evaluation for accuracy, reproducibility, standardization of acquisition and reporting, and practicality of performance as part of CCTA analysis is ongoing [77].

With delayed enhancement images obtained approximately 10 min after gadolinium-based contrast administration, gadolinium clears from normal myocardium, but

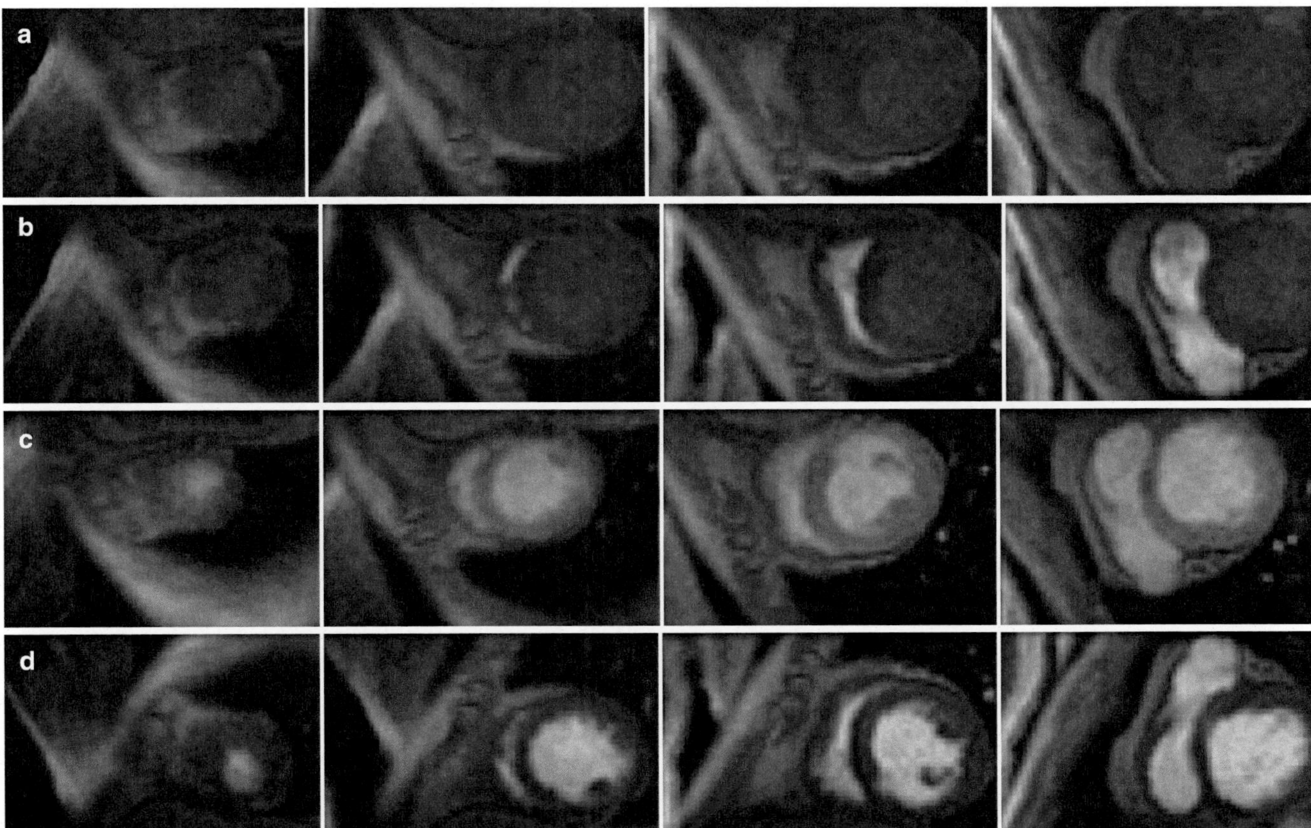

Fig. 26.2 First pass myocardial perfusion study with serial short axis images demonstrating the progression of gadolinium enhancement. Panel (**a**) Pre-gadolinium. Panel (**b**) Right ventricular chamber enhancement. Panel (**c**) Right and left ventricular chamber enhancement. Panel (**d**) Ventricular myocardial enhancement

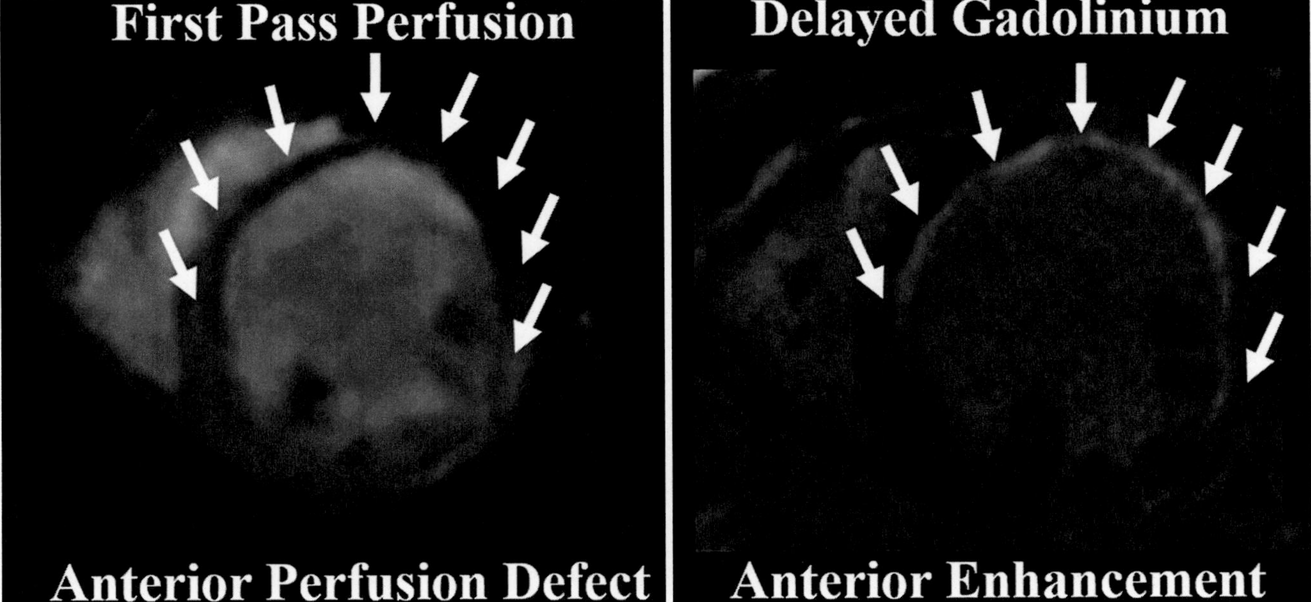

Fig. 26.3 First pass perfusion (*left panel*) and delayed gadolinium enhancement images (*right panel*) demonstrating decreased signal intensity in a subendocardial distribution involving the anteroseptal, anterior, and anterolateral walls (*left panel arrows*) with matching areas of delayed contrast enhancement (*right panel arrows*) consistent with an anterolateral myocardial infarction

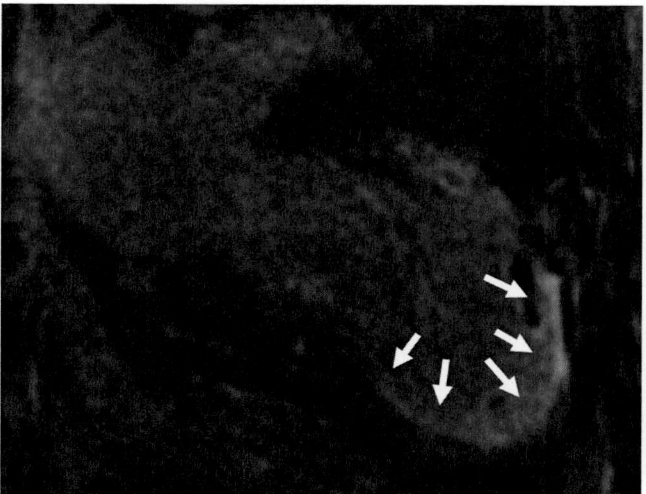

Fig. 26.4 Delayed gadolinium enhancement view showing a myocardial infarct (*arrows*) with extensive involvement of the mid anterior wall and apex due to mid occlusion of a wraparound left anterior descending coronary artery

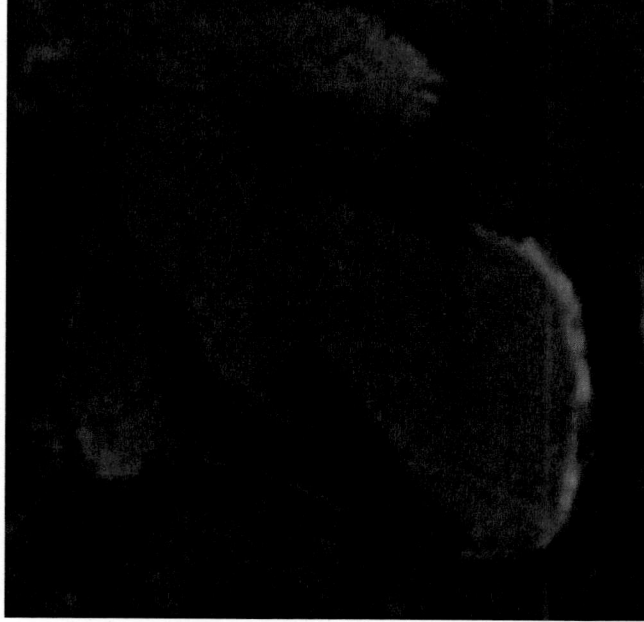

Fig. 26.5 Delayed gadolinium enhancement 2 chamber view demonstrating transmural myocardial enhancement and wall thinning due to infarction involving the mid to distal left anterior descending coronary artery distribution

enhances areas of fibrosis or inflammation [78]. Delayed enhancement imaging using iodinated contrast agent with CCTA is also able to image fibrosis associated with myocardial infarction, but is currently less well established [79, 80].

Delayed gadolinium enhancement may be useful in assessing a variety of cardiomyopathic processes. Myocardial infarction related delayed contrast enhancement typically occurs in the anatomic distribution of coronary arteries with

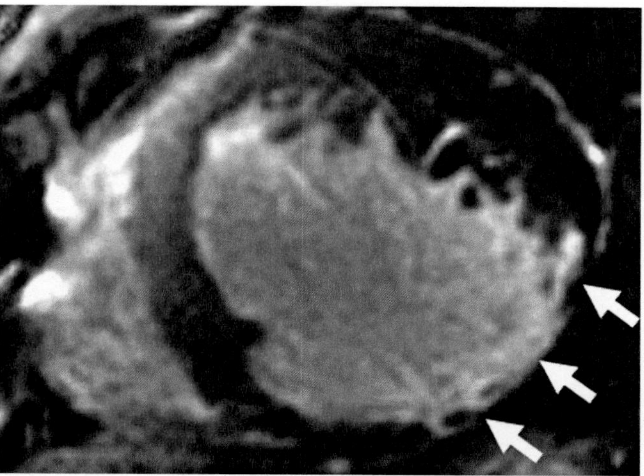

Fig. 26.6 Transmural inferolateral myocardial infarction (*arrows*) on a delayed gadolinium enhancement short axis view

subendocardial delayed enhancement and increasing degrees of transmural extension depending on the extent of infarct [81]. There may be areas of peri-infarct tissue heterogeneity representing areas of viable myocardium and fibrosis. These heterogeneous areas may increase the propensity for the development of ventricular tachycardia [82]. Microvascular obstruction is usually depicted as a subendocardial non-enhancing area due to tissue necrosis which is completely surrounded by delayed enhancement [83].

In ischemic cardiomyopathy, gadolinium delayed enhancement images can assess for areas of viability prior to potential revascularization. Specifically, in patients with ischemic cardiomyopathy, delayed hyperenhancement correlates with lack of viability defined by thallium single photon emission computed tomography [84]. Soon after acute myocardial infarction, gadolinium delayed enhancement CMR provides assessment of infarct size which correlates well with clinical infarct indices [85]. The degree of wall thickening correlates with degree of myocardial non-enhancement on delayed images after recent myocardial infarction and predicts improvement in wall thickening as assessed by follow-up examinations [86].

In addition to late gadolinium enhancement, techniques for assessment of tissue damage associated with acute myocardial infarction include pre-contrast T1-mapping and T2 weighted imaging for edema. Pre-contrast T1 mapping may be helpful in assessment of the extent of myocardial injury in acute myocardial infarction [87, 88]. Late gadolinium enhancement may underestimate the extent of acute myocardial infarction compared to T2 weighted sequences, particularly in patients with acute reperfusion [89]. Hypointensity on T2 weighted imaging is a marker of hemorrhage and is associated with infarct extent, microvascular obstruction, depression of ventricular function, and

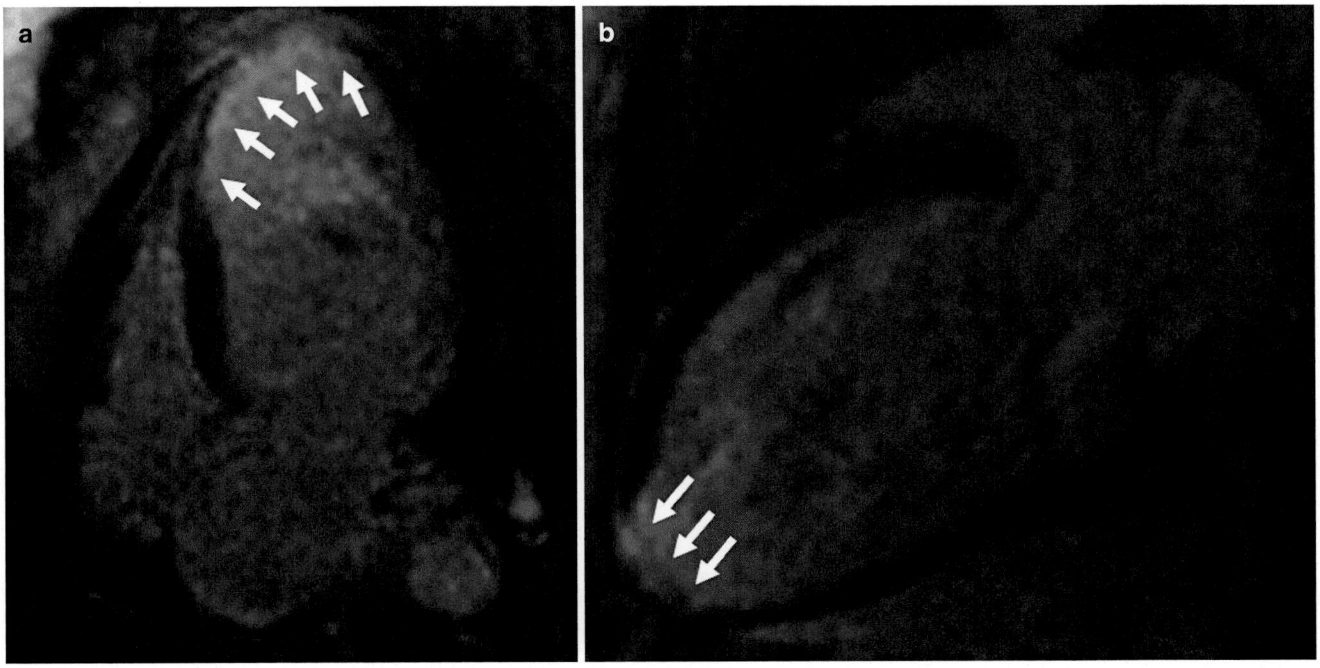

Fig. 26.7 Delayed contrast enhancement views showing wall thinning and delayed contrast enhancement associated with a myocardial infarct. Panel (**a**) 4 chamber view demonstrating apical and mid septal wall thinning and delayed gadolinium enhancement (*arrows*). Panel (**b**) 2 chamber view demonstrating the apical wall thinning and delayed gadolinium enhancement (*arrows*)

prognosis [90]. T2* imaging can provide identification and quantification of post infarction and post reperfusion intramyocardial hemorrhage and is associated with microvascular obstruction [91].

Characterization of Non-ischemic Cardiomyopathic Processes

The same sequences used to characterize ischemic cardiomyopathy can be utilized in the assessment of non-ischemic cardiomyopathic processes. Delayed contrast enhancement may be useful in differentiating ischemic from non-ischemic dilated cardiomyopathy. A delayed enhancement subendocardial to transmural infarct pattern in the distribution of a coronary artery is more likely consistent with ischemic cardiomyopathy as opposed to other patterns such as sub-epicardial and mid wall fibrosis [81].

Interpretation of gadolinium delayed contrast enhancement has become more complex as it has been recognized to occur in a variety of cardiovascular disease processes associated with fibrosis or inflammation. Interpretation of delayed enhancement requires correlation of the individual patient's medical history and the posed clinical question with the pattern of delayed enhancement. Assessment of the sensitivity and specificity of delayed enhancement patterns for diagnoses of specific disease processes requires greater investigation.

Mid-wall fibrosis can occur in dilated non-ischemic cardiomyopathy, and has been associated with worse prognosis and ventricular arrhythmias [92, 93]. The presence and degree of gadolinium enhancement can predict remodeling response to beta-blockers in both ischemic and non-ischemic cardiomyopathy [93]. The presence of late gadolinium enhancement is an independent predictor of malignant arrhythmias and of increased overall mortality, heart failure and hospitalization [94–96]. The extent of fibrosis can be quantified in dilated non-ischemic cardiomyopathy, extent of fibrosis has been shown to be a predictor of malignant arrhythmias and prognosis [97, 98].

Myocardial T1 mapping allows assessment of diffuse myocardial fibrosis and can be performed with non-contrast (native T1) and post-contrast (extracellular volume measurement) sequences [99, 100]. Non-contrast (native T1) studies demonstrate myocyte and interstitial disease. Post-contrast assessment of extracellular volume fraction is a marker of interstitial myocardial collagen content and is elevated in fibrotic and infiltrative myocardial disease processes. This novel modality has the potential for early detection and disease monitoring for the clinical disease staging of cardiomyopathic processes. In non-ischemic dilated cardiomyopathy, native T1 mapping can identify diffuse fibrosis compared to normal myocardium [101]. Post-contrast T1 mapping for the calculation of extracellular volume can be identified in severe dilated cardiomyopathy and in some patients with early dilated cardiomyopathy [98].

Preliminary assessment of extracellular volume by equilibrium contrast enhanced CCTA in cardiomyopathic processes is being investigated [102, 103].

Hypertrophic Cardiomyopathy

In hypertrophic cardiomyopathy, CMR and CCTA can be useful for defining phenotype, function, and potential etiology of ischemia. CMR can characterize regional wall thickness, indexed ventricular mass, ejection fraction, fibrosis, valvular function and hemodynamic data including gradients (Video 2) [104–108]. Late gadolinium enhancement by CMR correlates with the amount of myocardial fibrosis on histologic examination (Fig. 26.8) [109]. The presence of gadolinium enhancement in the substrate of hypertrophic cardiomyopathy provides prognostic risk information for all-cause and cardiac mortality [110]. Serial studies in patients with late gadolinium enhancement may demonstrate rapid progression [111, 112].

The presence and quantitative extent of late gadolinium enhancement in hypertrophic cardiomyopathy is predictive of the development of systolic dysfunction and sudden cardiac death events [113]. In comparison to non-ischemic dilated cardiomyopathy, the dilated phase of hypertrophic cardiomyopathy has a greater extent of delayed enhancement, predominantly in the septal and anterior walls [114]. In apical hypertrophic cardiomyopathy, echocardiographic assessment of the apex can be challenging. CMR can identify apical variants including an apical pouch as well as the presence of apical delayed gadolinium enhancement [115]. The presence and extent of late gadolinium enhancement is an independent predictor of prognosis in the apical variant of hypertrophic cardiomyopathy [116, 117]. In children with hypertrophic cardiomyopathy, the presence and extent of late gadolinium enhancement is predictive of adverse events similar to adults [118].

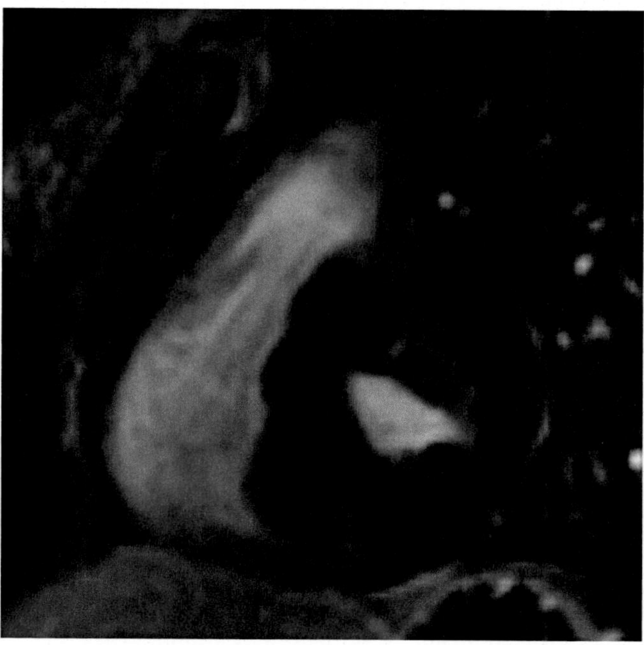

Fig. 26.8 Short axis delayed gadolinium enhancement view demonstrating contrast enhancement in hypertrophic cardiomyopathy

Delayed gadolinium enhancement has relevance for electrophysiology and interventional cardiology procedures in hypertrophic cardiomyopathy patients. The extent of fibrosis in hypertrophic cardiomyopathy is a predictor of inducibility of ventricular tachycardia during electrophysiology exams [119]. Areas of late gadolinium enhancement correlate with areas of abnormal depolarization and repolarization and the origin of ventricular tachycardia in patients with hypertrophic cardiomyopathy and clinical ventricular tachycardia [120]. Preoperative and follow-up studies may be useful in patients undergoing surgical myocardial resection or coronary artery septal embolization [106, 121]. CMR can image location and extent of myocardial infarction created by ventricular septal ablation [122, 123]. Preliminary studies of native T1 and post-contrast T1 mapping demonstrate that the presence of diffuse fibrosis can be detected non-invasively [101, 124, 125].

CCTA can assess regional wall thickness comparable to CMR. CCTA delayed enhancement imaging can detect dense areas of fibrosis in hypertrophic cardiomyopathy, but can underestimate total delayed enhancement [126]. Angina in hypertrophic cardiomyopathy can be due to multiple etiologies. Stress imaging can be associated with false positive findings for epicardial coronary artery disease. CCTA is therefore useful in the assessment for epicardial coronary artery disease in hypertrophic cardiomyopathy [127].

Amyloidosis

Amyloid infiltrative cardiomyopathy occurs due to myocardial amyloid deposition associated with a spectrum of disease processes including hematologic, chronic inflammatory, hereditary and senescent etiologies. CMR delayed gadolinium enhancement can detect amyloid accumulation in the interstitium reflective of amyloid burden (Figs. 26.9 and 26.10) [128, 129]. Diffuse myocardial amyloid is a predictor of mortality [130]. In systemic amyloid, the presence of delayed enhancement is associated with worse prognosis [131, 132]. Patterns of delayed gadolinium enhancement may differ depending on etiology, with a transmural pattern more likely to be associated with transthyretin-related amyloidosis than light-chain amyloidosis [133]. Assessment of diffuse amyloid can be challenging as it may be associated with inability to null myocardium. The pre contrast assessment myocardium nulling is important in amyloid, as there may be limited ability to null myocardium before contrast infusion in diffuse amyloid. This is important to the interpretation of inability to null myocardium on post contrast imaging [134].

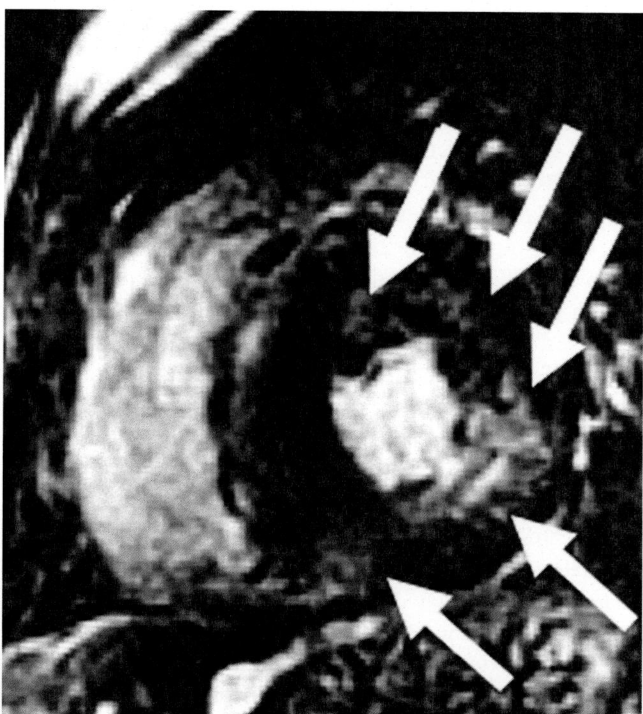

Fig. 26.9 Short axis delayed gadolinium contrast view demonstrating diffuse, patchy delayed enhancement (*arrows*) associated with familial ATTR cardiac amyloidosis

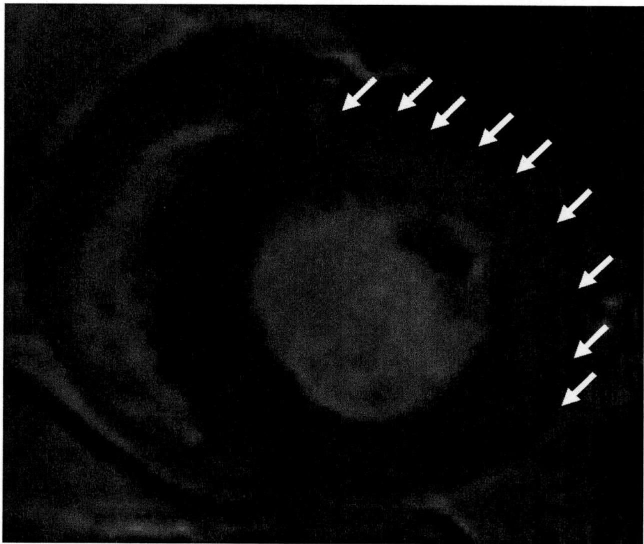

Fig. 26.10 Short axis delayed gadolinium image demonstrating enhancement (*arrows*) due senile systemic ATTR amyloidosis

Anderson-Fabry Disease

Anderson-Fabry disease is an X-linked storage disease due to abnormal sphingolipid metabolism which can lead to significant ventricular myocardial thickening and can therefore mimic hypertrophic cardiomyopathy and cardiac amyloidosis. CMR can visualize involvement through use of delayed gadolinium enhancement imaging in storage diseases such as Anderson-Fabry disease [135]. Native T1 mapping can demonstrate abnormalities before left ventricular wall thickening has occurred and correlates with early systolic and diastolic abnormalities as defined by echocardiography [136]. In disease follow-up, CMR has documented decreased left ventricular mass and wall thickness and reduced myocardial T2 relaxation times with therapy [137].

Sarcoidosis

Cardiac sarcoidosis can occur as part of systemic involvement or can exist with solely cardiac involvement. Gadolinium enhanced CMR can identify inflammation and fibrosis associated with cardiac sarcoidosis (Fig. 26.11) [138]. CMR delayed contrast enhancement in patients with systemic sarcoid has been associated with a higher rate of sudden cardiac death and ventricular tachyarrhythmias [139–141]. A decrease in delayed contrast enhancement has been reported with steroid therapy [142]. A significant degree of delayed gadolinium enhancement has also been associated with a lack of ventricular functional improvement and poor outcomes with steroid therapy [143].

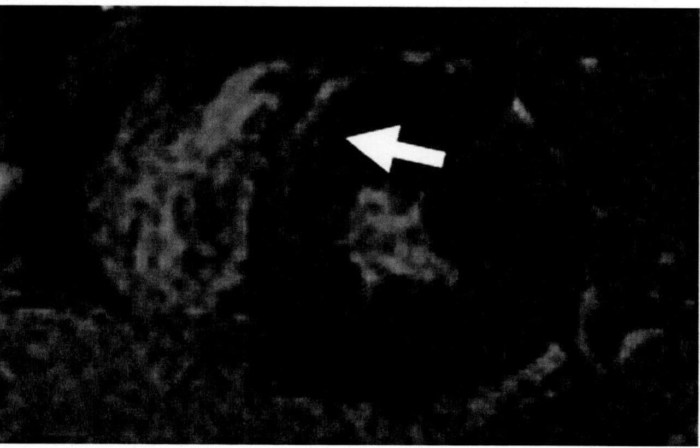

Fig. 26.11 Short axis delayed gadolinium enhancement view demonstrating cardiac sarcoidosis with involvement of the right ventricular aspect of the basal septum (*arrow*)

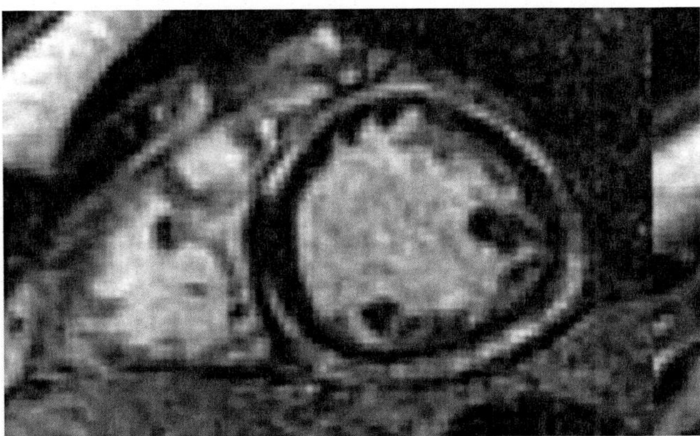

Fig. 26.12 Short axis delayed gadolinium enhancement images demonstrate subepicardial enhancement associated with acute myocarditis

Myocarditis

CMR has become an important modality for the diagnosis and characterization of acute and chronic myocarditis. The Lake Louise Consensus Criteria have been created based on early and delayed gadolinium enhancement and edema imaging (Fig. 26.12) [144]. Delayed gadolinium enhancement can be seen in acute and chronic myocarditis. A combined approach with early and delayed gadolinium enhancement and edema imaging can be useful for diagnosis and characterization of acute myocarditis and differentiation from acute myocardial infarction [145–147]. Additional findings of pericardial effusion and or pericardial delayed enhancement can be seen associated with perimyocarditis. Acute myocarditis findings may vary in regard to delayed gadolinium enhancement presence and pattern with variable correlation with histologic findings characterized by biopsy [148]. Late gadolinium enhancement is also useful in the diagnosis and characterization of chronic myocarditis.

T1 imaging is being assessed along with multiple other CMR indices. In patients with severe subacute myocarditis, late gadolinium enhancement coupled with T1 post-contrast imaging had better diagnostic accuracy than standard Lake Louise indices for myocarditis [149]. Studies preliminarily assessing the relative value of T1 and T2 for differentiation of acute versus chronic myocarditis have demonstrated variable results as to the superiority of T1 versus T2 imaging sequences [150–152].

CMR can be useful for assessment of prognosis in the setting of myocarditis. In children with myocarditis, the presence of late gadolinium enhancement in children predicted poor outcome [153]. In patients with clinical suspicion of myocarditis, a normal CMR predicted good prognosis which is independent of symptoms and other clinical findings [154]. In acute myocarditis, CMR evidence of edema was indicative of reversibility [155]. Data on CCTA comparison to CMR are limited, but preliminarily have demonstrated that in acute myocarditis, delayed contrast enhancement CT correlated with CMR enhancement [156–158].

CMR can detect early changes in autoimmune processes causing myocarditis, including early changes of edema and subclinical perimyocardial involvement through delayed gadolinium enhancement [159, 160]. Combined CMR modalities of T2-weighted and early and late enhancement are preliminarily being assessed for cardiac involvement in systemic lupus erythematosus [161]. In contrast, CCTA can be used to assess for coronary artery involvement with systemic lupus erythematosis due to vasculitis [162].

Myocarditis and cardiomyopathy can occur due to viral, bacterial, fungal, or parasitic infection. Gadolinium enhancement associated with the inflammatory process in Chagas disease has also been reported [163]. In Chagas disease, the extent of myocardial fibrosis correlates with disease severity, and delayed enhancement imaging can detect involvement in the early subclinical phase of disease [164].

Endocardial fibrosis is a rare form of restrictive cardiomyopathy, which is challenging from the etiologic, diagnostic and therapeutic standpoints with multiple potential associations including ischemic, congenital, hematologic, autoimmune and infectious disease processes [165–169]. This processes can occur in complex and potentially multifactorial scenarios. CMR is helpful in the diagnosis of subendocardial fibrosis due to the ability to differentiate tissue characteristics including normal myocardium, fibrosis, edema, and thrombi (Fig. 26.13).

Hemochromatosis

CMR properties associated with myocardial iron content can be useful for the assessment in primary hereditary causes of iron overload as well as secondary transfusion- dependent

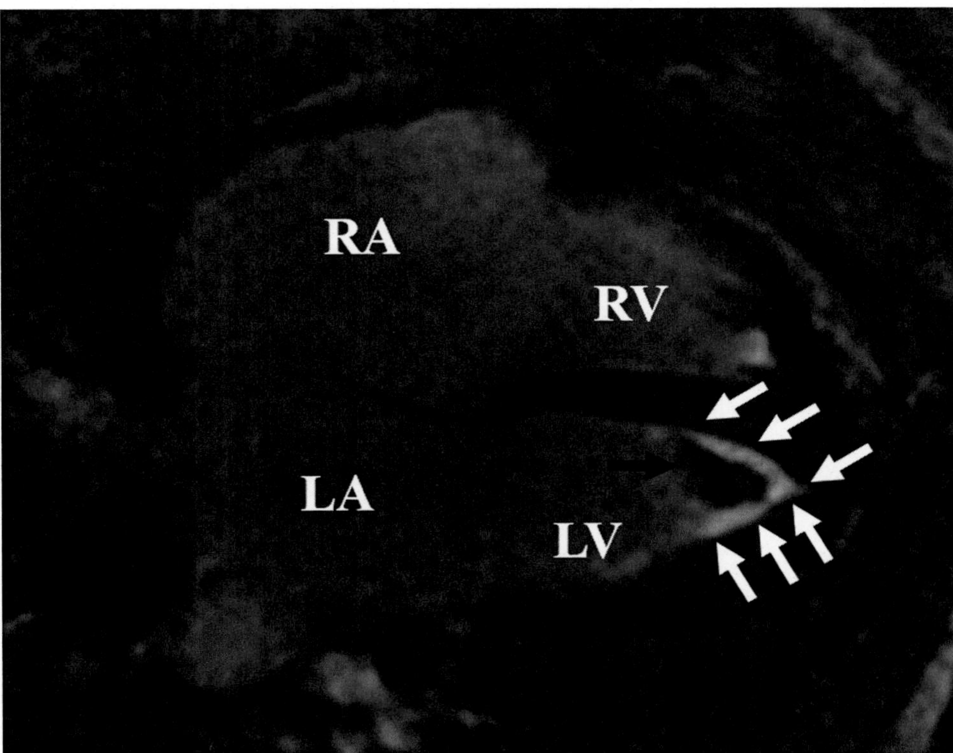

Fig. 26.13 Restrictive cardiomyopathy with endomyocardial fibrosis in a patient with a history of parasitic infection in the setting of rheumatoid arthritis. A 4 chamber delayed gadolinium enhancement image shows endomyocardial fibrosis which is most prominent in the mid to apical left ventricle (*white arrows*). A large wall-contoured mural thrombus is present at the left ventricular apex (*black arrow*). Additionally, biatrial enlargement is present. *LA* left atrium, *LV* left ventricle, *RA* right atrium, *RV* right ventricle

anemias. T2* relaxation times are useful for quantification myocardial iron overload, serial surveillance for iron overload, and assessment of response to treatment [170–172].

Muscular Dystrophies

CMR can detect evidence of cardiac involvement in Duchenne muscular dystrophy. In young patients with Duchenne muscular dystrophy, abnormal strain patterns occur and increase with age [173]. Abnormal post contrast T1 findings can be seen, even in some patients with normal left ventricular ejection fraction and no evidence of delayed gadolinium enhancement. Therefore, post contrast T1 sequences could potentially be useful for detection of early cardiac involvement [174]. In Duchenne muscular dystrophy carriers, increased ventricular volumes, myocardial mass reduction, regional myocardial thinning, depression of ejection fraction, and late gadolinium enhancement are common [175, 176]. In other muscular dystrophies such as Becker-Kiener and limb-girdle muscular dystrophy, depressed ejection fraction late gadolinium enhancement has been reported [177–179]. CMR can be useful to detect early structural and functional abnormalities in myotonic muscular dystrophy [180]. In myotonic muscular dystrophy, the presence of delayed gadolinium enhancement had a high prevalence in patients without evidence of ECG, arrhythmia monitoring or echo abnormalities [181]. Additionally, post-contrast myocardial T1 abnormalities have been seen in myotonic muscular dystrophy compared to control subjects [182].

Takotsubo (Stress-Mediated) Cardiomyopathy

CMR can be useful in differentiating Takotsubo (stress-mediated) cardiomyopathy from other etiologies in patients presenting with ECG changes, cardiac enzyme elevation, and regional wall motion abnormalities with no evidence of obstructive epicardial coronary artery disease. Areas of mid to apical reversible wall motion abnormities correlate with evidence of edema on T2 weighted imaging and typically occur without delayed contrast enhancement [183]. Late gadolinium enhancement has been reported, in the subacute phase of Takotsubo cardiomyopathy and was associated with greater severity and longer recovery than in those patients without enhancement [184, 185].

Arrhythmogenic Right Ventricular Cardiomyopathy/Dysplasia (ARVC/D)

ARVC/D is associated with ventricular arrhythmias and sudden cardiac death [186, 187]. Diagnosis is challenging and involves multiple possible factors, including clinical symptoms, family history, ECG and electrophysiologic findings, ventricular anatomy and function, and ventricular tissue characteristics [188, 189]. Imaging for abnormalities associated with ARVC/D can be missed with multiple imaging modalities. CMR has become the diagnostic modality most commonly used to assess for ARVC/D, as CMR can differentiate tissue characteristics, as well as provide assessment of right ventricular size, shape, and function (Fig. 26.14, Video 3). It is also important to note that the differential diagnosis of right ventricular enlargement and wall motion abnormalities includes right ventricular cardiomyopathy due to pressure or volume overload due to shunts, aortic valve, left ventricular, mitral valve, pulmonary vein, pulmonary artery, pulmonary valve, and tricuspid valve abnormalities. CMR can comprehensively and systematically assess for these etiologies of right ventricular cardiomyopathy in order to differentiate them from ARVC/D. As CMR may be problematic in patients with non-MR conditional devices, comprehensive diagnosis should be considered in patients suspected of having ARVC prior to device placement.

The initial focus of CMR identification of ARVC/D related to characterization of intramyocardial fat, but this

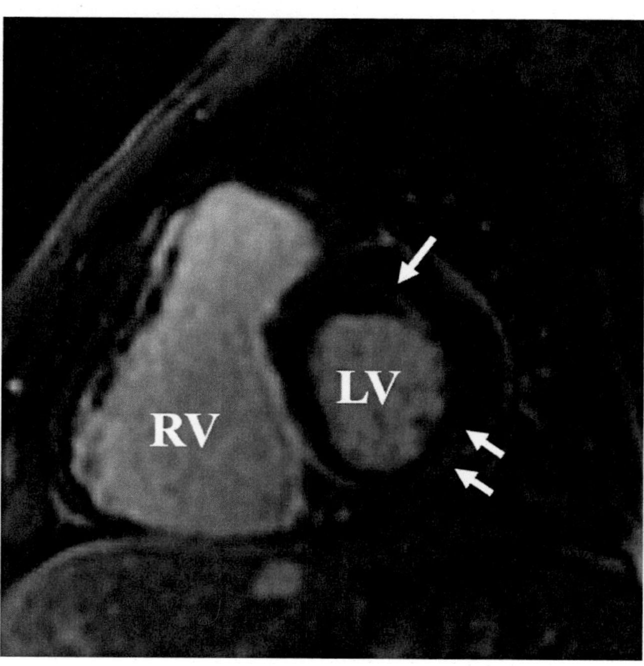

Fig. 26.14 Short axis delayed contrast enhancement view of arrhythmogenic right ventricular cardiomyopathy/dysplasia with right ventricular enlargement and evidence of left ventricular involvement demonstrated by late gadolinium enhancement of the left ventricular myocardium (*arrows*). *LV* left ventricle, *RV* right ventricle

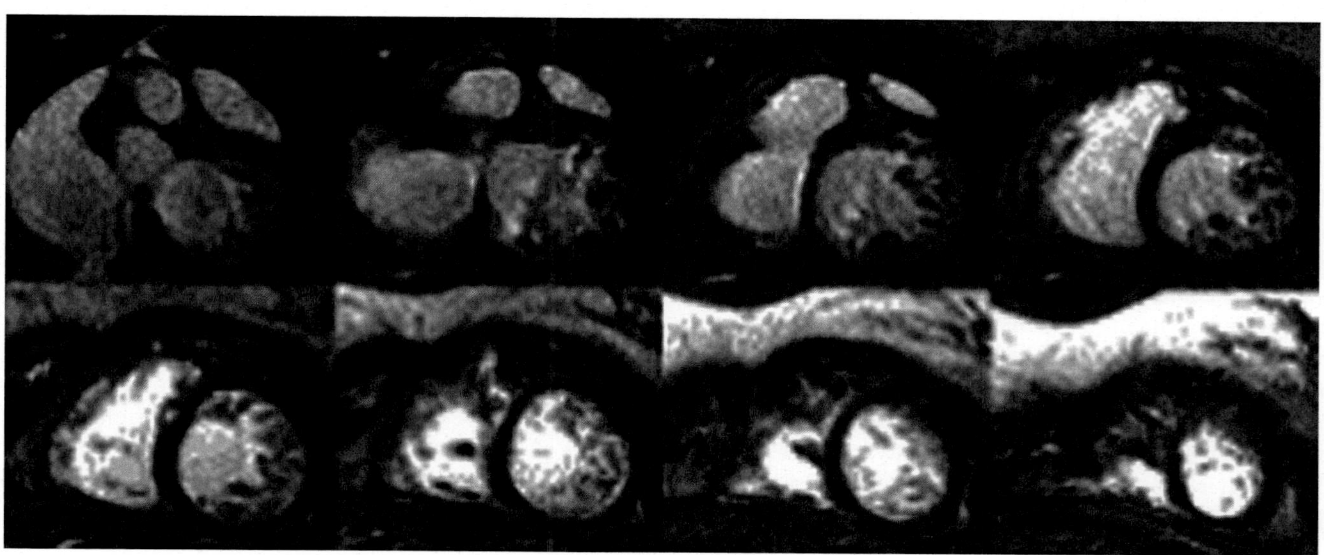

Fig. 26.15 Short axis, delayed enhancement views show deep trabeculation in a case of ventricular non-compaction. Delayed enhancement images were obtained with an inversion time chosen to null myocardial signal, which would normally suppress or darken myocardium. In this case, there is bright signal from contrast in the blood pool interdigitating into the bands of non-compacted myocardium

finding may also be present in normal subjects [190]. Initially, there was over-diagnosis of ARVC/D, partially due to focus on fat involvement and thinning of the right ventricle [191]. Subsequent focus has shifted to right ventricular size, shape, and function, with assessment for global and regional right ventricular wall motion abnormalities, scalloping of the ventricle, increased trabeculation, and delayed enhancement [192, 193]. Delayed enhancement due to fibrofatty infiltrates in ARVC/D can be challenging to visualize though due to the thin wall of the right ventricle [194]. Delayed enhancement can be seen in the left ventricle in ARVC/D. The revised 2010 ARVC/D Task Force criteria include major and minor CMR criteria related to right ventricular size and regional wall motion [189]. CMR involvement as defined by ARVC/D Task Force criteria as well as fatty infiltration, delayed enhancement and left ventricular involvement in conjunction with electrocardiographic abnormalities on ECG and Holter in ARVC/D mutation carriers was associated with the development of sustained ventricular arrhythmias [195].

CMR is useful in identifying mimics of ARVC/D and alternative etiologies of cardiomyopathy [196, 197] CMR findings can help to differentiate such disease processes as Brugada syndrome and cardiac sarcoidosis from ARVC/D. CMR assessment for structural changes associated with Brugada syndrome has only demonstrated subtle anatomic findings in comparison to normal volunteers, therefore CMR may be useful in differentiating ARVC/D from Brugada syndrome [198, 199]. Some CMR features may be useful in differentiating ARVC/D from sarcoidosis. ARVC/D demonstrates greater right ventricular volumes and lower right ventricular ejection fraction, while sarcoid patients have septal delayed gadolinium enhancement and a greater degree of left ventricular involvement as differentiating features [200].

Ventricular Non-compaction

CMR also provides excellent imaging of intraventricular ventricular structures such as trabeculae and is helpful in the diagnosis of ventricular non-compaction (Fig. 26.15). Familial and sporadic cases occur, with clinical manifestations including congestive heart failure, ventricular arrhythmias and thromboembolic events [201]. Criteria including percentage of non-compacted left ventricular myocardial mass, the ratio of non-compacted to compacted myocardium, and location of non-compaction are useful in differentiating ventricular non-compaction from other conditions including hypertrophic cardiomyopathy, dilated cardiomyopathy, hypertensive heart disease, and hypertrophy associated with aortic stenosis [202–204]. The degree of non-compaction may correlate with the occurrence of clinical sustained ventricular tachycardia [205]. Delayed gadolinium enhancement can occur and patterns can be heterogeneous. The presence and extent of late gadolinium enhancement has been associated with severity of disease [206, 207]. CCTA can also accurately assess the degree of non-compacted to compacted myocardium [208, 209].

Assessment of Atrial Myopathy

Similar to ventricular myopathy, atrial myopathy as evidenced by atrial enlargement, depression of atrial function, and focal and diffuse fibrosis, can be characterized by CMR. Imaging challenges exist though, due to the complex shape and thin walls of the atria. Normal ranges for right and left atrial volume by CMR have been determined [210, 211] Assessment of atrial function can be achieved based on volumetric assessment and strain imaging [212–214]. CCTA and CMR atrial volumes are comparable in persistent atrial fibrillation [215]. Atrial myopathy as evidenced by atrial delayed gadolinium enhancement is associated with older age, history of atrial fibrillation and structural heart disease [216]. The degree of delayed contrast enhancement associated with decreased left atrial function and is an independent factor associated with previous occurrence of stroke [217, 218]. Delayed gadolinium atrial enhancement can also be visualized in infiltrative processes involving the atrial such as amyloid [219].

Assessment of structure and function is important to the treatment of supraventricular arrhythmias, as sequelae of atrial myopathy include atrial tachycardia, atrial flutter, and atrial fibrillation. CCTA and CMR provide similar assessment of pulmonary veins before atrial fibrillation ablation [220]. In addition to atrial volumes and function, CMR can characterize pulmonary vein location, shape, complexity, and variation to help in the pre-operative planning, procedural facilitation, and postoperative follow-up for atrial fibrillation ablation procedures [221–226]. Large pulmonary vein size by CMR correlates with recurrence of atrial fibrillation after pulmonary vein isolation [227]. Similar to CCTA, the integration of real time catheter-based electro- anatomic maps and 3-D CMR angiography images obtained pre-procedure facilitates the performance of ablation procedures (Fig. 26.16) [228–230]. Integration of intracardiac echo and CMR images can allow for mapping and ablation with real time localization of esophageal position and catheter tissue contact (Fig. 26.17) [231]. Similar to cardiovascular CCTA, CMR has been used to diagnose and provide surveillance for pulmonary vein stenosis, a potential complication of atrial fibrillation ablation [232–235].

Delayed gadolinium enhancement can assess preablation scar due to atrial myopathy and post procedure scar created by ablation lesions. In comparison to myopathy related fibrosis, ablation scar has greater density [236]. The greater the preablation delayed gadolinium enhancement due to atrial myopathy, the greater the recurrence postablation [237]. The greater the scar created by ablation the lower the recurrence rate [238]. Acute ablation lesions can display hyperenhancement as well as areas of no reflow phenomena. Areas of initial no reflow were better predictors of scar at 3 months and lack of arrhythmia recurrence compared to acutely hyperenhanced areas [239]. In preliminary studies, diffuse atrial fibrosis assessment though T1 mapping correlated with catheter–based tissue mapping voltage, atrial fibrillation and atrial fibrillation arrhythmia recurrence [240, 241].

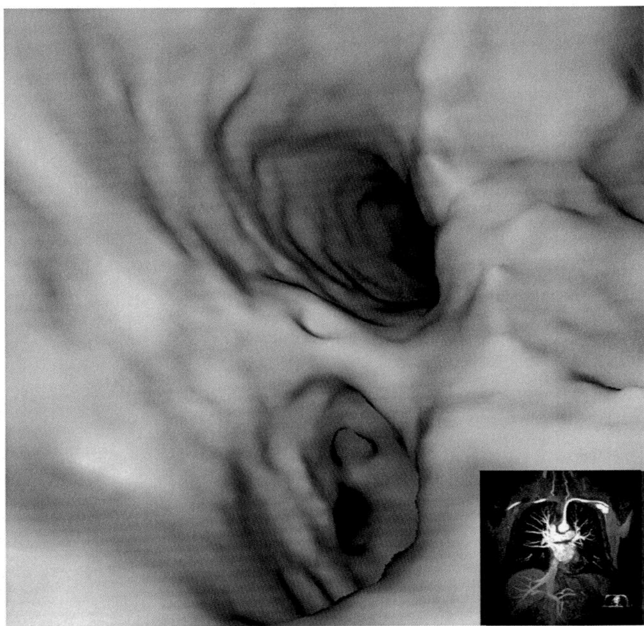

Fig. 26.16 Endovascular view of the left upper and left lower pulmonary veins obtained from reconstruction of a MR angiogram (*lower right panel*) for use with integration with electroanatomic mapping to facilitate atrial fibrillation ablation

An important component of imaging related to atrial myopathy and atrial fibrillation therapies is evaluation of the left atrial appendage for atrial thrombi. Left atrial appendage size, morphology and function can be assessed with CMR [242, 243]. Although CMR can identify atrial appendage thrombi, the technology can misidentify poor contrast filling of the appendage as thrombus and can overestimate the size of thrombi [244, 245]. CMR studies show low diagnostic accuracy for detection of atrial thrombi related to limitations in spatial resolution [246]. CCTA has excellent negative predictive value, but limited positive predictive value and therefore transesophageal echo remains the gold standard for assessment of atrial appendage thrombi [247]. In regard to left atrial appendage occlusion procedures for prophylaxis against stroke, CMR has been shown to be useful for the planning and follow-up. CMR can quantify the left atrial appendage with appendage ostial diameter and appendage long-axis diameter, and can assess for appendage occlusion after device placement [248]. CCTA provides superior image resolution for detailed assessment of the multiple morphologies of the appendage for planning of atrial appendage occlusion techniques [249, 250].

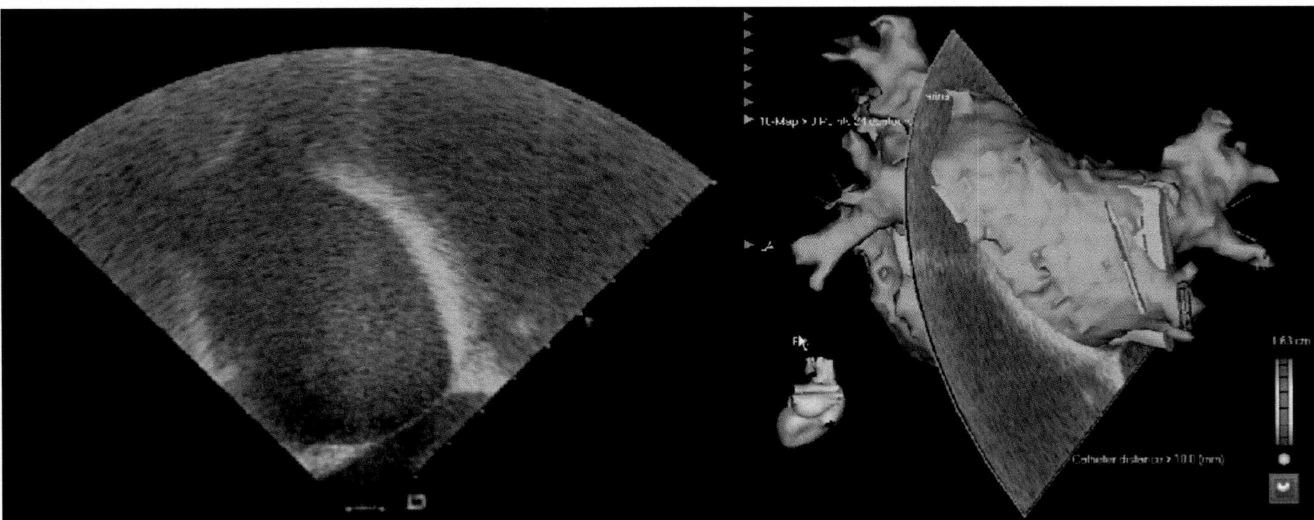

Fig. 26.17 Volume rendered MR angiography integration with intracardiac echo images for atrial fibrillation ablation

Congenital and Acquired Valvular Heart Disease

Echocardiography is the first line modality for assessment of valvular heart disease. As adjuncts to transthoracic and transesophageal echocardiography, both CMR and CT have complementary roles in order to define anatomy and pathophysiology challenging to visualize or quantitate with echocardiography. The strengths of CT relate predominantly to anatomy, while CMR is helpful with tissue characteristics, anatomy, and physiology. Transesophageal echocardiography remains the gold standard for the diagnosis of endocarditis, as with transthoracic echo, CMR and CCTA, small and hypermobile vegetations and leaflet perforations can be missed. Image quality issues exist with all modalities due to artifacts associated with mechanical and bioprosthetic valves. Issues particular to CMR include contraindications to imaging ball and cage valves, dephasing artifacts, and signal void with imaging of calcium. Issues particular to CT relate to beam hardening artifacts. Tomographic imaging with CMR and CCTA allows assessment of adjacent structures for fistulas, abscesses, aneurysms, pseudoaneurysms, and stigmata of embolic phenomena [251–253]. The use of 18F fluorodeoxyglucose PET/CT in the setting of prosthetic valve endocarditis has preliminarily demonstrated increased sensitivity compared with echocardiography, CMR, and CCTA [254].

Aortic Valve

In the assessment of aortic valve stenosis, CMR can be used to quantitate effective aortic valve orifice area, which is comparable to transthoracic and transesophageal echo [255–257]. Transvalvular mean pressure gradients though can be underestimated compared to transthoracic echocardiography [258]. In the setting of cardiomyopathy associated with severe aortic stenosis, late gadolinium enhancement can be visualized correlating with abnormalities of diastolic and systolic dysfunction [259, 260]. The degree of fibrosis provides prognostic assessment of all cause mortality and correlates inversely with the degree of functional improvement after aortic valve replacement and [261].

In assessment and planning for transcatheter aortic valve implantation (TAVI), CCTA is the gold standard for characterization of preprocedure anatomy [262]. CMR can be used, with some limitations due to signal void associated with calcium. It is helpful for post procedure assessment of aortic regurgitation. In comparison to CCTA, CMR can quantitate aortic anatomy for TAVI, but is limited when prosthetic valves are present due to ferromagnetic artifact associated with struts [263]. CMR can also document reverse remodeling including decrease in late gadolinium enhancement post TAVI [264].

CCTA and CMR provide the ability to assess valve morphology to differentiate bicuspid valves from tricuspid valves. These modalities can also identify associated findings including aortopathy, coarctation, or patent ductus arteriosus. CMR [265–269].

The spectrum of issues related to prosthetic valves, including pannus, thrombus, paravalvular leak, abscess, mycotic aneurysm and pseudoaneurysm can be visualized with both CMR and CCTA, with choice depending on relative concerns about image quality related to the specific type of valve. In prosthetic valve assessment, retrospectively gated CT can be used to assess mechanical valve motion and can be helpful to identify and characterize restricted motion due to pannus or thrombus. In mechanical valve models, CT can identify limited mechanical leaflet closure similar to fluoroscopy and can assess for abnormal leaflet motion including frozen leaflets [270]. CT can visualize pannus formation with some limitation due to beam hardening artifact [271–273]. CCTA can be potentially performed as a replacement for invasive coronary angiography in order to decrease embolic risk from thrombus or vegetation, before prosthetic valve reoperation. In patients with previously known coronary artery disease and in some patients with no previous known coronary artery disease though imaging may be non-diagnostic [274].

A strength of CMR is assessment of the physiology of regurgitant valvular disease through steady state free precession functional imaging, ventricular volumes, and regurgitant fraction with velocity encoded imaging (Fig. 26.18, Video 4) [275]. CMR aortic regurgitant orifice correlates with regurgitant volume and regurgitant fraction

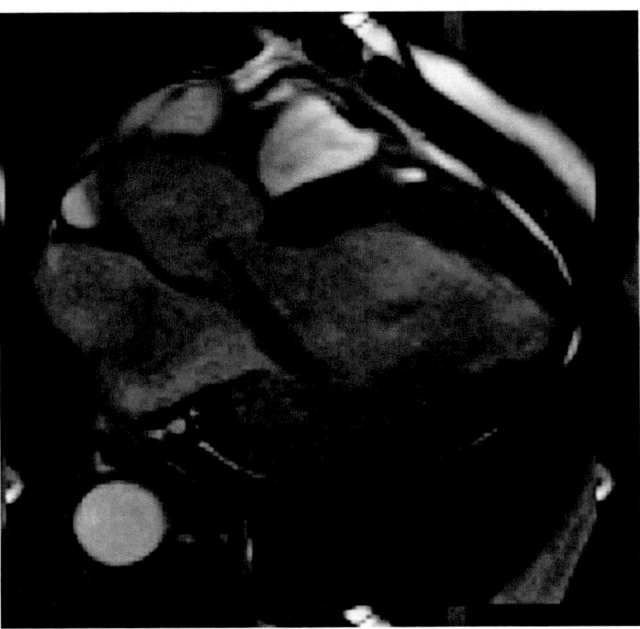

Fig. 26.18 Mild aortic regurgitation with an eccentric jet

by CMR phase velocity mapping [276]. Two-D echo may have difficulties with eccentric jets compared to CMR and 3-D echo [277]. CCTA can provide more limited information regarding aortic regurgitation. Preliminarily, CCTA assessment of regurgitant orifice area correlated with degree of aortic regurgitation by CMR [278]. CCTA volumetric assessment of aortic regurgitation is extrapolated from right and left ventricular stroke volume and must occur in isolation from other valvular lesions for assessment [279].

CMR is useful for assessment of aortic valve regurgitation after TAVI. CMR assessment of aortic valve regurgitant volume and regurgitant fraction after TAVI demonstrates that echocardiography can underestimate the degree of aortic regurgitation [280–283]. After TAVI, CMR can more accurately classify the degree of paravalvular leak and can provide greater prognostic significance than transthoracic echo [284]. CMR assessment of aortic regurgitation effect on ventricular remodeling after TAVI shows that mild to moderate aortic regurgitation is common. Degrees of aortic regurgitation beyond mild lead to prevention of positive remodeling with TAVI. For prediction of post TAVI aortic regurgitation, both CMR and CCTA demonstrate that larger annuli are associated with post procedure regurgitation [285]. For assessment of TAVI perivalvular leak, CCTA is helpful as an adjunct to echo for procedural planning. For surgically placed valves, it can be challenging to differentiate paravalvular leak from residual surgical suture material on CCTA.

Mitral Valve

The mitral valve has complex morphology and motion. Due to its saddle shape and subvalvular apparatus, volumetric assessment of mitral regurgitation is challenging with all modalities. Mitral regurgitant fraction can be extrapolated from CMR phase contrast velocity mapping of aortic outflow volume and left ventricular stroke volume [286, 287]. CMR measurement of anatomic regurgitant orifice correlated with CMR regurgitant fraction and volume as well as with cardiac catheterization regurgitant fraction and volume [288]. With mitral valve prolapse, CMR assessment and quantification of valvular characteristics of anterior leaflet length, posterior leaflet displacement, posterior leaflet thickness, and the presence of flail leaflet were predictors of the degree of mitral regurgitation [289]. Negative remodeling with CMR delayed gadolinium enhancement can be seen in primary mitral regurgitation [290]. In ischemic mitral regurgitation, the degree of basal fibrosis on CMR was a predictor of postoperative ejection fraction and adverse outcome [291]. For percutaneous mitral valve clip repair for mitral regurgitation, CMR performed pre and post procedure was feasible and demonstrated decreases in left ventricular volumes, mitral annular diameter, myocardial mass, and left atrial size [292]. In prosthetic valve mitral regurgitation, CMR can assess jet size and density for assessment of severe MR with transesophageal echo as a reference [293].

CCTA can assess mitral valve, mitral annular and subvalvular morphology, valve function, and definition of the coronary artery and coronary venous 3-D anatomy in the region of the mitral annulus [294–298]. Planimetry of the mitral valve area can be performed in patients with mitral stenosis [299]. CCTA can also provide volumetric assessment of ventricular function and myocardial mass in the setting of mitral regurgitation comparable to CMR [300].

Pulmonary Valve

CMR is useful for assessment of pulmonary valve regurgitation or stenosis as well as the effect of these valvular abnormalities on the right ventricle and pulmonary arteries. These factors are particularly important in the assessment, treatment and follow-up of patients with abnormalities of the pulmonary valve and right ventricular outflow tract such as those with tetralogy of Fallot (Fig. 26.19). CMR can provide assessment of valve morphology and motion, right ventricular morphology, volumes, and function, velocity encoded imaging for calculation of fractional regurgitation, and angiographic assessment of the pulmonary arteries [301–303]. CMR also has been utilized for the follow-up of percutaneous pulmonary valve replacement [304].

Tricuspid Valve

The tricuspid valve has complex anatomy making assessment with CMR challenging. There are limited CMR data related to assessment of annular dimensions, valve geometry, and the effect of tricuspid regurgitation on right ventricular function [305–307]. CCTA has additional issues related to the heterogeneity of contrast in the right atrium and right ventricle. Preliminary study of tricuspid annular geometry using CCTA is being performed [308].

Congenital Heart Disease

The ability of CMR to provide comprehensive assessment of cardiovascular structure and function, as well as an extracardiac vasculature and thoracic structure, makes it useful in the diagnosis, facilitation of treatment, and follow-up of patients with congenital heart disease [309–312]. CMR can assess simple and complex congenital heart disease in the

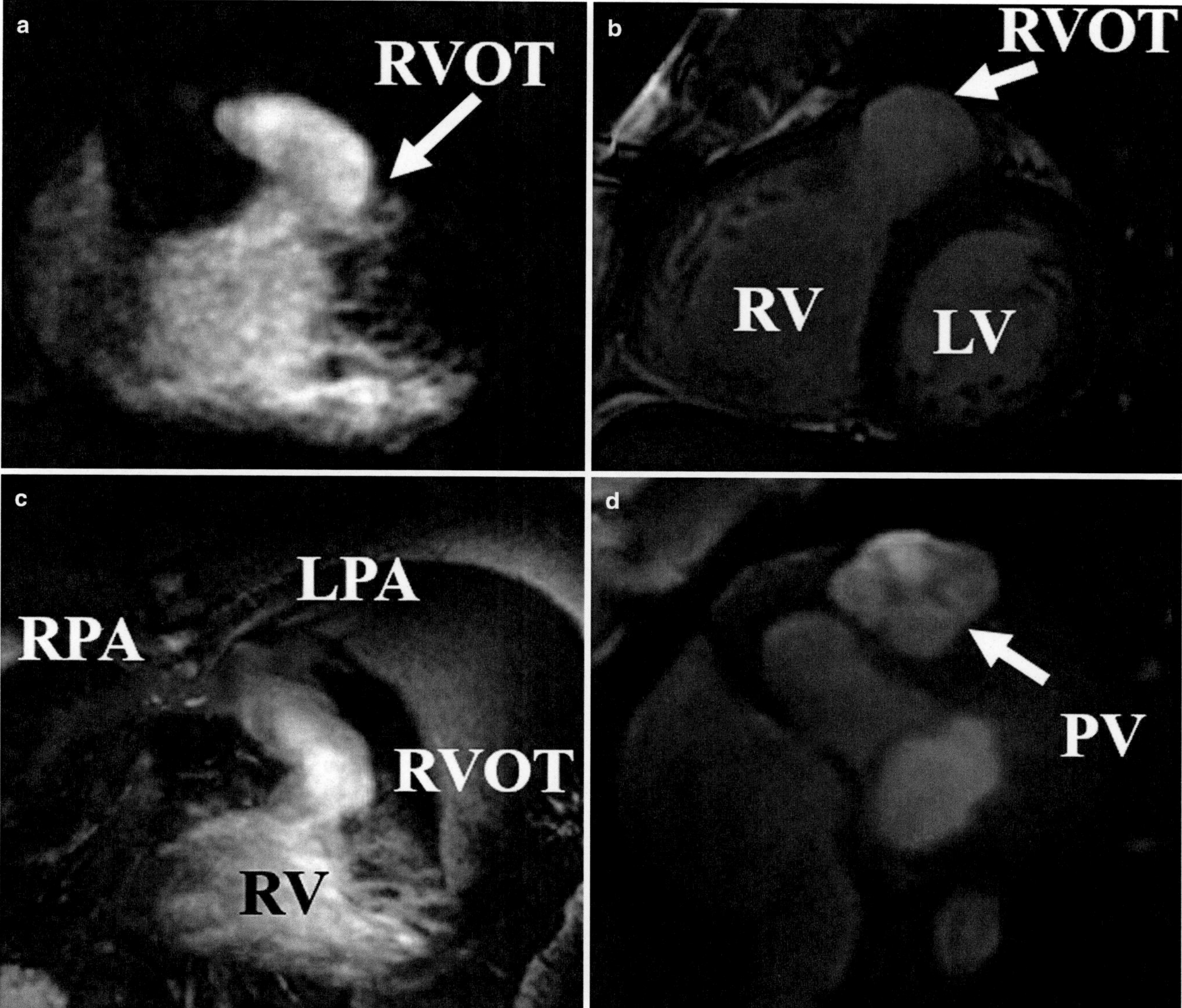

Fig. 26.19 Reconstructed right ventricular outflow tract in the setting of repaired tetralogy of Fallot. Panel (**a**): MR angiogram showing the patch reconstruction of the right ventricular outflow tract. Panel (**b**): Delayed gadolinium short axial view demonstrating enhancement of the patch reconstruction of the right ventricular outflow tract. Panel (**c**): MR angiogram showing the reconstructed right ventricular outflow tract and pulmonary arteries. The branch pulmonary arteries are patent and without evidence of stenoses. Panel (**d**): Coaxial view of the pulmonary valve with severe regurgitation (regurgitant fraction of 48 %). *LV* left ventricle, *LPA* left pulmonary artery, *PV* pulmonary valve, *RPA* right pulmonary artery, *RV* right ventricle, *RVOT* right ventricular outflow tract

native state or after interventional or surgical treatment. As many congenital heart disease patients have implanted cardiac devices or other surgical prosthetic materials, CMR imaging challenges exist which may contraindicate imaging or lead to artifacts limiting interpretation. Artifacts associated with sternotomy wires can affect imaging of structures adjacent to the sternum.

CMR is useful in pre-procedure planning for interventional and surgical approaches to congenital heart disease as well as post procedural follow-up [313–315]. Cardiac shunts can be accurately assessed over the spectrum of pulmonary to systemic shunt ratios [310]. Delayed enhancement imaging can be used to assess the location and degree of fibrosis associated with cardiomyopathy or surgical patches (Fig. 26.20) [316]. Novel approaches providing faster imaging sequences performed without breath hold in a more operator-independent manner should increase the utility of CMR for the assessment of congenital heart

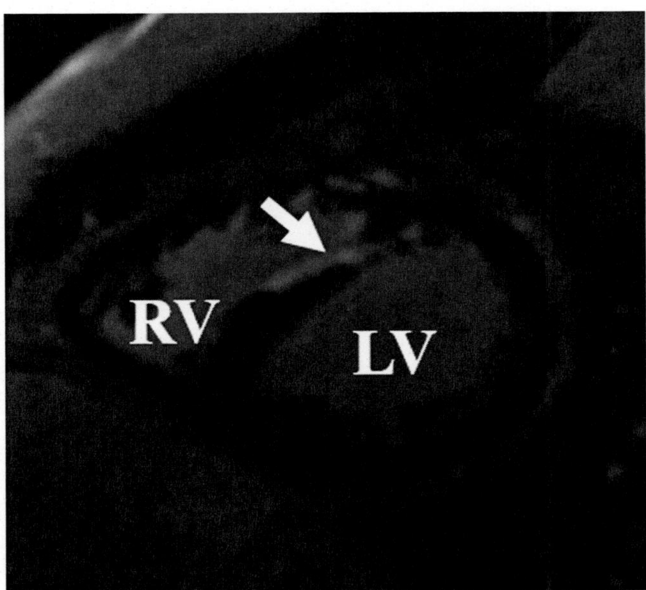

Fig. 26.20 A short axis delayed gadolinium view showing enhancement of a ventricular septal defect patch (*arrow*) associated with repair of tetralogy of Fallot. *LV* left ventricle, *RV* right ventricle

disease. Real time cardiac catheterization guided by magnetic resonance in compatible lab settings is being investigated for use in the assessment and treatment of congenital heart disease [317, 318].

Tetralogy of Fallot

CMR can be used for diagnosis of cardiovascular findings in tetralogy of Fallot. All routes of pulmonary blood flow in patients with pulmonary stenosis or pulmonary atresia including pulmonary artery flow and aorto pulmonary collaterals are important for surgical decisions and planning [319, 320]. CMR can provide characterization of these factors similarly to invasive angiography [321].

In follow-up of right ventricular outflow reconstruction in tetralogy of Fallot, quantitation of pulmonary fractional regurgitation and right ventricular volumes are important for decisions to intervene with interventional cardiology or surgical approaches [322]. Ventricular dysfunction late after surgical repair of tetralogy of Fallot is associated with worse prognosis [323]. Definition of right ventricle and outflow tract anatomy and geometry is potentially more challenging after surgical reconstruction due to artifacts. CMR can assess right ventricular indexed volumes and phase contrast velocity encoded imaging can quantify pulmonary regurgitant fraction in repaired tetralogy of Fallot [324]. Ventricular volumes can be measured by short axis slices or axial slices with better reproducibility seen with use of axial slices after operation for tetralogy of Fallot [325]. After surgical repair, phase contrast velocity CMR can assess for differential regurgitant fraction of right and left pulmonary arteries [326, 327]. Differences in measurement of pulmonary regurgitation depend on whether expiratory breath hold, inspiratory breath hold, or imaging without breath-hold is performed. Expiratory breath hold led to the lowest level of pulmonary regurgitation possibly due to changes in airway pressure [328]. Transthoracic echocardiogram is limited compared to CMR for assessment of pulmonic regurgitation in patients with repaired tetralogy of Fallot [329].

Late gadolinium enhancement can be utilized to visualize biventricular fibrosis after tetralogy of Fallot repair and has correlated with ventricular dysfunction, poor exercise tolerance and elevation of neurohormonal factors [330]. Restrictive right ventricular physiology has been associated with the degree of late gadolinium enhancement of the operated right ventricular outflow tract [331]. Biventricular negative remodeling has been seen with assessment of diffuse fibrosis with T1 post contrast imaging [332].

The strengths of CCTA for assessment of tetralogy of Fallot include detailed assessment of pulmonary vascular anatomy and assessment of coronary artery anatomy in relation to other structures for anomalous course prior to surgery [333–335]. Although radiation exposure is a concern particularly in the pediatric population, dose sparing protocols can allow for sub-millisievert exposures [336]. Preliminary study has demonstrated assessment of right ventricular volumes and ejection fraction comparable to CMR [337]. CCTA can be used for rapid prototyping of models for assessment and planning of patch repair of ventricular septal defects in tetralogy of Fallot [333].

Single Ventricle Physiology

There are a spectrum of congenital syndromes with single ventricle physiology with surgical interventions including creation of Fontan circulation and a host of other cavo- pulmonary surgeries. MR angiography can define these circuits, assess for baffle and conduit stenoses or leaks, and identify additional anomalous circulation (Fig. 26.21, Video 5). CMR provides quantification of cavo-pulmonary flow through phase contrast velocity mapping assessment of flow in the superior and inferior vena cava and left and right pulmonary arteries [338]. Time resolved 3-D magnetic resonance can assess vascular anatomy and flow dynamics of cavo-pulmonary circuits including Fontan circulation [339]. In contradistinction, CCTA can be challenging to use for

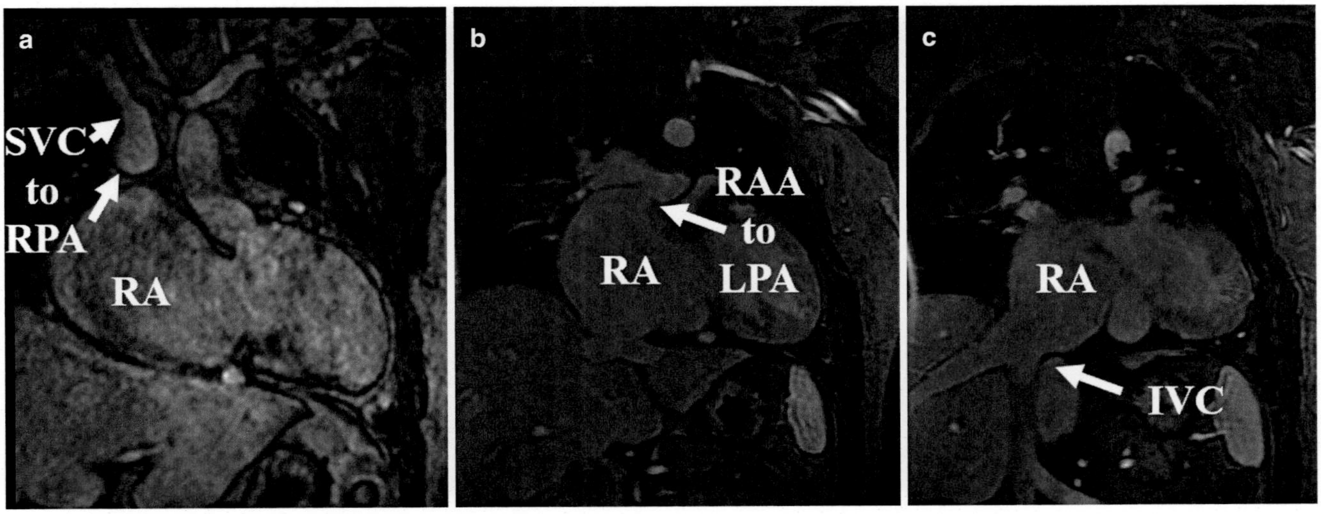

Fig. 26.21 MR angiography views of pulmonary atresia and hypoplastic right ventricle, status post Fontan. Panel (**a**): The superior vena cava connection to the right pulmonary artery (*arrow*) is patent. The right atrium is severely enlarged. Panel (**b**): The anastomosis of the right atrium to the left pulmonary artery via the right atrial appendage is patent. Panel (**c**): There is a normal connection of the inferior vena cava to the right atrium. *IVC* inferior vena cava, *LPA* left pulmonary artery, *RA* right atrium, *RAA* right atrial appendage, *RPA* right pulmonary artery

opacification of the Fontan circulation with upper extremity venous contrast injection and may require specialized injection protocols including delayed contrast imaging or simultaneous upper and lower extremity venous contrast injection [340, 341].

CMR indexed end-diastolic ventricular volume is a predictor of outcome in patients with Fontan anatomy [342]. Assessment of superior and inferior vena cava flow in Fontan patients in the context of quantification of geometry has been used to assess fluid dynamic power loss in Fontan circuits [343–345]. In late Fontan survivors, ventricular delayed gadolinium enhancement has been identified with its extent associated with ventricular enlargement and dysfunction, increased ventricular mass and non-sustained ventricular tachycardia [346].

Transposition of the Great Arteries

In the setting of transposition of the great arteries, CCTA and CMR are helpful in 3-D definition of the anatomic and physiologic relationships of the pulmonary arteries, aorta, cardiac chambers, valves, and thoracic visceral and skeletal structures. In the assessment and reporting the findings, it is essential to define the atrioventricular valves and cardiac chambers by morphology and physiologic function. A spectrum of uses in the setting of native and operated transposition syndromes exist, including initial diagnosis and characterization, planning of atrial switch procedures for D transposition of the great arteries, assessment of ventricular structure and function related to pulmonary artery banding (Figs. 26.22 and 26.23), and evaluation and follow-up of arterial switch procedures.

Assessment of function of the morphologic right ventricle in the systemic position is important for surgical decisions in transposition of the great arteries. In the setting of D-transposition of the great arteries status post atrial switch, the extent of late gadolinium enhancement of the morphologic right ventricle in the systemic position is associated with decreased ejection fraction and is a predictor of adverse outcome [347]. In young adults status post previous atrial switch, CMR demonstrated no evidence of inducible ischemia [348]. In congenitally corrected transposition of the great arteries or surgically palliated D-transposition of the great arteries with atrial switch, dobutamine CMR can be used to assess for follow-up for dysfunction due to right ventricular pressure overload [349]. Additionally, as the morphologic left ventricle is in the pulmonary position, CMR can assess ventricular wall thickness, volumes, ejection fraction, and response to pulmonary artery banding for potential arterial switch operations. CMR can also define issues related to surgical baffles [350, 351]. Additional congenital anomalies in the setting of transposition of the great arteries can also be identified with CMR (Fig. 26.24) [352].

CCTA is also useful in the diagnosis, procedural and surgical planning and follow-up of congenital heart disease related to transposition of the great arteries. Large and small

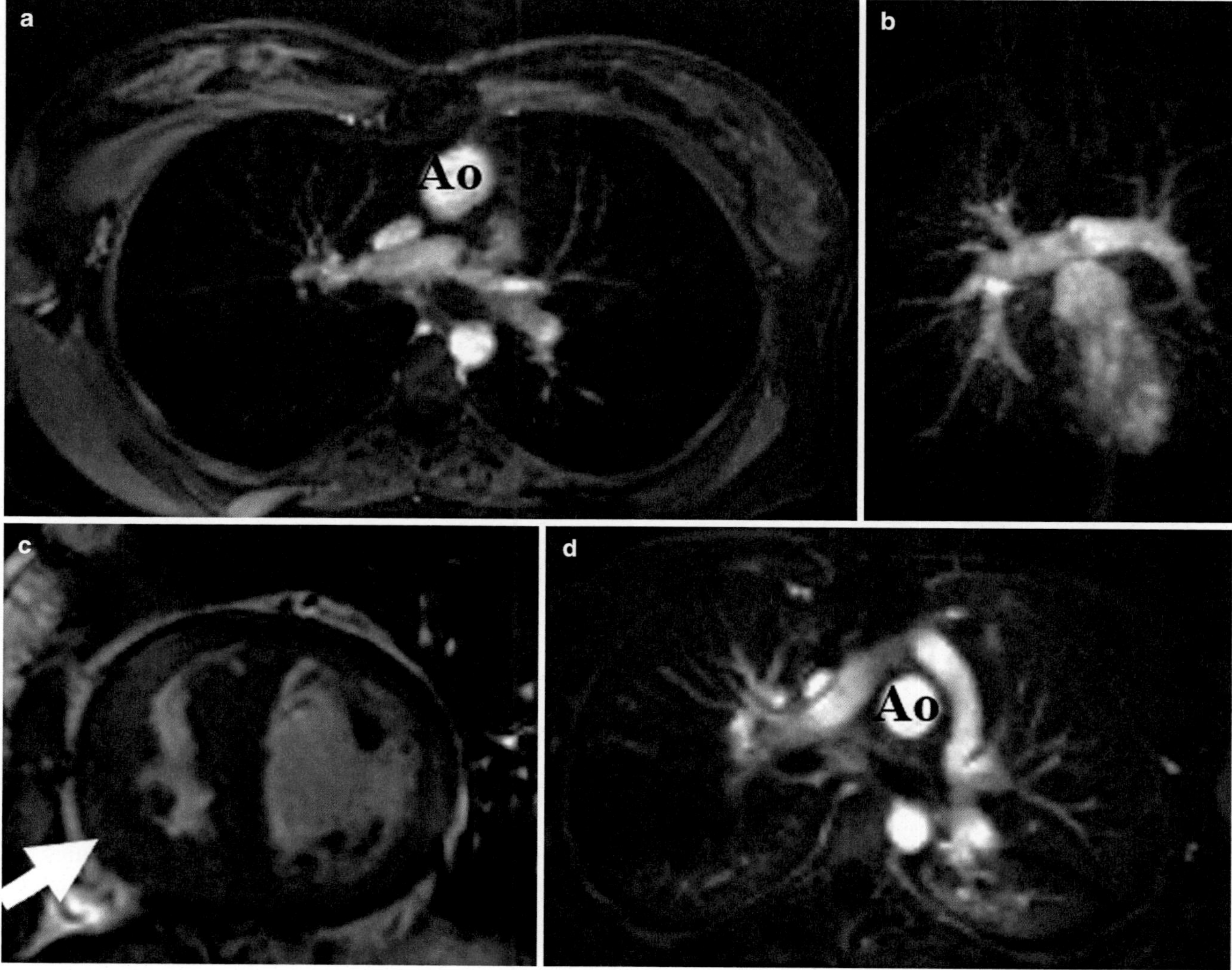

Fig. 26.22 Transposition of the great arteries (D-type), status post previous atrial baffle procedure in childhood, with subsequent pulmonary artery banding in preparation for an arterial switch operation. Panel (**a**): An axial view demonstrates the anterior position of the aorta. Panel (**b**): MR angiogram status post pulmonary artery banding. Panel (**c**): Due to the pulmonary artery banding, there is hypertrophy of the previously thin morphologic left ventricular myocardium in the venous position (*arrow*). Panel (**d**): After arterial switch, the neoaorta is located posterior to the main pulmonary artery. Ao aorta

Fig. 26.24 Multiple views of unrepaired congenitally corrected transposition of the great arteries with additional anomalies including a left-sided superior vena cava and partial anomalous pulmonary venous return. Panel (**a**): An axial view demonstrating the anterior and leftward position of the aorta in relation to the pulmonary artery (L-transposed great arteries). Panel (**b**): A 4 chamber view demonstrating the right atrium leading to the morphologic left ventricle (pulmonary ventricle) and left atrium leading to morphologic right ventricle (systemic ventricle). Panel (**c**): A 4 chamber view demonstrating continuity between the morphologic left ventricle and main pulmonary artery. Panel (**d**): A long axis view demonstrating continuity between the morphologic right ventricle and aorta. Panel (**e**): MR angiogram demonstrating bilateral superior vena cavae. The right upper pulmonary vein drains anomalously into the right superior vena cava. *Ao* aorta, *AV* atrioventricular, *LA* left atrium, *LV* left ventricle, *PA* pulmonary artery, *RA* right atrium, *RV* right ventricle, *SVC* superior vena cava

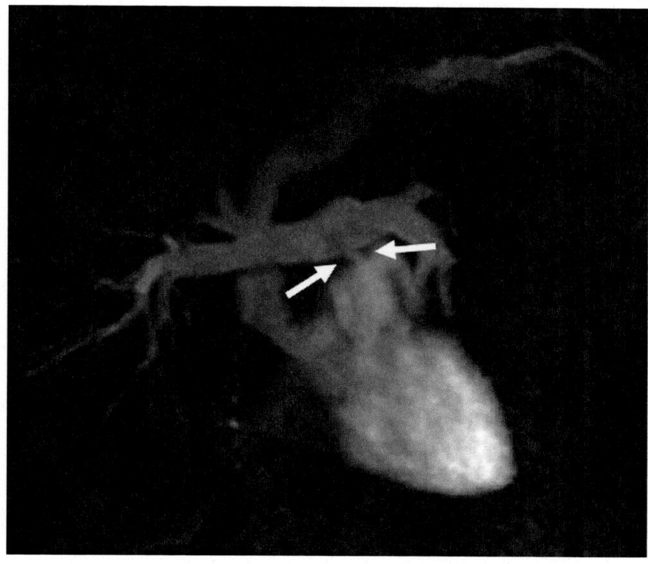

Fig. 26.23 MR angiogram demonstrating narrowing of the main pulmonary artery (*arrows*) due to surgical banding in the setting of D-transposition of the great arteries

vessel anatomy can be characterized, particularly assessment of coronary artery anomalies in relation to other cardiothoracic structure in the presurgical and postoperative states. CCTA is useful for evaluation of baffles associated with atrial switch procedures [353]. After arterial switch, CCTA is assess reimplanted coronary arteries for coronary artery stenoses and for anomalous courses with potential coronary artery compression [354].

Ebstein Anomaly

CMR and CCTA can be useful adjuncts to echocardiography for the evaluation of Ebstein anomaly (Fig. 26.25, Video 6). CMR measurement of right to left heart volumes and quantification of functional and atrialized right ventricular volumes and total right/left volume index can help to determine the severity of Ebstein anomaly [355–357]. CCTA can identify other cardiothoracic findings of large and small vessels including anomalous coronary arteries [358].

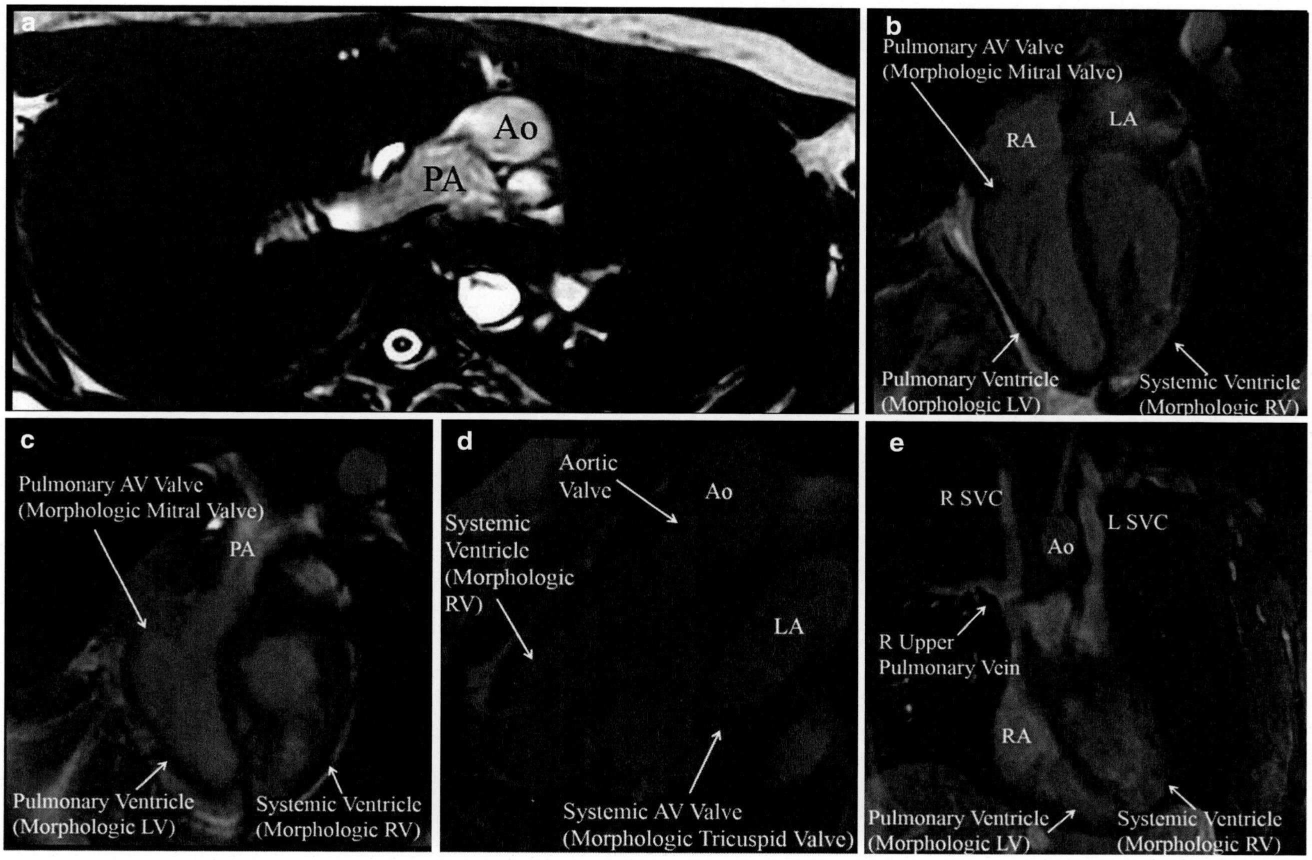

Septal Defects

For planning and follow-up of percutaneous closure of secundum atrial septal defects, CMR can assess atrial septal margins, maximal and minimal defect dimensions comparable to transesophageal echo (Figs. 26.26 and 26.27) [314, 359]. Additional data include coaxial velocity encoded CMR atrial septal defect flow, size and shape [360]. In assessment of Qp/Qs, CMR is comparable to cardiac catheterization [361]. Three-D MRA can characterize partial anomalous pulmonary venous return associated with atrial septal defects [320, 362, 363].

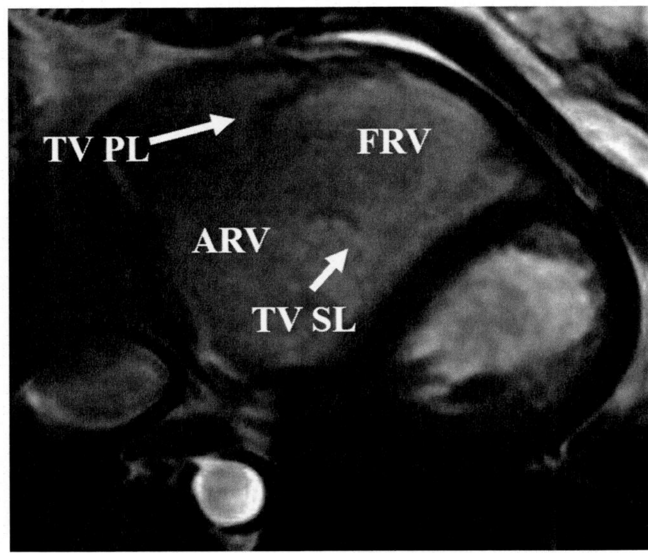

Fig. 26.25 CMR view of Ebstein anomaly. An axial steady state free precession view demonstrating apical displacement of the tricuspid leaflets, therefore dividing the right ventricle into functional and atrialized portions. Apical displacement of the septal leaflet and posterior leaflet is shown (*arrow*). *ARV* atrialized right ventricle, *FRV* functional right ventricle, *TV PL* tricuspid valve posterior leaflet, *TV SL* tricuspid valve septal leaflet

CCTA can be useful for preprocedure interventional and surgical planning as well as assessment of percutaneous closure for atrial septal defect sizing and characteristics including complex and multiple defects, assessment of coronary arteries and assessment of partial anomalous pulmonary venous return associated with atria septal defects [364–366]. Post-intervention assessment includes percutaneous closure device location for diagnosis of malposition or extension into systemic or pulmonary veins and assessment of right ventricular remodeling after closure [367, 368].

For ventricular septal defects, CMR and CCTA can provide pre-procedure interventional and surgical planning through definition of size, location, 3-D relationships to other structures, and identification of other cardiovascular anomalies [369]. CMR and CCTA imaging can be integrated with fluoroscopy for guidance of percutaneous closure interventions [370]. CMR can provide assessment of Qp:Qs, characterization of location and extent of myocardial infarct scar associated post-infarct ventricular septal defects, and can quantify sequelae of complex surgeries such as atrioventricular septal defect closure with flow dynamic characteristics of AV valve regurgitation after repair [371]. Multimodality imaging with CCTA and CMR can be useful adjuncts in complex scenarios (Fig. 26.28, Videos 7 and 8) [372].

Cardiac Masses

CMR is helpful in the evaluation of cardiac masses due to the ability to comprehensively assess tissue characteristics, as well as involvement of a mass in relation to surrounding

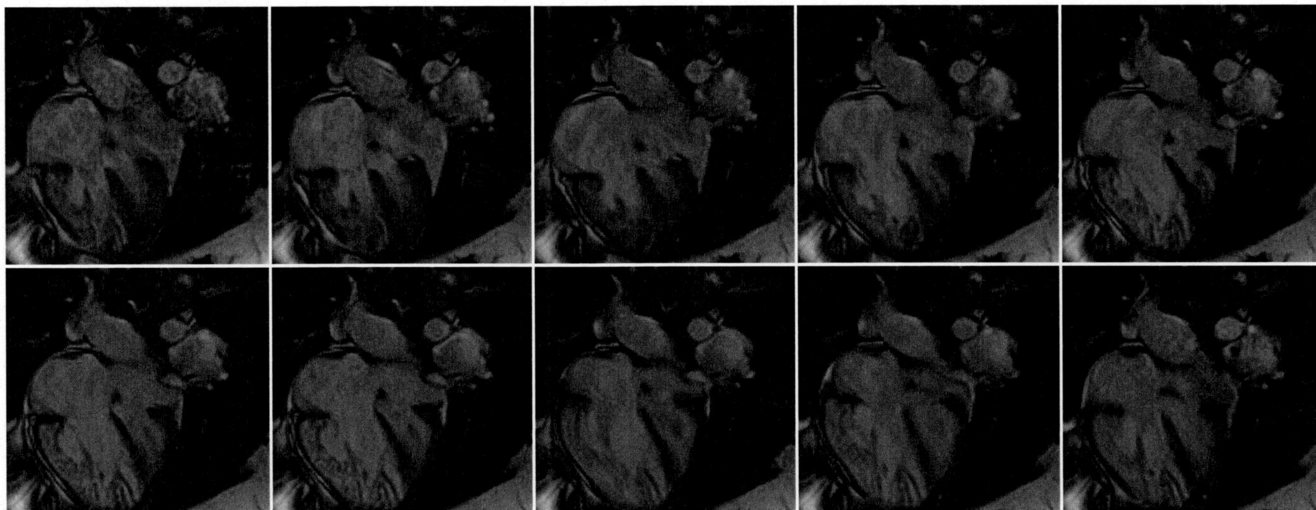

Fig. 26.26 CMR 4 chamber images demonstrating a large secundum atrial septal defect, with right ventricular enlargement and hypertrophy and right atrial enlargement

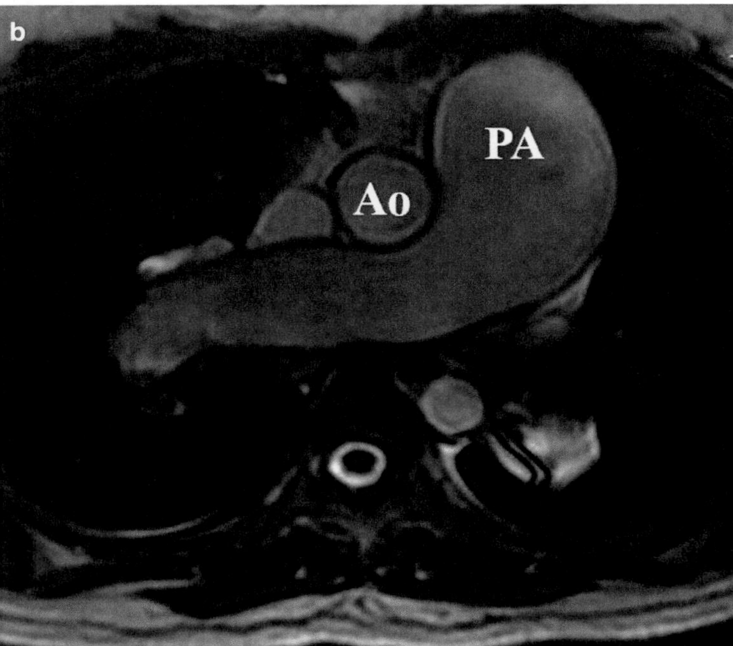

Fig. 26.27 Eisenmenger syndrome due to a large secundum atrial septal defect. Panel (**a**): A 4 chamber view shows the secundum atrial septal defect (*arrows*), right atrial enlargement, and right ventricular enlargement. Panel (**b**): An axial view demonstrates significant pulmonary artery enlargement due to pulmonary hypertension. *Ao* aorta, *ASD* atrial septal defect, *LA* left atrium, *LV* left ventricle, *PA* pulmonary artery, *RA* right atrium, *RV* right ventricle

cardiac and thoracic structures. Anatomic definition of masses include: number of masses, shape, morphology of the connection to the heart, intracameral, subendocardial, myocardial, epicardial, pericardial, or extracardiac location, and presence of invasion of the mass into structures (Figs. 26.29, 26.30, 26.31 and 26.32, Video 9). CMR is especially useful in assessment of the tissue of masses based on T1 and T2 characteristics as well as the presence, degree and location of perfusion and delayed gadolinium enhancement [373]. Mass location, tissue characteristics, and presence of pericardial or pleural involvement are important factors for evaluating and staging benign or malignant cardiac neoplasms when findings are compared to actual histologic examination [374].

Benign tumors, primary malignant tumors, and metastatic malignant tumors, have been identified with CMR, including fibromas, lipomas, myxomas, mesotheliomas, sarcomas, lymphomas, melanomas, and metastatic carcinomas [375–385]. Tumor mimics can also be identified including lipomatous hypertrophy of the interatrial septum, prominent crista terminalis, Chiari network, and thrombus [377, 386, 387]. Although CMR is useful, histologic tissue analysis remains the gold standard for diagnosis [388]. Due to its excellent spatial resolution, CCTA can provide assessment of cardiac mass morphology, location, with some ability tissue characterization based on Hounsfield Units and contrast enhancement. It is useful in situations in which application of CMR is challenging or contraindicated [389]. CCTA can be particularly useful in assessing the relationship of the coronary arteries to cardiac and extracardiac masses.

Assessment of Pericardial Disease

Pericardial disease includes a spectrum of processes due to infectious, inflammatory, malignant, ischemic, and traumatic etiologies. Echocardiography is an important imaging modality for initial assessment of the presence and hemodynamic effects of pericardial effusion and pericardial thickening. Tomographic processes including CMR and CCTA can provide additional assessment through biventricular morphology and function related to pericardial disease processes, regional assessment of pericardial fluid and pericardial thickening. The strength of CMR includes the ability to define tissue characteristics related to T1 and T2 weighting, delayed gadolinium assessment of pericardial inflammation (Fig. 26.33), and tagging to assess for areas of adhesion [390–392]. CCTA provides more limited tissue characterization, but is useful for assessing the degree and location of pericardial calcification, Hounsfield density estimation of the hematocrit of effusion, pericardial fat, relationship of calcified pericardium to the coronary arteries, and assessment for other thoracic disease [393].

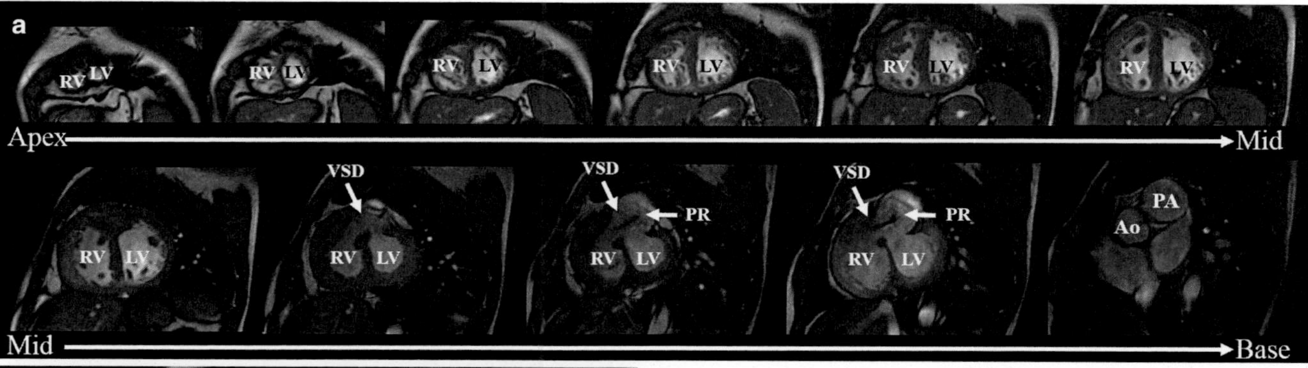

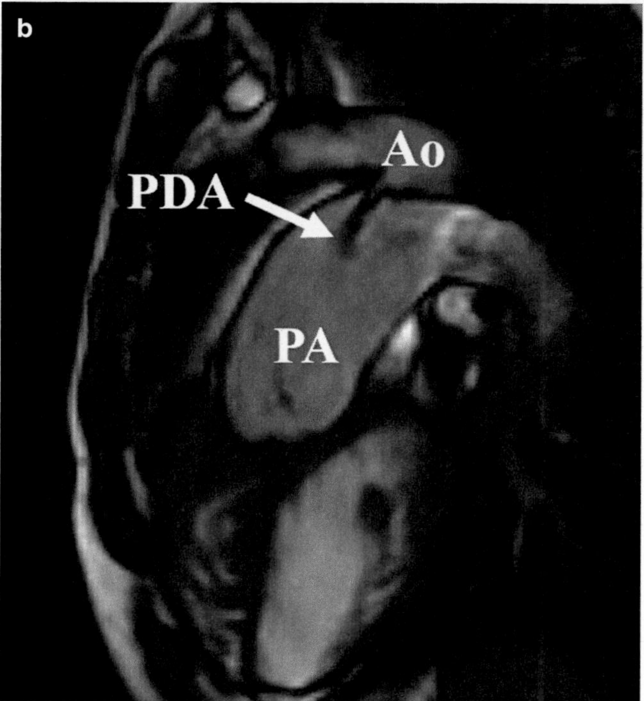

Fig. 26.28 Unoperated congenital heart disease with Eisenmenger syndrome due to a double outlet right ventricle with a large ventricular septal defect. Panel (**a**): Serial short axis steady state free precession views from apex to base show the double outlet right ventricle with a large ventricular septal defect. There is moderate dilatation and hypertrophy of right ventricle and a D-shaped septum due to right ventricular volume and pressure overload. A severe regurgitant jet of pulmonary regurgitation is preferentially directed towards the right ventricle. Panel (**b**): A steady state free precession view shows a patent ductus arteriosus. *Ao* aorta, *LV* left ventricle, *PA* pulmonary artery, *PDA* patent ductus arteriosus, *PR* pulmonary regurgitation, *RV* right ventricle, *VSD* ventricular septal defect

Vascular Disease

CMR and MR angiography are reliable for the detection of aortic aneurysm and aortic dissection. Gated CMR is particularly helpful for evaluation of the aortic root for aneurysm, dissection, and aortic valve function. Contrast enhanced black blood MR is particularly helpful for evaluating aortic plaque, ulceration and intramural hemorrhage.

Carotid MRA is generally effective in diagnosing stenosis. Carotid plaque MR evaluation can measure wall thickness and volume and analyze plaque components including lipid core, fibrosis, calcium, and dynamic contrast enhancement via k-trans measurement. In addition to congenital aortic lesions such as coarctation of the aorta (Fig. 26.34) and Marfan syndrome, CMR can diagnose acquired vascular and valvular heart disease including aneurysm, dissection, and wall abnormalities such as penetrating ulcers, calcification, or thrombus with ability to assess all aortic segments (Fig. 26.35, Video 10) [394–396]. CMR and CCTA may be particularly useful in assessment of aortic grafts particularly for endoleak with some studies favoring CMR, although CCTA can be useful when calcified plaque is present [397–399]. Clinically useful abdominal aorta and branch images

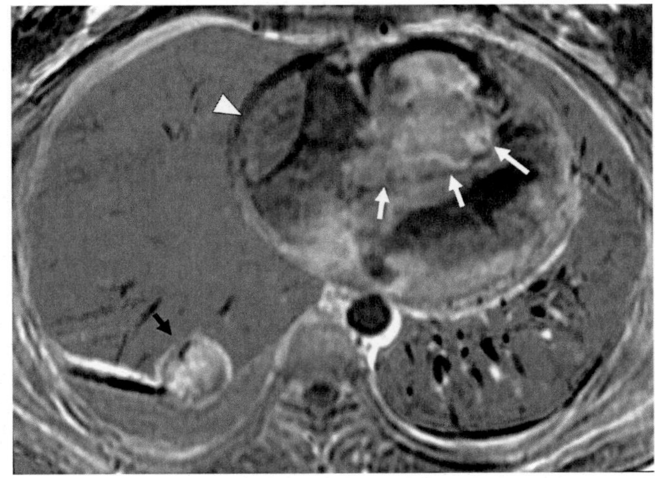

Fig. 26.29 A large, broad-based mass is present arising from the right ventricle (*white arrows*). There is also an enhancing mass in the right atrium (*arrowhead*). A right lower lobe enhancing lung mass is present (*black arrow*), likely representing a metastasis. A right pleural effusion is also present. The diagnosis was metastatic angiosarcoma

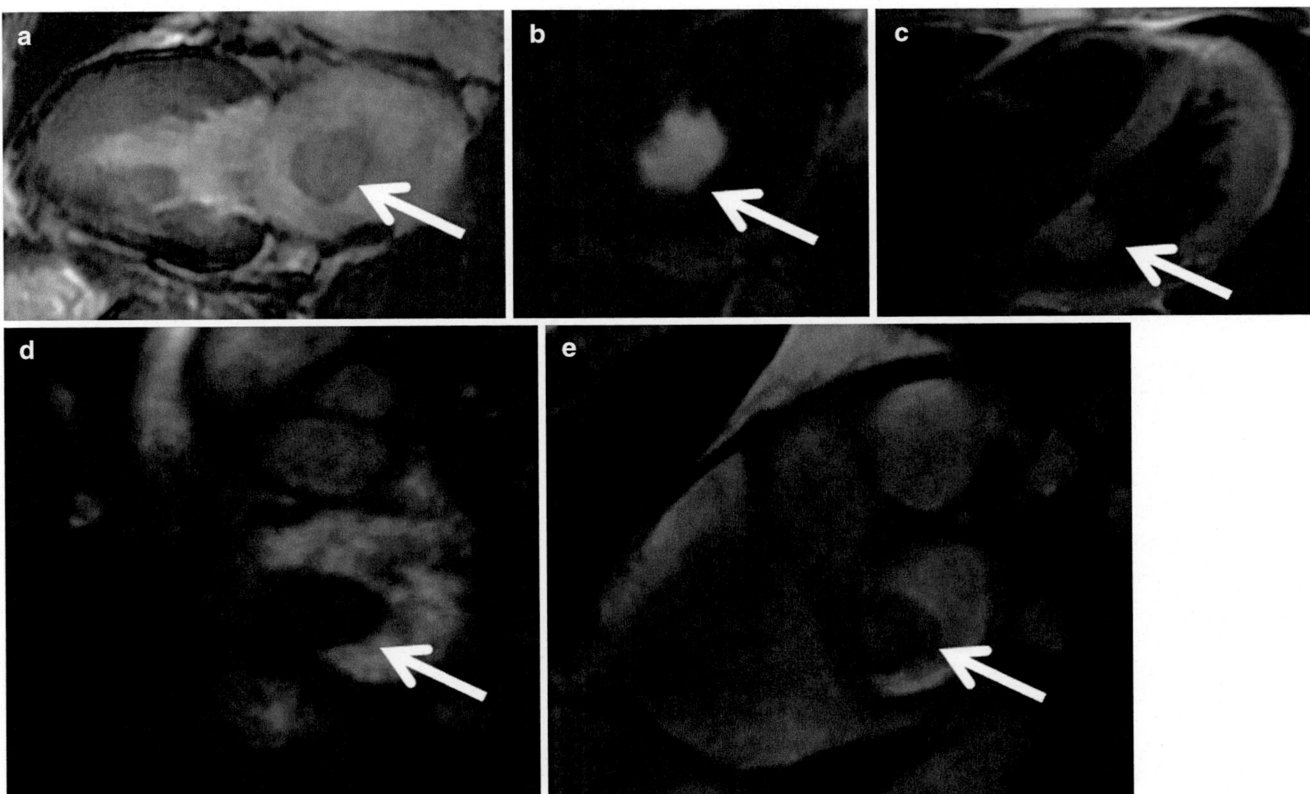

Fig. 26.30 A CMR study from a patient with a left atrial mass (*arrows*) with characteristics most consistent with myxoma. Panel (**a**): Within the left atrium there was a 3.3 × 1.8 × 2.4 cm intracameral mass along the interatrial septum at the fossa ovalis. Panel (**b**): The mass was hyperintense on the T2-weighted images. Panel (**c**): The mass was isointense to muscle on T1-weighted images. Panel (**d**): The mass demonstrated heterogeneous enhancement immediately post contrast. Panel (**e**): There was heterogeneous enhancement on delayed contrast images. There was no evidence of myocardial invasion, pericardial effusion or pleural effusions. The diagnosis of left atrial myxoma with organized thrombus formation was confirmed based on the surgical histological evaluation

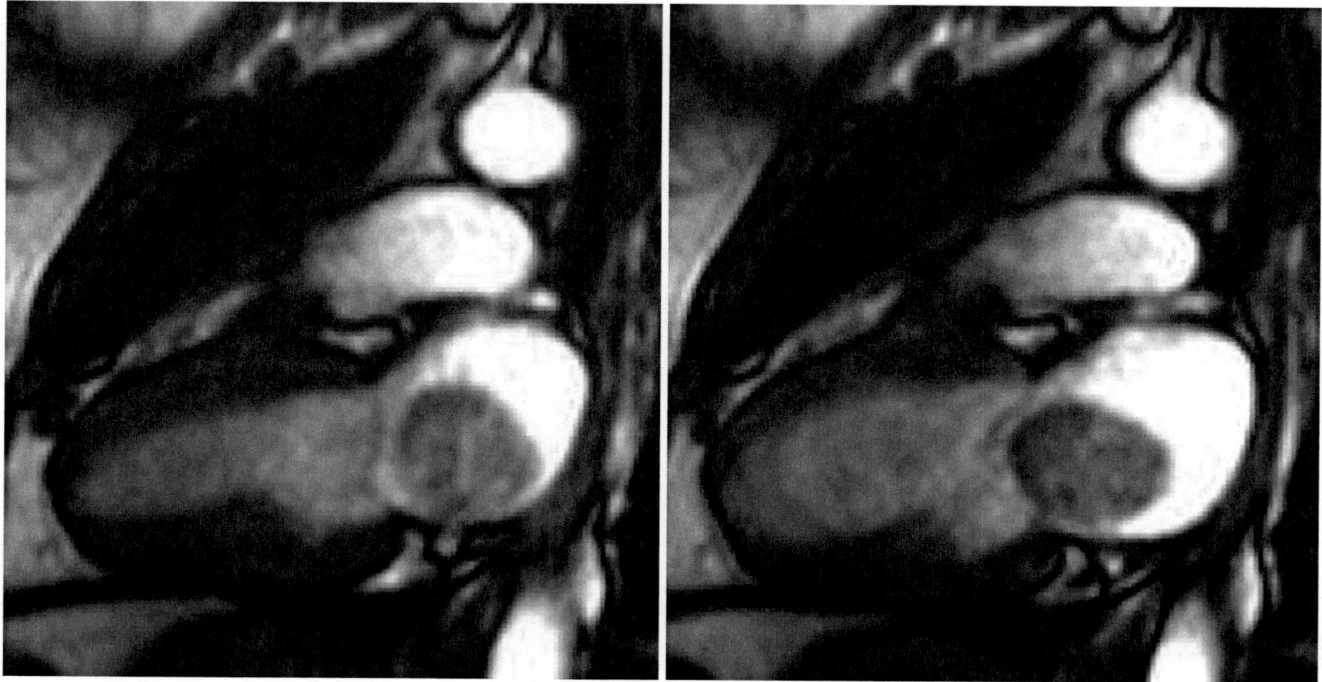

Fig. 26.31 Large atrial myxoma which obstructs the mitral valve during atrial systole

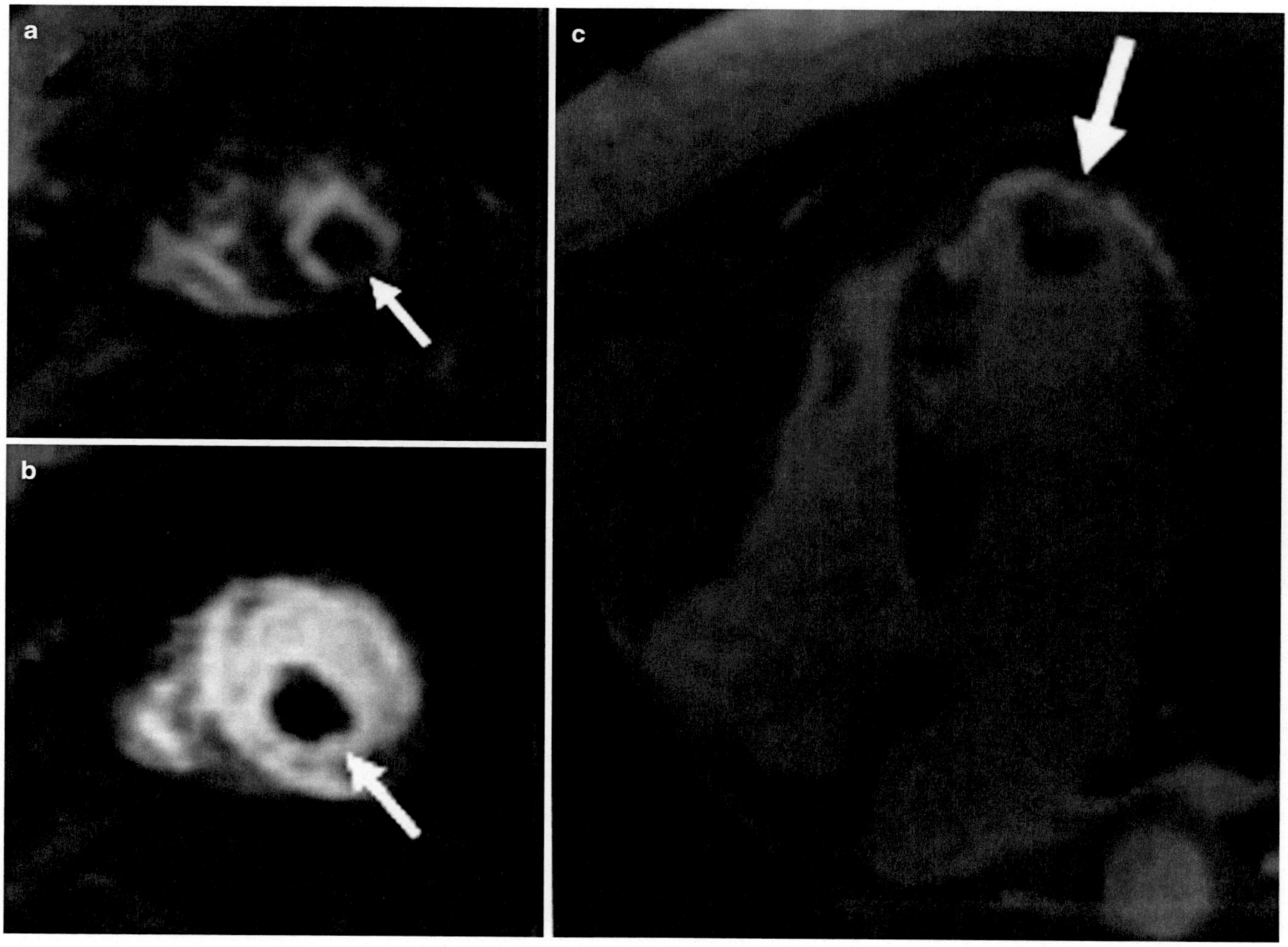

Fig. 26.32 Chronic myocardial infarction with an apical aneurysm and an apical thrombus (*arrows*). Panel (**a**): Short axis first pass perfusion image. Panel (**b**): Short axis functional image. Panel (**c**): Delayed gadolinium enhancement 4 chamber view

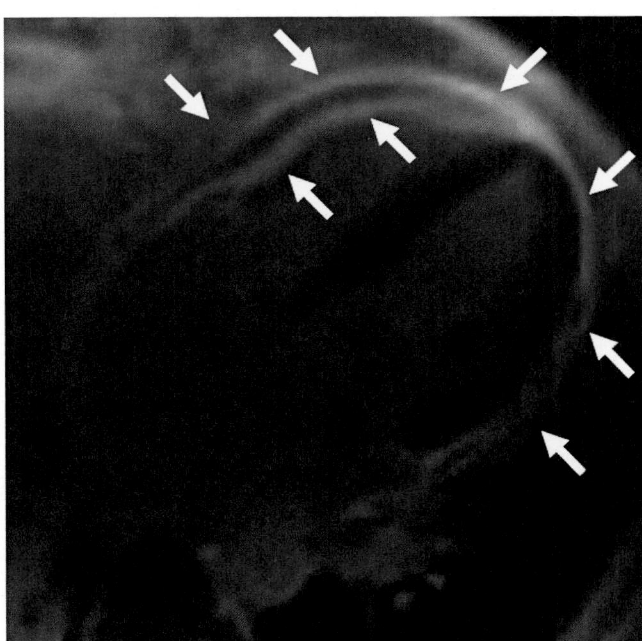

Fig. 26.33 A 4 chamber view demonstrating pericardial delayed gadolinium enhancement (*arrows*) associated with pericarditis

are readily obtained with either MRA or CCTA. Either may be performed for the evaluation of vascular anomalies and renal artery stenosis. CCTA may be preferred due to superior resolution and reliability. Clinically useful extremity vessel images are also readily obtained with either MRA or CCTA. In addition to arterial system abnormalities, CMR and CCTA can identify congenital and acquired abnormalities of the systemic veins such as left-sided superior vena cava with a connection to an aneurysmal coronary sinus, interrupted inferior vena cava, and superior vena cava compression.

Summary

Both CCTA and CMR are robust imaging modalities for characterization of cardiovascular substrates. Decisions related to performing CMR versus CCTA require information including patient age, allergy history, clinical stability to be in the MR environment for the amount of time necessary for study, history of claustrophobia, history of ferromagnetic devices, implant or deposits, devices, renal function, cardiac rhythm and rate, strengths and limitations of other imaging modalities, and the posed clinical question. CMR provides assessment for the diagnosis and treatment of cardiovascular disease, including cardiovascular structure, function, tissue characterization, myocardial perfusion, and metabolism. Applications include the assessment of coronary artery disease, cardiomyopathic substrates, congenital heart disease, thoracic vasculature, valvular function, masses, pericardial disease and assessment of aortic and branch vessel anatomy. Advances in technology will continue to lead to novel clinical and research applications.

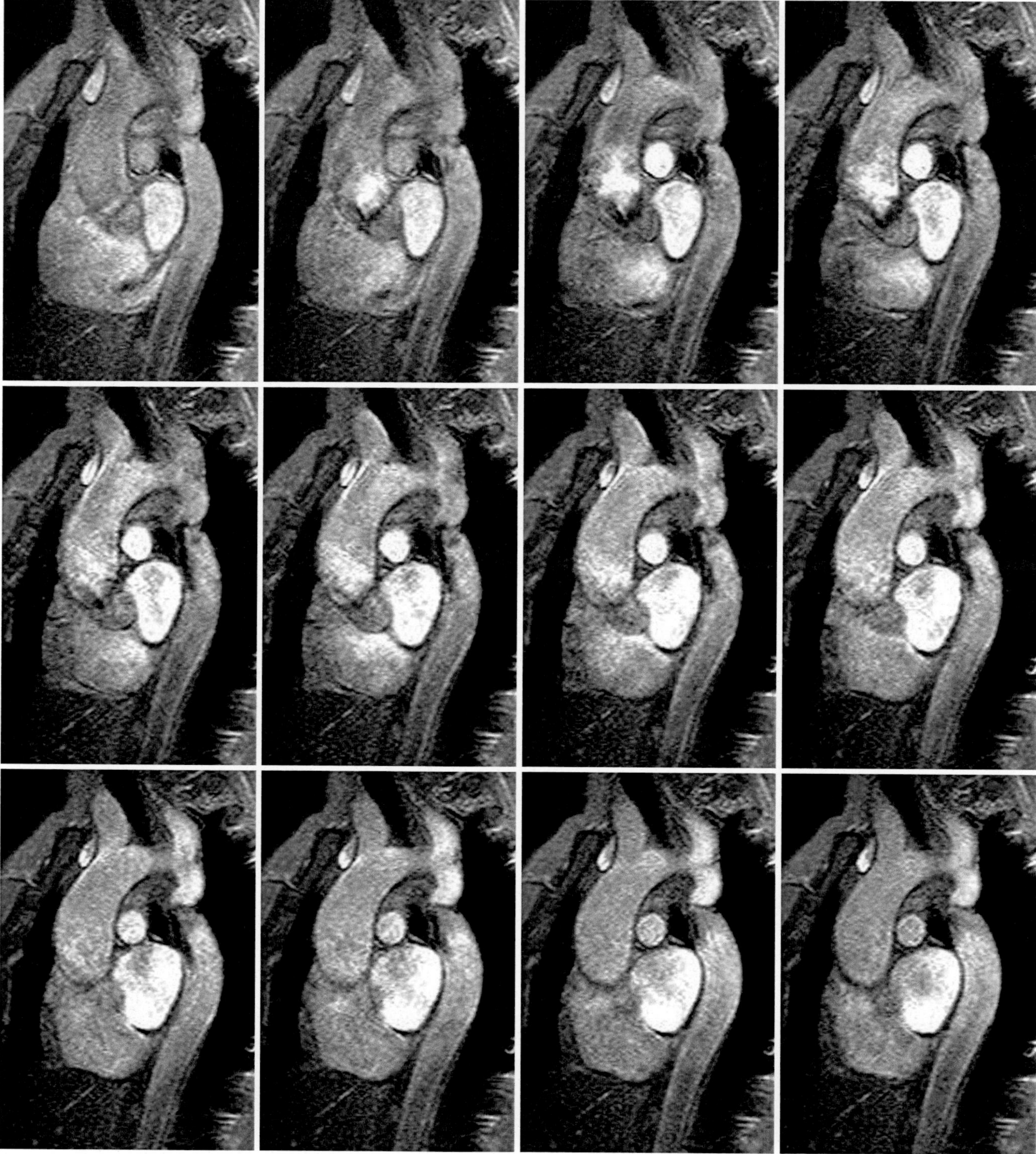

Fig. 26.34 Serial sagittal slices demonstrating coarctation of the aorta

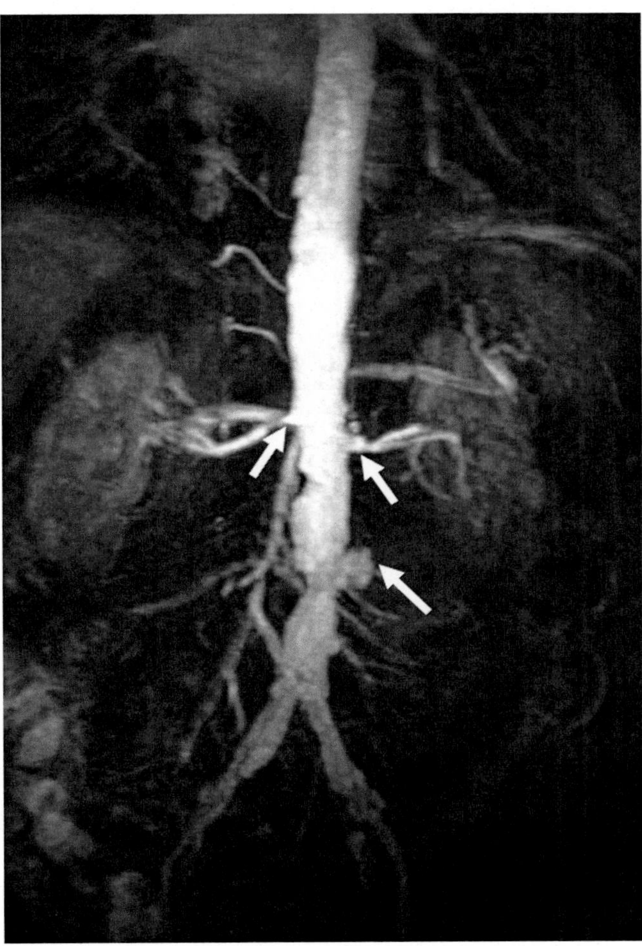

Fig. 26.35 MR angiogram demonstrates multifocal plaques, bilateral renal artery stenosis (*upper arrows*), and a saccular aneurysm of infrarenal aorta (*lower arrow*)

References

1. Hendel RC, Patel MR, Kramer CM, Poon M, Hendel RC, Carr JC, et al. ACCF/ACR/SCCT/SCMR/ASNC/NASCI/SCAI/SIR 2006 appropriateness criteria for cardiac computed tomography and cardiac magnetic resonance imaging: a report of the American College of Cardiology Foundation Quality Strategic Directions Committee Appropriateness Criteria Working Group, American College of Radiology, Society of Cardiovascular Computed Tomography, Society for Cardiovascular Magnetic Resonance, American Society of Nuclear Cardiology, North American Society for Cardiac Imaging, Society for Cardiovascular Angiography and Interventions, and Society of Interventional Radiology. J Am Coll Cardiol. 2006;48(7):1475–97.
2. Wolk MJ, Bailey SR, Doherty JU, Douglas PS, Hendel RC, Kramer CM, et al. ACCF/AHA/ASE/ASNC/HFSA/HRS/SCAI/SCCT/SCMR/STS 2013 multimodality appropriate use criteria for the detection and risk assessment of stable ischemic heart disease: a report of the American College of Cardiology Foundation Appropriate Use Criteria Task Force, American Heart Association, American Society of Echocardiography, American Society of Nuclear Cardiology, Heart Failure Society of America, Heart Rhythm Society, Society for Cardiovascular Angiography and Interventions, Society of Cardiovascular Computed Tomography, Society for Cardiovascular Magnetic Resonance, and Society of Thoracic Surgeons. J Am Coll Cardiol. 2014;63(4):380–406.
3. Einstein AJ, Henzlova MJ, Rajagopalan S. Estimating risk of cancer associated with radiation exposure from 64-slice computed tomography coronary angiography. JAMA. 2007;298(3):317–23.
4. Ergun I, Keven K, Uruc I, Ekmekci Y, Canbakan B, Erden I, et al. The safety of gadolinium in patients with stage 3 and 4 renal failure. Nephrol Dial Transpl Off Publ Eur Dial Transpl Assoc Eur Renal Assoc. 2006;21(3):697–700.
5. Sadowski EA, Bennett LK, Chan MR, Wentland AL, Garrett AL, Garrett RW, et al. Nephrogenic systemic fibrosis: risk factors and incidence estimation. Radiology. 2007;243(1):148–57.
6. Thomsen HS, Morcos SK, Almen T, Bellin MF, Bertolotto M, Bongartz G, et al. Nephrogenic systemic fibrosis and gadolinium-based contrast media: updated ESUR Contrast Medium Safety Committee guidelines. Eur Radiol. 2013;23(2):307–18.
7. Nayak KS, Cunningham CH, Santos JM, Pauly JM. Real-time cardiac MRI at 3 tesla. Magn Reson Med. 2004;51(4):655–60.
8. McGee KP, Debbins JP, Boskamp EB, Blawat L, Angelos L, King KF. Cardiac magnetic resonance parallel imaging at 3.0 Tesla: technical feasibility and advantages. J Magn Reson Imaging JMRI. 2004;19(3):291–7.
9. Gharib AM, Elagha A, Pettigrew RI. Cardiac magnetic resonance at high field: promises and problems. Curr Probl Diagn Radiol. 2008;37(2):49–56.
10. Suttie JJ, Delabarre L, Pitcher A, van de Moortele PF, Dass S, Snyder CJ, et al. 7 Tesla (T) human cardiovascular magnetic resonance imaging using FLASH and SSFP to assess cardiac function: validation against 1.5 T and 3 T. NMR Biomed. 2012;25(1):27–34.
11. von Knobelsdorff-Brenkenhoff F, Tkachenko V, Winter L, Rieger J, Thalhammer C, Hezel F, et al. Assessment of the right ventricle with cardiovascular magnetic resonance at 7 Tesla. J Cardiovasc Magn Reson Off J Soc Cardiovasc Magn Reson. 2013;15:23.
12. Klix S, Els A, Paul K, Graessl A, Oezerdem C, Weinberger O, et al. On the subjective acceptance during cardiovascular magnetic resonance imaging at 7.0 Tesla. PLoS One. 2015;10(1), e0117095.
13. Raff GL, Gallagher MJ, O'Neill WW, Goldstein JA. Diagnostic accuracy of noninvasive coronary angiography using 64-slice spiral computed tomography. J Am Coll Cardiol. 2005;46(3):552–7.
14. Shellock FG. Prosthetic heart valves and annuloplasty rings: assessment of magnetic field interactions, heating, and artifacts at 1.5 Tesla. J Cardiovasc Magn Reson Off J Soc Cardiovasc Magn Reson. 2001;3(4):317–24.
15. Martin ET, Coman JA, Shellock FG, Pulling CC, Fair R, Jenkins K. Magnetic resonance imaging and cardiac pacemaker safety at 1.5-Tesla. J Am Coll Cardiol. 2004;43(7):1315–24.
16. Gimbel JR. Magnetic resonance imaging of implantable cardiac rhythm devices at 3.0 tesla. Pacing Clin Electrophysiol PACE. 2008;31(7):795–801.
17. Shinbane JS, Colletti PM, Shellock FG. MR in patients with pacemakers and ICDs: defining the issues. J Cardiovasc Magn Reson Off J Soc Cardiovasc Magn Reson. 2007;9(1):5–13.
18. Shinbane JS, Colletti PM, Shellock FG. Magnetic resonance imaging in patients with cardiac pacemakers: era of "MR Conditional" designs. J Cardiovasc Magn Reson Off J Soc Cardiovasc Magn Reson. 2011;13:63.
19. Wilkoff BL, Bello D, Taborsky M, Vymazal J, Kanal E, Heuer H, et al. Magnetic resonance imaging in patients with a pacemaker system designed for the magnetic resonance environment. Heart Rhythm Off J Heart Rhythm Soc. 2011;8(1):65–73.
20. Bailey WM, Rosenthal L, Fananapazir L, Gleva M, Mazur A, Rinaldi CA, et al. Clinical safety of the ProMRI pacemaker system in patients subjected to head and lower lumbar 1.5-T magnetic resonance imaging scanning conditions. Heart Rhythm Off J Heart Rhythm Soc. 2015;12(6):1183–91.

21. Gold MR, Sommer T, Schwitter J, Al Fagih A, Albert T, Merkely B, et al. Full-body MRI in patients with an implantable cardioverter-defibrillator: primary results of a randomized study. J Am Coll Cardiol. 2015;65(24):2581–8.
22. Shinbane JS, Colletti PM, Shellock FG. MR imaging in patients with pacemakers and other devices: engineering the future. JACC Cardiovasc Imaging. 2012;5(3):332–3.
23. Colletti PM, Shinbane JS, Shellock FG. "MR-conditional" pacemakers: the radiologist's role in multidisciplinary management. AJR Am J Roentgenol. 2011;197(3):W457–9.
24. Francis JM, Pennell DJ. Treatment of claustrophobia for cardiovascular magnetic resonance: use and effectiveness of mild sedation. J Cardiovasc Magn Reson Off J Soc Cardiovasc Magn Reson. 2000;2(2):139–41.
25. Eshed I, Althoff CE, Hamm B, Hermann KG. Claustrophobia and premature termination of magnetic resonance imaging examinations. J Magn Reson Imaging JMRI. 2007;26(2):401–4.
26. Chia JM, Fischer SE, Wickline SA, Lorenz CH. Performance of QRS detection for cardiac magnetic resonance imaging with a novel vectorcardiographic triggering method. J Magn Reson Imaging JMRI. 2000;12(5):678–88.
27. Dimick RN, Hedlund LW, Herfkens RJ, Fram EK, Utz J. Optimizing electrocardiograph electrode placement for cardiac-gated magnetic resonance imaging. Invest Radiol. 1987; 22(1):17–22.
28. Counter SA, Olofsson A, Grahn HF, Borg E. MRI acoustic noise: sound pressure and frequency analysis. J Magn Reson Imaging JMRI. 1997;7(3):606–11.
29. Budoff MJ, Achenbach S, Duerinckx A. Clinical utility of computed tomography and magnetic resonance techniques for noninvasive coronary angiography. J Am Coll Cardiol. 2003; 42(11):1867–78.
30. Plein S, Greenwood JP, Ridgway JP, Cranny G, Ball SG, Sivananthan MU. Assessment of non-ST-segment elevation acute coronary syndromes with cardiac magnetic resonance imaging. J Am Coll Cardiol. 2004;44(11):2173–81.
31. Yang Q, Li K, Liu X, Bi X, Liu Z, An J, et al. Contrast-enhanced whole-heart coronary magnetic resonance angiography at 3.0-T: a comparative study with X-ray angiography in a single center. J Am Coll Cardiol. 2009;54(1):69–76.
32. Liu Z, Yang Q, Zhao Y, Jin L, Jerecic R, Xu D, et al. Use of coronary anatomy and late enhancement information both derived from contrast-enhanced whole-heart coronary MRA at 3 T for the assessment of ischemic left ventricular dysfunction. Clin Imaging. 2011;35(3):222–4.
33. Yang Q, Li K, Liu X, Du X, Bi X, Huang F, et al. 3.0T whole-heart coronary magnetic resonance angiography performed with 32-channel cardiac coils: a single-center experience. Circ Cardiovasc Imaging. 2012;5(5):573–9.
34. Stauder NI, Klumpp B, Stauder H, Blumenstock G, Fenchel M, Kuttner A, et al. Assessment of coronary artery bypass grafts by magnetic resonance imaging. Br J Radiol. 2007;80(960): 975–83.
35. Achenbach S, Kessler W, Moshage WE, Ropers D, Zink D, Kroeker R, et al. Visualization of the coronary arteries in three-dimensional reconstructions using respiratory gated magnetic resonance imaging. Coron Artery Dis. 1997;8(7):441–8.
36. Kessler W, Achenbach S, Moshage W, Zink D, Kroeker R, Nitz W, et al. Usefulness of respiratory gated magnetic resonance coronary angiography in assessing narrowings>or=50 % in diameter in native coronary arteries and in aortocoronary bypass conduits. Am J Cardiol. 1997;80(8):989–93.
37. So NM, Lam WW, Li D, Chan AK, Sanderson JE, Metreweli C. Magnetic resonance coronary angiography with 3D TrueFISP: breath-hold versus respiratory gated imaging. Br J Radiol. 2005;78(926):116–21.
38. Norgaard BL, Leipsic J, Gaur S, Seneviratne S, Ko BS, Ito H, et al. Diagnostic performance of noninvasive fractional flow reserve derived from coronary computed tomography angiography in suspected coronary artery disease: the NXT trial (Analysis of Coronary Blood Flow Using CT Angiography: Next Steps). J Am Coll Cardiol. 2014;63(12):1145–55.
39. Min JK, Leipsic J, Pencina MJ, Berman DS, Koo BK, van Mieghem C, et al. Diagnostic accuracy of fractional flow reserve from anatomic CT angiography. JAMA. 2012;308(12):1237–45.
40. Nakazato R, Park HB, Berman DS, Gransar H, Koo BK, Erglis A, et al. Noninvasive fractional flow reserve derived from computed tomography angiography for coronary lesions of intermediate stenosis severity: results from the DeFACTO study. Circ Cardiovasc Imaging. 2013;6(6):881–9.
41. Koo BK, Erglis A, Doh JH, Daniels DV, Jegere S, Kim HS, et al. Diagnosis of ischemia-causing coronary stenoses by noninvasive fractional flow reserve computed from coronary computed tomographic angiograms. Results from the prospective multicenter DISCOVER-FLOW (Diagnosis of Ischemia-Causing Stenoses Obtained Via Noninvasive Fractional Flow Reserve) study. J Am Coll Cardiol. 2011;58(19):1989–97.
42. Wong DT, Ko BS, Cameron JD, Leong DP, Leung MC, Malaiapan Y, et al. Comparison of diagnostic accuracy of combined assessment using adenosine stress computed tomography perfusion+computed tomography angiography with transluminal attenuation gradient+computed tomography angiography against invasive fractional flow reserve. J Am Coll Cardiol. 2014;63(18):1904–12.
43. Naghavi M, Libby P, Falk E, Casscells SW, Litovsky S, Rumberger J, et al. From vulnerable plaque to vulnerable patient: a call for new definitions and risk assessment strategies: part I. Circulation. 2003;108(14):1664–72.
44. Naghavi M, Libby P, Falk E, Casscells SW, Litovsky S, Rumberger J, et al. From vulnerable plaque to vulnerable patient: a call for new definitions and risk assessment strategies: part II. Circulation. 2003;108(15):1772–8.
45. Yeon SB, Sabir A, Clouse M, Martinezclark PO, Peters DC, Hauser TH, et al. Delayed-enhancement cardiovascular magnetic resonance coronary artery wall imaging: comparison with multislice computed tomography and quantitative coronary angiography. J Am Coll Cardiol. 2007;50(5):441–7.
46. Nikolaou K, Becker CR, Muders M, Babaryka G, Scheidler J, Flohr T, et al. Multidetector-row computed tomography and magnetic resonance imaging of atherosclerotic lesions in human ex vivo coronary arteries. Atherosclerosis. 2004;174(2):243–52.
47. Fayad ZA, Fuster V, Nikolaou K, Becker C. Computed tomography and magnetic resonance imaging for noninvasive coronary angiography and plaque imaging: current and potential future concepts. Circulation. 2002;106(15):2026–34.
48. Kim WY, Stuber M, Bornert P, Kissinger KV, Manning WJ, Botnar RM. Three-dimensional black-blood cardiac magnetic resonance coronary vessel wall imaging detects positive arterial remodeling in patients with nonsignificant coronary artery disease. Circulation. 2002;106(3):296–9.
49. Viles-Gonzalez JF, Poon M, Sanz J, Rius T, Nikolaou K, Fayad ZA, et al. In vivo 16-slice, multidetector-row computed tomography for the assessment of experimental atherosclerosis: comparison with magnetic resonance imaging and histopathology. Circulation. 2004;110(11):1467–72.
50. Kuo YS, Kelle S, Lee C, Hinojar R, Nagel E, Botnar R, et al. Contrast-enhanced cardiovascular magnetic resonance imaging of coronary vessel wall: state of art. Expert Rev Cardiovasc Ther. 2014;12(2):255–63.
51. Post JC, van Rossum AC, Bronzwaer JG, de Cock CC, Hofman MB, Valk J, et al. Magnetic resonance angiography of anomalous coronary arteries. A new gold standard for delineating the proximal course? Circulation. 1995;92(11):3163–71.

52. Bunce NH, Rahman SL, Keegan J, Gatehouse PD, Lorenz CH, Pennell DJ. Anomalous coronary arteries: anatomic and functional assessment by coronary and perfusion cardiovascular magnetic resonance in three sisters. J Cardiovasc Magn Reson Off J Soc Cardiovasc Magn Reson. 2001;3(4):361–9.
53. Sato Y, Matsumoto N, Komatsu S, Kunimasa T, Yoda S, Tani S, et al. Anomalous origin of the right coronary artery: depiction at whole-heart coronary magnetic resonance angiography. Int J Cardiol. 2008;127(2):274–5.
54. Shinbane JS, Shriki J, Fleischman F, Hindoyan A, Withey J, Lee C, et al. Anomalous coronary arteries: cardiovascular computed tomographic angiography for surgical decisions and planning. World J Pediatr Congenit Heart Surg. 2013;4(2):142–54.
55. Buchthal SD, den Hollander JA, Merz CN, Rogers WJ, Pepine CJ, Reichek N, et al. Abnormal myocardial phosphorus-31 nuclear magnetic resonance spectroscopy in women with chest pain but normal coronary angiograms. N Engl J Med. 2000; 342(12):829–35.
56. Johnson BD, Shaw LJ, Buchthal SD, Bairey Merz CN, Kim HW, Scott KN, et al. Prognosis in women with myocardial ischemia in the absence of obstructive coronary disease: results from the National Institutes of Health-National Heart, Lung, and Blood Institute-Sponsored Women's Ischemia Syndrome Evaluation (WISE). Circulation. 2004;109(24):2993–9.
57. Cranney GB, Lotan CS, Dean L, Baxley W, Bouchard A, Pohost GM. Left ventricular volume measurement using cardiac axis nuclear magnetic resonance imaging. Validation by calibrated ventricular angiography. Circulation. 1990;82(1):154–63.
58. Rumberger JA, Behrenbeck T, Bell MR, Breen JF, Johnston DL, Holmes Jr DR, et al. Determination of ventricular ejection fraction: a comparison of available imaging methods. The Cardiovascular Imaging Working Group. Mayo Clin Proc. 1997;72(9):860–70.
59. Scharhag J, Schneider G, Urhausen A, Rochette V, Kramann B, Kindermann W. Athlete's heart: right and left ventricular mass and function in male endurance athletes and untrained individuals determined by magnetic resonance imaging. J Am Coll Cardiol. 2002;40(10):1856–63.
60. Rominger MB, Bachmann GF, Geuer M, Puzik M, Boedeker RH, Ricken WW, et al. Accuracy of right and left ventricular heart volume and left ventricular muscle mass determination with cine MRI in breath holding technique. RoFo. 1999; 170(1):54–60.
61. Ioannidis JP, Trikalinos TA, Danias PG. Electrocardiogram-gated single-photon emission computed tomography versus cardiac magnetic resonance imaging for the assessment of left ventricular volumes and ejection fraction: a meta-analysis. J Am Coll Cardiol. 2002;39(12):2059–68.
62. Grothues F, Moon JC, Bellenger NG, Smith GS, Klein HU, Pennell DJ. Interstudy reproducibility of right ventricular volumes, function, and mass with cardiovascular magnetic resonance. Am Heart J. 2004;147(2):218–23.
63. Bodi V, Sanchis J, Nunez J, Mainar L, Lopez-Lereu MP, Monmeneu JV, et al. Prognostic value of a comprehensive cardiac magnetic resonance assessment soon after a first ST-segment elevation myocardial infarction. JACC Cardiovasc Imaging. 2009;2(7):835–42.
64. Eitel I, de Waha S, Wohrle J, Fuernau G, Lurz P, Pauschinger M, et al. Comprehensive prognosis assessment by CMR imaging after ST-segment elevation myocardial infarction. J Am Coll Cardiol. 2014;64(12):1217–26.
65. Mordini FE, Haddad T, Hsu LY, Kellman P, Lowrey TB, Aletras AH, et al. Diagnostic accuracy of stress perfusion CMR in comparison with quantitative coronary angiography: fully quantitative, semiquantitative, and qualitative assessment. JACC Cardiovasc Imaging. 2014;7(1):14–22.
66. Heer T, Reiter S, Hofling B, Pilz G. Diagnostic performance of non-contrast-enhanced whole-heart magnetic resonance coronary angiography in combination with adenosine stress perfusion cardiac magnetic resonance imaging. Am Heart J. 2013; 166(6):999–1009.
67. Cheng AS, Pegg TJ, Karamitsos TD, Searle N, Jerosch-Herold M, Choudhury RP, et al. Cardiovascular magnetic resonance perfusion imaging at 3-tesla for the detection of coronary artery disease: a comparison with 1.5-tesla. J Am Coll Cardiol. 2007; 49(25):2440–9.
68. Jahnke C, Nagel E, Gebker R, Kokocinski T, Kelle S, Manka R, et al. Prognostic value of cardiac magnetic resonance stress tests: adenosine stress perfusion and dobutamine stress wall motion imaging. Circulation. 2007;115(13):1769–76.
69. Dall'Armellina E, Morgan TM, Mandapaka S, Ntim W, Carr JJ, Hamilton CA, et al. Prediction of cardiac events in patients with reduced left ventricular ejection fraction with dobutamine cardiovascular magnetic resonance assessment of wall motion score index. J Am Coll Cardiol. 2008;52(4):279–86.
70. Kuijpers D, Ho KY, van Dijkman PR, Vliegenthart R, Oudkerk M. Dobutamine cardiovascular magnetic resonance for the detection of myocardial ischemia with the use of myocardial tagging. Circulation. 2003;107(12):1592–7.
71. Costa MA, Shoemaker S, Futamatsu H, Klassen C, Angiolillo DJ, Nguyen M, et al. Quantitative magnetic resonance perfusion imaging detects anatomic and physiologic coronary artery disease as measured by coronary angiography and fractional flow reserve. J Am Coll Cardiol. 2007;50(6):514–22.
72. Shah R, Heydari B, Coelho-Filho O, Murthy VL, Abbasi S, Feng JH, et al. Stress cardiac magnetic resonance imaging provides effective cardiac risk reclassification in patients with known or suspected stable coronary artery disease. Circulation. 2013;128(6):605–14.
73. Lipinski MJ, McVey CM, Berger JS, Kramer CM, Salerno M. Prognostic value of stress cardiac magnetic resonance imaging in patients with known or suspected coronary artery disease: a systematic review and meta-analysis. J Am Coll Cardiol. 2013;62(9):826–38.
74. Miller CD, Case LD, Little WC, Mahler SA, Burke GL, Harper EN, et al. Stress CMR reduces revascularization, hospital readmission, and recurrent cardiac testing in intermediate-risk patients with acute chest pain. JACC Cardiovasc Imaging. 2013;6(7):785–94.
75. Jogiya R, Morton G, De Silva K, Reyes E, Hachamovitch R, Kozerke S, et al. Ischemic burden by 3-dimensional myocardial perfusion cardiovascular magnetic resonance: comparison with myocardial perfusion scintigraphy. Circ Cardiovasc Imaging. 2014;7(4):647–54.
76. Bettencourt N, Chiribiri A, Schuster A, Ferreira N, Sampaio F, Pires-Morais G, et al. Direct comparison of cardiac magnetic resonance and multidetector computed tomography stress-rest perfusion imaging for detection of coronary artery disease. J Am Coll Cardiol. 2013;61(10):1099–107.
77. Morris PD, van de Vosse FN, Lawford PV, Hose DR, Gunn JP. "Virtual" (computed) fractional flow reserve: current challenges and limitations. JACC Cardiovasc Interv. 2015;8(8):1009–17.
78. Kim RJ, Fieno DS, Parrish TB, Harris K, Chen EL, Simonetti O, et al. Relationship of MRI delayed contrast enhancement to irreversible injury, infarct age, and contractile function. Circulation. 1999;100(19):1992–2002.
79. Gerber BL, Belge B, Legros GJ, Lim P, Poncelet A, Pasquet A, et al. Characterization of acute and chronic myocardial infarcts by multidetector computed tomography: comparison with contrast-enhanced magnetic resonance. Circulation. 2006;113(6):823–33.
80. Sato A, Nozato T, Hikita H, Akiyama D, Nishina H, Hoshi T, et al. Prognostic value of myocardial contrast delayed enhancement

with 64-slice multidetector computed tomography after acute myocardial infarction. J Am Coll Cardiol. 2012;59(8):730–8.

81. McCrohon JA, Moon JC, Prasad SK, McKenna WJ, Lorenz CH, Coats AJ, et al. Differentiation of heart failure related to dilated cardiomyopathy and coronary artery disease using gadolinium-enhanced cardiovascular magnetic resonance. Circulation. 2003;108(1):54–9.
82. Schmidt A, Azevedo CF, Cheng A, Gupta SN, Bluemke DA, Foo TK, et al. Infarct tissue heterogeneity by magnetic resonance imaging identifies enhanced cardiac arrhythmia susceptibility in patients with left ventricular dysfunction. Circulation. 2007;115(15):2006–14.
83. Lardo AC, Cordeiro MA, Silva C, Amado LC, George RT, Saliaris AP, et al. Contrast-enhanced multidetector computed tomography viability imaging after myocardial infarction: characterization of myocyte death, microvascular obstruction, and chronic scar. Circulation. 2006;113(3):394–404.
84. Ansari M, Araoz PA, Gerard SK, Watzinger N, Lund GK, Massie BM, et al. Comparison of late enhancement cardiovascular magnetic resonance and thallium SPECT in patients with coronary disease and left ventricular dysfunction. J Cardiovasc Magn Reson Off J Soc Cardiovasc Magn Reson. 2004;6(2):549–56.
85. Ingkanisorn WP, Rhoads KL, Aletras AH, Kellman P, Arai AE. Gadolinium delayed enhancement cardiovascular magnetic resonance correlates with clinical measures of myocardial infarction. J Am Coll Cardiol. 2004;43(12):2253–9.
86. Ichikawa Y, Sakuma H, Suzawa N, Kitagawa K, Makino K, Hirano T, et al. Late gadolinium-enhanced magnetic resonance imaging in acute and chronic myocardial infarction. Improved prediction of regional myocardial contraction in the chronic state by measuring thickness of nonenhanced myocardium. J Am Coll Cardiol. 2005;45(6):901–9.
87. Stork A, Muellerleile K, Bansmann PM, Graessner J, Kaul M, Kemper J, et al. Value of T2-weighted, first-pass and delayed enhancement, and cine CMR to differentiate between acute and chronic myocardial infarction. Eur Radiol. 2007;17(3):610–7.
88. Dall'Armellina E, Piechnik SK, Ferreira VM, Si QL, Robson MD, Francis JM, et al. Cardiovascular magnetic resonance by non contrast T1-mapping allows assessment of severity of injury in acute myocardial infarction. J Cardiovasc Magn Reson Off J Soc Cardiovasc Magn Reson. 2012;14:15.
89. Ubachs JF, Engblom H, Erlinge D, Jovinge S, Hedstrom E, Carlsson M, et al. Cardiovascular magnetic resonance of the myocardium at risk in acute reperfused myocardial infarction: comparison of T2-weighted imaging versus the circumferential endocardial extent of late gadolinium enhancement with transmural projection. J Cardiovasc Magn Reson Off J Soc Cardiovasc Magn Reson. 2010;12:18.
90. Eitel I, Kubusch K, Strohm O, Desch S, Mikami Y, de Waha S, et al. Prognostic value and determinants of a hypointense infarct core in T2-weighted cardiac magnetic resonance in acute reperfused ST-elevation-myocardial infarction. Circ Cardiovasc Imaging. 2011;4(4):354–62.
91. O'Regan DP, Ahmed R, Karunanithy N, Neuwirth C, Tan Y, Durighel G, et al. Reperfusion hemorrhage following acute myocardial infarction: assessment with T2* mapping and effect on measuring the area at risk. Radiology. 2009;250(3):916–22.
92. Assomull RG, Prasad SK, Lyne J, Smith G, Burman ED, Khan M, et al. Cardiovascular magnetic resonance, fibrosis, and prognosis in dilated cardiomyopathy. J Am Coll Cardiol. 2006; 48(10):1977–85.
93. Bello D, Shah DJ, Farah GM, Di Luzio S, Parker M, Johnson MR, et al. Gadolinium cardiovascular magnetic resonance predicts reversible myocardial dysfunction and remodeling in patients with heart failure undergoing beta-blocker therapy. Circulation. 2003;108(16):1945–53.
94. Perazzolo Marra M, De Lazzari M, Zorzi A, Migliore F, Zilio F, Calore C, et al. Impact of the presence and amount of myocardial fibrosis by cardiac magnetic resonance on arrhythmic outcome and sudden cardiac death in nonischemic dilated cardiomyopathy. Heart Rhythm Off J Heart Rhythm Soc. 2014;11(5):856–63.
95. Kuruvilla S, Adenaw N, Katwal AB, Lipinski MJ, Kramer CM, Salerno M. Late gadolinium enhancement on cardiac magnetic resonance predicts adverse cardiovascular outcomes in nonischemic cardiomyopathy: a systematic review and meta-analysis. Circ Cardiovasc Imaging. 2014;7(2):250–8.
96. Wu KC, Weiss RG, Thiemann DR, Kitagawa K, Schmidt A, Dalal D, et al. Late gadolinium enhancement by cardiovascular magnetic resonance heralds an adverse prognosis in nonischemic cardiomyopathy. J Am Coll Cardiol. 2008;51(25):2414–21.
97. Neilan TG, Coelho-Filho OR, Danik SB, Shah RV, Dodson JA, Verdini DJ, et al. CMR quantification of myocardial scar provides additive prognostic information in nonischemic cardiomyopathy. JACC Cardiovasc Imaging. 2013;6(9):944–54.
98. aus dem Siepen F, Buss SJ, Messroghli D, Andre F, Lossnitzer D, Seitz S, et al. T1 mapping in dilated cardiomyopathy with cardiac magnetic resonance: quantification of diffuse myocardial fibrosis and comparison with endomyocardial biopsy. Eur Heart J Cardiovasc Imaging. 2015;16(2):210–6.
99. Moon JC, Messroghli DR, Kellman P, Piechnik SK, Robson MD, Ugander M, et al. Myocardial T1 mapping and extracellular volume quantification: a Society for Cardiovascular Magnetic Resonance (SCMR) and CMR Working Group of the European Society of Cardiology consensus statement. J Cardiovasc Magn Reson Off J Soc Cardiovasc Magn Reson. 2013;15:92.
100. Iles L, Pfluger H, Phrommintikul A, Cherayath J, Aksit P, Gupta SN, et al. Evaluation of diffuse myocardial fibrosis in heart failure with cardiac magnetic resonance contrast-enhanced T1 mapping. J Am Coll Cardiol. 2008;52(19):1574–80.
101. Puntmann VO, Voigt T, Chen Z, Mayr M, Karim R, Rhode K, et al. Native T1 mapping in differentiation of normal myocardium from diffuse disease in hypertrophic and dilated cardiomyopathy. JACC Cardiovasc Imaging. 2013;6(4):475–84.
102. Treibel TA, Bandula S, Fontana M, White SK, Gilbertson JA, Herrey AS, et al. Extracellular volume quantification by dynamic equilibrium cardiac computed tomography in cardiac amyloidosis. J Cardiovasc Comput Tomogr. 2015;9:585–92.
103. Saeed M, Hetts SW, Jablonowski R, Wilson MW. Magnetic resonance imaging and multi-detector computed tomography assessment of extracellular compartment in ischemic and non-ischemic myocardial pathologies. World J Cardiol. 2014;6(11):1192–208.
104. Dong SJ, MacGregor JH, Crawley AP, McVeigh E, Belenkie I, Smith ER, et al. Left ventricular wall thickness and regional systolic function in patients with hypertrophic cardiomyopathy. A three-dimensional tagged magnetic resonance imaging study. Circulation. 1994;90(3):1200–9.
105. Devlin AM, Moore NR, Ostman-Smith I. A comparison of MRI and echocardiography in hypertrophic cardiomyopathy. Br J Radiol. 1999;72(855):258–64.
106. Schulz-Menger J, Strohm O, Waigand J, Uhlich F, Dietz R, Friedrich MG. The value of magnetic resonance imaging of the left ventricular outflow tract in patients with hypertrophic obstructive cardiomyopathy after septal artery embolization. Circulation. 2000;101(15):1764–6.
107. Teraoka K, Hirano M, Ookubo H, Sasaki K, Katsuyama H, Amino M, et al. Delayed contrast enhancement of MRI in hypertrophic cardiomyopathy. Magn Reson Imaging. 2004;22(2):155–61.
108. Moon JC, McKenna WJ, McCrohon JA, Elliott PM, Smith GC, Pennell DJ. Toward clinical risk assessment in hypertrophic cardiomyopathy with gadolinium cardiovascular magnetic resonance. J Am Coll Cardiol. 2003;41(9):1561–7.

109. Moravsky G, Ofek E, Rakowski H, Butany J, Williams L, Ralph-Edwards A, et al. Myocardial fibrosis in hypertrophic cardiomyopathy: accurate reflection of histopathological findings by CMR. JACC Cardiovasc Imaging. 2013;6(5):587–96.
110. Bruder O, Wagner A, Jensen CJ, Schneider S, Ong P, Kispert EM, et al. Myocardial scar visualized by cardiovascular magnetic resonance imaging predicts major adverse events in patients with hypertrophic cardiomyopathy. J Am Coll Cardiol. 2010; 56(11):875–87.
111. Choi HM, Kim KH, Lee JM, Yoon YE, Lee SP, Park EA, et al. Myocardial fibrosis progression on cardiac magnetic resonance in hypertrophic cardiomyopathy. Heart. 2015;101(11):870–6.
112. Todiere G, Aquaro GD, Piaggi P, Formisano F, Barison A, Masci PG, et al. Progression of myocardial fibrosis assessed with cardiac magnetic resonance in hypertrophic cardiomyopathy. J Am Coll Cardiol. 2012;60(10):922–9.
113. Chan RH, Maron BJ, Olivotto I, Pencina MJ, Assenza GE, Haas T, et al. Prognostic value of quantitative contrast-enhanced cardiovascular magnetic resonance for the evaluation of sudden death risk in patients with hypertrophic cardiomyopathy. Circulation. 2014;130(6):484–95.
114. Matoh F, Satoh H, Shiraki K, Saitoh T, Urushida T, Katoh H, et al. Usefulness of delayed enhancement magnetic resonance imaging to differentiate dilated phase of hypertrophic cardiomyopathy and dilated cardiomyopathy. J Card Fail. 2007;13(5):372–9.
115. Kebed KY, Al Adham RI, Bishu K, Askew JW, Klarich KW, Araoz PA, et al. Evaluation of apical subtype of hypertrophic cardiomyopathy using cardiac magnetic resonance imaging with gadolinium enhancement. Am J Cardiol. 2014;114(5):777–82.
116. Hen Y, Iguchi N, Utanohara Y, Takada K, Machida H, Takayama M, et al. Prognostic value of late gadolinium enhancement on cardiac magnetic resonance imaging in Japanese hypertrophic cardiomyopathy patients. Circulation J Off J Jpn Circulation Soc. 2014;78(4):929–37.
117. Hanneman K, Crean AM, Williams L, Moshonov H, James S, Jimenez-Juan L, et al. Cardiac magnetic resonance imaging findings predict major adverse events in apical hypertrophic cardiomyopathy. J Thorac Imaging. 2014;29(6):331–9.
118. Chaowu Y, Shihua Z, Jian L, Li L, Wei F. Cardiovascular magnetic resonance characteristics in children with hypertrophic cardiomyopathy. Circ Heart Fail. 2013;6(5):1013–20.
119. Fluechter S, Kuschyk J, Wolpert C, Doesch C, Veltmann C, Haghi D, et al. Extent of late gadolinium enhancement detected by cardiovascular magnetic resonance correlates with the inducibility of ventricular tachyarrhythmia in hypertrophic cardiomyopathy. J Cardiovasc Magn Reson Off J Soc Cardiovasc Magn Reson. 2010;12:30.
120. Sakamoto N, Kawamura Y, Sato N, Nimura A, Matsuki M, Yamauchi A, et al. Late gadolinium enhancement on cardiac magnetic resonance represents the depolarizing and repolarizing electrically damaged foci causing malignant ventricular arrhythmia in hypertrophic cardiomyopathy. Heart Rhythm Off J Heart Rhythm Soc. 2015;12(6):1276–84.
121. White RD, Obuchowski NA, Gunawardena S, Lipchik EO, Lever HM, Van Dyke CW, et al. Left ventricular outflow tract obstruction in hypertrophic cardiomyopathy: presurgical and postsurgical evaluation by computed tomography magnetic resonance imaging. Am J Card Imaging. 1996;10(1):1–13.
122. Yuan J, Qiao S, Zhang Y, You S, Duan F, Hu F, et al. Follow-up by cardiac magnetic resonance imaging in patients with hypertrophic cardiomyopathy who underwent percutaneous ventricular septal ablation. Am J Cardiol. 2010;106(10):1487–91.
123. Valeti US, Nishimura RA, Holmes DR, Araoz PA, Glockner JF, Breen JF, et al. Comparison of surgical septal myectomy and alcohol septal ablation with cardiac magnetic resonance imaging in patients with hypertrophic obstructive cardiomyopathy. J Am Coll Cardiol. 2007;49(3):350–7.
124. Hussain T, Dragulescu A, Benson L, Yoo SJ, Meng H, Windram J, et al. Quantification and significance of diffuse myocardial fibrosis and diastolic dysfunction in childhood hypertrophic cardiomyopathy. Pediatr Cardiol. 2015;36(5):970–8.
125. Ellims AH, Iles LM, Ling LH, Hare JL, Kaye DM, Taylor AJ. Diffuse myocardial fibrosis in hypertrophic cardiomyopathy can be identified by cardiovascular magnetic resonance, and is associated with left ventricular diastolic dysfunction. J Cardiovasc Magn Reson Off J Soc Cardiovasc Magn Reson. 2012;14:76.
126. Zhao L, Ma X, Feuchtner GM, Zhang C, Fan Z. Quantification of myocardial delayed enhancement and wall thickness in hypertrophic cardiomyopathy: multidetector computed tomography versus magnetic resonance imaging. Eur J Radiol. 2014;83(10):1778–85.
127. Shariat M, Thavendiranathan P, Nguyen E, Wintersperger B, Paul N, Rakowski H, et al. Utility of coronary CT angiography in outpatients with hypertrophic cardiomyopathy presenting with angina symptoms. J Cardiovasc Comput Tomogr. 2014; 8(6):429–37.
128. Maceira AM, Joshi J, Prasad SK, Moon JC, Perugini E, Harding I, et al. Cardiovascular magnetic resonance in cardiac amyloidosis. Circulation. 2005;111(2):186–93.
129. Maceira AM, Prasad SK, Hawkins PN, Roughton M, Pennell DJ. Cardiovascular magnetic resonance and prognosis in cardiac amyloidosis. J Cardiovasc Magn Reson Off J Soc Cardiovasc Magn Reson. 2008;10:54.
130. White JA, Kim HW, Shah D, Fine N, Kim KY, Wendell DC, et al. CMR imaging with rapid visual T1 assessment predicts mortality in patients suspected of cardiac amyloidosis. JACC Cardiovasc Imaging. 2014;7(2):143–56.
131. Syed IS, Glockner JF, Feng D, Araoz PA, Martinez MW, Edwards WD, et al. Role of cardiac magnetic resonance imaging in the detection of cardiac amyloidosis. JACC Cardiovasc Imaging. 2010;3(2):155–64.
132. Austin BA, Tang WH, Rodriguez ER, Tan C, Flamm SD, Taylor DO, et al. Delayed hyper-enhancement magnetic resonance imaging provides incremental diagnostic and prognostic utility in suspected cardiac amyloidosis. JACC Cardiovasc Imaging. 2009;2(12):1369–77.
133. Vogelsberg H, Mahrholdt H, Deluigi CC, Yilmaz A, Kispert EM, Greulich S, et al. Cardiovascular magnetic resonance in clinically suspected cardiac amyloidosis: noninvasive imaging compared to endomyocardial biopsy. J Am Coll Cardiol. 2008;51(10): 1022–30.
134. Dungu JN, Valencia O, Pinney JH, Gibbs SD, Rowczenio D, Gilbertson JA, et al. CMR-based differentiation of AL and ATTR cardiac amyloidosis. JACC Cardiovasc Imaging. 2014;7(2): 133–42.
135. Moon JC, Sachdev B, Elkington AG, McKenna WJ, Mehta A, Pennell DJ, et al. Gadolinium enhanced cardiovascular magnetic resonance in Anderson-Fabry disease. Evidence for a disease specific abnormality of the myocardial interstitium. Eur Heart J. 2003;24(23):2151–5.
136. Pica S, Sado DM, Maestrini V, Fontana M, White SK, Treibel T, et al. Reproducibility of native myocardial T1 mapping in the assessment of Fabry disease and its role in early detection of cardiac involvement by cardiovascular magnetic resonance. J Cardiovasc Magn Reson Off J Soc Cardiovasc Magn Reson. 2014;16:99.
137. Imbriaco M, Pisani A, Spinelli L, Cuocolo A, Messalli G, Capuano E, et al. Effects of enzyme-replacement therapy in patients with Anderson-Fabry disease: a prospective long-term cardiac magnetic resonance imaging study. Heart. 2009;95(13):1103–7.
138. Smedema JP, Snoep G, van Kroonenburgh MP, van Geuns RJ, Dassen WR, Gorgels AP, et al. Evaluation of the accuracy of gadolinium-enhanced cardiovascular magnetic resonance in the

diagnosis of cardiac sarcoidosis. J Am Coll Cardiol. 2005;45(10):1683–90.
139. Nadel J, Lancefield T, Voskoboinik A, Taylor AJ. Late gadolinium enhancement identified with cardiac magnetic resonance imaging in sarcoidosis patients is associated with long-term ventricular arrhythmia and sudden cardiac death. Eur Heart J Cardiovasc Imaging. 2015;16(6):634–41.
140. Crawford T, Mueller G, Sarsam S, Prasitdumrong H, Chaiyen N, Gu X, et al. Magnetic resonance imaging for identifying patients with cardiac sarcoidosis and preserved or mildly reduced left ventricular function at risk of ventricular arrhythmias. Circ Arrhythm Electrophysiol. 2014;7(6):1109–15.
141. Greulich S, Deluigi CC, Gloekler S, Wahl A, Zurn C, Kramer U, et al. CMR imaging predicts death and other adverse events in suspected cardiac sarcoidosis. JACC Cardiovasc Imaging. 2013;6(4):501–11.
142. Shimada T, Shimada K, Sakane T, Ochiai K, Tsukihashi H, Fukui M, et al. Diagnosis of cardiac sarcoidosis and evaluation of the effects of steroid therapy by gadolinium-DTPA-enhanced magnetic resonance imaging. Am J Med. 2001;110(7):520–7.
143. Ise T, Hasegawa T, Morita Y, Yamada N, Funada A, Takahama H, et al. Extensive late gadolinium enhancement on cardiovascular magnetic resonance predicts adverse outcomes and lack of improvement in LV function after steroid therapy in cardiac sarcoidosis. Heart. 2014;100(15):1165–72.
144. Friedrich MG, Sechtem U, Schulz-Menger J, Holmvang G, Alakija P, Cooper LT, et al. Cardiovascular magnetic resonance in myocarditis: a JACC White Paper. J Am Coll Cardiol. 2009;53(17):1475–87.
145. Abdel-Aty H, Boye P, Zagrosek A, Wassmuth R, Kumar A, Messroghli D, et al. Diagnostic performance of cardiovascular magnetic resonance in patients with suspected acute myocarditis: comparison of different approaches. J Am Coll Cardiol. 2005;45(11):1815–22.
146. Laissy JP, Hyafil F, Feldman LJ, Juliard JM, Schouman-Claeys E, Steg PG, et al. Differentiating acute myocardial infarction from myocarditis: diagnostic value of early- and delayed-perfusion cardiac MR imaging. Radiology. 2005;237(1):75–82.
147. Monney PA, Sekhri N, Burchell T, Knight C, Davies C, Deaner A, et al. Acute myocarditis presenting as acute coronary syndrome: role of early cardiac magnetic resonance in its diagnosis. Heart. 2011;97(16):1312–8.
148. Francone M, Chimenti C, Galea N, Scopelliti F, Verardo R, Galea R, et al. CMR sensitivity varies with clinical presentation and extent of cell necrosis in biopsy-proven acute myocarditis. JACC Cardiovasc Imaging. 2014;7(3):254–63.
149. Radunski UK, Lund GK, Stehning C, Schnackenburg B, Bohnen S, Adam G, et al. CMR in patients with severe myocarditis: diagnostic value of quantitative tissue markers including extracellular volume imaging. JACC Cardiovasc Imaging. 2014;7(7):667–75.
150. Ferreira VM, Piechnik SK, Dall'Armellina E, Karamitsos TD, Francis JM, Ntusi N, et al. T(1) mapping for the diagnosis of acute myocarditis using CMR: comparison to T2-weighted and late gadolinium enhanced imaging. JACC Cardiovasc Imaging. 2013;6(10):1048–58.
151. Hinojar R, Foote L, Arroyo Ucar E, Jackson T, Jabbour A, Yu CY, et al. Native T1 in discrimination of acute and convalescent stages in patients with clinical diagnosis of myocarditis: a proposed diagnostic algorithm using CMR. JACC Cardiovasc Imaging. 2015;8(1):37–46.
152. Bohnen S, Radunski UK, Lund GK, Kandolf R, Stehning C, Schnackenburg B, et al. Performance of t1 and t2 mapping cardiovascular magnetic resonance to detect active myocarditis in patients with recent-onset heart failure. Circ Cardiovasc Imaging. 2015;8(6):e003073.
153. Sachdeva S, Song X, Dham N, Heath DM, DeBiasi RL. Analysis of clinical parameters and cardiac magnetic resonance imaging as predictors of outcome in pediatric myocarditis. Am J Cardiol. 2015;115(4):499–504.
154. Schumm J, Greulich S, Wagner A, Grun S, Ong P, Bentz K, et al. Cardiovascular magnetic resonance risk stratification in patients with clinically suspected myocarditis. J Cardiovasc Magn Reson Off J Soc Cardiovasc Magn Reson. 2014;16:14.
155. Vermes E, Childs H, Faris P, Friedrich MG. Predictive value of CMR criteria for LV functional improvement in patients with acute myocarditis. Eur Heart J Cardiovasc Imaging. 2014;15(10):1140–4.
156. Dambrin G, Laissy JP, Serfaty JM, Caussin C, Lancelin B, Paul JF. Diagnostic value of ECG-gated multidetector computed tomography in the early phase of suspected acute myocarditis. A preliminary comparative study with cardiac MRI. Eur Radiol. 2007;17(2):331–8.
157. Boussel L, Gamondes D, Staat P, Elicker BM, Revel D, Douek P. Acute chest pain with normal coronary angiogram: role of contrast-enhanced multidetector computed tomography in the differential diagnosis between myocarditis and myocardial infarction. J Comput Assist Tomogr. 2008;32(2):228–32.
158. Axsom K, Lin F, Weinsaft JW, Min JK. Evaluation of myocarditis with delayed-enhancement computed tomography. J Cardiovasc Comput Tomogr. 2009;3(6):409–11.
159. Puntmann VO, D'Cruz D, Smith Z, Pastor A, Choong P, Voigt T, et al. Native myocardial T1 mapping by cardiovascular magnetic resonance imaging in subclinical cardiomyopathy in patients with systemic lupus erythematosus. Circ Cardiovasc Imaging. 2013;6(2):295–301.
160. Hoey ET, Gulati GS, Ganeshan A, Watkin RW, Simpson H, Sharma S. Cardiovascular MRI for assessment of infectious and inflammatory conditions of the heart. AJR Am J Roentgenol. 2011;197(1):103–12.
161. Abdel-Aty H, Siegle N, Natusch A, Gromnica-Ihle E, Wassmuth R, Dietz R, et al. Myocardial tissue characterization in systemic lupus erythematosus: value of a comprehensive cardiovascular magnetic resonance approach. Lupus. 2008;17(6):561–7.
162. Shriki J, Shinbane JS, Azadi N, Su TI, Hirschbein J, Quismorio Jr FP, et al. Systemic lupus erythematosus coronary vasculitis demonstrated on cardiac computed tomography. Curr Probl Diagn Radiol. 2014;43(5):294–7.
163. Bocchi EA, Kalil R, Bacal F, de Lourdes HM, Meneghetti C, Magalhaes A, et al. Magnetic resonance imaging in chronic Chagas' disease: correlation with endomyocardial biopsy findings and Gallium-67 cardiac uptake. Echocardiography. 1998;15(3):279–88.
164. Rochitte CE, Oliveira PF, Andrade JM, Ianni BM, Parga JR, Avila LF, et al. Myocardial delayed enhancement by magnetic resonance imaging in patients with Chagas' disease: a marker of disease severity. J Am Coll Cardiol. 2005;46(8):1553–8.
165. Bukhman G, Ziegler J, Parry E. Endomyocardial fibrosis: still a mystery after 60 years. PLoS Negl Trop Dis. 2008;2(2), e97.
166. Kobayashi Y, Giles JT, Hirano M, Yokoe I, Nakajima Y, Bathon JM, et al. Assessment of myocardial abnormalities in rheumatoid arthritis using a comprehensive cardiac magnetic resonance approach: a pilot study. Arthritis Res Ther. 2010;12(5):R171.
167. Francone M, Iacucci I, Mangia M, Carbone I. Endomyocardial disease related to idiopathic hypereosinophilic syndrome: a cardiac magnetic resonance evaluation. Pediatr Cardiol. 2010;31(6):921–2.
168. Alter P, Maisch B. Endomyocardial fibrosis in Churg-Strauss syndrome assessed by cardiac magnetic resonance imaging. Int J Cardiol. 2006;108(1):112–3.
169. Syed IS, Martinez MW, Feng DL, Glockner JF. Cardiac magnetic resonance imaging of eosinophilic endomyocardial disease. Int J Cardiol. 2008;126(3):e50–2.

170. Wood JC, Origa R, Agus A, Matta G, Coates TD, Galanello R. Onset of cardiac iron loading in pediatric patients with thalassemia major. Haematologica. 2008;93(6):917–20.
171. Carpenter JP, He T, Kirk P, Roughton M, Anderson LJ, de Noronha SV, et al. On T2* magnetic resonance and cardiac iron. Circulation. 2011;123(14):1519–28.
172. Wood JC. Use of magnetic resonance imaging to monitor iron overload. Hematol Oncol Clin North Am. 2014;28(4):747–64, vii.
173. Hor KN, Wansapura J, Markham LW, Mazur W, Cripe LH, Fleck R, et al. Circumferential strain analysis identifies strata of cardiomyopathy in Duchenne muscular dystrophy: a cardiac magnetic resonance tagging study. J Am Coll Cardiol. 2009;53(14):1204–10.
174. Soslow JH, Damon BM, Saville BR, Lu Z, Burnette WB, Lawson MA, et al. Evaluation of post-contrast myocardial t1 in duchenne muscular dystrophy using cardiac magnetic resonance imaging. Pediatr Cardiol. 2015;36(1):49–56.
175. Lang SM, Shugh S, Mazur W, Sticka JJ, Rattan MS, Jefferies JL, et al. Myocardial fibrosis and left ventricular dysfunction in Duchenne muscular dystrophy carriers using cardiac magnetic resonance imaging. Pediatr Cardiol. 2015;36(7):1495–501.
176. Schelhorn J, Schoenecker A, Neudorf U, Schemuth H, Nensa F, Nassenstein K, et al. Cardiac pathologies in female carriers of Duchenne muscular dystrophy assessed by cardiovascular magnetic resonance imaging. Eur Radiol. 2015;25(10):3066–72.
177. Wahbi K, Meune C, el Hamouda H, Stojkovic T, Laforet P, Becane HM, et al. Cardiac assessment of limb-girdle muscular dystrophy 2I patients: an echography, Holter ECG and magnetic resonance imaging study. Neuromuscul Disord NMD. 2008;18(8):650–5.
178. Yilmaz A, Gdynia HJ, Baccouche H, Mahrholdt H, Meinhardt G, Basso C, et al. Cardiac involvement in patients with Becker muscular dystrophy: new diagnostic and pathophysiological insights by a CMR approach. J Cardiovasc Magn Reson Off J Soc Cardiovasc Magn Reson. 2008;10:50.
179. Yilmaz A, Gdynia HJ, Mahrholdt H, Sechtem U. Cardiovascular magnetic resonance reveals similar damage to the heart of patients with Becker and limb-girdle muscular dystrophy but no cardiac symptoms. J Magn Reson Imaging JMRI. 2009;30(4):876–7.
180. Hermans MC, Faber CG, Bekkers SC, de Die-Smulders CE, Gerrits MM, Merkies IS, et al. Structural and functional cardiac changes in myotonic dystrophy type 1: a cardiovascular magnetic resonance study. J Cardiovasc Magn Reson Off J Soc Cardiovasc Magn Reson. 2012;14:48.
181. Petri H, Ahtarovski KA, Vejlstrup N, Vissing J, Witting N, Kober L, et al. Myocardial fibrosis in patients with myotonic dystrophy type 1: a cardiovascular magnetic resonance study. J Cardiovasc Magn Reson Off J Soc Cardiovasc Magn Reson. 2014;16(1):59.
182. Turkbey EB, Gai N, Lima JA, van der Geest RJ, Wagner KR, Tomaselli GF, et al. Assessment of cardiac involvement in myotonic muscular dystrophy by T1 mapping on magnetic resonance imaging. Heart Rhythm Off J Heart Rhythm Soc. 2012;9(10):1691–7.
183. Iacucci I, Carbone I, Cannavale G, Conti B, Iampieri I, Rosati R, et al. Myocardial oedema as the sole marker of acute injury in Takotsubo cardiomyopathy: a cardiovascular magnetic resonance (CMR) study. Radiol Med. 2013;118(8):1309–23.
184. Avegliano G, Huguet M, Costabel JP, Ronderos R, Bijnens B, Kuschnir P, et al. Morphologic pattern of late gadolinium enhancement in Takotsubo cardiomyopathy detected by early cardiovascular magnetic resonance. Clin Cardiol. 2011; 34(3):178–82.
185. Naruse Y, Sato A, Kasahara K, Makino K, Sano M, Takeuchi Y, et al. The clinical impact of late gadolinium enhancement in Takotsubo cardiomyopathy: serial analysis of cardiovascular magnetic resonance images. J Cardiovasc Magn Reson Off J Soc Cardiovasc Magn Reson. 2011;13:67.
186. Corrado D, Thiene G, Nava A, Rossi L, Pennelli N. Sudden death in young competitive athletes: clinicopathologic correlations in 22 cases. Am J Med. 1990;89(5):588–96.
187. Tabib A, Loire R, Chalabreysse L, Meyronnet D, Miras A, Malicier D, et al. Circumstances of death and gross and microscopic observations in a series of 200 cases of sudden death associated with arrhythmogenic right ventricular cardiomyopathy and/or dysplasia. Circulation. 2003;108(24):3000–5.
188. McKenna WJ, Thiene G, Nava A, Fontaliran F, Blomstrom-Lundqvist C, Fontaine G, et al. Diagnosis of arrhythmogenic right ventricular dysplasia/cardiomyopathy. Task Force of the Working Group Myocardial and Pericardial Disease of the European Society of Cardiology and of the Scientific Council on Cardiomyopathies of the International Society and Federation of Cardiology. Br Heart J. 1994;71(3):215–8.
189. Marcus FI, McKenna WJ, Sherrill D, Basso C, Bauce B, Bluemke DA, et al. Diagnosis of arrhythmogenic right ventricular cardiomyopathy/dysplasia: proposed modification of the task force criteria. Circulation. 2010;121(13):1533–41.
190. di Cesare E. MRI assessment of right ventricular dysplasia. Eur Radiol. 2003;13(6):1387–93.
191. Bomma C, Rutberg J, Tandri H, Nasir K, Roguin A, Tichnell C, et al. Misdiagnosis of arrhythmogenic right ventricular dysplasia/cardiomyopathy. J Cardiovasc Electrophysiol. 2004;15(3):300–6.
192. Casolo G, Di Cesare E, Molinari G, Knoll P, Midiri M, Fedele F, et al. Diagnostic work up of arrhythmogenic right ventricular cardiomyopathy by cardiovascular magnetic resonance (CMR). Consensus statement La Radiologia Medica. 2004;108(1–2):39–55.
193. Bluemke DA, Krupinski EA, Ovitt T, Gear K, Unger E, Axel L, et al. MR imaging of arrhythmogenic right ventricular cardiomyopathy: morphologic findings and interobserver reliability. Cardiology. 2003;99(3):153–62.
194. Tandri H, Saranathan M, Rodriguez ER, Martinez C, Bomma C, Nasir K, et al. Noninvasive detection of myocardial fibrosis in arrhythmogenic right ventricular cardiomyopathy using delayed-enhancement magnetic resonance imaging. J Am Coll Cardiol. 2005;45(1):98–103.
195. te Riele AS, Bhonsale A, James CA, Rastegar N, Murray B, Burt JR, et al. Incremental value of cardiac magnetic resonance imaging in arrhythmic risk stratification of arrhythmogenic right ventricular dysplasia/cardiomyopathy-associated desmosomal mutation carriers. J Am Coll Cardiol. 2013;62(19):1761–9.
196. Quarta G, Husain SI, Flett AS, Sado DM, Chao CY, Tome Esteban MT, et al. Arrhythmogenic right ventricular cardiomyopathy mimics: role of cardiovascular magnetic resonance. J Cardiovasc Magn Reson Off J Soc Cardiovasc Magn Reson. 2013;15:16.
197. Liu T, Pursnani A, Sharma UC, Vorasettakarnkij Y, Verdini D, Deeprasertkul P, et al. Effect of the 2010 task force criteria on reclassification of cardiovascular magnetic resonance criteria for arrhythmogenic right ventricular cardiomyopathy. J Cardiovasc Magn Reson Off J Soc Cardiovasc Magn Reson. 2014;16:47.
198. Wilde AA, Antzelevitch C, Borggrefe M, Brugada J, Brugada R, Brugada P, et al. Proposed diagnostic criteria for the Brugada syndrome: consensus report. Circulation. 2002;106(19):2514–9.
199. Papavassiliu T, Wolpert C, Fluchter S, Schimpf R, Neff W, Haase KK, et al. Magnetic resonance imaging findings in patients with Brugada syndrome. J Cardiovasc Electrophysiol. 2004;15(10): 1133–8.
200. Steckman DA, Schneider PM, Schuller JL, Aleong RG, Nguyen DT, Sinagra G, et al. Utility of cardiac magnetic resonance imaging to differentiate cardiac sarcoidosis from arrhythmogenic right ventricular cardiomyopathy. Am J Cardiol. 2012;110(4):575–9.
201. Carrilho-Ferreira P, Almeida AG, Pinto FJ. Non-compaction cardiomyopathy: prevalence, prognosis, pathoetiology, genetics, and risk of cardioembolism. Curr Heart Fail Rep. 2014;11(4): 393–403.

202. Petersen SE, Selvanayagam JB, Wiesmann F, Robson MD, Francis JM, Anderson RH, et al. Left ventricular non-compaction: insights from cardiovascular magnetic resonance imaging. J Am Coll Cardiol. 2005;46(1):101–5.
203. Cheng H, Zhao S, Jiang S, Lu M, Yan C, Ling J, et al. Comparison of cardiac magnetic resonance imaging features of isolated left ventricular non-compaction in adults versus dilated cardiomyopathy in adults. Clin Radiol. 2011;66(9):853–60.
204. Grothoff M, Pachowsky M, Hoffmann J, Posch M, Klaassen S, Lehmkuhl L, et al. Value of cardiovascular MR in diagnosing left ventricular non-compaction cardiomyopathy and in discriminating between other cardiomyopathies. Eur Radiol. 2012;22(12): 2699–709.
205. Choudhary P, Hsu CJ, Grieve S, Smillie C, Singarayar S, Semsarian C, et al. Improving the diagnosis of LV non-compaction with cardiac magnetic resonance imaging. Int J Cardiol. 2015;181:430–6.
206. Wan J, Zhao S, Cheng H, Lu M, Jiang S, Yin G, et al. Varied distributions of late gadolinium enhancement found among patients meeting cardiovascular magnetic resonance criteria for isolated left ventricular non-compaction. J Cardiovasc Magn Reson Off J Soc Cardiovasc Magn Reson. 2013;15:20.
207. Nucifora G, Aquaro GD, Pingitore A, Masci PG, Lombardi M. Myocardial fibrosis in isolated left ventricular non-compaction and its relation to disease severity. Eur J Heart Fail. 2011; 13(2):170–6.
208. Melendez-Ramirez G, Castillo-Castellon F, Espinola-Zavaleta N, Meave A, Kimura-Hayama ET. Left ventricular noncompaction: a proposal of new diagnostic criteria by multidetector computed tomography. J Cardiovasc Comput Tomogr. 2012;6(5):346–54.
209. Sidhu MS, Uthamalingam S, Ahmed W, Engel LC, Vorasettakarnkij Y, Lee AM, et al. Defining left ventricular noncompaction using cardiac computed tomography. J Thorac Imaging. 2014;29(1):60–6.
210. Maceira AM, Cosin-Sales J, Roughton M, Prasad SK, Pennell DJ. Reference left atrial dimensions and volumes by steady state free precession cardiovascular magnetic resonance. J Cardiovasc Magn Reson Off J Soc Cardiovasc Magn Reson. 2010;12:65.
211. Maceira AM, Cosin-Sales J, Roughton M, Prasad SK, Pennell DJ. Reference right atrial dimensions and volume estimation by steady state free precession cardiovascular magnetic resonance. J Cardiovasc Magn Reson Off J Soc Cardiovasc Magn Reson. 2013;15:29.
212. Jahnke C, Fischer J, Mirelis JG, Kriatselis C, Gerds-Li JH, Gebker R, et al. Cardiovascular magnetic resonance imaging for accurate sizing of the left atrium: predictability of pulmonary vein isolation success in patients with atrial fibrillation. J Magn Reson Imaging JMRI. 2011;33(2):455–63.
213. Kowallick JT, Morton G, Lamata P, Jogiya R, Kutty S, Hasenfuss G, et al. Quantification of atrial dynamics using cardiovascular magnetic resonance: inter-study reproducibility. J Cardiovasc Magn Reson Off J Soc Cardiovasc Magn Reson. 2015;17:36.
214. Vardoulis O, Monney P, Bermano A, Vaxman A, Gotsman C, Schwitter J, et al. Single breath-hold 3D measurement of left atrial volume using compressed sensing cardiovascular magnetic resonance and a non-model-based reconstruction approach. J Cardiovasc Magn Reson Off J Soc Cardiovasc Magn Reson. 2015;17:47.
215. Agner BF, Kuhl JT, Linde JJ, Kofoed KF, Akeson P, Rasmussen BV, et al. Assessment of left atrial volume and function in patients with permanent atrial fibrillation: comparison of cardiac magnetic resonance imaging, 320-slice multi-detector computed tomography, and transthoracic echocardiography. Eur Heart J Cardiovasc Imaging. 2014;15(5):532–40.
216. Cochet H, Mouries A, Nivet H, Sacher F, Derval N, Denis A, et al. Age, atrial fibrillation, and structural heart disease are the main determinants of left atrial fibrosis detected by delayed-enhanced magnetic resonance imaging in a general cardiology population. J Cardiovasc Electrophysiol. 2015;26(5):484–92.
217. Habibi M, Lima JA, Khurram IM, Zimmerman SL, Zipunnikov V, Fukumoto K, et al. Association of left atrial function and left atrial enhancement in patients with atrial fibrillation: cardiac magnetic resonance study. Circ Cardiovasc Imaging. 2015;8(2), e002769.
218. Daccarett M, Badger TJ, Akoum N, Burgon NS, Mahnkopf C, Vergara G, et al. Association of left atrial fibrosis detected by delayed-enhancement magnetic resonance imaging and the risk of stroke in patients with atrial fibrillation. J Am Coll Cardiol. 2011;57(7):831–8.
219. Kwong RY, Heydari B, Abbasi S, Steel K, Al-Mallah M, Wu H, et al. Characterization of cardiac amyloidosis by atrial late gadolinium enhancement using contrast-enhanced cardiac magnetic resonance imaging and correlation with left atrial conduit and contractile function. Am J Cardiol. 2015;116:622–9.
220. Hamdan A, Charalampos K, Roettgen R, Wellnhofer E, Gebker R, Paetsch I, et al. Magnetic resonance imaging versus computed tomography for characterization of pulmonary vein morphology before radiofrequency catheter ablation of atrial fibrillation. Am J Cardiol. 2009;104(11):1540–6.
221. Hauser TH, McClennen S, Katsimaglis G, Josephson ME, Manning WJ, Yeon SB. Assessment of left atrial volume by contrast enhanced magnetic resonance angiography. J Cardiovasc Magn Reson Off J Soc Cardiovasc Magn Reson. 2004; 6(2):491–7.
222. Lickfett L, Kato R, Tandri H, Jayam V, Vasamreddy CR, Dickfeld T, et al. Characterization of a new pulmonary vein variant using magnetic resonance angiography: incidence, imaging, and interventional implications of the "right top pulmonary vein". J Cardiovasc Electrophysiol. 2004;15(5):538–43.
223. Kato R, Lickfett L, Meininger G, Dickfeld T, Wu R, Juang G, et al. Pulmonary vein anatomy in patients undergoing catheter ablation of atrial fibrillation: lessons learned by use of magnetic resonance imaging. Circulation. 2003;107(15):2004–10.
224. Mansour M, Holmvang G, Sosnovik D, Migrino R, Abbara S, Ruskin J, et al. Assessment of pulmonary vein anatomic variability by magnetic resonance imaging: implications for catheter ablation techniques for atrial fibrillation. J Cardiovasc Electrophysiol. 2004;15(4):387–93.
225. Nori D, Raff G, Gupta V, Gentry R, Boura J, Haines DE. Cardiac magnetic resonance imaging assessment of regional and global left atrial function before and after catheter ablation for atrial fibrillation. J Interv Card Electrophysiol. 2009;26(2):109–17.
226. Mahabadi AA, Samy B, Seneviratne SK, Toepker MH, Bamberg F, Hoffmann U, et al. Quantitative assessment of left atrial volume by electrocardiographic-gated contrast-enhanced multidetector computed tomography. J Cardiovasc Comput Tomogr. 2009;3(2):80–7.
227. Hauser TH, Essebag V, Baldessin F, McClennen S, Yeon SB, Manning WJ, et al. Prognostic value of pulmonary vein size in prediction of atrial fibrillation recurrence after pulmonary vein isolation: a cardiovascular magnetic resonance study. J Cardiovasc Magn Reson Off J Soc Cardiovasc Magn Reson. 2015;17:49.
228. Dickfeld T, Calkins H, Zviman M, Kato R, Meininger G, Lickfett L, et al. Anatomic stereotactic catheter ablation on three-dimensional magnetic resonance images in real time. Circulation. 2003;108(19):2407–13.
229. Dickfeld T, Calkins H, Zviman M, Meininger G, Lickfett L, Roguin A, et al. Stereotactic magnetic resonance guidance for anatomically targeted ablations of the fossa ovalis and the left atrium. J Interv Card Electrophysiol. 2004;11(2):105–15.
230. Bertaglia E, Brandolino G, Zoppo F, Zerbo F, Pascotto P. Integration of three-dimensional left atrial magnetic resonance images into a real-time electroanatomic mapping system: validation of a registration method. Pacing Clin Electrophysiol PACE. 2008;31(3):273–82.

231. Aleong R, Heist EK, Ruskin JN, Mansour M. Integration of intracardiac echocardiography with magnetic resonance imaging allows visualization of the esophagus during catheter ablation of atrial fibrillation. Heart Rhythm Off J Heart Rhythm Soc. 2008;5(7):1088.
232. Robbins IM, Colvin EV, Doyle TP, Kemp WE, Loyd JE, McMahon WS, et al. Pulmonary vein stenosis after catheter ablation of atrial fibrillation. Circulation. 1998;98(17):1769–75.
233. Taylor GW, Kay GN, Zheng X, Bishop S, Ideker RE. Pathological effects of extensive radiofrequency energy applications in the pulmonary veins in dogs. Circulation. 2000;101(14):1736–42.
234. Dill T, Neumann T, Ekinci O, Breidenbach C, John A, Erdogan A, et al. Pulmonary vein diameter reduction after radiofrequency catheter ablation for paroxysmal atrial fibrillation evaluated by contrast-enhanced three-dimensional magnetic resonance imaging. Circulation. 2003;107(6):845–50.
235. Arentz T, Jander N, von Rosenthal J, Blum T, Furmaier R, Gornandt L, et al. Incidence of pulmonary vein stenosis 2 years after radiofrequency catheter ablation of refractory atrial fibrillation. Eur Heart J. 2003;24(10):963–9.
236. Fukumoto K, Habibi M, Gucuk Ipek E, Khurram IM, Zimmerman SL, Zipunnikov V, et al. Comparison of preexisting and ablation-induced late gadolinium enhancement on left atrial magnetic resonance imaging. Heart Rhythm Off J Heart Rhythm Soc. 2015;12(4):668–72.
237. Oakes RS, Badger TJ, Kholmovski EG, Akoum N, Burgon NS, Fish EN, et al. Detection and quantification of left atrial structural remodeling with delayed-enhancement magnetic resonance imaging in patients with atrial fibrillation. Circulation. 2009;119(13):1758–67.
238. Peters DC, Wylie JV, Hauser TH, Nezafat R, Han Y, Woo JJ, et al. Recurrence of atrial fibrillation correlates with the extent of post-procedural late gadolinium enhancement: a pilot study. JACC Cardiovasc Imaging. 2009;2(3):308–16.
239. McGann C, Kholmovski E, Blauer J, Vijayakumar S, Haslam T, Cates J, et al. Dark regions of no-reflow on late gadolinium enhancement magnetic resonance imaging result in scar formation after atrial fibrillation ablation. J Am Coll Cardiol. 2011; 58(2):177–85.
240. Beinart R, Khurram IM, Liu S, Yarmohammadi H, Halperin HR, Bluemke DA, et al. Cardiac magnetic resonance T1 mapping of left atrial myocardium. Heart Rhythm Off J Heart Rhythm Soc. 2013;10(9):1325–31.
241. Ling LH, McLellan AJ, Taylor AJ, Iles LM, Ellims AH, Kumar S, et al. Magnetic resonance post-contrast T1 mapping in the human atrium: validation and impact on clinical outcome after catheter ablation for atrial fibrillation. Heart Rhythm Off J Heart Rhythm Soc. 2014;11(9):1551–9.
242. Heist EK, Refaat M, Danik SB, Holmvang G, Ruskin JN, Mansour M. Analysis of the left atrial appendage by magnetic resonance angiography in patients with atrial fibrillation. Heart Rhythm Off J Heart Rhythm Soc. 2006;3(11):1313–8.
243. Muellerleile K, Sultan A, Groth M, Steven D, Hoffmann B, Adam G, et al. Velocity encoded cardiovascular magnetic resonance to assess left atrial appendage emptying. J Cardiovasc Magn Reson Off J Soc Cardiovasc Magn Reson. 2012;14:39.
244. Ohyama H, Hosomi N, Takahashi T, Mizushige K, Osaka K, Kohno M, et al. Comparison of magnetic resonance imaging and transesophageal echocardiography in detection of thrombus in the left atrial appendage. Stroke J Cereb Circ. 2003;34(10):2436–9.
245. Ohyama H, Mizushige K, Hosomi N. Magnetic resonance imaging of left atrial thrombus. Heart. 2002;88(3):233.
246. Mohrs OK, Nowak B, Petersen SE, Welsner M, Rubel C, Magedanz A, et al. Thrombus detection in the left atrial appendage using contrast-enhanced MRI: a pilot study. AJR Am J Roentgenol. 2006;186(1):198–205.
247. Budoff MJ, Shittu A, Hacioglu Y, Gang E, Li D, Bhatia H, et al. Comparison of transesophageal echocardiography versus computed tomography for detection of left atrial appendage filling defect (thrombus). Am J Cardiol. 2014;113(1):173–7.
248. Mohrs OK, Schraeder R, Petersen SE, Scherer D, Nowak B, Kauczor HU, et al. Percutaneous left atrial appendage transcatheter occlusion (PLAATO): planning and follow-up using contrast-enhanced MRI. AJR Am J Roentgenol. 2006;186(2):361–4.
249. van Rosendael PJ, Katsanos S, van den Brink OW, Scholte AJ, Trines SA, Bax JJ, et al. Geometry of left atrial appendage assessed with multidetector-row computed tomography: implications for transcatheter closure devices. EuroIntervention. 2014;10(3):364–71.
250. Poulter RS, Tang J, Jue J, Ibrahim R, Nicolaou S, Mayo J, et al. Cardiac computed tomography follow-up of left atrial appendage exclusion using the Amplatzer Cardiac Plug device. Can J Cardiol. 2012;28(1):119.e1–3.
251. Thadani SR, Dyverfeldt P, Gin A, Chitsaz S, Rao RK, Hope MD. Comprehensive evaluation of culture-negative endocarditis with use of cardiac and 4-dimensional-flow magnetic resonance imaging. Tex Heart Inst J. 2014;41(3):351–2.
252. Harris KM, Ang E, Lesser JR, Sonnesyn SW. Cardiac magnetic resonance imaging for detection of an abscess associated with prosthetic valve endocarditis: a case report. Heart Surg Forum. 2007;10(3):E186–7.
253. Feuchtner GM, Stolzmann P, Dichtl W, Schertler T, Bonatti J, Scheffel H, et al. Multislice computed tomography in infective endocarditis: comparison with transesophageal echocardiography and intraoperative findings. J Am Coll Cardiol. 2009;53(5): 436–44.
254. Saby L, Laas O, Habib G, Cammilleri S, Mancini J, Tessonnier L, et al. Positron emission tomography/computed tomography for diagnosis of prosthetic valve endocarditis: increased valvular 18 F-fluorodeoxyglucose uptake as a novel major criterion. J Am Coll Cardiol. 2013;61(23):2374–82.
255. John AS, Dill T, Brandt RR, Rau M, Ricken W, Bachmann G, et al. Magnetic resonance to assess the aortic valve area in aortic stenosis: how does it compare to current diagnostic standards? J Am Coll Cardiol. 2003;42(3):519–26.
256. Malyar NM, Schlosser T, Barkhausen J, Gutersohn A, Buck T, Bartel T, et al. Assessment of aortic valve area in aortic stenosis using cardiac magnetic resonance tomography: comparison with echocardiography. Cardiology. 2008;109(2):126–34.
257. Garcia J, Kadem L, Larose E, Clavel MA, Pibarot P. Comparison between cardiovascular magnetic resonance and transthoracic Doppler echocardiography for the estimation of effective orifice area in aortic stenosis. J Cardiovasc Magn Reson Off J Soc Cardiovasc Magn Reson. 2011;13:25.
258. Garcia J, Capoulade R, Le Ven F, Gaillard E, Kadem L, Pibarot P, et al. Discrepancies between cardiovascular magnetic resonance and Doppler echocardiography in the measurement of transvalvular gradient in aortic stenosis: the effect of flow vorticity. J Cardiovasc Magn Reson Off J Soc Cardiovasc Magn Reson. 2013;15:84.
259. Hoffmann R, Altiok E, Friedman Z, Becker M, Frick M. Myocardial deformation imaging by two-dimensional speckle-tracking echocardiography in comparison to late gadolinium enhancement cardiac magnetic resonance for analysis of myocardial fibrosis in severe aortic stenosis. Am J Cardiol. 2014;114(7):1083–8.
260. Lee SP, Park SJ, Kim YJ, Chang SA, Park EA, Kim HK, et al. Early detection of subclinical ventricular deterioration in aortic stenosis with cardiovascular magnetic resonance and echocardiography. J Cardiovasc Magn Reson Off J Soc Cardiovasc Magn Reson. 2013;15:72.
261. Azevedo CF, Nigri M, Higuchi ML, Pomerantzeff PM, Spina GS, Sampaio RO, et al. Prognostic significance of myocardial fibrosis

quantification by histopathology and magnetic resonance imaging in patients with severe aortic valve disease. J Am Coll Cardiol. 2010;56(4):278–87.

262. Holmes Jr DR, Mack MJ, Kaul S, Agnihotri A, Alexander KP, Bailey SR, et al. 2012 ACCF/AATS/SCAI/STS expert consensus document on transcatheter aortic valve replacement. J Am Coll Cardiol. 2012;59(13):1200–54.
263. Crouch G, Bennetts J, Sinhal A, Tully PJ, Leong DP, Bradbrook C, et al. Early effects of transcatheter aortic valve implantation and aortic valve replacement on myocardial function and aortic valve hemodynamics: insights from cardiovascular magnetic resonance imaging. J Thorac Cardiovasc Surg. 2015;149(2): 462–70.
264. Fairbairn TA, Steadman CD, Mather AN, Motwani M, Blackman DJ, Plein S, et al. Assessment of valve haemodynamics, reverse ventricular remodelling and myocardial fibrosis following transcatheter aortic valve implantation compared to surgical aortic valve replacement: a cardiovascular magnetic resonance study. Heart. 2013;99(16):1185–91.
265. Rossi A, van der Linde D, Yap SC, Lapinskas T, Kirschbaum S, Springeling T, et al. Ascending aorta dilatation in patients with bicuspid aortic valve stenosis: a prospective CMR study. Eur Radiol. 2013;23(3):642–9.
266. Malaisrie SC, Carr J, Mikati I, Rigolin V, Yip BK, Lapin B, et al. Cardiac magnetic resonance imaging is more diagnostic than 2-dimensional echocardiography in determining the presence of bicuspid aortic valve. J Thorac Cardiovasc Surg. 2012;144(2): 370–6.
267. Buchner S, Hulsmann M, Poschenrieder F, Hamer OW, Fellner C, Kobuch R, et al. Variable phenotypes of bicuspid aortic valve disease: classification by cardiovascular magnetic resonance. Heart. 2010;96(15):1233–40.
268. Murphy DJ, McEvoy SH, Iyengar S, Feuchtner G, Cury RC, Roobottom C, et al. Bicuspid aortic valves: diagnostic accuracy of standard axial 64-slice chest CT compared to aortic valve image plane ECG-gated cardiac CT. Eur J Radiol. 2014;83(8): 1396–401.
269. Alkadhi H, Leschka S, Trindade PT, Feuchtner G, Stolzmann P, Plass A, et al. Cardiac CT for the differentiation of bicuspid and tricuspid aortic valves: comparison with echocardiography and surgery. AJR Am J Roentgenol. 2010;195(4):900–8.
270. Sucha D, Symersky P, Vonken EJ, Provoost E, Chamuleau SA, Budde RP. Multidetector-row computed tomography allows accurate measurement of mechanical prosthetic heart valve leaflet closing angles compared with fluoroscopy. J Comput Assist Tomogr. 2014;38(3):451–6.
271. Symersky P, Budde RP, de Mol BA, Prokop M. Comparison of multidetector-row computed tomography to echocardiography and fluoroscopy for evaluation of patients with mechanical prosthetic valve obstruction. Am J Cardiol. 2009;104(8): 1128–34.
272. Tsai IC, Lin YK, Chang Y, Fu YC, Wang CC, Hsieh SR, et al. Correctness of multi-detector-row computed tomography for diagnosing mechanical prosthetic heart valve disorders using operative findings as a gold standard. Eur Radiol. 2009;19(4):857–67.
273. Ueda T, Teshima H, Fukunaga S, Aoyagi S, Tanaka H. Evaluation of prosthetic valve obstruction on electrocardiographically gated multidetector-row computed tomography – identification of subprosthetic pannus in the aortic position. Circ J Off J Jpn Circ Soc. 2013;77(2):418–23.
274. Tanis W, Sucha D, Laufer W, Habets J, van Herwerden LA, Symersky P, et al. Multidetector-row computed tomography for prosthetic heart valve dysfunction: is concomitant non-invasive coronary angiography possible before redo-surgery? Eur Radiol. 2015;25(6):1623–30.
275. Gelfand EV, Hughes S, Hauser TH, Yeon SB, Goepfert L, Kissinger KV, et al. Severity of mitral and aortic regurgitation as assessed by cardiovascular magnetic resonance: optimizing correlation with Doppler echocardiography. J Cardiovasc Magn Reson Off J Soc Cardiovasc Magn Reson. 2006;8(3):503–7.
276. Debl K, Djavidani B, Buchner S, Heinicke N, Fredersdorf S, Haimerl J, et al. Assessment of the anatomic regurgitant orifice in aortic regurgitation: a clinical magnetic resonance imaging study. Heart. 2008;94(3), e8.
277. Ewe SH, Delgado V, van der Geest R, Westenberg JJ, Haeck ML, Witkowski TG, et al. Accuracy of three-dimensional versus two-dimensional echocardiography for quantification of aortic regurgitation and validation by three-dimensional three-directional velocity-encoded magnetic resonance imaging. Am J Cardiol. 2013;112(4):560–6.
278. Ko SM, Park JH, Shin JK, Kim JS. Assessment of the regurgitant orifice area in aortic regurgitation with dual-source CT: Comparison with cardiovascular magnetic resonance. J Cardiovasc Comput Tomogr. 2015;9(4):345–53.
279. Feuchtner GM, Spoeck A, Lessick J, Dichtl W, Plass A, Leschka S, et al. Quantification of aortic regurgitant fraction and volume with multi-detector computed tomography comparison with echocardiography. Acad Radiol. 2011;18(3):334–42.
280. Frick M, Meyer CG, Kirschfink A, Altiok E, Lehrke M, Brehmer K, et al. Evaluation of aortic regurgitation after transcatheter aortic valve implantation: aortic root angiography in comparison to cardiac magnetic resonance. EuroIntervention. 2015;10(11): Epub ahead of print.
281. Sherif MA, Abdel-Wahab M, Beurich HW, Stocker B, Zachow D, Geist V, et al. Haemodynamic evaluation of aortic regurgitation after transcatheter aortic valve implantation using cardiovascular magnetic resonance. EuroIntervention. 2011;7(1):57–63.
282. Merten C, Beurich HW, Zachow D, Mostafa AE, Geist V, Toelg R, et al. Aortic regurgitation and left ventricular remodeling after transcatheter aortic valve implantation: a serial cardiac magnetic resonance imaging study. Circ Cardiovasc Interv. 2013;6(4):476–83.
283. Ribeiro HB, Le Ven F, Larose E, Dahou A, Nombela-Franco L, Urena M, et al. Cardiac magnetic resonance versus transthoracic echocardiography for the assessment and quantification of aortic regurgitation in patients undergoing transcatheter aortic valve implantation. Heart. 2014;100(24):1924–32.
284. Hartlage GR, Babaliaros VC, Thourani VH, Hayek S, Chrysohoou C, Ghasemzadeh N, et al. The role of cardiovascular magnetic resonance in stratifying paravalvular leak severity after transcatheter aortic valve replacement: an observational outcome study. J Cardiovasc Magn Reson Off J Soc Cardiovasc Magn Reson. 2014;16:93.
285. Jabbour A, Ismail TF, Moat N, Gulati A, Roussin I, Alpendurada F, et al. Multimodality imaging in transcatheter aortic valve implantation and post-procedural aortic regurgitation: comparison among cardiovascular magnetic resonance, cardiac computed tomography, and echocardiography. J Am Coll Cardiol. 2011;58(21):2165–73.
286. Chan KM, Wage R, Symmonds K, Rahman-Haley S, Mohiaddin RH, Firmin DN, et al. Towards comprehensive assessment of mitral regurgitation using cardiovascular magnetic resonance. J Cardiovasc Magn Reson Off J Soc Cardiovasc Magn Reson. 2008;10:61.
287. Shanks M, Siebelink HM, Delgado V, van de Veire NR, Ng AC, Sieders A, et al. Quantitative assessment of mitral regurgitation: comparison between three-dimensional transesophageal echocardiography and magnetic resonance imaging. Circ Cardiovasc Imaging. 2010;3(6):694–700.
288. Buchner S, Debl K, Poschenrieder F, Feuerbach S, Riegger GA, Luchner A, et al. Cardiovascular magnetic resonance for direct assessment of anatomic regurgitant orifice in mitral regurgitation. Circ Cardiovasc Imaging. 2008;1(2):148–55.

289. Delling FN, Kang LL, Yeon SB, Kissinger KV, Goddu B, Manning WJ, et al. CMR predictors of mitral regurgitation in mitral valve prolapse. JACC Cardiovasc Imaging. 2010;3(10):1037–45.
290. Van De Heyning CM, Magne J, Pierard LA, Bruyere PJ, Davin L, De Maeyer C, et al. Late gadolinium enhancement CMR in primary mitral regurgitation. Eur J Clin Invest. 2014; 44(9):840–7.
291. Takeda K, Matsumiya G, Hamada S, Sakaguchi T, Miyagawa S, Yamauchi T, et al. Left ventricular basal myocardial scarring detected by delayed enhancement magnetic resonance imaging predicts outcomes after surgical therapies for patients with ischemic mitral regurgitation and left ventricular dysfunction. Circ J Off J Jpn Circ Soc. 2011;75(1):148–56.
292. Krumm P, Zuern CS, Wurster TH, Mangold S, Klumpp BD, Henning A, et al. Cardiac magnetic resonance imaging in patients undergoing percutaneous mitral valve repair with the MitraClip system. Clin Res Cardiol Off J German Cardiac Soc. 2014;103(5):397–404.
293. Simprini LA, Afroz A, Cooper MA, Klem I, Jensen C, Kim RJ, et al. Routine cine-CMR for prosthesis-associated mitral regurgitation: a multicenter comparison to echocardiography. J Heart Valve Dis. 2014;23(5):575–82.
294. Feuchtner GM, Alkadhi H, Karlo C, Sarwar A, Meier A, Dichtl W, et al. Cardiac CT angiography for the diagnosis of mitral valve prolapse: comparison with echocardiography1. Radiology. 2010;254(2):374–83.
295. Koo HJ, Yang DH, Oh SY, Kang JW, Kim DH, Song JK, et al. Demonstration of mitral valve prolapse with CT for planning of mitral valve repair. Radiographics Rev Publ Radiol Soc North Am Inc. 2014;34(6):1537–52.
296. Smith T, Gurudevan S, Cheng V, Trento A, Derobertis M, Thomson L, et al. Assessment of the morphological features of degenerative mitral valve disease using 64-slice multi detector computed tomography. J Cardiovasc Comput Tomogr. 2012; 6(6):415–21.
297. Choure AJ, Garcia MJ, Hesse B, Sevensma M, Maly G, Greenberg NL, et al. In vivo analysis of the anatomical relationship of coronary sinus to mitral annulus and left circumflex coronary artery using cardiac multidetector computed tomography: implications for percutaneous coronary sinus mitral annuloplasty. J Am Coll Cardiol. 2006;48(10):1938–45.
298. Mao S, Shinbane JS, Girsky MJ, Child J, Carson S, Oudiz RJ, et al. Coronary venous imaging with electron beam computed tomographic angiography: three-dimensional mapping and relationship with coronary arteries. Am Heart J. 2005;150(2):315–22.
299. Messika-Zeitoun D, Serfaty JM, Laissy JP, Berhili M, Brochet E, Iung B, et al. Assessment of the mitral valve area in patients with mitral stenosis by multislice computed tomography. J Am Coll Cardiol. 2006;48(2):411–3.
300. Guo YK, Yang ZG, Ning G, Rao L, Dong L, Pen Y, et al. Sixty-four-slice multidetector computed tomography for preoperative evaluation of left ventricular function and mass in patients with mitral regurgitation: comparison with magnetic resonance imaging and echocardiography. Eur Radiol. 2009;19(9):2107–16.
301. Lewis MJ, O'Connor DS, Rozenshtien A, Ye S, Einstein AJ, Ginns JM, et al. Usefulness of magnetic resonance imaging to guide referral for pulmonary valve replacement in repaired tetralogy of Fallot. Am J Cardiol. 2014;114(9):1406–11.
302. Vliegen HW, van Straten A, de Roos A, Roest AA, Schoof PH, Zwinderman AH, et al. Magnetic resonance imaging to assess the hemodynamic effects of pulmonary valve replacement in adults late after repair of tetralogy of fallot. Circulation. 2002;106(13):1703–7.
303. Shah R, Shriki J, Shinbane JS. Cardiovascular magnetic resonance depiction of quadricuspid pulmonary valve with associated pulmonary regurgitation and pulmonary artery aneurysm. Tex Heart Inst J. 2014;41(3):349–50.
304. Secchi F, Resta EC, Cannao PM, Tresoldi S, Butera G, Carminati M, et al. Four-year cardiac magnetic resonance (CMR) follow-up of patients treated with percutaneous pulmonary valve stent implantation. Eur Radiol. 2015;25:3606–13.
305. Cho IJ, Oh J, Chang HJ, Park J, Kang KW, Kim YJ, et al. Tricuspid regurgitation duration correlates with cardiovascular magnetic resonance-derived right ventricular ejection fraction and predict prognosis in patients with pulmonary arterial hypertension. Eur Heart J Cardiovasc Imaging. 2014;15(1):18–23.
306. Maffessanti F, Gripari P, Pontone G, Andreini D, Bertella E, Mushtaq S, et al. Three-dimensional dynamic assessment of tricuspid and mitral annuli using cardiovascular magnetic resonance. Eur Heart J Cardiovasc Imaging. 2013;14(10):986–95.
307. Kim HK, Kim YJ, Park EA, Bae JS, Lee W, Kim KH, et al. Assessment of haemodynamic effects of surgical correction for severe functional tricuspid regurgitation: cardiac magnetic resonance imaging study. Eur Heart J. 2010;31(12):1520–8.
308. van Rosendael PJ, Joyce E, Katsanos S, Debonnaire P, Kamperidis V, van der Kley F, et al. Tricuspid valve remodelling in functional tricuspid regurgitation: multidetector row computed tomography insights. Eur Heart J Cardiovasc Imaging. 2016;17:96–105.
309. Fratz S, Hess J, Schuhbaeck A, Buchner C, Hendrich E, Martinoff S, et al. Routine clinical cardiovascular magnetic resonance in paediatric and adult congenital heart disease: patients, protocols, questions asked and contributions made. J Cardiovasc Magn Reson Off J Soc Cardiovasc Magn Reson. 2008;10:46.
310. Arheden H, Holmqvist C, Thilen U, Hanseus K, Bjorkhem G, Pahlm O, et al. Left-to-right cardiac shunts: comparison of measurements obtained with MR velocity mapping and with radionuclide angiography. Radiology. 1999;211(2):453–8.
311. Sorensen TS, Korperich H, Greil GF, Eichhorn J, Barth P, Meyer H, et al. Operator-independent isotropic three-dimensional magnetic resonance imaging for morphology in congenital heart disease: a validation study. Circulation. 2004;110(2):163–9.
312. Kilner PJ, Geva T, Kaemmerer H, Trindade PT, Schwitter J, Webb GD. Recommendations for cardiovascular magnetic resonance in adults with congenital heart disease from the respective working groups of the European Society of Cardiology. Eur Heart J. 2010;31(7):794–805.
313. Haramati LB, Glickstein JS, Issenberg HJ, Haramati N, Crooke GA. MR imaging and CT of vascular anomalies and connections in patients with congenital heart disease: significance in surgical planning. Radiographics Rev Publ Radiol Soc North Am Inc. 2002;22(2):337–47; discussion 48–9.
314. Durongpisitkul K, Tang NL, Soongswang J, Laohaprasitiporn D, Nanal A. Predictors of successful transcatheter closure of atrial septal defect by cardiac magnetic resonance imaging. Pediatr Cardiol. 2004;25(2):124–30.
315. Taylor AM, Dymarkowski S, Hamaekers P, Razavi R, Gewillig M, Mertens L, et al. MR coronary angiography and late-enhancement myocardial MR in children who underwent arterial switch surgery for transposition of great arteries. Radiology. 2005;234(2):542–7.
316. Harris MA, Johnson TR, Weinberg PM, Fogel MA. Delayed-enhancement cardiovascular magnetic resonance identifies fibrous tissue in children after surgery for congenital heart disease. J Thorac Cardiovasc Surg. 2007;133(3):676–81.
317. Geva T, Marshall AC. Magnetic resonance imaging-guided catheter interventions in congenital heart disease. Circulation. 2006;113(8):1051–2.
318. Tzifa A, Krombach GA, Kramer N, Kruger S, Schutte A, von Walter M, et al. Magnetic resonance-guided cardiac interventions using magnetic resonance-compatible devices: a preclinical study and first-in-man congenital interventions. Circ Cardiovasc Interv. 2010;3(6):585–92.

319. Geva T, Greil GF, Marshall AC, Landzberg M, Powell AJ. Gadolinium-enhanced 3-dimensional magnetic resonance angiography of pulmonary blood supply in patients with complex pulmonary stenosis or atresia: comparison with x-ray angiography. Circulation. 2002;106(4):473–8.
320. Prasad SK, Soukias N, Hornung T, Khan M, Pennell DJ, Gatzoulis MA, et al. Role of magnetic resonance angiography in the diagnosis of major aortopulmonary collateral arteries and partial anomalous pulmonary venous drainage. Circulation. 2004; 109(2):207–14.
321. Bernardes RJ, Marchiori E, Bernardes PM, Monzo Gonzaga MB, Simoes LC. A comparison of magnetic resonance angiography with conventional angiography in the diagnosis of tetralogy of Fallot. Cardiol Young. 2006;16(3):281–8.
322. Oosterhof T, van Straten A, Vliegen HW, Meijboom FJ, van Dijk AP, Spijkerboer AM, et al. Preoperative thresholds for pulmonary valve replacement in patients with corrected tetralogy of Fallot using cardiovascular magnetic resonance. Circulation. 2007; 116(5):545–51.
323. Ghai A, Silversides C, Harris L, Webb GD, Siu SC, Therrien J. Left ventricular dysfunction is a risk factor for sudden cardiac death in adults late after repair of tetralogy of Fallot. J Am Coll Cardiol. 2002;40(9):1675–80.
324. Rebergen SA, Chin JG, Ottenkamp J, van der Wall EE, de Roos A. Pulmonary regurgitation in the late postoperative follow-up of tetralogy of Fallot. Volumetric quantitation by nuclear magnetic resonance velocity mapping. Circulation. 1993;88(5 Pt 1): 2257–66.
325. Fratz S, Schuhbaeck A, Buchner C, Busch R, Meierhofer C, Martinoff S, et al. Comparison of accuracy of axial slices versus short-axis slices for measuring ventricular volumes by cardiac magnetic resonance in patients with corrected tetralogy of fallot. Am J Cardiol. 2009;103(12):1764–9.
326. Kang IS, Redington AN, Benson LN, Macgowan C, Valsangiacomo ER, Roman K, et al. Differential regurgitation in branch pulmonary arteries after repair of tetralogy of Fallot: a phase-contrast cine magnetic resonance study. Circulation. 2003;107(23):2938–43.
327. Lee C, Lee CH, Kwak JG, Kim SH, Shim WS, Lee SY, et al. Factors associated with right ventricular dilatation and dysfunction in patients with chronic pulmonary regurgitation after repair of tetralogy of Fallot: analysis of magnetic resonance imaging data from 218 patients. J Thorac Cardiovasc Surg. 2014; 148(6):2589–95.
328. Johansson B, Babu-Narayan SV, Kilner PJ. The effects of breath-holding on pulmonary regurgitation measured by cardiovascular magnetic resonance velocity mapping. J Cardiovasc Magn Reson Off J Soc Cardiovasc Magn Reson. 2009;11:1.
329. Mercer-Rosa L, Yang W, Kutty S, Rychik J, Fogel M, Goldmuntz E. Quantifying pulmonary regurgitation and right ventricular function in surgically repaired tetralogy of Fallot: a comparative analysis of echocardiography and magnetic resonance imaging. Circ Cardiovasc Imaging. 2012;5(5):637–43.
330. Babu-Narayan SV, Kilner PJ, Li W, Moon JC, Goktekin O, Davlouros PA, et al. Ventricular fibrosis suggested by cardiovascular magnetic resonance in adults with repaired tetralogy of fallot and its relationship to adverse markers of clinical outcome. Circulation. 2006;113(3):405–13.
331. Munkhammar P, Carlsson M, Arheden H, Pesonen E. Restrictive right ventricular physiology after tetralogy of Fallot repair is associated with fibrosis of the right ventricular outflow tract visualized on cardiac magnetic resonance imaging. Eur Heart J Cardiovasc Imaging. 2013;14(10):978–85.
332. Kozak MF, Redington A, Yoo SJ, Seed M, Greiser A, Grosse-Wortmann L. Diffuse myocardial fibrosis following tetralogy of Fallot repair: a T1 mapping cardiac magnetic resonance study. Pediatr Radiol. 2014;44(4):403–9.
333. Ma XJ, Tao L, Chen X, Li W, Peng ZY, Chen Y, et al. Clinical application of three-dimensional reconstruction and rapid prototyping technology of multislice spiral computed tomography angiography for the repair of ventricular septal defect of tetralogy of Fallot. Genet Mol Res GMR. 2015;14(1):1301–9.
334. Lin MT, Wang JK, Chen YS, Lee WJ, Chiu HH, Chen CA, et al. Detection of pulmonary arterial morphology in tetralogy of Fallot with pulmonary atresia by computed tomography: 12 years of experience. Eur J Pediatr. 2012;171(3):579–86.
335. Vastel-Amzallag C, Le Bret E, Paul JF, Lambert V, Rohnean A, El Fassy E, et al. Diagnostic accuracy of dual-source multislice computed tomographic analysis for the preoperative detection of coronary artery anomalies in 100 patients with tetralogy of Fallot. J Thorac Cardiovasc Surg. 2011;142(1):120–6.
336. Bardo DM, Asamato J, Mackay CS, Minette M. Low-dose coronary artery computed tomography angiogram of an infant with tetralogy of fallot using a 256-slice multidetector computed tomography scanner. Pediatr Cardiol. 2009;30(6):824–6.
337. Raman SV, Cook SC, McCarthy B, Ferketich AK. Usefulness of multidetector row computed tomography to quantify right ventricular size and function in adults with either tetralogy of Fallot or transposition of the great arteries. Am J Cardiol. 2005;95(5):683–6.
338. Whitehead KK, Sundareswaran KS, Parks WJ, Harris MA, Yoganathan AP, Fogel MA. Blood flow distribution in a large series of patients having the Fontan operation: a cardiac magnetic resonance velocity mapping study. J Thorac Cardiovasc Surg. 2009;138(1):96–102.
339. Goo HW, Yang DH, Park IS, Ko JK, Kim YH, Seo DM, et al. Time-resolved three-dimensional contrast-enhanced magnetic resonance angiography in patients who have undergone a Fontan operation or bidirectional cavopulmonary connection: initial experience. J Magn Reson Imaging JMRI. 2007;25(4):727–36.
340. Park EA, Lee W, Chung SY, Yin YH, Chung JW, Park JH. Optimal scan timing and intravenous route for contrast-enhanced computed tomography in patients after Fontan operation. J Comput Assist Tomogr. 2010;34(1):75–81.
341. Greenberg SB, Bhutta ST. A dual contrast injection technique for multidetector computed tomography angiography of Fontan procedures. Int J Cardiovasc Imaging. 2008;24(3):345–8.
342. Rathod RH, Prakash A, Kim YY, Germanakis IE, Powell AJ, Gauvreau K, et al. Cardiac magnetic resonance parameters predict transplantation-free survival in patients with fontan circulation. Circ Cardiovasc Imaging. 2014;7(3):502–9.
343. Ovroutski S, Nordmeyer S, Miera O, Ewert P, Klimes K, Kuhne T, et al. Caval flow reflects Fontan hemodynamics: quantification by magnetic resonance imaging. Clin Res Cardiol Off J German Cardiac Soc. 2012;101(2):133–8.
344. Restrepo M, Mirabella L, Tang E, Haggerty CM, Khiabani RH, Fynn-Thompson F, et al. Fontan pathway growth: a quantitative evaluation of lateral tunnel and extracardiac cavopulmonary connections using serial cardiac magnetic resonance. Ann Thorac Surg. 2014;97(3):916–22.
345. Haggerty CM, Restrepo M, Tang E, de Zelicourt DA, Sundareswaran KS, Mirabella L, et al. Fontan hemodynamics from 100 patient-specific cardiac magnetic resonance studies: a computational fluid dynamics analysis. J Thorac Cardiovasc Surg. 2014;148(4):1481–9.
346. Rathod RH, Prakash A, Powell AJ, Geva T. Myocardial fibrosis identified by cardiac magnetic resonance late gadolinium enhancement is associated with adverse ventricular mechanics and ventricular tachycardia late after Fontan operation. J Am Coll Cardiol. 2010;55(16):1721–8.
347. Rydman R, Gatzoulis MA, Ho SY, Ernst S, Swan L, Li W, et al. Systemic right ventricular fibrosis detected by cardiovascular magnetic resonance is associated with clinical outcome, mainly

new-onset atrial arrhythmia, in patients after atrial redirection surgery for transposition of the great arteries. Circ Cardiovasc Imaging. 2015;8(5):e002628.
348. Tobler D, Motwani M, Wald RM, Roche SL, Verocai F, Iwanochko RM, et al. Evaluation of a comprehensive cardiovascular magnetic resonance protocol in young adults late after the arterial switch operation for d-transposition of the great arteries. J Cardiovasc Magn Reson Off J Soc Cardiovasc Magn Reson. 2014;16:98.
349. Tulevski II, van der Wall EE, Groenink M, Dodge-Khatami A, Hirsch A, Stoker J, et al. Usefulness of magnetic resonance imaging dobutamine stress in asymptomatic and minimally symptomatic patients with decreased cardiac reserve from congenital heart disease (complete and corrected transposition of the great arteries and subpulmonic obstruction). Am J Cardiol. 2002;89(9):1077–81.
350. Fogel MA, Hubbard A, Weinberg PM. Mid-term follow-up of patients with transposition of the great arteries after atrial inversion operation using two- and three-dimensional magnetic resonance imaging. Pediatr Radiol. 2002;32(6):440–6.
351. Johansson B, Babu-Narayan SV, Kilner PJ, Cannell TM, Mohiaddin RH. 3-dimensional time-resolved contrast-enhanced magnetic resonance angiography for evaluation late after the mustard operation for transposition. Cardiol Young. 2010;20(1):1–7.
352. Shinbane JS, Shriki J, Hindoyan A, Ghosh B, Chang P, Farvid A, et al. Unoperated congenitally corrected transposition of the great arteries, nonrestrictive ventricular septal defect, and pulmonary stenosis in middle adulthood: do multiple wrongs make a right? World J Pediatr Congenit Heart Surg. 2012;3(1):123–9.
353. Cook SC, McCarthy M, Daniels CJ, Cheatham JP, Raman SV. Usefulness of multislice computed tomography angiography to evaluate intravascular stents and transcatheter occlusion devices in patients with d-transposition of the great arteries after mustard repair. Am J Cardiol. 2004;94(7):967–9.
354. Ou P, Mousseaux E, Azarine A, Dupont P, Agnoletti G, Vouhe P, et al. Detection of coronary complications after the arterial switch operation for transposition of the great arteries: first experience with multislice computed tomography in children. J Thorac Cardiovasc Surg. 2006;131(3):639–43.
355. Yalonetsky S, Tobler D, Greutmann M, Crean AM, Wintersperger BJ, Nguyen ET, et al. Cardiac magnetic resonance imaging and the assessment of ebstein anomaly in adults. Am J Cardiol. 2011;107(5):767–73.
356. Hosch O, Sohns JM, Nguyen TT, Lauerer P, Rosenberg C, Kowallick JT, et al. The total right/left-volume index: a new and simplified cardiac magnetic resonance measure to evaluate the severity of Ebstein anomaly of the tricuspid valve: a comparison with heart failure markers from various modalities. Circ Cardiovasc Imaging. 2014;7(4):601–9.
357. Hosch O, Ngyuen TT, Lauerer P, Schuster A, Kutty S, Staab W, et al. BNP and haematological parameters are markers of severity of Ebstein's anomaly: correlation with CMR and cardiopulmonary exercise testing. Eur Heart J Cardiovasc Imaging. 2015; 16(6):670–5.
358. Aggarwala G, Thompson B, van Beek E, Jagasia D. Multislice computed tomography angiography of Ebstein anomaly and anomalous coronary artery. J Cardiovasc Comput Tomogr. 2007;1(3):168–9.
359. Teo KS, Disney PJ, Dundon BK, Worthley MI, Brown MA, Sanders P, et al. Assessment of atrial septal defects in adults comparing cardiovascular magnetic resonance with transoesophageal echocardiography. J Cardiovasc Magn Reson Off J Soc Cardiovasc Magn Reson. 2010;12:44.
360. Thomson LE, Crowley AL, Heitner JF, Cawley PJ, Weinsaft JW, Kim HW, et al. Direct en face imaging of secundum atrial septal defects by velocity-encoded cardiovascular magnetic resonance in patients evaluated for possible transcatheter closure. Circ Cardiovasc Imaging. 2008;1(1):31–40.
361. Weber C, Weber M, Ekinci O, Neumann T, Deetjen A, Rolf A, et al. Atrial septal defects type II: noninvasive evaluation of patients before implantation of an Amplatzer Septal Occluder and on follow-up by magnetic resonance imaging compared with TEE and invasive measurement. Eur Radiol. 2008;18(11):2406–13.
362. Riesenkampff EM, Schmitt B, Schnackenburg B, Huebler M, Alexi-Meskishvili V, Hetzer R, et al. Partial anomalous pulmonary venous drainage in young pediatric patients: the role of magnetic resonance imaging. Pediatr Cardiol. 2009;30(4):458–64.
363. Ferrari VA, Scott CH, Holland GA, Axel L, Sutton MS. Ultrafast three-dimensional contrast-enhanced magnetic resonance angiography and imaging in the diagnosis of partial anomalous pulmonary venous drainage. J Am Coll Cardiol. 2001;37(4):1120–8.
364. Tada N, Takizawa K, Mizutani Y, Suzuki S, Sakurai M, Arai T, et al. Multiple atrial septal defects in multidetector-row computed tomography. JACC Cardiovasc Interv. 2014;7(6):e61–2.
365. Kivisto S, Hanninen H, Holmstrom M. Partial anomalous pulmonary venous return and atrial septal defect in adult patients detected with 128-slice multidetector computed tomography. J Cardiothorac Surg. 2011;6:126.
366. Amat F, Le Bret E, Sigal-Cinqualbre A, Coblence M, Lambert V, Rohnean A, et al. Diagnostic accuracy of multidetector spiral computed tomography for preoperative assessment of sinus venosus atrial septal defects in children. Interact Cardiovasc Thorac Surg. 2011;12(2):179–82.
367. Berbarie RF, Anwar A, Dockery WD, Grayburn PA, Hamman BL, Vallabhan RC, et al. Measurement of right ventricular volumes before and after atrial septal defect closure using multislice computed tomography. Am J Cardiol. 2007;99(10):1458–61.
368. Marini D, Ou P, Boudjemline Y, Kenny D, Bonnet D, Agnoletti G. Midterm results of percutaneous closure of very large atrial septal defects in children: role of multislice computed tomography. EuroIntervention. 2012;7(12):1428–34.
369. Artis NJ, Thomson J, Plein S, Greenwood JP. Percutaneous closure of postinfarction ventricular septal defect: cardiac magnetic resonance-guided case selection and postprocedure evaluation. Can J Cardiol. 2011;27(6):869.e3–5.
370. Ratnayaka K, Raman VK, Faranesh AZ, Sonmez M, Kim JH, Gutierrez LF, et al. Antegrade percutaneous closure of membranous ventricular septal defect using X-ray fused with magnetic resonance imaging. JACC Cardiovasc Interv. 2009;2(3):224–30.
371. Calkoen EE, Westenberg JJ, Kroft LJ, Blom NA, Hazekamp MG, Rijlaarsdam ME, et al. Characterization and quantification of dynamic eccentric regurgitation of the left atrioventricular valve after atrioventricular septal defect correction with 4D Flow cardiovascular magnetic resonance and retrospective valve tracking. J Cardiovasc Magn Reson Off J Soc Cardiovasc Magn Reson. 2015;17:18.
372. Schueler R, Sinning JM, Zimmer S, Nickenig G, Hammerstingl C. Multimodality imaging for interventional planning and device closure of an atypical ventricular septal defect occurring late after myocardial infarction. Eur Heart J. 2014;35(15):1007.
373. Grizzard JD, Ang GB. Magnetic resonance imaging of pericardial disease and cardiac masses. Magn Reson Imaging Clin N Am. 2007;15(4):579–607, vi.
374. Hoffmann U, Globits S, Schima W, Loewe C, Puig S, Oberhuber G, et al. Usefulness of magnetic resonance imaging of cardiac and paracardiac masses. Am J Cardiol. 2003;92(7):890–5.
375. Brechtel K, Reddy GP, Higgins CB. Cardiac fibroma in an infant: magnetic resonance imaging characteristics. J Cardiovasc Magn Reson Off J Soc Cardiovasc Magn Reson. 1999;1(2):159–61.
376. Kamiya H, Ohno M, Iwata H, Ohsugi S, Sawada K, Koike A, et al. Cardiac lipoma in the interventricular septum: evaluation by computed tomography and magnetic resonance imaging. Am Heart J. 1990;119(5):1215–7.

377. Salanitri JC, Pereles FS. Cardiac lipoma and lipomatous hypertrophy of the interatrial septum: cardiac magnetic resonance imaging findings. J Comput Assist Tomogr. 2004;28(6):852–6.
378. Matsuoka H, Hamada M, Honda T, Kawakami H, Abe M, Shigematsu Y, et al. Morphologic and histologic characterization of cardiac myxomas by magnetic resonance imaging. Angiology. 1996;47(7):693–8.
379. Watanabe AT, Teitelbaum GP, Henderson RW, Bradley Jr WG. Magnetic resonance imaging of cardiac sarcomas. J Thorac Imaging. 1989;4(2):90–2.
380. Inoko M, Iga K, Kyo K, Kondo H, Tamura T, Izumi C, et al. Primary cardiac angiosarcoma detected by magnetic resonance imaging but not by computed tomography. Intern Med. 2001;40(5):391–5.
381. Tahara T, Takase B, Yamagishi T, Takayama E, Miyazaki K, Arakawa K, et al. A case report on primary cardiac non-Hodgkin's lymphoma: an approach by magnetic resonance and thallium-201 imaging. J Cardiovasc Magn Reson Off J Soc Cardiovasc Magn Reson. 1999;1(2):163–7.
382. Schrem SS, Colvin SB, Weinreb JC, Glassman E, Kronzon I. Metastatic cardiac liposarcoma: diagnosis by transesophageal echocardiography and magnetic resonance imaging. J Am Soc Echocardiography Off Publ Am Soc Echocardiography. 1990;3(2):149–53.
383. Mousseaux E, Meunier P, Azancott S, Dubayle P, Gaux JC. Cardiac metastatic melanoma investigated by magnetic resonance imaging. Magn Reson Imaging. 1998;16(1):91–5.
384. Testempassi E, Takeuchi H, Fukuda Y, Harada J, Tada S. Cardiac metastasis of colon adenocarcinoma diagnosed by magnetic resonance imaging. Acta Cardiol. 1994;49(2):191–6.
385. Weinsaft JW, Kim HW, Shah DJ, Klem I, Crowley AL, Brosnan R, et al. Detection of left ventricular thrombus by delayed-enhancement cardiovascular magnetic resonance prevalence and markers in patients with systolic dysfunction. J Am Coll Cardiol. 2008;52(2):148–57.
386. Gaudio C, Di Michele S, Cera M, Nguyen BL, Pannarale G, Alessandri N. Prominent crista terminalis mimicking a right atrial mixoma: cardiac magnetic resonance aspects. Eur Rev Med Pharmacol Sci. 2004;8(4):165–8.
387. Hong YJ, Hur J, Kim YJ, Lee HJ, Nam JE, Kim HY, et al. The usefulness of delayed contrast-enhanced cardiovascular magnetic resonance imaging in differentiating cardiac tumors from thrombi in stroke patients. Int J Cardiovasc Imaging. 2011;27 Suppl 1:89–95.
388. Beroukhim RS, Prakash A, Buechel ER, Cava JR, Dorfman AL, Festa P, et al. Characterization of cardiac tumors in children by cardiovascular magnetic resonance imaging: a multicenter experience. J Am Coll Cardiol. 2011;58(10):1044–54.
389. Rajiah P, Kanne JP, Kalahasti V, Schoenhagen P. Computed tomography of cardiac and pericardiac masses. J Cardiovasc Comput Tomogr. 2011;5(1):16–29.
390. Klein AL, Abbara S, Agler DA, Appleton CP, Asher CR, Hoit B, et al. American Society of Echocardiography clinical recommendations for multimodality cardiovascular imaging of patients with pericardial disease: endorsed by the Society for Cardiovascular Magnetic Resonance and Society of Cardiovascular Computed Tomography. J Am Soc Echocardiography Off Publ Am Soc Echocardiography. 2013;26(9):965–1012.e15.
391. Bogaert J, Francone M. Cardiovascular magnetic resonance in pericardial diseases. J Cardiovasc Magn Reson Off J Soc Cardiovasc Magn Reson. 2009;11:14.
392. Taylor AM, Dymarkowski S, Verbeken EK, Bogaert J. Detection of pericardial inflammation with late-enhancement cardiac magnetic resonance imaging: initial results. Eur Radiol. 2006;16(3):569–74.
393. Rifkin RD, Mernoff DB. Noninvasive evaluation of pericardial effusion composition by computed tomography. Am Heart J. 2005;149(6):1120–7.
394. Muzzarelli S, Meadows AK, Ordovas KG, Higgins CB, Meadows JJ. Usefulness of cardiovascular magnetic resonance imaging to predict the need for intervention in patients with coarctation of the aorta. Am J Cardiol. 2012;109(6):861–5.
395. Dormand H, Mohiaddin RH. Cardiovascular magnetic resonance in Marfan syndrome. J Cardiovasc Magn Reson Off J Soc Cardiovasc Magn Reson. 2013;15:33.
396. Hartnell GG. Imaging of aortic aneurysms and dissection: CT and MRI. J Thorac Imaging. 2001;16(1):35–46.
397. Cantisani V, Ricci P, Grazhdani H, Napoli A, Fanelli F, Catalano C, et al. Prospective comparative analysis of colour-Doppler ultrasound, contrast-enhanced ultrasound, computed tomography and magnetic resonance in detecting endoleak after endovascular abdominal aortic aneurysm repair. Eur J Vasc Endovasc Surg Off J Eur Soc Vasc Surg. 2011;41(2):186–92.
398. Dudeck O, Schnapauff D, Herzog L, Lowenthal D, Bulla K, Bulla B, et al. Can early computed tomography angiography after endovascular aortic aneurysm repair predict the need for reintervention in patients with type II endoleak? Cardiovasc Intervent Radiol. 2015;38(1):45–52.
399. Muller-Wille R, Borgmann T, Wohlgemuth WA, Zeman F, Pfister K, Jung EM, et al. Dual-energy computed tomography after endovascular aortic aneurysm repair: the role of hard plaque imaging for endoleak detection. Eur Radiol. 2014;24(10):2449–57.

Cardiovascular CT in the Emergency Department

27

Asim Rizvi and James K. Min

Abstract

Acute-onset chest pain is one of the most common presentations in the emergency department (ED) and despite a thorough, time intensive, and costly ED evaluation utilizing the standard strategy, there is a non-negligible clinical risk of missed acute coronary syndrome (ACS) with 2–5 % of these patients being discharged inappropriately. The resultant consequences are, increased risk of short and long term mortality. This chapter discusses the current role of cardiac computed tomography in the evaluation of patients with acute chest pain in the ED and evaluates the current evidence supporting accuracy and safety of cardiac computed tomography, as well as it's ability to reduce ED cost.

Keywords

Acute coronary syndrome • Cardiac • Chest pain • Emergency department • Coronary computed tomography angiography

Current State of the Literature

Acute chest pain is one of the most frequent reasons for patient visits to the emergency department (ED) in the United States and a large amount of expense and time is spent in the workup of these patients. It is estimated that as many as 6 million people per year visit the ED with chest pain [1]; however, only a small minority of these patients ultimately receive a diagnosis of acute coronary syndrome (ACS) as the etiology of their chest pain [2]. Although most of these patients do not have a life-threatening underlying condition, a large proportion of these patients undergo routine evaluation of acute chest pain that includes hospital admission or observation unit stay to rule out ACS with the use of serial electrocardiography (ECG) and cardiac biomarker assessment. Such an approach is costly, time-consuming and puts additional strain on already limited resources.

A. Rizvi, MD • J.K. Min, MD, FACC (✉)
Dalio Institute of Cardiovascular Imaging,
NewYork-Presbyterian Hospital and Weill Cornell Medical College,
413 E. 69th Street Suite 108, New York, NY 10021, USA
e-mail: jkm2001@med.cornell.edu

Diagnosis of ACS

The term ACS describes clinical manifestations of acute myocardial ischemia induced by coronary artery disease (CAD). The American Heart Association (AHA) differentiates among ACS that involve myocardial infarction (MI) with acute ST segment elevation (STEMI), MI without ST segment elevation (non-STEMI), and unstable angina (UA) [3–5]. The diagnosis of STEMI is clear by ECG alone, but diagnosis of non-STEMI and UA is more challenging and requires additional data to risk stratify patients appropriately [6]. The third universal definition of MI, published in 2012, states that the diagnostic criteria for MI require a rise and/or fall of cardiac biomarkers (preferably troponins) with at least one value above the 99th percentile of the upper reference limit. In addition, patient should have symptoms of ischemia with new ECG changes and imaging evidence of a new loss of viable myocardium or new regional wall motion

M.J. Budoff, J.S. Shinbane (eds.), *Cardiac CT Imaging: Diagnosis of Cardiovascular Disease*,
DOI 10.1007/978-3-319-28219-0_27

abnormality, or the identification of an intracoronary thrombus by angiography or autopsy [7]. However, the initial standard ED evaluation of patients with acute chest pain [8] does not often provide a firm diagnosis for appropriate triage decision and to safely rule out ACS based on negative cardiac troponin and ECG.

Risk Assessment in the Emergency Department

Patients with acute chest pain are generally stratified into high, intermediate, or low risk categories during their early clinical assessment in the ED. This risk assessment work-up traditionally includes patient's history of prior cardiovascular events, repeated physical examinations, and serial electrocardiographic and biochemical marker measurements [9–11]. Patients who are at high-risk of ACS or have STEMI based on ECG findings should be admitted and treated promptly as per guidelines [8]. Patients who are at low to intermediate risk carry a 5–20 % risk of an ACS and the current standard of care for these patients includes serial ECG and cardiac troponin measurements followed by stress testing with or without imaging to exclude myocardial ischemia [8]. This approach leads to prolonged hospital stay and significant cost burden and eventually only 2–8 % of this patient group is diagnosed with ACS [12].

Multiple risk stratification models based upon multivariable regression techniques have been created in order to help clinicians in therapeutic decision making and includes the Thrombolysis in Myocardial Infarction (TIMI) risk score, Global Registry of Acute Coronary Events (GRACE) risk score, and the Platelet Glycoprotein IIb/IIIa in Unstable Angina: Receptor Suppression Using Integrillin Therapy (PURSUIT) risk model [13–15]. The TIMI risk score is a simple and easily applied scoring system that has been validated for patients who present to the ED, and aids in assessing the likelihood of developing an adverse cardiac outcome (death, reinfarction, or recurrent severe ischemia requiring revascularization) within 14 days of presentation in patients presenting with UA and NSTEMI [14].

Despite these clinical risk scores, uncertainty often exists as to the etiology of a patient's symptoms and the potential adverse prognosis associated with them. This uncertainty emphasizes the need for diagnostic strategies that facilitate rapid and reliable early triage of patients who are at low-to-intermediate risk for ACS [16].

Supporting Evidence for Cardiac CT Use in the Emergency Department

With improvements in imaging capabilities, coronary computed tomography angiography (CCTA) has emerged as a new and promising imaging modality for the detection and assessment of coronary stenosis and atherosclerotic plaque, and has become integral in the assessment of patients with suspected ACS. Several single-center and multicenter studies have demonstrated the feasibility, safety, and accuracy of cardiac CT in the ED to exclude the presence of CAD [9, 17–30]. Most patients with ACS have significant coronary stenosis, and ACS is rare in the absence of coronary atherosclerosis [31, 32]. Therefore, the detection of obstructive CAD may be effective in identifying patients with ACS and the exclusion of coronary atherosclerosis may be helpful in ruling out ACS.

Given the excellent predictive value, CCTA allows for improved risk stratification of patients and appropriate triage, and can be considered an alternative to standard ED evaluation of acute chest pain patients. Furthermore, CCTA has been shown to reduce length of stay in the hospital. A meta-analysis comparing CCTA to standard care triage of acute chest pain in a total of 3266 low-to intermediate risk patients presenting to the ED noted that only 1.3 % overall MIs occurred mostly during the index hospitalization. In addition, length of stay in the hospital was significantly reduced with CCTA compared to standard care strategy. It was also found that CCTA significantly increased invasive coronary angiography (8.4 % versus 6.3 %) and revascularization (4.6 % versus 2.6 %). This meta-analysis included three major multicenter trials, CT-STAT [28], ACRIN-PA [30], and ROMICAT II [29], which have been pivotal in demonstrating the safe use of CCTA for early triage of patients in the ED [33]. In each of these trials, patients with no ECG changes and a negative initial troponin were randomized to either CCTA or standard treatment with serial cardiac markers and ECGs.

The CT-STAT (Coronary Computed Tomographic Angiography for Systematic Triage of Acute Chest Pain Patients to Treatment) is a multicenter trial of low risk ED patients that prospectively included 699 patients who were either randomly allocated to CCTA (n =361) versus myocardial perfusion imaging (MPI) (n=338). The investigators sought to compare the efficiency, cost, and safety of using CCTA in the evaluation of patients with acute chest pain and low risk of ACS [28]. The primary outcome of the study was time to diagnosis. The investigators also showed a cost reduction in patients randomized to CCTA. Those in the CCTA arm had a 54 % reduction in time to diagnosis and 38 % reduction in costs. There was no difference in major adverse cardiac events (MACE) between the two study groups [28].

The ACRIN-PA (American College of Radiology Imaging Network- Pennsylvania) multicenter trial was designed to evaluate the safety of CCTA strategy, defined as the absence of MI or cardiac death during 30-day follow-up, in low-to-intermediate risk patients in the ED [30]. This trial included 1370 patients randomized in a 2:1 ratio to CCTA versus standard of care. The trial concluded that utilization of CCTA early in the ED was safe and of the 640 patients with negative CCTA examinations, none of them died or had a myocardial infarction within 30 days of presentation. They also found that early CCTA led to a shorter mean hospital stay (18 versus 24.8 h) and subsequently more frequent ED discharge when compared to standard of care (50 % versus 23 %) [30].

The ROMICAT II (Rule Out Myocardial Infarction Using Computer Assisted Tomography) trial is a multicenter comparative effectiveness trial that randomized patients to early implementation of CCTA versus standard ED evaluation in 1000 low-to-intermediate risk patients recruited from nine centers in the United States with suspected ACS [29]. The primary endpoint was length of stay. Approximately 8 % of the study patients developed ACS. The study showed that early CCTA utilization decreased the mean length of stay in the hospital by 7.6 h compared to standard ED evaluation and patients were more often discharged directly from the ED (47 vs. 12 %). Additionally, there were no missed cardiac events within 72 h, making CCTA a viable alternative for low-intermediate risk patients in the ED. However, increased diagnostic testing and higher radiation exposure was observed in the CCTA group. While there was a reduction in ED costs with an early CCTA strategy, there was no overall reduction in the cost of care during index hospitalization or 28-day follow-up [29].

In aggregate, these studies support the use of CCTA as an efficient and safe alternative to the more traditional triaging methods for low and low-to-intermediate risk patients as an option to exclude obstructive CAD as the etiology of chest pain, while allowing for a faster ED discharge and ED cost savings. However, such use of CCTA has been associated with increases in downstream invasive coronary angiography (ICA) and coronary revascularization, and the benefit of this approach requires further study.

Appropriate Use and Guidelines

The use of CCTA in patients presenting to the ED with acute chest pain and low-to-intermediate risk of ACS is supported by the current literature, as previously discussed. The Society of Cardiovascular Computed Tomography (SCCT) has recently published guidelines for the use of CCTA in the diagnosis of acute chest pain in patients with suspected ACS in the ED [34]. A summary of these guidelines is presented in Tables 27.1 and 27.2.

The ACCF/SCCT/ACR/AHA/ASE/ASNC/NASCI/SCAI/SCMR 2010 Appropriate Use Criteria for Cardiac Computed Tomography lists the use of CCTA as appropriate for "detection of CAD in symptomatic patients without known heart disease—acute symptoms with suspicion of ACS (urgent presentation) (Appropriate, score 7)" in patients with the following [35]:

- Normal ECG and cardiac biomarkers and low pretest probability of CAD
- Normal ECG and cardiac biomarkers and intermediate pretest probability of CAD
- ECG uninterpretable and low pretest probability of CAD
- ECG uninterpretable and intermediate pretest probability of CAD
- Non-diagnostic ECG or equivocal cardiac biomarkers and low pretest probability of CAD
- Non-diagnostic ECG or equivocal cardiac biomarkers and intermediate pretest probability of CAD

Evolution of Coronary CT Angiography Technology

Since the introduction of CT as a tool for medical imaging, there has been a desire to apply this technology for imaging of the heart. Electron-beam CT (EBCT) had been proposed earlier to the introduction of multi-detector row CT (MDCT) scanners, for the evaluation of patients arriving in the ED with acute chest pain. EBCT had better temporal but inferior spatial resolution as compared to MDCT, and this approach relied on the total coronary calcium score, called the Agatston score [36] as a measure of overall plaque burden, and showed high sensitivity but low specificity for the detection of obstructive CAD. Technologic development continued to 16-detector row and subsequently the 64-detector row MDCT scanners in 2002 and 2005, respectively, which were used to obtain ECG-synchronized images of the heart at high spatial and temporal resolution [37], to quantify coronary artery calcium [38], and to detect coronary artery stenosis [37, 39]. These scanners were capable of image acquisition with high spatial resolution (0.5–0.8 mm isotropic resolution), high temporal resolution (350–400 ms), and sufficient Z-axis coverage (20–40 mm). Scan times with these scanners were less than 10 s when only the heart is evaluated and less than 20 s when the entire thorax is imaged with ECG synchronization. The field of CCTA has continued to improve since 2005 with the introduction of MDCT scanners capable of even greater spatial resolution (up to 0.23 mm in-plane resolution), higher temporal resolution (via dual-source and high-pitch helical technology), and increased volume coverage (through 256- or 320-detector arrays). Broader 256- or 320- detector arrays allow complete volume coverage of the heart in a single heartbeat, thus reducing limitations concerning arrhythmia, and high and variable heart rates [37, 38, 40].

Table 27.1 Society of cardiovascular computed tomography (SCCT) guidelines on the use of CCTA for patients presenting with acute chest pain in the ED [34]

I. **Site Requirements**
Equipment
Required equipment:
≥64 detector rows scanner that is equipped with coronary artery-specific capabilities Advanced cardiac life support (ACLS) equipment to be present in the patient preparation and scanner areas Image interpretation platforms with three-dimensional post-processing software Prior year CCTA, with a minimum volume of 300 scans per year CT laboratory accreditation
Recommended equipment:
Scanner that is equipped to perform prospectively triggered axial scanning protocols in appropriate patients should be available for radiation dose reduction
Quality assurance program goals:
Achieving a diagnostic-quality scan rate of ≥95 % Quarterly median radiation dose rate within target reference level, established by the SCCT guidelines on radiation dose and dose-optimization strategies in cardiovascular CT Quarterly review of CCTA interpretation compared with invasive angiography, achieving at least 75 % per-patient accuracy
Staffing requirements:
At least one technologist is required with prior volume experience of at least 100 CCTA scans Current ACLS certification is required for technologists performing scans without the immediate proximity of an ACLS-certified nurse For beta-blocker premedication of patients, properly trained ACLS-certified nursing staff is required For prompt response to urgent or emergent complications, rapid response team and/or ACLS-certified physician must be available Scanner operation and availability, and staffing-service hours must satisfy ED minimum requirements
II. Interpreting Physician Requirements
Requirements:
At least one physician with a minimum of 2 years of clinical experience and/or at least 300 prior CCTA scan interpretations All other interpreting physicians must attain and maintain level-2 or the equivalent CCTA certification Interpreting physicians must be promptly available in person or by phone for consultation about patient preparation and scan protocol Interpreting physicians must be trained in the best-practice protocol selection of the scanners in use A qualified physician must interpret all non-cardiac anatomy on all scans
Recommendations:
Certification Board of Cardiovascular Computed Tomography certification or American College of Radiology Board certification or dedicated fellowship training in advanced cardiac imaging
III. Patient Selection
Appropriate indications:
Patients with acute chest pain with clinically suspected coronary ischemia ECG negative or indeterminate for myocardial ischemia Low to intermediate pretest likelihood by risk stratification tools (e.g., Thrombolysis in Myocardial Infarction [TIMI] grade of low [0–2] or intermediate [3–4]) Equivocal or inadequate previous functional testing during index ED hospitalization or within the previous 6 months
Uncertain indications:
High clinical likelihood of ACS by clinical assessment and standard risk criteria (e.g., TIMI grade >4) Previously known CAD (prior myocardial infarction, prior ischemia, prior revascularization, coronary artery calcium score >400)
Relative contraindications:

In case of history of allergic reaction to iodinated contrast without history of anaphylaxis or allergic reaction after adequate steroid/antihistamine preparation, alternative testing should be preferred
Glomerular filtration rate (GFR) <60
Previous substantial volume of contrast within 24 h
Factors leading to potentially non-diagnostic scans (vary with scanner technology and site capabilities)
  Heart rate is greater than the site maximum for reliable diagnostic scans after beta-blockers
  Contraindications to beta-blockers and inadequate heart rate control
  Atrial fibrillation or other markedly irregular rhythm
  Body mass index >39 kg/m^2

Absolute contraindications:
ACS: definite GFR <30 unless on chronic dialysis or evidence of acute tubular necrosis Previous anaphylaxis after iodinated contrast administration Previous episode of contrast allergy after adequate steroid/antihistamine preparation Inability to cooperate, including inability to raise arms Pregnancy or uncertain pregnancy status in premenopausal women

Patient preparation, scan protocol, and reporting should follow the SCCT guidelines. In addition, interpretation of the CCTA should be tailored according to the needs of the ED

Table 27.2 An example of management recommendations [34]

Sample management recommendations to emergency department physicians
Stenosis 0–25 % (ACS unlikely): Reasonable to discharge the patient Follow-up at physician's discretion
Stenosis 26–49 % (ACS unlikely): Reasonable to discharge the patient Outpatient follow-up is recommended for preventive measures
Stenosis 50–69 % (ACS possible): Further evaluation of the patient is indicated before discharge
Stenosis >70 % (ACS likely): Admit the patient for further evaluation

Coronary Artery Calcium Quantification

Prior to discussion of CCTA in the evaluation of acute chest pain patients presenting to the ED, the role of non-contrast coronary artery calcium (CAC) scanning is worthy to mention. CAC scan is relatively cheaper and faster to conduct and interpret. Due to the strong correlation of CAC to overall coronary artery atherosclerotic disease burden, there has been interest to use CAC scan in low-to-intermediate risk patients and to exclude CAD in patients with CAC score of zero. An American College of Cardiology Foundation/American Heart Association consensus statement endorsed the use of CAC testing for low-risk symptomatic patients as a "filter" for further cardiovascular testing. It is recommended that CAC scoring may be used in a binary fashion such that CAC of zero excludes CAD and no further testing is performed as compared to CAC >0, for which additional functional stress testing for obstructive CAD can be considered [41].

In contrast, a recent analysis from the CONFIRM registry demonstrated that CCTA findings were superior to CAC scoring for adverse cardiovascular outcomes in 10,037 low-to-intermediate risk patients, albeit stable rather than acute in presentation, undergoing both CAC and CCTA. CCTA occasionally demonstrated significant luminal stenosis of ≥50 % in patients with zero CAC score (3.5 % incidence). The investigators concluded that in symptomatic patients with a CAC score of 0, obstructive CAD is possible and is associated with increased cardiovascular events [42].

The major disadvantage of CAC scan is the inability to visualize non-calcified plaque, which may be present in a large proportion of patients. Moreover, non-calcified plaque carries with it important prognostic value that can be readily assessed by CCTA but not by CAC scan. Therefore, CAC scan is not widely considered a first-line test because of its inability to rule out stenosis by non-calcified plaque and low specificity for obstructive CAD, and CCTA may be a preferable option for most patients with acute chest pain.

Detection of Coronary Plaque by CCTA

CCTA is a contrast-enhanced CT scan used for non-invasive evaluation of the coronary arteries. The prognostic value and cost-effectiveness of CCTA have been described by many studies [43–55]. As opposed to non-contrast coronary calcium scoring, contrast-enhanced CCTA can identify calcified, non-calcified, and partially calcified (calcified and non-calcified) lesions of the coronary arteries. There is supporting evidence that the manual quantification of the coronary plaque volumes by CCTA for non-calcified and partially calcified plaques correlate closely with invasive intravascular ultrasound [56–59]. The detection of non-calcified plaque is more challenging compared to calcified plaque detection, and optimal image quality is required that can be achievable by using 64-slice scanners.

Beyond high-grade coronary stenoses, specific coronary plaque features are linked with ACS and other adverse cardiovascular events. Studies have shown that potentially vulnerable plaques have distinct features that include large plaque volume, large necrotic core size, attenuated fibrous caps, and positive arterial remodeling (growth of atherosclerotic plaque into the vessel wall rather than the vessel lumen) [60, 61]. Furthermore, the presence of "spotty" plaque calcifications has been associated with acute MI. CCTA can assess some of these "adverse" features of potentially vulnerable plaques [62]. Therefore, CCTA assessment of plaque may prove prognostically useful when including identification of adverse plaque features. The "adverse" plaque features associated with ACS and other adverse cardiovascular events to date include low attenuation plaque, positive remodeling, spotty calcifications, and the "napkin-ring sign". Studies have demonstrated the characteristics of coronary plaque in patients presenting with ACS [63–66]. Patients with ACS had greater portions of non-calcified plaque, had larger plaque volumes, presented more often with "spotty" calcifications, and included plaques with greater positive remodeling and lower CT attenuation than patients with stable angina [63, 64, 66]. Furthermore, the presence of a napkin-ring sign has also been shown to be a sign of high-risk coronary plaque [64, 67, 68].

Beyond these plaque features that require generally arduous measurements, prior investigations have also shown that major adverse cardiac events (MACE) were associated with more easily identifiable characteristics, including a higher amount of non-calcified plaque in non-obstructive CAD. Conversely, the amount of calcified plaque was not significantly associated with an increased risk for MACE [51].

Non-coronary CCTA Findings

A multitude of additional information proffered by CCTA may be of benefit in the acute and long-term assessment of the ED patients. This includes evaluation of non-coronary cardiac findings, including left ventricle volume and ejection fraction; left ventricular mass; right heart dimensions and function; and great vessel pathology; as well as non-cardiac thoracic pathology of a patient's chest pain [69–75]. Furthermore, identification of pulmonary nodules as a non-cardiac incidental finding can improve follow-up related to potentially adverse findings [76–79].

The assessment of non-cardiac thoracic pathology by utilizing CCTA may include aortic dissection, pulmonary embolism, pneumonia, pericardial disease, abscesses, effusions, and cancer [45, 80, 81]. In this regard, some investigators have considered whether acute chest pain needs to be evaluated with a "triple rule-out" protocol which effectively increases the Z-axis coverage of the CT scan, and allows for exclusion of ACS, aortic dissection, and pulmonary embolus in a single scan; but there is no clear clinical benefit to this extended approach which has the disadvantage of significantly increased radiation dose, higher imaging costs, and longer interpretation and reporting time. Thus, routine use of a "triple rule-out" protocol is not currently recommended [34].

Diagnostic Accuracy of CCTA

Prospective multicenter diagnostic performance have demonstrated the ability of CCTA to accurately detect coronary stenosis when compared to invasive coronary angiography (ICA) as a reference standard. In the ACCURACY (Assessment by Coronary Computed Tomographic Angiography of Individuals Undergoing Invasive Coronary Angiography) trial [18], 230 patients underwent both CCTA and ICA for non-emergent typical or atypical chest pain. The study investigators demonstrated CCTA to have a sensitivity of 95 %, specificity of 83 %, positive predictive value of 64 %, and negative predictive value of 99 % for prediction of obstructive CAD with >50 % stenosis by ICA. The high negative predictive value of 99 % at both the patient and the vessel level demonstrated that cardiac CT is an effective non-invasive alternative to ICA to rule out obstructive CAD [18]. Furthermore, a meta-analysis of 40 ACCURACY studies concluded that in comparison with ICA, the sensitivity and specificity of CCTA to detect ≥50 % stenosis were 99 % and 89 %, respectively at per patient level, and 90 % and 97 %, respectively at per segment level [82]. Particularly germane to the topic at hand, CCTA in low-to-intermediate risk patients suspected to have ACS retains its very high sensitivity (92 %) and negative predictive value (99 %), with MACE at 30 days, 6 months, or at 1 year equal to zero or minimal in patients who were discharged with a normal CCTA or when CCTA demonstrated mild non-obstructive disease [25, 26, 83].

The ability of CCTA to rapidly exclude obstructive CAD among ED patients helps in identifying patients who can be safely and rapidly discharged from the ED relative to standard of care [33, 84]. The American College of Cardiology (ACC)/ American Heart Association (AHA) guidelines have incorporated CCTA among current noninvasive tests for use in low-to-intermediate risk patients with suspected ACS. However, current literature still lacks a standardized approach to guide ED patient management based on cardiac CT findings.

Radiation Risk

Although CCTA has evolved as a useful diagnostic imaging modality in the assessment of CAD, the potential risks due to ionizing radiation exposure associated with CCTA have raised concerns, particularly with regard to potential long-term risks of radiation-induced malignancy, and has led to the "As Low As Reasonably Achievable (ALARA)" principle of radiation protection [85]. In spite of the fact that the increased risk of malignancy from CCTA remains controversial, the ALARA principle prevails in clinical practice. The clinical usefulness of CCTA for the rapid evaluation of chest pain in the ED must be weighed against the radiation exposure. Improvements in CCTA technology, including prospective ECG triggering, tube voltage reduction to 100 kV or less in non-obese patients, use of iterative image reconstruction, and high-pitch helical acquisition, have allowed for substantial reduction of radiation doses by CCTA to <1 mSv. These 1 mSv scans, though theoretically attractive, are still not routine due to certain challenges such as higher heart rates and arrhythmias, and large body habitus.

Indications

The use of cardiac CT to rule out ACS, especially in low-to-intermediate risk patients, is supported by the recent SCCT guidelines [34], which recommends CCTA in the setting of acute chest pain in patients with low-to-intermediate likelihood of ACS with negative initial electrocardiographic and biochemical markers, and TIMI grade ≤4. The indications according to these guidelines are as follows [34]:

Appropriate Indications

- Patients with acute chest pain with clinically suspected coronary ischemia
- ECG negative or indeterminate for myocardial ischemia
- Low-to-intermediate pretest likelihood by risk stratification tools (e.g., TIMI grade of low [0–2] or intermediate [3–4])
- Equivocal or inadequate previous functional testing during index ED hospitalization or within the previous 6 months

Uncertain Indications

- High clinical likelihood of ACS by clinical assessment and standard risk criteria (e.g., TIMI grade >4)
- Previously known CAD (prior MI, prior ischemia, prior revascularization, coronary artery calcium score >400)

Moreover, the ACCF/SCCT/ACR/AHA/ASE/ASNC/NASCI/SCAI/SCMR 2010 Appropriate Use Criteria for Cardiac Computed Tomography lists the use of CCTA as appropriate for "detection of CAD in symptomatic patients without known heart disease—acute symptoms with suspicion of ACS (urgent presentation) (Appropriate, score 7)" [35], as previously discussed.

Contraindications

CCTA is contraindicated in patients with severe renal impairment because of the high risk of contrast-induced nephropathy (CIN). In addition, pregnancy is a contraindication due to radiation exposure. Prior contrast reactions are a relative contraindication; such patients can frequently be pre-treated with the use of a steroid and anti-histamine medications one day prior to the CT examination. The absolute and relative contraindications to CCTA according to SCCT recently published guidelines include the following [34]:

Absolute Contraindications

- ACS: definite
- GFR <30 unless on chronic dialysis or evidence of acute tubular necrosis
- Previous anaphylaxis after iodinated contrast administration
- Previous episode of contrast allergy after adequate steroid/antihistamine preparation
- Inability to cooperate, including inability to raise arms
- Pregnancy or uncertain pregnancy status in premenopausal women

Relative Contraindications

- Alternative testing should be preferred in these cases: history of allergic reaction to iodinated contrast without history of anaphylaxis or allergic reaction after adequate steroid/antihistamine preparation
- Glomerular filtration rate (GFR) <60
- Previous substantial volume of contrast within 24 h (this will vary with the GFR)
- Factors leading to potentially nondiagnostic scans (vary with scanner technology and site capabilities)
  - Heart rate is greater than the site maximum for reliable diagnostic scans after beta-blockers
  - Contraindications to beta-blockers and inadequate heart rate control
  - Atrial fibrillation or other markedly irregular rhythm
  - Body mass index >39 kg/m^2

Summary of Strengths

CCTA is unique from prior forms of imaging in that it does not require stress provocation to determine burden of CAD. Multiple single-center and multicenter trials have established CCTA as a noninvasive diagnostic test with excellent sensitivity (97.2 %) and good specificity (87.4 %) for the detection of obstructive CAD with >50 % stenosis [17, 18]. The major strength of CCTA is its high negative predictive value for stenosis (99 %). In addition, CCTA is highly sensitive (90 %) and specific (92 %) for the detection of calcified and non-calcified coronary atherosclerotic plaque [57, 59, 86].

Summary of Limitations

A significant limitation of the CCTA is its lower specificity that may be attributable to a spatial resolution of about 0.5 mm. This non-ideal specificity of CCTA is concerning and could lead to increased downstream testing and, possibly, ICA with revascularization, thus warranting further improvements in CCTA technology. Another important limitation is that patients with extensive coronary calcification may have non-diagnostic scans because of calcium "blooming" and "beam hardening" artifacts. Cardiac dysrhythmias and inadequate heart rate control during imaging are other factors leading to sub-optimal scans for diagnostic purposes.

Moreover, assessment of CAD by cardiac CT requires ionizing radiation exposure and administration of contrast dye, compared to other modalities (e.g., exercise treadmill, rest echocardiography, exercise or pharmacologic stress echocardiography, rest or stress cardiac magnetic resonance imaging). Patients with significant contrast dye allergies or renal insufficiency are not candidates for CCTA. Morbid obesity can compromise image quality and thus reduce diagnostic accuracy or require higher doses of radiation. Higher heart rates and arrhythmias can cause misregistration artifacts, leading to poor visualization of the coronary arteries.

Future Directions

Chest pain is so commonly encountered in the practice of medicine and future advancements in CCTA technology are expected to improve the overall accuracy of CT-determined stenosis in comparison with reference standard fractional flow reserve (FFR) measurements during ICA. Currently, investigators are interested in changing the face of how ACS is diagnosed and managed by improving the specificity of qualitative determination of coronary stenosis by fractional flow reserve derived from CT, or FFR_{CT}, a novel non-invasive method that applies computational fluid dynamics for the calculation of FFR from typically acquired CCTA studies. This technique has been demonstrated to have higher diagnostic performance for ischemia-causing lesions than any other functional imaging method [87]. Importantly, given its ability to obviate the requirement for use of adenosine or for additional scanning, this technique offers the added safety to not require increased radiation doses. In the future, it is expected that the maturation of dual-energy CT may further improves stenosis assessment and diagnostic accuracy in patients with heavy coronary calcifications, and may allow for further radiation reduction. In aggregate, noninvasive coronary imaging by CT is likely here to stay.

References

1. Niska R, Bhuiya F, Xu J. National Hospital Ambulatory Medical Care Survey: 2007 emergency department summary. Natl Health Stat Rep. 2007;2010(26):1–31.
2. Graff LG, Dallara J, Ross MA, Joseph AJ, Itzcovitz J, Andelman RP, et al. Impact on the care of the emergency department chest pain patient from the chest pain evaluation registry (CHEPER) study. Am J Cardiol. 1997;80(5):563–8.
3. Braunwald E, Antman EM, Beasley JW, Califf RM, Cheitlin MD, Hochman JS, et al. ACC/AHA 2002 guideline update for the management of patients with unstable angina and non-ST-segment elevation myocardial infarction – summary article: a report of the American College of Cardiology/American Heart Association task force on practice guidelines (Committee on the Management of Patients With Unstable Angina). J Am Coll Cardiol. 2002;40(7):1366–74.
4. Luepker RV, Apple FS, Christenson RH, Crow RS, Fortmann SP, Goff D, et al. Case definitions for acute coronary heart disease in epidemiology and clinical research studies: a statement from the AHA Council on Epidemiology and Prevention; AHA Statistics Committee; World Heart Federation Council on Epidemiology and Prevention; the European Society of Cardiology Working Group on Epidemiology and Prevention; Centers for Disease Control and Prevention; and the National Heart, Lung, and Blood Institute. Circulation. 2003;108(20):2543–9.
5. Ornato JP, American College of Cardiology/American Heart A. Management of patients with unstable angina and non-ST-segment elevation myocardial infarction: update ACC/AHA guidelines. Am J Emerg Med. 2003;21(4):346–51.
6. Kaul P, Newby LK, Fu Y, Hasselblad V, Mahaffey KW, Christenson RH, et al. Troponin T and quantitative ST-segment depression offer complementary prognostic information in the risk stratification of acute coronary syndrome patients. J Am Coll Cardiol. 2003; 41(3):371–80.
7. Vafaie M, Katus HA. Myocardial infarction. New universal definition and its implementation in clinical practice. Herz. 2013; 38(8):821–7.
8. Wright RS, Anderson JL, Adams CD, Bridges CR, Casey Jr DE, Ettinger SM, et al. 2011 ACCF/AHA focused update incorporated into the ACC/AHA 2007 guidelines for the management of patients with unstable angina/non-ST-elevation myocardial infarction: a report of the American College of Cardiology Foundation/ American Heart Association Task Force on Practice Guidelines developed in collaboration with the American Academy of Family Physicians, Society for Cardiovascular Angiography and Interventions, and the Society of Thoracic Surgeons. J Am Coll Cardiol. 2011;57(19):e215–367.
9. Goldstein JA, Gallagher MJ, O'Neill WW, Ross MA, O'Neil BJ, Raff GL. A randomized controlled trial of multi-slice coronary computed tomography for evaluation of acute chest pain. J Am Coll Cardiol. 2007;49(8):863–71.
10. Tosteson AN, Goldman L, Udvarhelyi IS, Lee TH. Cost-effectiveness of a coronary care unit versus an intermediate care unit for emergency department patients with chest pain. Circulation. 1996;94(2):143–50.
11. Goodacre S, Calvert N. Cost effectiveness of diagnostic strategies for patients with acute, undifferentiated chest pain. Emerg Med J. 2003;20(5):429–33.
12. Roger VL, Go AS, Lloyd-Jones DM, Benjamin EJ, Berry JD, Borden WB, et al. Heart disease and stroke statistics – 2012 update: a report from the American Heart Association. Circulation. 2012;125(1):e2–220.
13. Granger CB, Goldberg RJ, Dabbous O, Pieper KS, Eagle KA, Cannon CP, et al. Predictors of hospital mortality in the global registry of acute coronary events. Arch Intern Med. 2003;163(19): 2345–53.
14. Antman EM, Cohen M, Bernink PJ, McCabe CH, Horacek T, Papuchis G, et al. The TIMI risk score for unstable angina/non-ST elevation MI: a method for prognostication and therapeutic decision making. JAMA. 2000;284(7):835–42.
15. Invasive compared with non-invasive treatment in unstable coronary-artery disease: FRISC II prospective randomised multicentre study. FRagmin and Fast Revascularisation during InStability in Coronary artery disease Investigators. Lancet. 1999;354(9180): 708–15.
16. Pollack Jr CV, Sites FD, Shofer FS, Sease KL, Hollander JE. Application of the TIMI risk score for unstable angina and non-ST elevation acute coronary syndrome to an unselected emergency department chest pain population. Acad Emerg Med. 2006;13(1): 13–8.
17. Miller JM, Rochitte CE, Dewey M, Arbab-Zadeh A, Niinuma H, Gottlieb I, et al. Diagnostic performance of coronary angiography by 64-row CT. N Engl J Med. 2008;359(22):2324–36.
18. Budoff MJ, Dowe D, Jollis JG, Gitter M, Sutherland J, Halamert E, et al. Diagnostic performance of 64-multidetector row coronary computed tomographic angiography for evaluation of coronary artery stenosis in individuals without known coronary artery disease: results from the prospective multicenter ACCURACY (Assessment by Coronary Computed Tomographic Angiography of Individuals Undergoing Invasive Coronary Angiography) trial. J Am Coll Cardiol. 2008;52(21):1724–32.
19. Johnson TR, Nikolaou K, Wintersperger BJ, Knez A, Boekstegers P, Reiser MF, et al. ECG-gated 64-MDCT angiography in the differential diagnosis of acute chest pain. AJR Am J Roentgenol. 2007;188(1):76–82.
20. Gallagher MJ, Ross MA, Raff GL, Goldstein JA, O'Neill WW, O'Neil B. The diagnostic accuracy of 64-slice computed tomography coronary angiography compared with stress nuclear imaging in emergency department low-risk chest pain patients. Ann Emerg Med. 2007;49(2):125–36.
21. Rubinshtein R, Halon DA, Gaspar T, Jaffe R, Karkabi B, Flugelman MY, et al. Usefulness of 64-slice cardiac computed tomographic angiography for diagnosing acute coronary syndromes and predicting clinical outcome in emergency department patients with chest pain of uncertain origin. Circulation. 2007;115(13):1762–8.
22. Johnson TR, Nikolaou K, Becker A, Leber AW, Rist C, Wintersperger BJ, et al. Dual-source CT for chest pain assessment. Eur Radiol. 2008;18(4):773–80.

23. Takakuwa KM, Halpern EJ. Evaluation of a "triple rule-out" coronary CT angiography protocol: use of 64-Section CT in low-to-moderate risk emergency department patients suspected of having acute coronary syndrome. Radiology. 2008;248(2):438–46.
24. Ueno K, Anzai T, Jinzaki M, Yamada M, Kohno T, Kawamura A, et al. Diagnostic capacity of 64-slice multidetector computed tomography for acute coronary syndrome in patients presenting with acute chest pain. Cardiology. 2009;112(3):211–8.
25. Hollander JE, Chang AM, Shofer FS, McCusker CM, Baxt WG, Litt HI. Coronary computed tomographic angiography for rapid discharge of low-risk patients with potential acute coronary syndromes. Ann Emerg Med. 2009;53(3):295–304.
26. Hollander JE, Chang AM, Shofer FS, Collin MJ, Walsh KM, McCusker CM, et al. One-year outcomes following coronary computerized tomographic angiography for evaluation of emergency department patients with potential acute coronary syndrome. Acad Emerg Med. 2009;16(8):693–8.
27. Hansen M, Ginns J, Seneviratne S, Slaughter R, Premaranthe M, Samardhi H, et al. The value of dual-source 64-slice CT coronary angiography in the assessment of patients presenting to an acute chest pain service. Heart Lung Circ. 2010;19(4):213–8.
28. Goldstein JA, Chinnaiyan KM, Abidov A, Achenbach S, Berman DS, Hayes SW, et al. The CT-STAT (Coronary Computed Tomographic Angiography for Systematic Triage of Acute Chest Pain Patients to Treatment) trial. J Am Coll Cardiol. 2011; 58(14):1414–22.
29. Hoffmann U, Truong QA, Schoenfeld DA, Chou ET, Woodard PK, Nagurney JT, et al. Coronary CT angiography versus standard evaluation in acute chest pain. N Engl J Med. 2012;367(4): 299–308.
30. Litt HI, Gatsonis C, Snyder B, Singh H, Miller CD, Entrikin DW, et al. CT angiography for safe discharge of patients with possible acute coronary syndromes. N Engl J Med. 2012;366(15): 1393–403.
31. Diver DJ, Bier JD, Ferreira PE, Sharaf BL, McCabe C, Thompson B, et al. Clinical and arteriographic characterization of patients with unstable angina without critical coronary arterial narrowing (from the TIMI-IIIA Trial). Am J Cardiol. 1994;74(6):531–7.
32. Roe MT, Harrington RA, Prosper DM, Pieper KS, Bhatt DL, Lincoff AM, et al. Clinical and therapeutic profile of patients presenting with acute coronary syndromes who do not have significant coronary artery disease. The Platelet Glycoprotein IIb/IIIa in Unstable Angina: Receptor Suppression Using Integrilin Therapy (PURSUIT) Trial Investigators. Circulation. 2000;102(10):1101–6.
33. Hulten E, Pickett C, Bittencourt MS, Villines TC, Petrillo S, Di Carli MF, et al. Outcomes after coronary computed tomography angiography in the emergency department: a systematic review and meta-analysis of randomized, controlled trials. J Am Coll Cardiol. 2013;61(8):880–92.
34. Raff GL, Chinnaiyan KM, Cury RC, Garcia MT, Hecht HS, Hollander JE, et al. SCCT guidelines on the use of coronary computed tomographic angiography for patients presenting with acute chest pain to the emergency department: a report of the Society of Cardiovascular Computed Tomography Guidelines Committee. J Cardiovasc Comput Tomogr. 2014;8(4):254–71.
35. Taylor AJ, Cerqueira M, Hodgson JM, Mark D, Min J, O'Gara P, et al. ACCF/SCCT/ACR/AHA/ASE/ASNC/NASCI/SCAI/SCMR 2010 appropriate use criteria for cardiac computed tomography. A report of the American College of Cardiology Foundation Appropriate Use Criteria Task Force, the Society of Cardiovascular Computed Tomography, the American College of Radiology, the American Heart Association, the American Society of Echocardiography, the American Society of Nuclear Cardiology, the North American Society for Cardiovascular Imaging, the Society for Cardiovascular Angiography and Interventions, and the Society for Cardiovascular Magnetic Resonance. J Cardiovasc Comput Tomogr. 2010;4(6):407.e1–33.
36. Agatston AS, Janowitz WR, Hildner FJ, Zusmer NR, Viamonte Jr M, Detrano R. Quantification of coronary artery calcium using ultrafast computed tomography. J Am Coll Cardiol. 1990;15(4): 827–32.
37. Ohnesorge B, Flohr T, Becker C, Kopp AF, Schoepf UJ, Baum U, et al. Cardiac imaging by means of electrocardiographically gated multisection spiral CT: initial experience. Radiology. 2000; 217(2):564–71.
38. Kopp AF, Ohnesorge B, Becker C, Schroder S, Heuschmid M, Kuttner A, et al. Reproducibility and accuracy of coronary calcium measurements with multi-detector row versus electron-beam CT. Radiology. 2002;225(1):113–9.
39. Achenbach S, Ulzheimer S, Baum U, Kachelriess M, Ropers D, Giesler T, et al. Noninvasive coronary angiography by retrospectively ECG-gated multislice spiral CT. Circulation. 2000;102(23):2823–8.
40. Laudon DA, Vukov LF, Breen JF, Rumberger JA, Wollan PC, Sheedy 2nd PF. Use of electron-beam computed tomography in the evaluation of chest pain patients in the emergency department. Ann Emerg Med. 1999;33(1):15–21.
41. Greenland P, Bonow RO, Brundage BH, Budoff MJ, Eisenberg MJ, Grundy SM, et al. ACCF/AHA 2007 clinical expert consensus document on coronary artery calcium scoring by computed tomography in global cardiovascular risk assessment and in evaluation of patients with chest pain: a report of the American College of Cardiology Foundation Clinical Expert Consensus Task Force (ACCF/AHA Writing Committee to Update the 2000 Expert Consensus Document on Electron Beam Computed Tomography) developed in collaboration with the Society of Atherosclerosis Imaging and Prevention and the Society of Cardiovascular Computed Tomography. J Am Coll Cardiol. 2007;49(3):378–402.
42. Villines TC, Hulten EA, Shaw LJ, Goyal M, Dunning A, Achenbach S, et al. Prevalence and severity of coronary artery disease and adverse events among symptomatic patients with coronary artery calcification scores of zero undergoing coronary computed tomography angiography: results from the CONFIRM (Coronary CT Angiography Evaluation for Clinical Outcomes: An International Multicenter) registry. J Am Coll Cardiol. 2011; 58(24):2533–40.
43. Motoyama S, Sarai M, Harigaya H, Anno H, Inoue K, Hara T, et al. Computed tomographic angiography characteristics of atherosclerotic plaques subsequently resulting in acute coronary syndrome. J Am Coll Cardiol. 2009;54(1):49–57.
44. Nance Jr JW, Schlett CL, Schoepf UJ, Oberoi S, Leisy HB, Barraza Jr JM, et al. Incremental prognostic value of different components of coronary atherosclerotic plaque at cardiac CT angiography beyond coronary calcification in patients with acute chest pain. Radiology. 2012;264(3):679–90.
45. Min JK, Shaw LJ, Devereux RB, Okin PM, Weinsaft JW, Russo DJ, et al. Prognostic value of multidetector coronary computed tomographic angiography for prediction of all-cause mortality. J Am Coll Cardiol. 2007;50(12):1161–70.
46. Gaemperli O, Valenta I, Schepis T, Husmann L, Scheffel H, Desbiolles L, et al. Coronary 64-slice CT angiography predicts outcome in patients with known or suspected coronary artery disease. Eur Radiol. 2008;18(6):1162–73.
47. Hadamitzky M, Freissmuth B, Meyer T, Hein F, Kastrati A, Martinoff S, et al. Prognostic value of coronary computed tomographic angiography for prediction of cardiac events in patients with suspected coronary artery disease. JACC Cardiovasc Imaging. 2009;2(4):404–11.
48. Carrigan TP, Nair D, Schoenhagen P, Curtin RJ, Popovic ZB, Halliburton S, et al. Prognostic utility of 64-slice computed tomography in patients with suspected but no documented coronary artery disease. Eur Heart J. 2009;30(3):362–71.
49. Chow BJ, Wells GA, Chen L, Yam Y, Galiwango P, Abraham A, et al. Prognostic value of 64-slice cardiac computed tomography severity of coronary artery disease, coronary atherosclerosis, and

left ventricular ejection fraction. J Am Coll Cardiol. 2010; 55(10):1017–28.
50. Kristensen TS, Kofoed KF, Kuhl JT, Nielsen WB, Nielsen MB, Kelbaek H. Prognostic implications of nonobstructive coronary plaques in patients with non-ST-segment elevation myocardial infarction: a multidetector computed tomography study. J Am Coll Cardiol. 2011;58(5):502–9.
51. Russo V, Zavalloni A, Bacchi Reggiani ML, Buttazzi K, Gostoli V, Bartolini S, et al. Incremental prognostic value of coronary CT angiography in patients with suspected coronary artery disease. Circ Cardiovasc Imaging. 2010;3(4):351–9.
52. Min JK, Feignoux J, Treutenaere J, Laperche T, Sablayrolles J. The prognostic value of multidetector coronary CT angiography for the prediction of major adverse cardiovascular events: a multicenter observational cohort study. Int J Cardiovasc Imaging. 2010;26(6): 721–8.
53. Petretta M, Daniele S, Acampa W, Imbriaco M, Pellegrino T, Messalli G, et al. Prognostic value of coronary artery calcium score and coronary CT angiography in patients with intermediate risk of coronary artery disease. Int J Cardiovasc Imaging. 2012;28(6): 1547–56.
54. Alexanderson E, Canseco-Leon N, Inarra F, Meave A, Dey D. Prognostic value of cardiovascular CT: is coronary artery calcium screening enough? The added value of CCTA. J Nucl Cardiol. 2012;19(3):601–8.
55. American College of Cardiology Foundation Task Force on Expert Consensus D, Mark DB, Berman DS, Budoff MJ, Carr JJ, Gerber TC, et al. ACCF/ACR/AHA/NASCI/SAIP/SCAI/SCCT 2010 expert consensus document on coronary computed tomographic angiography: a report of the American College of Cardiology Foundation Task Force on Expert Consensus Documents. J Am Coll Cardiol. 2010;55(23):2663–99.
56. Schepis T, Marwan M, Pflederer T, Seltmann M, Ropers D, Daniel WG, et al. Quantification of non-calcified coronary atherosclerotic plaques with dual-source computed tomography: comparison with intravascular ultrasound. Heart. 2010;96(8):610–5.
57. Leber AW, Becker A, Knez A, von Ziegler F, Sirol M, Nikolaou K, et al. Accuracy of 64-slice computed tomography to classify and quantify plaque volumes in the proximal coronary system: a comparative study using intravascular ultrasound. J Am Coll Cardiol. 2006;47(3):672–7.
58. Leber AW, Knez A, Becker A, Becker C, von Ziegler F, Nikolaou K, et al. Accuracy of multidetector spiral computed tomography in identifying and differentiating the composition of coronary atherosclerotic plaques: a comparative study with intracoronary ultrasound. J Am Coll Cardiol. 2004;43(7):1241–7.
59. Petranovic M, Soni A, Bezzera H, Loureiro R, Sarwar A, Raffel C, et al. Assessment of nonstenotic coronary lesions by 64-slice multidetector computed tomography in comparison to intravascular ultrasound: evaluation of nonculprit coronary lesions. J Cardiovasc Comput Tomogr. 2009;3(1):24–31.
60. Narula J, Strauss HW. The popcorn plaques. Nat Med. 2007; 13(5):532–4.
61. Narula J, Garg P, Achenbach S, Motoyama S, Virmani R, Strauss HW. Arithmetic of vulnerable plaques for noninvasive imaging. Nat Clin Pract Cardiovasc Med. 2008;5 Suppl 2:S2–10.
62. Maurovich-Horvat P, Ferencik M, Voros S, Merkely B, Hoffmann U. Comprehensive plaque assessment by coronary CT angiography. Nat Rev Cardiol. 2014;11(7):390–402.
63. Motoyama S, Kondo T, Sarai M, Sugiura A, Harigaya H, Sato T, et al. Multislice computed tomographic characteristics of coronary lesions in acute coronary syndromes. J Am Coll Cardiol. 2007; 50(4):319–26.
64. Pflederer T, Marwan M, Schepis T, Ropers D, Seltmann M, Muschiol G, et al. Characterization of culprit lesions in acute coronary syndromes using coronary dual-source CT angiography. Atherosclerosis. 2010;211(2):437–44.
65. Hoffmann U, Moselewski F, Nieman K, Jang IK, Ferencik M, Rahman AM, et al. Noninvasive assessment of plaque morphology and composition in culprit and stable lesions in acute coronary syndrome and stable lesions in stable angina by multidetector computed tomography. J Am Coll Cardiol. 2006;47(8):1655–62.
66. Ferencik M, Schlett CL, Ghoshhajra BB, Kriegel MF, Joshi SB, Maurovich-Horvat P, et al. A computed tomography-based coronary lesion score to predict acute coronary syndrome among patients with acute chest pain and significant coronary stenosis on coronary computed tomographic angiogram. Am J Cardiol. 2012;110(2): 183–9.
67. Maurovich-Horvat P, Hoffmann U, Vorpahl M, Nakano M, Virmani R, Alkadhi H. The napkin-ring sign: CT signature of high-risk coronary plaques? JACC Cardiovasc Imaging. 2010;3(4):440–4.
68. Narula J, Achenbach S. Napkin-ring necrotic cores: defining circumferential extent of necrotic cores in unstable plaques. JACC Cardiovasc Imaging. 2009;2(12):1436–8.
69. Lin FY, Devereux RB, Roman MJ, Meng J, Jow VM, Jacobs A, et al. Cardiac chamber volumes, function, and mass as determined by 64-multidetector row computed tomography: mean values among healthy adults free of hypertension and obesity. JACC Cardiovasc Imaging. 2008;1(6):782–6.
70. Raman SV, Shah M, McCarthy B, Garcia A, Ferketich AK. Multi-detector row cardiac computed tomography accurately quantifies right and left ventricular size and function compared with cardiac magnetic resonance. Am Heart J. 2006;151(3):736–44.
71. Yamamuro M, Tadamura E, Kubo S, Toyoda H, Nishina T, Ohba M, et al. Cardiac functional analysis with multi-detector row CT and segmental reconstruction algorithm: comparison with echocardiography, SPECT, and MR imaging. Radiology. 2005;234(2):381–90.
72. Henneman MM, Schuijf JD, Jukema JW, Holman ER, Lamb HJ, de Roos A, et al. Assessment of global and regional left ventricular function and volumes with 64-slice MSCT: a comparison with 2D echocardiography. J Nucl Cardiol. 2006;13(4):480–7.
73. Gilkeson RC, Markowitz AH, Balgude A, Sachs PB. MDCT evaluation of aortic valvular disease. AJR Am J Roentgenol. 2006; 186(2):350–60.
74. Gilard M, Cornily JC, Pennec PY, Joret C, Le Gal G, Mansourati J, et al. Accuracy of multislice computed tomography in the preoperative assessment of coronary disease in patients with aortic valve stenosis. J Am Coll Cardiol. 2006;47(10):2020–4.
75. Jongbloed MR, Lamb HJ, Bax JJ, Schuijf JD, de Roos A, van der Wall EE, et al. Noninvasive visualization of the cardiac venous system using multislice computed tomography. J Am Coll Cardiol. 2005;45(5):749–53.
76. Lehman SJ, Abbara S, Cury RC, Nagurney JT, Hsu J, Goela A, et al. Significance of cardiac computed tomography incidental findings in acute chest pain. Am J Med. 2009;122(6):543–9.
77. Machaalany J, Yam Y, Ruddy TD, Abraham A, Chen L, Beanlands RS, et al. Potential clinical and economic consequences of noncardiac incidental findings on cardiac computed tomography. J Am Coll Cardiol. 2009;54(16):1533–41.
78. Lee CI, Tsai EB, Sigal BM, Plevritis SK, Garber AM, Rubin GD. Incidental extracardiac findings at coronary CT: clinical and economic impact. AJR Am J Roentgenol. 2010;194(6):1531–8.
79. Koonce J, Schoepf JU, Nguyen SA, Northam MC, Ravenel JG. Extra-cardiac findings at cardiac CT: experience with 1,764 patients. Eur Radiol. 2009;19(3):570–6.
80. Kim TJ, Han DH, Jin KN, Won LK. Lung cancer detected at cardiac CT: prevalence, clinicoradiologic features, and importance of full-field-of-view images. Radiology. 2010;255(2):369–76.
81. Ostrom MP, Gopal A, Ahmadi N, Nasir K, Yang E, Kakadiaris I, et al. Mortality incidence and the severity of coronary atherosclerosis assessed by computed tomography angiography. J Am Coll Cardiol. 2008;52(16):1335–43.
82. Mowatt G, Cook JA, Hillis GS, Walker S, Fraser C, Jia X, et al. 64-Slice computed tomography angiography in the diagnosis and

assessment of coronary artery disease: systematic review and meta-analysis. Heart. 2008;94(11):1386–93.
83. Hoffmann U, Bamberg F, Chae CU, Nichols JH, Rogers IS, Seneviratne SK, et al. Coronary computed tomography angiography for early triage of patients with acute chest pain: the ROMICAT (Rule Out Myocardial Infarction using Computer Assisted Tomography) trial. J Am Coll Cardiol. 2009;53(18):1642–50.
84. Cheezum MK, Bittencourt MS, Hulten EA, Scirica BM, Villines TC, Blankstein R. Coronary computed tomographic angiography in the emergency room: state of the art. Expert Rev Cardiovasc Ther. 2014;12(2):241–53.
85. Abbara S, Arbab-Zadeh A, Callister TQ, Desai MY, Mamuya W, Thomson L, et al. SCCT guidelines for performance of coronary computed tomographic angiography: a report of the Society of Cardiovascular Computed Tomography Guidelines Committee. J Cardiovasc Comput Tomogr. 2009;3(3):190–204.
86. Achenbach S, Moselewski F, Ropers D, Ferencik M, Hoffmann U, MacNeill B, et al. Detection of calcified and noncalcified coronary atherosclerotic plaque by contrast-enhanced, submillimeter multidetector spiral computed tomography: a segment-based comparison with intravascular ultrasound. Circulation. 2004; 109(1):14–7.
87. Min JK, Leipsic J, Pencina MJ, Berman DS, Koo BK, van Mieghem C, et al. Diagnostic accuracy of fractional flow reserve from anatomic CT angiography. JAMA. 2012;308(12): 1237–45.

Index

M.J. Budoff, J.S. Shinbane (eds.), *Cardiac CT Imaging: Diagnosis of Cardiovascular Disease*,
DOI 10.1007/978-3-319-28219-0

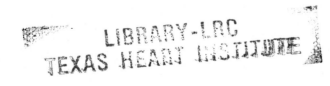

Printed in the United States
By Bookmasters